Instructor Resources for Success

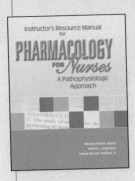

Instructor's Resource Manual
ISBN: 0131100173
This manual contains a wealth of material to help faculty plan and manage the pharmacology for nurses course. It includes information on how to teach pharmacology using a pathophysiologic approach, chapter overviews, detailed lecture suggestions and outlines, learning objectives, a complete test bank with NCLEX-RN questions, answers to the textbook critical thinking exercises, teaching tips, and more for each chapter. The IRM also guides faculty how to assign and use the text-specific Companion Website, www.prenhall.com/adams, and the free student CD-ROM that accompany the textbook.

Instructor's Resource CD-ROM
ISBN: 0130498394
This cross-platform CD-ROM provides an electronic version of the Instructor's Resource Manual, as well as illustrations and notes in PowerPoint for use in classroom lectures. It also contains the Test-Gen electronic test bank, answers to the textbook critical thinking exercises, and animations from the Student CD-ROM. This supplement is available to faculty **free** upon adoption of the textbook.

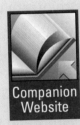

Companion Website Syllabus Manager
www.prenhall.com/adams
Faculty adopting this textbook have **free** access to the online Syllabus Manager on the Companion Website, www.prenhall.com/adams. Syllabus Manager offers a whole host of features that facilitate the students' use of the Companion Website, and allows faculty to post syllabi and course information online for their students. For more information or a demonstration of Syllabus Manager, please contact a Prentice Hall Sales Representative.

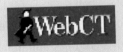

Online Course Management Systems
Also available are online companions to help faculty manage their course, both in the classroom and online. The online course management solutions feature online grade book, communications, syllabi posting, interactive modules, electronic test bank, PowerPoint images, animations, assessment activities and more. For more information about adopting an online course management system to accompany *Pharmacology for Nurses: A Pathophysiologic Approach*, please contact your Prentice Hall Health Sales Representative or go online to the appropriate website below and select a course.
WebCT: http://cms.prenhall.com/webct/index.html
Blackboard: http//cms.prenhall.com/blackboard/index.html
CourseCompass: http//cms.prenhall.com/coursecompass/index.html

Brief Contents

Pharmacology for Nurses
A Pathophysiologic Approach

Michael Patrick Adams, PhD, RT(R)
Associate Dean of Health, Mathematics, and Science
Pasco-Hernando Community College

Dianne L. Josephson, RN, MSN
Nursing Education Consultant

Leland Norman Holland, Jr., PhD
Associate Academic Dean
Southeastern University

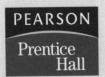

PEARSON
Prentice Hall

Upper Saddle River, New Jersey 07458

Library of Congress Cataloging-in-Publication Data

Adams, Michael (date)
  Pharmacology for nurses : a pathophysiologic approach / Michael Adams, Norman Holland, Dianne Josephson.
    p. ; cm.
  ISBN 0–13–028148–4
 1. Pharmacology. 2. Nurses.
  [DNLM: 1. Drug Therapy–nursing. 2. Pharmacology–Nurses' Instruction. WB 330 A215p
2004] I. Holland, Norman (date). II. Josephson, Dianne L. III. Title.
  RM301.A32 2004
  615'. 1–dc22

               2003020618

Publisher: Julie Levin Alexander
Assistant to the Publisher: Regina Bruno
Editor-in-Chief: Maura Connor
Executive Editor: Barbara Krawiec
Assistant Editor: Sladjana Repic
Developmental Editor: Elena M. Mauceri
Editorial Assistant: Jennifer Dwyer
Director of Production & Manufacturing: Bruce Johnson
Managing Production Editor: Patrick Walsh
Production Liaison: Mary C. Treacy
Production Editor: Amy Hackett, Carlisle Communications
Manufacturing Manager: Ilene Sanford
Manufacturing Buyer: Pat Brown
Design Director: Cheryl Asherman
Senior Design Coordinator: Maria Guglielmo Walsh
Manager of Media Production: Amy Peltier
Senior Media Editor: John J. Jordan
New Media Product Manager: Stephen Hartner
Media Development Editor: Sheba Jalaluddin
Senior Marketing Manager: Nicole Benson
Marketing Assistant: Janet Ryerson
Channel Marketing Manager: Rachele Triano
Composition: Carlisle Communications Ltd.
Illustrator: Precision Graphics
Cover Printer: Lehigh Press
Printer/Binder: Von Hoffmann Press

DEDICATION

I dedicate this book to my wife, Kim, and my daughter, Kimberly Michelle Valiance, who supported me through the endless hours of creativity and preparation that culminated in this work.

               —MPA

I dedicate this book to the memory of my parents, Judy and Jim Diaz. I also want to acknowledge my husband, Rick, for enduring yet another writing project, and my children, Jennifer, Jeff, and Bethany—you are my life.

               —DLJ

I would like to acknowledge the willful encouragement of Farrell and Norma Jean Stalcup. I dedicate this book to my beloved wife, Karen, and my two wonderful children, Alexandria Noelle, my double-deuce daughter, and Caleb Jaymes, my number-one son.

               —LNH

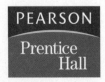

10 9 8 7 6 5 4
ISBN 0–13–028148–4

Detailed Contents

When students are asked which subject in their nursing program is the most challenging, pharmacology always appears near the top of the list. The study of pharmacology demands that students apply knowledge from a wide variety of the natural and applied sciences. To successfully predict drug action requires a thorough knowledge of anatomy, physiology, chemistry, and pathology as well as the social sciences of psychology and sociology. Lack of proper application of pharmacology can result in immediate and direct harm to the patient; thus, the stakes in learning the subject are high.

Pharmacology cannot be made easy, but it can be made understandable, if the proper connections are made to knowledge learned in these other disciplines. The vast majority of drugs in clinical practice are prescribed for specific diseases, yet many pharmacology textbooks fail to recognize the complex interrelationships between pharmacology and pathophysiology. When drugs are learned in isolation from their associated diseases or conditions, students have difficulty connecting pharmacotherapy to therapeutic goals and patient wellness. The pathophysiology approach of this textbook gives the student a clearer picture of the importance of pharmacology to disease, and ultimately to patient care. The approach and rationale of this textbook focus on a holistic perspective to patient care, which clearly shows the benefits and limitations of pharmacotherapy in curing or preventing illness. Although difficult and challenging, the study of pharmacology is truly a fascinating, lifelong journey.

Approach and Rationale

Disease and Body System Approach

Pharmacology for Nurses: A Pathophysiologic Approach is organized according to body systems (units) and diseases (chapters). Complete information on the drug classifications used to treat the disease(s) is presented in the chapters. Specially designed headings cue students to each classification discussion. The writing style is clear and succinct.

A pathophysiology approach clearly places the drugs in context with how they are used therapeutically. The student is able to easily locate all relevant anatomy, physiology, pathology, and pharmacology in the same chapter in which the drugs are discussed. This approach provides the student with a clear view of the connection between pharmacology and pathophysiology, and the content learned in the medical-surgical nursing course. **PharmFacts** features, which are included in each disease chapter, present pertinent facts and statistics related to the disease, providing a social and economic perspective of the disease.

Prototype Approach

The vast number of drugs available in clinical practice is staggering. To facilitate learning, a prototype approach is used in which the one or two most representative drugs in each classification are introduced in detail. Students are less intimidated when they can focus their learning on one representative drug in each class. **Prototype Drug** boxes are used to clearly indicate these important medications. Within these boxes, the actions and uses of the drug are succinctly presented, including **administration alerts** which highlight vital information related to the administration of that drug. **Adverse effects** and **drug-drug**, **herb-drug**, and **food-drug interactions** are also included.

Focused Nursing Process Coverage

This textbook provides a focused Nursing Process approach, which allows students to quickly find the content that is essential for them to know for safe, effective drug therapy.

Nursing Considerations sections appear within each drug class discussion. These sections discuss the major needs of the patient, including general assessments, interventions, and patient teaching for the classification.

Nursing Process Focus flowcharts provide a succinct, easy-to-read view of the most commonly prescribed drug class for the disease. Need-to-know nursing actions are presented in a format that reflects the "flow" of the Nursing Process: nursing assessment, potential nursing diagnoses, planning, interventions, patient education and discharge planning, and evaluation. Rationales for interventions are included in parentheses. The Nursing Process Focus flowcharts identify clearly what nursing actions are most important.

Some prototype drugs have important nursing actions that are specific to that drug; in these instances, the authors have provided a Nursing Process Focus flowchart in the text devoted solely to the prototype drug. A Nursing Process Focus flowchart for every prototype drug can be found on the companion website (www.prenhall. com/adams). The ⊕ icon is provided at the bottom of each Prototype Drug box to remind the student that this content can be found on the companion website.

Patient education is an important nursing intervention. Patient education information in the Nursing Considerations sections and each Nursing Process Focus flowchart assists the nurse in imparting essential information to the patient and caregiver.

Integrated rationales for nursing actions provide the physiology of the drug action to answer the "why" of nursing interventions. This is key to developing critical-thinking skills.

Pharmacology as a Visual Discipline

For nearly all students, learning is a highly visual process. *Pharmacology for Nurses: A Pathophysiologic Approach* is the first nursing pharmacology textbook to incorporate

Mechanism in Action animations, which use computer simulations to clearly demonstrate drug action at the molecular, tissue, and system levels. MediaLink tabs with CD-ROM icons can be found in the margin next to appropriate Prototype Drug boxes. This marginal tab indicates that the full-color animation, including audio narrations that describe each step of the mechanism, is provided on the included student CD-ROM. Additional animations, which illustrate important pharmacologic concepts such as agonists and antagonists, can also be found on the CD-ROM. The textbook also incorporates generous use of artwork to illustrate and summarize key concepts, including drug action.

Holistic Pharmacology

Pharmacology for Nurses: A Pathophysiologic Approach examines pharmacology from a holistic perspective.

The **Special Considerations** features present pharmacology and nursing issues related to **cultural, ethnic, age, gender,** and **psychosocial** aspects. These features remind students that a drug's efficacy is affected as much by its pharmacokinetics as by the uniqueness of the individual. In addition, **pediatric** and **geriatric** considerations are integrated throughout the textbook.

Natural Therapies features present a popular herbal or dietary supplement that may be considered along with conventional drugs. Although the authors do not recommend the use of these alternative treatments in lieu of conventional medicines, the majority of patients use complementary and alternative therapies and the nurse must become familiar with how they affect patient health. **Herb-drug interactions** are also included within the Prototype Drug boxes. Nonpharmacologic methods for controlling many diseases are also integrated into the chapters, and include **lifestyle and dietary modifications**.

A Note about Terminology

The term "healthcare provider" is used to denote the physician, nurse practitioner, and any other health professional that is legally authorized to prescribe drugs.

Key Features of the Textbook

The fundamental structure of the textbook includes:

- Units organized by body system, and chapters organized by disease. All classes of drugs used to treat a particular disease are discussed in one chapter, placing the drugs in context with how they are used therapeutically, providing a key link to content learned in medical-surgical nursing courses.

- Disease chapters that each provide essential concepts in anatomy, physiology, and pathology that are relevant to drug therapy.

- An interdisciplinary approach to the subject that is applicable for the student preparing to practice as a professional nurse. The textbook may also serve as a

review for those searching for a concise, current refresher on drug action.

Unique chapter features and elements include the following:

- **Drugs at a Glance** presents a quick way for students to see the drug classifications (and prototype drugs) used to treat the disease(s) discussed in the chapter.

- **MediaLink** features summarize the chapter content-related technology resources available to students.

- Learning **objectives** and a listing of **key terms** and page numbers are in each chapter. Each key term appears in bold blue type the first time it is introduced in the text.

- Numbered **Key Concept** headings, which are a concise means of communicating the most important pharmacologic concepts, allow students to quickly identify key ideas. Within the chapter, these numbered concepts appear as brief headings; then at the end of the chapter, they are expanded into statements that provide a succinct **Key Concepts** list that the student should understand before moving on to the next chapter. The use of numbering helps students easily locate that section within the textbook if they require further review.

- **Nursing Considerations** sections within the drug classification discussions provide nursing information related to patient care, including integrated rationales for nursing actions.

- **Prototype Drug** boxes provide detailed information on one or two of the most common drugs in each classification, including actions and uses, administration alerts, and the most common adverse effects as well as drug-drug, food-drug, and herb-drug interactions. This textbook includes 150 Prototype Drug boxes.

- The remaining drugs in the class appear in brief **drug tables** that give students an overview of the drugs within each classification, with adult dosages provided. This minimizes repetition of information in drug handbooks. Drugs that are highlighted as prototypes within the chapter are identified with a prototype icon 💊 . For additional resources and drug-related updates, students can visit the Prentice Hall *Nurse's Drug Guide* online at www.prenhall.com/drugguides.

- **MediaLink tabs** in the margins indicate that **Mechanism in Action animations** (which show how the prototype drugs act within the body), as well as other animations and activities, can be found on the included CD-ROM and companion website.

- **Nursing Process Focus** flowcharts provide a succinct summary of nursing actions related to the broad pharmacologic classification or the prototype drug. **Rationales** for nursing actions are provided in parentheses.

- Cross-reference icons 🔗 are used to indicate related content that can be found in another section of the textbook.

- The generous use of artwork is a highly visual process used to enhance student learning.

- **Special Considerations** features present pharmacology and nursing issues related to **cultural, ethnic, age, gender,** and **psychosocial aspects**. In addition, **pediatric** and **geriatric** considerations are integrated throughout the textbook.

- **Natural Therapies** features provide coverage of frequently used herbs and supplements.

- **PharmFacts** features put the disease in a social and economic perspective by providing relevant statistics related to the disease.

- Chapter Review sections include the following:

  - **Key Concepts** provide a concise wrap-up of the essential ideas presented in the chapter, numbered to correspond to Key Concept sections within the chapter.

  - **Review Questions** provide a way for students to test their knowledge. Students can easily scan through the chapter to check their answers.

  - **Critical Thinking Questions** help the student apply essential components of nursing practice through **scenario-based** questions. Answers are provided in Appendix D.

  - **EXPLORE MediaLink** features guide the student to resources, interactive exercises, and animations for that chapter on the student CD-ROM and companion website.

- A comprehensive appendices section provides the following resources:

  - Complete glossary of key terms
  - Canadian drugs and their U.S. equivalents
  - Top 200 drugs ranked by number of prescriptions
  - Bibliography and references for each chapter
  - Answers to critical-thinking questions
  - Index, with special treatment of diseases, prototype drugs, classifications, and generic and trade names of drugs

Comprehensive Teaching-Learning Package

To enhance the teaching and learning process, an attractive media-focused supplements package for both students and faculty has been developed for *Pharmacology for Nurses: A Pathophysiologic Approach*. The various components of the package are also described on the inside front cover of this textbook. The full complement of supplemental teaching materials is available to all qualified instructors from your Prentice Hall Health Sales Representative.

Student CD-ROM.   The student CD-ROM is packaged **FREE** with every copy of the textbook. It includes:

- Animations of selected prototype drugs and their mechanism of action within the body, showing how drug action occurs at the molecular, tissue, and sys-

tem levels, including audio narrative of the drug action; these animations build upon the drug action discussions in the Prototype Drug boxes in the textbook

- Additional animations that show other concepts that are important to pharmacology, such as the actions of agonists and antagonists in the body

- Audio glossary with pronunciations of every key term in the textbook

- Chapter objectives

- Simulated NCLEX review, with multiple-choice questions that emphasize the application of care and patient education related to drug administration; immediate feedback is provided, with rationales for correct and incorrect answers

- Access to the companion website, which is described in the following text (internet connection required)

Student Workbook.   A Student Workbook for *Pharmacology for Nurses: A Pathophysiologic Approach* has been developed for the textbook. The workbook contains a variety of question types and a large number of practice questions and learning activities, including fill-ins, matching, multiple choice, case studies, and dosage calculations. MediaLinks refer students to the student CD-ROM and companion website. Other study aids may be found at the companion website.

Instructor's Resource Manual.   This manual contains a wealth of material to help faculty plan and manage the pharmacology course. It includes lecture suggestions and outlines, learning objectives, a complete test bank, teaching tips, and more for each chapter. The IRM also guides faculty on how to assign and use the text-specific companion website (www.prenhall.com/adams) and the CD-ROM that accompany the textbook.

Instructor's Resource CD-ROM.   This CD-ROM provides many resources in an electronic format. First, the CD-ROM includes the complete test bank in Test-Gen format. Second, it includes a comprehensive collection of images from the textbook and discussion point slides in PowerPoint format, so faculty can easily import these photographs and illustrations into classroom lecture presentations. Finally, the CD-ROM provides instructors with access to the same animations that appear on the student CD-ROM, so faculty can incorporate these visual accents into lectures.

Companion Website and Syllabus Manager®. Students and faculty will both benefit from the **FREE** companion website at www.prenhall.com/adams. This website serves as a text-specific, interactive online workbook to *Pharmacology for Nurses: A Pathophysiologic Approach*. The companion website includes:

- MediaLinks: internet links and exercises that correspond to MediaLink tabs within the textbook

- Nursing Care Plan exercises: essay modules in which students will be asked to complete their own drug care plans for specific disorders/drug therapies

- Prototype-specific Nursing Process Focus flowcharts

- Dosage calculation exercises

- Audio glossary

- Case study exercises, which present patient scenarios with critical-thinking exercises that challenge the student to apply newly acquired knowledge to patients in the hospital, extended care, and home care settings

- Drug Guide Toolbox, with links to the most current Prentice Hall nurses' drug guide—available online

- Expanded versions of the end-of-chapter Key Concepts summaries

- More NCLEX review

Instructors adopting this textbook for their courses have **FREE** access to an online Syllabus Manager with a whole host of features to facilitate the students' use of this companion website and allow faculty to post syllabi online for students. For more information or a demonstration of Syllabus Manager, please contact your Prentice Hall Health Sales Representative or go online to www.prenhall.com/demo.

 Online Course Management Systems. Also available are online companions to help faculty manage their course, both in the classroom and online. The online course management solutions feature online grade book, communications, syllabi posting, interactive modules, electronic test bank, PowerPoint images, animations, assessment activities and more. For more information about adopting an online course management system to accompany *Pharmacology for Nurses: A*

Pathophysiologic Approach, please contact your Prentice Hall Health Sales Representative or go online to the appropriate website below and select a course.
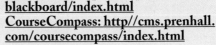
WebCT: http://cms.prenhall.com/webct/index.html
Blackboard: http//cms.prenhall.com/blackboard/index.html
CourseCompass: http//cms.prenhall.com/coursecompass/index.html

Acknowledgments

When authoring a textbook such as this, a huge number of dedicated and talented professionals are needed to bring the initial vision to reality. At the top of our list is Elena Mauceri, Publishing Consultant, who worked tirelessly for several years to coordinate, review, and pull this project along; truly this work would not have reached outstanding quality without her efforts. Maura Connor, Editor-in-Chief, is responsible for helping us to sculpt the original vision for the text. Our Editor, Barbara Krawiec, supplied the expert guidance and leadership to keep everyone on task and to be certain it reached its fruition (on time). Providing the necessary expertise for our comprehensive supplement package was Sladjana Repic, Assistant Editor. Sheba Jalaluddin and Jennifer Dwyer, Editorial Assistants, did an outstanding job of managing the myriad office details. Sheba's work to coordinate the CD-ROM and companion website content was invaluable.

The design staff at Prentice Hall, especially Cheryl Asherman, Design Director, and Maria Guglielmo, Design Coordinator, created a magnificent text design. Patrick Walsh, Managing Production Editor, provided expertise on art and photography issues. Overseeing the production process with finesse was Mary Treacy, Production Editor at Prentice Hall. Amy Hackett and the staff at Carlisle Publisher Services provided expert and professional guidance in all aspects of the art and production process.

Contributors

This textbook is a culmination of writing provided by many writers. Of particular note are Rita Plyer, whose contributions were valuable to the initial vision for this text, and Robert (Rob) Koch, whose clear nursing perspectives and guidance were invaluable to us during the critical final stages of the book. The authors wish to extend their special thanks to the many other nurse contributors who provided their unique knowledge and wisdom to this project. Their willingness to make such sacrifices to meet our deadlines is so appreciated. Their dedication to quality nursing education is very evident in this text.

Text Contributors

Ellise D. Adams, CNM, MSN, CD(DONA), ICCE
Calhoun Community College
Decatur, Alabama

Jeanine Brice, MSN, RN
Pasco-Hernando Community College
New Port Richey, Florida

Marti Burton, RN, BS
Canadian Valley Technology Center
El Reno, Oklahoma

Karen Stuart Champion, RN, MS
Indian River Community College
Fort Pierce, Florida

Janice M. Dieber, EdD
St. George, Utah

Marianne Fasano, RN, BSN, MEd
Pasco-Hernando Community College
New Port Richey, Florida

Ethlyn Gibson, MSN, RN, C
Tacoma General Hospital
Tacoma, Washington

Donna Hallas, PhD, APRN, BC, CPNP
Pace University
Pleasantville, New York

Robert Koch, DNS, RN
Loewenberg School of Nursing, University of Memphis
Memphis, Tennessee

Catherine McJannet, RN, MN, CEN
Southwestern College
Chula Vista, California

Barbara McNeil, RN, MSN, Med, CS
College of Lake County
Grayslake, Illinois

Terrilynn Fox Quillen, RN, BS
Greenwood, Indiana

Betty Kehl Richardson, PhD, APRN, BC, CNAA, LPC, LMFT
Austin Community College
Austin, Texas

Claudia R. Stoffel, MSN, RN
Paducah Community College
Paducah, Kentucky

Patricia R. Teasley, MSN, RN, CS
Central Texas College
Killeen, Texas

Carol Urban, RN, MSN
George Mason University
Fairfax, Virginia

Debra J. Walden, MNSc, RN
Arkansas State University
State University, Arkansas

Frances M. Warrick, MS, RN
El Centro College
Dallas, Texas

Jennifer Whitley, RN, MSN, CNOR
Corporate University
Huntsville Hospital
Huntsville, Alabama

Patricia Moran Woodbery, MSN, ARNP-CS
Valencia Community College
Orlando, Florida

Supplement and Media Contributors

Student CD-ROM

Janice M. Dieber, EdD
St. George, Utah

Donna Hallas, PhD, APRN, BC, CPNP
Pace University
Pleasantville, New York

Betty Kehl Richardson, PhD, APRN, BC, CNAA, LPC, LMFT
Austin Community College
Austin, Texas

Janelle Hernden Sorrell, RN, BS
Northwest-Shoals Community College
Muscle Shoals, Alabama

Daryle Wane, APRN, BC, MS
Pasco-Hernando Community College
New Port Richey, Florida

Martina M. Ware, MSN, RN
Montgomery County Community College
Blue Bell, Pennsylvania

Frances M. Warrick, MS, RN
El Centro College
Dallas, Texas

Jennifer Whitley, RN, MSN, CNOR
Corporate University
Huntsville Hospital
Huntsville, Alabama

Patricia Moran Woodbery, MSN, ARNP-CS
Valencia Community College
Orlando, Florida

Companion Website

Betty Kehl Richardson, PhD, APRN, BC, CNAA, LPC, LMFT
Austin Community College
Austin, Texas

Susan Parnell Scholtz, DNSc, RN
St. Luke's School at Moravian College
Bethlehem, Pennsylvania

Claudia R. Stoffel, MSN, RN
Paducah Community College
Paducah, Kentucky

Patricia R. Teasley, MSN, RN, CS
Central Texas College
Killeen, Texas

Daryle Wane, APRN, BC, MS
Pasco-Hernando Community College
New Port Richey, Florida

Frances M. Warrick, MS, RN
El Centro College
Dallas, Texas

Jennifer Whitley, RN, MSN, CNOR
Corporate University
Huntsville Hospital
Huntsville, Alabama

Student Workbook

Ellise D. Adams, CNM, MSN, CD(DONA), ICCE
Calhoun Community College
Decatur, Alabama

Carol Ann Alexander, MSN, RN
Palm Beach Community College
Lake Worth, Florida

Darcus Margarette Kottwitz, MSN, RN
Fort Scott Community College
Fort Scott, Kansas

Janelle Hernden Sorrell, RN, BS
Northwest-Shoals Community College
Muscle Shoals, Alabama

Jonna Swithers White, MSN, RN
Tennessee State University, School of Nursing
Nashville, Tennessee

Patricia Moran Woodbery, MSN, ARNP-CS
Valencia Community College
Orlando, Florida

Instructor's Resource Manual and Instructor's Resource CD-ROM

Connie S. Dempsey, BSN, MSN, RN
Stark State College of Technology
Canton, Ohio

Linda F. Garner, PhD, RN
Baylor University Louise Herrington School of Nursing
Dallas, Texas

Christine Cloutier Mihal, MSN, RN, C
Felician College
Lodi, New Jersey

Daryle Wane, APRN, BC, MS
Pasco-Hernando Community College
New Port Richey, Florida

Reviewers

We are grateful to all the educators who reviewed the manuscript of this textbook. Their insights, suggestions, and eye for detail helped us to prepare a more relevant and useful book, one that focuses on the essential components of learning in the field of pharmacology.

Ellise D. Adams, CNM, MSN, CD(DONA), ICCE
Calhoun Community College
Decatur, Alabama

William Baker, RN, MS, MSEd
Mt. Carmel College of Nursing
Columbus, Ohio

Jean Krajicek Bartek, PhD, APRN
University of Nebraska Medical Center College of Nursing
Omaha, Nebraska

Ilene Borze, RN, MS
Gateway Community College
Phoenix, Arizona

Joyce Campbell, RN, MSN, CCRN, FNP-C
Chattanooga State Technical Community College
Chattanooga, Tennessee

Karen Stuart Champion, RN, MS
Indian River Community College
Fort Pierce, Florida

Pattie Garrett Clark, RN, MSN
Abraham Baldwin College
Tifton, Georgia

Isabelita Duncan, MSN, RN, CS, CNRN
Sinclair Community College
Dayton, Ohio

Rebecca Ensminger, RN, MSN
Valencia Community College
Orlando, Florida

Nancy Fairchild, MS, CAES, RN
Boston College School of Nursing
Chestnut Hill, Massachusetts

William Farnsworth, MSN, ABD
University of Texas at El Paso
El Paso, Texas

Ethlyn Gibson, MSN, RN, C
Tacoma General Hospital
Tacoma, Washington

Diane Greslick, RN, MSN
St. Joseph's College of Maine
Standish, Maine

Donna Hallas, PhD, APRN, BC, CPNP
Pace University
Pleasantville, New York

Johnelle Keck, MSN, RN
Emporia State University
Emporia, Kansas

Mary Kishman, PhD(c), RN
College of Mount St. Joseph
Cincinnati, Ohio

Barbara Kinsman, RN, MSN
Corning Community College
Corning, New York

Mary Beth Kiefner, MS, RN
Illinois Central College
Peoria, Illinois

Robert Koch, DNS, RN
Loewenberg School of Nursing, University of Memphis
Memphis, Tennessee

Darlene Lacy, PhD, RNC
University of Mary Hardin-Baylor
Belton, Texas

Carol Ann Lammon, RN, PhD
Capstone College of Nursing, The University of Alabama
Tuscaloosa, Alabama

Kari R. Lane, RN, BSN, MSN
South Dakota State University
Brookings, South Dakota

L. Renee Lewis, MS, RN, CCRN
Rose State College
Midwest City, Oklahoma

Joni D. Marsh, MN, ARNP
Intercollegiate College of Nursing
Spokane, Washington

Edwina A. McConnell, RN, PhD, FRNCA
Madison, Wisconsin

Catherine McJannet, RN, MN, CEN
Southwestern College
Chula Vista, California

Barbara McNeil, RN, MSN, Med, CS
College of Lake County
Grayslake, Illinois

Ann Miller, MSN, Med, BSN, RN
Central Methodist College
Fayette, Missouri

Carolyn Roe, RN, MSN
Kalamazoo Valley Community College
Kalamazoo, Michigan

Lyndi Shadbolt, MS, BSN, RN
Amarillo College
Amarillo, Texas

About the Authors

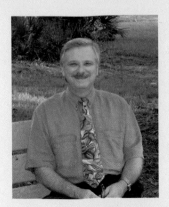

Michael Patrick Adams, PhD, RT(R), is the Associate Dean for Health, Mathematics, and Science at Pasco-Hernando Community College. He is an accomplished educator, author, and national speaker. The National Institute for Staff and Organizational Development in Austin, Texas, named Dr. Adams a Master Teacher. He has been registered by the American Registry of Radiologic Technologists for over 30 years. Dr. Adams obtained his Masters degree in Pharmacology from Michigan State University and his Doctorate in Education at the University of South Florida.

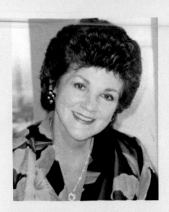

Dianne L. Josephson, RN, MSN, is a nurse educator and author, and is currently self-employed as a nursing education consultant and legal consulting expert. Her past employment experience includes Hotel Dieu Hospital in El Paso, Texas, where she worked as a nurse manager, supervisor, and patient/staff educator; and the El Paso Community College, where she served as a nursing faculty member and clinical mentor, and participated in curriculum development. She has advanced training as a bereavement facilitator through the American Academy of Bereavement. Ms. Josephson is a member of the Intravenous Nurses Association, and is listed in *Who's Who in American Nursing*, *Notable Women of Texas*, *The National Dean's List*, and *The Society of Nursing Professionals*. She has been listed as a Sigma Theta Tau International Media Guide Expert in the areas of infusion therapy, pharmacology, and bereavement support since 1998.

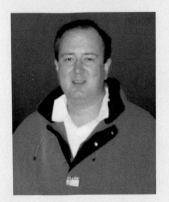

Leland Norman Holland, Jr., PhD, serves as Associate Academic Dean at Southeastern University in Lakeland, Florida. He is an active member in the Department of Natural Science where he teaches biological chemistry in the pre-med program. He has taught pharmacology for the last 12 years at both the undergraduate and graduate level preparing students for various health professions including medicine, nursing, dentistry, and health education. He comes to the teaching profession after spending several years doing basic science research at the VA Hospital in Augusta, Georgia, and the Medical College of Georgia where he received his PhD in Pharmacology.

PHARMACOLOGY WITH THE RIGHT DOSE OF...
Pathophysiology...

The organization by **body systems and diseases** clearly places the drugs in context with how they are used therapeutically. The student is able to easily locate all relevant anatomy, physiology, pathology, and pharmacology in the same chapter in which the drugs are discussed.

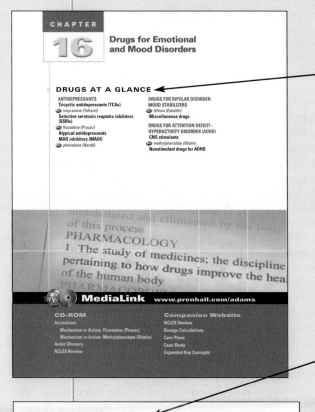

Drugs at a Glance
This feature presents a quick way for students to see the classifications and prototypes that are covered in the chapter, organized by disorder.

Disease and Body System Approach
This approach gives students a clear understanding of the role of pharmacology related to disease and patient care.

PharmFacts
The **PharmFacts** feature puts the disease in a social and economic context.

Prototype Drugs...

Within each drug classification discussion, a prototype, or representative, drug is highlighted. This approach allows the student to focus their learning on one representative drug in the classification.

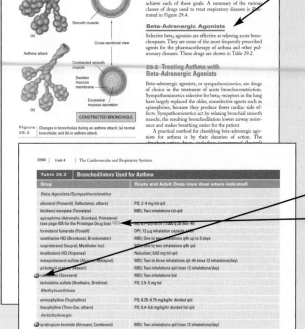

Drug Classification Discussion
Written clearly and succinctly, the text has specially-designed headings that cue students to each classification discussion.

Drug Tables
Drug tables, organized by classification, summarize the drugs used to treat each disease, and provide the most important information for each drug in a user-friendly format. Drugs that are highlighted as prototypes within that chapter are also identified with a **prototype icon**. Drugs that are highlighted as prototypes in other chapters are also identified with a **cross-reference icon** and page number for easy reference.

Prototype Drug Boxes
Focusing in detail on the one or two most representative drugs in each classification, **Prototype Drug** boxes highlight key information about the drugs that represent the classification.

Provides a focused nursing process approach, allowing students to quickly find the content that is essential for safe, effective drug therapy.

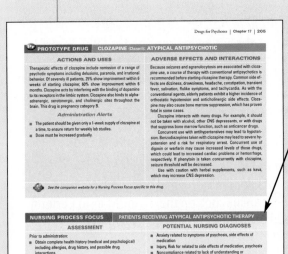

Nursing Considerations

Nursing Considerations sections appear within each drug class discussion. These sections discuss the major needs of the patient, including general assessments, interventions, and patient teaching for the classification.

Nursing Process Focus flowcharts

The **Nursing Process Focus** "flowcharts" present succinct, pharmacology-oriented information focused on the classification or prototype drug. Need-to-know nursing actions are presented in a format that reflects the "flow" of the nursing process: **assessment, nursing diagnoses, planning, implementation** with **interventions** and **patient education/discharge planning**, and **evaluation**. The Nursing Process Focus flowcharts identify clearly what nursing actions are most important.

Rationales for nursing interventions are placed in parentheses to highlight this important aspect of developing critical thinking skills.

Media Resources...

Media resources are integrated throughout. **Animations** *that clearly demonstrate drug action for 40 prototype drugs, plus content enhancements and activities are included.*

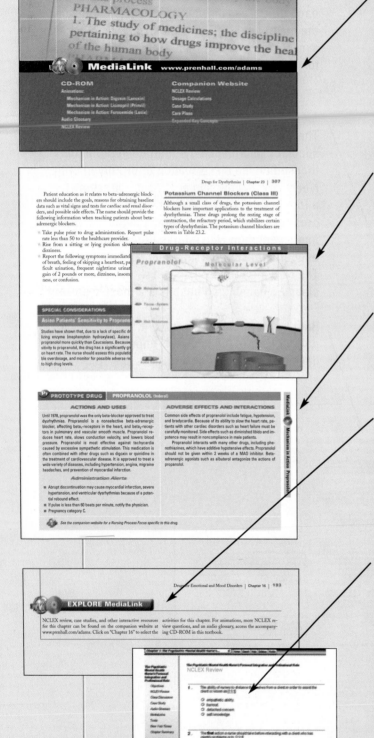

MediaLink

MediaLink, included at the beginning of each chapter, identifies specific animations, MediaLinks, and other resources available to the student on the accompanying **FREE** CD-ROM and Companion Website. MediaLink serves as a gateway to additional learning.

Mechanism in Action Animations

State-of-the-art animations on the **FREE** CD-ROM show drug action at the system, tissue, and molecular levels for 40 prototype drugs. Visualization adds clarity and reinforces drug action discussions in the chapters.

MediaLink Margin Tabs

MediaLink tabs in the margins cue the student to view animations on the CD-ROM or to perform specific activities on the Companion Website.

EXPLORE MediaLink

EXPLORE MediaLink appears at the end of each chapter. This feature guides the student to resources, interactive exercises, and animations for that chapter on the free Student CD-ROM and Companion Website.

NCLEX Review

Both the Student CD-ROM and the Companion Website offer students numerous opportunities for practicing NCLEX questions. The CD-ROM includes multiple-choice **NCLEX-RN Review** questions that emphasize application of care and client education related to drug administration, with **automatic grading,** and **rationales for right *and* wrong answers.** The NCLEX review module on the Companion Website allows students to e-mail their results directly to instructors. Students will also find the **audio glossary** and objectives useful for review.

Plus, all the best tools for student success...

Consistent features and elements ensure that the students have all the tools they need to succeed in pharmacology.

KEY TERMS

attention deficit-hyperactivity disorder (ADHD) *page 188*	monoamine oxidase inhibitor (MAOI) *page 179*	serotonin syndrome (SES) *page 178*
bipolar disorder (manic depression) *page 184*	mood disorder *page 173*	tricyclic antidepressant (TCA) *page 175*
depression *page 173*	mood stabilizer *page 185*	tyramine *page 180*
electroconvulsive therapy (ECT) *page 174*	selective serotonin reuptake inhibitor (SSRI) *page 177*	
mania *page 184*		

OBJECTIVES

After reading this chapter, the student should be able to:

1. Identify the two major categories of mood disorders and their symptoms.
2. Explain the etiology of clinical depression.
3. Discuss the nurse's role in the pharmacologic management of patients with depression, bipolar disorder, or attention deficit-hyperactivity disorder.
4. Identify symptoms of attention deficit-hyperactivity disorder.
5. For each of the drug classes listed in Drugs at a Glance, know representative drug examples, explain their mechanism of action, primary actions, and important adverse effects.
6. Categorize drugs used for mood and emotional disorders based on their classification and drug action.
7. Use the Nursing Process to care for patients receiving drug therapy for mood and emotional disorders.

Key Terms

Key terms, with the page number on which the first reference to the word can be found. Key terms are shown in blue boldface type throughout the text, and are defined at their first use. A Glossary of terms and definitions is also provided at the end of the text. An audio glossary is provided on the **FREE** CD-ROM, with pronunciations of the key terms in the text.

Drugs for Emotional and Mood Disorders | *Chapter 16* | **189**

AGENTS FOR ATTENTION DEFICIT-HYPERACTIVITY DISORDER

The traditional drugs used to treat ADHD in children have been CNS stimulants. These drugs stimulate specific areas of the central nervous system that heighten alertness and increase focus. Recently, a non-CNS stimulant was approved to treat ADHD. Agents for treating ADHD are shown in Table 16.4.

CNS Stimulants

CNS stimulants are the main course of treatment for ADHD. Stimulants reverse many of the symptoms, helping patients to focus on tasks. The most widely prescribed drug for ADHD is methylphenidate (Ritalin). Other CNS stimulants that are rarely prescribed include d- and l-amphetamine racemic mixture (Adderall), dextroamphetamine (Dexedrine), methamphetamine (Desoxyn), or pemoline (Cylert).

16.10 Pharmacotherapy of ADHD

Patients taking CNS stimulants must be carefully monitored. CNS stimulants used to treat ADHD may create paradoxical hyperactivity. Adverse reactions include insomnia, nervousness, anorexia, and weight loss. Occasionally, a patient may suffer from dizziness, depression, irritability, nausea, or abdominal pain. These are Schedule II controlled substances and pregnancy category C.

Non-CNS stimulants have been tried for ADHD; however, they exhibit less efficacy. Clonidine (Catapres) is some-

times prescribed when patients are extremely aggressive, active, or have difficulty falling asleep. Atypical antidepressants such as bupropion (Wellbutrin) and tricyclics such as desipramine (Norpramin) and imipramine (Tofranil)

SPECIAL CONSIDERATIONS

Zero Tolerance in Schools

Methylphenidate is an effective drug to treat ADHD and is often promoted by teachers and school counselors as an adjunct to improving academic performance and social adjustment. However, most schools have a "zero drug tolerance" policy which creates a hostile environment for students who must take this drug. Zero tolerance policies generally prohibit the possession of any drug and define the school's right to search and seizure and the right to demand that students submit to random drug testing, or screening as a condition of participating in sports and extracurricular activities. Schools maintain the right to suspend the students found in violation of such policies. In some districts, possession of scheduled drugs may also result in arrest and prosecution of the student.

Methylphenidate is a Schedule II controlled substance considered to have a high abuse potential. Students who take this drug should be made aware of the academic and social consequences of unauthorized possession of this medication. Most schools have strict guidelines regarding medication administration and require original prescriptions and containers of drug to be supplied to the school health office. Students should carry an official notice from the healthcare provider regarding methylphenidate therapy that may be produced in the event of random drug testing.

Objectives

Objectives provide the student with a listing of knowledge they can expect to have upon completion of the chapter.

Key Concepts

Through the use of numbered **Key Concept headings**, the student is able to quickly identify key ideas.

---

192 Unit 3 | The Nervous System

CHAPTER REVIEW

Key Concepts

The numbered key concepts provide a succinct summary of the important points from the corresponding numbered section within the chapter. If any of these points are not clear, refer to the numbered section within the chapter for review. Expanded versions can be found on the companion website.

16.1 Depression has many causes and methods of classification. The identification of depression and its etiology is essential for proper treatment.

16.2 Major depression may be treated with medications, psychotherapeutic techniques, or electroconvulsive therapy.

16.3 Antidepressants act by correcting neurotransmitter imbalances in the brain. The two basic mechanisms of action are blocking the enzymatic breakdown of norepinephrine and slowing the reuptake of serotonin.

16.4 Tricyclic antidepressants are older medications used mainly for the treatment of major depression, obsessive-compulsive disorders, and panic attacks.

16.5 SSRIs act by selectively blocking the reuptake of serotonin in nerve terminals. Because of fewer side effects, a).

SSRIs are drugs of choice in the pharmacotherapy of depression.

16.6 MAOIs are usually prescribed in cases when other antidepressants have not been successful. They have more serious side effects than other antidepressants.

16.7 Patients with bipolar disorder may also have signs of depression, but also mania, a state characterized by excessive psychomotor activity and irritability.

16.8 Mood stabilizers such as lithium (Eskalith) are used to treat both the manic and depressive stages of bipolar disorder.

16.9 Attention deficit-hyperactivity disorder (ADHD) is a common condition occurring primarily in children and is characterized by difficulty paying attention, hyperactivity, and impulsiveness.

16.10 The most efficacious drugs for symptoms of ADHD are the CNS stimulants such as methylphenidate (Ritalin). A newer, nonstimulant drug, atomoxetine (Stratter has shown promise in patients with ADHD.

Review Questions

1. Identify the classes of drugs used to treat major depression. Which class is the most effective? Which exhibits the fewest side effects?
2. A sexually active man insists upon discontinuing his SSRI due to his inability to achieve erections during intercourse. What are his options for controlling depression?
3. A patient with bipolar disorder becomes physically abusive during manic episodes and denies his behavior is abnormal. What advice would you give, and what treatment options are available?
4. The frustrated parents of a 9-year-old insist that their son be medicated for ADHD. What assessment would be needed? What therapeutic options are available?

Critical Thinking Questions

1. A 10-year-old girl has been diagnosed with ADHD. Her parents have been reluctant to agree with the pediatrician's recommendation for pharmacologic management; however, the child's behavior in school has deteriorated. A school nurse notes that the child has been placed on amphetamine (Adderall), not methylphenidate (Ritalin). After reviewing the dosing schedule, the nurse identifies the developmental considerations that might support the use of Adderall. Discuss these.

2. A 66-year-old female patient has been diagnosed with clinical depression following the death of her husband. She says that she has not been able to sleep for weeks and

that she is "living on coffee and cigarettes." The healthcare provider prescribes fluoxetine (Prozac). The patient seeks reassurance from the nurse regarding when she should begin feeling "more like myself." How should the nurse respond?

3. A 26-year-old mother of three children comes to the prenatal clinic suspecting a fourth pregnancy. She tells the nurse that she got "real low" after her third baby and that she was prescribed sertraline (Zoloft). She tells the nurse that she is really afraid of "going crazy" if she has to stop taking the drug because of this pregnancy. What concerns should the nurse have?

Key Concept Summary

Key Concept summary provides expanded versions of the shorter numbered headings from within the chapter. These statements provide a succinct summary of the "key concepts" that the student should understand before moving onto the next chapter. The use of numbering helps the student easily locate that section within the text if they require further review.

Review Questions

Review Questions provide a way for students to test their knowledge.

Critical Thinking Questions

Scenario-based critical thinking questions foster this essential component of effective nursing practice. Answers are provided as an appendix in the text.

…and the most current content and up-to-date drug information.

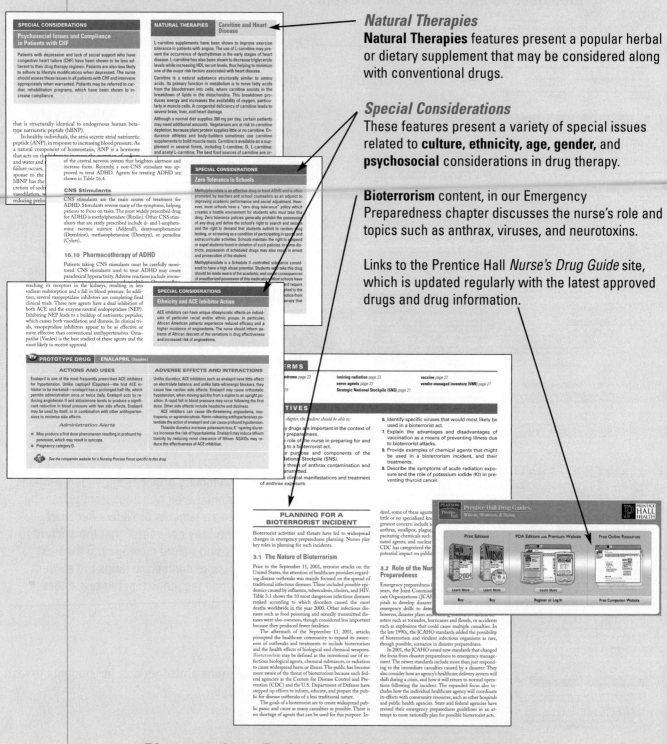

Natural Therapies
Natural Therapies features present a popular herbal or dietary supplement that may be considered along with conventional drugs.

Special Considerations
These features present a variety of special issues related to **culture, ethnicity, age, gender,** and **psychosocial** considerations in drug therapy.

Bioterrorism content, in our Emergency Preparedness chapter discusses the nurse's role and topics such as anthrax, viruses, and neurotoxins.

Links to the Prentice Hall *Nurse's Drug Guide* site, which is updated regularly with the latest approved drugs and drug information.

Pharmacology. Pathophysiology. Prototype Drugs.
Focused Nursing Process. Media.
…Plus built-in tools and current content.

The *best* medicine for nursing success!

Special Features

■ *PharmFacts*

■ *Prototype Drugs*

■ *Special Considerations*

Core Concepts in Pharmacology

More drugs are being administered to consumers than ever before. Over 3 billion prescriptions are dispensed each year in the United States, and the number is rapidly approaching 4 billion. The purpose of this chapter is to introduce the subject of pharmacology and to emphasize the role of government in ensuring that drugs, herbals, and other natural alternatives are safe and effective for public use.

metabolized and eliminated by the bod
of this process
PHARMACOLOGY
1. The study of medicines; the disciplin
pertaining to how drugs improve the he
of the human body
PHARMACOPEIA

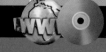 **MediaLink** www.prenhall.com/adams

CD-ROM
Audio Glossary
NCLEX Review

Companion Website
NCLEX Review
Case Study
Expanded Key Concepts
Challenge Your Knowledge

biologics *page 4*
clinical investigation *page 7*
clinical phase trials *page 7*
complementary and alternative
    therapies *page 4*
drug *page 4*

Food and Drug Administration
    (FDA) *page 6*
formulary *page 5*
medication *page 4*
NDA review *page 8*
pharmacology *page 4*

pharmacopoeia *page 5*
pharmacotherapy *page 4*
postmarketing surveillance *page 8*
preclinical investigation *page 7*
therapeutics *page 4*

OBJECTIVES

After reading this chapter, the student should be able to:

1. Identify key events in the history of pharmacology.
2. Explain the interdisciplinary nature of pharmacology, giving examples of subject areas needed to learn the discipline well.
3. Compare and contrast therapeutics and pharmacology.
4. Compare and contrast traditional drugs, biologics, and alternative therapies.
5. Identify the advantages and disadvantages of prescription and over-the-counter (OTC) drugs.

6. Identify key U.S. drug regulations that have ensured the safety and efficacy of medications.
7. Discuss the role of the U.S. Food and Drug Administration (FDA) in the drug approval process.
8. Explain the four stages of approval for therapeutic and biologic drugs.
9. Discuss how the FDA has increased the speed at which new drugs reach consumers.
10. Describe the Canadian drug approval process and identify similarities between how drugs are approved in the United States.

1.1 History of Pharmacology

The story of pharmacology is rich and exciting, filled with accidental discoveries and landmark events. Its history likely began when a human first used a plant to relieve symptoms of disease. One of the oldest forms of healthcare, herbal medicine has been practiced in virtually every culture dating to antiquity. The Babylonians recorded the earliest surviving "prescriptions" on clay tablets in 3000 B.C. At about the same time, the Chinese recorded the *Pen Tsao* (Great Herbal), a 40-volume compendium of plant remedies dating to 2700 B.C. The Egyptians followed in 1500 B.C. by archiving their remedies on a document known as the Eber's Papyrus.

Little is known about pharmacology during the Dark Ages. Although it is likely that herbal medicine continued to be practiced, few historical events related to this topic were recorded. Pharmacology, and indeed medicine, could not advance until the discipline of science was eventually viewed as legitimate by the religious doctrines of the era.

The first recorded reference to the word *pharmacology* was found in a text entitled, "Pharmacologia sen Manuductio and Materiam Medicum," by Samuel Dale in 1693. Before this date, the study of herbal remedies was called "Materia Medica," a term that persisted into the early 20th century.

Although the exact starting date is obscure, modern pharmacology is thought to have begun in the early 1800s. At that time, chemists were making remarkable progress in isolating specific substances from complex mixtures. This enabled chemists to isolate the active agents morphine, colchicine, curare, cocaine, and other early pharmacological agents from their natural products. Pharmacologists could then study their effects in animals more precisely, using standardized amounts. Indeed, some of the early researchers used themselves as test subjects. Frederich Serturner, who first isolated morphine from opium in 1805, injected himself and three friends with a huge dose (100 mg) of his new product. He and his cohorts suffered acute morphine intoxication for several days afterward.

Pharmacology as a distinct discipline was officially recognized when the first department of pharmacology was established in Estonia in 1847. John Jacob Abel, who is considered the father of American pharmacology due to his many contributions to the field, founded the first pharmacology department in the United States at the University of Michigan in 1890.

In the 20th century, the pace of change in all areas of medicine became exponential. Pharmacologists no longer needed to rely upon the slow, laborious process of isolating active agents from scarce natural products; they could synthesize drugs in the laboratory. Hundreds of new drugs could be synthesized and tested in a relatively short time. More importantly, it became possible to understand how drugs produced their effects, down to their molecular mechanism of action.

The current practice of pharmacology is extremely complex and far advanced compared with its early, primitive history. The nurses and other health professionals who practice it, however, must never forget its early roots: the application of products to relieve human suffering. Whether it is a substance extracted from the Pacific yew tree, one isolated from a fungus, or one created totally in a laboratory, the central purpose of pharmacology is to focus on the patient and to improve the quality of life.

1.2 Pharmacology: The Study of Medicines

The word **pharmacology** is derived from two Greek words, *pharmakon*, which means "medicine, drug," and *logos*, which means "study." Thus, pharmacology is most simply defined as the study of medicines.

Pharmacology is an expansive subject ranging from understanding how drugs are administered, to where they travel in the body, to the actual responses produced. To learn the discipline well, nursing students need a firm understanding of concepts from various foundation areas such as anatomy and physiology, chemistry, microbiology, and pathophysiology.

Over 10,000 brand name, generic drugs, and combination agents are currently available. Each has its own characteristic set of therapeutic applications, interactions, side effects, and mechanisms of action. Many drugs are prescribed for more than one disease and most produce multiple effects on the body. Further complicating the study of pharmacology is the fact that drugs may elicit different responses depending on individual patient factors such as age, sex, body mass, health status, and genetics. Indeed, learning the applications of existing medications and staying current with new drugs introduced every year is an enormous challenge for the nurse. The task, however, is a critical one for both the patient and the healthcare practitioner. If applied properly, drugs can dramatically improve the quality of life. If applied improperly, the consequences of improper drug action can be devastating.

1.3 Pharmacology and Therapeutics

It is obvious that a thorough study of pharmacology is important to healthcare providers who prescribe drugs on a daily basis. Although state or provincial laws sometimes limit the kinds of drugs marketed and the methods used to dispense them, *all* nurses are directly involved with patient care and are active in educating, managing, and monitoring the proper use of drugs. This applies not only for nurses in clinics, hospitals, and home healthcare settings, but also for nurses who teach and for new students entering the nursing profession. In all of these cases, a thorough knowledge of pharmacology is necessary for them to perform their duties. As nursing students progress toward their chosen specialty, pharmacology is at the core of patient care and is integrated into every step of the nursing process. Learning pharmacology is a gradual, continuous process that does not end with graduation. Never does one completely master every facet of drug action and application. That is one of the motivating challenges of the nursing profession.

Another important area of study for the nurse, sometimes difficult to distinguish from pharmacology, is the study of therapeutics. Therapeutics is slightly different from the field of pharmacology, although the disciplines are closely connected. **Therapeutics** is the branch of medicine concerned with the prevention of disease and treatment of suffering. **Pharmacotherapy**, or pharmacotherapeutics is the application of drugs for the purpose of disease prevention and treatment of suffering. Drugs are just one of many tools available to the nurse for preventing or treating human suffering.

1.4 Classification of Therapeutic Agents as Drugs, Biologics, and Alternative Therapies

Substances applied for therapeutic purposes fall into one of the following three general categories.

- Drugs or medications
- Biologics
- Alternative therapies

A **drug** is a chemical agent capable of producing biological responses within the body. These responses may be desirable (therapeutic) or undesirable (adverse). After a drug is administered, it is called a **medication**. From a broad perspective, drugs and medications may be considered a part of the body's normal activities, from the essential gases that we breathe to the foods that we eat. Because drugs are defined so broadly, it is necessary to clearly separate them from other substances such as foods, household products, and cosmetics. Many agents such as antiperspirants, sunscreens, toothpaste, and shampoos might alter the body's normal activities, but they are not considered medically therapeutic, as are drugs.

While most modern drugs are synthesized in a laboratory, **biologics** are agents naturally produced in animal cells, microorganisms, or by the body itself. Examples of biologics include hormones, monoclonal antibodies, natural blood products and components, interferon, and vaccines. Biologics are used to treat a wide variety of illnesses and conditions.

Other therapeutic approaches include **complementary and alternative therapies.** These involve natural plant extracts, herbs, vitamins, minerals, dietary supplements, and many techniques considered by some to be unconventional. Such therapies include acupuncture, hypnosis, biofeedback, and massage. Because of their great popularity, herbal and alternative therapies are featured throughout this text, where they show promise in treating a disease or condition. Herbal therapies are presented in Chapter 11 ∞ .

1.5 Prescription and Over-the-Counter Drugs

Legal drugs are obtained either by a prescription or over the counter (OTC). There are major differences between the two methods of dispensing drugs. To obtain prescription drugs, an order must be given authorizing the patient to receive the drug. The advantages to requiring an authorization are numerous. The healthcare provider has an opportunity to examine the patient and determine a specific diagnosis. The practitioner can maximize therapy by ordering the proper drug for the patient's condition, and by controlling the amount and frequency of drug to be dispensed. In addition, the healthcare provider has an opportunity to teach the patient the proper use of the drug and what side effects to expect. In a few instances, a high margin of safety observed over many years can prompt a change in the status of a drug from prescription to OTC.

In contrast to prescription drugs, OTC drugs do not require a physician's order. In most cases, patients may treat themselves safely if they carefully follow instructions included with the medication. If patients do not follow these guidelines, OTC drugs can have serious adverse effects.

Patients prefer to take OTC drugs for many reasons. They may be obtained more easily than prescription drugs. No appointment with a physician is required, thus saving time and money. Without the assistance of a healthcare provider, however, choosing the proper drug for a specific problem can be challenging for a patient. OTC drugs may react with foods, herbal products, prescription medications, or other OTC drugs. Patients may not be aware that some drugs can impair their ability to function safely. Self-treatment is sometimes ineffective, and the potential for harm may increase if the disease is allowed to progress.

1.6 Drug Regulations and Standards

Until the 19th century, there were few standards or guidelines to protect the public from drug misuse. The archives of drug regulatory agencies are filled with examples of early medicines, including rattlesnake oil for rheumatism; epilepsy treatment for spasms, hysteria, and alcoholism; and fat reducers for a slender, healthy figure. Many of these early concoctions proved ineffective, though harmless. At their worst, some contained hazardous levels of dangerous or addictive substances. It became quite clear that drug regulations were needed to protect the public.

PHARMFACTS — Consumer Spending on Prescription Drugs

- Spending on prescription drugs comprises about 9% of total healthcare costs.
- Between 1990 and 2000, prescription drug expenditures increased by more than 200%.
- The average number of prescription drugs taken per year increased from 7.8 prescriptions per person in 1993 to 10.9 prescriptions per person in 2001.
- The average cost of a prescription drug in 2000 was $45.79. This is a 108% increase from 1990, when the average was $22.06 per prescription.
- Total pharmaceutical expenditures in the United States increased 19%, from $146 billion in 2000 to $175 billion in 2001.

The first standard commonly used by pharmacists was the formulary, or list of drugs and drug recipes. In the United States, the first comprehensive publication of drug standards, called the *U.S. Pharmacopoeia* (*USP*), was established in 1820. A pharmacopoeia is a medical reference summarizing standards of drug purity, strength, and directions for synthesis. In 1852, a national professional society of pharmacists called the American Pharmaceutical Association (APhA) was founded. From 1852 to 1975, two major compendia maintained drug standards in the United States, the *U.S. Pharmacopoeia* and the *National Formulary* (*NF*) established by the APhA. All drug products were covered in the *USP*; pharmaceutic ingredients were the focus of the *NF*. In 1975, the two merged into a single publication, the *U.S. Pharmacopoeia—National Formulary* (*USP-NF*). The current document of about 2,400 pages contains 3,777 drug monographs in 164 chapters. Official monographs and interim revision announcements for the *USP-NF* are published regularly, with the full bound version printed every 5 years. Today, the USP label can be found on many medications verifying the purity and exact amounts of ingredients found within the container. Sample labels are illustrated in Figure 1.1.

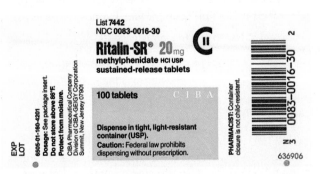
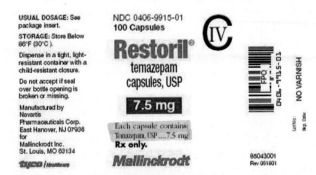

Figure 1.1 | Examples of USP labels *Source: Courtesy of Novartis Pharmaceuticals Corporation and Mallinckrodt Pharmaceuticals.*

In the early 1900s, the United States began to develop and enforce tougher drug legislation to protect the public. In 1902, the Biologics Control Act helped to standardize the quality of serums and other blood-related products. The Pure Food and Drug Act of 1906 gave the government power to control the labeling of medicines. In 1912, the Sherley Amendment prohibited the sale of drugs labeled with false therapeutic claims that were intended to defraud the consumer. In 1938, Congress passed the Food, Drug, and Cosmetic Act. This was the first law preventing the sale of drugs that had not been thoroughly tested before marketing. Later amendments to this law required drug companies to prove the safety and efficacy of any drug before it could be sold within the United States. In reaction to the rising popularity of dietary supplements, Congress passed the Dietary Supplement Health and Education Act of 1994 in an attempt to control misleading industry claims. A brief timeline of major events in U.S. drug regulation is shown in Figure 1.2.

1.7 The Role of the Food and Drug Administration

Much has changed in the regulation of drugs in the past 100 years. In 1988, the Food and Drug Administration (FDA) was officially established as an agency of the U.S. Department of Health and Human Services. The Center for Drug Evaluation and Research (CDER), a branch of the FDA, exercises control over whether prescription drugs and OTC drugs may be used for therapy. The CDER states its mission as facilitating the availability of safe, effective drugs; keeping unsafe or ineffective drugs off the market; improving the health of Americans; and providing clear, easily understandable drug information for safe and effective use. Any pharmaceutical laboratory, whether private, public, or academic, must solicit FDA approval before marketing a drug.

Another branch of the FDA, the Center for Biologics Evaluation and Research (CBER), regulates the use of bi-

TIMELINE	REGULATORY ACTS, STANDARDS, AND ORGANIZATIONS
1820	A group of physicians established the first comprehensive publication of drug standards called the **U.S. Pharmacopeia (USP)**.
1852	A group of pharmacists founded a national professional society called the **American Pharmaceutical Association (APhA)**. The APhA then established the **National Formulary (NF)**, a standardized publication focusing on pharmaceutical ingredients. The *USP* continued to catalogue all drug related substances and products.
1862	This was the beginning of the **Federal Bureau of Chemistry**, established under the administration of President Lincoln. Over the years and with added duties, it gradually became the Food and Drug Administration (FDA).
1902	Congress passed the **Biologics Control Act** to control the quality of serums and other blood-related products.
1906	**The Pure Food and Drug Act** gave the government power to control the labeling of medicines.
1912	**The Sherley Amendment** made medicines safer by prohibiting the sale of drugs labeled with false therapeutic claims.
1938	Congress passed the **Food, Drug, and Cosmetic Act**. It was the first law preventing the marketing of drugs not thoroughly tested. This law now provides for the requirement that drug companies must submit a New Drug Application (NDA) to the FDA prior to marketing a new drug.
1944	Congress passed the **Public Health Service Act**, covering many health issues including biological products and the control of communicable diseases.
1975	The *U.S. Pharmacopeia* and *National Formulary* announced their union. The **USP-NF** became a single standardized publication.
1986	Congress passed the **Childhood Vaccine Act.** It authorized the FDA to acquire information about patients taking vaccines, to recall biologics, and to recommend civil penalties if guidelines regarding biologic use were not followed.
1988	The **FDA** was officially established as an agency of the **U.S. Department of Health and Human Services**.
1992	Congress passed the **Prescription Drug User Fee Act.** It required that nongeneric drug and biologic manufacturers pay fees to be used for improvements in the drug review process.
1994	Congress passed the **Dietary Supplement Health and Education Act** that requires clear labeling of dietary supplements. This act gives the FDA the power to remove supplements that cause a significant risk to the public.
1997	The **FDA Modernization Act** reauthorized the Prescription Drug User Fee Act. This act represents the largest reform effort of the drug review process since 1938.

Figure 1.2 | A historical timeline of regulatory acts, standards, and organizations

ologics including serums, vaccines, and blood products. One historical achievement involving biologics is the 1986 Childhood Vaccine Act. This act authorized the FDA to acquire information about patients taking vaccines, to recall biologics, and to recommend civil penalties if guidelines regarding biologics were not followed.

The FDA also oversees administration of herbal products and dietary supplements through the Center for Food Safety and Applied Nutrition (CFSAN). Herbal products and dietary supplements are regulated by the Dietary Supplement Health and Education Act of 1994. This act does not provide the same degree of protection for consumers as the Food, Drug, and Cosmetic Act of 1938. For example, herbal and dietary supplements may be marketed without prior approval from the FDA. This act is discussed in detail in Chapter 11 ⊝ .

1.8 Stages of Approval for Therapeutic and Biologic Drugs

The amount of time spent by the FDA in the review and approval process for a particular drug depends on several checkpoints along a well-developed and organized plan. Therapeutic drugs and biologics are reviewed in four phases. These phases, summarized in Figure 1.3, are as follows:

1. Preclinical investigation
2. Clinical investigation

3. Review of the New Drug Application (NDA)
4. Postmarketing surveillance

Preclinical investigation involves extensive laboratory research. Scientists perform many tests on human and microbial cells cultured in the laboratory. Studies are performed in several species of animals to examine the drug's effectiveness at different doses, and to look for adverse effects. Extensive testing on cultured cells and in animals is essential because it allows the pharmacologist to predict whether the drug will cause harm to humans. Because laboratory tests do not always reflect the way a *human* responds, preclinical investigation results are always inconclusive. Animal testing may overestimate or underestimate the actual risk to humans.

Clinical investigation, the second stage of drug testing, takes place in three different stages termed *clinical phase trials.* Clinical phase trials are the longest part of the drug approval process. Clinical pharmacologists first perform tests on healthy volunteers to determine proper dosage and to assess for adverse effects. Large groups of selected patients with the particular disease are then given the medication. Clinical investigators from different medical specialties address concerns such as whether the drug is effective, worsens other medical conditions, interacts unsafely with existing medications, or affects one type of patient more than others.

Clinical phase trials are an essential component of drug evaluations due to the variability of responses among

New Drug Development Timeline

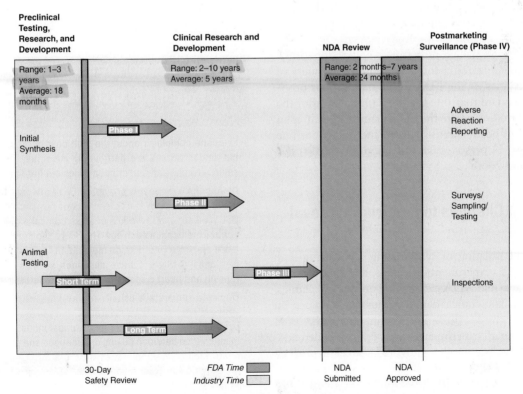

Figure 1.3 | A new drug development timeline, with the four phases of drug approval

patients. If a drug appears to be effective and without serious side effects, approval for marketing may be accelerated, or the drug may be used immediately in special cases with careful monitoring. If the drug shows promise but precautions are noted, the process is delayed until the pharmaceutical company remedies the concerns. In any case, a NDA must be submitted before a drug is allowed to proceed to the next stage of the approval process.

The **NDA review** is the third stage of the drug approval process. During this stage, clinical phase III trials and animal testing may continue depending on the results obtained from preclinical testing. By law, the FDA is permitted 6 months to initially review a NDA. If the NDA is approved, the process continues to the final stage. If the NDA is rejected, the process is suspended until noted concerns are addressed by the pharmaceutical company. The average NDA review time for new medications is approximately 17–24 months.

Postmarketing surveillance, the final stage of the drug approval process, begins after clinical trials and the NDA review have been completed. The purpose of stage IV testing is to survey for harmful drug effects in a larger population. Some adverse effects take longer to appear and are not identified until a drug is circulated to large numbers of people. One example is the diabetes drug, troglitazone (Rezulin), which was placed on the market in 1997. In 1998, Britain banned its use after discovering at least one death and several cases of liver failure in diabetic patients taking the medication. The FDA became aware of a number of cases in the United States where Rezulin was linked with liver failure and heart failure. Rezulin was recalled in March 2000 after healthcare providers asked the FDA to reconsider its therapeutic benefits versus its identified risks.

The FDA holds public meetings annually to receive feedback from patients and professional and pharmaceutical organizations regarding the effectiveness and safety of new drug therapies. If the FDA discovers a serious problem, it will mandate that the drug be withdrawn from the market. The situation where the FDA banned Rezulin is an ideal example of postmarketing surveillance in action. The FDA withdrew 11 prescription drugs from the market between 1997 and 2000.

1.9 Recent Changes to the Drug Approval Process

The process of isolating or synthesizing a new drug and testing it in cells, experimental animals, and humans can take many years. The NDA can include dozens of volumes of experimental and clinical data that must be examined in the drug review process. Some NDAs contain over 100,000 pages. Even after all experiments have been concluded and clinical data have been gathered, the FDA review process can take several years.

Expenses associated with development of a new drug can cost pharmaceutical manufacturers millions of dollars.

A recent study estimated the cost to bring a new drug to market at $802 million. These companies are often critical of the regulatory process, and are anxious to get the drug marketed to recoup their research and development expenses. The public is also anxious to receive new drugs, particularly for diseases that have a high mortality rate. While the criticisms of manufacturers and the public are certainly understandable—and sometimes justified—the fundamental priority of the FDA is to ensure that drugs are safe. Without an exhaustive review of scientific data, the public could be exposed to dangerous medications, or those that are ineffective in treating disease.

In the early 1990s, due to pressures from organized consumer groups and various drug manufacturers, governmental officials began to plan how to speed up the drug review process. Reasons identified for the delay in the FDA drug approval process included outdated guidelines, poor communication, and insufficient staff to handle the workload.

In 1992, FDA officials, members of Congress, and representatives from pharmaceutical companies negotiated the Prescription Drug User Fee Act on a 5-year trial basis. This act required drug and biologic manufacturers to provide yearly product user fees. This added income allowed the FDA to hire more employees and to restructure its organization to more efficiently handle the processing of a greater number of drug applications. The result of restructuring was a resounding success. From 1992 to 1996, the FDA approved double the number of drugs while cutting some review times by as much as half. In 1997, the FDA Modernization Act reauthorized the Prescription Drug

SPECIAL CONSIDERATIONS

How Prescription Drug Costs Affect Senior Citizens

Everyone complains about the high cost of prescription drugs, but senior citizens are particularly impacted. The facts about senior citizens and prescription drugs are hard to ignore:

Americans over age 65 are only 13% of the population, but account for about 34% of all prescriptions dispensed and 40% of all OTC medications. Over 80% of all seniors take at least one prescribed medication each day. The average older person is taking more than four prescription medications at once, plus two OTC medications. Many of these medicines, such as those for hypertension and heart disease, are taken on a permanent basis.

Because seniors are usually retired, they are less likely than younger people to have insurance that covers the cost of prescription medications. On a fixed annual income, many seniors must choose between buying medications and purchasing adequate food or material necessities. The annual drug spending per senior grew from an average of $559 in 1992 to over $1,200 in 2000.

MediaLink

Canadian Drug Regulations

PHARMFACTS — Time Length for New Drug Approvals

- It takes about 11 years of research and development before a drug is submitted to FDA for review.
- Phase I clinical trials take about 1 year and involve 20 to 80 normal, healthy volunteers.
- Phase II clinical trials last about 2 years and involve 100 to 300 volunteer patients with the disease.
- Phase III clinical trials take about 3 years and involve 1,000 to 3,000 patients in hospitals and clinic agencies.
- For every 5,000 chemicals that enter preclinical testing, only 5 make it to human testing. Of these five potential drugs, only one is finally approved.
- Since the 1992 Prescription Drug User Fee Act was passed, more than 700 drugs and biologics have come to the market.

User Fee Act. Nearly 700 employees were added to the FDA's drug and biologics program, and over $300 million was collected in user fees.

1.10 Canadian Drug Standards

As in the United States, drug testing and risk assessment in Canada is a major priority. The Health Protection Branch (HPB) of the Canadian government serves under the auspices of the Department of Health and Welfare. The HPB's task is to protect Canadians from the potential health hazards of marketed products, imported goods, and environmental agents. The deputy minister enforces regulations concerned with consumer protection issues such as the Food and Drugs Act and the Tobacco Act.

Health Canada is the federal department working in partnership with provincial and territorial governments. It also coordinates its efforts with other federal departments to ensure proper management of health and safety issues.

The Health Products and Food Branch (HPFB) of Health Canada regulates the use of therapeutic substances through several national programs, the Therapeutic Products Programme (TPP), the Office of Natural Health Products, and the Food Directorate. The TPP covers such drugs as pharmaceuticals, narcotic, controlled and restricted drugs, and biologics. Some natural health products and food-based products called nutraceuticals are also regulated. The Office of Natural Products limits its focus to natural substances, for example, homeopathic and herbal remedies. The Food Directorate regulates nutraceuticals.

The Canadian Food and Drugs Act is an important regulatory document specifying that drugs cannot be marketed without a Notice of Compliance (NOC) and Drug Identification Number (DIN) from Health Canada. Amended guidelines date back to 1953, stating that the use of foods, drugs, cosmetics, and therapeutic devices must follow established guidelines. Any drug that does not comply with standards established by recognized pharmacopoeias and formularies in the United States, Europe, Britain, or France cannot be labeled, packaged, sold, or advertised in Canada.

The drug approval process in Canada is illustrated in Table 1.1. Many similarities exist between how drugs are regulated in both Canada and the United States. These include the fact that both governments have realized a need to monitor natural products, dietary supplements and herbs, and newly developed traditional drug therapies.

Table 1.1	Steps of Approval for Drugs Marketed within Canada
Step 1	Preclinical studies or experiments in culture, living tissue, and small animals are performed, followed by extensive clinical trials or testing done in humans.
Step 2	A drug company completes a *drug submission* to Health Canada. This report details important safety and effectiveness information including how the drug product will be produced and packaged, expected therapeutic benefits and adverse reactions.
Step 3	A committee of drug experts including medical and drug scientists reviews the drug submission to identify potential benefits and drug risks.
Step 4	Health Canada reviews information about the drug product and passes on important details to health practitioners and consumers.
Step 5	Health Canada issues a Notice of Compliance (NOC) and Drug Identification Number (DIN). Both permit the manufacturer to market the drug product.
Step 6	Health Canada monitors the effectiveness and concerns of the drug after it has been marketed. This is done by regular inspection, notices, newsletters, and feedback from consumers and healthcare professionals.

CHAPTER REVIEW

Key Concepts

The numbered key concepts provide a succinct summary of the important points from the corresponding numbered section within the chapter. If any of these points are not clear, refer to the numbered section within the chapter for review. Expanded versions can be found on the companion website.

1.1 The history of pharmacology began thousands of years ago with the use of plant products to treat disease.

1.2 Pharmacology is the study of medicines. It includes how drugs are administered and how the body responds.

1.3 The fields of pharmacology and therapeutics are closely connected. Pharmacotherapy is the application of drugs to prevent disease and ease suffering.

1.4 Therapeutic agents may be classified as traditional drugs, biologics, or alternative therapies.

1.5 Drugs are available by prescription or over the counter (OTC). Prescription drugs require an order from a healthcare provider.

1.6 Drug regulations were created to protect the public from drug misuse, and to assume continuous evaluation of safety and effectiveness.

1.7 The regulatory agency responsible for ensuring that drugs and medical devices are safe and effective is the Food and Drug Administration (FDA).

1.8 There are four stages of approval for therapeutic and biologic drugs. These progress from cellular and animal testing to use of the experimental drug in patients with the disease.

1.9 Once criticized for being too slow, the FDA has streamlined the process to get new drugs to market more quickly.

1.10 Drug standards also ensure the effectiveness and safety of drugs for Canadian consumers.

Review Questions

1. Explain how the use of drugs has evolved since ancient times.

2. Explain why a patient might seek treatment from an OTC drug, instead of a more effective prescription drug.

3. How does the FDA ensure the safety and effectiveness of drugs? How has this process changed in recent years?

4. In many respects, the role of the FDA continues long after the initial drug approval. Explain the continued involvement of the FDA.

EXPLORE MediaLink

NCLEX review, case studies, and other interactive resources for this chapter can be found on the companion website at www.prenhall.com/adams. Click on "Chapter 1" to select the activities for this chapter. For animations, more NCLEX review questions, and an audio glossary, access the accompanying CD-ROM in this textbook.

Drug Classes and Schedules

The student beginning the study of pharmacology is quickly confronted with hundreds of drugs having specific dosages, side effects, and mechanisms of action. Without a means of grouping or organizing this information, most students would be overwhelmed by the vast amounts of new data. Drugs can be classified by a number of different methods which provide logical systems for identifying drugs and determining the limitations of their use. This chapter presents methods of grouping drugs: by therapeutic or pharmacologic classification, and by drug schedules.

metabolized and eliminated by the body.
of this process

PHARMACOLOGY
1. The study of medicines; the discipline pertaining to how drugs improve the hea
of the human body

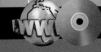 **MediaLink** www.prenhall.com/adams

CD-ROM
Audio Glossary
NCLEX Review

Companion Website
NCLEX Review
Case Study
Expanded Key Concepts
Challenge Your Knowledge

OBJECTIVES

After reading this chapter, the student should be able to:

1. Explain the basis for placing drugs into therapeutic and pharmacological classes.
2. Discuss the prototype approach to drug classification.
3. Describe what is meant by a drug's mechanism of action.
4. Distinguish between a drug's chemical name, generic name, and trade name.
5. Explain why generic drug names are preferred to trade name drugs.
6. Discuss why drugs are sometimes placed on a restrictive list, and the controversy surrounding this issue.
7. Explain the meaning of a controlled substance.
8. Explain the U.S. Controlled Substance Act of 1970 and the role of the U.S. Drug Enforcement Agency in controlling drug abuse and misuse.
9. Identify the five drug schedules and give examples of drugs at each level.
10. Explain how drugs are scheduled according to Parts III and IV of the Canadian Food and Drugs Act and the Narcotic Control Act.

2.1 Therapeutic and Pharmacologic Classification of Drugs

One useful method of organizing drugs is based on their therapeutic usefulness in treating particular diseases. This is referred to as a therapeutic classification. Drugs may also be organized by pharmacologic classification. A drug's pharmacologic classification refers to the way an agent works at the molecular, tissue, and body system level. Both types of classification are widely used in categorizing the thousands of available drugs.

Table 2.1 shows the method of therapeutic classification, using cardiac care as an example. Many different types of drugs affect cardiovascular function. Some drugs influence blood clotting while others lower blood cholesterol or prevent the onset of stroke. Drugs may be used to treat elevated blood pressure, heart failure, abnormal rhythm,

chest pain, heart attack, or circulatory shock. Thus, drugs that treat cardiac disorders may be placed in several types of therapeutic classes, for example, anticoagulants, antihyperlipidemics, and antihypertensives.

A therapeutic classification need not be complicated. For example, it is appropriate to simply classify a medication as a "drug used for stroke" or a "drug used for shock." The key to therapeutic classification is to clearly state what a particular drug does clinically. Other examples of therapeutic classifications include antidepressants, antipsychotics, drugs for erectile dysfunction, and antineoplastics.

The pharmacologic classification addresses a drug's mechanism of action, or *how* a drug produces its effect in the body. Table 2.2 shows a variety of pharmacologic classifications using hypertension as an example. A diuretic treats hypertension by lowering plasma volume. Calcium channel blockers treat this disorder by decreasing cardiac

Table 2.1	Organizing Drug Information by Therapeutic Classification
Therapeutic Focus: Cardiac Care / Drugs Affecting Cardiovascular Function	
Therapeutic Usefulness	**Therapeutic Classification**
influencing blood clotting	anticoagulants
lowering blood cholesterol	antihyperlipidemics
lowering blood pressure	antihypertensives
restoring normal cardiac rhythm	antidysrhythmics
treating angina	antianginals

Table 2.2	Organizing Drug Information by Pharmacologic Classification
Focus on How a Therapy Is Applied: Pharmacotherapy for Hypertension May Be Achieved by:	
Mechanism of Action	**Pharmacologic Classification**
lowering plasma volume	diuretic
blocking heart calcium channels	calcium channel blocker
blocking hormonal activity	angiotensin-converting enzyme inhibitor
blocking stress-related activity	adrenergic antagonist
dilating peripheral blood vessels	vasodilator

contractility. Other drugs block intermediates of the renin-angiotensin pathway. Notice that each example describes *how* hypertension might be controlled. A drug's pharmacologic classification is more specific than a therapeutic classification and requires an understanding of biochemistry and physiology. In addition, pharmacologic classifications may be described with varying degrees of complexity, sometimes taking into account drugs' chemical names.

When classifying drugs, it is common practice to select a single drug from a class and compare all other medications to this representative drug. A **prototype drug** is the well-understood drug model from which other drugs in a pharmacological class are compared. By learning the prototype drug, students may predict the actions and adverse effects of other drugs in the same class. For example, by knowing the effects of penicillin V, students can extend this knowledge to the other drugs in the penicillin class of antibiotics. The original drug prototype is not always the most widely used drug in its class. Newer drugs in the same class may be more effective, have a more favorable safety profile, or have a longer duration of action. These factors may sway healthcare providers from using the original prototype drug. In addition, healthcare providers and pharmacology textbooks sometimes differ as to which drug should be the prototype. In any case, becoming familiar with the drug prototypes and keeping up with newer and more popular drugs is an essential part of mastering drugs and drug classes.

2.2 Chemical, Generic, and Trade Names for Drugs

A major challenge in studying pharmacology is learning thousands of drug names. Adding to this difficulty is the fact that most drugs have multiple names. The three basic types of drug names are chemical, generic, and trade names.

Chemical names are assigned, using standard nomenclature established by the International Union of Pure and Applied Chemistry (IUPAC). A drug has only one chemical name, which is sometimes helpful in predicting a substance's physical and chemical properties. Although chemical names convey a clear and concise meaning about the nature of a drug, they are often complicated and difficult to remember or pronounce. For example, few nurses know the

chemical name for diazepam: 7-chloro-1,3-dihydro-1-methyl-5-phenyl-2H-1,4-benzodiazepin-2-one. In only a few cases, usually when the name is brief and easily remembered, will nurses use chemical names. Examples of useful chemical names include lithium carbonate, calcium gluconate, and sodium chloride.

More practically, drugs are sometimes classified by a *portion* of their chemical structure, known as the chemical group name. Examples are antibiotics such as fluoroquinolones and cephalosporins. Other common examples include phenothiazines, thiazides, and benzodiazepines. Although they may seem complicated when first encountered, knowledge of chemical group names will become invaluable as the nursing student begins to learn and understand major drug classes and actions.

The **generic name** of a drug is assigned by the U.S. Adopted Name Council. With few exceptions, generic names are less complicated and easier to remember than chemical names. Many organizations, including the FDA, the U.S. Pharmacopoeia, and the World Health Organization routinely describe a medication by its generic name. Because there is only one generic name for each drug, healthcare providers often use this name, and students generally must memorize it.

A drug's **trade name** is assigned by the company marketing the drug. The name is usually selected to be short and easy to remember. The trade name is sometimes called the proprietary, or product or brand name. The term **proprietary** suggests ownership. In the United States, a drug developer is given exclusive rights to name and market a drug for 17 years after a new drug application is submitted to the FDA. Because it takes several years for a drug to be approved, the amount of time spent in approval is usually subtracted from the 17 years. For example, if it takes 7 years for a drug to be approved, competing companies will not be allowed to market a generic equivalent drug for another 10 years. The rationale is that the developing company should be allowed sufficient time to recoup the millions of dollars in research and development costs in designing the new drug. After 17 years, competing companies may sell a generic equivalent drug, sometimes using a different name, which the FDA must approve.

Trade names may be a challenge for students to learn because of the dozens of product names containing similar

MediaLink ◯ Therapeutic Drug Classes

MediaLink ◯ IUPAC

Table 2.3	Examples of Brand Name Products Containing Popular Generic Substances
Generic Substance	**Brand Names**
aspirin	Acetylsalicylic Acid, Acuprin, Anacin, Aspergum, Bayer, Bufferin, Ecotrin, Empirin, Excedrin, Maprin, Norgesic, Salatin, Salocol, Salsprin, Supac, Talwin, Triaphen-10, Vanquish, Verin, ZORprin
diphenhydramine	Allerdryl, Benadryl, Benahist, Bendylate, Caladryl, Compoz, Diahist, Diphenadril, Eldadryl, Fenylhist, Fynex, Hydramine, Hydril, Insomnal, Noradryl, Nordryl, Nytol, Tusstat, Wehdryl
ibuprofen	Advil, Amersol, Apsifen, Brufen, Haltran, Medipren, Midol 200, Motrin, Neuvil, Novoprofen, Nuprin, Pamprin-IB, Rufen, Trendar

ingredients. In addition, **combination drugs** contain more than one active generic ingredient. This poses a problem in trying to match one generic name with one product name. As an example, refer to Table 2.3 and consider the drug diphenhydramine (generic name), also called Benadryl (one of many trade names). Diphenhydramine is an antihistamine. Low doses of diphenhydramine may be purchased OTC; higher doses require a prescription. When looking for diphenhydramine, the nurse may find it listed under many trade names, such as Allerdryl and Compoz, provided alone or in combination with other active ingredients. Ibuprofen and aspirin are also examples of drugs with many different trade names. The rule of thumb is that the active ingredients in a drug are described by their generic name. When referring to a drug, the generic name is usually written in lowercase, whereas the trade name is capitalized.

2.3 Differences between Brand Name Drugs and Their Generic Equivalents

During its 17 years of exclusive rights to a new drug, the pharmaceutical company determines the price of the medication. Because there is no competition, the price is generally quite high. The developing company sometimes uses legal tactics to extend their exclusive rights, since this can bring hundreds of millions of dollars per year in profits for a popular medicine. Once the exclusive rights end, competing companies market the generic drug for less money and consumer savings may be considerable. In some states, pharmacists may routinely substitute a generic drug when the prescription calls for a brand name. In other states, the pharmacist must dispense drugs directly as written by a healthcare provider or obtain approval before providing a generic substitute.

The companies marketing brand name drugs often lobby aggressively against laws that might restrict the routine use of their brand name products. The lobbyists claim that significant differences exist between a trade name drug and its generic equivalent, and that switching to the generic drug may be harmful for the patient. Consumer advocates, on the other hand, argue that generic substitutions should always be permitted because of the cost savings to patients.

Are there really differences between a brand name drug and its generic equivalent? The answer is unclear. Despite the fact that the dosages may be identical, drug formulations are not always the same. The two drugs may have different inert ingredients. For example, if in tablet form, the active ingredients may be more tightly compressed in one of the preparations.

The key to comparing brand name drugs and their generic equivalents lies in measuring the bioavailability of the two preparations. **Bioavailability** is the physiologic ability of the drug to reach its target cells and produce its effect. Bioavailability may indeed be affected by inert ingredients and tablet compression. Anything that affects absorption of a drug, or its distribution to the target cells, can certainly affect drug action. Measuring how long a drug takes to exert its effect gives pharmacologists a crude measure of bioavailability. For example, if a patient is in circulatory shock and it takes the generic equivalent drug 5 minutes longer to produce its effect, that is indeed significant; however, if a generic medication for arthritis pain relief takes 45 minutes to act, compared with the brand name drug which takes 40 minutes, it probably does not matter which drug is prescribed.

PHARMFACTS | **Marketing and Promotional Spending**

- When generic versions of paclitaxel (Taxol) became available, various legal tactics by Bristol-Myers Squibb delayed their entry to market. The estimated additional cost to consumers for 2 more years of patent extension was over $1 billion.
- Promotional spending on prescription drugs rose to $15.7 billion in 2000, up from $13.9 billion in 1999 and $9.2 billion in 1996.
- Spending on consumer drug advertisements on television and in print media increased to $2.5 billion in 2000, up from $1.85 billion in 1999 and $791 million in 1996.
- Consumer advocates claim that promotional advertisements drive up demand for the newer, more expensive drugs, instead of using the older, less costly drugs that might be equally effective.

Table 2.4	Negative Formulary List in Florida
Generic Name	**Brand Name Equivalent**
conjugated estrogen	Premarin
chlorpromazine	Thorazine
dicumarol	Dicumarol
digitoxin	Crystodigin
digoxin*	Lanoxin
levothyroxine sodium	Synthroid
pancrelipase	Pancrease
phenytoin*	Dilantin
quinidine gluconate*	Quinaglute
theophylline	Theo-Dur
warfarin*	Coumadin

*Removed from the Negative Formulary List by the Florida legislature in 2001.

To address this issue, some states have compiled a negative formulary list. In Florida, for example, drugs found on a negative formulary list must be dispensed exactly as written without allowing generic substitution by the pharmacist. In theory, these are drugs prescribed for critical conditions, in which small differences in bioavailability could adversely affect patient outcomes. In addition, they may be drugs in which research has shown significant differences in bioavailability among different formulations. The pharmaceutical companies that market brand name drugs often lobby to get medications added to these lists. The Florida list is shown in Table 2.4.

2.4 Controlled Substances and Drug Schedules

Some drugs are frequently abused or have a high potential for addiction. Technically, addiction refers to the overwhelming feeling that drives someone to use a drug repeatedly. Dependence is a related term, often defined as a physiological or psychological need for a substance. Physical dependence refers to an altered physical condition caused by the nervous system adapting to repeated drug use. In this case, when the drug is no longer available, the individual expresses physical signs of discomfort known as withdrawal. In contrast, when an individual is psychologically dependent, there are few signs of physical discomfort when the drug is withdrawn; however, the individual feels an intense compelling desire to continue drug use. These concepts are discussed in detail in Chapter 12 ⌖ .

Drugs that cause dependency are restricted for use in situations of medical necessity, if at all. According to law, drugs that have a significant potential for abuse are placed into five categories called schedules. These scheduled drugs are classified according to their potential for abuse: Schedule I

drugs have the highest potential for abuse, and Schedule V drugs have the lowest potential for abuse. Schedule I drugs have little to no therapeutic value or are intended for research purposes only. Drugs in the other four schedules may be dispensed only in cases when therapeutic value has been determined. Schedule V is the only category in which some drugs may be dispensed without a prescription, because the quantities of the controlled drug are so low that the possibility of causing dependence is extremely remote. Table 2.5 shows the five drug schedules with examples. Not all drugs with an abuse potential are regulated or placed into schedules. Tobacco, alcohol, and caffeine are significant examples.

In the United States, controlled substances are drugs whose use is restricted by the Controlled Substances Act of 1970 and later revisions. The Controlled Substances Act is also called the Comprehensive Drug Abuse Prevention and Control Act. Hospitals and pharmacies must register with the Drug Enforcement Administration (DEA) and then

PHARMFACTS	Extent of Drug Abuse

- In 2001, over 8 million people reported driving under the influence of illegal drugs during the previous year.
- In 2001, over 3 million teenagers had smoked cigarettes during the past month. Although it is illegal in the United States to sell tobacco to underaged youths, in 2001, almost 2 million youths aged 12 to 17 who smoked cigarettes purchased them personally.
- From 1994 to 2001, emergency department mentions of abused substances such as GHB, Ketamine, and MDMA rose over 2,000%.
- In 2001, almost 17 million Americans abused or were dependent on either alcohol or illicit drugs.

Table 2.5	U.S. Drug Schedules and Examples			
Drug Schedule	**Abuse Potential**	**Dependency Potential**		**Examples (Therapeutic Use)**
		Physical	**Psychological**	
I	highest	high	high	heroin, LSD, marijuana, and methaqualone (limited or no therapeutic use)
II	high	high	high	morphine, PCP, cocaine, methadone, and methamphetamine (used therapeutically with prescription; some drugs no longer used)
III	moderate	moderate	high	anabolic steroids, codeine and hydrocodone with aspirin or Tylenol, and some barbiturates (used therapeutically with prescription)
IV	lower	lower	lower	Darvon, Talwin, Equanil, Valium, and Xanax (used therapeutically with prescription)
V	lowest	lowest	lowest	over-the-counter cough medicines with codeine (used therapeutically without prescription)

use their assigned registration numbers to purchase scheduled drugs. They must maintain complete records of all quantities purchased and sold. Drugs with higher abuse potential have more restrictions. For example, a special order form must be used to obtain Schedule II drugs, and orders must be written and signed by the healthcare provider. Telephone orders to a pharmacy are not permitted. Refills for Schedule II drugs are not permitted; patients must visit their healthcare provider first. Those convicted of unlawful manufacturing, distributing, and dispensing of controlled substances face severe penalties.

2.5 Canadian Regulations Restricting Drugs of Abuse

In Canada, controlled substances are those drugs subject to guidelines outlined in Part III, Schedule G of the Canadian Food and Drugs Act. According to these guidelines, a healthcare provider may only dispense these medications to patients suffering from specific diseases or illnesses. Regulated drugs include amphetamines, barbiturates, methaqualone, and anabolic steroids. Controlled drugs must be labeled clearly with the letter C on the outside of the container.

Restricted drugs not intended for human use are covered in Part IV, Schedule H of the Canadian Food and Drugs Act. These are drugs used in the course of a chemical or analytical procedure for medical, laboratory, industrial, educational, or research purposes. They include hallucinogens such as LSD (lysergic acid diethylamide), MDMA (Ecstasy), and DOM (STP).

Schedule F drugs are those drugs requiring a prescription for their sale. Examples are methylphenidate (Ritalin), diazepam (Valium), and chlordiazepoxide (Librium). Drugs such as morphine, heroin, cocaine, and cannabis are covered under the Canadian Narcotic Control Act and amended schedules. According to Canadian law, narcotic drugs must be labeled clearly with the letter N on the outside of the container.

Throughout Canada, both prescription and nonprescription drugs must meet specific criteria for public distribution and use. The Health Protection Branch, Department of National Health and Welfare, has proposed that all drugs used for medicinal purposes be grouped into three schedules as summarized in Table 2.6. Nonprescription drugs are provided according to guidelines and acts established by the respective Canadian provinces. Pharmacies must monitor those drugs used specifically to treat self-limiting discomforts such as cold, flu, mild gastrointestinal, or other symptoms. Other nonprescription drugs may be sold without monitoring.

Table 2.6	Three-Schedule System for Drugs Sold in Canada
Drug Schedule	**Drug Type**
I	all prescription drugs
	drugs with no potential for abuse: Schedule F
	controlled drugs: Schedule G
	narcotic drugs
II	all nonprescription drugs monitored for sale by pharmacists
III	all nonprescription drugs not monitored for sale by pharmacists

CHAPTER REVIEW

Key Concepts

The numbered key concepts provide a succinct summary of the important points from the corresponding numbered section within the chapter. If any of these points are not clear, refer to the numbered section within the chapter for review. Expanded versions can be found on the companion website.

2.1 Drugs may be organized by their therapeutic or pharmacologic classification.

2.2 Drugs have chemical, generic, and trade names. A drug has only one chemical or generic name but may have multiple trade names.

2.3 Generic drugs are less expensive than brand name drugs, but they may differ in their bioavailability, the ability of the drug to reach its target tissue and produce its action.

2.4 Drugs with a potential for abuse are restricted by the Controlled Substances Act and are categorized into schedules. Schedule I drugs are the most tightly controlled, Schedule V drugs have less potential for addiction and are less tightly controlled.

2.5 Canadian regulations restrict drugs with a potential for abuse and label them as C (controlled) or N (narcotic).

Review Questions

1. What is the difference between therapeutic and pharmacologic classifications? Identify the following classifications as therapeutic or pharmacologic: beta-adrenergic blocker, oral contraceptive, laxative, folic acid antagonist, antianginal agent.

2. What is a prototype drug, and how does it differ from other drugs in the same class?

3. A pharmacist decides to switch from a trade name drug that was ordered by the physician to a generic equivalent drug. What advantages does this have for the patient? What disadvantages might be caused by the switch?

4. Why are certain drugs placed in schedules? What extra precautions are required of healthcare providers when prescribing scheduled drugs?

 ## EXPLORE MediaLink

NCLEX review, case studies, and other interactive resources for this chapter can be found on the companion website at www.prenhall.com/adams. Click on "Chapter 2 " to select the activities for this chapter. For animations, more NCLEX review questions, and an audio glossary, access the accompanying CD-ROM in this textbook.

Emergency Preparedness

It is important that nursing students understand the role that drugs play in preventing or controlling global disease outbreaks. Drugs are the most powerful tools available to the medical community for countering worldwide epidemics and bioterrorist threats. If medical personnel could not identify, isolate, or treat the causes of global diseases, a major incident could easily overwhelm healthcare resources and produce a catastrophic loss of life. Drugs are a major component of emergency preparedness plans. This chapter discusses the role of pharmacology in the prevention and treatment of diseases or conditions that might develop in the context of a biological, chemical, or nuclear attack.

metabolized and eliminated by the body
of this process
PHARMACOLOGY
1. The study of medicines; the disciplin
pertaining to how drugs improve the he
of the human body
PHARMACOPEI

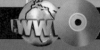

MediaLink   www.prenhall.com/adams

CD-ROM
Audio Glossary
NCLEX Review

Companion Website
NCLEX Review
Case Study
Expanded Key Concepts
Challenge Your Knowledge

OBJECTIVES

After reading this chapter, the student should be able to:

1. Explain why drugs are important in the context of emergency preparedness.
2. Discuss the role of the nurse in preparing for and responding to a bioterrorist act.
3. Identify the purpose and components of the Strategic National Stockpile (SNS).
4. Explain the threat of anthrax contamination and how it is transmitted.
5. Discuss the clinical manifestations and treatment of anthrax exposure.

6. Identify specific viruses that would most likely be used in a bioterrorist act.
7. Explain the advantages and disadvantages of vaccination as a means of preventing illness due to bioterrorist attacks.
8. Provide examples of chemical agents that might be used in a bioterrorism incident, and their treatments.
9. Describe the symptoms of acute radiation exposure and the role of potassium iodide (KI) in preventing thyroid cancer.

PLANNING FOR A BIOTERRORIST INCIDENT

Bioterrorist activities and threats have led to widespread changes in emergency preparedness planning. Nurses play key roles in planning for such incidents.

3.1 The Nature of Bioterrorism

Prior to the September 11, 2001, terrorist attacks on the United States, the attention of healthcare providers regarding disease outbreaks was mainly focused on the spread of traditional infectious diseases. These included possible epidemics caused by influenza, tuberculosis, cholera, and HIV. Table 3.1 shows the 10 most dangerous infectious diseases ranked according to which disorders caused the most deaths worldwide in the year 2000. Other infectious diseases such as food poisoning and sexually transmitted diseases were also common, though considered less important because they produced fewer fatalities.

The aftermath of the September 11, 2001, attacks prompted the healthcare community to expand its awareness of outbreaks and treatments to include bioterrorism and the health effects of biological and chemical weapons. Bioterrorism may be defined as the intentional use of infectious biological agents, chemical substances, or radiation to cause widespread harm or illness. The public has become more aware of the threat of bioterrorism because such federal agencies as the Centers for Disease Control and Prevention (CDC) and the U.S. Department of Defense have stepped up efforts to inform, educate, and prepare the public for disease outbreaks of a less traditional nature.

The goals of a bioterrorist are to create widespread public panic and cause as many casualties as possible. There is no shortage of agents that can be used for this purpose. In-

deed, some of these agents are easily obtainable and require little or no specialized knowledge to disseminate. Areas of greatest concern include acutely infectious diseases such as anthrax, smallpox, plague, and hemorrhagic viruses; incapacitating chemicals such as nerve gas, cyanide, and chlorinated agents; and nuclear and radiation emergencies. The CDC has categorized the biological threats, based on their potential impact on public health, as shown in Table 3.2.

3.2 Role of the Nurse in Emergency Preparedness

Emergency preparedness is not a new concept. For over 30 years, the Joint Commission on Accreditation of Healthcare Organizations (JCAHO) has required accredited hospitals to develop disaster plans and to conduct periodic emergency drills to determine readiness. Until recently, however, disaster plans and training focused on natural disasters such as tornados, hurricanes and floods, or accidents such as explosions that could cause multiple casualties. In the late 1990s, the JCAHO standards added the possibility of bioterrorism and virulent infectious organisms as rare, though possible, scenarios in disaster preparedness.

In 2001, the JCAHO issued new standards that changed the focus from disaster preparedness to emergency management. The newer standards include more than just responding to the immediate casualties caused by a disaster: They also consider how an agency's healthcare delivery system will shift during a crisis, and how it will return to normal operations following the incident. The expanded focus also includes how the individual healthcare agency will coordinate its efforts with community resources, such as other hospitals and public health agencies. State and federal agencies have revised their emergency preparedness guidelines in an attempt to more rationally plan for possible bioterrorist acts.

Table 3.1	The 10 Most Dangerous Infectious Diseases in the World, 2000		
Disease	**Cause**	**Target**	**Deaths per Year (millions)**
influenza	*Haemophilus influenzae*	respiratory system	3.7
tuberculosis	*Mycobacterium tuberculosis*	lungs	2.9
cholera	*Vibrio cholerae*	digestive tract	2.5
AIDS	human immuno-deficiency virus	immune response	2.3
malaria	*Plasmodium falciparum*	blood disorder	1.5
measles	rubeola virus	lungs and meninges	0.96
hepatitis B	hepatitis B virus (HBV)	liver	0.605
whooping cough	*Bordetella pertussis*	respiratory system	0.41
tetanus	*Clostridium tetani*	entire body (infections)	0.275
dengue fever	flavivirus	entire body (fever)	0.14

Source: World Health Organization Data, www.ac-reunion.fr/pedagogie/anglaislp/OurFood/General_bacteriology.html

Table 3.2	Categories of Infectious Agents	
Category	**Description**	**Examples**
A	agents that can be easily disseminated or transmitted person to person; cause high mortality, with potential for major public health impact; might cause public panic and social disruption; and require special action for public health preparedness	*Bacillus anthracis* (anthrax) *Clostridium botulinum* toxin (botulism) *Francisella tularensis* (tularemia) variola major (smallpox) viral hemorrhagic fevers such as Marburg and Ebola *Yersinia pestis* (plague)
B	moderately easy to disseminate; cause moderate morbidity and low mortality; and require specific enhancements of CDC's diagnostic capacity and enhanced disease surveillance	*Brucella* species (brucellosis) *Burkholderia mallei* (glanders) *Burkholderia pseudomallei* (melioidosis) *Chlamydia psittaci* (psittacosis) *Coxiella burnetii* (Q fever) epsilon toxin of *Clostridium perfringens* food safety threats such as *Salmonella* and *E. coli* ricin toxin from *Ricinus communis* *Staphylococcus* enterotoxin B viral encephalitis water safety threats such as *Vibrio cholerae* and *Cryptosporidium parvum*
C	emerging pathogens that could be engineered for mass dissemination in the future because of their availability, ease of production and dissemination, and potential for high morbidity and mortality rates and major health impacts	hantaviruses multidrug-resistant tuberculosis Nipah virus (NiV) tick-borne encephalitis viruses yellow fever

Source: www.bt.cdc.gov/Agent/agentlist.asp

Planning for bioterrorist acts requires close cooperation among all the different healthcare professionals. Nurses are central to the effort. Because a bioterrorist incident may occur in any community without advance warning, nurses must be prepared to immediately respond. The following elements underscore the key roles of nurses in meeting the challenges of a potential bioterrorist event.

■ *Education* Nurses must maintain a current knowledge and understanding of emergency management relating to bioterrorist activities.

■ *Resources* Nurses must maintain a current listing of health and law enforcement contacts and resources in their local community that would assist in the event of bioterrorist activity.

■ *Diagnosis and treatment* Nurses must be aware of the early signs and symptoms of chemical and biological agents, and their immediate treatment.

■ *Planning* Nurses should be involved in developing emergency management plans.

3.3 Strategic National Stockpile

Should a chemical or biological attack occur, it would likely be rapid and unexpected, and produce multiple casualties. Although planning for such an event is an important part of disaster preparedness, individual healthcare agencies and local communities could easily be overwhelmed by such a crisis. Shortages of needed drugs, medical equipment, and supplies would be expected.

The **Strategic National Stockpile (SNS)**, formerly called the National Pharmaceutical Stockpile, is a program designed to ensure the immediate deployment of essential medical materials to a community in the event of a large-scale chemical or biological attack. Managed by the CDC, the stockpile consists of the following materials.

■ Antibiotics
■ Vaccines
■ Medical, surgical, and patient support supplies such as bandages, airway supplies, and IV equipment

The SNS has two components. The first is called a push package, which consists of a preassembled set of supplies and pharmaceuticals designed to meet the needs of an unknown biological or chemical threat. There are eight, fully stocked, 50-ton push packages stored in climate-controlled warehouses throughout the United States. They are in locations where they can reach any community in the United States within 12 hours after an attack. The decision to deploy the push package is based on an assessment of the situation by federal government officials.

The second SNS component consists of a **vendor-managed inventory (VMI)** package. VMI packages are shipped, if necessary, after the chemical or biological threat has been more clearly identified. The materials consist of supplies and pharmaceuticals more specific to the chemical or biological agent used in the attack. VMI packages are designed to arrive within 24 to 36 hours.

The stockpiling of antibiotics and vaccines by local hospitals, clinics, or individuals for the purpose of preparing for a bioterrorist act is not recommended. Pharmaceuticals have a finite expiration date, and keeping large stores of drugs can be costly. Furthermore, stockpiling could cause drug shortages and prevent the delivery of these pharmaceuticals to communities where they may be needed most.

AGENTS USED IN BIOTERRORISM ACTS

Bioterrorists could potentially use any biological, chemical, or physical agent to cause widespread panic and serious illness. Knowing which agents are most likely to be used in an incident helps nurses to plan and implement emergency preparedness policies.

3.4 Anthrax

One of the first threats following the terrorist attacks on the World Trade Center was **anthrax**. In fall 2001, five people died as a result of exposure to anthrax, presumably due to purposeful, bioterrorist actions. At least 13 U.S. citizens were infected, several governmental employees were threatened, and the U.S. Postal Service was interrupted for several weeks. There was initial concern that anthrax outbreaks might disrupt many other essential operations throughout the country.

Anthrax is caused by the bacterium *Bacillus anthracis*, which normally affects domestic and wild animals. A wide variety of hoofed animals are affected by the disease, including cattle, sheep, goats, horses, donkeys, pigs, American bison, antelopes, elephants, and lions. If transmitted to humans by exposure to an open wound, through contaminated food, or by inhalation, *B. anthracis* can cause serious damage to body tissues. Symptoms of anthrax infection usually appear in 1 to 6 days after exposure. Depending on how the bacterium is transmitted, specific types of anthrax "poisoning" may be observed, each characterized by hallmark symptoms. Clinical manifestations of anthrax are summarized in Table 3.3.

B. anthracis causes disease by the emission of two types of toxins, edema toxin and lethal toxin. These toxins cause necrosis and accumulation of exudate, which produces pain, swelling, and restriction of activity, the general symptoms associated with almost every form of anthrax. Another component, the anthrax binding receptor, allows the bacterium to bind to human cells and act as a "doorway" for both types of toxins to enter.

Further ensuring its chance for spreading, *B. anthracis* is spore forming. Anthrax spores can remain viable in soil for hundreds, and perhaps thousands, of years. Anthrax spores are resistant to drying, heat, and some harsh chemicals. These spores are the main cause for public health concern, because they are responsible for producing inhalation anthrax, the most dangerous form of the disease. After entry into the lungs, *B. anthracis* spores are ingested by macrophages and carried to lymphoid tissue resulting in tissue necrosis, swelling, and hemorrhage. One of the main body areas affected is the mediastinum, which is a potential site for tissue injury and fluid accumulation. Meningitis is also a common pathology. If treatment is delayed, inhalation anthrax is lethal in almost every case.

B. anthracis is found in contaminated animal products such as wool, hair, dander, and bonemeal, but it can also be packaged in other forms making it transmissible through the air or by direct contact. Terrorists have delivered it in the form of a fine powder, making it less obvious to detect. The powder can be inconspicuously spread on virtually any surface, making it a serious concern for public safety.

The antibiotic ciprofloxacin (Cipro) has traditionally been used for anthrax prophylaxis and treatment. For prophylaxis, the usual dosage is 500 mg PO, every 12 hours for

Table 3.3	Clinical Manifestations of Anthrax	
Type	**Description**	**Symptoms**
cutaneous anthrax	most common but least complicated form of anthrax; almost always curable if treated within the first few weeks of exposure; results from direct contact of contaminated products with an open wound or cut	small skin lesions develop and turn into black scabs; inoculation takes less than 1 week; cannot be spread by person-to-person contact
gastrointestinal anthrax	rare form of anthrax; without treatment, can be lethal in up to 50% of cases; results from eating anthrax-contaminated food, usually meat	sore throat, difficulty swallowing, cramping, diarrhea, and abdominal swelling
inhalation anthrax	least common, but the most dangerous form of anthrax; can be successfully treated if identified within the first few days after exposure; results from inhaling anthrax spores	initially fatigue and fever for several days, followed by persistent cough and shortness of breath; without treatment, death can result within 4–6 days

MediaLink Anthrax Vaccine Immunization Program (AVIP)

MediaLink Other Biological Threats

60 days. If exposure has been confirmed, ciprofloxacin should be immediately administered at a usual dose of 400 mg IV, every 12 hours. Other antibiotics are also effective against anthrax, including penicillin, vancomycin, ampicillin, erythromycin, tetracycline, and doxycycline. In the case of inhalation anthrax, the FDA has approved the use of ciprofloxacin and doxycycline in combination for treatment.

Many members of the public have become intensely concerned about bioterrorism threats and have asked their healthcare provider to provide them with ciprofloxacin. The public should be discouraged from seeking the prophylactic use of antibiotics in cases when anthrax exposure has not been confirmed. Indiscriminate, unnecessary use of antibiotics can be expensive, cause significant side effects, and promote the appearance of resistant bacterial strains. The student should refer to Chapter 32 to review the precautions and guidelines regarding the appropriate use of antibiotics .

Although anthrax immunization (vaccination) has been licensed by the FDA for 30 years, it has not been widely used because of the extremely low incidence of this disease in the United States prior to September 2001. The vaccine has been prepared from proteins from the anthrax bacteria, dubbed "protective antigens." Anthrax vaccine works the same way as other vaccines: by causing the body to make protective antibodies and thus preventing the onset of disease and symptoms. Immunization for anthrax consists of three subcutaneous injections given 2 weeks apart, followed by three additional subcutaneous injections given at 6, 12, and 18 months. Annual booster injections of the vaccine are recommended. At this time, the CDC recommends vaccination for only select populations: laboratory personnel who work with anthrax, military personnel deployed to high-risk areas, and those who deal with animal products imported from areas with a high incidence of the disease.

There is an ongoing controversy regarding the safety of the anthrax vaccine, and whether it is truly effective in preventing the disease. Until these issues are resolved, the use of anthrax immunization will likely remain limited to select groups. Vaccines and the immune response are discussed in more detail in Chapter 31 .

3.5 Viruses

In 2002, the public was astounded as researchers announced that they had "built" a poliovirus, a threat that U.S. health officials thought was essentially eradicated in 1994. Although virtually eliminated in the Western Hemisphere, at least 27 countries reported polio transmission as late as 1998. The infection still persists among infants and children in areas with contaminated drinking water or food, mainly in underdeveloped regions of India, Pakistan, Afghanistan, western and central Africa, and the Dominican Republic. In the United States, polio remains a potential threat in 1 of 300,000 to 500,000 patients who are vaccinated with the oral poliovirus vaccine.

The current concern is that bioterrorists will culture the poliovirus and release it into regions where people have not been vaccinated. An even more dangerous threat is that a mutated strain, for which there is no effective vaccine, might be developed. Because the genetic code of the poliovirus is small (around 7,500 base pairs), it can be manufactured in a relatively simple laboratory. Once the virus is isolated, hundreds of different mutant strains could be produced in a very short time.

In addition to polio, smallpox is considered a potential biohazard. Once thought to be eradicated from the planet in the 1970s, the variola virus that causes this disease has been harbored in research labs in several countries. Much of its genetic code (200,000 base pairs) has been sequenced, and is public information. The disease is spread person to person as an aerosol or droplets or by contact with contaminated objects such as clothing or bedding. Only a few viral particles are needed to cause infection. If released into an unvaccinated population, as many as one in three could die from the virus.

There are no effective therapies for treating patients infected by most types of viruses that could be used in a bioterrorist attack. For some viruses, however, it is possible to create a vaccine that could stimulate the body's immune system in a manner that can be remembered at a later date. In the case of smallpox, a stockpile of the vaccine exists in enough quantity to administer to every person in the United States. The variola vaccine provides a high level of protection if given prior to exposure, or up to 3 days later. Protection may last from 3 to 5 years. The following are contraindications to receiving the smallpox vaccine, unless the individual has confirmed face-to-face contact with an infected patient.

- Persons with (or a history of) atopic dermatitis or eczema
- Persons with acute, active, or exfoliative skin conditions
- Persons with altered immune states (e.g., HIV, AIDS, leukemia, lymphoma, immunosuppressive drugs)
- Pregnant and breastfeeding women
- Children younger than 1 year
- Persons who have a serious allergy to any component of the vaccine

One suggestion has been that multiple vaccines be created, mass produced, and stockpiled to meet the challenges of a terrorist attack. Another suggestion has called for mass vaccination of the public, or at least those healthcare providers and law enforcement employees who might be exposed to infected patients.

Vaccines have side effects, some of which are quite serious. In the case of smallpox vaccination, for example, it is estimated that there might be as many as 250 deaths for every million people inoculated. If given to every person in the United States (approximately 285 million), possible deaths from smallpox vaccination could exceed 71,000. In addition, terrorists having some knowledge of genetic structure could create a modified strain of the virus that renders existing vaccines totally ineffective. It appears, then, that mass vaccination is not an appropriate solution until research can produce safer and more effective vaccines.

3.6 Toxic Chemicals

Although chemical warfare agents have been available since World War I, medicine has produced few drug antidotes. Many treatments provide minimal help, other than to relieve some symptoms and provide comfort following exposure. Most chemical agents used in warfare were created to cause mass casualties; others were designed to cause so much discomfort that soldiers would be too weak to con-

tinue fighting. Potential chemicals that could be used in a terrorist act include nerve gases, blood agents, choking and vomiting agents, and those that cause severe blistering. Table 3.4 provides a summary of selected chemical agents and known antidotes and first-aid treatments.

The chemical category of main pharmacologic significance is **nerve agents**. Exposure to these acutely toxic chemicals can cause convulsions and loss of consciousness within seconds, and respiratory failure within minutes. Almost all signs of exposure to nerve gas agents relate to overstimulation of the neurotransmitter acetylcholine (Ach) at both central and peripheral sites located throughout the body.

Acetylcholine is normally degraded by the enzyme, acetylcholinesterase (AchE), in the synaptic space. Nerve agents block AchE, increasing the action of acetylcholine in the synaptic space; therefore, all symptoms of nerve gas exposure such as salivation, increased sweating, muscle twitching, involuntary urination and defecation, confusion, convulsions, and death are the direct result of Ach overstimulation. To remedy this condition, nerve agent antidote and mark I injector kits that contain the anticholinergic drug atropine or a related medication are available in cases when nerve agent release is expected. Atropine blocks the attachment of Ach to receptor sites and prevents the overstimulation caused by the nerve agent. Neurotransmitters, synapses, and autonomic receptors are discussed in detail in Chapter 13 ∞ .

3.7 Ionizing Radiation

In addition to biological and chemical weapons, it is possible that bioterrorists could develop nuclear bombs capable of mass destruction. In such a scenario, the greatest number of casualties would occur due to the physical blast itself. Survivors, however, could be exposed to high levels of **ionizing radiation** from hundreds of different radioisotopes created by the nuclear explosion. Some of these radioisotopes emit large amounts of radiation and persist in the environment for years. As was the case in the 1986 Chernobyl nuclear accident in the Ukraine, the resulting radioisotopes could travel through wind currents, to land thousands of miles away from the initial explosion. Smaller scale radiation exposure could occur through terrorist attacks upon nuclear power plants or by the release of solid or liquid radioactive materials into public areas.

The acute effects of ionizing radiation have been well documented and depend primarily on the dose of radiation that the patient receives. The **acute radiation syndrome**, sometimes called radiation sickness, can occur within hours or days after extreme doses. Immediate symptoms are nausea, vomiting, and diarrhea. Later symptoms include weight loss, anorexia, fatigue, and bone marrow suppression. Patients who survive the acute exposure are at high risk for developing various cancers, particularly leukemia.

Table 3.4	Chemical Warfare Agents and Treatments	
Category	**Signs of Discomfort/Fatality**	**Antidotes/First Aid**
Nerve Agents		
GA—Tabun (liquid) GB—Sarin (gaseous liquid) GD—Soman (liquid) VX (gaseous liquid)	Depending on the nerve agent, symptoms may be slower to appear and cumulative depending on exposure time: miosis, runny nose, difficulty breathing, excessive salivation, nausea, vomiting, cramping, involuntary urination and defecation, twitching and jerking of muscles, headaches, confusion, convulsion, coma, death.	Nerve agent antidote and mark I injector kits with atropine are available. Flush eyes immediately with water. Apply sodium bicarbonate or 5% liquid bleach solution to the skin. Vomiting should not be induced.
Blood Agents		
hydrogen cyanide (liquid)	Red eyes, flushing of the skin, nausea, headaches, weakness, hypoxic convulsions, death	Flush eyes and wash skin with water. For inhalation of mist, oxygen and amyl nitrate may be given. For ingestion of cyanide liquid, 1% sodium thiosulfate may be given to induce vomiting.
cyanogen chloride (gas)	Loss of appetite, irritation of the respiratory tract, pulmonary edema, death	Oxygen and amyl nitrate may be given. Give patient milk or water. Do not induce vomiting.
Choking/Vomiting Agents		
phosgene (gas)	Dizziness, burning eyes, thirst, throat irritation, chills, respiratory and circulatory failure, cyanosis, frostbite-type lesions	Provide fresh air. Administer oxygen. Flush eyes with normal saline or water. Keep patient warm and calm.
Adamsite—DM (crystalline dispensed in aerosol)	Irritating to the eyes and respiratory tract, tightness of the chest, nausea, and vomiting	Rinse nose and throat with saline, water, or 10% solution of sodium bicarbonate. Treat the skin with borated talcum powder.
Blister/Vesicant Agents		
phosgene oxime (crystalline or liquid)	Destruction of mucous membranes, eye tissue, and skin (subcutaneous edema), followed by scab formation	Flush affected area with copious quantities of water. If ingested, do not induce vomiting.
mustard-lewisite mixture—HL, nitrogen mustard—HN-1, HN-2, HN-3, sulfur mustard agents	Irritating to the eyes, nasal membranes, and lungs; nausea and vomiting; formation of blisters on the skin; cytotoxic reactions in hematopoietic tissues including bone marrow, lymph nodes, spleen, and endocrine glands	Flush affected area with water. Treat the skin with 5% solution of sodium hypochlorite or household bleach. Give milk to drink. Do not induce vomiting. Skin contact with lewisite may be treated with 10% solution of sodium carbonate.

Source: Chemical Fact Sheets at the U.S. Army Center for Health Promotion and Preventative Medicine website, http://chemistry.about.com/gi/dynamic/offsite.htm?site = http%3A%2F%2Fchppm-www.apgea.army.mil%2Fdts%2Fdtchemfs.htm

Symptoms of nuclear and radiation exposure remain some of the most difficult to treat pharmacologically. Apart from the symptomatic treatment of radiation sickness, taking potassium iodide (KI) tablets after an incident or an attack is the only recognized therapy specifically designed for radiation exposure. Following a nuclear explosion, one of the resultant radioisotopes is iodine-131. Because iodine is naturally concentrated in the thyroid gland, I-131 will immediately enter the thyroid and damage thyroid cells. For example, following the Chernobyl nuclear disaster, the incidence of thyroid cancer in the Ukraine jumped from 4 to 6 cases per million people to 45 cases per million. If taken prior to, or immediately following, a nuclear incident, KI can prevent up to 100% of the radioactive iodine from entering the thyroid gland. It is effective even if taken 3 to 4 hours after radiation exposure. Generally, a single 130 mg dose is necessary.

Unfortunately, KI only protects the thyroid gland from I-131. It has no protective effects on other body tissues, and it offers no protection against the dozens of other harmful radioisotopes generated by a nuclear blast. Like vaccines and antibiotics, the stockpiling of KI by local healthcare agencies or individuals is not recommended. Interestingly, I-131 is also a medication used to shrink the size of overactive thyroid glands. Thyroid medications are presented in Chapter 39 ∞ .

PHARMFACTS	**Potential Chemical and Biological Agents for Terrorist Attacks**

- Robert Stevens, the 63-year-old employee of American Media who died in Florida on October 5, 2001, was the first person to die from anthrax in the United States in 25 years.
- In 1979, accidental release of anthrax from a research lab in the Soviet Union killed 68 people. The problem was traced to a faulty air filter.
- The Ebola virus causes death by hemorrhagic fever in up to 90% of the patients who show clinical symptoms of infection.
- Ebola viruses are found in central Africa. Although the source of the viruses in nature remains unknown, monkeys (like humans) appear to be susceptible to infection and serve as sources of virus if infected.
- Widespread public smallpox vaccinations ceased in the United States in 1972.
- It is estimated that 7 million to 8 million doses of smallpox vaccine is in storage at the CDC. This stock cannot be easily replenished, since all vaccine production facilities were dismantled after 1980, and new vaccine production requires 24 to 36 months.
- Most of the nerve agents were originally produced in a search for insecticides, but because of their toxicity, they were evaluated for military use.
- Chemicals used in bioterrorist acts need not be sophisticated or difficult to obtain: Toxic industrial chemicals such as chlorine, phosgene, and hydrogen cyanide are used in commercial manufacturing and are readily available.

MediaLink Potassium Iodide (KI)

CHAPTER REVIEW

Key Concepts

The numbered key concepts provide a succinct summary of the important points from the corresponding numbered section within the chapter. If any of these points are not clear, refer to the numbered section within the chapter for review. Expanded versions can be found on the companion website.

3.1 Bioterrorism is the deliberate use of a biological or physical agent to cause panic and mass casualties. The health aspects of biological and chemical agents have become important public issues.

3.2 Nurses play key roles in emergency preparedness, including education, resources, diagnosis and treatment, and planning.

3.3 The Strategic National Stockpile (SNS) is used to rapidly deploy medical necessities to communities experiencing a chemical or biological attack. The two components are the push package and the vendor managed inventory.

3.4 Anthrax can enter the body through ingestion, inhalation, or by the cutaneous route. Antibiotic therapy can be successful if given prophylactically or within a short time after exposure.

3.5 Viruses such as polio, smallpox, and the hemorrhagic fevers are potential biological weapons. If available, vaccines are the best treatments.

3.6 Chemicals and neurotoxins are potential bioterrorist threats for which there are no specific antidotes.

3.7 Potassium iodide (KI) may be used to block the effects of acute radiation exposure on the thyroid gland, but is not effective for protecting other organs.

Review Questions

1. Why is the medical community opposed to the mass vaccination of the general public for potential bioterrorist threats such as anthrax and smallpox?

2. Why does the protective effect of KI not extend to body tissues other than the thyroid gland?

3. Explain the differences between the Strategic National Stockpile (SNS) and the vendor-managed inventory (VMI).

4. Why do nurses play such a central role in emergency preparedness?

EXPLORE MediaLink

NCLEX review, case studies, and other interactive resources for this chapter can be found on the companion website at www.prenhall.com/adams. Click on "Chapter 3" to select the activities for this chapter. For animations, more NCLEX review questions, and an audio glossary, access the accompanying CD-ROM in this textbook.

Principles of Drug Administration

The primary role of the nurse in drug administration is to ensure that prescribed medications are delivered in a safe manner. Drug administration is an important component of providing comprehensive nursing care that incorporates all aspects of the nursing process. In the course of drug administration, nurses will collaborate closely with physicians, pharmacists, and, of course, their patients. The purpose of this chapter is to introduce the roles and responsibilities of the nurse in delivering medications safely and effectively.

metabolized and eliminated by the body.
of this process
PHARMACOLOGY
1. The study of medicines; the discipline pertaining to how drugs improve the heal of the human body

 **MediaLink** www.prenhall.com/adams

CD-ROM
Audio Glossary
NCLEX Review

Companion Website
NCLEX Review
Case Study
Expanded Key Concepts
Challenge Your Knowledge

OBJECTIVES

After reading this chapter, the student should be able to:

1. Discuss drug administration as a component of safe, effective nursing care, utilizing the nursing process.

2. Describe the roles and responsibilities of the nurse regarding drug administration.

3. Explain how the five rights of drug administration impact patient safety.

4. Give specific examples of how the nurse can increase patient compliance in taking medications.

5. Interpret drug orders that contain abbreviations.

6. Compare and contrast the three systems of measurement used in pharmacology.

7. Explain the proper methods to administer enteral, topical, and parenteral drugs.

8. Compare and contrast the advantages and disadvantages of each route of drug administration.

NURSING MANAGEMENT OF DRUG ADMINISTRATION

4.1 Medication Knowledge, Understanding, and Responsibilities of the Nurse

Whether administering drugs or supervising drug use, the nurse is expected to understand the pharmacotherapeutic principles for all medications received by each patient. Given the large number of different drugs and the potential consequences of medication errors, this is indeed an enormous task. The nurse's responsibilities include knowledge and understanding of the following:

- What drug is ordered
  - Name (generic and trade) and drug classification
  - Intended or proposed use
  - Effects on the body
  - Contraindications
  - Special considerations, (e.g., how age, weight, body fat distribution, and individual pathophysiologic states affect pharmacotherapeutic response)
  - Side effects
- Why the medication has been prescribed for this particular patient
- How the medication is supplied by the pharmacy
- How the medication is to be administered, including dosage ranges
- What nursing process considerations related to the medication apply to this patient

Before any drug is administered, the nurse must obtain and process pertinent information regarding the patient's medical history, physical assessment, disease processes, and learning needs and capabilities. Growth and developmental factors must always be considered. It is important to remember that a large number of variables influence a patient's response to medications. Having a firm understanding of these variables can increase the success of pharmacotherapy.

A major goal in studying pharmacology is to limit the number and severity of adverse drug events. Many adverse effects are preventable. Professional nurses can routinely avoid many serious adverse drug effects in their patients by applying their experience and knowledge of pharmacotherapeutics to clinical practice. Some adverse effects, however, are not preventable. It is vital that the nurse be prepared to recognize and respond to potential adverse effects of medications.

Allergic and anaphylactic reactions are particularly serious effects that must be carefully monitored and prevented, when possible. An **allergic reaction** is an acquired hyperresponse of body defenses to a foreign substance (allergen). Signs of allergic reactions vary in severity and include skin rash with or without itching, edema, nausea, diarrhea, runny nose, or reddened eyes with tearing. Upon discovering that the patient is allergic to a product, it is the nurse's responsibility to alert all personnel by documenting the allergy in the medical record, and by applying labels to the chart and medication administration record (MAR). An appropriate, agency-approved bracelet should be placed on the patient to alert all caregivers of the specific drug allergy.

Information related to drug allergy must be communicated to the physician and pharmacist so the medication regimen can be evaluated for cross-sensitivity between various pharmacologic products.

Anaphylaxis is a severe type of allergic reaction that involves the massive, systemic release of histamine and other chemical mediators of inflammation that can lead to life-threatening shock. Symptoms such as acute dyspnea and the sudden appearance of hypotension or tachycardia following drug administration are indicative of anaphylaxis, which must receive immediate treatment. The pharmacotherapy of allergic reactions and anaphylaxis is covered in Chapters 30 and 26, respectively⊚ .

4.2 The Rights of Drug Administration

The traditional **five rights of drug administration** form the operational basis for the safe delivery of medications. The five rights offer simple and practical guidance for nurses to use during drug preparation, delivery, and administration, and focus on individual performance. The five rights are as follows:

- Right patient
- Right medication
- Right dose
- Right route of administration
- Right time of delivery

Additional rights have been added over the years, depending on particular academic curricula or agency policies. Additions to the original five rights include considerations such as the right to refuse medication, the right to receive drug education, the right preparation, and the right documentation. Ethical and legal considerations regarding the five rights are discussed in Chapter 9⊚ .

The **three checks of drug administration** that nurses use in conjunction with the five rights help to ascertain patient safety and drug effectiveness. Traditionally these checks incorporate the following:

- Checking the drug with the MAR or the medication information system when removing it from the medication drawer, refrigerator, or controlled substance locker
- Checking the drug when preparing it; pouring it, taking it out of the unit dose container, or connecting the IV tubing to the bag
- Checking the drug before administering it to the patient

Despite all attempts to provide safe drug delivery, errors continue to occur, some of which are fatal. Although the nurse is held accountable for preparing and administering medications, safe drug practices are a result of multidisciplinary endeavors. Responsibility for accurate drug administration lies with multiple individuals, including physicians, pharmacists, and other healthcare professionals. Factors contributing to medication errors are presented in Chapter 9⊚ .

4.3 Patient Compliance and Successful Pharmacotherapy

Compliance is a major factor affecting pharmacotherapeutic success. As it relates to pharmacology, **compliance** is taking a medication in the manner prescribed by the practitioner or, in the case of OTC drugs, following the instructions on the

---

PHARMFACTS | **Potentially Fatal Drug Reactions**

Toxic Epidermal Necrolysis (TEN)

- Severe and deadly drug-induced allergic reaction
- Characterized by widespread epidermal sloughing, caused by massive disintegration of keratinocytes
- Severe epidermal detachment involving the top layer of the skin and mucous membranes
- Multisystem organ involvement and death if the reaction is not recognized and diagnosed
- Occurs when the liver fails to properly break down a drug, which then cannot be excreted normally
- Associated with use of some anticonvulsants (phenytoin [Dilantin], carbamazepine [Tegretol]), the antibiotic trimethoprim/sulfamethoxazole Bactrim, Septra), and other drugs, but can occur with the use of any prescription or OTC preparation, including ibuprofen (Advil, Motrin)
- Risk of death decreased if the offending drug is quickly withdrawn and supportive care is maintained
- Skin sloughing of 30% or more of the body

Stevens-Johnson Syndrome (SJS)

- Usually prompted by the same or similar drugs as TEN
- Begins within 1 to 14 days of pharmacotherapy
- Nonspecific upper respiratory infection (URI) with chills, fever, and malaise usually signals the start of SJS
- Generalized blisterlike lesions following within a few days
- Skin sloughing of 10% of the body.

SPECIAL CONSIDERATIONS

The Challenges of Pediatric Drug Administration

Administering medication to infants and young children requires special knowledge and techniques. The nurse must have knowledge of growth and developmental patterns. When possible, give the child a choice regarding the use of a spoon, dropper, or syringe. Present a matter-of-fact attitude in giving a child medications: Using threats or dishonesty is unacceptable. Oral medications that must be crushed for the child to swallow them can be mixed with honey, flavored syrup, jelly, or fruit puree to avoid unpleasant tastes. Medications should not be mixed with certain dietary products, such as potatoes, milk, or fruit juices, to mask the taste, because the child may develop an unpleasant association with these items and refuse to consume them in the future. To prevent nausea, medications can be preceded and followed with sips of a carbonated beverage that is poured over crushed ice.

label. Patient noncompliance ranges from not taking the medication at all, to taking it at the wrong time or in the wrong manner.

Although the nurse may be extremely conscientious in applying all the principles of effective drug administration, these strategies are of little value unless the patient agrees that the prescribed drug regimen is personally worthwhile. Before administering the drug, the nurse should use the nursing process to formulate a personalized care plan that will best enable the patient to become an active participant in his or her care (see Chapter 8) . This allows the patient to accept or reject the pharmacologic course of therapy, based on accurate information that is presented in a manner that addresses individual learning styles. It is imperative to remember that a responsible, well-informed adult always has the legal option of refusal to take any medication.

In the plan of care, it is important to address essential information that the patient must know regarding the prescribed medications. This includes factors such as the name of the drug, why it has been ordered, expected drug actions, associated side effects, and potential interactions with other medications, foods, herbal supplements, or alcohol. Patients need to be reminded that they share an active role in ensuring their own medication effectiveness and safety.

Many factors can influence whether patients comply with pharmacotherapy. The drug may be too expensive or not approved by the patient's health insurance plan. Patients sometimes forget doses of medications, especially when they must be taken three or four times per day. Patients often discontinue the use of drugs that have annoying side effects or those that impair major lifestyle choices. Adverse effects that often prompt noncompliance are headache, dizziness, nausea, diarrhea, or impotence.

PHARMFACTS | **Grapefruit Juice and Drug Interactions**

- Grapefruit juice may not be safe for people who take certain medications.
- Chemicals (most likely flavonoids) in grapefruit juice lower the activity of specific enzymes in the intestinal tract that normally break down medications. This allows a larger amount of medication to reach the bloodstream, resulting in increased drug activity.
- Drugs that may be affected by grapefruit juice include midazolam (Versed), cyclosporine (Sandimmune, Neoral), antihyperlipidemics such as lovastatin (Mevacor) and simvastatin (Zocor), certain antihistamines such as astemizole (Hismanal), erythromycin, certain antifungals such as itraconazole (Sporanox), ketoconazole (Nizoral), and mibefradil (Posicor).
- Grapefruit juice should be consumed at least 2 hours before or 5 hours after taking a medication that may interact with it.
- Some drinks that are flavored with fruit juice could contain grapefruit juice, even if grapefruit is not part of the name of the drink. Check the ingredients label.

Patients often take medications in an unexpected manner, sometimes self-adjusting their doses. Some patients believe that if one tablet is good, two must be better. Others believe they will become dependent on the medication if it is taken as prescribed; thus, they take only half the required dose. Patients are usually reluctant to admit or report noncompliance to the nurse for fear of being reprimanded or feeling embarrassed. Because the reasons for noncompliance are many and varied, the nurse must be vigilant in questioning patients about their medications. When pharmacotherapy fails to produce the expected outcomes, non-compliance should be considered a possible explanation.

4.4 Drug Orders and Time Schedules

Healthcare providers use accepted abbreviations to communicate the directions and times for drug administration. Table 4.1 lists common abbreviations that relate to universally scheduled times.

A **STAT order** refers to any medication that is needed immediately, and is to be given only once. It is often associated with emergency medications that are needed for life-threatening situations. The term STAT comes from *statim*, the Latin word meaning "immediately". The physician normally notifies the nurse of any STAT order, so it can be obtained from the pharmacy and administered immediately. The time frame between writing the order and administering the drug should be 5 minutes or less. Although not as urgent, an **ASAP** (as soon as possible) **order** should be available for administration to the patient within 30 minutes of the written order.

The **single order** is for a drug that is to be given only once, and at a specific time, such as a preoperative order. A **PRN order** (Latin: *pro re nata*) is administered *as required* by the patient's condition. The nurse makes the judgment, based on patient assessment, as to when such a medication is to be administered. Orders not written as STAT, ASAP, NOW, or PRN are called **routine orders**. These are usually carried out within 2 hours of the time the order is written by the physician. A **standing order** is written in advance of a situation, which is to be carried out under specific circumstances. An example of a standing order is a set of postoperative PRN prescriptions that are written for all patients who have undergone a specific surgical procedure. A common standing order for patients who have had a tonsillectomy is "Tylenol elixir 325 mg PO q6h PRN sore throat". Because of the legal implications of putting all patients into a single treatment category, standing orders are no longer permitted in some facilities.

Agency policies dictate that drug orders be reviewed by the attending physician within specific time frames, usually at least every 7 days. Prescriptions for narcotics and other scheduled drugs are often automatically discontinued after 72 hours, unless specifically reordered by the physician. Automatic stop orders do not generally apply when the number of doses, or an exact period of time, is specified.

Some medications must be taken at specific times. If a drug causes stomach upset, it is usually administered *with*

Table 4.1	Drug Administration Abbreviations		
Abbreviation	**Meaning**	**Abbreviation**	**Meaning**
ac	before meals	qd	every day[1]
ad lib	as desired/as directed	qh	every hour
AM	morning	qhs	bedtime (every night)[2]
bid	twice per day	qid	four times per day
cap	capsule	qod	every other day[3]
/d	per day	q2h	every 2 hours (even)
gtt	drop	q4h	every 4 hours (even)
h or hr	hour	q6h	every 6 hours (even)
hs	hour of sleep/bedtime	q8h	every 8 hours (even)
no	number	q12h	every 12 hours
pc	after meals; after eating	Rx	take
PM	afternoon	STAT	immediately; at once
PRN	when needed/necessary	tab	tablet
q	every	tid	three times per day

The Institute for Safe Medical Practices recommends the following changes, to avoid medication errors:[1] for qd, use "daily" or "every day";[2] for qhs, use "nightly";[3] for qod, use "every other day."

meals to prevent epigastric pain, nausea, or vomiting. Other medications should be administered *between* meals because food interferes with absorption. Some CNS drugs and antihypertensives are best administered *at bedtime*, because they may cause drowsiness. Sildenafil (Viagra) is unique in that it should be taken 30 to 60 minutes prior to expected sexual intercourse, to achieve an effective erection. The nurse must pay careful attention to educating patients about the timing of their medications, to enhance compliance and to increase the potential for therapeutic success.

Once medications are administered, the nurse must correctly document that they have been given to the patient. It is necessary to include the drug name, dosage, time administered, any assessments, and the nurse's signature. If a medication is refused or omitted, this fact must be recorded on the appropriate form within the medical record. It is customary to document the reason, when possible. Should the patient voice any concerns or complaints about the medication, these are also included.

4.5 Systems of Measurement

Dosages are labeled and dispensed according to their weight or volume. Three systems of measurement are used in pharmacology: metric, apothecary, and household.

The most common system of drug measurement uses the metric system. The volume of a drug is expressed in terms of the liter (L) or milliliter (ml). The cubic centimeter (cc) is a common measurement of volume that is equivalent to 1 ml of fluid. The metric weight of a drug is stated in terms of kilograms (kg), grams (g), milligrams (mg), or micrograms (mcg or μg).

The apothecary and household systems are older systems of measurement. Although most physicians and pharmacies use the metric system, these older systems are still encountered. Until the metric system totally replaces the other systems, the nurse must recognize dosages based on all three systems of measurement. Approximate equivalents between metric, apothecary, and household units of volume and weight are listed in Table 4.2.

Because Americans are very familiar with the teaspoon, tablespoon, and cup, it is important for the nurse to be able to convert between the household and metric systems of measurement. In the hospital, a glass of fluid is measured in milliliters or cubic centimeters—an 8 ounce glass of water is recorded as 240 ml (cc). If a patient being discharged is ordered to drink 2400 ml of fluid per day, the nurse may instruct the patient to drink ten 8 ounce glasses or 10 cups of fluid per day. Likewise, when a child is to be given a drug that is administered in elixir form, the nurse should explain that 5 ml of the drug is the same as 1 teaspoon. The nurse should encourage the use of accurate medical dosing devices at home, such as oral dosing syringes, oral droppers, cylindrical spoons, and medication cups. These are preferred over the traditional household measuring spoon because they are more accurate. Eating utensils that are commonly referred to as teaspoons or tablespoons often do not hold the volume that their names imply.

ROUTES OF DRUG ADMINISTRATION

The three broad categories of routes of drug administration are enteral, topical, and parenteral, and subsets are within each of these. Each route has both advantages and

Table 4.2	Metric, Apothecary, and Household Approximate Measurement Equivalents	
Metric	**Apothecary**	**Household**
1 ml	15–16 minims	15–16 drops
4–5 ml (cc)	1 fluid dram	1 teaspoon or 60 drops
15–16 ml	4 fluid drams	1 Tablespoon or 3–4 teaspoons
30–32 ml	8 fluid drams or 1 fluid ounce	2 Tablespoons
240–250 ml	8 fluid ounces (1/2 pint)	1 glass or cup
500 ml	1 pint	2 glasses or 2 cups
1 liter	32 fluid ounces or 1 quart	4 glasses or 4 cups or 1 quart
1 mg	1/60 grain	-
60–64 mg	1 grain	-
300–325 mg	5 grains	-
1 gram	15–16 grains	-
1 kg	-	2.2 pounds
To convert grains to grams: Divide grains by 15 or 16		
To convert grams to grains: Multiply grams by 15 or 16		
To convert minims to milliliters: Divide minims by 15 or 16		

disadvantages. While some drugs are formulated to be given by several routes, others are specific to only one route. Pharmacokinetic considerations, such as how the route of administration affects drug absorption and distribution, are discussed in Chapter 5 ⊂⊃ .

Certain protocols and techniques are common to all methods of drug administration. The student should review the drug administration guidelines in the following list before proceeding to subsequent sections that discuss specific routes of administration.

■ Review the medication order and check for drug allergies.
■ Wash hands and apply gloves, if indicated.
■ Use aseptic technique when preparing and administering parenteral medications.
■ Identify the patient by asking the person to state his or her full name (or by asking the parent or guardian), checking the identification band, and comparing this information with the MAR.
■ Ask the patient about known allergies.
■ Inform the patient of drug name and method of administration.
■ Position the patient for the appropriate route of administration.
■ For enteral drugs, assist the patient to a sitting position.
■ If the drug is prepackaged (unit dose), remove from its packaging at the bedside when possible.
■ Unless specifically instructed to do so in the orders, do not leave drugs at bedside.
■ Document the medication administration and any pertinent patient responses on the MAR.

4.6 Enteral Drug Administration

The **enteral route** includes drugs given orally, and those administered through nasogastric or gastrostomy tubes. Oral drug administration is the most common, most convenient, and usually the least costly of all routes. It is also considered the safest route because the skin barrier is not compromised. In cases of overdose, medications remaining in the stomach can be retrieved by inducing vomiting. Oral preparations are available in tablet, capsule, and liquid forms. Medications administered by the enteral route take advantage of the vast absorptive surfaces of the oral mucosa, stomach, or small intestine.

Tablets and Capsules

Tablets and capsules are the most common forms of drugs. Patients prefer tablets or capsules over other routes and forms because of their ease of use. In some cases, tablets may be scored for more individualized dosing.

Some patients, particularly children, have difficulty swallowing tablets and capsules. Crushing tablets or opening capsules and sprinkling the drug over food or mixing it with juice will make it more palatable and easier to swallow. However, the nurse should not crush tablets or open capsules unless the manufacturer specifically states this is permissible. Some drugs are inactivated by crushing or opening, while others severely irritate the stomach mucosa and cause nausea or vomiting. Occasionally, drugs should not be crushed because they irritate the oral mucosa, are extremely bitter, or contain dyes that stain the teeth. Most drug guides provide lists of drugs that may

Table 4.3	Enteral Drug Administration
Drug Form	**Administration Guidelines**
A. tablet, capsule, or liquid	1. Assess that patient is alert and has ability to swallow. 2. Place tablets or capsules into medication cup. 3. If liquid, shake the bottle to mix the agent, and measure the dose into the cup at eye level. 4. Hand the patient the medication cup. 5. Offer a glass of water to facilitate swallowing the medication. Milk or juice may be offered if not contraindicated. 6. Remain with patient until all medication is swallowed.
B. sublingual	1. Assess that patient is alert and has ability to hold medication under tongue. 2. Place sublingual tablet under tongue. 3. Instruct patient not to chew or swallow the tablet, or move the tablet around with tongue. 4. Instruct patient to allow tablet to dissolve completely before swallowing saliva. 5. Remain with patient to determine that all of the medication has dissolved. 6. Offer a glass of water, if patient desires.
C. buccal	1. Assess that patient is alert and has ability to hold medication between the gums and the cheek. 2. Place buccal tablet between the gum line and the cheek. 3. Instruct patient not to chew or swallow the tablet, or move the tablet around with tongue. 4. Instruct patient to allow tablet to dissolve completely before swallowing saliva. 5. Remain with patient to determine that all of the medication has dissolved. 6. Offer a glass of water, if patient desires.
D. nasogastric and gastrostomy	1. Administer liquid forms when possible to avoid clogging the tube. 2. If solid, crush finely into powder and mix thoroughly with at least 30 ml of warm water until dissolved. 3. Assess and verify tube placement. 4. Turn off feeding, if applicable to patient. 5. Aspirate stomach contents and measure the residual volume. If greater than 100 ml for an adult, check agency policy. 6. Return residual via gravity and flush with water. 7. Pour medication into syringe barrel and allow to flow into the tube by gravity. Give each medication separately, flushing between with water. 8. Keep head of bed elevated for 1 hour to prevent aspiration. 9. Reestablish continual feeding, as scheduled. Keep head of bed elevated 45 degrees to prevent aspiration.

not be crushed (Wilson, Shannon, Stang, 2003). Guidelines for administering tablets or capsules are given in Table 4.3A.

The strongly acidic contents within the stomach can present a destructive obstacle to the absorption of some medications. To overcome this barrier, tablets may have a hard, waxy coating that enables them to resist the acidity. These **enteric coated** tablets are designed to dissolve in the alkaline environment of the small intestine. It is important that the nurse not crush enteric-coated tablets, as the medication would then be directly exposed to the stomach environment.

Studies have clearly demonstrated that compliance declines as the number of doses per day increases. With this in mind, pharmacologists have attempted to design new drugs so that they may be administered only once or twice daily. **Sustained-release** tablets or capsules are designed to dissolve very slowly. This releases the medication over an extended time and results in a longer duration of action for the medication. Also called extended-release (XR), long-acting (LA), or slow-release (SR) medications, these forms allow for the convenience of once or twice a day dosing. Extended-release medications must not be crushed or opened.

Giving medications by the oral route has certain disadvantages. The patient must be conscious and able to swallow properly. Certain types of drugs, including proteins, are inactivated by digestive enzymes in the stomach and small intestine. Medications absorbed from the stomach and small intestine first travel to the liver, where they may be inactivated before they ever reach their target organs. This process, called first-pass metabolism, is discussed in Chapter 5 ☞ . The significant variation in the motility of the GI tract and in its ability to absorb medications can create differences in bioavailability. In addition, children and some adults have an aversion to swallowing large tablets and capsules, or to taking oral medications that are distasteful.

Sublingual and Buccal Drug Administration

For sublingual and buccal administration, the tablet is not swallowed, but kept in the mouth. The mucosa of the oral cavity contains a rich blood supply that provides an excellent absorptive surface for certain drugs. Medications given by this route are not subjected to destructive digestive enzymes, nor do they undergo hepatic first-pass metabolism.

For the **sublingual route**, the medication is placed under the tongue and allowed to dissolve slowly. Because of the rich blood supply in this region, the sublingual route results in a rapid onset of action. Sublingual dosage forms are most often formulated as rapidly disintegrating tablets, or as soft gelatin capsules filled with liquid drug.

When multiple drugs have been ordered, the sublingual preparations should be administered after oral medications have been swallowed. The patient should be instructed not to move the drug with the tongue, nor to eat or drink anything until the medication has completely dissolved. The sublingual mucosa is not suitable for extended-release formulations because it is a relatively small area and is constantly being bathed by a substantial amount of saliva. Table 4.3B and Figure 4.1A present important points regarding sublingual drug administration.

To administer by the **buccal route**, the tablet or capsule is placed in the oral cavity between the gum and the cheek. The patient must be instructed not to manipulate the medication with the tongue, otherwise it could get displaced to the sublingual area where it would be more rapidly absorbed, or to the back of the throat where it could be swallowed. The buccal mucosa is less permeable to most medications than the sublingual area, providing for slower absorption. The buccal route is preferred over the sublingual route for sustained-release delivery because of its greater mucosal surface area. Drugs formulated for buccal administration generally do not cause irritation and are small enough to not cause discomfort to the patient. Like the sublingual route, drugs administered by the buccal route avoid first-pass metabolism by the liver and the enzymatic processes of the stomach and small intestine. Table 4.3C and Figure 4.1B provide important guidelines for buccal drug administration.

Nasogastric and Gastrostomy Drug Administration

Patients with a nasogastric tube or enteral feeding mechanism such as a gastrostomy tube may have their medications administered through these devices. A nasogastric (NG) tube is a soft, flexible tube inserted by way of the nasopharynx with the tip lying in the stomach. A gastrostomy (G) tube is surgically placed directly into the patient's stomach. Generally, the NG tube is used for short-term treatment, whereas the G tube is inserted for patients requiring long-term care. Drugs administered through these tubes are usually in liquid form. Although solid drugs can be crushed or dissolved, they tend to cause clogging within the tubes. Sustained-release release drugs should not be crushed and administered through NG or G tubes. Drugs administered by this route are exposed to the same physiologic processes as those given orally. Table 4.3D gives important guidelines for administering drugs through NG or G tubes.

4.7 Topical Drug Administration

Topical drugs are those applied locally to the skin or the membranous linings of the eye, ear, nose, respiratory tract, urinary tract, vagina, and rectum. These applications include the following:

- *Dermatologic preparations* Drugs applied to the skin; the topical route most commonly used. Formulations include creams, lotions, gels, powders, and sprays.
- *Instillations and irrigations* Drugs applied into body cavities or orifices. These include the eyes, ears, nose, urinary bladder, rectum, and vagina.
- *Inhalations* Drugs applied to the respiratory tract by inhalers, nebulizers, or positive pressure breathing apparatuses. The most common indication for inhaled drugs is bronchoconstriction due to bronchitis or asthma; however, a number of illegal, abused drugs are taken by this route because it provides a very rapid onset of drug action (see Chapter 12) ☞ . Additional details on inhalation drug administration can be found in Chapter 29 ☞ .

Many drugs are applied topically to produce a *local* effect. For example, antibiotics may be applied to the skin to treat skin infections. Antineoplastic agents may be instilled into the urinary bladder via catheter to treat tumors of the bladder mucosa. Corticosteroids are sprayed into the nostrils to reduce inflammation of the nasal mucosa due to allergic rhinitis. Local, topical delivery produces fewer side effects compared with the same drug given orally or parenterally. This is because, when given topically, these drugs are absorbed very slowly and amounts reaching the general circulation are minimal.

Some drugs are given topically to provide for slow release and absorption of the drug to the general circulation. These agents are given for their *systemic* effects. For example, a nitroglycerin patch is not applied to the skin to treat a local skin condition, but to treat a systemic condition;

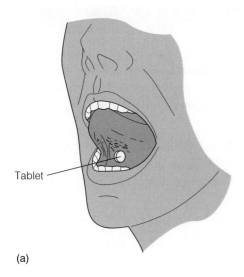

(a)

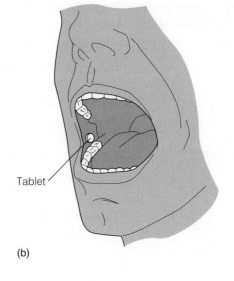

(b)

Figure 4.1 | (a) Sublingual drug administration; (b) buccal drug administration

coronary artery disease. Likewise, prochlorperazine (Compazine) suppositories are inserted rectally not to treat a disease of the rectum, but to alleviate nausea.

The distinction between topical drugs given for local effects and those given for systemic effects is an important one for the nurse. In the case of local drugs, absorption is undesirable and may cause side effects. For systemic drugs, absorption is essential for the therapeutic action of the drug. With either type of topical agent, drugs should not be applied to abraded or denuded skin, unless directed to do so.

Transdermal Delivery System

The use of transdermal patches provides an effective means of delivering certain medications. Examples include nitroglycerin for angina pectoris and scopolamine (Transderm-Scop) for motion sickness. Although transdermal patches contain a specific amount of drug, the rate of delivery and the actual dose received may be variable. Patches are changed on a regular basis, using a site rotation routine, which should be documented in the MAR. Before applying a transdermal patch, the nurse should verify that the previous patch has been removed and disposed of appropriately. Drugs to be administered by this route avoid the first-pass effect in the liver and bypass digestive enzymes. Table 4.4A and Figure 4.2 illustrate the major points of transdermal drug delivery.

Ophthalmic Administration

The ophthalmic route is used to treat local conditions of the eye and surrounding structures. Common indications include excessive dryness, infections, glaucoma, and dilation of the pupil during eye examinations. Ophthalmic drugs are available in the form of eye irrigations, drops, ointments, and medicated disks. Figure 4.3 and Table 4.4B give guidelines for adult administration. Although the procedure is the same with a child, it is advisable to enlist the help of an adult caregiver. In some cases, the infant or toddler may need to be immobilized with arms wrapped to prevent accidental injury to the eye during administration. For the young child, demonstrating the procedure using a doll facilitates cooperation and decreases anxiety.

Otic Administration

The otic route is used to treat local conditions of the ear, including infections and soft blockages of the auditory canal. Otic medications include eardrops and irrigations, which are usually ordered for cleaning purposes. Administration to infants and young children must be performed carefully to avoid injury to sensitive structures of the ear. Figure 4.4 and Table 4.4C present key points in administering otic medications.

Nasal Administration

The nasal route is used for both local and systemic drug administration. The nasal mucosa provides an excellent absorptive surface for certain medications. Advantages of this route include ease of use and avoidance of the first-pass effect and digestive enzymes. Nasal spray formulations of corticosteroids have revolutionized the treatment of allergic rhinitis due to their high safety margin when administered by this route.

Although the nasal mucosa provides an excellent surface for drug delivery, there is the potential for damage to the cilia within the nasal cavity, and mucosal irritation is common. In addition, unpredictable mucus secretion among some individuals may affect drug absorption from this site.

Drops or sprays are often used for their local **astringent effect**, which is to shrink swollen mucous membranes or to loosen secretions and facilitate drainage. This brings immediate relief from the nasal congestion caused by the common cold. The nose also provides the route to reach the

Table 4.4	Topical Drug Administration
Drug Form	**Administration Guidelines**
A. transdermal	1. Obtain transdermal patch, and read manufacturer's guidelines: Application site and frequency of changing differ according to medication. 2. Apply gloves before handling, to avoid absorption of the agent by the nurse. 3. Remove previous medication or patch, and cleanse area. 4. If using a transdermal ointment, apply the ordered amount of medication in an even line directly on the premeasured paper that accompanies the medication tube. 5. Press patch or apply medicated paper to clean, dry, and hairless skin. 6. Rotate sites to prevent skin irritation. 7. Label patch with date, time, and initials.
B. ophthalmic	1. Instruct patient to lie supine, or sit with head slightly tilted back. 2. With nondominant hand, pull lower lid down gently to expose the conjunctival sac, creating a pocket. 3. Ask patient to look upward. 4. Hold eyedropper 1/4–1/8 inch above the conjunctival sac. Do not hold dropper over eye as this may stimulate the blink reflex. 5. Instill prescribed number of drops into the center of the pocket. Avoid touching eye or conjunctival sac with tip of eyedropper. 6. If applying ointment, apply a thin line of ointment evenly along inner edge of lower lid margin, from inner to outer canthus. 7. Instruct the patient to close eye gently. Apply gentle pressure with finger to the nasolacrimal duct at the inner canthus for 1–2 minutes, to avoid overflow drainage into nose and throat, thus minimizing risk of absorption into the systemic circulation. 8. With tissue, remove excess medication around eye. 9. Replace dropper. Do not rinse eyedropper.
C. otic	1. Instruct patient to lie on side or to sit with head tilted so that affected ear is facing up. 2. If necessary, clean the pinna of the ear and the meatus with a clean washcloth to prevent any discharge from being washed into the ear canal during the instillation of the drops. 3. Hold dropper 1/4 inch above ear canal, and instill prescribed number of drops into the side of the ear canal, allowing the drops to flow downward. Avoid placing drops directly on the tympanic membrane. 4. Gently apply intermittent pressure to the tragus of the ear three or four times. 5. Instruct patient to remain on side for up to 10 minutes to prevent loss of medication. 6. If cotton ball is ordered, presoak with medication and insert it into the outermost part of ear canal. 7. Wipe any solution that may have dripped from the ear canal with a tissue.
D. nasal drops	1. Ask the patient to blow the nose to clear nasal passages. 2. Draw up the correct volume of drug into dropper. 3. Instruct the patient to open and breathe through the mouth. 4. Hold the tip of the dropper just above the nostril and, without touching the nose with the dropper, direct the solution laterally toward the midline of the superior concha of the ethmoid bone—not the base of the nasal cavity, where it will run down the throat and into the eustachian tube. 5. Ask the patient to remain in position for 5 minutes. 6. Discard any remaining solution that is in the dropper.

Table 4.4	Topical Drug Administration (Continued)
Drug Form	**Administration Guidelines**
E. vaginal	1. Instruct the patient to assume a supine position with knees bent and separated.
	2. Place water-soluble lubricant into medicine cup.
	3. Apply gloves; open suppository and lubricate the rounded end.
	4. Expose the vaginal orifice by separating the labia with nondominant hand.
	5. Insert the rounded end of the suppository about 8–10 cm along the posterior wall of the vagina, or as far as it will pass.
	6. If using a cream, jelly, or foam, gently insert applicator 5 cm along the posterior vaginal wall and slowly push the plunger until empty. Remove the applicator and place on a paper towel.
	7. Ask the patient to lower legs and remain lying in the supine or side-lying position for 5–10 minutes following insertion.
F. rectal suppositories	1. Instruct the patient to lie on left side (Sims' position).
	2. Apply gloves; open suppository and lubricate the rounded end.
	3. Lubricate the gloved forefinger of the dominant hand with water-soluble lubricant.
	4. Inform the patient when the suppository is to be inserted; instruct the patient to take slow, deep breaths and deeply exhale during insertion, to relax the anal sphincter.
	5. Gently insert the lubricated end of suppository into the rectum, beyond the anal-rectal ridge to ensure retention.
	6. Instruct the patient to remain in the Sims' position or lie supine to prevent expulsion of the suppository.
	7. Instruct the patient to retain the suppository for at least 30 minutes to allow absorption to occur, unless the suppository is administered to stimulate defecation.

nasal sinuses and the eustachian tube. Proper positioning of the patient prior to instilling nose drops for sinus disorders depends on which sinuses are being treated. The same holds true for treatment of the eustachian tube. Table 4.4D and Figure 4.5 illustrate important facts related to nasal drug administration.

Vaginal Administration

The vaginal route is used to deliver medications for treating local infections and to relieve vaginal pain and itching. Vaginal medications are inserted as suppositories, creams, jellies, or foams. It is important that the nurse explain the purpose of treatment and provide for privacy and patient dignity. Before inserting vaginal drugs, the nurse should instruct the patient to empty her bladder, to lessen both the discomfort during treatment and the possibility of irritating or injuring the vaginal lining. The patient should be offered a perineal pad following administration. Table 4.4E and Figure 4.6 provide guidelines regarding vaginal drug administration.

Rectal Administration

The rectal route may be used for either local or systemic drug administration. It is a safe and effective means of delivering drugs to patients who are comatose or who are experiencing nausea and vomiting. Rectal drugs are normally in suppository form, although a few laxatives and diagnostic agents are given via enema. Although absorption is slower than by other routes, it is steady and reliable provided the medication can be retained by the patient. Venous blood from the lower rectum is not transported by way of the liver; thus, the first-pass effect is avoided, as are the digestive enzymes of the upper GI tract. Table 4.4F gives selected details regarding rectal drug administration.

4.8 Parenteral Drug Administration

Parenteral administration refers to the dispensing of medications by routes other than oral or topical. The **parenteral route** delivers drugs via a needle into the skin layers, subcutaneous tissue, muscles, or veins. More advanced parenteral delivery includes administration into arteries, body cavities (such as intrathecal), and organs (such as intracardiac). Parenteral drug administration is much more invasive than topical or enteral. Because of the potential for introducing pathogenic microbes directly into the blood or body tissues, aseptic techniques must be strictly applied. The nurse is expected to identify and use appropriate materials for parenteral drug delivery, including specialized equipment and techniques involved in the preparation and administration of injectable products. The nurse must know the correct anatomical locations for parenteral administration, and safety procedures regarding hazardous equipment disposal.

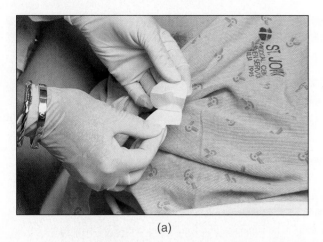

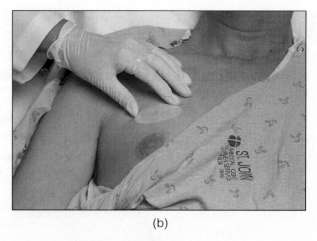

(a)

(b)

Figure 4.2 | Transdermal patch administration: (a) protective coating removed from patch; (b) patch immediately applied to clean, dry, hairless skin and labeled with date, time, and initials *Source: Pearson Education/PH College.*

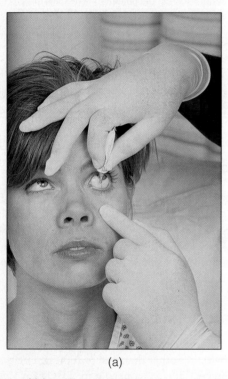

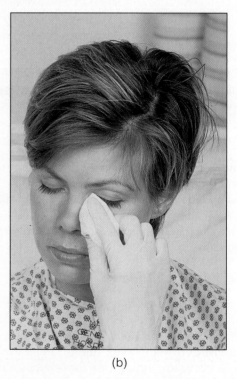

(a)

(b)

Figure 4.3 | (a) Instilling an eye ointment into the lower conjunctival sac; (b) pressing on the nasolacrimal duct *Source: ©Jenny Thomas Photography.*

Intradermal and Subcutaneous Administration

Injection into the skin delivers drugs to the blood vessels that supply the various layers of the skin. Drugs may be injected either intradermally or subcutaneously. The major difference between these methods is the depth of injection. An advantage of both methods is that they offer a means of administering drugs to patients who are unable to take them orally. Drugs administered by these routes avoid the hepatic first-pass effect and digestive enzymes. Disadvantages are that

only small volumes can be administered, and injections can cause pain and swelling at the injection site.

An **intradermal (ID)** injection is administered into the dermis layer of the skin. Because the dermis contains more blood vessels than the deeper subcutaneous layer, drugs are more easily absorbed. It is usually employed for allergy and disease screening or for local anesthetic delivery prior to venous cannulation. Intradermal injections are limited to very small volumes of drug, usually only 0.1 to 0.2 ml. The usual sites for ID injections are the nonhairy skin surfaces

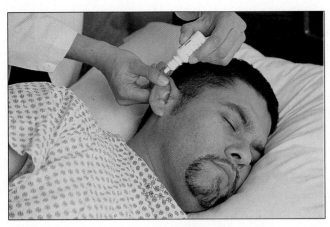

Figure 4.4 | Instilling eardrops *Source: ©Elena Dorfman.*

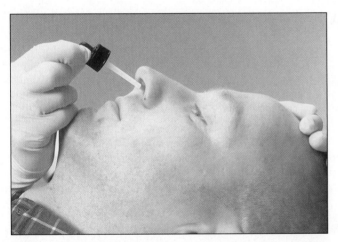

Figure 4.5 | Nasal drug administration *Source: Pearson Education/PH College.*

of the upper back, over the scapulae, the high upper chest, and the inner forearm. Guidelines for intradermal injections are given in Table 4.5A and Figure 4.7.

A **subcutaneous (SC or SQ)** injection is delivered to the deepest layers of the skin. Insulin, heparin, vitamins, some vaccines, and other medications are given in this area because the sites are easily accessible and provide rapid absorption. Body sites that are ideal for SC injections include the following:

- Outer aspect of the upper arms, in the area above the triceps muscle
- Middle two-thirds of the anterior thigh area
- Subscapular areas of the upper back
- Upper dorsogluteal and ventrogluteal areas
- Abdominal areas, above the iliac crest and below the diaphragm, 1.5 to 2 inches out from the umbilicus

Subcutaneous doses are small in volume, usually ranging from 0.5 to 1 ml. The needle size varies with the patient's quantity of body fat. The length is usually one half the size of a pinched/bunched skinfold that can be grasped between the thumb and forefinger. It is important to rotate injection sites in an orderly and documented manner, to promote absorption, minimize tissue damage, and alleviate discomfort. For insulin, however, rotation should be within an anatomical area to promote reliable absorption and maintain consistent blood glucose levels. When performing SC injections, it is not necessary to aspirate prior to the injection. Note that tuberculin syringes and insulin syringes are not interchangeable, so the nurse should not substitute one for the other. Table 4.5B and Figure 4.8 include important information regarding SC drug administration.

Intramuscular Administration

An **intramuscular (IM)** injection delivers medication into specific muscles. Because muscle tissue has a rich blood supply, medication moves quickly into blood vessels to

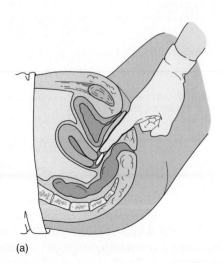

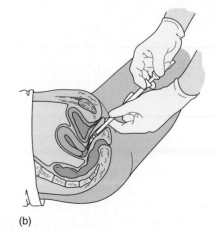

(a)   (b)

Figure 4.6 | Vaginal drug administration: (a) instilling a vaginal suppository; (b) using an applicator to instill a vaginal cream *Source: Pearson Education/PH College.*

Table 4.5	**Parenteral Drug Administration**
Drug Form	**Administration Guidelines**
A. intradermal route	1. Prepare medication in a tuberculin or 1 cc syringe, using a 25–27 gauge, 3/8–5/8 inch needle.
	2. Apply gloves and cleanse injection site with antiseptic swab in a circular motion. Allow to air dry.
	3. With thumb and index finger of nondominant hand, spread skin taut.
	4. Insert needle, with bevel facing upward, at angle of 10–15 degrees.
	5. Advance needle until entire bevel is under skin; do not aspirate.
	6. Slowly inject medication to form small wheal or bleb.
	7. Withdraw needle quickly, and pat site gently with sterile 2 × 2 gauze pad. Do not massage area.
	8. Instruct the patient not to rub or scratch the area.
B. subcutaneous route	1. Prepare medication in a 1–3 cc syringe using a 23–25 gauge, 1/2–5/8 inch needle. For heparin, the recommended needle is 3/8 inch and 25–26 gauge.
	2. Choose site, avoiding areas of bony prominence, major nerves, and blood vessels. For heparin, check with agency policy for the preferred injection sites.
	3. Check previous rotation sites and select a new area for injection.
	4. Apply gloves and cleanse injection site with antiseptic swab in a circular motion.
	5. Allow to air dry.
	6. Bunch the skin between thumb and index finger of nondominant hand or spread taut if there is substantial subcutaneous tissue.
	7. Insert needle at 45 or 90 degree angle depending on body size: 90 degrees if obese; 45 degrees if average weight. If the patient is very thin, gather skin at area of needle insertion and administer at 90 degree angle.
	8. For nonheparin injections, aspirate by pulling back on plunger. If blood appears, withdraw the needle, discard the syringe, and prepare a new injection. For heparin, do not aspirate, as this can damage surrounding tissues and cause bruising.
	9. Inject medication slowly.
	10. Remove needle quickly, and gently massage site with antiseptic swab. For heparin, do not massage the site, as this may cause bruising or bleeding.
C. intramuscular route: ventrogluteal site	1. Prepare medication using a 20–23 gauge, 1.5 inch needle.
	2. Apply gloves and cleanse injection site with antiseptic swab in a circular motion. Allow to air dry.
	3. Locate site by placing the hand with heel on the greater trochanter and thumb toward umbilicus. Point to the anterior iliac spine with the index finger spreading the middle finger to point toward the iliac crest (forming a V). Injection of medication is given within the V-shaped area of the index and third finger.
	4. Insert needle with smooth, dartlike movement at a 90 degree angle within V-shaped area.
	5. Aspirate, and observe for blood. If blood appears, withdraw the needle, discard the syringe, and prepare a new injection.
	6. Inject medication slowly and with smooth, even pressure on the plunger.
	7. Remove needle quickly.
	8. Apply pressure to site with a dry, sterile 2 × 2 gauze and massage vigorously to create warmth and promote absorption of the medication into the muscle.
D. intravenous route	1. To add drug to an IV fluid container:
	a. Verify order and compatibility of drug with IV fluid.
	b. Prepare medication in a 5–20 ml syringe using a 1–1.5 inch, 19–21 gauge needle.
	c. Apply gloves and assess injection site for signs and symptoms of inflammation or extravasation.
	d. Locate medication port on IV fluid container and cleanse with antiseptic swab.
	e. Carefully insert needle or access device into port and inject medication.

Table 4.5	Parenteral Drug Administration (Continued)
Drug Form	**Administration Guidelines**

D. intravenous route *(continued)*	f. Withdraw needle and mix solution by rotating container end to end.
	
	g. Hang container and check infusion rate.
	
	2. To add drug to an IV bolus (IV push) using existing IV line or IV lock (reseal):
	
	  a. Verify order and compatibility of drug with IV fluid.
	
	  b. Determine the correct rate of infusion.
	
	  c. Determine if IV fluids are infusing at proper rate (IV line) and that IV site is adequate.
	
	  d. Prepare drug in a syringe with 25–26 gauge needle.
	
	  e. Apply gloves and assess injection site for signs and symptoms of inflammation or extravasation.
	
	  f. Select injection port, on tubing, closest to insertion site (IV line).
	
	  g. Cleanse tubing or lock port with antiseptic swab and insert needle into port.
	
	  h. If administering medication through an existing IV line, occlude tubing by pinching just above the injection port.
	
	  i. Slowly inject medication over designated time; not usually faster that 1 mL/min, unless specified.
	
	  j. Withdraw syringe. Release tubing and ensure proper IV infusion if using an existing IV line.
	
	  k. If using an IV lock, check agency policy for use of saline flush before and after injecting medications.

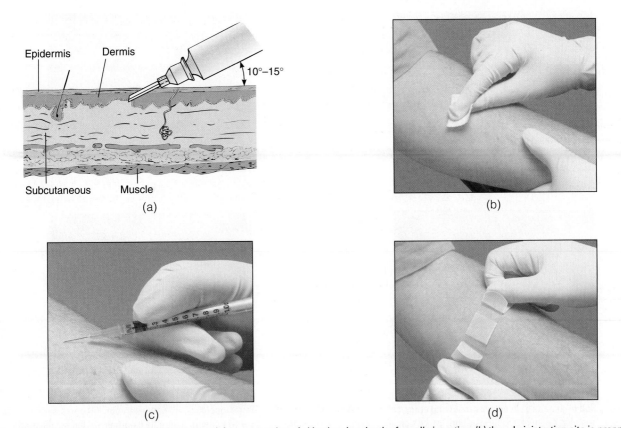

Figure 4.7 | Intradermal drug administration: (a) cross-section of skin showing depth of needle insertion; (b) the administration site is prepped; (c) the needle is inserted, bevel up at 10–15 degrees; (d) the needle is removed and the puncture site is covered with an adhesive bandage *Source: Pearson Education/PH College.*

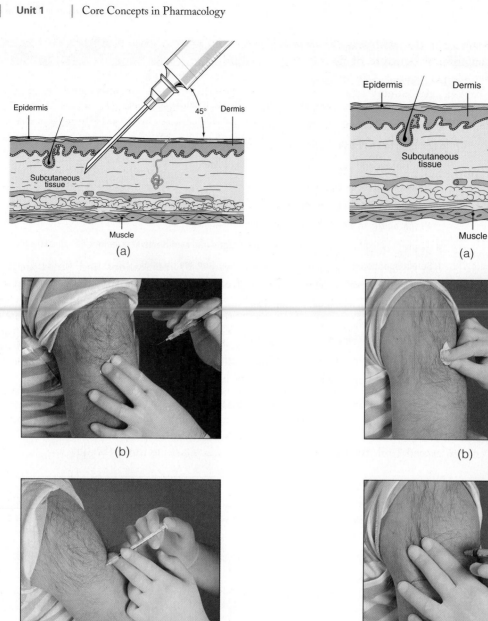

(a)

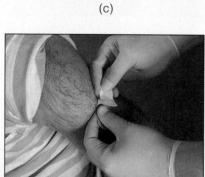

(b)

(c)

(d)

Figure 4.8 Subcutaneous drug administration: (a) cross-section of skin showing depth of needle insertion; (b) the administration site is prepped; (c) the needle is inserted at a 45 degree angle; (d) the needle is removed and the puncture site is covered with an adhesive bandage *Source: Pearson Education/PH College.*

(a)

(b)

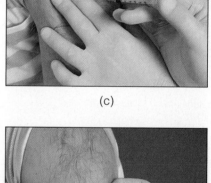

(c)

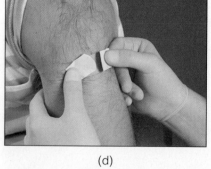

(d)

Figure 4.9 Intramuscular drug administration: (a) cross-section of skin showing depth of needle insertion; (b) the administration site is prepped; (c) the needle is inserted at a 90 degree angle; (d) the needle is removed and the puncture site is covered with an adhesive bandage *Source: Pearson Education/PH College.*

produce a more rapid onset of action than with oral, ID, or SC administration. The anatomical structure of muscle permits this tissue to receive a larger volume of medication than the subcutaneous region. An adult with well-developed muscles can safely tolerate up to 4 ml of medication in a large muscle, although only 2 to 3 ml is recommended. The deltoid and triceps muscles should receive a maximum of 1 ml.

A major consideration for the nurse regarding IM drug administration is the selection of an appropriate injection site. Injection sites must be located away from bone, large blood vessels, and nerves. The size and length of needle are determined by body size and muscle mass, the type of drug to be administered, the amount of adipose tissue overlying the muscle, and the age of the patient. Information regarding IM injections is given in Table 4.5C and Figure 4.9. The four common sites for intramuscular injections are as follows:

- *Ventrogluteal site* The preferred site for IM injections. This area provides the greatest thickness of gluteal muscles, contains no large blood vessels or nerves, is sealed off by bone, and contains less fat than the buttock area, thus eliminating the need to determine the depth of subcutaneous fat. It is a suitable site for children and infants over 7 months of age.
- *Deltoid site* Used in well-developed teens and adults for volumes of medication not to exceed 1 ml. Because the radial nerve lies in close proximity, the deltoid is not generally used, except for small volume vaccines, such as for hepatitis B in adults.
- *Dorsogluteal site* Used for adults and for children who have been walking for at least 6 months. The site is safe as long as the nurse appropriately locates the injection landmarks to avoid puncture or irritation of the sciatic nerve and blood vessels.
- *Vastus lateralis site* Usually thick and well developed in both adults and children, the middle third of the muscle is the site for IM injections.

Intravenous Administration

Intravenous (IV) medications and fluids are administered directly into the bloodstream and are immediately available for use by the body. The IV route is used when a very rapid onset of action is desired. Like other parenteral routes, IV medications bypass the enzymatic process of the digestive system and the first-pass effect of the liver. The three basic types of IV administration are as follows:

- *Large-volume infusion* For fluid maintenance, replacement, or supplementation. Compatible drugs may be mixed into a large-volume IV container with fluids such as normal saline or Ringer's lactate. Table 4.5D and Figure 4.10 illustrate this technique.

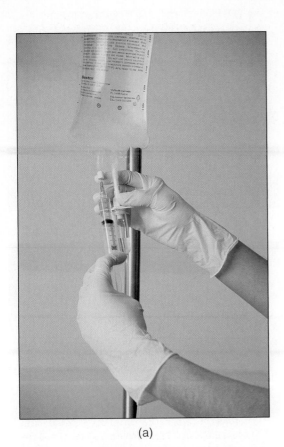

(a)

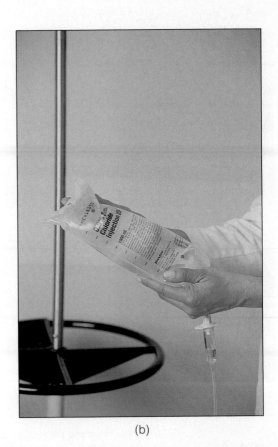

(b)

Figure 4.10 | Adding a drug to an existing infusion: (a) inserting a drug through the injection port of an infusion container; (b) rotating the IV bag to distribute the drug *Source: ©Elena Dorfman.*

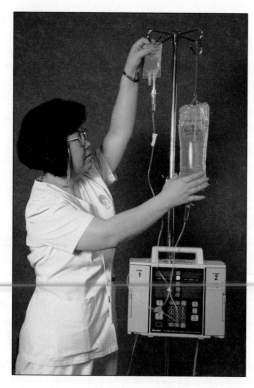

- *Intermittent infusion* Small amount of IV solution that is arranged tandem or piggy-backed to the primary large-volume infusion. Used to instill adjunct medications, such as antibiotics or analgesics over a short time period. This is illustrated in Figure 4.11.
- *IV bolus (push) administration* Concentrated dose delivered directly to the circulation via syringe to administer single-dose medications. Bolus injections may be given through an intermittent injection port or by direct IV push. Details on the bolus administration technique are given in Table 4.5D and Figure 4.12.

Although the IV route offers the fastest onset of drug action, it is also the most dangerous. Once injected, the medication cannot be retrieved. If the drug solution or the needle is contaminated, pathogens have a direct route to the bloodstream and body tissues. Patients who are receiving IV injections must be closely monitored for adverse reactions. Some adverse reactions occur immediately after injection; others may take hours or days to appear. Antidotes for drugs that can cause potentially dangerous or fatal reactions must always be readily available.

Figure 4.11 | An intermittent IV infusion given piggy-back to the primary infusion *Source: Pearson Education/PH College.*

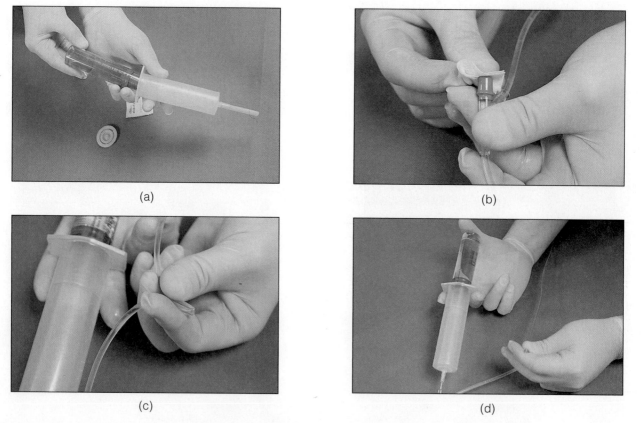

(a)

(b)

(c)

(d)

Figure 4.12 | Intravenous bolus administration: (a) the drug is prepared; (b) the administration port is cleaned; (c) line is pinched; (d) drug is administered *Source: Pearson Education/PH College.*

CHAPTER REVIEW

Key Concepts

The numbered key concepts provide a succinct summary of the important points from the corresponding numbered section within the chapter. If any of these points are not clear, refer to the numbered section within the chapter for review. Expanded versions can be found on the companion website.

4.1 The nurse must have a comprehensive knowledge of the actions and side effects of drugs before they are administered to limit the number and severity of adverse drugs events.

4.2 The five rights and three checks are guidelines to safe drug administration, which is a collaborative effort among nurses, physicians, and other healthcare professionals.

4.3 For pharmacologic compliance, the patient must understand and personally accept the value associated with the prescribed drug regimen. Understanding the reasons for noncompliance can help the nurse increase the success of pharmacotherapy.

4.4 There are established orders and time schedules by which medications are routinely administered. Documentation of drug administration and reported side effects are important responsibilities of the nurse.

4.5 Systems of measurement used in pharmacology include the metric, apothecary, and household systems. Although the metric system is most commonly used, the nurse must be able to convert dosages among the 3 systems of measurement.

4.6 The enteral route includes drugs given orally, and those administered through nasogastric or gastrostomy tubes. This is the most common route of drug administration

4.7 Topical drugs are applied locally to the skin or membranous linings of the eye, ear, nose, respiratory tract, urinary tract, vagina, and rectum.

4.8 Parenteral administration is the dispensing of medications via a needle, usually into the skin layers (ID), subcutaneous tissue (SC or SQ), muscles (IM) or veins (IV).

Review Questions

1. Why is it that errors continue to occur in spite of the fact that the nurse follows the five rights and three checks of drug administration?

2. What strategies can the nurse employ to ensure drug compliance for a patient who is refusing to take his or her medication?

3. Compare the oral, topical, IM, SC, and IV routes. Which has the fastest onset of drug action? Which routes avoid the hepatic first-pass effect? Which require strict aseptic technique?

4. What are the advantages of the metric system of measurement over the household or apothecary systems?

 ## EXPLORE MediaLink

NCLEX review, case studies, and other interactive resources for this chapter can be found on the companion website at www.prenhall.com/adams. Click on "Chapter 4" to select the activities for this chapter. For animations, more NCLEX review questions, and an audio glossary, access the accompanying CD-ROM in this textbook.

Pharmacokinetics

Medications are given to achieve a desirable effect. To produce this therapeutic effect, the drug must reach its target cells. For some medications, such as topical agents used to treat skin conditions, this is an easy task. For others, however, the process of reaching target cells in sufficient quantities to cause a physiological change may be challenging. Drugs are exposed to a myriad of different barriers and destructive processes after they enter the body. The purpose of this chapter is to examine factors that act upon the drug, as it attempts to reach its target cells.

MediaLink www.prenhall.com/adams

CD-ROM

Animation: Cytochrome

Audio Glossary

NCLEX Review

Companion Website

NCLEX Review

Case Study

Expanded Key Concepts

Challenge Your Knowledge

OBJECTIVES

After reading this chapter, the student should be able to:

1. Explain the applications of pharmacokinetics to clinical practice.
2. Identify the four components of pharmacokinetics.
3. Explain how substances travel across plasma membranes.
4. Discuss factors affecting drug absorption.
5. Explain the metabolism of drugs and its applications to pharmacotherapy.
6. Discuss how drugs are distributed throughout the body.
7. Describe how plasma proteins affect drug distribution.
8. Identify major processes by which drugs are excreted.
9. Explain how enterohepatic recirculation might affect drug activity.
10. Explain the applications of a drug's plasma half-life (t$_{1/2}$) to pharmacotherapy.
11. Explain how a drug reaches and maintains its therapeutic range in the plasma.
12. Differentiate between loading and maintenance doses.

5.1 Pharmacokinetics: How the Body Handles Medications

The term **pharmacokinetics** is derived from the root words *pharmaco*, which means "medicines," and *kinetics*, which means "movement or motion." Pharmacokinetics is thus the study of drug movement throughout the body. In practical terms, it describes how the body handles medications. Pharmacokinetics is a core subject in pharmacology, and a firm grasp of this topic allows nurses to better understand and predict the actions and side effects of medications in their patients.

Drugs face numerous obstacles in reaching their target cells. For most medications, the greatest barrier is crossing the many membranes that separate the drug from its target cells. A drug taken by mouth, for example, must cross the plasma membranes of the mucosal cells of the gastrointestinal tract and the capillary endothelial cells to enter the bloodstream. To leave the bloodstream, it must again cross capillary cells, travel through interstitial fluid, and enter target cells by passing through their plasma membranes. Depending on the mechanism of action, the drug may also need to enter cellular organelles such as the nucleus, which are surrounded by additional membranes. These are just some of the membranes and barriers that a drug must successfully penetrate, before it can elicit a response.

While seeking their target cells and attempting to pass through the various membranes, drugs are subjected to numerous physiological processes. For medications given by the enteral route, stomach acid and digestive enzymes often act to break down the drug molecules. Enzymes in the liver and other organs may chemically change the drug molecule to make it less active. If seen as foreign by the body, phagocytes may attempt to remove the drug, or an immune response may be triggered. The kidneys, large intestine, and other organs attempt to excrete the medication from the body.

These examples illustrate pharmacokinetic processes: how the body handles medications. The many processes of pharmacokinetics are grouped into four categories: absorption, distribution, metabolism, and excretion, as illustrated in Figure 5.1.

5.2 The Passage of Drugs through Plasma Membranes

Pharmacokinetic variables depend on the ability of a drug to cross plasma membranes. With few exceptions, drugs must penetrate these membranes to produce their effects. Like other chemicals, drugs primarily use two processes to cross body membranes.

- *Diffusion or passive transport* Movement of a chemical from an area of higher concentration to an area of lower concentration
- *Active transport* Movement of a chemical against a concentration or electrochemical gradient

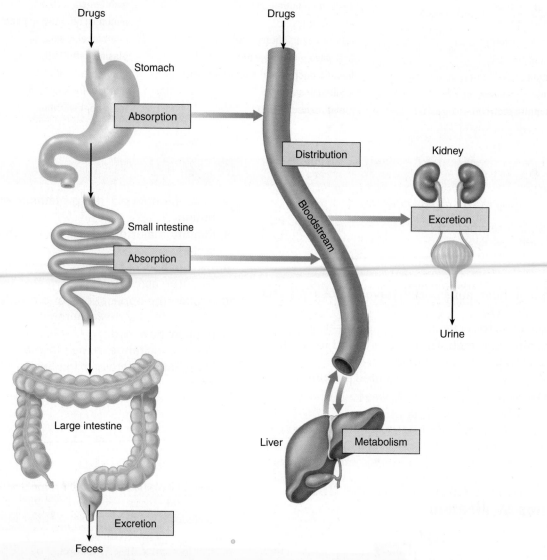

Figure 5.1 | The four processes of pharmacokinetics: absorption, distribution, metabolism, and excretion

Plasma membranes consist of a lipid bilayer, with proteins and other molecules interspersed in the membrane. This lipophilic membrane is relatively impermeable to large molecules, ions, and polar molecules. These physical characteristics have direct application to pharmacokinetics. For example, drug molecules that are small, nonionized, and lipid soluble will usually pass through plasma membranes by simple diffusion and more easily reach their target cells. Small water-soluble agents such as urea, alcohol, and water can enter through pores in the plasma membrane. Large molecules, ionized drugs, and water-soluble agents, however, will have more difficulty crossing plasma membranes. These agents may use other means to gain entry, such as carrier proteins or active transport. In some cases, the drug may not need to enter the cell to produce its effects: Once bound to the plasma membrane, some drugs activate a second messenger within the cell, which produces the physiologic change (See Chapter 6)⊙⊙ .

5.3 Absorption of Medications

Absorption is a process involving the movement of a substance from its site of administration, across body membranes, to circulating fluids. Absorption may occur across the skin and associated mucous membranes, or drugs may move across membranes that line the gastrointestinal or respiratory tract. Most drugs, with the exception of a few topical medications, intestinal antiinfectives, and some radiologic contrast agents, must be absorbed to produce an effect.

Absorption is the primary pharmacokinetic factor determining the length of time it takes a drug to produce its effect. In general, the more rapid the absorption, the faster the onset of drug action. Drugs that are used in critical care are designed to be absorbed within seconds or minutes. At the other extreme are drugs such as the contraceptive Norplant, which is enclosed in plastic tubes and implanted under the skin, where it is absorbed slowly over several years.

Absorption is conditional on many factors. Drugs administered IV have the most rapid onset of action. Drugs in elixir or syrup formulations are absorbed faster than tablets or capsules. Drugs administered in high doses are generally absorbed faster and have a more rapid onset of action than those given in low concentrations. Digestive motility, exposure to enzymes in the digestive tract, and blood flow to the site of drug administration also affect absorption.

The degree of ionization of a drug affects its absorption. A drug's ability to become ionized depends on the surrounding pH. Aspirin provides an excellent example of the effects of ionization on absorption, as depicted in Figure 5.2. In the acid environment of the stomach, aspirin is in its *nonionized* form and thus readily absorbed and distributed by the bloodstream. As aspirin enters the alkaline environment of the small intestine, however, it becomes ionized. In its ionized form, aspirin is not as likely to be absorbed and distributed to target cells. Unlike acidic drugs, medications that are weakly basic are in their *nonionized* form in an alkaline environment; therefore, basic drugs would be absorbed and distributed better in alkaline environments such as in the small intestine. The pH of the local environment directly influences drug absorption through its ability to ionize the drug. In simplest terms, it may help the student to remember that acids are absorbed in acids, and bases are absorbed in bases.

Drug-drug or food-drug interactions may influence absorption. Many examples of these interactions have been discovered. For example, administering tetracyclines with food or drugs containing calcium, iron, or magnesium can significantly delay absorption of the antibiotic. High-fat meals can slow stomach motility significantly and delay the absorption of oral medications taken with the meal. Dietary supplements may also affect absorption. Common ingredients in herbal weight-loss products such as aloe leaf, guar gum, senna, and yellow dock exert a laxative effect that may decrease intestinal transit time and reduce drug absorption (Scott & Elmer, 2002). The nurse must be aware of drug interactions and advise patients to avoid known combinations of foods and medications that significantly impact drug action.

5.4 Distribution of Medications

Distribution involves how pharmacologic agents are transported throughout the body. The simplest factor determining distribution is the amount of blood flow to body tissues. The heart, liver, kidneys, and brain receive the most blood supply. Skin, bone, and adipose tissue receive a lower blood flow; therefore, it is more difficult to deliver high concentrations of drugs to these areas.

The physical properties of the drug greatly influence how it moves throughout the body after administration. Lipid solubility is an important characteristic, because it determines how quickly a drug is absorbed, mixes within the bloodstream, crosses membranes, and becomes local-

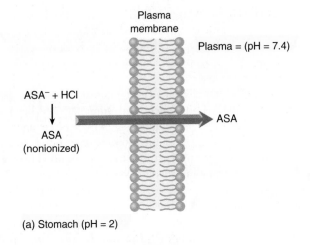

(a) Stomach (pH = 2)

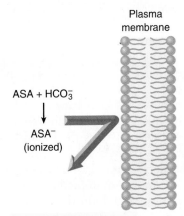

(b) Small intestine (pH = 8)

Figure 5.2 Effect of pH on drug absorption: (a) a weak acid such as aspirin (ASA) is in a nonionized form in an acidic environment and absorption occurs; (b) in a basic environment, aspirin is mostly in an ionized form and absorption is prevented

ized in body tissues. Lipid-soluble agents are not limited by the barriers that normally stop water-soluble drugs; thus, they are more completely distributed to body tissues.

Some tissues have the ability to accumulate and store drugs after absorption. The bone marrow, teeth, eyes, and adipose tissue have an especially high **affinity**, or attraction for certain medications. Examples of agents that are attracted to adipose tissue are thiopental (Pentothal), diazepam (Valium), and lipid-soluble vitamins. Tetracycline binds to calcium salts and accumulates in the bones and teeth. Once stored in tissues, drugs may remain in the body for many months.

Not all drug molecules in the plasma will reach their target cells, because many drugs bind reversibly to plasma proteins, particularly albumin, to form **drug-protein complexes**. Drug-protein complexes are too large to cross capillary membranes; thus, the drug is not available for distribution to body tissues. Drugs bound to proteins circulate in the plasma until they are released or displaced from the drug-protein complex. Only unbound (free) drugs can reach their target cells. This concept is illustrated in Figure 5.3. Some drugs, such as the anticoagulant warfarin (Coumadin) are highly bound; 99% of the drug in the plasma exists in drug-protein complexes and is unavailable to reach target cells.

Drugs and other chemicals compete with each other for plasma protein binding sites, and some agents have a greater affinity for these binding sites than other agents. Drug-drug and drug-food interactions may occur when one agent displaces another from plasma proteins. The displaced medication can immediately reach high levels in the blood and produce adverse effects. An example is the drug warfarin (Coumadin). After administration, 99% of the warfarin molecules are bound to plasma proteins. Drugs such as aspirin or cimetidine (Tagamet) displace warfarin from the drug-protein complex, thus raising blood levels of free warfarin and dramatically enhancing the risk of hemorrhage. Most drug guides give the percentage of medication bound to plasma proteins; when giving multiple drugs that are highly bound, the nurse should monitor the patient closely for adverse effects.

The brain and placenta possess special anatomical barriers that inhibit many chemicals and medications from entering. These barriers are referred to as the **blood-brain barrier** and **fetal-placental barrier**. Some medications such as sedatives, antianxiety agents, and anticonvulsants readily cross the blood-brain barrier to produce their actions on the central nervous system. On the other hand, most antitumor medications can not cross this barrier, making brain cancers difficult to treat.

The fetal-placental barrier serves an important protective function, because it prevents potentially harmful substances from passing from the mother's bloodstream to the fetus. Substances such as alcohol, cocaine, caffeine, and certain prescription medications, however, easily cross the placental barrier and could potentially harm the fetus. Because of this, no prescription medication, OTC drug or herbal therapy should be taken by a patient who is pregnant without first consulting with a healthcare provider. The healthcare provider should always question female patients in the childbearing years regarding their pregnancy status before prescribing a drug. Chapter 7 presents a list of drug pregnancy categories to assess fetal risk ⊗ .

5.5 Metabolism of Medications

Metabolism, also called biotransformation, is the process of chemically converting a drug to a form that is usually more easily removed from the body. Metabolism involves a study of the complex biochemical pathways and reactions that alter drugs, nutrients, vitamins, and minerals. The liver is the primary site of drug metabolism, although the kidneys and cells of the intestinal tract also have high metabolic rates.

Many types of biochemical reactions occur to medications as they pass through the liver, including hydrolysis, oxidation, and reduction. During metabolism, the addition

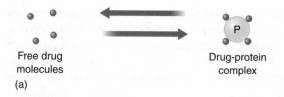

Free drug molecules ⇌ Drug-protein complex

(a)

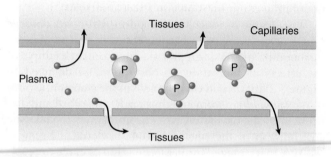

Tissues — Capillaries

Plasma

Tissues

(b)

Figure 5.3 | Plasma protein binding and drug availability: (a) drug exists in a free state or bound to plasma protein; (b) drug-protein complexes are too large to cross membranes

of side chains, known as **conjugates**, makes drugs more water-soluble and more easily excreted by the kidneys.

Most metabolism in the liver is accomplished by the **hepatic microsomal enzyme system**. This enzyme complex is sometimes called the P-450 system, named after cytochrome P-450, which is a key component of the system. As it relates to pharmacotherapy, the primary actions of the hepatic microsomal enzymes are to inactivate drugs and accelerate their excretion. In some cases, however, metabolism can produce a chemical alteration that makes the resulting molecule *more* active than the original. For example, the narcotic analgesic codeine undergoes biotransformation to morphine, which has significantly greater ability to relieve pain. In fact, some agents, known as **prodrugs**, have no pharmacologic activity unless they are first metabolized to their active form by the body. Examples of prodrugs include benazepril (Lotensin) and losartan (Cozaar).

Changes in the function of the hepatic microsomal enzymes can significantly affect drug metabolism. A few drugs have the ability to increase metabolic activity in the liver, a process called enzyme induction. For example, phenobarbital causes the liver to synthesize more microsomal enzymes. By doing so, phenobarbital will increase the rate of its own metabolism, as well as that of other drugs metabolized in the liver. In these patients, higher doses of medication may be required to achieve therapeutic effect.

Certain patients have decreased hepatic metabolic activity, which may alter drug action. Hepatic enzyme activity is generally reduced in infants and elderly patients; therefore, pediatric and geriatric patients are more sensitive to drug therapy than middle-age patients. Patients with severe liver damage, such as that caused by cirrhosis, will require reductions in drug dosage because of the decreased metabolic activity. Certain genetic disorders have been recognized in which patients lack specific metabolic enzymes; drug dosages in these patients must be adjusted accordingly. The nurse should pay careful attention to laboratory values that may indicate liver disease, so that doses may be adjusted accordingly.

Metabolism has a number of additional therapeutic consequences. As illustrated in Figure 5.4, drugs absorbed after oral administration cross directly into the hepatic portal circulation, which carries blood to the liver before it is distributed to other body tissues. As blood passes through the liver circulation, some drugs can be completely metabolized to an inactive form before they ever reach the general circulation. This first-pass effect is an important mechanism, since a large number of oral drugs are rendered inactive by hepatic metabolic reactions. Alternate routes of delivery that bypass the first-pass effect (e.g., sublingual, rectal, or parenteral routes) may need to be considered for these drugs.

5.6 Excretion of Medications

Drugs are removed from the body by the process of excretion. The rate at which medications are excreted determines their concentration in the bloodstream and tissues. This is important because the concentration of drugs in the bloodstream determines their duration of action. Pathologic states, such as liver disease or renal failure, often increase the duration of drug action in the body because they interfere with natural excretion mechanisms. Dosing regimens must be carefully adjusted in these patients.

Although drugs are removed from the body by numerous organs and tissues, the primary site of excretion is the kidney. In an average-size person, approximately 180 L of blood are filtered by the kidneys each day. Free drugs, water-soluble agents, electrolytes, and small molecules are easily filtered at the glomerulus. Proteins, blood cells, conjugates, and drug-protein complexes are not filtered because of their large size.

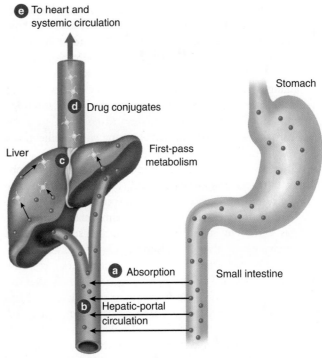

Figure 5.4 First-pass effect: (a) drugs are absorbed; (b) drugs enter hepatic portal circulation and go directly to liver; (c) hepatic microsomal enzymes metabolize drugs to inactive forms; (d) drug conjugates, leaving liver; (e) distribution to general circulation

Upon filtration, chemicals and drugs are subjected to the process of reabsorption in the renal tubule. Mechanisms of reabsorption are the same as absorption elsewhere in the body. Nonionized and lipid-soluble drugs cross renal tubular membranes easily and return to the circulation; ionized and water-soluble drugs generally remain in the filtrate for excretion.

Drug-protein complexes and substances too large to be filtered at the glomerulus are sometimes secreted into the distal tubule of the nephron. For example, only 10% of a dose of penicillin G is filtered at the glomerulus; 90% is secreted into the renal tubule. As with metabolic enzyme activity, secretion mechanisms are less active in infants and older adults.

Certain drugs may be excreted more quickly if the pH of the filtrate changes. Weak acids such as aspirin are excreted faster when the filtrate is slightly alkaline, because aspirin is ionized in an alkaline environment, and the drug will remain in the filtrate and be excreted in the urine. Weakly basic drugs such as diazepam (Valium) are excreted faster with a slightly acidic filtrate, because they are ionized in this environment. This relationship between pH and drug excretion can be used to advantage in critical care situations. To speed the renal excretion of acidic drugs such as aspirin in an overdosed patient, nurses can administer sodium bicarbonate. Sodium bicarbonate will make the urine more basic, which ionizes more aspirin, causing it to be excreted more readily. The excretion of diazepam, on the other hand, can be enhanced by giving ammonium chloride, to acidify the filtrate.

SPECIAL CONSIDERATIONS

Adverse Drug Effects and the Elderly

Adverse drug effects are more commonly recorded in elderly patients than in young adults or middle-age patients, because the geriatric population takes more drugs simultaneously (an average of seven) than other age groups. In addition, chronic diseases that affect pharmacokinetics are present more often in the elderly. A recent study by Doucet et al. (2002) of over 2,800 inpatients over age 70 found 500 adverse drug events at the time of admission. Over 60% of the adverse drug events were caused by drug-drug interactions. Of these, over 46% were considered "preventable," because the drug-drug interaction was known. Excess doses were administered in almost 15% of the patients; healthcare providers often forgot to adjust doses for pharmacokinetic variables that change with aging.

Alteration of kidney function can dramatically affect pharmacokinetics. Patients with renal failure will have diminished ability to excrete medications and may retain drugs for an extended time. Doses for these patients must be reduced, to avoid drug toxicity. Because small to moderate changes in renal status can cause rapid increases in serum drug levels, the nurse must constantly monitor kidney function in patients receiving drugs that may be nephrotoxic, or during pharmacotherapy with medications that have a narrow margin of safety.

Other organs can serve as important sites of excretion. Drugs that can easily be changed into a gaseous form are especially suited for excretion by the respiratory system. The rate of respiratory excretion is dependent on factors that affect gas exchange, including diffusion, gas solubility, and pulmonary blood flow. The elimination of volatile anesthetics following surgery is primarily dependent on respiratory activity. The faster the breathing rate, the greater the excretion. Conversely, the respiratory removal of water-soluble agents such as alcohol is more dependent on blood flow to the lungs. The greater the blood flow into lung capillaries, the greater the excretion. In contrast to other methods of excretion, the lungs excrete most drugs in their original unmetabolized form.

Glandular activity is another elimination mechanism. Water-soluble drugs may be secreted into the saliva, sweat, or breast milk. The "funny taste" that patients sometimes experience when given IV drugs is an example of agents secreted into the saliva. Another example of glandular excretion is the garlic smell that can be detected when standing next to a perspiring person who has recently eaten garlic. Excretion into breast milk is of considerable importance for basic drugs such as morphine or codeine, as these can achieve high concentrations and potentially affect the nursing infant. Nursing mothers should always check with their healthcare provider before taking any prescription medication, OTC drug, or herbal supplement. Pharmacology of the pregnant or breastfeeding patient is discussed in Chapter 7 ⬡ .

Some drugs are secreted in the bile, a process known as biliary excretion. In many cases, drugs secreted into bile will enter the duodenum and eventually leave the body in the feces. However, most bile is circulated back to the liver by **enterohepatic recirculation**, as illustrated in Figure 5.5. A percentage of the drug may be recirculated numerous times with the bile. Biliary reabsorption is extremely influential in prolonging the activity of cardiac glycosides, certain antibiotics, and phenothiazines. Recirculated drugs are ultimately metabolized by the liver and excreted by the kidneys. Recirculation and elimination of drugs through biliary excretion may continue for several weeks after therapy has been discontinued.

5.7 Drug Plasma Concentration and Therapeutic Response

The therapeutic response of most drugs is directly related to their level in the plasma. Although the concentration of

the medication at its *target tissue* is more predictive of drug action, this quantity is impossible to measure in most cases. For example, it is possible to conduct a laboratory test that measures the serum level of the bipolar drug lithium carbonate (Eskalith) by taking a blood sample; it is a far different matter to measure the quantity of this drug in neurons within the CNS. Indeed, it is common practice for nurses to monitor the plasma levels of certain drugs that have a low safety profile.

Several important pharmacokinetic principles can be illustrated by measuring the serum level of a drug following a single-dose administration. These pharmacokinetic values are shown graphically in Figure 5.6. This figure demonstrates two plasma drug levels. First is the **minimum effective concentration**, the amount of drug required to produce a therapeutic effect. Second is the **toxic concentration**, the level of drug that will result in serious adverse effects. The plasma drug concentration between the minimum effective concentration and the toxic concentration is called the **therapeutic range** of the drug. These values have great clinical significance. For example, if the patient has a severe headache and is given half of an aspirin tablet, the plasma level will remain below the minimum effective concentration, and the patient will not experience pain relief. Two or three tablets will increase the plasma level of aspirin into the therapeutic range, and the pain will subside. Taking six or more tablets may result in adverse effects, such as GI bleeding or tinnitus. For each drug administered, the nurse's goal is to keep its plasma concentration in the therapeutic range. For some drugs, this therapeutic range is quite wide; for other medications, the difference between a minimum effective dose and a toxic dose can be dangerously narrow.

5.8 Plasma Half-life and Duration of Drug Action

The most common description of a drug's duration of action is its **plasma half-life** ($t_{1/2}$), defined as the length of time required for a medication to decrease concentration in the plasma by one-half after administration. Some drugs have a half-life of only a few minutes, while others have a half-life of several hours or days. The greater the half-life, the longer it takes a medication to be excreted. For example, a drug with a $t_{1/2}$ of 10 hours would take longer to be excreted and thus produce a longer effect in the body than a drug with a $t_{1/2}$ of 5 hours.

The plasma half-life of a drug is an essential pharmacokinetic variable that has important clinical applications. Drugs with relatively short half-lives, such as aspirin ($t_{1/2} = $ 15 to 20 minutes) must be given every 3 to 4 hours. Drugs with longer half-lives, such as felodipine (Plendil) ($t_{1/2} = $ 10 hours), need only be given once a day. If a patient has extensive renal or hepatic disease, the plasma half-life of a drug will increase, and the drug concentration may reach toxic levels. In these patients, medications must be given less frequently, or the dosages must be reduced.

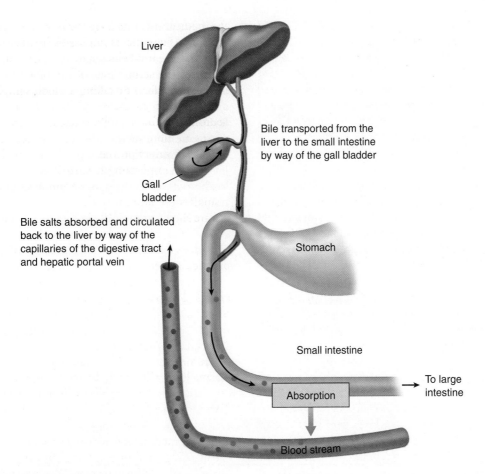

Figure 5.5 | Enterohepatic recirculation

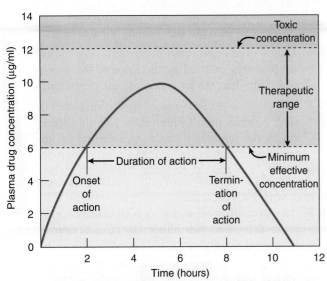

Figure 5.6 | Single-dose drug administration: pharmacokinetic values for this drug are as follows: onset of action = 2 hours; duration of action = 6 hours; termination of action = 8 hours after administration; peak plasma concentration = 10 µg/ml; time to peak drug effect = 5 hours; $t_{1/2}$ = 4 hours

5.9 Loading Doses and Maintenance Doses

Few drugs are administered as a single dose. Repeated doses result in an accumulation of drug in the bloodstream, as shown in Figure 5.7. Eventually, a plateau will be reached where the level of drug in the plasma is maintained continuously within the therapeutic range. At this level, the amount administered has reached equilibrium with the amount of drug being eliminated, resulting in a continuous therapeutic level of drug being distributed to body tissues. Theoretically, it takes approximately four half-lives to reach this equilibrium. If the medication is given as a continuous infusion, the plateau can be reached quickly and be maintained with little or no fluctuation in drug plasma levels.

The plateau may be reached faster by administration of loading doses followed by regular maintenance doses. A **loading dose** is a higher amount of drug, often given only once or twice, which is administered to "prime" the bloodstream with a level sufficient to quickly induce a therapeutic response. Before plasma levels can drop back toward zero, intermittent **maintenance doses** are given to keep

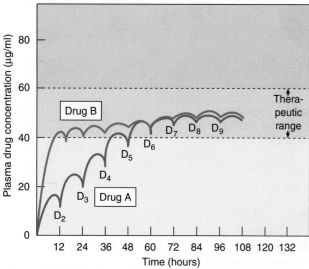

Figure 5.7 | Multiple-dose drug administration: drug A (—) and drug B (—) are administered every 12 hours; drug B reaches the therapeutic range faster, because the first dose is a loading dose

the plasma drug concentration in the therapeutic range. Although blood levels of the drug fluctuate with this approach, the equilibrium state can be reached almost as rapidly as with a continuous infusion. Loading doses are particularly important for drugs with prolonged half-lives, and for situations in which it is critical to raise drug plasma levels quickly, as might be the case when administering an antibiotic for a severe infection. In Figure 5.7, notice that it takes almost five doses (48 hours) before a therapeutic level is reached using a routine dosing schedule. With a loading dose, a therapeutic level is reached within 12 hours.

CHAPTER REVIEW

Key Concepts

The numbered key concepts provide a succinct summary of the important points from the corresponding numbered section within the chapter. If any of these points are not clear, refer to the numbered section within the chapter for review. Expanded versions can be found on the companion website.

5.1 Pharmacokinetics focuses on the movement of drugs throughout the body after they are administered.

5.2 The physiological properties of plasma membranes determine movement of drugs throughout the body. The four topics of pharmacokinetics are absorption, metabolism, distribution, and excretion.

5.3 Absorption is the process of moving a drug from the site of administration to the bloodstream. Absorption depends upon size of the drug molecule, its lipid solubility, degree of ionization and interactions with food or other medications.

5.4 Distribution represents how drugs are transported throughout the body. Distribution depends upon the formation of drug-protein complexes and special barriers such as the placenta or brain barriers.

5.5 Metabolism is a process that changes a drug's activity and makes it more likely to be excreted. Changes in hepatic metabolism can significantly affect drug action.

5.6 Excretion processes remove drugs from the body. Drugs are primarily excreted by the kidneys, but may be excreted into bile, the lung, or glandular secretions.

5.7 The therapeutic response of most drugs depends on their concentration in the plasma. The difference between the minimum effective concentration and the toxic concentration is called the therapeutic range.

5.8 Plasma half-life represents the duration of action for most drugs.

5.9 Repeated dosing allows a plateau drug plasma level to be reached. Loading doses allow a therapeutic drug level to be reached rapidly.

Review Questions

1. Describe the types of obstacles drugs face from the time they are administered, until they reach their target cells.

2. Why is $t_{1/2}$ important to the nurse?

3. How does the ionization of a drug affect its distribution in the body?

4. Explain why drugs that are metabolized through the first-pass effect may need to be administered by the parenteral route.

5. Explain how onset of action, duration of action, and the time to peak effect can be estimated from a single-dose response curve.

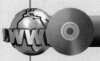

EXPLORE MediaLink

NCLEX review, case studies, and other interactive resources for this chapter can be found on the companion website at www.prenhall.com/adams. Click on "Chapter 5" to select the activities for this chapter. For animations, more NCLEX review questions, and an audio glossary, access the accompanying CD-ROM in this textbook.

Pharmacodynamics

I n clinical practice, nurses quickly learn that medications do not affect all patients in the same way: A dose that produces a dramatic response in one patient may have no effect on another. In some cases, the differences among patients are predictable, based on the pharmacokinetic principles discussed in Chapter 5. In other cases, the differences in response are not easily explained. Despite this patient variability, healthcare providers must choose optimal doses while avoiding unnecessary adverse effects. This is not an easy task given the wide variation of patient responses within a population. This chapter examines the mechanisms by which drugs affect patients, and how the nurse can apply these principles to clinical practice.

metabolized and eliminated by the bod
of this process
PHARMACOLOGY
1. The study of medicines; the discipli
pertaining to how drugs improve the he
of the human body
PHARMACOPEL

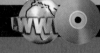 **MediaLink** www.prenhall.com/adams

CD-ROM

Animation:
  Agonist
Audio Glossary
NCLEX Review

Companion Website

NCLEX Review
Case Study
Expanded Key Concepts
Challenge Your Knowledge

OBJECTIVES

After reading this chapter, the student should be able to:

1. Apply principles of pharmacodynamics to clinical practice.
2. Discuss how frequency response curves may be used to explain how patients respond differently to medications.
3. Explain the importance of the median effective dose (ED$_{50}$) to clinical practice.
4. Compare and contrast median lethal dose (LD$_{50}$) and median toxicity dose (TD$_{50}$).
5. Discuss how a drug's therapeutic index is related to its margin of safety.
6. Identify the significance of the graded dose-response relationship to clinical practice.
7. Compare and contrast the terms potency and efficacy.
8. Distinguish between an agonist, partial agonist, and antagonist.
9. Explain the relationship between receptors and drug action.
10. Explain possible future developments in the field of pharmacogenetics.

6.1 Pharmacodynamics and Interpatient Variability

The term **pharmacodynamics** is comprised of the root words *pharmaco*, which means "medicine," and *dynamics*, which means "change." In simplest terms, pharmacodynamics refers to how a drug *changes* the body. A more complete definition explains pharmacodynamics as the branch of pharmacology concerned with the mechanisms of drug action and the relationships between drug concentration and responses in the body.

Pharmacodynamics has important clinical applications. Healthcare providers must be able to predict whether a drug will produce a significant change in patients. Although clinicians often begin therapy with average doses taken from a drug guide, intuitive experience often becomes the practical method for determining which doses of medications will be effective in a given patient. Knowledge of therapeutic indexes, dose-response relationships, and drug-receptor interactions will help the nurse provide safe and effective treatment.

Interpatient variability in responses to drugs can best be understood by examining a frequency distribution curve. A **frequency distribution curve**, shown in Figure 6.1, is a graphical representation of the number of patients responding to a drug action at different doses. Notice the wide range in doses that produced the patient responses shown on the curve. A few patients responded to the drug at very low doses. As the dose was increased, more and

more patients responded. Some patients required very high doses to elicit the desired response. The peak of the curve indicates the largest number of patients responding to the drug. The curve does not show the *magnitude* of response, only whether a measurable response occurred among the patients. As an example, think of the given response to an antihypertensive drug as being a reduction of 20 mm in systolic blood pressure. A few patients experienced the desired 20 mm reduction at a dose of only 10 mg of drug. A 50 mg dose gave the largest number of patients a 20 mm reduction in blood pressure; however, a few patients needed as much as 90 mg of drug to produce the same 20 mm reduction.

The dose in the middle of the frequency distribution curve represents the drug's **median effective dose (ED$_{50}$)**. The ED$_{50}$ is the dose required to produce a specific therapeutic response in 50% of a group of patients. Drug guides sometimes report the ED$_{50}$ as the average or standard dose.

The interpatient variability shown in Figure 6.1 has important clinical implications. First, the nurse should realize that the standard or average dose predicts a satisfactory therapeutic response for only *half* the population. In other words, many patients will require more or less than the average dose for optimum pharmacotherapy. Using the systolic blood pressure example, assume that a large group of patients is given the average dose of 50 mg. Some of these patients will experience toxicity at this level because they only needed 10 mg to achieve blood pressure reduction. Other patients in this group will probably have no reduction in blood pressure. By observing the patient, taking

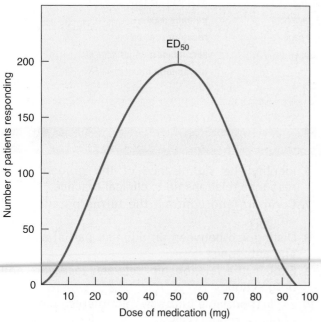

Figure 6.1 | Frequency Distribution Curve: Interpatient variability in drug response

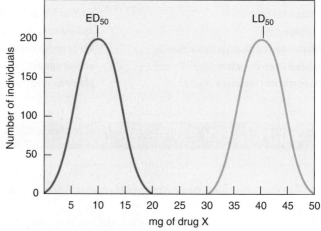

(a) Drug X : TI = $\dfrac{LD_{50}}{ED_{50}} = \dfrac{40}{10} = 4$

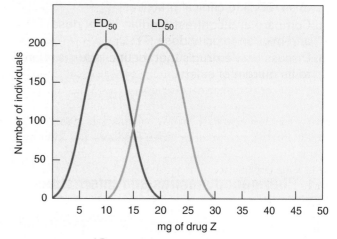

(b) Drug Z : TI = $\dfrac{LD_{50}}{ED_{50}} = \dfrac{20}{10} = 2$

Figure 6.2 | Therapeutic index: (a) drug X has a therapeutic index of 4; (b) drug Z has a therapeutic index of 2

vital signs, and monitoring associated laboratory data, the skill of the nurse is critical in determining whether the average dose is effective for the patient. It is not enough to simply memorize an average dose for a drug; the nurse must know when and how to adjust this dose to obtain the optimum therapeutic response.

6.2 Therapeutic Index and Drug Safety

Administering a dose that produces an optimum therapeutic response for each individual patient is only one component of effective pharmacotherapy. The nurse must also be able to predict whether the dose they are giving is safe for the patient.

Frequency distribution curves can also be used to represent the safety of a drug. For example, the **median lethal dose** (LD_{50}) is often determined in preclinical trials, as part of the drug development process discussed in Chapter 1 🔗. The LD_{50} is the dose of drug that will be lethal in 50% of a group of animals. As with ED_{50}, a group of animals will exhibit considerable variability in lethal dose; what may be a nontoxic dose for one animal may be lethal for another.

To examine the safety of a particular drug, the LD_{50} can be compared to the ED_{50}, as shown in Figure 6.2A. In this example, 10 mg of drug X is the average *effective* dose, and 40 mg is the average *lethal* dose. The ED_{50} and LD_{50} are used to calculate an important value in pharmacology, a drug's **therapeutic index**, the ratio of a drug's LD_{50} to its ED_{50}.

$$\text{Therapeutic index} = \frac{\text{median lethal dose } LD_{50}}{\text{median effective dose } ED_{50}}$$

The larger the difference between the two doses, the greater the therapeutic index. In Figure 6.2A, the thera-

peutic index is 4 (40 mg ÷ 10 mg). Essentially, this means that it would take an error in magnitude of *approximately* 4 times the average dose to be lethal to a patient. Thus, the therapeutic index is a measure of a drug's safety margin: the higher the value, the safer the medication.

As another example, the therapeutic index of a second drug is shown in Figure 6.2B. Drug Z has the same ED_{50} as drug X, but shows a different LD_{50}. The therapeutic index for drug Z is only 2 (20 mg ÷ 10 mg). The difference between an effective dose and a lethal dose is very small for drug Z; thus, the drug has a narrow safety margin. The therapeutic index offers the nurse practical information on the safety of a drug, and a means to compare one drug to another.

Because the LD_{50} cannot be experimentally determined in humans, the **median toxicity dose** (TD_{50}) is a more practical value in a clinical setting. The TD_{50} is the dose that will produce a given toxicity in 50% of a group of patients. The TD_{50} value may be extrapolated from animal data or based on adverse effects recorded in patient clinical trials.

6.3 The Graded Dose-Response Relationship and Therapeutic Response

In the previous examples, frequency distribution curves were used to graphically visualize patient differences in responses to medications in a *population*. It is also useful to visualize the variability in responses observed within a *single patient*.

The graded dose-response relationship is a fundamental concept in pharmacology. The graphical representation of this relationship is called a dose-response curve, as illustrated in Figure 6.3. By observing and measuring the patient's response obtained at different doses of the drug, one can explain several important clinical relationships.

The three distinct phases of a dose-response curve indicate essential pharmacodynamic principles that have relevance to clinical practice. Phase 1 occurs at the lowest doses. The flatness of this portion of the curve indicates that few target cells have been affected yet by the drug. Phase 2 is the straight-line portion of the curve. This portion often shows a linear relationship between the amount of drug administered and the degree of response obtained from the patient. For example, if the dose is doubled, twice as much response is obtained. This is the most desirable range of doses for pharmacotherapeutics, since giving more drug results in proportionately more effect; a lower drug dose gives less effect. In phase 3, a plateau is reached in which increasing the drug dose produces no additional therapeutic response. This may occur for a number of reasons. One explanation is that all the receptors for the drug are occupied. It could also mean that the drug has brought 100% relief, such as when a migraine headache has been terminated; giving higher doses produces no additional relief. In phase 3, although increasing the dose does not result in more therapeutic effect, the nurse should be mindful that increasing the dose may produce adverse effects.

6.4 Potency and Efficacy

Within a pharmacologic class, not all drugs are equally effective at treating a disorder. For example, some antineoplastic drugs kill more cancer cells than others, some antihypertensive agents lower blood pressure to a greater degree than others; and some analgesics are more effective at relieving severe pain than others in the same class. Furthermore, drugs in the same class are effective at different doses; one antibiotic may be effective at a dose of 1 mg/kg, whereas another is most effective at 100 mg/kg. Nurses need a method to compare one drug to another, so that they can administer treatment effectively.

There are two fundamental ways to compare medications within therapeutic and pharmacologic classes. First is the concept of potency. A drug that is more potent will produce a therapeutic effect at a lower dose, compared to another drug in the same class. Consider two agents, drug X and drug Y, which both produce a 20 mm drop in blood pressure. If drug X produced this effect at a dose of 10 mg, and drug X at 60 mg, then drug X is said to be more potent. Thus, potency is a way to compare the doses of two independently administered drugs in terms of how much is needed to produce a particular response. A useful way to visualize the concept of potency is by examining dose-response curves. Compare the two drugs shown in Figure 6.4A. In this example, drug A is more potent because it requires a lower dose to produce the same response.

The second method used to compare drugs is called efficacy, which is the magnitude of maximal response that can be produced from a particular drug. In the example in Figure 6.4B, drug A is more efficacious because it produces a higher maximal response.

Which is more important to the success of pharmacotherapy, potency or efficacy? Perhaps the best way to understand these concepts is to use the specific example of headache pain. Two common OTC analgesics are ibuprofen (200 mg) and aspirin (650 mg). The fact that ibuprofen relieves pain at a lower dose indicates that this agent is *more potent* than aspirin. At recommended doses, however, both are equally effective at relieving headache pain, thus, they have the *same efficacy*. If the patient is experiencing severe pain, however, neither aspirin nor ibuprofen has sufficient efficacy to bring relief. Narcotic analgesics such as morphine have a greater efficacy than aspirin or ibuprofen and could effectively treat this type of pain. From a pharmacotherapeutic perspective, efficacy is almost always more important than potency. In the previous example, the average dose is unimportant to the patient, but headache relief is essential. As another comparison, the patient with cancer is much more concerned about how many cancer cells have been killed (efficacy) than what dose the nurse administered (potency). Although the nurse will often hear claims that one drug is more potent than another, a more compelling concern is which drug is more efficacious.

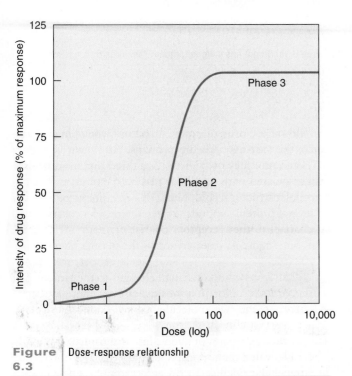

Figure 6.3 | Dose-response relationship

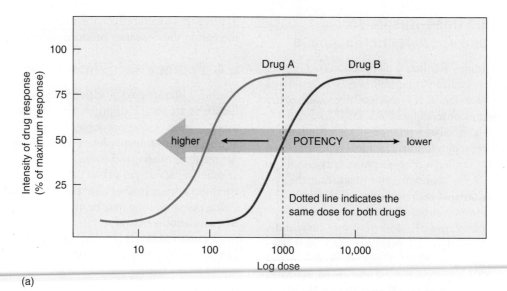

(a)

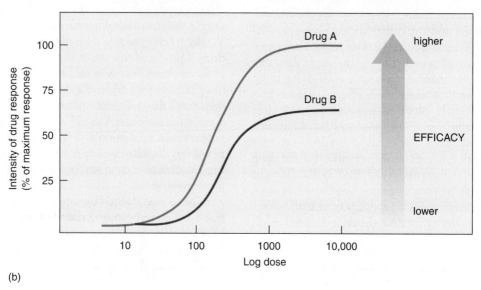

(b)

Figure 6.4 | Potency and efficacy: (a) drug A has a higher potency than drug B; (b) drug A has a higher efficacy than drug B

6.5 Cellular Receptors and Drug Action

Drugs act by modulating or changing existing physiological and biochemical processes. To effect such changes requires that the drug interact with specific molecules and chemicals normally found in the body. A cellular macromolecule to which a medication binds to initiate its effects is called a **receptor**. The concept of a drug binding to a receptor to cause a change in body chemistry or physiology is a fundamental theory in pharmacology. Receptor theory explains the mechanisms by which most drugs produce their effects. It is important to understand, however, that these receptors do not exist in the body solely to bind drugs. Their normal function is to bind endogenous molecules such as hormones, neurotransmitters, and growth factors.

Although a drug receptor can be any type of macromolecule, the vast majority are proteins. As shown in Figure 6.5, a receptor may be depicted as a three-dimensional protein associated with a cellular plasma membrane. The extracellular structural component of a receptor often consists of several protein subunits arranged around a central canal or channel. Other receptors consist of many membrane-spanning segments inserted across the plasma membrane.

A drug attaches to its receptor in a specific manner, much like a lock and key. Small changes to the structure of a drug, or its receptor, may weaken or even eliminate binding between the two molecules. Once bound, drugs may trigger a series of **second messenger** events within the cell, such as the conversion of adenosine triphosphate (ATP) to cyclic adenosine monophosphate (cyclic AMP), the release of intracellular calcium, or the activation of specific G pro-

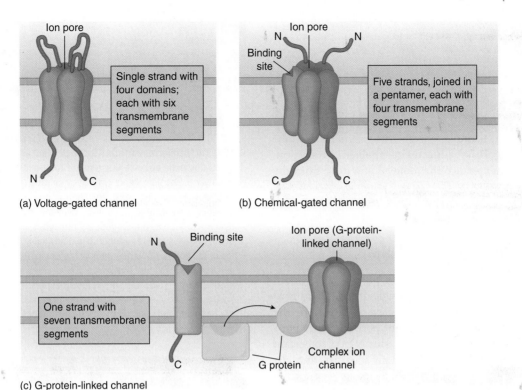

(a) Voltage-gated channel

Ion pore

Single strand with four domains; each with six transmembrane segments

(b) Chemical-gated channel

Ion pore

N   N

Binding site

Five strands, joined in a pentamer, each with four transmembrane segments

C   C

(c) G-protein-linked channel

N

Binding site

Ion pore (G-protein-linked channel)

One strand with seven transmembrane segments

C

G protein

Complex ion channel

Figure 6.5 | Cellular receptors

teins and associated enzymes. These biochemical cascades initiate the drug's action by either stimulating or inhibiting a normal activity of the cell.

Not all receptors are bound to plasma membranes; some are intracellular molecules such as DNA or enzymes in the cytoplasm. By interacting with these types of receptors, medications are able to inhibit protein synthesis or regulate events such as cell replication and metabolism. Examples of agents that bind intracellular components include steroid medications, vitamins, and hormones.

Receptors and their associated drug mechanisms are extremely important in therapeutics. Receptor *subtypes* are being discovered and new medications are being developed at a faster rate than any other time in history. These subtypes permit the "fine-tuning" of pharmacology. For example, the first medications affecting the autonomic nervous system affected all autonomic receptors. It was discovered that two basic receptor types existed in the body, alpha and beta, and drugs were then developed that affected only one type. The result was more specific drug action, with fewer adverse effects. Still later, several subtypes of alpha and beta receptors, including alpha-1, alpha-2, beta-1, and beta-2, were discovered that allowed even more specificity in pharmacotherapy. In recent years, researchers have further divided and refined these subtypes. It is likely that receptor research will continue to result in the development of new medications that activate very specific receptors and thus direct drug action that avoids unnecessary adverse effects.

Some drugs act independently of cellular receptors. These agents are associated with other mechanisms, such as changing the permeability of cellular membranes, depressing membrane excitability, or altering the activity of cellular pumps. Actions such as these are often described as **nonspecific cellular responses**. Ethyl alcohol, general anesthetics, and osmotic diuretics are examples of agents that act by nonspecific mechanisms.

6.6 Types of Drug-Receptor Interactions

When a drug binds to a receptor, several therapeutic consequences can result. In simplest terms, a specific activity of the cell is either enhanced or inhibited. The actual biochemical mechanism underlying the therapeutic effect, however, may be extremely complex. In some cases, the mechanism of action is not known.

When a drug binds to its receptor, it may produce a response that *mimics* the effect of the endogenous regulatory molecule. For example, when the drug bethanechol (Urecholine) is administered, it binds to acetylcholine receptors in the autonomic nervous system and produces the same actions as acetylcholine. A drug that produces the same type of response as the endogenous substance is called an **agonist**. Agonists sometimes produce a greater maximal response than the endogenous chemical. The term **partial agonist** describes a medication that produces a weaker, or less efficacious, response than an agonist.

A second possibility is that a drug will occupy a receptor and *prevent* the endogenous chemical from acting. This drug is called an **antagonist**. Antagonists often compete with agonists for the receptor binding sites. For example, the drug atropine competes with acetylcholine for specific receptors in the autonomic nervous system. If the dose is high enough, atropine will inhibit the effects of acetylcholine, because acetylcholine cannot bind to its receptors.

Not all antagonism is associated with receptors, *Functional* antagonists inhibit the effects of an agonist, not by competing for a receptor, but by changing pharmacokinetic factors. For example, antagonists may slow the absorption of a drug. By speeding up metabolism or excretion, an antagonist can enhance the removal of a drug from the body. The relationships that occur between agonists and antagonists explain many of the drug-drug and drug-food interactions that occur in the body.

6.7 Pharmacology of the Future: Customizing Drug Therapy

Until recently, it was thought that single drugs should provide safe and effective treatment to every patient in the same way. Unfortunately, a significant portion of the population either develops unacceptable side effects to certain drugs or is unresponsive to them. Many scientists and clinicians are now discarding the one-size-fits-all approach to drug therapy, which was designed to treat an entire population without addressing important interpatient variation.

With the advent of the Human Genome Project and other advances in medicine, pharmacologists are hopeful that future drugs can be customized for patients with specific genetic similarities. In the past, unpredictable and unexplained drug reactions have been labeled idiosyncratic responses. It is hoped that, by taking a DNA test before receiving a drug, these idiosyncratic side effects can someday be avoided.

SPECIAL CONSIDERATIONS

Enzyme Deficiency in Certain Ethnic Populations

Pharmacogenetics has identified a number of people who are deficient in the enzyme glucose-6-phosphate dehydrogenase (G6PD). This enzyme is essential in carbohydrate metabolism. Males of Mediterranean and African descent are more likely to express this deficiency. It is estimated to affect 400 million people worldwide. The disorder is caused by mutations in the DNA structure that encode for G6PD, resulting in one or more amino acid changes in the protein molecule. Following administration of certain drugs, such as primaquine, sulfonamides, or nitrofurantoin, an acute hemolysis of red blood cells occurs due to the breaking of chemical bonds in the hemoglobin molecule. Up to 50% of the circulating RBCs may be destroyed. Genetic typing does not always predict toxicity; thus, the nurse must observe patients carefully following the administration of these medications. Fortunately, there are good alternative choices for these medications.

Pharmacogenetics is the area of pharmacology that examines the role of heredity in drug response. The greatest advances in pharmacogenetics have been the identification of subtle genetic differences in drug-metabolizing enzymes. Genetic differences in these enzymes are responsible for a significant portion of drug-induced toxicity. It is hoped that the use of pharmacogenetic information may someday allow for customized drug therapy. Although therapies based on a patient's genetically based response may not be cost effective at this time, pharmacogenetics may radically change the way pharmacotherapy will be practiced in the future.

CHAPTER REVIEW

Key Concepts

The numbered key concepts provide a succinct summary of the important points from the corresponding numbered section within the chapter. If any of these points are not clear, refer to the numbered section within the chapter for review. Expanded versions can be found on the companion website.

6.1 Pharmacodynamics is the area of pharmacology concerned with how drugs produce *change* in patients, and the differences in patient responses to medications.

6.2 The therapeutic index, expressed mathematically as $TD_{50} \div ED_{50}$, is a value representing the margin of safety of a drug. The higher the therapeutic index, the safer the drug.

6.3 The graded dose-response relationship describes how the therapeutic response from a drug changes as the medication dose is increased.

6.4 Potency, the dose of medication required to produce a particular response, and efficacy, the magnitude of maximal response to a drug, are means of comparing medications.

6.5 Drug receptor theory is used to explain the mechanism of action of many medications.

6.6 Agonists, partial agonists, and antagonists are substances that compete with drugs for receptor binding, and can cause drug-drug and drug-food interactions.

6.7 In the future, pharmacotherapy will likely be customized to match the genetic makeup of each patient.

Review Questions

1. If the ED_{50} is the dose required to produce an effective response in 50% of a group of patients, what happens in the "other" 50% of the patients after a dose has been administered?

2. Explain why a drug with a high therapeutic index is safer than one with a low therapeutic index.

3. On a dose-response curve, compare two drugs, drug D and drug E. Illustrate drug D as being more potent, but drug E as being more efficacious.

4. Two drugs are competing for a receptor on a mast cell that will cause the release of histamine when activated. Compare the effects of an agonist on this receptor to an antagonist. Which would likely be called an antihistamine, the agonist or the antagonist?

EXPLORE MediaLink

NCLEX review, case studies, and other interactive resources for this chapter can be found on the companion website at www.prenhall.com/adams. Click on "Chapter 6" to select the activities for this chapter. For animations, more NCLEX review questions, and an audio glossary, access the accompanying CD-ROM in this textbook.

Pharmacology and the Nurse-Patient Relationship

Drug Administration throughout the Lifespan

Beginning with conception, and continuing throughout the lifespan, the organs and systems within the body undergo predictable physiologic alterations that influence the absorption, metabolism, distribution, and elimination of medications. Healthcare providers must recognize such changes to ensure that drugs are delivered in a safe and effective manner to patients of all ages. The purpose of this chapter is to examine how principles of developmental physiology and lifespan psychology apply to drug administration.

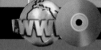 **MediaLink** www.prenhall.com/adams

CD-ROM
Audio Glossary
NCLEX Review

Companion Website
NCLEX Review
Case Study
Expanded Key Concepts
Challenge Your Knowledge

OBJECTIVES

After reading this chapter, the student should be able to:

1. Understand basic concepts of human growth and development.
2. Explain how physical, cognitive, and psychomotor development influences pharmacotherapeutics.
3. Match the five pregnancy categories with their definitions.
4. Identify the importance of teaching the breast-feeding mother about prescription and OTC drugs, as well as the use of herbal products.

5. Describe physiological and biochemical changes that occur in the older adult, and how these affect pharmacotherapy.
6. Discuss the nursing and pharmacologic implications associated with each of the following developmental age groups: prenatal, infancy, toddlerhood, preschool, school age, adolescence, young adulthood, middle adulthood, and older adulthood.

7.1 Pharmacotherapy across the Lifespan

Growth is a term that characterizes the progressive increase in physical (bodily) size. Development refers to the functional evolution of the physical, psychomotor, and cognitive capabilities of a living being. Stages of growth and physical development usually go hand in hand, in a predictable sequence, whereas psychomotor and cognitive development have a tendency to be more variable in nature.

Healthcare providers must understand *normal* growth and developmental patterns, to provide optimum care. It is from this benchmark that *deviations* from the norm can be recognized, so that health pattern impairments can be appropriately addressed. For pharmacotherapy to achieve its desired outcomes, such knowledge is essential.

The development of a person is a complex process interweaving the biophysical with the psychosocial, ethnocultural, and spiritual components to make each individual a unique human being. This whole-person view is essential to holistic care. The very nature of pharmacology requires that the nurse consider the individuality of each patient and the specifics of age, growth, and development in relation to pharmacokinetics and pharmacodynamics.

7.2 Drug Administration during Pregnancy and Lactation

The prenatal stage is the time span from conception to birth. This stage is subdivided into the embryonic period (conception to 8 weeks) and the fetal period (8 to 40 weeks or birth). In terms of pharmacotherapy, this is a strategic stage, because the nurse must take into consideration the health and welfare of both the pregnant mother and the child in utero (Fig. 7.1). Pharmacologically, the focus must be to eliminate potentially toxic agents that may harm the mother or unborn child. Agents that cause fetal malformations are termed teratogens. The baseline incidence of teratogenic events is approximately 3% of all pregnancies.

During the first trimester (0 to 3 months) of pregnancy, when the skeleton and major organs begin to develop, the fetus is at greatest risk for developmental anomalies. Drugs and other chemicals derived from foods ingested by the mother may cross the placental barrier and affect the developing fetus. An in-depth health history and prenatal assessment are vital so that potentially hazardous substances can be eliminated, alternative drugs substituted, or dosages adjusted. Preexisting conditions such as diabetes, coagulation defects, epilepsy, or HIV infection must also be taken into consideration. The mother needs to be informed about the risks, to both herself and her unborn child, related to the use of drugs, alcohol, tobacco, alternative therapies, and OTC medications. From a medical, nursing, and pharmacologic standpoint, the primary considerations during this period must be the safety of the mother and the delivery of a healthy baby.

During the second trimester (4 to 6 months) of pregnancy, the development of the major organs has progressed considerably; however, exposure to certain substances taken by the mother can still cause considerable harm to the fetus. The nurse-patient relationship is vital during this time, especially in terms of teaching. A woman who is pregnant can mistakenly believe that her unborn baby is safe from anything she consumes, because the "baby is fully formed and just needs time to grow." During prenatal visits, the

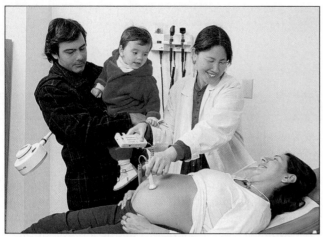

Figure 7.1 | Pharmacotherapy of the pregnant patient *Source: © Jenny Thomas Photography.*

nurse must be vigilant in assessing and evaluating each patient, so that any mistaken beliefs can be clarified.

During the last trimester (7 to 9 months) of pregnancy, blood flow to the placenta increases and placental vascular membranes become thinner. Such alterations allow the transfer of more substances from the maternal circulation to the fetal blood. As a result, the fetus will receive larger doses of medications and other substances taken by the mother. Because the fetus lacks mature metabolic enzymes and efficient excretion mechanisms, medications will have a prolonged duration of action within the unborn child.

During all stages of pregnancy, the nurse should help the mother to assess all medications or dietary supplements to determine if they are necessary. The physician may need to adjust dosages. Certain conditions of the mother, such as diabetes, hypertension, or infections, can jeopardize the health of both the mother and the unborn child; thus, pharmacotherapy may be indicated. Impairments in the functioning of the mother's liver or kidneys may have a profound impact on maternal and fetal safety. Healthcare providers must consider these factors, so to minimize the risk of toxicity to the mother and child. Through careful assessments, the nurse contributes to this risk-benefit analysis, which is essential for protecting both the mother and her baby.

The FDA has developed drug pregnancy categories that rate medications as to their risks during pregnancy. Table 7.1 shows the five pregnancy categories, which guide the healthcare team and the patient in selecting drugs that are least hazardous for the fetus. Nurses who routinely work with women who are pregnant must memorize the drug pregnancy categories for medications commonly prescribed for their patients. Examples of category D or X drugs that have been associated with teratogenic effects include testosterone (Andro), estrogens (Premarin), ergotamine (Ergostat), all angiotensin-converting enzyme (ACE) inhibitors, methotrexate (Amethopterin), thalidomide (Thalomid), tetracycline (Achromycin), valproic acid (Depakote), and

warfarin (Coumadin). In addition, alcohol, nicotine and illicit drugs such as cocaine also affect the unborn child.

It is impossible to experimentally test drugs for teratogenicity in human subjects during clinical trials. Although drugs are tested in pregnant laboratory animals, the structure of the human placenta is unique. Pregnancy drug categories are extrapolated from this animal data and may be crude approximations of the actual risk to a human fetus. No prescription drug, OTC medication, or herbal product should be taken during pregnancy unless the physician verifies that the therapeutic benefits to the mother clearly outweigh the potential risks for the unborn.

The current A, B, C, D, and X pregnancy labeling system is simplistic and gives no specific clinical information to help guide nurses or their patients as to whether a medication is truly safe. The system does not indicate how the dose should be adjusted during pregnancy or lactation. Most drugs are category C, as very high doses often produce teratogenic effects in animals. The FDA is in the process of updating these categories to provide more descriptive information on the risks and benefits of taking each medication. The new labels will include pharmacokinetic and pharmacodynamic information that will suggest optimum doses for the childbearing patient. To gather this information, the FDA is encouraging all pregnant women who are taking medication to join a pregnancy registry that will survey drug effects on both the patient and the fetus or newborn. Evaluation of a large number of pregnancies is needed to determine the effects of medicine on babies.

Breastfeeding is highly recommended as a means of providing nutrition, emotional bonding, and immune protection to the neonate. It is imperative, however, to teach the mother that many prescription medications, OTC drugs, and herbal products are excreted in breast milk and

---

PHARMFACTS | **Possible Fetal Effects Caused by Drug Use During Pregnancy**

- Marijuana: low birthweight babies, increased risk of birth defects, increased risk of leukemia, increased behavioral problems, and decreased attention span
- Cocaine: increased risk of miscarriage, premature delivery, malformations of fetal limbs and kidneys, later learning difficulties
- Heroin: increased risk of miscarriage, low birthweight babies, babies born with neonatal abstinence syndrome (diarrhea, fever, sneezing, yawning, tremors, seizures, irregular breathing, and irritability)
- Tobacco: increased risk of stillbirths, premature delivery, low birthweight babies, increased risk of sudden infant death syndrome (SIDS)
- Alcohol: alcohol-related birth defects ranging from miscarriage and stillbirth to fetal alcohol syndrome (small stature, joint problems, and problems with attention, memory, intelligence, coordination, and problem solving)

Source: Data from Prevention Source, Vancouver, BC.

Table 7.1	FDA Pregnancy Categories
Category	**Definition**
A	Adequate, well-controlled studies in pregnant women have not shown an increased risk of fetal abnormalities.
B	Animal studies have revealed no evidence of harm to the fetus; however, there are no adequate, well-controlled studies in pregnant women. or Animal studies have shown an adverse effect, but adequate, well-controlled studies in pregnant women have failed to demonstrate a risk to the fetus.
C	Animal studies have shown an adverse effect and there are no adequate, well-controlled studies in pregnant women. or No animal studies have been conducted and there are no adequate, well-controlled studies in pregnant women.
D	Studies, either adequate, well-controlled or observational, in pregnant women have demonstrated a risk to the fetus; however, the benefits of therapy may outweigh the potential risk.
X	Studies, either adequate, well-controlled or observational, in animals or pregnant women have demonstrated positive evidence of fetal abnormalities. The use of the product is contraindicated in women who are or may become pregnant.

Source: U.S. Food and Drug Administration, 2001.

have the potential to affect her child (Fig. 7.2). The same guidelines for drug use apply during the breastfeeding period as during pregnancy—drugs should only be taken if the benefits to the mother clearly outweigh the potential risks to the infant. The nurse should explore the possibility of postponing pharmacotherapy until the baby is weaned, or perhaps selecting an alternative, nonpharmacologic treatment. If a drug is indicated, it is sometimes useful to administer it immediately after breastfeeding, so that the longest possible time elapses before the next feeding. The nurse can assist the mother in protecting the child's safety by teaching her to avoid illicit drugs, alcohol, and tobacco products during breastfeeding.

The American Academy of Pediatrics (AAP) Committee on Drugs provides guidance on which drugs should be avoided during breastfeeding to protect the child's safety. Medications that pass into breast milk are indicated in drug guides. Nurses who work with women who are pregnant or breastfeeding should give careful attention to this information. Selected drugs that enter the breast milk and have been shown to produce adverse effects are shown in Table 7.2.

7.3 Drug Administration during Infancy

Infancy is the period from birth to 12 months of age. During this time, nursing care and pharmacotherapy are directed toward safety of the infant, proper dosing of prescribed drugs, and teaching parents how to administer medications properly.

When an infant is ill, it is sometimes traumatic for the parents. Having knowledge of growth and development, the nurse can assist the parents in caring for the baby (Fig. 7.3). The nurse must stress the importance of holding and cuddling the baby, and if the baby is on fluid restrictions due to vomiting or diarrhea, to offer a pacifier. Medications administered at home to infants are often given via droppers into the eyes, ears, nose, or mouth. Oral medications should be administered slowly to avoid aspiration. If rectal suppositories are administered, the buttocks should be held together for 5 to 10 minutes to prevent expulsion of the drug before absorption has occurred.

Special considerations must be observed when administering IM or IV injections to infants. Unlike adults, infants lack well-developed muscle masses, so the smallest needle appropriate for the drug should be used. The vastus lateralis is the preferred site for IM injections, because it has few nerves and is relatively well developed in infants. The gluteal site is usually contraindicated because of potential damage to the sciatic nerve, which may result in permanent disability. Because of the lack of choices for injection sites, the nurse must take care not to overuse a particular location, as inflammation and excessive pain may result. For IV sites, the feet and scalp often provide good venous access.

Medications for infants are often prescribed in milligrams per kilogram per day (mg/kg/24h), rather than according to the baby's age in weeks or months. An alternate method of calculating doses is to use the infant's body surface area (BSA). Because the liver and kidneys of infants are immature, drugs will have a greater impact due to their

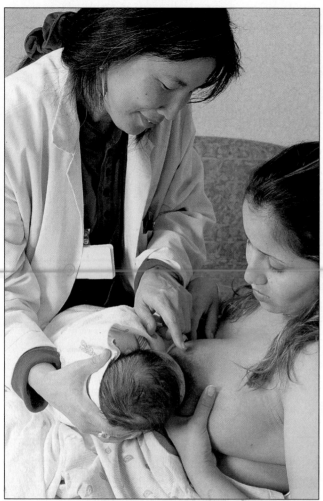

Figure 7.2 | Pharmacotherapy of the breastfeeding mother
Source: © Jenny Thomas Photography.

prolonged duration of action. For these reasons, it is important to consider age and size in determining safe dosages of medications for infants.

From early infancy, the natural immunity a child receives from the mother in utero slowly begins to decline. The child's developing immune system must then take over. Childhood diseases that were once damaging or fatal can now be controlled through routine immunizations. The nurse plays a key role in educating parents about the importance of keeping their child's immunizations current. Vaccinations are discussed in Chapter 30 .

7.4 Pharmacotherapy of Toddlers

Toddlerhood ranges from 1 to 3 years of age. During this period, a toddler displays a tremendous sense of curiosity. The child begins to explore, wants to try new things, and tends to place everything in the mouth. This becomes a major concern for medication and household product safety. The nurse must be instrumental in teaching parents that poisons come in all shapes, sizes, and forms and include

medicines, cosmetics, cleaning supplies, arts and crafts materials, plants, and food products that are improperly stored. Parents should be instructed to request child-resistant containers from the pharmacist, and to stow all medications in secure cabinets.

Toddlers can swallow liquids and may be able to chew solid medications. When prescription drugs are supplied as flavored elixirs, it is important to stress that the child not be given access to the medications. Drugs must never be left at the bedside or within easy reach of the child. To a child who has access to a bottle of cherry-flavored acetaminophen (Tylenol), the tasty liquid may produce a fatal overdose. Nurses should educate parents about the following means to protect their children from poisoning.

- Read and carefully follow directions on the label before using drugs and household products.
- Store all drugs and harmful agents out of the reach of children and in locked cabinets.
- Keep all household products and drugs in their original containers. Never put chemicals in empty food or drink containers.
- Always ask for medication to be placed in child-resistant containers.
- Never tell children that medicine is candy.
- Keep a bottle of syrup of ipecac in the home to induce vomiting. **Do not give this medication unless instructed to do so by a healthcare provider.**
- Keep the Poison Control Center number near the phones and call immediately on suspicion of a poisoning.
- Never leave medication unattended in a child's room or in areas where the child plays.

Administration of medications to toddlers can be challenging for the nurse. At this stage, the child is rapidly developing increased motor ability and learning to assert independence, but has extremely limited ability to reason or understand the relationship of medicines to health. Giving long, detailed explanations to the toddler will prolong the procedure and create additional anxiety. Short, concrete explanations followed by immediate drug administration are best for this age group. Physical comfort in the form of touching, hugging, or verbal praise following drug administration is important.

Oral medications that taste bad should be mixed with a vehicle such as jam, syrup, or fruit puree, if possible. The medication may be followed with a carbonated beverage or mint-flavored candy. Nurses should teach parents to avoid placing medicine in milk, orange juice, or cereals because the child may associate these healthy foods with bad-tasting medications. Pharmaceutical companies often formulate pediatric medicines in sweet syrups to increase the ease of drug administration.

IM injections for toddlers may be given into the vastus lateralis muscle. IV injections may use scalp or feet veins; additional peripheral site options become available in late toddlerhood. Suppositories may be difficult to administer due to the resistance of the child. For any of these invasive

Table 7.2	Selected Drugs Associated with Adverse Effects during Breastfeeding
Drug	**Reported Effect or Reasons for Concern**
amphetamine	irritability, poor sleeping pattern
cocaine	cocaine intoxication: irritability, vomiting, diarrhea, tremulousness, seizures
heroin	tremors, restlessness, vomiting, poor feeding
phencyclidine	potent hallucinogen
acebutolol (Sectral)	hypotension; bradycardia; tachypnea
atenolol (Tenormin)	cyanosis; bradycardia
bromocriptine (Parlodel)	suppresses lactation; may be hazardous to the mother
aspirin (salicylates)	metabolic acidosis
ergotamine (Ergostat)	vomiting, diarrhea, convulsions (doses used in migraine medications)
lithium (Eskalith)	one-third to one-half therapeutic blood concentration in infants
phenindione	anticoagulant: increased prothrombin and partial thromboplastin time
phenobarbital (Luminal)	sedation; infantile spasms after weaning from milk containing phenobarbital, methemoglobinemia
primidone (Mysoline)	sedation, feeding problems
sulfasalazine (Azulfidine)	bloody diarrhea

Source: From "The Transfer of Drugs and Other Chemicals into Human Breast Milk" by American Academy of Pediatrics, Committee on Drugs, 2001, Pediatrics, 3, pp. 776–782. Reprinted by permission.

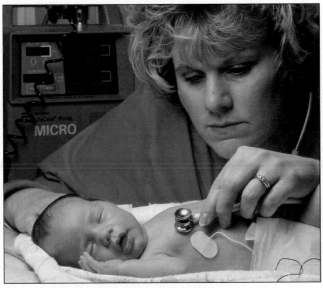

Figure 7.3 | Pharmacotherapy of the infant
Source: PearsonEducation/PH College.

administration procedures, having a parent in close proximity will usually reduce the toddler's anxiety and increase cooperation.

7.5 Pharmacotherapy of Preschoolers and School-age Children

The preschool child ranges in age from 3 to 5 years. During this period, the child begins to refine gross and fine mo-

PHARMFACTS | Poisoning

According to the National Emergency Medical Association (NEMA):

- Each year, 2 million Americans are poisoned.
- Poisoning can be prevented through education and awareness.
- Many poisonings occur in children under 6 years.
- Adults can be poisoned by taking the wrong dose of medication, confusing different medications, or splashing a poison on the skin or in the eyes accidentally.

tor skills and develop language abilities. The child initiates new activities and becomes more socially involved with other children.

Preschoolers can sometimes comprehend the difference between health and illness and that medications are administered to help them feel better. Nonetheless, medications and other potentially dangerous products must still be safely stowed out of the child's reach.

In general, principles of medication administration that pertain to the toddler also apply to this age group. Preschoolers cooperate in taking oral medications, if they are crushed or mixed with food or flavored beverages. After a child is walking for about a year, the dorsogluteal site may be used for IM injections, as it causes less pain than the vastus lateralis site. The scalp veins can no longer be used for IV access; peripheral veins are used for IV injections.

Like the toddler, preschoolers often physically resist medication administration, and a long, detailed explanation of the procedure will promote additional anxiety. A brief explanation followed quickly by medication administration is usually the best method. Uncooperative children may need to be restrained, and patients over 4 years of age may require two adults to administer the medication. Before and after medication procedures, the child may benefit from opportunities to play-act troubling experiences with dolls. When the child plays the role of doctor or nurse by giving a "sick" doll a pill or injection, comforting the doll, and explaining that the doll will now feel better, the little actor feels safer and more in control of the situation.

The school-age child is between 6 and 12 years of age. Some refer to this period as the middle childhood years. This is the time in a child's life when there is progression away from the family-centered environment to the larger peer relationship environment. Rapid physical, mental, and social development occur and early ethical-moral development begins to take shape. Thinking processes become progressively logical and more consistent.

During this time, most children remain relatively healthy, with immune system development well under way. Respiratory infections and gastrointestinal upsets are the most common complaints. Because the child feels well most of the time, there is little concept of illness or the risks involved with ingesting a harmful substance offered to the child by a peer or older person.

The nurse is usually able to gain considerable cooperation from school age children. Longer, more detailed explanations may be of value, because the child has developed some reasoning ability and can understand the relationship between the medicine and feeling better. When children are old enough to welcome choices, they can be offered limited dosing alternatives to provide a sense of control and encourage cooperation. The option of taking one medication before another or the chance to choose which drink will fol-

low a chewable tablet helps to distract children from the issue of whether they will take the medication at all. It also makes an otherwise strange or unpleasant experience a little more enjoyable. Making children feel that they are willing participants in medication administration, rather than victims, is an important foundation for compliance. Praise for cooperation is appropriate for any pediatric patient, and will set the stage for successful medication administration in the future (Fig. 7.4).

School-age children can take chewable tablets, and may swallow tablets or capsules. Many still resist injections; however, an experienced pediatric nurse can usually administer parenteral medications quickly and compassionately, without the need for restraining the child. The ventrogluteal site is preferred for IM injections, although the muscles of older children are developed enough for the nurse to use other sites.

7.6 Pharmacotherapy of Adolescents

Adolescence is the time between ages 13 and 16 years. A person in this age group is able to think in abstract terms and come to logical conclusions based on a given set of observations. Rapid physical growth and psychologic maturation have a great impact on personality development. The adolescent relates stongly to peers, wanting and needing their support, approval, and presence. Physical appearance and conformity with peers in terms of behavior, dress, and social interactions is important.

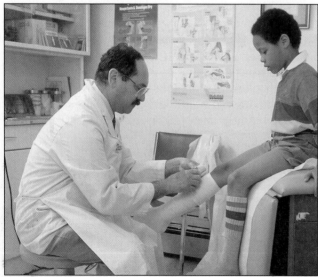

Figure 7.4 | Pharmacotherapy of younger school-age children
Source: PearsonEducation/PH College.

SPECIAL CONSIDERATIONS

Pediatric Drug Research and Labeling

An estimated 75% of the medications prescribed for children contain no specific dosing information for pediatric patients. Without specific labeling information, healthcare providers have largely based their doses on the smaller weight of the child. Children, however, are not merely small adults; they have unique differences in physiology and biochemistry that may place them at risk to drug therapy.

Inclusion of children in clinical trials is an expensive and potentially risky process. Costs for testing drugs in large numbers of children in different age groups may reach as much as $35 million (Heinrich, 2001). Manufacturers also faced liability and malpractice issues associated with testing new medications in children.

In 1997, Congress provided financial incentives for pharmaceutical manufacturers to test drugs in children. In return for comprehensive testing in children, the FDA granted the company an additional 6 months of exclusive marketing rights for the drug. As a result of this effort, over 28 drugs have been investigated in children, and 18 drug labels have been changed to incorporate the results of the research findings. Drugs that now have more specific pediatric labeling include ibuprofen (Motrin), ranitidine (Zantac), fluvoxamine (Luvox), etodolac (Lodine), and midazolam (Versed). The legislation is reauthorized until 2007, and extended to include the study of "off-patent" drugs in children and the establishment of an Office of Pediatric Therapeutics at the FDA.

The most common needs for pharmacotherapy in this age group is for skin problems, headaches, menstrual symptoms, and sports-related injuries. There is an increased need for contraceptive information and counseling with sexually related health problems. Since bulimia occurs in this population, the nurse should carefully question adolescents about their eating habits and their use of OTC appetite suppressants or laxatives. Tobacco use and illicit drug experimentation may be prevalent in this population. Teenage athletes may use amphetamines to delay the onset of fatigue, as well as anabolic steroids to increase muscle strength and endurance. The nurse assumes a key role in educating adolescent patients about the hazards of tobacco use and illicit drugs.

The adolescent has a need for privacy and control in drug administration. The nurse should seek complete cooperation, and communicate with the teen more in the manner of an adult, than as a child. Teens usually appreciate thorough explanations of their treatment, and ample time should be allowed for them to ask questions. Adolescents are often reluctant to admit their lack of knowledge, so the nurse should carefully explain important information regarding their medications and expected side effects, even if the patient claims to understand. Teens are easily embarrassed and the nurse should be sensitive to their need for self-expression, privacy, and individuality, particularly when parents, siblings, or friends are present.

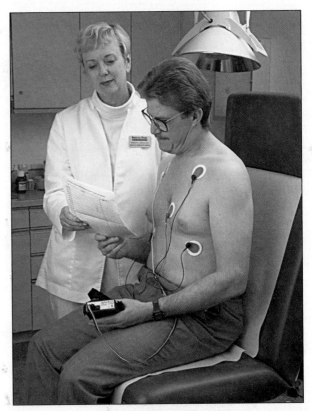

Figure 7.5 | Pharmacotherapy of middle-age adults
Source: PearsonEducation/PH College.

7.7 Pharmacotherapy of Young and Middle-age Adults

When considering adult health, it is customary to divide this period of life into three stages: young adulthood (18 to 40 years), middle adulthood (40 to 65 years), and older adulthood (over 65 years). Within each of these divisions are similar biophysical, psychosocial, and spiritual characteristics that impact nursing and pharmacotherapy.

The health status of younger adults is generally good; absorption, metabolic, and excretion mechanisms are at their peak. There is minimal need for prescription drugs unless chronic diseases such as diabetes or immune-related conditions exist. The use of vitamins, minerals, and herbal remedies is prevalent in young adulthood. Prescription drugs are usually related to contraception, or agents needed during pregnancy and delivery. Medication compliance is positive within this age range, as there is clear comprehension of benefit in terms of longevity and feeling well.

Substance abuse is a cause for concern in the 18 to 24 age group, with alcohol, tobacco products, amphetamines, and illicit drugs (marijuana and cocaine) being a problem. For young adults who are sexually active, with multiple partners, prescription medications for the treatment of herpes, gonorrhea, syphilis, and HIV infections may be necessary.

The physical status for the middle-age adult is on par with the young adult until about 45 years of age. During this period of life, numerous transitions occur that often result in excessive stress. Middle-aged adults are sometimes referred to as the "sandwich generation," because they are often caring for aging parents as well as children and grandchildren. Because of the pressures of work and family, they often take medication to control health alterations that could best be treated with positive lifestyle modifications. The nurse must emphasize the importance of lifestyle choices, such as limiting lipid intake, maintaining optimum weight, and exercising, to overall health (Fig. 7.5).

Health impairments related to cardiovascular disease, hypertension, obesity, arthritis, cancer, and anxiety begin to surface in middle age. The use of drugs to treat hypertension, hyperlipidemia, digestive disorders, erectile dysfunction, and arthritis are becoming more common. Respiratory disorders related to lifelong tobacco use or exposure to secondhand smoke and environmental toxins may develop that require drug therapies. Adult onset diabetes mellitus often emerges during this time of life. The use of antidepressants and antianxiety agents is prominent in the over-50 population.

7.8 Pharmacotherapy of Older Adults

During the 20th century, an improved quality of life and the ability to effectively treat many diseases contributed to increased longevity. As individuals age, however, the number of chronic health disorders they experience increases, and more drugs are prescribed to treat them. The taking of multiple drugs concurrently, known as polypharmacy, has become commonplace among older adults. Polypharmacy dramatically increases the risk for drug interactions and side effects.

Although predictable, physiological, and psychosocial changes occur with aging, significant variability exists among patients. For example, although cognitive decline and memory loss certainly occur with age, these may occur in middle adulthood, older adulthood, or not at all. The nurse should avoid preconceived notions that elderly patients will have physical or cognitive impairment simply because they have reached a certain age. Careful assessment is always necessary (Fig. 7.6).

When administering medications to older adults, the nurse should offer the patient the same degree of independence and dignity that would be afforded middle-age adults, unless otherwise indicated. Like their younger counterparts, older patients have a need to understand why they are receiving a drug, and what outcomes are expected. Accommodations must be made for older adults who have certain impairments. Visual and auditory changes make it important for the nurse to provide drug instructions in large type, and to obtain patient feedback to be certain that medication instructions have been understood. Elderly patients with cognitive decline and memory loss can benefit from aids such as alarmed pill containers, medicine management boxes, and clearly written instructions. During assessment, the nurse should determine if the patient is capable of self-administering medications, or whether the assistance of a caregiver will be required. As long as small children are not present in the household, older patients with arthritis should be encouraged to ask the pharmacist for regular screw-cap medication bottles, for ease of opening.

Older patients experience more adverse effects from drug therapy than any other age group. Although some of these effects are due to polypharmacy, many of the adverse events are predictable, based on normal physiologic and biochemical processes that occur during aging. By understanding these changes, the nurse can avoid many adverse effects in older patients. Changes that affect pharmacotherapy of the older adult are as follows:

- Increased gastric pH and decreased peristaltic rate affect medication absorption. Often, when laxatives are used to compensate for slower peristalsis, medications may be rapidly excreted from the body before they can provide their full therapeutic benefit.
- The liver's production of enzymes decreases, resulting in reduced hepatic drug metabolism.

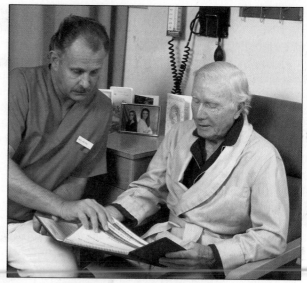

Figure 7.6 | Pharmacotherapy of the older adult
Source: PearsonEducation/PH College.

- The aging liver reduces albumin production, resulting in decreased plasma protein binding and increased levels of free drug in the bloodstream, thus increasing the potential for drug-drug interactions.
- Reduced blood flow to the kidneys and decreased nephron function reduce drug elimination, which increases serum drug levels and the potential for toxicity.
- The percentage of body water decreases, making the effects of dehydration more dramatic. Risk for toxicity is boosted by fluid deficit. Elderly patients who have reduced body fluid experience more orthostatic hypotension.
- The ratio of body fat to water increases, enhancing storage of fat-soluble drugs and vitamins. The ratio of fat to muscle increases, slowing metabolism.
- The aging cardiovascular system has decreased cardiac output and less efficient blood circulation which slow drug distribution. This makes it important to initiate pharmacotherapy with smaller dosages and slowly increase the amount to a safe, effective level.
- Immune system function diminishes with aging, so autoimmune diseases and infections occur more frequently in elderly clients. There is an increased need for influenza and pneumonia vaccinations.

MediaLink **Health and Aging**

CHAPTER REVIEW

Key Concepts

The numbered key concepts provide a succinct summary of the important points from the corresponding numbered section within the chapter. If any of these points are not clear, refer to the numbered section within the chapter for review. Expanded versions can be found on the companion website.

7.1 To contribute to safe and effective pharmacotherapy, it is essential for the nurse to comprehend and apply fundamental concepts of growth and development.

7.2 Pharmacotherapy during pregnancy should only be conducted when the benefits to the mother outweigh the potential risks to the unborn child. Pregnancy categories guide the healthcare provider in prescribing drugs for these patients. Breastfeeding patients must be aware that drugs and other substances can appear in milk and affect the infant.

7.3 During infancy, pharmacotherapy is directed toward the safety of the child and teaching the parents how to properly administer medications and care for the infant.

7.4 Drug administration to toddlers can be challenging; short, concrete explanations followed by immediate drug administration are usually best for the toddler.

7.5 Preschool and younger school-age children can begin to assist with medication administration.

7.6 Pharmacologic compliance in the adolescent is dependent on an understanding and respect for the uniqueness of the person in this stage of growth and development.

7.7 Young adults comprise the healthiest age group and generally need few prescription medications. Middle-age adults begin to suffer from stress-related illness such as hypertension.

7.8 Older adults take more medications and experience more adverse drug events than any other age group. For drug therapy to be successful, the nurse must make accommodations for age-related changes in physiologic and biochemical functions.

Review Questions

1. How is drug safety for the three trimesters of pregnancy determined?

2. What factors should be considered before administering medications to an infant? a toddler? a school-age child? an adolescent?

3. What physiological changes make it important to consider advanced age when prescribing or administering medication?

4. A patient who is on several medications for psychiatric disorders has just delivered her baby and is about to begin breastfeeding. What information should she receive before she is discharged from the ward?

Critical Thinking Questions

1. A 22-year-old pregnant patient is diagnosed with pyelonephritis and an antibiotic is prescribed. What information does the nurse need to have to safely administer the drug?

2. An 86-year-old male patient is confused and anxious. His daughter wonders if "a small dose" of diazepam (Valium) might help her father to be less anxious. Prior to responding to the daughter or consulting the prescribing authority, the nurse should review age-related concerns. What are the nurse's concerns?

3. An 8-month-old child is prescribed acetaminophen (Tylenol) elixir for management of fever. She is recovering from gastroenteritis and is still having several loose stools per day. The child spits some of the elixir on her shirt. Does the nurse repeat the dose? What are the implications of this child's age and physical condition for oral drug administration?

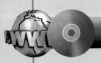

EXPLORE MediaLink

NCLEX review, case studies, and other interactive resources for this chapter can be found on the companion website at www.prenhall.com/adams. Click on "Chapter 7" to select the activities for this chapter. For animations, more NCLEX review questions, and an audio glossary, access the accompanying CD-ROM in this textbook.

The Nursing Process in Pharmacology

The Nursing Process, a systematic method of problem solving, forms the foundation of all nursing practice. The use of the Nursing Process is particularly essential during medication administration. By using the steps of the Nursing Process, nurses can ensure that the interdisciplinary practice of pharmacology results in safe, effective, and individualized medication administration and outcomes for all patients under their care.

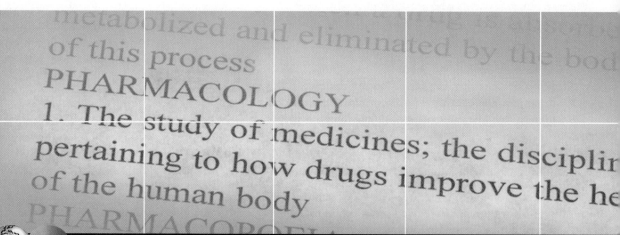

MediaLink   www.prenhall.com/adams

CD-ROM
Audio Glossary
NCLEX Review

Companion Website
NCLEX Review
Case Study
Expanded Key Concepts
Challenge Your Knowledge

OBJECTIVES

After reading this chapter, the student should be able to:

1. Explain the steps of the Nursing Process.
2. Identify assessment data to be gathered that is pertinent to medication administration.
3. Develop appropriate nursing diagnoses for patients receiving medications.
4. Set realistic goals and outcomes during the planning stage for patients receiving medications.
5. Discuss key intervention strategies to be carried out for patients receiving medications.
6. Evaluate the outcomes of medication administration.
7. When giving medications, apply the Nursing Process using the Nursing Process Focus flowcharts found in Chapters 13 through 48.

8.1 Review of the Nursing Process

Most nursing students enter a pharmacology course after taking a course on the fundamentals of nursing, during which the steps of the Nursing Process are discussed in detail. This section presents a brief review of those steps before discussing in detail how they can be applied to pharmacology. Students who are unfamiliar with the Nursing Process are encouraged to consult one of the many excellent fundamentals of nursing textbooks for a more detailed explanation.

Assessment, the first step in the Nursing Process, is an ongoing process that begins with the nurse's initial contact with the patient, and continues with every interaction thereafter. During the initial assessment, baseline data are gathered which will be used to compare to information obtained during later interactions. Assessment consists of gathering subjective data, which include what the patient says or perceives, and objective data gathered through physical assessment, laboratory tests, and other diagnostic sources.

Once the initial assessment data are gathered, the nurse makes clinical-based judgments about the patient and his or her responses to health and illness. Nursing diagnoses provide the basis for establishing goals and outcomes, planning interventions to meet those goals and outcomes, and helping nurses evaluate the effectiveness of the care given. Unlike medical diagnoses that focus on a disease or condition, nursing diagnoses focus on a patient's response to actual or potential health and life processes. The North American Nursing Diagnosis Association (NANDA) defines nursing diagnoses as:

> A clinical judgment about individual, family or community responses to actual or potential health/life processes. Per NANDA, nursing diagnoses provide the basis for selection of nursing interventions to achieve outcomes for which the nurse is accountable.

Nursing diagnoses are often the most challenging part of the Nursing Process. Sometimes the nurse identifies what is believed to be the patient's problem, only to discover from further assessment that the planned goals, outcomes, and interventions have not "solved" the problem. A key point to remember is that nursing diagnoses focus on the patient's problems, not the nurse's problems. A primary nursing role is to enable patients to become active participants in their own care. By verifying identified problems and their associated nursing diagnoses with the patient, the nurse encourages the patient to take a more active role in working toward solving these problems.

After a nursing diagnosis has been established, the nurse begins to plan ways to assist the patient to return to, or maintain, an optimum level of wellness as defined by that diagnosis. Short- or long-term goals are established that focus on what the patient will be able to do or achieve, not what the nurse will do. Outcomes are the objective measure of those goals. They specifically define what the patient will do, under what circumstances, and within a specified time frame. Goals and outcomes are also verified with the patient or caregiver, and are prioritized to address immediate needs first.

Planning links strategies, or interventions, to the established goals and outcomes. It is the formal written process that communicates with all members of the healthcare team what the nurse will do to assist the patient in meeting those goals. Each healthcare organization decides how this plan of care will be communicated and it may be nurse centered or interdisciplinary.

Interventions are designed to meet the patient's needs and ensure safe, effective care. As the nurse provides care, reassessment is ongoing and new data are compared to the earlier data. The nurse compares the data to established nursing diagnoses, goals, and outcomes and begins the process of evaluation. Established nursing diagnoses are reviewed while taking into consideration the patient's response to care. More assessment data are gathered as needed and goals and outcomes are considered as to whether they were met, partially met, or not met at all. The process comes full circle as new or modified diagnoses are established, goals and outcomes redefined, and new interventions planned.

Nursing has not always relied on such an organized approach to nursing care, but has always been concerned with delivering safe and effective care. The administration of medications requires the use of the Nursing Process to ensure the best possible outcomes for the patient. These steps will now be applied specifically to drug administration.

8.2 Assessment of the Patient Related to Drug Administration

A health history and physical assessment are usually completed during the initial meeting between a nurse and patient. Many pieces of data are gathered during this initial assessment, which have specific implications for the process of drug administration. Ongoing assessments after this time will provide additional data to help the nurse evaluate the outcomes of medication use. This section discusses pertinent assessment components and how they relate to drug administration.

The initial health history is tailored to the patient's clinical condition. A complete history is the most detailed, but the appropriateness of this history must be considered given the patient's condition. Often a problem-focused or "chief complaint" history is taken, focusing on the symptoms that led the patient to seek care. In any history, key components must be assessed that may affect the successful outcome of drug administration. Essential questions to ask in the initial history relate to allergies; past medical history; medications used currently and in the recent past; personal and social history such as the use of alcohol, tobacco, or caffeine; health risks such as the use of street drugs or illicit substances; and reproductive health questions such as the pregnancy status of women of childbearing age. Table 8.1 provides pertinent questions that may be asked during an initial health history that provide baseline data before the administration of medications. The health history is tailored to the patient's condition and all questions may not be appropriate during the initial assessment. Keep in mind that what is *not* being said may be of as much importance, or more, than what *is* said. For instance, a patient may deny or downplay any symptoms of pain while grimacing or guarding a certain area from being touched. Nurses must use their keen skills of observation during the history to gather such critical data.

Along with the health history, a physical assessment is completed to gather objective data on the patient's condition. Vital signs, height and weight, a head-to-toe physical assessment, and lab specimens may be obtained. These values provide the baseline data to compare with future assessments, and guide the healthcare provider in deciding which medications to prescribe. Many medications can affect the heart rate and blood pressure and these especially should be noted. Baseline electrolyte values are important

parameters to obtain because many medications affect electrolyte balance. Renal and hepatic function tests are essential for many patients, particularly older adults and those who are critically ill, as these will be used to determine the proper drug dosage.

Once pharmacotherapy is initiated, ongoing assessments are conducted to determine the effects of the medications. Assessment should first focus on determining whether the patient is experiencing the expected therapeutic benefits from the medications. For example, if a drug is given for symptoms of pain, is the pain subsiding? If an antibiotic is given for an infection, are the signs of that infection—elevated temperature, redness or swelling, drainage from infected sites, etc.—improving over time? If a patient is not experiencing the therapeutic effects of the medication, then further assessment must be done to determine the reason. Dosages and the scheduling of medications are reviewed and serum drug levels may be obtained.

Assessment during pharmacotherapy also focuses on any side or adverse effects the patient may be experiencing. Often these effects are manifested in dermatologic, cardiovascular, gastrointestinal, or neurologic symptoms. Here again, baseline data are compared with the current assessment to determine what changes have occurred since the initiation of pharmacotherapy. The Nursing Process Focus flowcharts provided in Chapters 13 through 48 illustrate key assessment data to be gathered associated with specific medications or classes of drugs.

Finally, an assessment of the ability of the patient to assume responsibility for their own drug administration is necessary. Will the patient require assistance obtaining or affording the prescribed medications, or with taking them safely? What kind of medication storage facilities exist and are they adequate to protect the patient, others in the home, and the efficacy of the medication? Does the patient understand the uses and effects of this medication and how it is properly taken? Would assessment data suggest that the use of this medication might present a problem, such as difficulty swallowing large capsules or an inability to administer medication when home anticoagulant therapy has been ordered parenterally?

After analyzing the assessment data, the nurse determines patient-specific nursing diagnoses appropriate for the drugs prescribed. These diagnoses will form the basis for the remaining steps of the Nursing Process.

8.3 Nursing Diagnoses for the Patient Receiving Medications

Assessment data are used to develop a list of problems, or nursing diagnoses, that address the patient's responses to health and life processes. These nursing diagnoses are used to set goals and plan care. They focus on the patient's problems and are prioritized by importance to the patient's clinical condition. Although the process of developing a nursing diagnosis is a challenging part of the Nursing Process, certain diagnoses often stand out as priorities. This section discusses common nursing diagnoses related to

Table 8.1	Health History Assessment Questions Pertinent to Drug Administration

Health History Component Areas	Pertinent Questions
chief complaint	• How do you feel? (Describe) • Are you having any pain? (Describe) • Are you experiencing other symptoms? (Especially pertinent to medications are: nausea, vomiting, headache, itching, dizziness, shortness of breath, nervousness or anxiousness, palpitations or heart "fluttering," weakness or fatigue)
allergies	• Are you allergic to any medications? • Are you allergic to any foods, environmental substances (e.g., pollen or "seasonal" allergies), tape, soaps, or cleansers? • What specifically happens when you experience an allergy?
past medical history	• Do you have a history of diabetes, heart or vascular conditions, respiratory conditions, neurologic conditions? • Do you have any dermatologic conditions? • How have these been treated in the past? Currently?
family history	• Has anyone in your family experienced difficulties with any medications? (Describe) • Does anyone in your family have any significant medical problems?
drug history	• What prescription medications are you currently taking? (List drug name, dosage, frequency of administration) • What nonprescription/OTC medications are you taking? (List name, dosage, frequency) • What drugs, prescription or OTC, have you taken within the past month or two? • Have you ever experienced any side effects or unusual symptoms with any medications? (Describe) • What do you know, or have been taught, about these medications? • Do you use any herbal or homeopathic remedies? Any nutritional substances or vitamins?
health management	• When was the last time you saw a healthcare provider? • What is your normal diet? • Do you have any trouble sleeping?
reproductive history	• Is there any possibility you are pregnant? (Ask *every* woman of childbearing age) • Are you breastfeeding?
personal-social history	• Do you smoke? • What is your normal alcohol intake? • What is your normal caffeine intake? • Do you have any religious or cultural beliefs or practices concerning medications or your health that we should know about? • What is your occupation? What hours do you work? • Do you have any concerns regarding insurance or the ability to afford medications?
health risk history	• Do you have any history of depression or other mental illness? • Do you use any street drugs or illicit substances?

Patients with Speaking, Visual, or Hearing Impairments

Speaking impairments may make obtaining responses from the patient difficult. Communication may be facilitated by having the patient write or draw responses. Clarify by paraphrasing the response back to the patient. Use gestures, body language, and yes/no questions if writing or drawing is difficult. Allow adequate time for responses. Be especially aware of nonverbal clues, such as grimacing, when performing interventions that may cause discomfort or pain.

Provide adequate lighting for patients with visual impairments and be aware of the phrasing of verbal communication and how phrasing affects the message conveyed. Remember that the nonverbal cues involved in communication may be missed by the patient. Paraphrase responses back to the patient to be sure they understood the message in the absence of nonverbal cues. Explain interventions in detail before implementing procedures or activities with the patient.

Patients with hearing impairments benefit from communication that is spoken clearly and slowly in a low-pitched voice. Sit near the patient and avoid speaking loudly or shouting, especially if hearing devices are used. Limit the amount of background noise when possible. Write or draw to clarify verbal communication and use nonverbal gestures and body language to aid communication. Allow adequate time for communication and responses. Alert other members of the healthcare team that the patient has a hearing impairment and may not hear a verbal answer to the nurse's call light given over an intercom system.

medication administration, and the development of appropriate nursing diagnosis statements.

Nursing diagnoses that focus on drug administration are the same as diagnoses written for other patient condition-specific responses. They may address actual problems, such as the treatment of pain; focus on potential problems such as a risk for fluid volume deficit; or concentrate on maintaining the patient's current level of wellness. The diagnosis is written as a one-, two-, or three-part statement depending on whether a wellness, risk, or actual problem has been identified. Actual and risk problems will include the diagnostic statement and a related factor, or inferred cause. Actual diagnoses will also contain a third part, the evidence gathered to support the chosen statement. There are many diagnoses appropriate to medication administration. Some problems are nursing specific that the nurse can manage independently, whereas other problems are multidisciplinary and require collaboration with other members of the healthcare team. For any of the medications given to a patient, there are often combinations of nursing-independent and collaborative diagnoses that can be established.

Two of the most common nursing diagnoses for medication administration are *Deficient Knowledge* and *Noncompliance*. Deficient knowledge may be that the patient has been given a new prescription and has no previous experience with the medication. It may also be applicable when a patient has not received adequate education about the drugs used in the treatment of his or her condition. When obtaining a medication history, the nurse should assess the patient's knowledge regarding the drugs currently being taken, and evaluate whether the drug education has been adequate. Sometimes a patient refuses to take a drug which has been prescribed or refuses to follow the directions correctly. Noncompliance assumes that the patient has been properly educated about the medication, and has made an informed decision not to take it. Because labeling a patient's response as noncompliant may have a negative impact on the nurse-patient relationship, it is vital that the nurse assess all possible factors leading to the noncompliance *before* establishing this diagnosis. Does the patient understand why the medication has been prescribed? Has dosing and scheduling information been explained? Are side effects causing the patient to refuse the medication? Do cultural, religious, social issues, or health beliefs have an impact on taking the medication? Is the noncompliance related to inadequate resources, either financial or social support? A thorough assessment of possible causes should be conducted before labeling the patient's response as noncompliant.

Nursing diagnoses applicable to drug administration are often collaborative problems that require communication with other healthcare providers. For example, fluid volume deficit related to diuretic drugs may require additional interventions such as medical orders by the physician to ensure that electrolytes and intravascular fluid volume remain within normal limits. Nurses may assist the patient with ambulation if weakness or postural hypotension occur secondary to this fluid volume deficit independent of medical orders. Table 8.2 provides an abbreviated list of some of the common nursing diagnoses appropriate to drug administration. Although the list contains actual nursing diagnoses, these may also be identified as risk diagnoses. This is not an exhaustive list of all NANDA-approved diagnoses, and the establishment of new diagnoses is ongoing. The nurse is encouraged to consult books on nursing diagnoses for more information on establishing, writing, and researching other nursing diagnoses that may apply to drug administration.

8.4 Setting Goals and Outcomes for Drug Administration

After the nurse has gathered patient assessment data and formulated nursing diagnoses, goals and outcomes are developed and priorities established, to assist the nurse in planning care, carrying out interventions, and evaluating the effectiveness of that care. Before administering and monitoring the effects of medications, nurses should establish clear goals and outcomes so that planned interventions ensure safe and effective use of these agents.

Goals are somewhat different than outcomes. Goals focus on what the patient should be able to achieve and do, based on the nursing diagnosis established from the assessment data. Outcomes provide the specific, measurable cri-

Table 8.2	Common Nursing Diagnoses Applicable to Drug Administration
NANDA-Approved Nursing Diagnoses	
Activity Intolerance	Mobility: Physical, Impaired
Airway Clearance, Ineffective	Nausea
Anxiety	Noncompliance
Aspiration, Risk for	Nutrition, Imbalanced
Breathing Pattern, Ineffective	Oral Mucous Membrane, Impaired
Cardiac Output, Decreased	Pain
Communication, Impaired Verbal	Poisoning, Risk for
Constipation	Self-Care Deficit
Coping, Ineffective	Sensory Perception, Disturbed
Diarrhea	Sexual Dysfunction
Falls, Risk for	Skin Integrity, Impaired
Fatigue	Sleep Pattern, Disturbed
Fluid Volume, Deficient	Suicide, Risk for
Fluid Volume, Excess	Swallowing, Impaired
Gas Exchange, Impaired	Therapeutic Regimen Management, Ineffective
Health Maintenance, Ineffective	Thermoregulation, Impaired
Hyperthermia	Thought Processes, Disturbed
Hypothermia	Tissue Perfusion, Ineffective
Infection, Risk for	Urinary Incontinence
Injury, Risk for	Urinary Retention
Knowledge, Deficient	

Source: Adapted from North American Nursing Diagnosis Association, 2003.

teria that will be used to evaluate the degree to which the goal was met. Both goals and outcomes are focused on what the patient will achieve or do, are realistic, and are verified with the patient or caregiver. Priorities are established based on the assessment data and nursing diagnoses, with high-priority needs addressed before low-priority items. Safe and effective administration of medications, with the best therapeutic outcome possible, is the overall goal of any nursing plan of care.

Goals may be focused for the short term or long term, depending on the setting and situation. In the acute care or ambulatory setting, short-term goals may be most appropriate whereas in the rehabilitation setting, long-term goals may be more commonly identified. For a patient with a thrombus in the lower extremity who has been placed on anticoagulant therapy, a short-term goal may be that the patient will not experience an increase in clot size as evidenced by improving circulation to the lower extremity distal to the

clot. A long-term goal might focus on teaching the patient to effectively administer parenteral anticoagulant therapy at home. Like assessment data, goals should focus first on the therapeutic outcomes of medications, then on the limitation or treatment of side effects. For the patient on pain medication, relief of pain is a priority established before treating the nausea, vomiting, or dizziness caused by the medication. The Nursing Process Focus flowcharts provided in Chapters 13 through 48 outline some of the common goals that might be developed with the patient.

Outcomes are the specific criteria used to measure attainment of the selected goals. They are written to include the subject (the patient in most cases), the actions required by that subject, under what circumstances, the expected performance, and the specific time frame in which the performance will be accomplished. In the example of the patient who will be taught to self-administer anticoagulant therapy at home, an outcome may be written as: Patient will

Non-English Speaking and Culturally Diverse Patients

Nurses should know, in advance, what translation services and interpreters are available in their healthcare facility to assist with communication. The nurse should use interpreter's services when available, validating with the interpreter that he or she is able to understand the patient. Many dialects are similar but not the same, and knowing another language is not the same as understanding the culture. Can the interpreter understand the patient's language and cultural expressions or nuances well enough for effective communication to occur? If a family member is interpreting, especially if a child is interpreting for a parent or relative, be sure that the interpreter first understands and repeats the information back to the nurse before explaining it in the patient's own language. This is especially important if the translation is a summary of what has been said rather than a line-by-line translation. Before an interpreter is available, or if one is unavailable, use pictures, simple drawings, nonverbal cues, and body language to communicate with the patient. Be aware of cultural-based nonverbal communication behaviors (e.g., use of personal space, eye contact, or lack of eye contact). Gender sensitivities related to culture (e.g., male nurse or physician for female patients) and the use of touch are often sensitive issues. In the United States, an informal and personal style is often the norm. When working with patients of other cultures, adopting a more formal style may be more appropriate.

demonstrate the injection of enoxaparin (Lovenox) using the preloaded syringe provided, given subcutaneously into the anterior abdominal areas, in 2 days (1 day prior to discharge). This outcome includes the subject (patient), actions (demonstrate injection), circumstances (using a preloaded syringe), performance (SC injection into the abdomen), and time frame (2 days from now—1 day before discharge home). Writing specific outcomes also gives the nurse a concrete time frame to work toward to assist the patient to meet the goals.

After goals and outcomes are identified based on the nursing diagnoses, a plan of care is written. Each agency determines whether this plan will be communicated as either nursing centered, interdisciplinary, or both. All plans should be patient focused and verified with the patient or caregiver. The goals and outcomes identified in the plan of care will assist the nurse, and other healthcare providers, in carrying out interventions and evaluating the effectiveness of that care.

8.5 Key Interventions for Drug Administration

After the plan of care has been written, making explicit any goals and outcomes based on established nursing diagnoses, the nurse implements this plan. Interventions are aimed at returning the patient to an optimum level of wellness and limiting adverse effects related to the patient's medical diagnosis or condition. Chapter 4 discusses interventions specific to drug administration, such as the five rights and the techniques of administering medications . This section focuses on other key intervention strategies that the nurse completes for a patient receiving medications.

Monitoring drug effects is a primary intervention that nurses perform. A thorough knowledge of the actions of each medication is necessary to carry out this monitoring process. The nurse should first monitor for the identified therapeutic effect. A lack of sufficient therapeutic effect suggests the need to reassess pharmacotherapy. Monitoring may require a reassessment of the patient's physical condition, vital signs, body weight, lab values, and/or serum drug levels. The patient's statements about pain relief, as well as objective data, such as a change in blood pressure, are used to monitor the therapeutic outcomes of pharmacotherapy. The nurse also monitors for side and adverse effects and attempts to prevent or limit these effects when possible. Some side effects may be managed by the nurse independently of medical orders, whereas others require collaboration with physicians to alleviate patient symptoms. For example, a patient with nausea and vomiting after receiving a narcotic pain reliever may be comforted by the nurse who provides small frequent meals, sips of carbonated beverages, or frequent changes of linen. However, the physician may need to prescribe an antiemetic drug to control the side effect of intense nausea.

Documentation of both therapeutic and adverse effects is completed during the intervention phase. This includes appropriate documentation of the administration of the medication, as well as the effects observed. Additional objective assessment data, such as vital signs, may be included in the documentation to provide more details about the specific drug effects. A patient's statements can provide subjective detail to the documentation. Each healthcare facility determines where, when, and how to document the administration of medications and any follow-up assessment data that have been gathered.

Patient teaching is a vital component of the nurse's interventions for a patient receiving medications. Knowledge deficit, and even noncompliance, are directly related to the type and quality of medication education that a patient has received. State nurse practice acts and regulating bodies such as the JCAHO consider teaching to be a primary role for nurses, giving it the weight of law and key importance in accreditation standards. Because the goals of pharmcotherapy are the safe administration of medications, with the best therapeutic outcomes possible, teaching is aimed at providing the patient with the information necessary to ensure this occurs. Every nurse-patient interaction can present an opportunity for teaching. Small portions of education given over time are often more effective than large amounts of information given on only one occasion. Discussing medications each time they are administered is an effective way to increase the amount of education accomplished. Providing written material also assists the patient to retain the information and review it later. Some medications come with a self-contained teaching program that includes videotapes. A word of caution on the use of audio and written material is necessary, however. The patient must be able to read and understand the material provided. Pharmacies may dispense patient education pamphlets that detail all of the effects of a medication and the monitoring required, but they are ineffective if the reading level is above what the patient can understand, or is in a language unfamiliar to the patient. Having the patient "teach" the nurse, or summarize key points after the teaching has been provided, is a safety check that may be used to verify that the patient understands the information.

Elderly and pediatric patients often present special challenges to patient teaching. Age-appropriate written or video materials, and teaching that is repeated slowly and provided in small increments, may assist the nurse in teaching these patients. It is often necessary to co-teach the patient's caregiver.

Table 8.3 summarizes key areas of teaching and provides sample questions the nurse might ask, or observations that can be made, to verify that teaching has been effective. The Nursing Process Focus flowcharts in Chapters 13 through 48 also supply information on specific drugs and drug classes that is important to include in patient teaching.

8.6 Evaluating the Effects of Drug Administration

Evaluation is the final step of the Nursing Process. It considers the effectiveness of the interventions in meeting established goals and outcomes. The process comes full circle as the nurse reassesses the patient, reviews the nursing diagnoses, makes necessary changes, reviews and rewrites goals and outcomes, and carries out further interventions to meet the goals and outcomes. When evaluating the effectiveness of drug administration, the nurse assesses for

Table 8.3	Important Areas of Teaching for a Patient Receiving Medications
Area of Teaching	**Important Questions and Observations**
therapeutic use and outcomes	• Can you tell me the name of your medicine and what the medicine is used for? • What will you look for to know that the medication is effective? (How will you know that the medicine is working?)
monitoring side and adverse effects	• Which side effects can you handle by yourself? (e.g., simple nausea, diarrhea) • Which side effects should you report to your healthcare provider? (e.g., extreme cases of nausea or vomiting, extreme dizziness, bleeding)
medication administration	• Can you tell me how much of the medication you are to take? (mg, number of tablets, ml of liquid, etc.) • Can you tell me how often you are to take it? • What special requirements are necessary when you take this medication? (e.g., take with a full glass of water; take on an empty stomach and remain upright for 30 minutes) • Is there a specific order in which you are to take your medications? (e.g., a bronchodilator before using a corticosteroid inhaler) • Can you show me how you will give yourself the medication? (e.g., eye drops, subcutaneous injections) • What special monitoring is required before you take this medication? (e.g., pulse rate) Can you demonstrate this for me? Based on that monitoring, when should you NOT take the medication? • Do you know how, or where, to store this medication? • What should you do if you miss a dose?
other monitoring and special requirements	• Are there any special tests you are to have related to this medication? (e.g., fingerstick glucose levels, therapeutic drug levels) • How often should these tests be done? • What other medications should you NOT take with this medication? • Are there any foods or beverages you must not have while taking this medication?

therapeutic effects and a minimal occurrence of side or adverse effects. The nurse also evaluates the effectiveness of teaching provided and notes areas where further drug education is needed. Evaluation is not the end of the process, but the beginning of another cycle as the nurse continues to work to ensure safe and effective medication use and active patient involvement in his or her care. It is a checkpoint where the nurse considers the overall goal of safe and effective administration of medications, with the best therapeutic outcome possible, and takes the steps necessary to ensure success. The Nursing Process acts as the overall framework to work toward this success.

CHAPTER REVIEW

Key Concepts

The numbered key concepts provide a succinct summary of the important points from the corresponding numbered section within the chapter. If any of these points are not clear, refer to the numbered section within the chapter for review. Expanded versions can be found on the companion website.

8.1 The Nursing Process is a systematic method of problem solving and consists of clearly defined steps: assessment, establishment of nursing diagnoses, planning care through the formulation of goals and outcomes, carrying out interventions, and evaluating the care provided.

8.2 Assessment of the patient receiving medications includes health history information, physical assessment data, lab values and other measurable data, and an assessment of medication effects, both therapeutic and side effects.

8.3 Nursing diagnoses are written to address the patient's responses related to drug administration. They are developed after an analysis of the assessment data, are focused on the patient's problems, and are verified with the patient or caregiver.

8.4 Goals and outcomes, developed from the nursing diagnoses, will direct the interventions required by the plan of care. Goals focus on what the patient should be able to achieve and outcomes provide the specific, measurable criteria that will be used to measure goal attainment.

8.5 Interventions are aimed at returning the patient to an optimum level of wellness through the safe and effective administration of medications. Key interventions required of the nurse include monitoring drug effects, documenting medications, and patient teaching.

8.6 Evaluation begins a new cycle as new assessment data are gathered and analyzed, nursing diagnoses are reviewed or rewritten, goals and outcomes refined, and new interventions carried out.

Review Questions

1. A patient visits an outpatient clinic for treatment of a sore throat that is diagnosed to be caused by *streptococcus* bacteria, and is given a prescription for an antibiotic. What pertinent medical history information would the nurse gather, given the short duration of this patient's visit that would ensure optimum outcomes from this prescription?

2. Develop two possible nursing diagnoses for the patient in question 1 related to the use or administration of the medication.

3. Write a pertinent goal for this patient related to antibiotic use. Write an outcome statement.

4. What essential areas should be covered when teaching this patient before discharge from the clinic?

5. This patient returns to the clinic in 3 days for a problem unrelated to the previous infection. What would the nurse evaluate at this time, to demonstrate success or areas that still need to be addressed, related to the antibiotic prescription?

Critical Thinking Questions

1. A 13-year-old patient who is a cheerleader from a rural community has been diagnosed with type 1 diabetes. She is supported by a single mother who is frustrated with her daughter's eating habits. The patient has lost weight since beginning her insulin regimen. The nurse notes that the patient and her mother, who is very well dressed, are both extremely thin. Identify additional data that the nurse would need to obtain before making the nursing diagnosis, *Noncompliance*.

2. Regarding the patient in question 1, her drug regimen is evaluated and the healthcare provider suggests a subcutaneous insulin pump to help control the patient's fluctuating blood glucose levels. Write three nursing diagnoses related to this new therapy.

3. A nursing student is assigned to a licensed preceptor who is administering oral medications. The student notes that the preceptor administers the drugs safely, but routinely fails to offer the patient information about the drug being administered. Discuss this action in relation to the concept of accountability.

EXPLORE MediaLink

NCLEX review, case studies, and other interactive resources for this chapter can be found on the companion website at www.prenhall.com/adams. Click on "Chapter 8" to select the activities for this chapter. For animations, more NCLEX review questions, and an audio glossary, access the accompanying CD-ROM in this textbook.

Legal and Ethical Issues Related to Drug Administration

Drug administration is one of the most important responsibilities of the nurse, and one that has obvious ethical and legal connections to nursing practice. Because nurses are regularly confronted with issues relating to legal practice, having a firm grasp of the applicable law is essential to provide for patient safety and to avoid litigation. Similarly, nurses are confronted by ethical dilemmas in their practice where professional judgment and experience, rather than laws, guide their decision making.

In simple terms, medical ethics is what a nurse *ought* to do, based on fundamental moral principles. Medical law is what a nurse *must* do, based on federal, state, or local legislation. In clinical practice, ethical and legal issues nearly always overlap. The differences between ethical decisions and legal decisions are often unclear. The purpose of this chapter is to examine medical ethics and law, as they relate to drug administration by the nurse. Specific legislation regulating drug use in the United States and Canada can be found in Chapter 2.

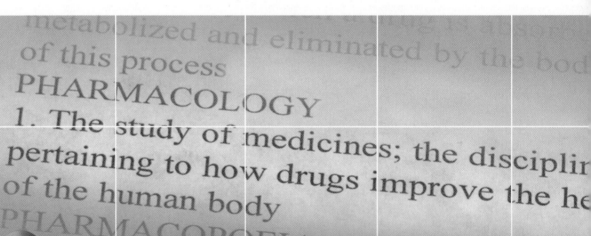

 MediaLink www.prenhall.com/adams

CD-ROM
Audio Glossary
NCLEX Review

Companion Website
NCLEX Review
Case Study
Expanded Key Concepts
Challenge Your Knowledge

KEY TERMS

autonomy *page 88*

beneficence *page 87*

ethical dilemma *page 88*

ethics *page 87*

fidelity *page 88*

justice *page 88*

medication administration record (MAR)
page 89

medication error *page 89*

nonmaleficence *page 87*

nurse practice act *page 88*

standards of care *page 89*

veracity *page 88*

OBJECTIVES

After reading this chapter, the student should be able to:

1. Explain how the ethical principles contained in the ANA Code of Ethics are used to guide nurses in their practice.
2. Apply general moral principles to the effective administration of medications.
3. Describe how nurse practice acts are designed to protect the public.
4. Discuss the standards of care in the application of the nursing process.
5. Explain the importance of documentation in the administration of medications.
6. Discuss factors contributing to medication errors.
7. Identify the process in reporting medication errors.
8. Describe strategies that the nurse may implement to prevent medication errors.

MEDICAL ETHICS ASSOCIATED WITH DRUG ADMINISTRATION

9.1 Medical Ethics and Nursing Practice

Ethics is the branch of philosophy dealing with the moral principles guiding a person's behavior or conduct. An individual's ethical principles are learned from family, religious affiliations, cultural traditions, role models, and close acquaintances. Although ethical principles are highly personal and individualized, certain commonalities guide individuals in a given culture as they seek to establish their ethical standards.

Professional ethics are an extension of personal ethics. For example, most nursing students enter school already having acquired a strong desire to help people in need, as a guiding moral principle. In nursing classes, this principle, and others, are reinforced and extended to include people who are terminally ill, critically injured, or of different cultural traditions.

In 1950, the American Nurses Association (ANA) published the Code of Ethics for Nursing. This initial attempt to guide nurses in their clinical practice was the basis for further standards of care in nursing. Periodic revisions are made to the code so that it remains reflective of current nursing practice. Table 9.1 shows the 2001 edition of the ANA Code of Ethics. A detailed examination of this code is important, but beyond the scope of this text. The student should review a fundamentals of nursing textbook for a complete discussion of the ANA's code.

9.2 Moral Principles Guiding Drug Administration

Moral principles are used by nurses daily to guide their decision making. Several of these fundamental moral principles have direct application to drug administration.

The most obvious moral principle that guides nurses is beneficence, the obligation to seek interventions that are beneficial or good for the patient. The individualized plan of care is designed to determine, implement, and evaluate what is best for the patient's health. Choosing the course of action that will lead to the most good for the patient, including drug administration, is the primary reason for the Nursing Process (Chapter 8) . If a medication will do no good for the patient, it should probably not be prescribed. Ongoing assessments are conducted to determine whether pharmacotherapy is right for the patient, and adjustments are made accordingly. Beneficence is a subjective principle: Professionals often disagree on what they believe is best for the patient. For example, a nurse may question the moral decision of the physician to prolong a terminally ill patient's life through chemotherapy or enteral feedings.

In addition to doing good for the patient, nurses must observe the moral principle of nonmaleficence, the obligation to not harm the patient. Although similar to beneficence, the two principles are somewhat different. For example, by administering a medication that was intended to be beneficial, the nurse may cause harm by not following proper drug administration procedures or by creating adverse effects in the patient that could have been avoided.

Table 9.1	ANA Code of Ethics

1. The nurse provides services with respect for human dignity and the uniqueness of the client unrestricted by considerations of social or economic status, personable attributes, or nature of health programs.

2. The nurse safeguards the client's right to privacy by judiciously protecting information of a confidential manner.

3. The nurse acts to safeguard the client and the public when healthcare and safety are affected by the incompetent, unethical, or illegal practice of any person.

4. The nurse assumes responsibility and accountability for individual nursing judgments and actions.

5. The nurse maintains competence in nursing.

6. The nurse exercises informed judgment and uses individual competence and qualifications as criteria in seeking consultation, accepting responsibilities, and delegating nursing activities to others.

7. The nurse participates in activities that contribute to the implement and improve standards of nursing.

8. The nurse participates in the profession's efforts to implement and improve standards of nursing.

9. The nurse participates in the profession's efforts to establish and maintain conditions of employment conducive to high quality nursing care.

10. The nurse participates in the profession's efforts to protect the public from misinformation and misrepresentation and to maintain the integrity of nursing.

11. The nurse collaborates with members of the health professions and other citizens in promoting community and national efforts to meet the health needs of the public.

Source: From American Nurses Association, Code of Ethics for Nurses with Interpretive Statement, Washington, DC. ©2001 American Nurses Publishing, American Nurses Association. Reprinted by permission.

Perhaps the nurse was too distracted to notice extravasation at the IV site or forgot to document a patient's allergy the last time the drug was given. Beneficence and nonmaleficence often go hand in hand.

Autonomy pertains to an individual's freedom and the right to make his or her own decisions. The moral principle of autonomy assumes that the patient has been given all the necessary information to make rational choices. Informed consent is a legal doctrine of this principle. The nurse is often called upon to use persuasion skills and logic to convince patients of the value of taking medications. It must be remembered that, unless otherwise incapacitated, adult patients have the right to refuse medications even if the nurse does not agree with the decision. For pediatric patients, the right of autonomy is given to the parents.

Veracity is the moral obligation to tell the truth. This becomes important when informing patients about medication effects and answering their questions truthfully and to the best of the nurse's ability. It also has great importance in reporting medication errors. The nurse who administers an incorrect medication or gives it at the wrong dosage must be truthful about the incident.

Other moral principles include **justice**, the obligation to be fair, and **fidelity**, the obligation to be faithful to agreements and fulfill promises. These have specific applications to decision making in nursing practice.

Occasionally, the nurse is confronted with situations where two moral principles appear to be in conflict. These situations, called **ethical dilemmas**, force the nurse to weigh the relative importance of each principle. For exam-ple, the physician orders morphine at a dose that the nurse considers unsafe. The nurse is faced with an ethical dilemma, because this person has an obligation to not harm the patient, which conflicts with an obligation to perform requested duties. Which is more important? Should the order of the physician be implemented despite the fact it *might* cause harm to the patient? If the nurse injects the morphine and the patient dies, who is responsible? If the nurse refuses to administer the medication and the patient suffers ill effects from not receiving the drug, who is responsible? The nurse must weigh the specific moral and legal issues to determine which principles are most important. In most ethical dilemmas, safeguarding the patient's health through beneficence or nonmaleficence is the most important guiding moral principle. Furthermore, although responsibility may be shared with others, nurses are always responsible for their actions (or lack of actions).

MEDICAL LAW ASSOCIATED WITH DRUG ADMINISTRATION

9.3 Nurse Practice Acts and Standards of Care

Each state has a **nurse practice act**, designed to protect the public by defining the legal scope of practice. The means of ensuring the enforcement of nurse practice acts is provided by state boards of nursing or by state nursing examiners. The nurse practice acts are important pieces of legislation because they include the definition of professional nursing, part of which includes the safe delivery of medications. The professional nurse must be qualified to administer medications, as defined in each nurse practice act.

Every practicing nurse and student nurse should consult the state's nurse practice act prior to implementing care to patients. Because these acts are frequently amended, and differ from state to state, practicing nurses should periodically review their current nurse practice act for changes and updates.

Standards of care are the skills and learning commonly possessed by members of a profession. In nursing, standards of care are defined by nurse practice acts and the rule of reasonable and prudent action. This rule defines the standard of care as the actions that a reasonable and prudent nurse with equivalent preparation would do under similar circumstances. In the previous morphine example, the nurse's actions would be legally judged by whether he or she acted within the state's nurse practice act and whether the actions were what a reasonable and prudent nurse would have done when faced with a similar dilemma.

9.4 Documentation of Drug Administration

Nurses are quite familiar with the saying, if the documentation is not completed, then the patient care is not finished. It is important for the nurse to accurately check the physician's orders for current medications against what is recorded on the **medication administration record (MAR)**. This helps to prevent errors that can occur in the transcription of the order from chart to MAR. Some facilities mandate that this check be conducted on every shift.

It is not good nursing practice to document medications on the MAR *before* they are given to the patient. Circumstances may occur that can prevent the patient from receiving the medication, thus making the MAR inaccurate.

It is the nurse's responsibility to document medication errors. In most cases, the physician is immediately notified about the error. Further orders are obtained from the physician, with close monitoring of the patient. An incident report is initiated by the nurse who discovered the error or by the person who witnessed the error. The incident report is given to the nursing manager, and is reviewed by the hospital's quality assurance department. A primary goal of this documentation and follow-through process is to identify common errors so that they may be prevented through training and inservice.

9.5 Medication Errors

According to the National Coordinating Council for Medication Error Reporting and Prevention (NCCMERP), a **medication error** is "any preventable event that may cause or lead to inappropriate medication use or patient harm while the medication is in the control of the health care professional, patient, or consumer." Medication

PHARMFACTS	Legal Considerations

- Each board of nursing has a provision of what and how the registered nurse administers as medications.
- Each provision is sourced and referenced with date.
- These provisions are updated and revised as needed by practicing nurses to state boards.
- To protect consumers, standards of care are adopted by individual nursing organizations, such as the Intravenous Nurses Society (INS).
- Many individual institutions adopt standards of care for their policies and procedures.
- Medication errors are classified by NCCMERP in two categories: medication errors that cause harm and those that do not.

errors impede pharmacotherapeutic outcomes and can cause serious illness or death. Furthermore, medication errors can lead to litigation against the nurse, physician, or healthcare agency. Despite extensive efforts on the part of healthcare providers, medication error rates in communities, hospitals, and homes are increasing.

Factors leading to medication errors include the following:

- Omission of one of the five rights of drug administration (Chapter 4) ⊖ .
- Failure to perform a system check within an agency. Both pharmacists and nurses must collaborate on checking the accuracy and appropriateness of drug orders before they are administered to patients.
- Failure to take into account patient variables, such as recent changes in renal or hepatic function. Nurses should always review recent laboratory data and other information in the patient's chart before administering medications.
- Giving medications based on verbal orders, over the phone or at bedside, that may be misinterpreted or go undocumented. Nurses should remind the prescriber that medication orders must be in writing before they can be administered.
- Giving medications based on an incomplete order or an illegible order, where the nurse is unsure of the correct drug, dosage, or administration method. Incomplete orders should be clarified with the prescriber before the medication is administered.

Because lack of knowledge about medications is a cause for errors, it is important that nurses remain current in pharmacotherapeutics. Nurses should never administer any medication about which they are unfamiliar, as it is considered an unsafe practice. There are many venues by which the nurse can obtain medication knowledge and updates. Current drug references should be available on every nursing unit. Other medication sources are available on the internet and in nursing journals. It is recommended that nurses familiarize themselves with research on medical errors and how they may be prevented.

9.6 Reporting Medication Errors

There has been some hesitation in reporting medication errors in the nursing profession. Most nurses fear humiliation from superiors and their peers when reporting medication errors, although, it is the nurse's ethical and legal responsibility to document such occurrences. Unreported errors may affect the health of patients and cause legal ramifications for the nurse. In severe cases, adverse reactions caused by medication errors may require the initiation of lifesaving interventions for the patient. After such an event, the patient may need intense supervision and additional medical treatments.

The Food and Drug Administration (FDA) is concerned with medication errors at the federal level. The FDA requests that nurses and other healthcare providers report medication errors in order to build a current database that can be used to assist other professionals in avoiding these mistakes. Medication errors, or situations that can lead to errors, may be reported in confidence directly to the FDA by telephone at 800–23-ERROR.

A second organization that has been established to provide assistance on the subject of medication errors is the National Coordinating Council for Medication Error Reporting and Prevention (NCCMERP). This organization was formed by the U.S. Pharmacopoeia Convention in 1995, to help examine interdisciplinary causes of medication errors and promote medication safety. The telephone number for NCCMERP is 800–822–8772.

9.7 Preventing Medication Errors

What can the nurse do in the clinical setting to prevent medication errors? The nurse can begin by using the four steps of the Nursing Process:

1. *Assessment* Ask the patient about allergies to food or medications, current health concerns, use of OTC medications, and herbal supplements. Ensure that the patient is receiving the right dose, at the right time, and by the right route. Assess renal and liver function, and for impairments of other body systems that may impact pharmacotherapy.

2. *Planning* Have the patient state the prescribed outcome of the medication, including the right time to take medication and the right dose.

3. *Implementation* Advise the patient to take medication as prescribed and to question the nurse if medications "look different" (different color, larger pill).

SPECIAL CONSIDERATIONS

Age-Related Issues in Drug Administration

The Pediatric Population

- Always check identification bracelets prior to drug administration.
- Most neonates' identification bracelets are on their ankles.
- Verify safe dose of medications prescribed prior to administration.
- Communication is essential in pediatric drug administration; notify physician if order is incomplete or not legible.

The Elderly Population

- Always check identification bracelets prior to drug administration, sometimes repeating patient's name. (This may not be as helpful in identifying this population of patients due to possible alteration in thought processes.)
- Asking this phrase may be helpful for alert patients: "Can you tell me your name?"
- Remember that medications have the ability to cause adverse effects in this population due to slowed ability to absorb and metabolize medications.
- Monitor drug levels and current lab values for prevention of adverse effects.

4. *Evaluation* Assess whether the expected outcomes of pharmacotherapy have been achieved and whether the patient encountered adverse reactions.

One of the best preventative practices is to educate patients about their medications. When patients are knowledgeable about the outcomes of pharmacotherapy errors decrease. Teaching methods can include written handouts and audiovisual teaching aids on medications (at a reading level and language the patient can understand), and contact information for healthcare providers who should be notified in the event of adverse reactions. Nurses should collaborate with other healthcare providers and agencies to seek means of medication error reduction. Examples of common errors that may be fixed by changing policies and procedures within an institution are as follows:

- Improper storage of medication
- Use of time-expired medications
- Transfer of doses from one container to another
- Overstocking of medications

CHAPTER REVIEW

Key Concepts

The numbered key concepts provide a succinct summary of the important points from the corresponding numbered section within the chapter. If any of these points are not clear, refer to the numbered section within the chapter for review. Expanded versions can be found on the companion website.

9.1 Ethics helps guide a person's behavior or conduct. The American Nurses Association publishes a list of ethical principles that nurses can use to guide their decision making.

9.2 Moral principles such as beneficence, nonmaleficence, veracity, autonomy, justice, and fidelity are important for the nurse to apply in drug administration.

9.3 Nurse practice acts are enacted by every state to define the scope of practice of professional nursing and to protect the public.

9.4 Documentation of drug administration, including any errors, should be completed immediately after the medication is taken by the patient.

9.5 A medication error is a preventable error that may cause or lead to an adverse reaction in the patient. Causes may include omitting of one of the five rights or giving medications based on verbal, illegible, or incomplete orders.

9.6 It is the ethical and legal responsibility of the nurse to report medication errors that might have occurred.

9.7 Finding strategies to prevent medication errors involves various processes, including the Nursing Process.

Review Questions

1. What are standards of care? How do they relate to the regulation of nursing practice?

2. Discuss the ANA Code of Ethics and its relationship to the administration of medications.

3. Explain the medical and legal responsibilities of the nurse in documenting medication errors.

4. What strategies can the nurse use to prevent medication errors?

Critical Thinking Questions

1. A registered nurse is assigned a team of eight patients. Six of these patients have medications scheduled for once-a-day dosing at 10 A.M. Explain how this nurse will be able to administer these drugs to the patients at the "right time."

2. A healthcare provider writes an order for Tylenol 3 PO q3–4h for mild pain. The nurse evaluates this order and is concerned that it is incomplete. Discuss the probable concern and describe what the nurse should do prior to administering this drug.

3. Advanced nurse practitioners have achieved prescriptive authority in several states. In many states, professional nursing organizations are responsible for establishing prescriptive authority. Describe the process that would be required to change a nursing practice related to drug administration.

4. A new nurse does not check an antibiotic dosage ordered by a healthcare provider on a pediatric unit. The nurse subsequently overdoses a 2-year-old patient before an experienced nurse notices the error during the shift change. Who is responsible for the error?

EXPLORE MediaLink

NCLEX review, case studies, and other interactive resources for this chapter can be found on the companion website at www.prenhall.com/adams. Click on "Chapter 9" to select the activities for this chapter. For animations, more NCLEX review questions, and an audio glossary, access the accompanying CD-ROM in this textbook.

Biosocial Aspects
of Pharmacotherapy

I t is convenient for a nurse to memorize an average drug dose, administer the medication, and expect all patients to achieve the same outcomes. Unfortunately, this is rarely the case. For pharmacotherapy to be successful, the needs of each individual patient must be assessed and evaluated. In Chapter 5, variables such as absorption, metabolism, plasma protein binding, and excretion mechanisms are examined in an attempt to explain how these modify patient responses to drugs. In Chapter 6, variability among patient responses is explained in terms of differences in drug-receptor interactions. Chapter 7 examines how these pharmacokinetic and pharmacodynamic factors change patient responses to drugs throughout the lifespan. This chapter examines additional psychological, social, and biologic variables that must be considered for optimum pharmacotherapy.

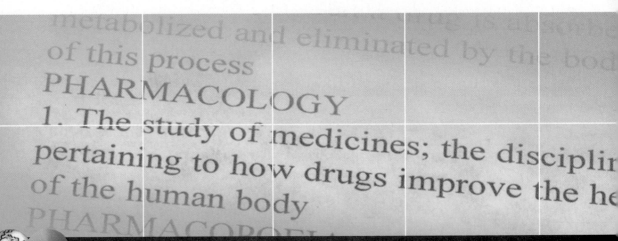

MediaLink www.prenhall.com/adams

CD-ROM
Audio Glossary
NCLEX Review

Companion Website
NCLEX Review
Case Study
Expanded Key Concepts
Challenge Your Knowledge

KEY TERMS

culture *page 95*
ethnic *page 95*
genetic polymorphism *page 96*

holistic *page 93*
psychology *page 94*

sociology *page 94*
spirituality *page 94*

OBJECTIVES

After reading this chapter, the student should be able to:

1. Describe fundamental concepts underlying a holistic approach to pharmacotherapy.
2. Describe the components of the human integration pyramid model.
3. Identify psychosocial and spiritual factors that can impact pharmacotherapeutics.
4. Explain how ethnicity can affect pharmacotherapeutic outcomes.
5. Identify examples of how cultural values and beliefs can influence pharmacotherapeutic outcomes.
6. Explain how community and environmental factors can affect healthcare outcomes.
7. Convey how genetic polymorphisms can influence pharmacotherapy.
8. Relate the implications of gender to the actions of certain drugs.

10.1 The Concept of Holistic Pharmacotherapy

To fully recognize the individuality and totality of the patient, each person must be viewed as an integrated biological, psychosocial, cultural, communicating whole, existing and functioning within the communal environment. Within the scope of nursing and pharmacology, the recipient of care must be regarded in such a **holistic** context for health to be impacted in a positive manner. Medicine has recently begun to use this "whole person" focus to better understand how established risk factors such as age, genetics, biologic characteristics, personal habits, lifestyle, and environment increase a person's likelihood of acquiring specific diseases. Pharmacology has taken the study of these characteristics one step further—to examine and explain how they influence pharmacotherapeutic outcomes.

The human integration pyramid (Fig. 10.1) is a model of six categories that compartmentalize the functional environment in which human beings exist, while maintaining an interrelated connection between them. This representation provides a useful approach to addressing the nursing and pharmacologic needs of patients within the collaborative practices of healthcare delivery. Where appropriate, concepts illustrated in the pyramid will be presented throughout this book, as they relate to the various drug categories. All levels of the pyramid are important and connected: Some are specific to certain drug classes and nursing activities, whereas others apply more diversely across the nursing-pharmacology spectrum.

By its very nature, modern (Western) medicine as it is practiced in the United States is seemingly incompatible with holistic medicine. Western medicine focuses on specific diseases, their causes, and treatments. Disease is viewed as a malfunction of a specific organ or system.

Sometimes, the disease is viewed even more specifically, and categorized as a change in DNA structure or a malfunction of one enzyme. Sophisticated technology is used to image and classify the specific structural or functional abnormality. Somehow, the total patient is lost in this focus of categorizing disease. Too often, it does not matter how or why the patient developed cancer, diabetes, or hypertension, or how they feel about it; the psychosocial and cultural dimensions are lost. Yet these dimensions can profoundly impact the success of pharmacotherapy. The nurse must consciously direct care toward a holistic treatment of each individual patient, in his or her psychosocial, spiritual, and communal context.

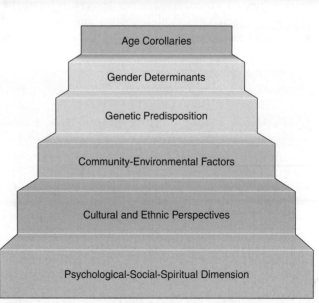

Figure 10.1 | The human integration pyramid care model

MediaLink Healthy People 2010

10.2 Psychosocial Influences on Pharmacotherapy

Whereas science and medicine are founded on objective, logical, critical deliberation, psychology and sociology are based more on intuitive and subjective considerations. Psychology is the science that deals with normal and abnormal mental processes and their impact on behavior. Sociology studies human behavior within the context of groups and societies. Spirituality incorporates the capacity to love, to convey compassion and empathy, to give and forgive, to enjoy life, and to find peace of mind and fulfillment in living. The spiritual life overlaps with components of the emotional, mental, physical, and social aspects of living.

From a healthcare perspective, every human being should be considered as an integrated psychological, social, and spiritual being. Health impairments related to an individual's psychosocial situation often require a blending of individualized nursing care and therapeutic drugs, in conjunction with psychotherapeutic counseling. The term "psycho-social-spiritual" is appearing more frequently in nursing literature. It is now acknowledged that when patients have strong spiritual or religious beliefs, these may greatly influence their perceptions of illness and their preferred modes of treatment. In many situations, these beliefs have a strong bearing on pharmacotherapy. When illness imposes threats to health, the patient commonly presents with psychological, social, and spiritual issues along with physical symptoms. Patients face concerns related to ill health, suffering, loneliness, despair, and death, and at the same time look for meaning, value, and hope in their situation. Such issues can have a great impact on wellness and preferred methods of medical treatment, nursing care, and pharmacotherapy.

The patient's psychosocial history is an essential component of the initial patient interview and assessment. This history delves into the personal life of the patient, with inquiries directed toward lifestyle preferences, religious beliefs, sexual practices, alcohol intake, and tobacco and nonprescription drug use. The nurse must show extreme sensitivity when gathering the data. If a trusting nurse-patient relationship is not quickly established, the patient will be reluctant to share important personal data that could affect nursing care.

The psychological dimension can exert a strong influence on pharmacotherapy. Patients who are convinced that their treatment is important and beneficial to their well-being will demonstrate better compliance with drug therapy. The nurse must ascertain the patient's goals in seeking treatment, and determine whether drug therapy is compatible with those goals. Past experiences with healthcare may lead a patient to distrust medications. Drugs may not be acceptable for the social environment of the patient. For example, having to take drugs at school or in the workplace may cause embarrassment; patients may fear that they will be viewed as weak, unhealthy, or dependent.

Patients who display positive attitudes toward their personal health and have high expectations regarding the results of their pharmacotherapy are more likely to achieve positive outcomes. The nurse plays a pivotal role in encouraging the patient's positive expectations. The nurse must always be forthright in explaining drug actions and potential side effects. Trivializing the limitations of pharmacotherapy or minimizing potential adverse effects can cause the patient to have unrealistic expectations regarding treatment. The nurse-patient relationship may be jeopardized and the patient may acquire an attitude of distrust. As discussed in Chapter 9 ∞, the patient has an ethical and legal right to receive accurate information regarding the benefits and effects of drug therapy.

10.3 Cultural and Ethnic Influences on Pharmacotherapy

Despite the apparent diverse cultural and ethnic differences among humans, we are, indeed, one species. It has been estimated that all humans share 99.8% of the same DNA sequences. The remaining 0.2% of the sequences that differ are shared among peoples with similar historic and geographic heritage.

SPECIAL CONSIDERATIONS

Alcoholism: Cultural and Environmental Influences

Alcoholism is considered a disease with both social and biological components. It clearly has a genetic basis that sensitizes some individuals to the action of ethanol. It also is known to develop in individuals who are exposed, from an early age, to situations when drinking is considered socially acceptable. It is supported by cultural customs, poverty, traumatic experiences, and other environmental factors. The nurse is often the key healthcare professional who is trained to identify these factors during patient assessment, and to refer the patient to the proper health or social agency for assistance. The condition must be considered and treated in a holistic and compassionate manner if the problem is to be controlled.

SPECIAL CONSIDERATIONS

Religious Affiliation and Disease Incidence

Religious affiliation is correlated with a reduction in the incidence of some diseases such as cancer and coronary artery disease. Religious and spiritual factors often figure into important decisions for patients facing terminal illness and death, for example, the employment of advance directives such as the living will and the durable power of attorney for healthcare. Considerations of the meaning, purpose, and value of human life are used to make choices about the desirability of CPR and aggressive life support, or whether and when to forgo life support and accept death as appropriate and natural under the circumstances.

- In 2000, the majority ethnic group in the United States was non-Hispanic whites at 71%.
- By 2025, the population of non-Hispanic whites is expected to decrease to 62%, and they fall to 55% by 2045.
- Sometime between 2050 and 2060, non-Hispanic white persons will themselves become a "minority," shrinking to less than half of all Americans.
- Whereas 89% of white non-Hispanics are covered by a health insurance plan, only 67% of Hispanics have such insurance. American Indians and Alaska Natives were less likely to have health insurance than other racial groups, with the exception of Hispanics.
- 80% of Caucasians report having a regular doctor. This percentage is reduced to 57% for Hispanics, 68% for Asian Americans, and 70% for African Americans.
- African American (13%) and Hispanic (14%) adults were more than twice as likely as Caucasian (6%) adults to report no regular source of care, or that the emergency room is the usual source of care.
- 65% of Caucasian medicare beneficiaries reported that they were vaccinated against the flu in the past 12 months. This number was reduced to 43% for African Americans and 49% for Hispanics.
- Among part-time workers, 64% of Caucasians reported having employer-based insurance. This number was reduced to 45% for African Americans and 40% for Hispanics.
- Among workers earning more than $15 per hour, 79% of Caucasians reported that they were provided employer-based insurance, compared with 67% of African Americans and 54% of Hispanics.

Source: www.census.gov, U.S. Census Results, 2000.

An **ethnic** group is a community of people having a common history and similar genetic heritage. Members of an ethnic group share distinctive social and cultural traditions, which are maintained from generation to generation. These beliefs include a shared perception of health and illness.

Culture is a set of beliefs, values, religious rituals, and customs shared by a group of people. In some respects, culture and ethnicity are similar, and many people use the words interchangeably. Ethnicity more often is used to refer to biologic and genetic similarities. For example, thousands of Africans were taken from their tribes and forcibly moved to America as part of the slave trade in the 1700s and 1800s. Over several hundred years, many African Americans have adopted the cultural norms of European Americans. Others have kept some of their African cultural traditions and beliefs that have been passed on from generation to generation. As a group, however, all African Americans share genetic similarities to those living in Africa today, and thus are considered as belonging to the same ethnic group.

Culture can be a dominant force influencing the relationship between the patient and the nurse. The practitioner-patient relationship is a cross-cultural encounter, with the patient bringing religious, and ideological beliefs that may challenge or conflict with what the healthcare provider believes to be in the best interests of the patient. The patient's definition of illness is, in fact, often based on cultural beliefs and values. It is also important to remember that diversity not only exists *between* different cultures but also *within* individual cultures. Examples include differences between age groups or between genders within a given culture.

Cultural sensitivity must be demonstrated by the nurse during the initial phase of the nursing process, when the nurse and patient first meet and culturally specific information is obtained during the medical history. Cultural competence requires knowledge of the values, beliefs, and practices of various peoples, along with an attitude of awareness, openness, and sensitivity. Understanding and respecting the beliefs of the patient are key to establishing and maintaining a positive therapeutic relationship that culminates in culturally sensitive nursing care. Therapeutic communication mandates that all healthcare providers bear in mind the cultural, racial, and social factors that make up each person, and how these impact behavior. Failure to take these beliefs seriously can undermine the patient's ability to trust the nurse, and may even persuade some patients to avoid seeking medical care when it is needed.

Culture and ethnicity can impact pharmacotherapy in many ways. The nurse must keep in mind the following variables when treating patients in different ethnic groups.

- *Diet* Every culture has a unique set of foods and spices, which have the potential to affect pharmacotherapy. For example, Asian diets tend to be high in carbohydrates and low on protein and fat. African American diets are higher in lipid content.
- *Alternative therapies* Many cultural groups believe in using herbs and other alternative therapies either along with or in place of modern medicines. Some of these folk remedies and traditional treatments have existed for thousands of years and helped to form the foundation for modern medical practice. Many Chinese go to herbalists to treat their illnesses. Native Americans often take great care in collecting, storing, and using herbs to treat and prevent disease. Certain Hispanic cultures use spices and herbs to maintain a balance of hot and cold, which is thought to promote wellness. Therapeutic massage, heat, and tea infusions are used by many cultures. The nurse needs to interpret how these herbal and alternative therapies will impact the desired pharmacotherapeutic outcomes.
- *Beliefs of health and disease* Each culture has distinct ways to view sickness and health. Some individuals seek the assistance of people in their community that they believe are blessed with healing powers. Native Americans may seek help from a tribal medicine man or Hispanics from a *curandero* (folk healer). African Americans sometimes know of neighbors who have gifts of healing through the use of laying on of hands. The nurse must understand that patients may place great trust in these alternative healers, and should not demean their belief system.

■ *Genetic differences* With the advent of DNA sequencing, hundreds of structural variants in metabolic enzymes have been discovered. Some of these appear more frequently in certain ethnic groups and have an impact on pharmacotherapeutics, as discussed in Section 10.5.

10.4 Community and Environmental Influences on Pharmacotherapy

A number of community and environmental factors have been identified that influence disease and its subsequent treatment. Population growth, complex technological advances, and evolving globalization patterns have all affected healthcare. Communities vary significantly in regard to urbanization levels, age distributions, socioeconomic levels, occupational patterns, and industrial growth. All of these have the potential to affect health and access to pharmacotherapy.

Access to healthcare is perhaps the most obvious community-related influence on pharmacotherapy. There are many potential obstacles to obtaining appropriate healthcare. Without an adequate health insurance plan, some people are reluctant to seek healthcare for fear of bankrupting the family unit. Older adults fear losing their retirement savings or being placed in a nursing home for the remainder of their lives. Families living in rural areas may have to travel great distances to obtain necessary treatment. Once treatment is rendered, the cost of prescription drugs may be far too high for patients on limited incomes. The nurse must be aware of these variables and have knowledge of social agencies in the local community that can assist in improving healthcare access.

Literacy is another community-related variable that can affect healthcare. Up to 48% of English-speaking patients do not have functional literacy—a basic ability to read, understand, and act on health information (Andrus & Roth, 2002). The functional illiteracy rate is even higher in certain populations, particularly non-English-speaking individuals and older patients. The nurse must be aware that these patients may not be able to read drug labels, understand written treatment instructions, or read brochures describing their disease or therapy. Functional illiteracy can result in a lack of understanding about the importance of pharmacotherapy and lead to poor compliance. The nurse must attempt to identify these patients and provide them with brochures, instructions, and educational materials that can be understood. For non-English-speaking patients or those for whom English is their second language, the nurse should have proper materials in the patient's primary language, or provide an interpreter who can help with accurate translations. The nurse should ask the patient to repeat important instructions, to ensure comprehension. The use of more graphical materials is appropriate for certain therapies.

For many patients, belief in a higher spiritual being is important to wellness; prayer is an essential component of daily life. When serious illness occurs, or when death is imminent, patients may find comfort and support from religious rituals and artifacts. For these patients, the nurse should provide proper spiritual support and contacts for community churches. The nurse may want to provide information regarding local ministers, priests, or rabbis who visit the hospital on a regular basis. Spiritual guidance may provide patients with positive expectations regarding their health, and improve compliance.

10.5 Genetic Influences on Pharmacotherapy

Although humans are 99.8% alike in their DNA sequences, the remaining 0.2% may result in significant differences in patients' ability to metabolize medications. These differences are created when a mutation occurs in the portion of DNA responsible for encoding a certain metabolic enzyme. A single base mutation in DNA may result in an amino acid change in the enzyme, which changes its function. Hundreds of such mutations have been identified. These changes in enzyme structure and function are called **genetic polymorphisms**. The change may result in either increased or decreased drug metabolism, depending on the exact type of genetic polymorphism. The study of these polymorphisms is called pharmacogenetics.

Genetic polymorphisms are most often identified in specific ethnic groups, because people in an ethnic group have been located in the same geographical area and have married others within the same ethnic group for hundreds of generations. This allows the genetic polymorphism to be amplified within that population.

PHARMFACTS | **Community Health Statistics in the United States**

- Americans who live in the suburbs fare significantly better in many key health measures than those who live in the most rural and most urban areas.
- Those who live in the suburbs of large metropolitan areas have the lowest infant mortality rates and are more likely to have health insurance and healthy lifestyles.
- Death rates for working-age adults are higher in the most rural and most urban areas.
- The highest death rates for children and young adults are in the most rural counties.
- Homicide rates are highest in the central counties of large metropolitan areas.
- Suburban residents are more likely to exercise during leisure time and more likely to have health insurance. Suburban women are the least likely to be obese.
- Both the most rural and most urban areas have a similarly high percent of residents without health insurance.
- Teenagers and adults in rural counties are the most likely to smoke.
- Residents of the most rural communities have the fewest visits for dental care.

Source: www.cdc.gov/nchs/

Table 10.1	Enzyme Polymorphisms of Importance to Pharmacotherapy	
Enzyme	**Result of Polymorphism**	**Drugs Using This Metabolic Enzyme/Pathway**
acetyltransferase	slow acetylation in Scandinavians, Jews, North African Caucasians Fast acetylation in Japanese	isoniazid, chlordiazepam, hydralazine, procainamide, caffeine
debrisoquin hydroxylase	poor metabolizers in Asians and African Americans	amitriptyline, imipramine, perphenazine, haloperidol, propranolol, metoprolol, codeine, morphine
mephenytoin hydroxylase	poor metabolizers in Asians and African Americans	diazepam, imipramine, barbiturates, warfarin

The relationship between genetic factors and drug response has been documented for decades. The first polymorphism was discovered in the enzyme acetyltransferase which metabolizes isoniazid (INH). The metabolic process, known as acetylation, occurs slowly in certain Caucasians. The slow clearance can cause the drug to build up to toxic levels in these patients, who are known as slow acetylators. The opposite effect, fast acetylation, is found in many Japanese.

In recent years, several other enzyme polymorphisms have been identified. Asian Americans are less likely to be able to metabolically convert codeine to morphine due to an inherent absence of the enzyme debrisoquin, a defect that interferes with the analgesic properties of codeine. In another example, some persons of African American descent receive decreased effects from beta-adrenergic antagonist drugs such as propranolol (Inderal), due to genetically influenced variances in plasma renin levels. Another set of oxidation enzyme polymorphisms have been found that alter the response to warfarin (Coumadin), diazepam (Valium), and several other medications. Table 10.1 summarizes the three most common polymorphisms. Expanding knowledge about the physiologic impact of heredity on pharmacologic treatment may someday allow for personalization of the treatment process.

10.6 Gender Influences on Pharmacotherapy

A person's gender influences many aspects of health maintenance, promotion, and treatment, as well as drug response. It is a substantiated fact, for example, that women pay more attention to changes in health patterns and seek healthcare earlier than their male counterparts. Conversely, many women do not seek medical attention for potential cardiac problems, because heart disease is considered to be a "man's disease." Alzheimer's disease affects both men and women, but studies in various populations have shown that between 1.5 and 3 times as many women as men suffer from the disease. Alzheimer's disease is becoming recognized as a major "women's health issue" comparable to osteoporosis, breast cancer, and fertility disorders.

Acceptance or rejection of the use of particular categories of medication may be gender based. Because of the side effects associated with certain medications, some patients do not take them appropriately—or take them at all. A common example is the use of certain antihypertensive agents in men. These may have, as a common side effect, male impotence. In certain instances, male patients have suffered a stroke because they abruptly stopped taking the drug and did not communicate this fact to their healthcare provider. With open communication, dilemmas regarding drug problems and side effects can be brought out into the open so alternative drug therapies can be considered. As with so many areas of healthcare, appropriate patient teaching by the nurse is a key aspect in preventing or alleviating pharmacologic-related health problems.

Local and systemic responses to some medications can differ between genders. These response differences may be based on differences in body composition such as the fat-to-muscle ratio. In addition, cerebral blood flow variances between males and females may alter the response to certain analgesics. Some of the benzodiazapines used for anxiety have slower elimination rates in women, and this difference becomes even more significant if the woman is concurrently taking oral contraceptives. There are numerous gender-related situations that the nurse must understand in order to monitor drug actions and effects appropriately.

Until recently, the vast majority of drug research studies were conducted using only male subjects. It was wrongly assumed that the conclusions of these studies applied in the same manner to females. Since 1993, the FDA has formalized policies that require the inclusion of subjects of both genders during drug development. This includes analyses of clinical data by gender, assessment of potential pharmacokinetic and pharmacodynamic differences between genders, and, where appropriate, conducting additional studies specific to women's health.

Also of issue is gender inequity regarding prescription drug coverage. A common example is employer health plans that exclude women's contraceptive medications. It was not until a federal district court ruling in June 2001 that exclusion of prescription of female contraceptives by an employer's healthcare provider was deemed sex discrimination.

CHAPTER REVIEW

Key Concepts

The numbered key concepts provide a succinct summary of the important points from the corresponding numbered section within the chapter. If any of these points are not clear, refer to the numbered section within the chapter for review. Expanded versions can be found on the companion website.

10.1 To deliver holistic treatment, the nurse must consider the patient's psychosocial and spiritual needs in a communal context.

10.2 The psychosocial domain must be considered when taking patient medical histories. Positive attitudes and high expectations toward therapeutic outcomes in the patient may increase the success of pharmacotherapy.

10.3 Culture and ethnicity are two interconnected perspectives that can impact nursing care and pharmacotherapy. Differences in diet, use of alternative therapies, percep-

tions of wellness, and genetic makeup can influence patient drug response.

10.4 Community and environmental factors affect health and impact the public's access to healthcare and pharmacotherapy. Inadequate access to healthcare resources and an inability to read or understand instructions may negatively impact treatment outcomes.

10.5 Genetic differences in metabolic enzymes that occur among different ethnic groups must be considered for effective pharmacotherapy. Small differences in the structure of enzymes can result in profound changes in drug metabolism.

10.6 Gender can influence many aspects of health maintenance, promotion, and treatment, as well as medication response.

Review Questions

1. Give examples of how cultural beliefs can influence a patient's symptoms.

2. What are three features of culturally sensitive care?

3. What influence can the nurse's own culture or cultural-ethnic background have on the attitudes toward the use of prescription drugs and alcohol?

4. Why is a particular enzyme polymorphism seen more frequently in one ethnic group versus another?

Critical Thinking Questions

1. A 72-year-old African American heart patient, who has been treated for atrial flutter, is taking warfarin sodium (Coumadin) 2.5 mg PO once a day. He comes to the outpatient clinical for his routine international normalized ratio (INR), which is no longer in the therapeutic range. The patient lives in the rural South and "keeps" a vegetable garden. What questions would a nurse need to ask in order to evaluate the cause of the decreased drug effectiveness?

2. An 82-year-old female patient is admitted to the emergency department. She has been taking furosemide (Lasix)

40 mg PO daily as part of a regimen for congestive heart failure. She is confused and dehydrated. What gender-related considerations should the nurse make when assessing this patient?

3. A 19-year-old male of Mexican descent presents to a health clinic for migrant farm workers. In broken English, he describes severe pain in his lower jaw. An assessment reveals two abscessed molars and other oral health problems. Discuss the probable reasons for this patient's condition.

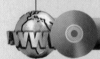

EXPLORE MediaLink

NCLEX review, case studies, and other interactive resources for this chapter can be found on the companion website at www.prenhall.com/adams. Click on "Chapter 10" to select the activities for this chapter. For animations, more NCLEX review questions, and an audio glossary, access the accompanying CD-ROM in this textbook.

CHAPTER 11

Herbal and Alternative Therapies

Herbal supplements and alternative therapies represent a multibillion-dollar industry. Sales of dietary supplements alone exceed $17 billion annually, with over 158 million consumers using them. Despite the fact that these therapies have not been subjected to the same scientific scrutiny as prescription medications, consumers have turned to these treatments for a variety of reasons. Many people have the impression that natural substances have more healing power than synthetic medications. The ready availability of herbal supplements at a reasonable cost has convinced many consumers to try them. This chapter examines the role of complementary and alternative therapies in the prevention and treatment of disease.

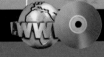

MediaLink   www.prenhall.com/adams

CD-ROM
Audio Glossary
NCLEX Review

Companion Website
NCLEX Review
Case Study
Expanded Key Concepts
Challenge Your Knowledge

KEY TERMS

OBJECTIVES

After reading this chapter, the student should be able to:

1. Explain the role of complementary and alternative medicine in patient wellness.
2. Discuss reasons why herbal and dietary supplements have increased in popularity.
3. Identify the parts of an herb that may contain active ingredients and the types of formulations made from these parts.
4. Describe the strengths and weaknesses of the Dietary Supplement Health and Education Act (DSHEA) of 1994.
5. Describe some adverse effects that may be caused by herbal preparations.
6. Discuss the role of the nurse in teaching patients about complementary and alternative therapies.
7. Identify common drug-herbal interactions.

11.1 Alternative Therapies

Complementary and alternative medicine (CAM) comprises an extremely diverse set of therapies and healing systems that are considered to be outside of mainstream healthcare. Although diverse, the major CAM systems have the following common characteristics.

- Focus on treating each person as an individual
- Consideration of the health of the whole person
- Integration of mind and body
- Promotion of disease prevention, self-care, and self-healing
- Recognition of the role of spirituality in health and healing

Because of its popularity, considerable attention has begun to focus on the effectiveness, or lack of effectiveness, of CAM. Although research into these alternative systems has begun to appear worldwide, few CAM therapies have been subjected to rigorous clinical and scientific study. It is likely that some of these therapies will be found ineffective, while others will become mainstream treatments. The line between what is defined as an alternative therapy and what is considered mainstream is constantly changing. Increasing numbers of healthcare providers are now accepting CAM therapies and recommending them to their patients. Table 11.1 lists many of these therapies.

Nurses have long known the value of CAM therapies in preventing and treating disease. Prayer, meditation, massage, and yoga, for example, have been used to treat both body and mind for centuries. From a pharmacology perspective, the value of CAM therapies lies in their ability to reduce the need for medications. For example, if a patient can find anxiety relief through herbal products, massage or biofeedback therapy, then the use of anxiolytic drugs may be reduced or eliminated. Reduction of drug dose leads to fewer adverse effects.

The nurse should be sensitive to the patient's need for alternative treatment and not be judgmental. Both advantages and limitations must be presented to patients so they may make rational and informed decisions on their treatment. Pharmacotherapy and alternative therapies can serve complementary and essential roles in the healing of the total patient.

11.2 Brief History of Therapeutic Natural Products

An **herb** is technically a **botanical** without woody tissue such as stems or bark. Over time, the terms *botanical* and *herb* have come to be used interchangeably to refer to any plant product with some useful application either as a food enhancer, such as flavoring, or as a medicine.

The use of botanicals has been documented for thousands of years. One of the earliest recorded uses of plant products was a prescription for garlic in 3000 B.C. Eastern and Western medicine have recorded thousands of herbs and herb combinations reputed to have therapeutic value. Some of the most popular herbal supplements and their primary uses are shown in Table 11.2.

With the birth of the pharmaceutical industry in the late 1800s, interest in herbal medicines began to wane. Synthetic drugs could be standardized and produced more cheaply than natural herbal products. Regulatory agencies required that products be safe and effective. The focus of healthcare was on diagnosing and treating specific diseases, rather than promoting wellness and holistic care. Most alternative therapies were no longer taught in medical or nursing schools; these healing techniques were criticized as being unscientific relics of the past.

Beginning in the 1970s and continuing to the present, alternative therapies and herbal medicine have experienced

Table 11.1	Complementary and Alternative Therapies
Healing Method	**Examples**
biological-based therapies	herbal therapies
	nutritional supplements
	special diets
alternate healthcare systems	naturopathy
	homeopathy
	chiropractic
	Native American medicine (e.g., sweat lodges, medicine wheel)
	Chinese traditional medicine (e.g., acupuncture, Chinese herbs)
manual healing	massage
	pressure-point therapies
	hand-mediated biofield therapies
mind-body interventions	yoga
	meditation
	hypnotherapy
	guided imagery
	biofeedback
	movement-oriented therapies (e.g., music, dance)
spiritual	shamans
	faith and prayer
others	bioelectromagnetics
	detoxifying therapies
	animal-assisted therapy

PHARMFACTS **Alternative Therapies in America**

Possibly the largest nonscientific study of attitudes toward alternative therapies surveyed 46,000 people and was reported in Consumer Reports, May 2000. Findings of this study are as follows:

- 65% did not use alternative therapies, primarily because they were satisfied with standard medical treatments.
- 35% used alternative therapies, primarily to relieve symptoms that were not successfully treated with conventional therapies.
- The most likely people trying alternatives were those in severe pain or with stress.
- For almost all medical conditions, respondents stated that prescription drugs were more effective than herbal therapies.
- For back pain and fibromyalgia, deep muscle massage was rated more effective than prescription drugs.
- 25% of those who tried alternatives did so on the recommendation of a doctor or nurse. Only 5% of doctors disapproved of alternative therapies.

a remarkable resurgence, such that the majority of adult Americans are currently taking botanicals on a regular basis or have taken them in the past. This increase in popularity is due to factors such as increased availability of herbal products, aggressive marketing by the herbal industry, increased attention to natural alternatives, and a renewed interest in preventive medicine. The gradual aging of the population has led to more patients seeking therapeutic alternatives for chronic conditions such as pain, arthritis, hormone replacement therapy, and prostate difficulties. In addition, the high cost of prescription medicines has driven patients to seek less expensive alternatives. Nurses have been instrumental in promoting self-care and recommending CAM therapies for patients.

11.3 Herbal Product Formulations

The pharmacologically active chemicals in an herbal product may be present in only one specific part of the plant, or in all parts. For example, the active chemicals in chamomile

Table 11.2	Best-Selling Herbal Supplements, in Rank Order	
Herb	**Medicinal Part**	**Primary Use(s)**
ginkgo	leaves and seeds	improve memory, reduce dizziness
echinacea	entire plant	enhance immune system, anti-inflammatory
garlic	bulbs	reduce blood cholesterol, reduce blood pressure, anticoagulation
ginseng	root	relieve stress, enhance immune system, decrease fatigue
soy	beans	source of protein, vitamins, and minerals; relief of menopausal symptoms, prevent cardiovascular disease, anticancer
saw palmetto	ripe fruit/berries	relieve urinary problems related to prostate enlargement
St. John's wort	flowers, leaves, stems	reduce depression, reduce anxiety, anti-inflammatory
valerian	roots	relieve stress, promote sleep
cranberry	berries/juice	prevent urinary tract infection
black cohosh	roots	relief of menopausal symptoms
kava kava	rhizome	reduce stress, promote sleep
milk thistle	seeds	antitoxin, protection against liver disease
evening primrose	seeds/oil	source of essential fatty acids, relief of premenstrual or menopausal symptoms, relief of rheumatoid arthritis and other inflammatory symptoms
grape seed	seeds/oil	source of essential fatty acids, antioxidant, restore microcirculation to tissues
bilberry	berry/leaf	terminate diarrhea, improve and protect vision, antioxidant

Source: Data from Information Resources, Inc., Chicago.

SPECIAL CONSIDERATIONS

Dietary Supplements and the Older Adult

Can dietary supplements improve the health of older adults? A growing body of evidence is showing that the use of supplements can positively influence seniors' health. Dietary supplements have been successfully used to enhance their immune systems, reduce short-term memory loss, lessen the risks of Alzheimer's disease, and improve overall health. Nutritional deficiencies greatly increase with age, and supplements help to prevent or eliminate these deficiencies in seniors. In addition, some research has shown that older adults who have low levels of folate and vitamin B_{12} have an increased risk of developing Alzheimer's disease. The nurse should assess the need for such supplements in all elderly patients. The nurse, however, should be aware that herbal and dietary supplements can be expensive; thus, they should not be automatically included in treatment plans. In addition, older adults should be educated as to the risks of megavitamin therapy.

are in the above ground portion that includes the leaves, stems, and flowers. For other herbs, such as ginger, the underground rhizomes and roots are used for their healing properties. If collecting herbs for home use, it is essential to know which portion of the plant contains the active chemicals.

Most drugs contain only one active chemical. This chemical can be standardized and measured, and the amount of drug received by the patient is precisely known. It is a common misunderstanding that herbs also contain one active ingredient, which can be extracted and delivered to patients in precise doses, like drugs. Herbs, however, may contain dozens of active chemicals, many of which have not yet been isolated, studied, or even identified. It is possible that some of these substances work together synergistically and may not have the same activity if isolated. Furthermore, the strength of an herbal preparation may vary depending on where it was grown and how it was collected and stored.

Some attempts have been made to standardize herbal extracts, using a marker substance such as the percent flavones in ginkgo or the percent lactones in kava kava. Some of these standardizations are shown in Table 11.3. Until science can

Table 11.3	**Standardization of Selected Herb Extracts**	
Herb	**Standardization**	**Percent**
black cohosh rhizome	triterpene glycosides	2.5
cascara sagrada bark	hydroxyanthracenic heterosides	20
echinacea purpurea herb	phenolics	4
ginger rhizome	pungent compounds	>10
ginkgo leaf	flavoglycosides	24–25
	lactones	6
ginseng root	ginseosides	20–30
kava kava rhizome	kavalactones	40–45
milk thistle root	silymarin	80
St. John's wort herb	hypericins	0.3–0.5
	hyperforin	3–5
saw palmetto fruit	total fatty acids	80–90

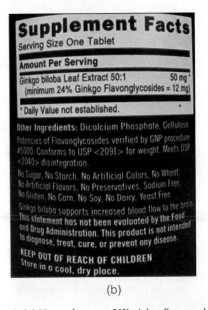

(a)   (b)

Figure 11.1 | Two ginkgo biloba labels: note the lack of standardization in (a) 60 mg of extract, 24% ginkgo flavone glycosides and 6% terpenes; and (b) 50:1 ginkgo leaf extract, 24% ginkgo flavonglycosides

better characterize these substances, however, it is best to conceptualize the active ingredient of an herb as being the herb itself. An example of the ingredients and standardization of ginkgo biloba is shown in Figure 11.1.

The two basic formulations of herbal products are solid and liquid. Solid products include pills, tablets, and capsules made from the dried herbs. Other solid products are salves and ointments that are administered topically. Liquid formulations are made by extracting the active chemicals from the plant using solvents such as water, alcohol, or glycerol. The liquids are then concentrated in various strengths and ingested. The various liquid formulations of herbal

preparations are described in Table 11.4. Figure 11.2 illustrates formulations of the popular herbal, ginkgo biloba.

11.4 Regulation of Herbal Products and Dietary Supplements

Since the passage of the Food, Drug and Cosmetic Act in 1936, Americans have come to expect that all approved prescription and OTC drugs have passed rigid standards of safety, prior to being marketed. Furthermore, it is expected that these drugs have been tested for efficacy and that they truly provide the medical benefits claimed by the

Table 11.4	Liquid Formulations of Herbal Products
Product	**Description**
tea	fresh or dried herbs are soaked in hot water for 5–10 minutes before ingestion; convenient
infusion	fresh or dried herbs are soaked in hot water for long periods, at least 15 minutes; stronger than teas
decoction	fresh or dried herbs are boiled in water for 30–60 minutes until much of the liquid has boiled off; very concentrated
tincture	extraction of active ingredients using alcohol by soaking the herb; alcohol remains as part of the liquid
extract	extraction of active ingredients using organic solvents to form a highly concentrated liquid or solid form; solvent may be removed or be part of the final product

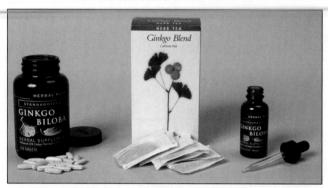

Figure 11.2 | Three different ginkgo formulations: tablets, tea bags, and liquid extract

manufacturer. Americans cannot and should not expect the same quality standards for herbal products. These products are regulated by a far less rigorous law, the Dietary Supplement Health and Education Act (DSHEA) of 1994.

According to the DSHEA, "dietary supplements" are specifically exempted from the Food, Drug and Cosmetic Act. Dietary supplements are products intended to enhance or supplement the diet such as botanicals, vitamins, minerals, or other extract or metabolite that is not already approved as a drug by the FDA. A major strength of the legislation is it gives the FDA the power to remove from the market any product that poses a "significant or unreasonable" risk to the public. It also requires these products to be clearly labeled as "dietary supplements." An example of an herbal label for black cohosh is shown in Figure 11.3.

Unfortunately, the DSHEA has several significant flaws that lead to a lack of standardization in the dietary supplement industry, and to less protection of the consumer.

- Dietary supplements do not have to be tested prior to marketing.
- Efficacy does not have to be demonstrated by the manufacturer.
- The manufacturer does not have to prove the safety of the dietary supplement: If it is to be removed from the market, the government has to prove that the dietary supplement is unsafe.
- Dietary supplements must state that the product is not intended to diagnose, treat, cure, or prevent any disease; however, the label may make claims about the product's effect on body structure and function, such as the following:
    Helps promote healthy immune systems
    Reduces anxiety and stress
    Helps to maintain cardiovascular function
    May reduce pain and inflammation
- The DSHEA does not regulate the accuracy of the label; the product may or may not contain the product listed, in the amounts claimed.

11.5 The Pharmacologic Actions and Safety of Herbal Products

A key concept to remember when dealing with alternative therapies is that "natural" is not synonymous with "better" or "safe." There is no question that some botanicals contain powerful active chemicals, perhaps that are more effective than currently approved medications. Thousands of years of experience, combined with current scientific research, have shown that some herbal remedies have therapeutic actions. Because a substance comes from a natural product, however, does not make it safe or effective. For example, poison ivy is natural but it certainly is not safe or therapeutic. Natural products may not offer an improvement over conventional therapy in treating certain disorders and, indeed, may be of no value whatsoever. Furthermore, a patient who substitutes an unproven alternative therapy for an established, effective medical treatment may delay healing and suffer irreparable harmful effects.

Some herbal products contain ingredients that may serve as agonists or antagonists to prescription drugs. When obtaining medical histories, nurses should include questions on dietary supplements. Patients taking medications with potentially serious adverse effects such as insulin, warfarin (Coumadin), or digoxin (Lanoxin) should be warned to never take any herbal product or dietary supplement without first discussing their needs with a physician. Drug interactions with selected herbs are shown in Table 11.5.

When using natural products, one must also beware of allergic reactions. Most herbal products contain a mixture of ingredients, many of which have not been identified. It is not unusual to find dozens of different chemicals in teas and infusions made from the flowers, leaves, or roots of a plant. Patients who have known allergies to food products or medicines should seek medical advice before taking a new herbal product. It is always wise to take the smallest amount possible when starting herbal therapy, even less than the recommended dose, to see if allergies or other adverse effects occur.

Nurses have an obligation to seek the latest medical information on herbal products, since there is a good possibility that their patients are using them to supplement traditional medicines. Patients should be advised to be skeptical of claims on the labels of dietary supplements and to seek health information from reputable sources. Nurses should never condemn a patient's use of alternative medicines, but instead should be supportive and seek to understand the patient's goals for taking the supplements. The healthcare provider will often need to educate patients on the role of CAM therapies in the treatment of their disorder and discuss which treatment or combination of treatments will best meet their health goals.

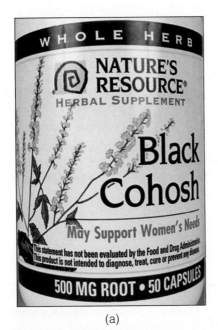
(a)

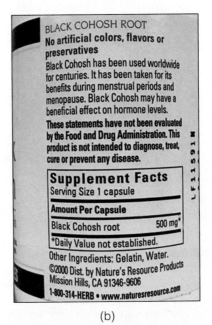
(b)

Figure 11.3 | Labeling of black cohosh: (a) front label with general health claim; and (b) back label with more health claims and FDA disclaimer

Table 11.5	Common Herb-Drug Interactions	
Common (*Scientific*) Name	**Interacts with**	**Comments**
echinacea (*Echinacea purpurea*)	amiodarone	Possible increased hepatotoxicity
	anabolic steroids	Possible increased hepatotoxicity
	ketoconazole	Possible increased hepatotoxicity
	methotrexate	Possible increased hepatotoxicity
feverfew (*Tanacetum parthenium*)	aspirin	Increased bleeding potential
	heparin	Increased bleeding potential
	NSAIDs	Increased bleeding potential
	warfarin	Increased bleeding potential
garlic (*Allium sativum*)	aspirin	Increased bleeding potential
	insulin	Additive hypoglycemic effects
	NSAIDs	Increased bleeding potential
	oral hypoglycemic agents	Additive hypoglycemic effects
	warfarin	Increased bleeding potential

(continued)

Table 11.5   **Common Herb-Drug Interactions (Continued)**

Common (*Scientific*) Name	Interacts with	Comments
ginger (*Zingiber officinalis*)	aspirin	Increased bleeding potential
	heparin	Increased bleeding potential
	NSAIDs	Increased bleeding potential
	warfarin	Increased bleeding potential
ginkgo (*Ginkgo biloba*)	anticonvulsants	May decrease anticonvulsant effectiveness
	aspirin	Increased bleeding potential
	heparin	Increased bleeding potential
	NSAIDs	Increased bleeding potential
	tricyclic antidepressants	May decrease seizure threshold
	warfarin	Increased bleeding potential
ginseng (*Panax quinquefolius/ Eleutherococcus senticosus*)	CNS depressants	Potentiate sedation
	digoxin	Increased toxicity
	diuretics	May attenuate diuretic effects
	insulin	Increased hypoglycemic effects
	MAO inhibitors	Hypertension, manic symptoms, headaches, nervousness
	oral hypoglycemic agents	Increased hypoglycemic effects
	warfarin	Decreased anticoagulant effects
goldenseal (*Hydrastis canadensis/Eleutherococcus senticosus*)	diuretics	May attenuate diuretic effects
kava kava (*Piper methysticum*)	barbiturates	Potentiate sedation
	benzodiazepines	Potentiate sedation
	CNS depressants	Potentiate sedation
	levodopa/carbidopa	Worsening of Parkinson's symptoms
	phenothiazines	Increased risk and severity of dystonic reactions
St. John's wort (*Hypericum perforatum*)	CNS depressants	Potentiate sedation
	cyclosporine	May decrease cyclosporine levels
	efavirenz	Decreased antiretroviral activity
	MAO inhibitors	May cause hypertensive crisis
	opiate analgesics	Increased sedation
	protease inhibitors	Decreased antiretroviral activity of indinavir
	reserpine	Antagonize hypotensive effects
	selective serotonin reuptake inhibitors	May cause serotonin syndrome[*]
	theophylline	Decreased theophylline efficacy
	tricyclic antidepressants	May cause serotonin syndrome[*]
	warfarin	Decreased anticoagulant effects
valerian (*Valeriana officinalis*)	barbiturates	Potentiate sedation
	benzodiazepines	Potentiate sedation
	CNS depressants	Potentiate sedation

[*]Serotonin syndrome: headache, dizziness, sweating, agitation

Source: Data modified from www.prenhall.com/drugguides

CHAPTER REVIEW

Key Concepts

The numbered key concepts provide a succinct summary of the important points from the corresponding numbered section within the chapter. If any of these points are not clear, refer to the numbered section within the chapter for review. Expanded versions can be found on the companion website.

11.1 Complementary and alternative medicine is a set of diverse therapies and healing systems used by many people for disease prevention and self-healing.

11.2 Natural products obtained from plants have been used as medicines for thousands of years.

11.3 Herbal products are available in a variety of formulations, some containing standarized extracts and others containing whole herbs.

11.4 Herbal products and dietary supplements are regulated by the Dietary Supplement Health and Education Act of 1994, which does not require safety or efficacy testing prior to marketing.

11.5 Natural products may have pharmacologic actions and result in adverse effects, including significant interactions with prescription medications.

Review Questions

1. When obtaining a medical history, the nurse finds the patient is taking St. John's wort. How might this affect the treatment plan for this patient who has been diagnosed with clinical depression?

2. How does the federal regulation of drugs differ from that of dietary supplements?

3. Using specific examples, give the types of claims or statements that are *not* allowed on a dietary supplement label, according to the DSHEA.

4. An 80-years-old patient is suffering from chronic back pain and has been unresponsive to nonnarcotic medications. Name complementary therapies the patient might consider to find pain relief.

Critical Thinking Questions

1. A 44-year-old breast cancer survivor is placed on tamoxifen (Nolvadex) 20 mg PO daily. Since receiving chemotherapy, the patient has not had a menstrual cycle. She is concerned about being menopausal and wonders about the possibility of using a soy-based product as a form of natural hormone replacement. How should the nurse advise the patient?

2. A 62-year-old male patient is recuperating from a myocardial infarction. He is on the anticoagulant warfarin sodium (Coumadin) and antidysrhythmic digitalis. He talks to his wife about starting garlic to help lower his blood lipid levels and ginseng because he has heard it helps in coronary artery disease. Discuss the potential concerns about the use of garlic and ginseng by this patient.

3. A 22-year-old female college student is brought to the emergency room. She has just experienced a seizure in her dormitory. Her apical pulse is 122 and blood pressure is 166/92 mm Hg. Her roommate states that she "has never done this before" and she takes no prescribed medications. What should the nurse consider when conducting the assessment?

 ## EXPLORE MediaLink

NCLEX review, case studies, and other interactive resources for this chapter can be found on the companion website at www.prenhall.com/adams. Click on "Chapter 11" to select the activities for this chapter. For animations, more NCLEX review questions, and an audio glossary, access the accompanying CD-ROM in this textbook.

DRUGS AT A GLANCE: ABUSED SUBSTANCES

CNS DEPRESSANTS
Sedatives
Barbiturates
Benzodiazepines
Opioids
Ethyl alcohol

CANNABINOIDS
Marijuana

HALLUCINOGENS
LSD
Other hallucinogens

CNS STIMULANTS
Amphetamines and methylphenidate
Cocaine
Caffeine

NICOTINE

MediaLink www.prenhall.com/adams

CD-ROM
Animation:
   Cocaine
Audio Glossary
NCLEX Review

Companion Website
NCLEX Review
Dosage Calculations
Case Study
Expanded Key Concepts
Challenge Your Knowledge

OBJECTIVES

After reading this chapter, the student should be able to:

1. Explain underlying causes of addiction.
2. Compare and contrast psychological and physical dependence.
3. Compare withdrawal syndromes for the various abused substance classes.
4. Discuss how nurses can recognize drug tolerance in patients.

5. Explain the major characteristics of abuse, dependence, and tolerance resulting from the following substances: alcohol, nicotine, marijuana, hallucinogens, CNS stimulants, sedatives, and opioids.
6. Describe the role of the nurse in delivering care to individuals who have substance abuse issues.

Substance abuse is the self-administration of a drug in a manner that does not conform to the norms within one's given culture or society. Throughout history, individuals have consumed both natural substances and prescription drugs to increase performance, assist with relaxation, alter psychological state, or to simply fit in with the crowd. Substance abuse has a tremendous economic, social, and public health impact on society. Although the terms *drug abuse* and *substance abuse* are sometimes used interchangeably, substance abuse is preferred, because many of these agents are not legal drugs or medications.

12.1 Overview of Substance Abuse

Abused substances belong to a number of diverse chemical classes. They have few structural similarities, but have in common an ability to affect the nervous system, particularly the brain. Some substances, such as opium, marijuana, cocaine, nicotine, caffeine, and alcohol, are obtained from natural sources. Others are synthetic or designer drugs, created in illegal laboratories for the express purpose of making fortunes in illicit drug trafficking.

Although the public often associates substance abuse with illegal drugs, this is not necessarily the case: Alcohol and nicotine are the two most commonly abused drugs. Legal, prescription medications such as methylphenidate (Ritalin) and meperidine (Demerol) are sometimes abused. Illegal substances that are frequently abused include marijuana, volatile inhalants such as aerosols and paint thinners, narcotic analgesics (opioids), sedatives, and hallucinogens such as lysergic acid diethylamide (LSD) and phencyclidine hydrochloride (PCP).

Several drugs once used therapeutically are now illegal due to their high potential for abuse. Cocaine was once widely used as a local anesthetic, but today nearly all the cocaine acquired by users is obtained illegally. LSD is now illegal, although in the 1940s and 1950s, it was used in psychotherapy. Phencyclidine was popular in the early 1960s as an anesthetic, but was withdrawn from the market in 1965 due to patients reporting hallucinations, delusions,

PHARMFACTS	Substance Abuse in the United States

- Each school year, 25% of high school students use an illegal drug on a monthly or more frequent basis.
- An estimated 2.4 million Americans have used heroin during their lives.
- About one in five Americans have lived with an alcoholic while growing up: Children of alcoholic parents are 4 times more likely to become alcoholics than children of nonalcoholic parents.
- Alcohol is an important factor in 68% of manslaughters, 54% of murders, 48% of robberies, and 44% of burglaries.
- Among youth between the ages of 12 and 17, over 7 million drank alcohol at least once in the past year. Girls are as likely as boys to drink alcohol.
- In 2002, 15% of eighth graders and almost 36% of twelfth graders reported using marijuana in the past year.
- In 2002, 5% of high school seniors reported using cocaine, down from 9.8% in 1999.
- In 2002, almost 4% of twelfth graders reported using LSD, down from 14% in 1997.
- In 2002, 15% of eighth graders reported using volatile inhalants, down from 21% in 1997.
- In 2002, 57% of twelfth graders and 31% of eighth graders reported they had tried smoking cigarettes.
- In 2002, 10% of twelfth graders reported they had ever used Ecstasy (MDMA).
- 28 million Americans have used illicit drugs at least once.

Source: www.nida.nih.gov

MediaLink Cocaine Animation

and anxiety after recovering from anesthesia. Many amphetamines once used for bronchodilation were discontinued in the 1980s after psychotic episodes were reported.

12.2 Neurobiological and Psychosocial Components of Substance Abuse

Addiction is an overwhelming compulsion that drives someone to repetitive drug-taking behavior, despite serious health and social consequences. It is impossible to accurately predict whether a person will become a substance abuser. Attempts to predict a person's addictive tendency using psychological profiles or genetic markers have largely been unsuccessful. Substance abuse depends on multiple complex, interacting variables. These variables focus on the following categories.

- *Agent or drug factors* Cost, availability, dose, mode of administration (e.g., oral, IV, inhalation), speed of onset/termination, and length of drug use
- *User factors* Genetic factors (e.g., metabolic enzymes, innate tolerance), propensity for risk-taking behavior, prior experiences with drugs, disease that may require a scheduled drug
- *Environmental factors* Social/community norms, role models, peer influences, educational opportunities

In the case of legal prescription drugs, addiction may begin with a legitimate need for pharmacotherapy. For example, narcotic analgesics may be indicated for pain relief or sedatives for a sleep disorder. These drugs may result in a favorable experience, such as pain relief or sleep, and patients will want to repeat these positive experiences.

It is a common misunderstanding, even among some health professionals, that the therapeutic use of scheduled drugs creates large numbers of addicted patients. In fact, prescription drugs rarely cause addiction, when used according to accepted medical protocols. The risk of addiction for prescription medications is primarily a function of the dose and the length of therapy. Because of this, medications having a potential for abuse are usually prescribed at the lowest effective dose and for the shortest time necessary to treat the medical problem. Nurses should administer these medications as prescribed for the relief of patient symptoms, without undue fear of producing dependency. As mentioned in Chapters 1 and 2 ⊕, numerous laws have been passed in an attempt to limit drug abuse and addiction.

12.3 Physical and Psychological Dependence

Whether a substance is addictive is related to how easily an individual can stop taking the agent on a repetitive basis. When a person has an overwhelming desire to take a drug and cannot stop, this is referred to as substance dependence. Substance dependence is classified by two categories, physical dependence and psychological dependence.

Physical dependence refers to an altered physical condition caused by the nervous system adapting to repeated substance use. Over time, the body's cells are tricked into believing that it is normal for the substance to be continually present. With physical dependence, uncomfortable symptoms known as withdrawal result when the agent is discontinued. Opioids, such as morphine and heroin, may produce physical dependence rather quickly with repeated doses, particularly when taken intravenously. Alcohol, sedatives, some stimulants, and nicotine are other examples of substances that may produce physical dependence easily with extended use.

In contrast, psychological dependence produces no signs of physical discomfort after the agent is discontinued. The user, however, has an overwhelming desire to continue substance use despite obvious negative economic, physical, or social consequences. This intense craving may be associated with the patient's home environment or social contacts. Strong psychological craving for a substance may continue for months or even years and is often responsible for relapses during substance abuse therapy, and a return to drug-seeking behavior. Psychological dependence usually requires relatively high doses for a prolonged time, such as with marijuana and antianxiety drugs; however, psychological dependence may develop quickly, perhaps after only one use, with crack—a potent, inexpensive form of cocaine.

12.4 Withdrawal Syndrome

Once a patient becomes physically dependent and the substance is discontinued, a withdrawal syndrome will occur. Symptoms of withdrawal syndrome may be particularly severe for patients who are physically dependent on alcohol and sedatives. Because of the severity of the symptoms, the process of withdrawal from these agents is best accomplished in a substance abuse treatment facility. Examples of the types of withdrawal syndromes experienced with different abused substances are shown in Table 12.1.

Prescription drugs may be used to reduce the severity of withdrawal symptoms. For example, alcohol withdrawal can be treated with a short-acting benzodiazepine such as oxazepam (Serax), and opioid withdrawal can be treated with methadone. Symptoms of nicotine withdrawal may be relieved by nicotine replacement therapy in the form of patches or chewing gum. No specific pharmacologic intervention is indicated for withdrawal from CNS stimulants, hallucinogens, marijuana, or inhalants.

With chronic substance abuse, patients will often associate their conditions and surroundings, including social contacts with other users, with the taking of the drug. Users tend to revert back to drug-seeking behavior when they return to the company of other substance abusers. Counselors often encourage users to refrain from associating with past social contacts or relationships with other substance abusers to lessen the possibility for relapse. The formation of new

Table 12.1	Withdrawal Symptoms of Selected Drugs of Abuse
Drug	**Symptoms**
opioids	excessive sweating, restlessness, dilated pupils, agitation, goosebumps, tremor, violent yawning, increased heart rate and blood pressure, nausea/vomiting, abdominal cramps and pain, muscle spasms with kicking movements, weight loss
barbiturates and similar sedative-hypnotics	insomnia, anxiety, weakness, abdominal cramps, tremor, anorexia, seizures, hallucinations, delirium
benzodiazepines	insomnia, restlessness, abdominal pain, nausea, sensitivity to light and sound, headache, fatigue, muscle twitches
alcohol	tremors, fatigue, anxiety, abdominal cramping, hallucinations, confusion, seizures, delirium
cocaine and amphetamines	mental depression, anxiety, extreme fatigue, hunger
nicotine	irritability, anxiety, restlessness, headaches, increased appetite, insomnia, inability to concentrate, decrease in heart rate and blood pressure
marijuana	irritability, restlessness, insomnia, tremor, chills, weight loss
hallucinogens	rarely observed; dependent upon specific drug

social contacts as a result of association with self-help groups such as Alcoholics Anonymous helps some patients transition to a drug-free lifestyle.

12.5 Tolerance

Tolerance is a biological condition that occurs when the body adapts to a substance after repeated administration. Over time, higher doses of the agent are required to produce the same initial effect. For example, at the start of pharmacotherapy, a patient may find that 2 mg of a sedative is effective at inducing sleep. After taking the medication for several months, the patient notices that it takes 4 mg or perhaps 6 mg to fall asleep. Development of drug tolerance is common for substances that affect the nervous system. Tolerance should be thought of as a natural consequence of continued drug use and not be considered evidence of addiction or substance abuse.

Tolerance does not develop at the same rate for all actions of a drug. For example, patients usually develop tolerance to the nausea and vomiting produced by narcotic analgesics after only a few doses. Tolerance to the mood-altering effects of these drugs and to their ability to reduce pain develops more slowly but eventually may be complete. Tolerance never develops to the drug's ability to constrict the pupils. Patients will often endure annoying side effects of drugs, such as the sedation caused by antihistamines, if they know that tolerance will develop quickly to these effects.

Once tolerance develops to a substance, it often extends to closely related drugs. This phenomenon is known as **cross-tolerance.** For example, a heroin addict will be tolerant to the analgesic effects of other opioids such as morphine or meperidine. Patients who have developed tolerance to alcohol will show tolerance to other CNS depressants such as barbiturates, benzodiazepines, and some general anesthetics. This has important clinical implications for the nurse, as doses of these related medications will have to be adjusted accordingly to obtain maximum therapeutic benefit.

SPECIAL CONSIDERATIONS
Pediatric Abuse of Volatile Inhalants

Many parents are concerned about their children smoking tobacco or marijuana, or becoming addicted to crack or amphetamines. Yet few parents consider that the most common sources of abused substances lie in their own homes. Inhaling volatile chemicals, known as huffing, is most prevalent in the 10- to 12-year-old group, and declines with age; one in five children has done this by the eighth grade. Virtually any organic compound can be huffed, including nail polish remover, spray paint, household glue, correction fluid, propane, gasoline, and even whipped cream propellants. These agents are readily available, inexpensive, legal, and can be used anytime and anywhere. Children can die after a single exposure, or suffer brain damage which may be manifested as slurred or slow speech, tremor, memory loss, or personality changes. Nurses who work with pediatric patients should be aware of the widespread nature of this type of abuse and advise parents to keep close watch on volatile substances.

The terms *immunity* and *resistance* are often confused with tolerance. These terms more correctly refer to the immune system and infections, and should not be used interchangeably with tolerance. For example, microorganisms become resistant to the effects of an antibiotic: They do not become tolerant. Patients become tolerant to the effects of pain relievers: They do not become resistant.

12.6 CNS Depressants

CNS depressants form a group of drugs that cause patients to feel sedated or relaxed. Drugs in this group include barbiturates, nonbarbiturate sedative-hypnotics, benzodiazepines, alcohol, and opioids. Although the majority of these are legal substances, they are controlled due to their abuse potential.

Sedatives

Sedatives, also known as tranquilizers, are primarily prescribed for sleep disorders and certain forms of epilepsy. The two primary classes of sedatives are the barbiturates and the nonbarbiturate sedative-hypnotics. Their actions, indications, safety profiles, and addictive potential are roughly equivalent. Physical dependence, psychological dependence, and tolerance develop when these agents are taken for extended periods at high doses. Patients sometimes abuse these drugs by faking prescriptions or by sharing their medication with friends. They are commonly combined with other drugs of abuse, such as CNS stimulants or alcohol. Addicts often alternate between amphetamines, which keep them awake for several days, and barbiturates, which are needed to help them relax and fall sleep.

Many sedatives have a long duration of action: Effects may last an entire day, depending on the specific drug. Patients may appear dull or apathetic. Higher doses resemble alcohol intoxication, with slurred speech and motor incoordination. Four commonly abused barbiturates are pentobarbital (Nembutal), amobarbital (Amytal), secobarbital (Seconal), and a combination of secobarbital and amobarbital (Tuinal). The medical use of barbiturates and nonbarbiturate sedative-hypnotics has declined markedly over the past 20 years. The use of barbiturates in treating sleep disorders is discussed in Chapter 14, and their use in epilepsy is presented in Chapter 15 ⊂⊃.

Overdoses of barbiturates and nonbarbiturate sedative-hypnotics are extremely dangerous. The drugs suppress the respiratory centers in the brain and the user may stop breathing or lapse into a coma. Death may result from barbiturate overdose. Withdrawal symptoms from these drugs resemble those of alcohol withdrawal and may be life-threatening.

Benzodiazepines are another group of CNS depressants that have a potential for abuse. They are one of the most widely prescribed classes of drugs, and have largely replaced the barbiturates for certain disorders. Their primary indication is anxiety (Chapter 14), although they are also used to prevent seizures (Chapter 15) and as muscle relaxants (Chapter 45) ⊂⊃. Popular benzodiazepines include alprazolam (Xanax), diazepam (Valium), temazepam (Restoril), triazolam (Halcion), and midazolam (Versed).

Although they are the most frequently prescribed drug class, benzodiazepine abuse is not common. Individuals abusing benzodiazepines may appear carefree, detached, sleepy, or disoriented. Death due to overdose is rare, even with high doses. Users may combine these agents with alcohol, cocaine, or heroin to augment their drug experience. If combined with these other agents, overdose may be lethal. The benzodiazepine withdrawal syndrome is less severe than that of barbiturates or alcohol.

Opioids

Opioids, also known as narcotic analgesics, are prescribed for severe pain, persistent cough, and diarrhea. The opioid class includes natural substances obtained from the unripe seeds of the poppy plant such as opium, morphine, and codeine, and synthetic drugs such as propoxyphene (Darvon), meperidine (Demerol), oxycodone (OxyContin), fentanyl (Duragesic, Sublimaze), methadone (Dolophine), and heroin. The therapeutic effects of the opioids are discussed in detail in Chapter 19 ⊂⊃.

The effects of *oral* opioids begin within 30 minutes and may last over a day. *Parenteral* forms produce immediate effects, including the brief, intense rush of euphoria sought by heroin addicts. Individuals experience a range of CNS effects from extreme pleasure to slowed body activities and profound sedation. Signs include constricted pupils, an increase in the pain threshold, and respiratory depression.

Addiction to opioids can occur rapidly, and withdrawal can produce intense symptoms. While extremely unpleasant, withdrawal from opioids is not life-threatening, compared to barbiturate withdrawal. Methadone is a narcotic sometimes used to treat opioid addiction. Although methadone has addictive properties of its own, it does not produce the same degree of euphoria as other opioids, and its effects are longer lasting. Heroin addicts are switched to methadone, to prevent unpleasant withdrawal symptoms. Since methadone is taken orally, patients are no longer exposed to serious risks associated with intravenous drug use, such as hepatitis and AIDS. Patients sometimes remain on methadone maintenance for a lifetime. Withdrawal from methadone is more prolonged than with heroin or morphine, but the symptoms are less intense.

Ethyl Alcohol

Ethyl alcohol, commonly known as alcohol, is one of the most commonly abused drugs. Alcohol is a legal substance for adults, and it is readily available as beer, wine, and liquor. The economic, social, and health consequences of alcohol abuse are staggering. Despite the enormous negative consequences associated with long-term use, small quantities of alcohol consumed on a daily basis have been found to reduce the risk of stroke and heart attack.

Alcohol is classified as a CNS depressant, because it slows the region of the brain responsible for alertness and wakefulness. Alcohol easily crosses the blood-brain barrier so its effects are observed within 5 to 30 minutes after consumption. Effects of alcohol are directly proportional to the amount consumed, and include relaxation, sedation, memory impairment, loss of motor coordination, reduced judgment, and decreased inhibition. Alcohol also imparts a characteristic odor to the breath and increases blood flow in certain areas of the skin, causing a flushed face, pink cheeks, or red nose. Although these symptoms are easily recognized, the nurse must be aware that other substances and disorders may cause similar effects. For example, many antianxiety agents, sedatives, and antidepressants can cause drowsiness, memory difficulties, and loss of motor coordination. Certain mouthwashes contain alcohol and cause the breath to smell alcoholic. During assessment, the skilled nurse must consider these factors before suspicion of alcohol use can be confirmed.

The presence of food in the stomach will slow the absorption of alcohol, thus delaying the onset of drug action. Metabolism, or detoxification of alcohol by the liver occurs at a slow, constant rate, which is not affected by the presence of food. The average rate is about 15 ml per hour—the practical equivalent of one alcoholic beverage per hour. If consumed at a higher rate, alcohol will accumulate in the blood and produce greater effects on the brain. Acute overdoses of alcohol produce vomiting, severe hypotension, respiratory failure, and coma. Death due to alcohol poisoning is not uncommon. The nurse should teach patients to never combine alcohol consumption with the use of other CNS depressants, as their effects are cumulative and profound sedation or coma may result.

Chronic alcohol consumption produces both psychologic and physiologic dependence and results in a large number of adverse health effects. The organ most affected by chronic alcohol abuse is the liver. Alcoholism is a common cause of cirrhosis, a debilitating and often fatal failure of the liver to perform its vital functions. Liver failure results in abnormalities in blood clotting and nutritional deficiencies, and sensitizes the patient to the effects of all medications metabolized by the liver. For alcoholic patients, the nurse should begin therapy with lower than normal doses until the adverse effects of the medication can be assessed.

The alcohol withdrawal syndrome is severe and may be life-threatening. The use of anticonvulsants in the treatment of alcohol withdrawal is discussed in Chapter 15 🔗 . Long-term treatment for alcohol abuse includes behavioral counseling and self-help groups such as Alcoholics Anonymous. Disulfiram (Antabuse) may be given to discourage relapses. Disulfiram inhibits acetaldehyde dehydrogenase, the enzyme that metabolizes alcohol. If alcohol is consumed while taking disulfiram, the patient becomes violently ill within 5–10 minutes, with headache, shortness of breath, nausea/vomiting, and other unpleasant symptoms. Disulfiram is only effective in highly motivated patients, since the success of pharmacotherapy is entirely dependent upon patient compliance. Alcohol sensitivity continues for up to 2 weeks after disulfiram has been discontinued. As a pregnancy category X drug, disulfiram should never be taken during pregnancy.

12.7 Cannabinoids

Cannabinoids are agents obtained from the hemp plant *Cannabis sativa,* which thrives in tropical climates. Cannabinoid agents are usually smoked, and include marijuana, hashish, and hash oil. Although over 61 cannabinoid chemicals have been identified, the ingredient responsible for most of the psychoactive properties is delta-9-tetrahydrocannabinol (THC).

Marijuana

Marijuana, also known as grass, pot, weed, reefer, or dope, is a natural product obtained from *C. sativa*. It is the most commonly used illicit drug in the United States.

Use of marijuana slows motor activity, decreases coordination, and causes disconnected thoughts, feelings of paranoia, and euphoria. It increases thirst and craving for food, particularly chocolate and other candies. One hallmark symptom of marijuana use is red or bloodshot eyes, caused by dilation of blood vessels. THC accumulates in the gonads.

When inhaled, marijuana produces effects that occur within minutes and last up to 24 hours. Because marijuana smoke is inhaled more deeply and held within the lungs for a longer time than cigarette smoke, marijuana smoke introduces 4 times more particulates (tar) into the lungs than tobacco smoke. Smoking marijuana on a daily basis may increase the risk of lung cancer and other respiratory disorders. Chronic use is associated with a lack of motivation in achieving or pursuing life goals.

Unlike many abused substances, marijuana produces little physical dependence or tolerance. Withdrawal symptoms are mild, if they are experienced at all. Metabolites of THC, however, remain in the body for months to years, allowing laboratory specialists to easily determine whether someone has taken marijuana. For several days after use, THC can also be detected in the urine. Despite numerous attempts to demonstrate therapeutic applications for marijuana, results have been controversial and the medical value of the drug remains to be proven.

12.8 Hallucinogens

Hallucinogens consist of a diverse class of chemicals that have in common the ability to produce an altered, dream-like state of consciousness. Sometimes called **psychedelics,** the prototype substance for this class is lysergic acid diethylamide (LSD). All hallucinogens are Schedule I drugs: They have no medical use.

LSD

For nearly all drugs of abuse, predictable symptoms occur in every user. Effects from hallucinogens, however, are highly variable and dependent upon the mood and expectations of the user, and the surrounding environment in which the substance is used. Two patients taking the same agent will report completely different symptoms, and the same patient may report different symptoms with each use. Users who take LSD or psilocybin (magic mushrooms, or shrooms) (Fig. 12.1) may experience symptoms such as laughter, visions, religious revelations, or deep personal insights. Common occurrences are hallucinations and after-images being projected onto people as they move. Users also report unusually bright lights and vivid colors. Some users hear voices; others report smells. Many experience a profound sense of truth and deep-directed thoughts. Unpleasant experiences can be terrifying and may include anxiety, panic attacks, confusion, severe depression, and paranoia.

LSD, also called acid, the beast, blotter acid, and California sunshine, is derived from a fungus that grows on rye

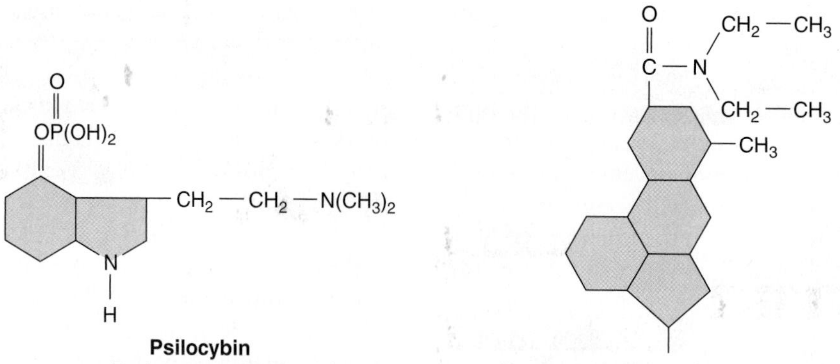

Figure 12.1 | Comparison of the chemical structures of psilocybin and LSD. Psilocybin (at left) is derived from a mushroom *Source: Pearson Education/PH College.*

and other grains. LSD is nearly always administered orally and can be manufactured in capsule, tablet, or liquid form. A common and inexpensive method for distributing LSD is to place drops of the drug on paper, often containing the images of cartoon characters or graphics related to the drug culture. After drying, the paper containing the LSD is ingested to produce the drug's effects.

LSD is distributed throughout the body immediately after use. Effects are experienced within an hour, and may last from 6 to 12 hours. It affects the central and autonomic nervous systems, increasing blood pressure, elevating body temperature, dilating pupils, and increasing the heart rate. Repeated use may cause impaired memory and inability to reason. In extreme cases, patients may develop psychoses. One unusual adverse effect is flashbacks, in which the user experiences the effects of the drug again, sometimes weeks, months, or years after the drug was initially taken. While tolerance is observed, little or no dependence occurs with the hallucinogens.

Other Hallucinogens

In addition to LSD, other hallucinogens that are abused include the following:

- *Mescaline* Found in the peyote cactus of Mexico and Central America (Fig. 12.2)
- *MDMA (3,4-methylenedioxymethamphetamine, XTC or Ecstasy)* An amphetamine originally synthesized for research purposes, but has since become extremely popular among teens and young adults
- *DOM (2,5 dimethoxy-4-methylamphetamine)* A recreational drug often linked with rave parties as a drug of choice having the name STP
- *MDA (3,4-methylenedioxyamphetamine)* Called the love drug due to a belief that it enhances sexual desires
- *Phenylcyclohexylpiperadine (PCP; angel dust or phencyclidine)* Produces a trancelike state that may last for days and results in severe brain damage
- *Ketamine (date rape drug or special coke)* produces unconsciousness and amnesia; primary legal use is as an anesthetic

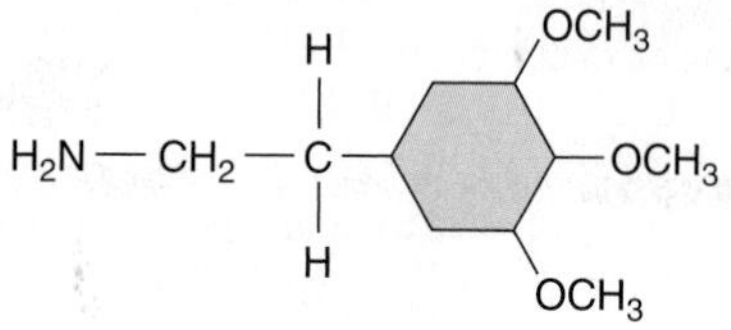

Figure 12.2 | The chemical structure of mescaline, derived from the peyote cactus *Source: Pearson Education/PH College.*

12.9 CNS Stimulants

Stimulants include a diverse family of drugs known for their ability to increase the activity of the CNS. Some are available by prescription for use in the treatment of narcolepsy, obesity, and attention deficit disorder. As drugs of abuse, CNS stimulants are taken to produce a sense of exhilaration, improve mental and physical performance, reduce appetite, prolong wakefulness, or simply "get high." Stimulants include the amphetamines, cocaine, methylphenidate, and caffeine.

Amphetamines and Methylphenidate

CNS stimulants have effects similar to the neurotransmitter norepinephrine (Chapter 13) ⊙ . Norepinephrine affects awareness and wakefulness by activating neurons in a part of the brain called the reticular formation. High doses of amphetamines give the user a feeling of self-confidence, euphoria, alertness, and empowerment; but just as short-term use induces favorable feelings, long-term use often results in feelings of restlessness, anxiety, and fits of rage, especially when the user is coming down from a high induced by the drug.

Most CNS stimulants affect cardiovascular and respiratory activity, resulting in increased blood pressure and increased respiration rate. Other symptoms include dilated pupils, sweating, and tremors. Overdoses of some stimulants lead to seizures and cardiac arrest.

NATURAL THERAPIES	Herbal Stimulants and Ephedra

Recovering from addiction may be a difficult experience. Individuals claim that discretionary use of some herbal stimulants may ease the symptoms associated with recovery. Examples are kola, damiana, Asiatic and Siberian ginseng, and gotu kola. These agents are thought to stimulate the CNS, providing just enough of an effect to reduce tension and the stresses associated with drug craving.

Ephedra is an herbal stimulant that has received considerable attention. In addition to its stimulant effects of increasing wakefulness and alertness, the herb affects the cardiovascular system to potentially cause increases in blood pressure and heart rate. Ephedra is an ingredient in a variety of products marketed as dietary supplements for weight loss, energy enhancement, and body-building purposes. It has been implicated in several deaths and serious adverse effects, such as heart attack and stroke, and may be removed from the U.S. market due to safety concerns. Nurses should advise their patients to never take this herbal stimulant until they have consulted with their physician.

Amphetamines and dextroamphetamines were once widely prescribed for depression, obesity, drowsiness, and congestion. In the 1960s it became recognized that the medical uses of amphetamines did not outweigh their risk for dependence. Due to the development of safer medications, the current therapeutic uses of these drugs are extremely limited. Most substance abusers obtain these agents from illegal laboratories, which can easily produce amphetamines and make tremendous profits.

Dextroamphetamine (Dexedrine) may be used for short-term weight loss, when all other attempts to reduce weight have been exhausted, and to treat narcolepsy. Methamphetamine, commonly called ice, is often used as a recreational drug for users who like the rush that it gives them. It usually is administered in powder or crystal form, but it may also be smoked. Methamphetamine is a Schedule II drug marketed under the trade name Desoxyn, although most abusers obtain it from illegal methamphetamine laboratories. A structural analog of methamphetamine, methcathinone (street name, Cat) is made illegally and snorted, taken orally, or injected IV. Methcathinone is a Schedule I agent.

Methylphenidate (Ritalin) is a CNS stimulant widely prescribed for children diagnosed with attention deficit disorder (ADD). Ritalin has a calming effect in children who are inattentive or hyperactive. It stimulates the alertness center in the brain and the child is able to focus on tasks for longer periods of time. This explains the paradoxical calming effects that this stimulant has on children, which is usually opposite that of adults. The therapeutic applications of methylphenidate are discussed in Chapter 16 ⬭ .

Ritalin is a Schedule II drug that has many of the same effects as cocaine and amphetamines. It is sometimes abused by adolescents and adults seeking euphoria. Tablets are crushed and used intranasally or dissolved in liquid and injected IV. Ritalin is sometimes mixed with heroin, a combination called a speedball.

Cocaine

Cocaine is a natural substance obtained from leaves of the coca plant, which grows in the Andes Mountain region of South America. Documentation suggests that the plant has been used by Andean cultures since 2500 B.C. Natives in this region chew the coca leaves, or make teas of the dried leaves. Because it is taken orally, absorption is slow, and the leaves contain only 1% cocaine, users do not suffer the ill effects caused by chemically pure extracts from the plant. In the Andean culture, use of coca leaves is not considered substance abuse because it is part of the social norms of that society.

Cocaine is a Schedule II drug that produces actions similar to the amphetamines, although its effects are usually more rapid and intense. It is the second most commonly abused illicit drug in the United States. Routes of administration include snorting, smoking, and injecting. In small doses, cocaine produces feelings of intense euphoria, a decrease in hunger, analgesia, illusions of physical strength, and increased sensory perception. Larger doses will magnify these effects and also cause rapid heartbeat, sweating, dilation of the pupils, and an elevated body temperature. After the feelings of euphoria diminish, the user is left with a sense of irritability, insomnia, depression, and extreme distrust. Some users report the sensation that insects are crawling under the skin. Users who snort cocaine develop a chronic runny nose, a crusty redness around the nostrils, and deterioration of the nasal cartilage. Overdose can result in dysrhythmias, convulsions, stroke, or death due to respiratory arrest. The withdrawal syndrome for amphetamines and cocaine is much less intense than that from alcohol or barbiturate abuse.

Caffeine

Caffeine is a natural substance found in the seeds, leaves, or fruits of more than 63 plant species throughout the world. Significant amounts of caffeine are consumed in chocolate, coffee, tea, soft drinks, and ice cream. Caffeine is sometimes added to OTC pain relievers because it has been shown to increase the effectiveness of these medications. Caffeine travels to almost all parts of the body after ingestion and several hours are needed for the body to metabolize and eliminate the drug. Caffeine has a pronounced diuretic effect.

Caffeine is considered a CNS stimulant because it produces increased mental alertness, restlessness, nervousness, irritability, and insomnia. The physical effects of caffeine include bronchodilation, increased blood pressure, increased production of stomach acid, and changes in blood glucose levels. Repeated use of caffeine may result in physical dependence and tolerance. Withdrawal symptoms include headaches, fatigue, depression, and impaired performance of daily activities.

12.10 Nicotine

Nicotine is sometimes considered a CNS stimulant and although it does increase alertness, its actions and long-term consequences place it into a class by itself. Nicotine is unique among abused substances in that it is legal, strongly addictive, and highly carcinogenic. Furthermore, use of tobacco can cause harmful effects to those in the immediate area due to secondhand smoke. Patients often do not consider tobacco use as substance abuse.

Tobacco Use and Nicotine

The most common method by which nicotine enters the body is through the inhalation of cigarette, pipe, or cigar smoke. Tobacco smoke contains over 1,000 chemicals, a significant number of which are carcinogens. The primary addictive substance present in cigarette smoke is nicotine. Effects of inhaled nicotine may last from 30 minutes to several hours.

Nicotine affects many body systems including the nervous, cardiovascular, and endocrine systems. Nicotine stimulates the CNS directly, causing increased alertness and ability to focus, feelings of relaxation, and light-headedness. The cardiovascular effects of nicotine include an accelerated heart rate and increased blood pressure, caused by activation of nicotinic receptors located throughout the autonomic nervous system (Chapter 13) ⊙ . These cardiovascular effects can be particularly serious in patients taking oral contraceptives: The risk of a fatal heart attack is 5 times greater in smokers than in nonsmokers. Muscular tremors may occur with moderate doses of nicotine and convulsions may result from very high doses. Nicotine affects the endocrine system by increasing the basal metabolic rate, leading to weight loss. Nicotine also reduces appetite. Chronic use leads to bronchitis, emphysema, and lung cancer.

Both psychologic and physical dependence occur relatively quickly with nicotine. Once started on tobacco, patients tend to continue their drug use for many years, despite overwhelming medical evidence that the quality of life will be adversely affected and their lifespan shortened. Discontinuation results in agitation, weight gain, anxiety, headache, and an extreme craving for the drug. Although nicotine replacement patches and gum assist patients in dealing with the unpleasant withdrawal symptoms, only 25% of patients who attempt to stop smoking remain tobacco-free a year later.

SPECIAL CONSIDERATIONS
Ethnic Groups and Smoking

The incidence of tobacco use varies among racial and ethnic groups. The highest rate is among American Indians and Alaska Natives. African Americans also have a high prevalence of smoking. The lowest prevalence is among Asian American and Hispanic women.

Smoking and other tobacco uses are major contributors of the three leading causes of death in African Americans—heart disease, cancer, and stroke. African American men are at least 50% more likely to develop lung cancer than white men. Cerebrovascular disease is twice as high among African American men compared to white men. African American women do not fare any better: The incidence of strokes are twice as high among African American women as among white women. Nurses should educate their ethnic minority patients, particularly African Americans, about their increased risk of disease.

12.11 The Nurse's Role in Substance Abuse

The nurse serves a key role in the prevention, diagnosis, and treatment of substance abuse. A thorough medical history must include questions about substance abuse. In the case of IV drug users, the nurse must consider the possibility of HIV infection, hepatitis, tuberculosis, and associated diagnoses. Patients are often reluctant to report their drug use, for fear of embarrassment or being arrested. The nurse must be knowledgeable about the signs of substance abuse and withdrawal symptoms, and develop a keen sense of perception during the assessment stage. A trusting nurse-patient relationship is essential to helping patients deal with their dependence.

It is often difficult for a healthcare provider not to condemn or stigmatize a patient for their substance abuse. Nurses, especially those in large cities, are all too familiar with the devastating medical, economic, and social consequences of heroin and cocaine abuse. The nurse must be firm in disapproving of substance abuse, yet compassionate in trying to help the patient receive treatment. A list of social agencies dealing with dependency should be readily available to provide patients. When possible, the nurse should attempt to involve family members and other close contacts in the treatment regimen. Educating the patient and family members about the long-term consequences of substance abuse is essential.

CHAPTER REVIEW

Key Concepts

The numbered key concepts provide a succinct summary of the important points from the corresponding numbered section within the chapter. If any of these points are not clear, refer to the numbered section within the chapter for review. Expanded versions can be found on the companion website.

12.1 A wide variety of different substances may be abused by individuals, all of which share the common characteristic of altering brain physiology and/or perception.

12.2 Addiction is an overwhelming compulsion to continue repeated drug use that has both neurobiological and psychosocial components.

12.3 Certain substances can cause both physical and psychological dependence, which result in continued drug-seeking behavior despite negative health and social consequences.

12.4 The withdrawal syndrome is a set of uncomfortable symptoms that occur when an abused substance is no longer available. The severity of the withdrawal syndrome varies among the different drug classes.

12.5 Tolerance is a biological condition that occurs with repeated use of certain substances, and results in higher doses being needed to achieve the same initial response. Cross-tolerance occurs between closely related drugs.

12.6 CNS depressants, which include sedatives, opioids, and ethyl alcohol, decrease the activity of the central nervous system.

12.7 Cannabinoids, which include marijuana, are the most frequently abused class of substances. They cause less physical dependence and tolerance than the CNS depressants.

12.8 Hallucinogens, including LSD, cause an altered state of thought and perception similar to that found in dreams. Their effects are extremely variable and unpredictable.

12.9 CNS stimulants, including amphetamines, methylphenidate, caffeine, and cocaine, increase the activity of the central nervous system and produce increased wakefulness.

12.10 Nicotine is a powerful and highly addictive cardiovascular and CNS stimulant that has serious adverse effects with chronic use.

12.11 The nurse serves an important role in educating patients about the consequences of drug abuse and in recommending appropriate treatment.

Review Questions

1. What is the difference between physical dependence and psychological dependence? How does a patient know when he or she is physically dependent on a substance?

2. Name three legal substances that are abused more commonly than illegal drugs. Are these natural or synthetic substances?

3. By examining and interviewing a patient, how can a nurse distinguish whether the patient is under the influence of marijuana or hallucinogens?

4. Name three classes of CNS stimulants and give examples for each group. Name three major systems in the body affected by stimulants.

Critical Thinking Questions

1. A 16-year-old male is hospitalized in the ICU following the ingestion of a high dose of MDMA (Ecstasy) at a street dance. His mother cannot understand why her son could have such serious renal and cardiovascular complications after "just one dose." The nurse is concerned that the mother lacks sufficient knowledge to be helpful. What teaching does the nurse conduct?

2. The wife of a 24-year-old professional football player is admitted to the ER after being beaten and verbally abused by her husband. She says that he is under a great deal of stress and has been working hard to maintain peak athletic fitness. She says she has noticed that her husband becomes irritable easily. What assessments and interventions should the nurse perform?

3. A 44-year-old businessman travels weekly for his company and has had difficulty sleeping in "one hotel after another." He consulted his healthcare provider and has been taking secobarbital (Seconal) nightly to help him sleep. The patient has called the nurse at the healthcare provider's office and says, "I have just got to have something stronger." What does the nurse consider as part of the assessment?

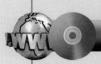

EXPLORE MediaLink

NCLEX review, case studies, and other interactive resources for this chapter can be found on the companion website at www.prenhall.com/adams. Click on "Chapter 12" to select the activities for this chapter. For animations, more NCLEX review questions, and an audio glossary, access the accompanying CD-ROM in this textbook.

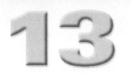

CHAPTER 13

Drugs Affecting the Autonomic Nervous System

DRUGS AT A GLANCE

**PARASYMPATHOMIMETICS
(MUSCARINIC AGONISTS)**

Pr *bethanechol (Urecholine)*

**ANTICHOLINERGICS
(MUSCARINIC BLOCKERS)**

Pr *atropine*

Other Prototypes:

benztropine (Cogentin): Chapter 18
donepezil (Aricept): Chapter 18
ipratropium (Atrovent, Combivent): Chapter 29

**SYMPATHOMIMETICS
(ADRENERGIC AGONISTS)**

Pr *phenylephrine (Neo-Synephrine)*

Other Prototypes:

norepinephrine (Levarterenol): Chapter 26
dopamine (Dopastat, Intropin): Chapter 26
salmeterol (Serevent): Chapter 29
oxymetazoline (Afrin and others): Chapter 31
epinephrine (Adrenalin): Chapter 31

**ADRENERGIC ANTAGONISTS
(ADRENERGIC BLOCKERS)**

Pr *prazosin (Minipress)*

Other Prototypes:

atenolol (Tenormin): Chapter 25
carvedilol (Coreg): Chapter 22
doxazosin (Cardura): Chapter 21
metoprolol (Lopressor): Chapter 25
propranolol (Inderal): Chapter 23
timolol (Timoptic): Chapter 48

metabolized and eliminated by the bod
of this process
PHARMACOLOGY
1. The study of medicines; the disciplir
pertaining to how drugs improve the he
of the human body
PHARMACOPEIA

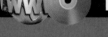 **MediaLink** www.prenhall.com/adams

CD-ROM
Audio Glossary
NCLEX Review

Companion Website
NCLEX Review
Case Study
Care Plans
Dosage Calculations
Nursing Process Focus
Expanded Key Concepts

OBJECTIVES

After reading this chapter, the student should be able to:

1. Identify the two fundamental divisions of the nervous system.
2. Identify the three primary functions of the nervous system.
3. Compare and contrast the actions of the sympathetic and parasympathetic nervous systems.
4. Explain the process of synaptic transmission and the neurotransmitters important to the autonomic nervous system.
5. Compare and contrast the types of responses that occur when a drug activates $alpha_1$-, $alpha_2$-, $beta_1$-, or $beta_2$-adrenergic receptors.
6. Describe the nurse's role in the pharmacologic management of patients receiving drugs affecting the autonomic nervous system.
7. For each of the drug classes listed in Drugs at a Glance, explain the mechanism of drug action, primary actions, and important adverse effects.
8. Use the Nursing Process to care for patients receiving parasympathomimetics, anticholinergics, sympathomimetics, and adrenergic blockers.

Neuropharmacology represents one of the largest, most complicated, and least understood branches of pharmacology. Nervous system drugs are used to treat a large and diverse set of conditions, including pain, anxiety, depression, schizophrenia, insomnia, and convulsions. By their action on nerves, medications are used to treat disorders affecting many body systems. Examples include abnormalities in heart rate and rhythm, hypertension, glaucoma, asthma, and even a runny nose.

The study of nervous system pharmacology extends over the next eight chapters of this textbook. Traditionally, the study of neuropharmacology begins with the autonomic nervous system. A firm grasp of autonomic physiology is necessary to understand nervous, cardiovascular, and respiratory pharmacology. This chapter serves dual purposes. First, it is a comprehensive review of autonomic nervous system physiology, a subject that is often covered superficially in anatomy and physiology classes. Second, it introduces the four fundamental classes of autonomic drugs.

13.1 The Peripheral Nervous System

The nervous system has two major divisions: the central nervous system (CNS) and the peripheral nervous system. The CNS consists of the brain and spinal cord. The peripheral nervous system consists of all nervous tissue outside the CNS, including sensory and motor neurons. The basic functions of the nervous system are as follows:

- Recognize changes in the internal and external environments
- Process and integrate the environmental changes that are perceived
- React to the environmental changes by producing an action or response

Figure 13.1 shows the functional divisions of the nervous system. In the peripheral nervous system, neurons either recognize changes to the environment (sensory division) or respond to these changes by moving muscles or secreting chemicals (motor division). The somatic nervous system consists of nerves that provide *voluntary* control over skeletal muscle. Nerves of the autonomic nervous system, on the other hand, give *involuntary* control over the contraction of smooth muscle and cardiac muscle, and the secretion of

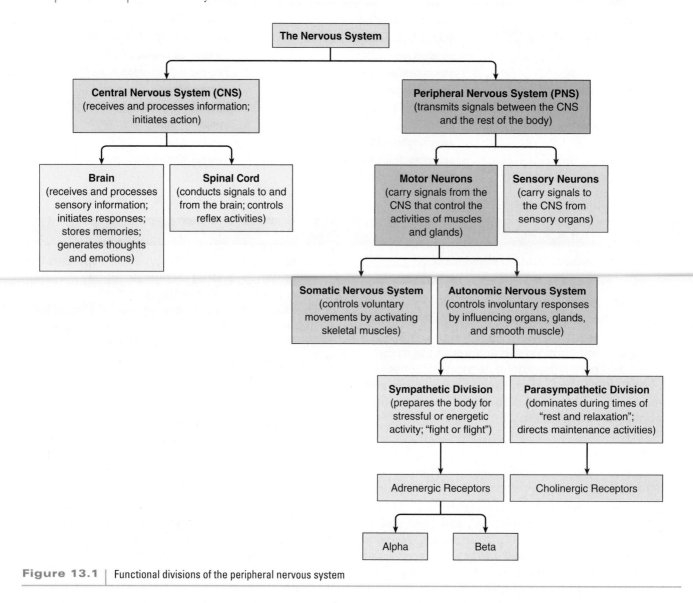

Figure 13.1 | Functional divisions of the peripheral nervous system

glands. Organs and tissues regulated by neurons from the autonomic nervous system include the heart, digestive tract, respiratory tract, reproductive tracts, arteries, salivary glands, and portions of the eye. Whereas only a few medications directly affect the somatic nervous system, a large number affect autonomic nerves.

13.2 The Autonomic Nervous System: Sympathetic and Parasympathetic Branches

The autonomic nervous system has two divisions: the sympathetic and the parasympathetic nervous systems. With a few exceptions, organs and glands receive nerves from both branches of the autonomic nervous system. The ultimate action of the smooth muscle or gland depends on which branch is sending the most signals at a given time. The major actions of the two divisions are shown in Figure 13.2. It is essential that the student learn these actions early in the study of pharmacology, because knowledge of autonomic effects is used to predict the actions and side effects of many drugs.

The sympathetic nervous system is activated under conditions of stress, and produces a set of actions called the fight-or-flight response. Activation of this system will ready the body for an immediate response to a potential threat. The heart rate and blood pressure increase, and more blood is shunted to skeletal muscles. The liver immediately produces more glucose for energy. The bronchi dilate to allow more air into the lungs and the pupils dilate for better vision.

Conversely, the parasympathetic nervous system is activated under nonstressful conditions and produces symptoms called the rest-and-digest response. Digestive processes are promoted, and heart rate and blood pressure decline. Not as much air is needed, so the bronchi constrict. Most of the actions of the parasympathetic division are opposite to those of the sympathetic division.

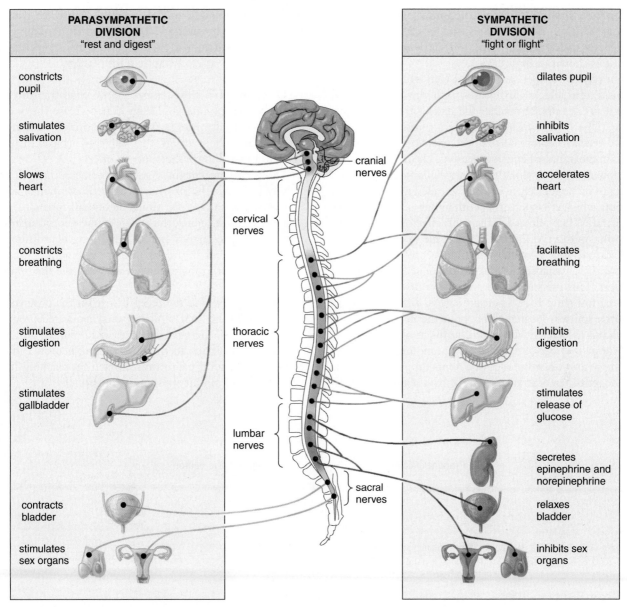

PARASYMPATHETIC DIVISION
"rest and digest"

constricts pupil

stimulates salivation

slows heart

constricts breathing

stimulates digestion

stimulates gallbladder

contracts bladder

stimulates sex organs

SYMPATHETIC DIVISION
"fight or flight"

dilates pupil

inhibits salivation

accelerates heart

facilitates breathing

inhibits digestion

stimulates release of glucose

secretes epinephrine and norepinephrine

relaxes bladder

inhibits sex organs

cranial nerves

cervical nerves

thoracic nerves

lumbar nerves

sacral nerves

Figure 13.2 | Effects of the sympathetic and parasympathetic nervous systems *Source: From Biology: A Guide to the Natural World, 2ed. (p 558) by David Krogh, 2002, Upper Saddle River, NJ, Prentice Hall. Reprinted by permission.*

A proper balance of the two autonomic branches is required for internal homeostasis. Under most circumstances, the two branches cooperate to achieve a balance of readiness and relaxation. Because they have mostly opposite effects, homeostasis may be achieved by changing one or both branches. For example, heart rate can be increased by either *increasing* the firing of sympathetic nerves, or by *decreasing* the firing of parasympathetic nerves. This allows the body a means of fine-tuning its essential organ systems.

The sympathetic and parasympathetic divisions are not always opposite in their effects. For example, the constriction of arterioles is controlled entirely by the sympathetic branch. Sympathetic stimulation causes constriction of arterioles, whereas lack of stimulation causes vasodilation. Sweat glands are controlled only by sympathetic nerves. In the male

reproductive system, the roles are complementary. Erection of the penis is a function of the parasympathetic division and ejaculation is controlled by the sympathetic branch.

13.3 Structure and Function of Synapses

For information to be transmitted throughout the nervous system, neurons must communicate with each other, and with muscles and glands. In the autonomic nervous system this involves the connection of two neurons, in series. As an action potential travels along the first nerve, it encounters a structure at the end called a synapse. The synapse contains a physical space called the synaptic cleft, which must be bridged for the impulse to reach the next nerve. The nerve carrying the original impulse is called the presynaptic neuron. The nerve on the other side of the synapse, waiting to receive the impulse, is the **postsynaptic neuron**. If this connection occurs outside the CNS, it is called a **ganglion**. The basic structure of a synapse is shown in Figure 13.3.

The physical space of the synaptic cleft is bridged by neurotransmitters which are released into the synaptic cleft when a nerve impulse reaches the end of the presynaptic neuron. The neurotransmitter diffuses across the synaptic cleft to reach receptors on the postsynaptic neuron, which results in the impulse being regenerated. The regenerated action potential travels along the postganglionic neuron until it reaches its target: a type of synapse called a neuroeffector junction, which is located on smooth muscle, cardiac muscle, or a gland. When released at the neuroeffector junction, the neurotransmitter induces the target tissue to elicit its characteristic response. Generally, the more neurotransmitter released into the synapse, the greater and longer lasting will be its effect. This process, called **synaptic transmission**, is illustrated in Figure 13.4. There are several different types of neurotransmitters located throughout the nervous system, and each is associated with particular functions.

A large number of drugs affect autonomic function by altering neurotransmitter activity. Some drugs are identical to endogenous neurotransmitters, or have a similar chemical structure, and are able to directly activate the gland or muscle. Others are used to block the activity of natural neurotransmitters. Following are the five general mechanisms by which drugs affect synaptic transmission.

- Drugs may affect the *synthesis* of the neurotransmitter in the presynaptic nerve. Drugs that decrease the amount of neurotransmitter synthesis will inhibit autonomic function. Those drugs that increase neurotransmitter synthesis will have the opposite effect.
- Drugs can prevent the *storage* of the neurotransmitter in vesicles within the presynaptic nerve. Prevention of neurotransmitter storage will inhibit autonomic function.
- Drugs can influence the *release* of the neurotransmitter from the presynaptic nerve. Promoting neurotransmitter release will stimulate autonomic function, whereas slowing neurotransmitter release will have the opposite effect.
- Drugs can *bind* to the receptor site on the postsynaptic neuron. Drugs that bind to postsynaptic receptors and stimulate the nerve will increase autonomic function. Drugs that attach to the postsynaptic neuron and prevent the natural neurotransmitter from reaching its receptors will inhibit autonomic function.

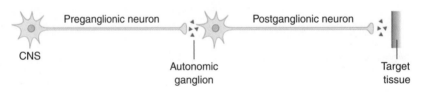

Figure 13.3 | Basic structure of an autonomic pathway

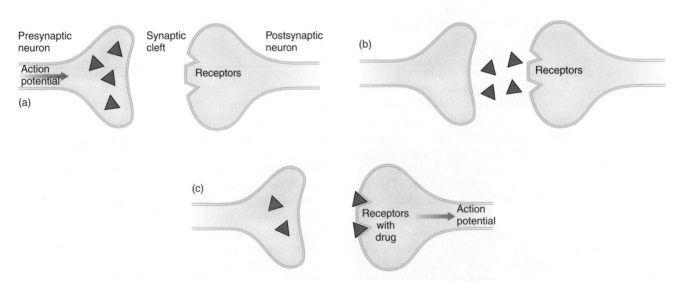

Figure 13.4 | Synaptic transmission: (a) action potential reaches synapse; (b) neurotransmitter released into synaptic cleft; and (c) neurotransmitter reaches receptors to regenerate action potential

- Drugs can *prevent the normal destruction or reuptake* of the neurotransmitter. Drugs that cause the neurotransmitter to remain in the synapse for a longer time will stimulate autonomic function.

It is important for the student to understand that autonomic drugs are not given to correct physiologic defects in the autonomic nervous system. Compared to other body systems, the autonomic nervous system itself has remarkably little disease. Rather, drugs are used to stimulate or inhibit *target organs* of the autonomic nervous system, such as the heart, lungs, or digestive tract. With few exceptions, the disorder lies in the target organ, not the autonomic nervous system. Thus, when an "autonomic drug" such as norepinephrine (Levarterenol) is administered, it does not correct an autonomic disease; it corrects disorders of target organs through its effects on autonomic nerves.

13.4 Acetylcholine and Cholinergic Transmission

The two primary neurotransmitters of the autonomic nervous system are **norepinephrine (NE)** and **acetylcholine (Ach)**. A detailed knowledge of the underlying physiology of these neurotransmitters is required for proper understanding of drug action. When reading the following sections, the student should refer to the sites of acetylcholine and norepinephrine action shown in Figure 13.5.

Nerves releasing acetylcholine are called **cholinergic** nerves. There are two types of cholinergic receptors that bind Ach, which are named after certain chemicals that bind to them.

- Preganglionic neurons ending in ganglia in both the sympathetic and parasympathetic nervous systems (nicotinic receptors)
- Postganglionic neurons ending in neuroeffector target tissues in the parasympathetic nervous system (muscarinic receptors)

Early research on laboratory animals found that the actions of Ach at the *ganglia* resemble those of nicotine, the active agent found in tobacco products. Because of this similarity, receptors for Ach in the ganglia are called **nicotinic** receptors. Nicotinic receptors are also present in skeletal muscle, which is controlled by the somatic nervous system. Because these receptors are present in so many locations, drugs affecting nicotinic receptors produce profound effects on both the autonomic and somatic nervous systems. Activation of these Ach receptors causes tachycardia, hypertension, and increased tone and motility in the digestive tract. Although nicotinic receptor blockers were some of the first drugs used to treat hypertension, the only current therapeutic application of these agents, known as ganglionic blockers, is to produce muscle relaxation during surgical procedures (Chapter 20)⚭.

Activation of acetylcholine receptors at *postganglionic* nerve endings in the parasympathetic nervous system results in the classic symptoms of parasympathetic stimulation shown in Figure 13.2. Early research discovered that these actions closely resemble those produced when a patient ingests the poisonous mushroom, *Amanita muscaria*. Because of this similarity, these Ach receptors were named **muscarinic** receptors. Unlike the nicotinic receptors that have few pharmacologic applications, a number of medications affect muscarinic receptors, and these are discussed in

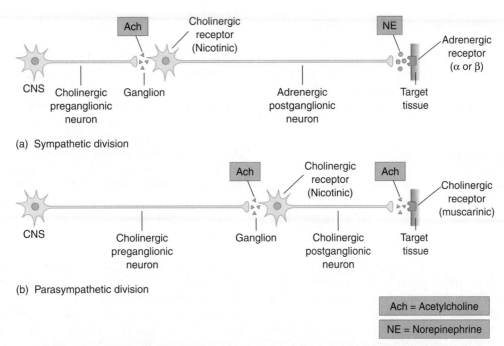

(a) Sympathetic division

(b) Parasympathetic division

Ach = Acetylcholine

NE = Norepinephrine

Figure 13.5 | Receptors in the autonomic nervous system: (a) sympathetic division; (b) parasympathetic division

Table 13.1	Types of Autonomic Receptors		
Neurotransmitter	**Receptor**	**Primary Locations**	**Responses**
acetylcholine (cholinergic)	muscarinic	parasympathetic target: organs other than the heart	stimulation of smooth muscle and gland secretions
		heart	decreased heart rate and force of contraction
	nicotinic	postganglionic neurons and neuromuscular junctions of skeletal muscle	stimulation of smooth muscle and gland secretions
norepinephrine (adrenergic)	alpha$_1$	all sympathetic target organs except the heart	constrict blood vessels, dilate pupils
	alpha$_2$	presynaptic adrenergic nerve terminals	inhibit release of norepinephrine
	beta$_1$	heart and kidneys	increased heart rate and force of contraction; release of renin
	beta$_2$	all sympathetic target organs except the heart	inhibition of smooth muscle

subsequent sections of this chapter. The locations of nicotinic and muscarinic receptors are illustrated in Figure 13.5. Table 13.1 summarizes the actions produced by the two types of Ach receptors.

The physiology of acetylcholine affords several mechanisms by which drugs may act. Acetylcholine is synthesized in the presynaptic nerve terminal from choline and acetyl coenzyme A. The enzyme that catalyzes this reaction is called acetylcholinesterase (AchE), or simply cholinesterase. (Note the suffix -erase can be thought of as wiping out the Ach.) Once synthesized, Ach is stored in vesicles in the presynaptic neuron. When an action potential reaches the nerve ending, Ach is released into the synaptic cleft, where it diffuses across to find nicotinic or muscarinic receptors. Ach in the synaptic cleft is rapidly destroyed by acetylcholinesterase, and choline is reformed. The choline is taken up by the presynaptic neuron to make more Ach, and the cycle is repeated. Drugs can affect the formation, release, receptor activation, or destruction of Ach.

13.5 Norepinephrine and Adrenergic Transmission

In the sympathetic nervous system, norepinephrine is the neurotransmitter released at almost all postganglionic nerves. Norepinephrine belongs to a class of endogenous agents called catecholamines, all of which are involved in neurotransmission. Other catecholamines include epinephrine (adrenaline) and dopamine. The receptors at the ends of postganglionic sympathetic neurons are called adrenergic, which comes from the word adrenaline.

Adrenergic receptors are of two basic types, alpha (α) and beta (β). These receptors are further divided into the subtypes beta$_1$, beta$_2$, alpha$_1$, and alpha$_2$. Activation of each type of subreceptor results in a characteristic set of physiological responses, which are summarized in Table 13.1.

The significance of these receptor subtypes to pharmacology cannot be overstated. Some drugs are selective and activate only one type of adrenergic receptor, whereas others affect all receptor subtypes. Furthermore, a drug may activate one type of receptor at low doses and begin to affect other receptor subtypes as the dose is increased. Committing the receptor types and their responses to memory is an essential step in learning autonomic pharmacology.

Norepinephrine is synthesized in the nerve terminal through a series of steps that require the amino acids phenylalanine and tyrosine. The final step of the synthesis involves the conversion of dopamine to norepinephrine. NE is stored in vesicles, until an action potential triggers its release into the synaptic cleft. NE then diffuses across the cleft to alpha- or beta-receptors on the effector organ. The reuptake of NE back into the presynaptic neuron terminates its action. Once reuptake occurs, NE in the nerve terminal may be returned to vesicles for future use, or destroyed enzymatically by monoamine oxidase (MAO). The primary method for termination of NE action is through reuptake. Many drugs affect autonomic function by influencing the synthesis, storage, release, reuptake, or destruction of NE.

The adrenal medulla is a tissue closely associated with the sympathetic nervous system that has a much different anatomical and physiological arrangement than the rest of the sympathetic branch. Early in embryonic life, the adrenal medulla is part of the neural tissue destined to become the sympathetic nervous system. The primitive tissue splits, however, and the adrenal medulla becomes its own functional division. The preganglionic neuron from the spinal cord terminates in the adrenal medulla, and releases the neurotransmitter epinephrine directly into the blood. Once released, epinephrine travels to target organs, where it elicits the classic fight-or-flight symptoms. The action of epinephrine is terminated through hepatic metabolism, rather than reuptake.

Other types of adrenergic receptors exist. Although dopamine was once thought to function only as a chemical precursor to norepinephrine, research has determined that dopamine serves a larger role as neurotransmitter. Five dopaminergic receptors (D_1 through D_5) have been discovered in the CNS. Dopaminergic receptors in the CNS are important to the action of certain antipsychotic medicines (Chapter 17) and in the treatment of Parkinson's disease (Chapter 18)⊂⊃. Dopamine receptors in the peripheral nervous system are located in the arterioles of the kidney and other viscera. Although these receptors likely have a role in autonomic function, their therapeutic importance has yet to be discovered.

AUTONOMIC DRUGS

13.6 Classification and Naming of Autonomic Drugs

Given the opposite actions of the sympathetic and parasympathetic nervous systems, autonomic drugs are classified based on one of four possible actions.

1. *Stimulation of the sympathetic nervous system* These drugs are called sympathomimetics or adrenergic agonists, and they produce the classic symptoms of the fight-or-flight response.

2. *Stimulation of the parasympathetic nervous system* These drugs are called parasympathomimetics or muscarinic agonists, and they produce the characteristic symptoms of the rest-and-digest response.

3. *Inhibition of the sympathetic nervous system* These drugs are called adrenergic antagonists or adrenergic blockers, and they produce actions *opposite* to those of the sympathomimetics.

4. *Inhibition of the parasympathetic nervous system* These drugs are called anticholinergics, parasympatholytics, or muscarinic blockers, and they produce actions *opposite* to those of the parasympathomimetics.

Students beginning their study of pharmacology often have difficulty understanding the terminology and actions of autonomic drugs. Upon examining the four drug classes, however, it is evident that only one group need be learned because the others are logical extensions of the first. If the fight-or-flight actions of the sympathomimetics are learned, the other three groups are either the same or opposite. For example, both the sympathomimetics and the anticholinergics increase heart rate and dilate the pupil. The other two groups, the parasympathomimetics and the adrenergic antagonists, have the opposite effects of slowing heart rate and constricting the pupils. Although this is an oversimplification and exceptions do exist, it is a timesaving means of learning the basic actions and adverse effects

of dozens of drugs affecting the autonomic nervous system. It should be emphasized again that mastering the actions and terminology of autonomic drugs early in the study of pharmacology will reap rewards later in the course when these drugs are applied to various systems.

Parasympathomimetics

Parasympathomimetics are drugs that activate the parasympathetic nervous system. These drugs induce the rest-and-digest response.

13.7 Clinical Applications of Parasympathomimetics

The classic parasympathomimetic is acetylcholine, the endogenous neurotransmitter at cholinergic synapses in the autonomic nervous system. Acetylcholine, however, has almost no therapeutic use because it is rapidly destroyed after administration and it produces many side effects. Recall that Ach is the neurotransmitter at the ganglia in both the parasympathetic and sympathetic divisions, and at the neuroeffector junctions in the parasympathetic nervous system, as well as in skeletal muscle. It is not surprising that administration of Ach or drugs that mimic Ach will have widespread and varied effects on the body.

Parasympathomimetics are divided into two subclasses, direct acting and indirect acting, based on their mechanism of action (see Table 13.2). Direct-acting agents, such as bethanechol (Urecholine), bind to cholinergic receptors to produce the rest-and-digest response. Because they are relatively resistant to the enzyme acetylcholinesterase, they have a longer duration of action than Ach. They are poorly absorbed across the GI tract and generally do not cross the blood-brain barrier. They have little effect on Ach receptors in ganglia. Because they are moderately selective to muscarinic receptors when used at therapeutic doses, they are sometimes called muscarinic agonists.

The indirect-acting parasympathomimetics, such as neostigmine (Prostigmin), inhibit the action of AchE. This inhibition allows endogenous Ach to avoid rapid destruction and remain on cholinergic receptors for a longer time, thus prolonging its action. These drugs are called cholinesterase inhibitors. Unlike the direct-acting agents, the cholinesterase inhibitors are nonselective and affect all Ach sites: autonomic ganglia, muscarinic receptors, skeletal muscle, and Ach sites in the CNS.

One of the first drugs discovered in this class, physostigmine (Antilirium), was obtained from the dried ripe seeds of *Physostigma venenosum*, a plant found in West Africa. The bean of this plant was used in tribal rituals. As research continued under secrecy during World War II, similar compounds were synthesized that produced potent neurologic effects that could be used during chemical warfare. This class of agents now includes organophosphate insecticides such as malathion and parathion, and toxic nerve gasses such as sarin. Nurses who work in agricultural areas may become quite familiar

Table 13.2	Parasympathomimetics	
Type	**Drug**	**Primary Use**
direct acting (muscarinic agonists)	bethanechol (Urecholine)	increase urination
	cevimeline HCl (Evoxac)	treatment of dry mouth
	pilocarpine (Isopto Carpine, Salagen)	glaucoma
indirect acting (cholinesterase inhibitors)	ambenonium (Mytelase)	myasthenia gravis
	donepezil (Aricept)	Alzheimer's disease
	edrophonium (Tensilon)	diagnosis of myasthenia gravis
	galantamine hydrobromide (Reminyl)	Alzheimer's disease
	neostigmine (Prostigmin)	myasthenia gravis, increase urination
	physostigmine (Antilirium)	glaucoma, treatment of anticholinergic overdose
	pyridostigmine (Mestinon)	myasthenia gravis
	rivastigmine (Exelon)	Alzheimer's disease
	tacrine (Cognex)	Alzheimer's disease

with the symptoms of acute poisoning with organophosphates. Poisoning results in intense stimulation of the parasympathetic nervous system, which may result in death, if untreated.

Because of their high potential for serious adverse effects, few parasympathomimetics are widely used in pharmacotherapy. Some have clinical applications in ophthalmology, because they reduce intraocular pressure in patients with glaucoma (Chapter 48) 👁. Others are used for their stimulatory effects on the smooth muscle of the bowel or urinary tract.

Several drugs in this class are used for their effects on acetylcholine receptors in skeletal muscle or in the CNS, rather than for their parasympathetic action. **Myasthenia gravis** is a disease characterized by destruction of nicotinic receptors on skeletal muscles. Administration of pyridostigmine (Mestinon) or neostigmine (Prostigmin) will stimulate skeletal muscle contraction and help to reverse the severe muscle weakness characteristic of this disease. In addition, tacrine (Cognex) is useful in treating Alzheimer's disease because of its ability to increase the amount of acetylcholine in receptors in the CNS (Chapter 18) 👁.

NURSING CONSIDERATIONS

The role of the nurse in drug therapy with parasympathomimetics involves careful monitoring of a patient's condition and providing education as it relates to the prescribed drug regimen. Both direct- and indirect-acting parasympathomimetics are contradindicated for patients with hypersensitivity. These drugs should not be used in patients with obstruction of the gastrointestinal and urinary systems because they increase muscular tone and contraction. Additionally, they should not be used in patients with active asthma, bradycardia, hypotension, or Parkinson's disease.

Indirect-Acting Parasympathomimetics

The indirect-acting agents are contraindicated for patients with mechanical obstruction of either the intestine or urinary tract due to their ability to intensify smooth muscle contractions. Smooth muscle contractions can also occur in the bronchi, so extreme caution must be exercised when treating patients with asthma or chronic obstructive pulmonary disease (COPD).

Due to the ability of these medications to inhibit acetylcholinesterase at many locations, Ach will accumulate at the muscarinic and the neuromuscular junctions and cause side effects such as profuse salivation, increased muscle tone, urinary frequency, bronchoconstriction, and bradycardia. Atropine should be available to counteract the increased levels of Ach by providing selective blockage of muscarinic cholinergic receptors. The nurse should monitor the patient for drug-induced insomnia. The nurse should also assess for pregnancy and breastfeeding status, as these agents are contraindicated for both situations.

For patients with myasthenia gravis, it is important to perform a baseline physical assessment of neuromuscular and respiratory function. Myasthenia gravis affects the muscles of the respiratory tract and other muscle groups due to the destruction of nictotinic receptors on the skeletal muscles. It is also important to assess the patient's swallowing ability prior to drug administration, due to decreased muscle strength caused by the disease process.

See "Nursing Process Focus: Patients Receiving Parasympathomimetic Therapy" for specific points the nurse should include when teaching patients about indirect-acting parasympathomimetics.

Direct-Acting Parasympathomimetics

Due to the stimulation of the CNS by these agents, several additional nursing actions are required. These include assessment of past medical history for any of the following:

Pr PROTOTYPE DRUG | BETHANECHOL (Urecholine)

ACTIONS AND USES

Bethanechol is a direct-acting parasympathomimetic that interacts with muscarinic receptors to cause actions typical of parasympathetic stimulation. Its effects are most noted in the digestive and urinary tracts, where it will stimulate smooth muscle contraction. These actions are useful in increasing smooth muscle tone and muscular contractions in the GI tract following general anesthesia. In addition, it is used to treat nonobstructive urinary retention in patients with atony of the bladder. Although poorly absorbed from the GI tract, it may be administered orally or by SC injection.

Administration Alerts

- Never administer by IM or IV.
- Oral and SC doses are *not* interchangeable.
- Monitor blood pressure, pulse, and respirations before administration and for at least 1 hour after SC administration.
- Pregnancy category C.

ADVERSE EFFECTS AND INTERACTIONS

The side effects of bethanechol are predicted from its parasympathetic actions. It should be used with extreme caution in patients with disorders that could be aggravated by increased contractions of the digestive tract, such as suspected obstruction, active ulcer, or inflammatory disease. The same caution should be exercised in patients with suspected urinary obstruction or COPD. Side effects include increased salivation, sweating, abdominal cramping, and hypotension that could lead to fainting. It should not be given to patients with asthma.

Drug interactions with bethanechol include increased effects from cholinesterase inhibitors and decreased effects from procainamide, quinidine, atropine, and epinephrine.

 See the companion website for a Nursing Process Focus specific to this drug.

angina pectoris, recent myocardial infarction, and dysrhythmias. The nurse should obtain history information for possible use of lithium and adenosine, because both drugs are contraindicated due to their interaction with nicotine. Lithium is a CNS agent that can produce significant muscarinic blockade to atropine. Adenosine is an antidysrhythmic agent, and its effect with nicotine can cause an increased risk of heart block. For mothers who are breastfeeding, the nurse should monitor the infant's respiratory patterns and any CNS changes prior to and after feedings. The nurse should monitor elderly patients for episodes of dizziness and sleep disturbances caused by CNS stimulation from the parasympathomimetic.

See "Nursing Process Focus: Patients Receiving Parasympathomimetic Therapy" for specific points the nurse should include when teaching patients about direct-acting parasympathomimetics.

Anticholinergics

Anticholinergics are drugs that inhibit parasympathetic impulses. By suppressing the parasympathetic division, symptoms of the fight-or-flight response are induced.

13.8 Clinical Applications of Anticholinergics

Agents that block the action of acetylcholine are known by a number of names, including anticholinergics, cholinergic blockers, muscarinic antagonists, and parasympatholytics (see Table 13.3). Although the term *anticholinergic* is most commonly used, the most accurate term for this class of

drugs is muscarinic antagonists, because at therapeutic doses, these drugs are selective for Ach muscarinic receptors, and thus have little effect on Ach nicotinic receptors.

Anticholinergics act by competing with acetylcholine for binding muscarinic receptors. When anticholinergics occupy these receptors, no response is generated at the neuroeffector organs. By suppressing the effects of Ach, symptoms of sympathetic nervous system activation predominate. Most therapeutic uses of the anticholinergics are predictable extensions of their parasympathetic-blocking actions: dilation of the pupils, increase in heart rate, drying of secretions, and relaxation of the bronchi. Note that these are also symptoms of sympathetic activation (fight or flight).

Historically, anticholinergics have been widely used for many different disorders. Extracted from the deadly nightshade plant, *Atropa belladonna*, references to these agents date back to the ancient Hindus, the Roman Empire, and the Middle Ages. Because of its extreme toxicity, extracts of belladonna were sometimes used for intentional poisoning. Acts of intentional poisoning included suicide as well as religious and beautification rituals. The name *belladonna* is Latin for "pretty woman." Roman women applied extracts of belladonna to the face to create the preferred female attributes of the time—pink cheeks and dilated doe-like eyes.

Therapeutic uses of anticholinergics include the following:

- *GI disorders* These agents decrease the secretion of gastric acid in peptic ulcer disease (chapter 36). They also slow intestinal motility and may be useful for reducing the cramping and diarrhea associated with irritable bowel syndrome (Chapter 37) .

NURSING PROCESS FOCUS | PATIENTS RECEIVING PARASYMPATHOMIMETIC THERAPY

ASSESSMENT

Prior to administration:
- Obtain complete health history including vital signs, allergies, and drug history for possible drug interactions.
- Assess reason for drug administration.
- Assess for contraindications of drug administration.
- Assess for urinary retention, urinary patterns initially and throughout therapy (direct acting).
- Assess muscle strength, and neuromuscular status, ptosis, diplopia, and chewing.

POTENTIAL NURSING DIAGNOSES

- Urinary Incontinence (direct acting)
- Impaired Physical Mobility (indirect acting)
- Deficient Knowledge, related to drug therapy
- Risk for Injury, related to side effects

PLANNING: PATIENT GOALS AND EXPECTED OUTCOMES

The patient will:
- Exhibit increased bowel/bladder function and tone by regaining normal pattern of elimination (direct acting)
- Exhibit a decrease in myasthenia gravis symptoms such as muscle weakness, ptosis, and diplopia (indirect acting)
- Demonstrate understanding of the drug's action by accurately describing drug side effects and precautions

IMPLEMENTATION

Interventions and (Rationales)	Patient Education/Discharge Planning
All Parasympathomimetics	
■ Monitor for adverse effects such as abdominal cramping, diarrhea, excessive salivation, difficulty breathing, and muscle cramping. (These may indicate cholinergic crisis that requires atropine.)	■ Instruct patient to report nausea, vomiting, diarrhea, rash, jaundice, or change in color of stool, or any other adverse reactions to the drug.
■ Monitor liver enzymes with initiation of therapy and weekly for 6 weeks (for possible hepatotoxicity).	■ Instruct patient to adhere to laboratory testing regimen for serum blood level tests of liver enzymes as directed.
■ Assess and monitor for appropriate self-care administration to prevent complications.	Instruct patient to: ■ Take drug as directed on regular schedule to maintain serum levels and control symptoms ■ Not chew or crush sustained-release tablets ■ Take oral parasympathomimetics on empty stomach to lessen incidence of nausea and vomiting and to increase absorption
Direct Acting	
■ Monitor intake and output ratio. Palpate abdomen for bladder distention. (These drugs have an onset of action of 60 minutes due to binding of the drug to cholinergic receptors on the smooth muscle of the bladder, which relaxes the bladder to stimulate urination.)	■ Advise patient to be near bathroom facilities after taking drug.
■ Monitor for blurred vision (a cholinergic effect).	■ Advise patient that blurred vision is a possible side effect and to take appropriate precautions. ■ Instruct patient not to drive or perform hazardous activities until effects of the drugs are known.
■ Monitor for orthostatic hypotension.	■ Instruct patient to avoid abrupt changes in position. Avoid prolonged standing in one place.
Indirect Acting	
■ Monitor muscle strength, and neuromuscular status, ptosis, diplopia, and chewing to determine if the therapeutic effect is achieved.	■ Instruct patient to report difficulty with vision or swallowing.

continued

NURSING PROCESS FOCUS: *Patients Receiving Parasympathomimetic Therapy (continued)*

Indirect Acting

■ Schedule medication around meal times. (This will achieve therapeutic effect and aid in chewing and swallowing.)	■ Instruct patient to take medication about 30 minutes before meal.
■ Schedule activities to avoid fatigue.	■ Instruct patient to plan activities according to muscle strength and fatigue. ■ Instruct patient to take frequent rest periods.
■ Monitor for muscle weakness. (This symptom, depending on time onset, indicates cholinergic crisis—overdose—OR myasthenic crisis—underdose.)	Instruct patient to: ■ Report any severe muscle weakness that occurs 1 hour after administration of medication ■ Report any muscle weakness that occurs 3 or more hours after medication administration, as this is a major symptom of myasthenic crisis

EVALUATION OF OUTCOME CRITERIA

Evaluate effectiveness of drug therapy by confirming that patient goals and expected outcomes have been met (see "Planning").

See Table 13.2 for a list of drugs to which these nursing applications apply.

SPECIAL CONSIDERATIONS

Impact of Anticholinergics on Male Sexual Function

A functioning autonomic nervous system is essential for normal male sexual health. The parasympathetic nervous system is necessary for erections, whereas the sympathetic division is responsible for the process of ejaculation. Anticholinergic drugs will block transmission of parasympathetic impulses and may interfere with normal erections. Adrenergic antagonists can interfere with the smooth muscle contractions in the seminal vesicles and penis, resulting in an inability to ejaculate.

For patients receiving autonomic medications, the nurse should include questions about sexual activity during the assessment process. For male patients who are not sexually active, these side effects may be unimportant. For patients who are sexually active, however, drug-induced sexual dysfunction may be a major cause of noncompliance. The patient should be informed to expect such side effects and to report them to their healthcare provider immediately. In most cases, alternative medications are available which do not affect sexual function. Inform the patient that supportive counseling is available.

NATURAL THERAPIES   Valerian

Valerian root (*Valeriana officinalis*) is a perennial native to Europe and North America, that is an herbal choice for nervous tension and anxiety. This natural product promotes rest without affecting REM sleep and has a reputation for calming an individual without causing side effects or discomfort. Its name comes from the Latin *valere,* which means "to be well." One thing that is *not well,* however, is its pungent odor, though many users claim that the smell is well worth the benefits. Valerian also is purported to reduce pain and headaches without the worry of dependency. There is no drug hangover, as is sometimes experienced with tranquilizers and sedatives. It is available as a tincture (alcohol mixture), tea, or extract. Sometimes it is placed in juice and consumed immediately before taking a nap or going to bed.

gics can decrease excessive respiratory secretions and reverse the bradycardia caused by anesthetics (Chapter 20).

■ *Asthma* A few agents, such as ipratropium (Atrovent), are useful in treating asthma, due to their ability to dilate the bronchi (Chapter 29).

The prototype drug, atropine, is used for several additional medical conditions due to its effective muscarinic receptor blockade. These applications include reversal of adverse muscarinic effects and treatment of muscarinic agonist poisoning, including that caused from overdose of bethanechol (Urecholine), cholinesterase inhibitors, or accidental ingestion of certain types of mushrooms or organophosphate pesticides.

■ *Ophthalmic procedures* May be used to cause mydriasis or cycloplegia during eye procedures (Chapter 48).

■ *Cardiac rhythm abnormalities* Can be used to accelerate the heart rate in patients experiencing bradycardia.

■ *Preanesthesia* Combined with other agents, anticholiner-

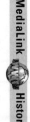

MediaLink   Historical Use of Belladonna

Table 13.3	Anticholinergics
Drug	**Primary Use**
atropine	Increase heart rate, dilate pupils
benztropine (Cogentin)	Parkinson's disease
cyclopentolate (Cyclogyl)	dilate pupils
dicyclomine (Bentyl, others)	irritable bowel syndrome
glycopyrrolate (Robinul)	produce a dry field prior to anesthesia, peptic ulcers
ipratropium (Atrovent)	asthma
oxybutynin (Ditropan)	incontinence
propantheline (Pro-Banthine)	irritable bowel syndrome, peptic ulcer
scopolamine (Hyoscine, Transderm-Scop)	motion sickness, irritable bowel syndrome, adjunct to anesthesia
trihexyphenydil (Artane, others)	Parkinson's disease

Some of the anticholinergics are used for their effects on the CNS, rather than their autonomic actions. Scopolamine (Hyoscine, Transderm-Scop) is used for sedation and motion sickness (Chapter 37); benztropine (Cogentin) is prescribed to reduce the muscular tremor and rigidity associated with Parkinson's disease; and donepezil (Aricept) has a slight memory enhancement effect in patients with Alzheimer's disease (Chapter 18).

Anticholinergics exhibit a relatively high incidence of side effects. Important adverse effects that limit their usefulness include tachycardia, CNS stimulation, and the tendency to cause urinary retention in men with prostate disorders. Adverse effects such as dry mouth and dry eyes occur due to blockade of muscarinic receptors on salivary glands and lacrimal glands, respectively. Blockade of muscarinic receptors on sweat glands can inhibit sweating, which may lead to hyperthermia. Photophobia can occur due to the pupil being unable to constrict in response to bright light. Symptoms of overdose (cholinergic crisis) include fever, visual changes, difficulty swallowing, psychomotor agitation, and/or hallucinations. (The nurse can easily recall the signs of cholinergic crisis by memorizing the following simile: "Hot as hades, blind as a bat, dry as a bone, mad as a hatter.") The development of safer, and sometimes more effective, drugs has greatly decreased the current use of anticholinergics. An exception is ipratropium (Atrovent), a relatively new anticholinergic used for patients with COPD. Because it is delivered via aerosol spray, this agent produces more localized action with fewer systemic side effects than atropine.

NURSING CONSIDERATIONS

The role of the nurse in anticholinergic therapy involves careful monitoring of a patient's condition and providing education as it relates to the prescribed drug regimen. The nurse should perform a thorough medical history, including medications the patient is currently taking that could cause drug-drug interactions. Antihistamines, in particular, can lead to excessive muscarinic blockade. The nurse should check for history of taking herbal supplements; some have atropine-like actions that potentiate the effects of the medication and can be harmful to the patient. For example, aloe, senna, buckthorn, and cascara sagrada may increase atropine's effect, particulary with chronic use of the herbs.

This classification of drugs should not be used if the patient has history of acute angle-closure glaucoma. Anticholinergics block muscarinic receptors in the eye, creating paralysis of the iris sphincter, which can increase intraocular pressure. Safety has not been established for pregnancy and lactating mothers. Anticholinergics may produce fetal tachycardia.

Anticholinergics are contraindicated in patients with cardiopulmonary conditions such as COPD, asthma, heart disease, and hypertension, because blockade of cardiac muscarinic receptors prevents the parasympathetic nervous system from slowing the heart. This can result in an acceleration of heart rate that may exacerbate these conditions. Patients with hyperthyroidism should not be given these medications, because in hyperthyroidism, the heart rate is generally high and administration of anticholinergics can cause dysrhythmias due to norepinephrine released from sympathetic nerves that regulate heart rate.

The nurse should also assess for baseline bowel and bladder function. Renal conditions are contraindicated due to anticholinergics' effect on bladder functioning. Gastrointestinal conditions such as ulcerative colitis and ileus are contraindicated, because blockade of muscarinic receptors in the intestine can decrease the tone and motility of intestinal smooth muscle, which can exacerbate intestinal conditions. The nurse should monitor patients with esophageal reflux and hiatal hernia, because anticholinergics reduce GI motility. Patients with gastroesophageal reflux disease (GERD) and hiatal hernia experience decreased muscle tone in the lower esophageal sphincter and delayed stomach emptying. Anticholinergics exacerbate these symptoms, increasing the risk of esophageal injury and aspiration. Patients with Down syndrome may be more sensitive to the effects of atropine due to structural differences

Pr PROTOTYPE DRUG | **ATROPINE** (Atropair, Atropisol)

ACTIONS AND USES

By occupying muscarinic receptors, atropine blocks the parasympathetic actions of Ach and induces symptoms of the fight-or-flight response. Most prominent are increased heart rate, bronchodilation, decreased motility in the GI tract, mydriasis, and decreased secretions from glands. At therapeutic doses, atropine has no effect on nicotinic receptors in ganglia or on skeletal muscle.

Although atropine has been used for centuries for a variety of purposes, its use has declined in recent decades because of the development of safer and more effective medications. Atropine may be used to treat hypermotility diseases of the GI tract such as irritable bowel syndrome, to suppress secretions during surgical procedures, to increase the heart rate in patients with bradycardia, and to dilate the pupil during eye examinations. Once widely used to cause bronchodilation in patients with asthma, atropine is now rarely prescribed for this disorder.

Administration Alerts

- May be given direct IV (push) or by infusion.
- May cause initial paradoxical bradycardia, lasting up to 2 minutes, especially at lower doses. May induce ventricular fibrillation in cardiac patients.
- Pregnancy category C.

ADVERSE EFFECTS AND INTERACTIONS

The side effects of atropine limit its therapeutic usefulness and are predictable extensions of its autonomic actions. Expected side effects include dry mouth, constipation, urinary retention, and an increased heart rate. Initial CNS excitement may progress to delirium and even coma. Atropine is usually contraindicated in patients with glaucoma, because the drug may increase pressure within the eye. Accidental poisoning has occurred in children who eat the colorful, purple berries of the deadly nightshade, mistaking them for cherries. Symptoms of poisoning are those of intense parasympathetic stimulation.

Drug interactions with atropine include an increased effect with antihistamines, tricyclic antidepressants, quinidine, and procainamide, and decreased effects with levodopa. Use with caution with herbal supplements, such as aloe, senna, buckthorn, and cascara sagrada, which may increase atropine's effect, particulary with chronic use of these herbs.

 See the companion website for a Nursing Process Focus specific to this drug.

---

in the CNS caused by chromosomal abnormality (trisomy). Patients with Down syndrome also tend to have disorders such as GERD and heart disease, which may be adversely affected by anticholinergics.

See "Nursing Process Focus: Patients Receiving Anticholinergic Therapy" for specific points the nurse should include when teaching patients about this class of drugs.

Sympathomimetics

Sympathomimetics stimulate the sympathetic nervous system and induce symptoms characteristic of the fight-or-flight response. These drugs have clinical applications in the treatment of shock and hypotension.

13.9 Clinical Applications of Sympathomimetics

The sympathomimetics, also known as adrenergic agonists, produce many of the same responses as the anticholinergics. However, because the sympathetic nervous system has alpha- and beta-subreceptors, the actions of many sympathomimetics are more specific and have wider therapeutic application (see Table 13.4).

Sympathomimetics may be classified as catecholamines or noncatecholamines. The catecholamines have a chemical structure similar to norepinephrine, a short duration of action, and must be administered parenterally. The noncatecholamines can be taken orally and have longer durations of action because they are not rapidly destroyed by monoamine oxidase.

Most sympathomimetics act by directly binding to and activating adrenergic receptors. Examples include the three endogenous catecholamines: epinephrine, norepinephrine, and dopamine. Other medications in this class act indirectly, by causing the release of norepinephrine from its vesicles on the presynaptic neuron or by inhibiting the reuptake or destruction of NE. Those that act by indirect mechanisms, such as amphetamine or cocaine, are used for their central effects on the brain rather than their autonomic effects. A few agents, such as ephedrine, act by both direct and indirect mechanisms.

Most effects of sympathomimetics are predictable based on their autonomic actions, dependent upon which adrenergic subreceptors are stimulated. Because the receptor responses are so different, the student will need to memorize the specific subclass(es) of receptors activated by each sympathomimetic. Therapeutic applications for the different receptor activations are as follows:

- Alpha$_1$-receptor agonists: treatment of nasal congestion or hypotension; causes mydriasis during ophthalmic examinations
- Alpha$_2$-receptor agonists: treatment of hypertension through nonautonomic (central-acting) mechanism

NURSING PROCESS FOCUS | PATIENTS RECEIVING ANTICHOLINERGIC THERAPY

ASSESSMENT

Prior to administration:
- Obtain complete health history, including drug history to determine possible drug interactions and allergies.
- Assess reason for drug administration.
- Assess for heart rate, blood pressure, temperature, and elimination patterns (initially and throughout therapy).

POTENTIAL NURSING DIAGNOSES

- Deficient Knowledge, related to drug therapy
- Decreased Cardiac Output
- Risk for Imbalanced Body Temperature
- Impaired Oral Mucous Membrane
- Constipation
- Urinary Retention

PLANNING: PATIENT GOALS AND EXPECTED OUTCOMES

The patient will:
- Exhibit a decrease in symptoms for which the medication is prescribed
- Demonstrate an understanding of the drug's action by accurately describing drug side effects and precautions
- Verbalize techniques to avoid hazardous side effects associated with anticholinergic therapy

IMPLEMENTATION

Interventions and (Rationales)	*Patient Education/Discharge Planning*
■ Monitor for signs of anticholinergic crisis resulting from overdosage: fever, tachycardia, difficulty swallowing, ataxia, reduced urine output, psychomotor agitation, confusion, hallucinations.	■ Instruct patients to report side effects related to therapy such as shortness of breath, cough, dysphagia, syncope, fever, anxiety, right upper quadrant pain, extreme lethargy, or dizziness.
■ Report significant changes in heart rate, blood pressure, or the development of dysrhythmias.	■ Instruct patient to monitor vital signs, ensuring proper use of home equipment.
■ Observe for side effects such as drowsiness, blurred vision, tachycardia, dry mouth, urinary hesitancy, and decreased sweating.	Instruct patient to: ■ Report side effects ■ Avoid driving and hazardous activities until effects of the drugs are known ■ Wear sunglasses to decrease the sensitivity to bright light
■ Provide comfort measures for dryness of mucous membranes such as apply lubricant to moisten lips and oral mucosa, assist in rinsing mouth, use artificial tears for dry eyes, as needed.	■ Instruct patient that oral rinses, sugarless gum or candy, and frequent oral hygiene may help relieve dry mouth. Avoid alcohol-containing mouthwashes that can further dry oral tissue.
■ Minimize exposure to heat or cold and strenuous exercise. (Anticholinergics can inhibit sweat gland secretions due to direct blockade of the muscarinic receptors on the sweat glands. Sweating is necessary for patients to cool down and this can increase their risk for hyperthermia.)	■ Advise patient to limit activity outside when the temperature is hot. Strenuous activity in a hot environment may cause heat stroke.
■ Monitor intake and output ratio. Palpate abdomen for bladder distention.	■ Instruct patient to notify healthcare provider if difficulty in voiding occurs.
■ Monitor patient for abdominal distention and auscultate for bowel sounds.	■ Advise patient to increase fluid and add bulk to the diet, if constipation becomes a problem.

EVALUATION OF OUTCOME CRITERIA

Evaluate effectiveness of drug therapy by confirming that patient goals and expected outcomes have been met (see "Planning").

⊂⊃ See Table 13.3 for a list of drugs to which these nursing actions apply.

Table 13.4	Sympathomimetics	
Drug	**Primary Receptor Subtype**	**Primary Use**
albuterol (Proventil, Ventolin)	beta$_2$	asthma
clonidine (Catapres)	alpha$_2$ in CNS	hypertension
dexmedetomidine HCl (Precedex)	alpha$_2$ in CNS	sedation
dobutamine (Dobutrex)	beta$_1$	cardiac stimulant
dopamine (Intropin)	alpha$_1$ and beta$_1$	shock
epinephrine (Adrenalin, Primatene, others)	alpha and beta	cardiac arrest, asthma
formoterol (Foradil)	beta$_2$	asthma, COPD
isoproterenol (Isuprel)	beta$_1$ and beta$_2$	asthma, dysrhythmias, heart failure
metaproterenol (Alupent)	beta$_2$	asthma
metaraminol (Aramine)	alpha$_1$ and beta$_1$	shock
methyldopa (Aldomet)	alpha$_2$ in CNS	hypertension
norepinephrine (Levarterenol, Levophed)	alpha$_1$ and beta$_1$	shock
oxymetazoline (Afrin and others)	alpha	nasal congestion
phenylephrine (Neo-Synephrine)	alpha	nasal congestion
pseudoephedrine (Sudafed and others)	alpha and beta	nasal congestion
ritodrine (Yutopar)	beta$_2$	slow uterine contraction
salmeterol (Serevent)	beta$_2$	decongestant
terbutaline (Brethine and others)	beta$_2$	asthma

■ Beta$_1$-receptor agonists: treatment of cardiac arrest, heart failure, and shock

■ Beta$_2$-receptor agonists: treatment of asthma and premature labor contractions

Some sympathomimetics are nonselective, stimulating more than one type of adrenergic receptor. For example, epinephrine stimulates all four types of adrenergic receptors and is used for cardiac arrest and asthma. Pseudoephedrine (Sudafed and others) stimulates both alpha$_1$- and beta$_2$-receptors and is used as a nasal decongestant. Isoproterenol (Isuprel) stimulates both beta$_1$- and beta$_2$-receptors and is used to increase the rate, force, and conduction speed of the heart, and occasionally for asthma. The nonselective drugs generally cause more autonomic-related side effects than the selective agents.

The side effects of the sympathomimetics are mostly extensions of their autonomic actions. Cardiovascular effects such as tachycardia, hypertension, and dysrhythmias are particularly troublesome and may limit therapy. Large doses can induce CNS excitement and seizures. Other sympathomimetic responses that may occur are dry mouth, nausea, and vomiting. Some of these agents cause anorexia, which has led to their historical use as appetite suppressants. Because of prominent cardiovascular side effects, sympathomimetics are now rarely used for this purpose.

Drugs in this class are found as prototypes in many other sections in this textbook. For additional prototypes of drugs in this class, see dopamine (Intropin) and norepinephrine (Levophed) in Chapter 26, oxymetazoline (Afrin) and epinephrine (Adrenalin) in Chapter 31, and salmeterol (Serevent) in Chapter 29.

NURSING CONSIDERATIONS

Since the purposes and indications of drugs within this class vary greatly, the Nursing Process Focus applies to all patients receiving sympathomimetic drugs. For specific nursing considerations, contraindications, and precautions, see Chapters 26, 29, and 31.

Adrenergic Antagonists

Adrenergic antagonists inhibit the sympathetic nervous system and produce many of the same rest-and-digest symptoms as the parasympathomimetics. They have wide therapeutic application in the treatment of hypertension.

13.10 Clinical Applications of Adrenergic Antagonists

Adrenergic antagonists act by directly blocking adrenergic receptors. The actions of these agents are specific to either alpha or beta blockade. Medications in this class have great therapeutic application: They are the most widely prescribed class of autonomic drugs (see Table 13.5).

Alpha-adrenergic antagonists, or simply alpha-blockers, are used for their effects on vascular smooth muscle. By relaxing vascular smooth muscle in small arteries, alpha$_1$-blockers such as doxazosin (Cardura) cause vasodilation that

Pr PROTOTYPE DRUG | PHENYLEPHRINE (Neo-Synephrine)

ACTIONS AND USES

Phenylephrine is a selective alpha-adrenergic agonist that is available in several different formulations, including intranasal, ophthalmic, IM, SC, and IV. All of its actions and indications are extensions of its sympathetic stimulation. When applied intranasally by spray or drops, it reduces nasal congestion by constricting small blood vessels in the nasal mucosa. Applied topically to the eye during ophthalmic examinations, phenylephrine can dilate the pupil, without causing significant cycloplegia. The parenteral administration of phenylephrine can reverse acute hypotension caused by spinal anesthesia or vascular shock. Because it lacks beta-adrenergic agonist activity, it produces relatively few cardiac side effects at therapeutic doses. Its longer duration of activity and lack of significant cardiac effects gives phenylephrine some advantages over epinephrine or norepinephrine in treating acute hypotension.

Administration Alerts

- Parenteral administration can cause tissue injury with extravasation.
- Phenylephrine ophthalmic drops may damage soft contact lenses.
- Pregnancy category C.

ADVERSE EFFECTS AND INTERACTIONS

When used topically or intranasally, side effects are uncommon. Intranasal use can cause burning of the mucosa and rebound congestion if used for prolonged periods (see Chapter 31). Ophthalmic preparations can cause narrow-angle glaucoma, secondary to their mydriatic effect. High doses can cause reflex bradycardia due to the elevation of blood pressure caused by stimulation of alpha$_1$-receptors. When used parenterally, the drug should be used with caution in patients with advanced coronary artery disease or hypertension. Anxiety, restlessness, and tremor may occur due to the drug's stimulation effect on the CNS. Patients with hyperthyroidism may experience a severe increase in basal metabolic rate, resulting in increased blood pressure and tachycardia. Drug interactions may occur with MAO inhibitors, causing a hypertensive crisis. Increased effects may also occur with tricyclic antidepressants. This drug is incompatible with iron preparations (ferric salts).

 See the companion website for a Nursing Process Focus specific to this drug.

Table 13.5	Adrenergic Antagonists	
Drug	**Primary Receptor Subtype**	**Primary Use**
acebutolol (Sectral)	beta$_1$	hypertension, dysrhythmias, angina
atenolol (Tenormin)	beta$_1$	hypertension, angina
carteolol (Cartrol)	beta$_1$ and beta$_2$	hypertension, glaucoma
carvedilol (Coreg)	alpha$_1$, beta$_1$, and beta$_2$	hypertension
doxazocin (Cardura)	alpha$_1$	hypertension
esmolol (Brevibloc)	beta$_1$	hypertension, dysrhythmias
metoprolol (Lopressor)	beta$_1$	hypertension
nadolol (Corgard)	beta$_1$ and beta$_2$	hypertension
phentolamine (Regitine)	alpha	severe hypertension
prazosin (Minipress)	alpha$_1$	hypertension
propranolol (Inderal)	beta$_1$ and beta$_2$	hypertension, dysrhythmias, heart failure
sotalol (Betapace)	beta$_1$ and beta$_2$	dysrhythmias
terazosin (Hytrin)	alpha$_1$	hypertension
timolol (Blocadren, Timoptic)	beta$_1$ and beta$_2$	hypertension, angina, glaucoma

results in decreased blood pressure. They may be used either alone or in combination with other agents in the treatment of hypertension (Chapter 21). A second use is in the treatment of benign prostatic hyperplasia, due to their ability to increase urine flow (Chapter 42). The most common adverse effect of alpha-blockers is orthostatic hypotension, which occurs when a patient abruptly changes from a recumbent to an upright position. Reflex tachycardia, nasal congestion, and impotence are other important side effects that occur due to increased parasympathetic activity.

NURSING PROCESS FOCUS   PATIENTS RECEIVING SYMPATHOMIMETIC THERAPY

ASSESSMENT

Prior to administration:
- Determine reason for drug administration.
- Monitor vital signs, urinary output, and cardiac output (initially and throughout therapy).
- For treatment of nasal congestion, assess the nasal mucosa for changes such as excoriation or bleeding.
- Obtain complete health history including allergies, drug history, and possible drug interactions.

POTENTIAL NURSING DIAGNOSES

- Deficient Knowledge, related to drug therapy
- Decreased Cardiac Output
- Ineffective Cardiopulmonary Tissue Perfusion
- Risk for Injury, related to side effect of drug therapy
- Ineffective Breathing Pattern, related to nasal congestion
- Disturbed Sleep Pattern

PLANNING: PATIENT GOALS AND EXPECTED OUTCOMES

The patient will:
- Exhibit a decrease in the symptoms for which the drug is being given
- Demonstrate understanding of the drug's action by accurately describing drug side effects and precautions
- Return demonstrate proper nasal/opthalmic drug instillation technique

IMPLEMENTATION

Interventions and (Rationales)	Patient Education/Discharge Planning
<ul><li>Closely monitor IV insertion sites for extravasation with IV administration. Use an infusion pump to deliver the medication.</li><li>Use a tuberculin syringe when administering SC—doses that are extremely small.</li><li>For metered dose inhalation, shake container well and wait at least 2 minutes between medications.</li><li>Instill only the prescribed number of drops when using ophthalmic solutions.</li></ul>	Instruct patient to:<ul><li>Use the drug strictly as prescribed, and not "double up" on doses</li><li>Take medication early in day to avoid insomnia</li></ul>
<ul><li>Monitor the patient for side effects. (Side effects of sympathomimetics may be serious and limit therapy.)</li></ul>	Instruct patient to:<ul><li>Immediately report shortness of breath, palpitations, dizziness, chest/arm pain or pressure, or other angina-like symptoms</li><li>Consult healthcare provider before attempting to use sympathomimetics to treat nasal congestion or eye irritation</li><li>Monitor blood pressure, pulse, and temperature to ensure proper use of home equipment</li></ul>
<ul><li>Monitor breathing patterns and observe for shortness of breath and/or audible wheezing.</li></ul>	<ul><li>Instruct patient to immediately report any difficulty breathing. Instruct patients with a history of asthma to consult their healthcare provider before using OTC drugs to treat nasal congestion.</li></ul>
<ul><li>Observe the patient's responsiveness to light. (Some sympathomimetics cause photosensitivity by affecting the pupillary light accommodation/response.)</li><li>Provide eye comfort by reducing exposure to bright light in the environment; shield the eyes with a rolled washcloth or eye bandages for severe photosensitivity.</li></ul>	<ul><li>Instruct patients using ophthalmic sympathomimetics that transient stinging and blurred vision upon instillation is normal. Headache and/or brow pain may also occur.</li><li>Instruct patient to avoid driving and other activities requiring visual acuity until blurring subsides.</li></ul>
<ul><li>For patients receiving nasal sympathomimetics, observe the nasal cavity. Monitor for rhinorrhea and epistaxis.</li></ul>	Instruct patient to:<ul><li>Observe nasal cavity for signs of excoriation or bleeding before instilling nasal spray or drops; review procedure for safe instillation of nasal sprays or eye drops</li><li>Limit OTC usage of sympathomimetics; inform patient about rebound nasal congestion</li></ul>

continued

NURSING PROCESS FOCUS: **Patients Receiving Sympathomimetic Therapy (continued)**

EVALUATION OF OUTCOME CRITERIA

Evaluate effectiveness of drug therapy by confirming that patient goals and expected outcomes have been met (see "Planning").

See Table 13.4 for a list of drugs to which these nursing actions apply.

Beta-adrenergic antagonists may block beta$_1$-receptors, beta$_2$-receptors, or both types. Regardless of their receptor specificity, the therapeutic applications of all beta-blockers relate to their effects on the cardiovascular system. Beta-blockers will decrease the rate and force of contraction of the heart, and slow electrical conduction through the atrioventricular node. Drugs that selectively block beta$_1$-receptors, such as atenolol (Tenormin), are called cardioselective agents. Because they have little effect on noncardiac tissue, they exert fewer side effects than nonselective agents such as propranolol.

The primary use of beta-blockers is in the treatment of hypertension. Although the exact mechanism by which beta-blockers reduce blood pressure is not completely understood, it is thought that the reduction may be due to the decreased cardiac output or suppression of renin release by the kidney. The student should refer to Chapter 21 for a more comprehensive description of the use of beta-blockers in hypertension management.

Beta-adrenergic antagonists have several other important therapeutic applications, discussions of which appear in many chapters in this textbook. By decreasing the cardiac workload, beta-blockers can ease the symptoms of angina pectoris (Chapter 25). By slowing electrical conduction across the myocardium, beta-blockers are able to treat certain types of dysrhythmias (Chapter 23). Other therapeutic uses include the treatment of heart failure (Chapter 22), myocardial infarction (Chapter 25), and narrow-angle glaucoma (Chapter 48).

NURSING CONSIDERATIONS

Because the purposes and indications of drugs within this class vary greatly, the Nursing Process Focus applies to all patients receiving adrenergic antagonist drugs. For specific nursing considerations, contraindications, and precautions, see Chapters 21, 25, and 48 for more information about alpha- and beta-adrenergic blockers.

Pr **PROTOTYPE DRUG** | **PRAZOSIN** (Minipress)

ACTIONS AND USES

Prazosin is a selective alpha$_1$-adrenergic antagonist that competes with norepinephrine at its receptors on vascular smooth muscle in arterioles and veins. Its major action is a rapid decrease in peripheral resistance that reduces blood pressure. It has little effect on cardiac output or heart rate and it causes less reflex tachycardia than some other drugs in this class. Tolerance may occur to its antihypertensive effect. Its most common use is in combination with other agents, such as beta-blockers or diuretics, in the pharmacotherapy of hypertension. Prazosin has a short half-life and is often taken two or three times per day.

Administration Alerts

- Increases urinary metabolites of vanillylmandelic acid (VMA) and norepinephrine, which are measured to screen for pheochromocytoma (adrenal tumor). Prazosin will cause false-positive results.
- Pregnancy category C.

ADVERSE EFFECTS AND INTERACTIONS

Like other alpha-blockers, prazosin has a tendency to cause orthostatic hypotension due to alpha$_1$ inhibition in vascular smooth muscle. In rare cases, this hypotension can be so severe as to cause unconsciousness about 30 minutes after the first dose. This is called the *first dose phenomenon*. To avoid this situation, the first dose should be very low, and given at bedtime. Dizziness, drowsiness, or lightheadedness may occur as a result of decreased blood flow to the brain due to the drug's hypotensive action. Reflex tachycardia may occur due to the rapid falls in blood pressure. The alpha blockade may also result in nasal congestion or inhibition of ejaculation.

Drug interactions include increased hypotensive effects with concurrent use of antihypertensives and diuretics.

 See the companion website for a Nursing Process Focus specific to this drug.

NURSING PROCESS FOCUS	PATIENTS RECEIVING ADRENERGIC ANTAGONIST THERAPY

ASSESSMENT

Prior to administration:
- Assess vital signs, urinary output, and cardiac output (initially and throughout therapy).
- Assess reason for drug administration.
- Obtain complete health history, including allergies, drug history, and possible drug interactions.

POTENTIAL NURSING DIAGNOSES

- Deficient Knowledge, related to drug administration and effects
- Disturbed Sensory Perception (Visual, Kinesthetic)
- Risk for Injury, related to dizziness, syncope
- Impaired Urinary Elimination
- Sexual Dysfunction

PLANNING: PATIENT GOALS AND EXPECTED OUTCOMES

The patient will:
- Exhibit a decrease in blood pressure with fewer of adverse effects
- Report a decrease in urinary symptoms such as hesitancy and difficulty voiding
- Demonstrate an understanding of the drug's action by accurately describing drug side effects and precautions, and importance of follow-up care

IMPLEMENTATION

Interventions and (Rationales)

- For prostatic hypertrophy, monitor for urinary hesitancy/feeling of incomplete bladder emptying, interrupted urinary stream.

- Monitor for syncope. (Alpha-adrenergic antagonists produce first dose syncope phenomenon, and may cause loss of consciousness.)

- Monitor vital signs, level of consciousness, and mood. (Adrenergic antagonists can exacerbate existing mental depression.)

- Monitor carefully for dizziness, drowsiness, or lightheadedness. (These are signs of decreased blood flow to the brain due to the drug's hypotensive action.)

- Observe for side effects which may include blurred vision, tinnitus, epistaxis, and edema.

- Monitor liver function (due to increased risk for liver toxicity).

Patient Education/Discharge Planning

- Instruct patient to report increased difficulty with urinary voiding to healthcare provider.

Instruct patient to:
- Take this medication at bedtime, and to take the first dose *immediately* before getting into bed
- Avoid abrupt changes in position
Warn patient about the first dose phenomenon; reassure that this effect diminishes with continued therapy.

- Instruct patient to immediately report any feelings of dysphoria.
- Interview patient regarding suicide potential; obtain a "no-self harm" verbal contract from the patient.

Instruct patient:
- To monitor vitals signs, especially blood pressure, ensuring proper use of home equipment
- Regarding the normotensive range of blood pressure; instruct patient to consult the nurse regarding "reportable" blood pressure readings
- To report dizziness or syncope that persists beyond the first dose, as well as paresthesias and other neurological changes

Instruct patient:
- That nasal congestion may be a side effect
- To report any adverse reactions to the healthcare provider
Warn patient about the potential danger of concomitant use of OTC nasal decongestants.

Instruct patient to:
- Adhere to a regular schedule of laboratory testing for liver function as ordered by the healthcare provider
- Report signs and symptoms of liver toxicity: nausea, vomiting, diarrhea, rash, jaundice, abdominal pain, tenderness or distention, or change in color of stool
Inform patient of the importance of ongoing medication compliance and follow-up.

continued

EVALUATION OF OUTCOME CRITERIA

Evaluate effectiveness of drug therapy by confirming that patient goals and expected outcomes have been met (see "Planning").

⌸ See Table 13.5 for a list of drugs to which these nursing actions apply.

CHAPTER REVIEW

Key Concepts

The numbered key concepts provide a succinct summary of the important points from the corresponding numbered section within the chapter. If any of these points are not clear, refer to the numbered section within the chapter for review. Expanded versions can be found on the companion website.

13.1 The peripheral nervous system is divided into a somatic portion, which is under voluntary control, and an autonomic portion, which is involuntary and controls smooth muscle, cardiac muscle, and glandular secretion.

13.2 Stimulation of the sympathetic division of the autonomic nervous system causes symptoms of the fight-or-flight response, whereas stimulation of the parasympathetic branch induces rest-and-digest responses.

13.3 Drugs can affect nervous transmission across a synapse by preventing the storage or release of the neurotransmitter, binding receptors for the neurotransmitter, or by preventing the destruction of the neurotransmitter.

13.4 Acetylcholine is the primary neurotransmitter released at cholinergic receptors (nicotinic and muscarinic) in both the sympathetic and parasympathetic nervous systems. It is also the neurotransmitter at nicotinic receptors in skeletal muscle.

13.5 Norepinephrine is the primary neurotransmitter released at adrenergic receptors, which are divided into alpha and beta subtypes.

13.6 Autonomic drugs are classified by which receptors they stimulate or block: sympathomimetics stimulate sympathetic nerves and parasympathomimetics stimulate parasympathetic nerves; adrenergic antagonists inhibit the sympathetic division, whereas anticholinergics inhibit the parasympathetic branch.

13.7 Parasympathomimetics act directly by stimulating cholinergic receptors or indirectly by inhibiting acetylcholinesterase. They have few therapeutic uses because of their numerous side effects.

13.8 Anticholinergics act by blocking the effects of acetylcholine at muscarinic receptors, and are used to dry secretions, treat asthma, and prevent motion sickness.

13.9 Sympathomimetics act by directly activating adrenergic receptors, or indirectly by increasing the release of norepinephrine from nerve terminals. They are primarily used for their effects on the heart, bronchial tree, and nasal passages.

13.10 Adrenergic antagonists are primarily used for hypertension and are the most widely prescribed class of autonomic drugs.

Review Questions

1. How would a person who is entering a fight benefit from the sympathetic effects of bronchodilation, slowed GI motility, and pupil dilation?

2. Why do the sympathomimetics produce many of the same symptoms as the anticholinergics?

3. Both parasympathomimetics and adrenergic blockers produce similar actions. Why are the adrenergic blockers used to treat hypertension, but the parasympathomimetics not used for this purpose?

4. A new drug has been developed that is classified as an adrenergic-receptor antagonist. Why is it important to know which type of adrenergic receptor is blocked, before administering this medication?

Critical Thinking Questions

1. A 24-year-old patient (gravida 3, para 1) is admitted to the labor and delivery unit stating that she is having contractions. She is 32 weeks' gestation. The obstetrician initially begins tocolysis with magnesium sulfate and then switches the patient to terbutaline (Brethine), 5 mg PO q4h around the clock. The nurse recognizes terbutaline as a beta$_2$-adrenergic agonist. What education does the patient require in relation to terbutaline therapy?

2. A 74-year-old female patient has undergone a retropubic urethral suspension. She required a Foley catheter for 4 days post-op and was still unable to void. She was re-catheterized and a bladder rehabilitation program was begun which included bethanechol (Urecholine). What nursing diagnosis should be considered as a part of this patient's plan of care given this new drug regimen?

3. A 42-year-old male patient has been diagnosed with having Parkinson's disease for 4 years. He is being treated with a regimen of amantadine (Symmetrel), an indirect-acting dopaminergic agent, and benztropine mesylate (Cogentin). The nurse recognizes this drug as an anticholinergic agent. Discuss the potential side effects of benztropine that the nurse should assess for in this patient.

 ## EXPLORE MediaLink

NCLEX review, case studies, and other interactive resources for this chapter can be found on the companion website at www.prenhall.com/adams. Click on "Chapter 13" to select the activities for this chapter. For animations, more NCLEX review questions, and an audio glossary, access the accompanying CD-ROM in this textbook.

CHAPTER 14

Drugs for Anxiety and Insomnia

◼ DRUGS AT A GLANCE

BENZODIAZEPINES

Ⓟ *lorazepam (Ativan)*

BARBITURATES

NONBENZODIAZEPINES, NONBARBITURATE CNS DEPRESSANTS

Ⓟ *zolpidem (Ambien)*

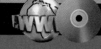

MediaLink www.prenhall.com/adams

CD-ROM
Audio Glossary
NCLEX Review

Companion Website
NCLEX Review
Dosage Calculations
Case Study
Care Plans
Expanded Key Concepts

KEY TERMS

anxiety *page 143*

anxiolytics *page 144*

electroencephalogram (EEG) *page 147*

generalized anxiety disorder (GAD) *page 143*

hypnotic *page 147*

insomnia *page 144*

limbic system *page 144*

obsessive-compulsive disorder (OCD) *page 144*

panic disorder *page 144*

phobias *page 144*

posttraumatic stress disorder (PTSD) *page 144*

rebound insomnia *page 147*

REM sleep *page 147*

reticular activating system (RAS) *page 144*

reticular formation *page 144*

sedative *page 147*

sedative-hypnotic *page 147*

situational anxiety *page 143*

sleep debt *page 147*

OBJECTIVES

After reading this chapter, the student should be able to:

1. Identify the major types of anxiety disorders.

2. Discuss factors contributing to anxiety and explain some nonpharmacologic therapies used to cope with this disorder.

3. Identify the regions of the brain associated with anxiety, sleep, and wakefulness.

4. Identify the three classes of medications used to treat anxiety and sleep disorders.

5. Explain the pharmacologic management of anxiety and insomnia.

6. Describe the nurse's role in the pharmacologic management of anxiety and insomnia.

7. Identify normal sleep patterns and explain how these might be affected by anxiety and stress.

8. Categorize drugs used for anxiety and insomnia based on their classification and mechanism of action.

9. For each of the classes listed in Drugs at a Glance, know representative drugs and explain their mechanisms of action, primary actions, and important adverse effects.

10. Use the Nursing Process to care for patients receiving drug therapy for anxiety and insomnia.

People experience nervousness and tension more often than any other symptoms. Seeking relief from these symptoms, patients often turn to a variety of pharmacologic and alternative therapies. Most healthcare providers agree that even though drugs do not cure the underlying problem, they can provide short-term help to calm patients who are experiencing acute anxiety, or who have simple sleep disorders. This chapter deals with drugs that treat anxiety, cause sedation, or help patients sleep.

ANXIETY DISORDERS

According to the *International Classification of Diseases*, 10th edition (ICD-10), **anxiety** is a state of "apprehension, tension, or uneasiness that stems from the anticipation of danger, the source of which is largely unknown or unrecognized." Anxious individuals can often identify at least some factors that bring on their symptoms. Most state that their feelings of anxiety are disproportionate to any factual dangers.

14.1 Types of Anxiety Disorders

The anxiety experienced by people faced with a stressful environment is called **situational anxiety**. To a certain degree, situational anxiety is beneficial because it motivates people to accomplish tasks in a prompt manner—if for no other reason than to eliminate the source of nervousness. Situational stress may be intense, though patients often learn coping mechanisms to deal with the stress without seeking conventional medical intervention. From an early age, ego defense mechanisms begin to develop that serve as defenses against anxiety.

Generalized anxiety disorder (GAD) is a difficult to control, excessive anxiety that lasts 6 months or more. It focuses on a variety of life events or activities, and interferes with normal, day-to-day functions. It is by far the most common type of stress disorder, and the one most frequently encountered by the nurse. Symptoms include restlessness, fatigue, muscle tension, nervousness, inability to focus or concentrate, an overwhelming sense of dread, and sleep disturbances. Autonomic signs of sympathetic nervous system activation include blood pressure elevation, heart palpitations, varying degrees of respiratory change, dry mouth, and increased reflexes. Parasympathetic responses may consist of abdominal cramping, diarrhea, fatigue, urinary urgency, and numbness and tingling of the extremities. Females are slightly more likely to experience GAD, and its prevalence is highest in the 20–35 age group.

A second category of anxiety, called panic disorder, is characterized by intense feelings of immediate apprehension, fearfulness, terror, or impending doom, accompanied by increased autonomic nervous system activity. Although panic attacks usually last less than 10 minutes, patients may describe them as seemingly endless. As much as 5% of the population will experience one or more panic attacks during their lifetime, with women being affected about twice as often as men.

Other categories of anxiety disorders include phobias, obsessive-compulsive disorder, and posttraumatic stress disorder. Phobias are fearful feelings attached to situations or objects. Common phobias include fear of snakes, spiders, crowds, or heights. Phobias compel a patient to avoid the fearful stimulus. Obsessive-compulsive disorder (OCD) involves recurrent, intrusive thoughts or repetitive behaviors that interfere with normal activities or relationships. Common examples include fear of exposure to germs and repetitive handwashing. Posttraumatic stress disorder (PTSD) is a type of anxiety that develops in response to re-experiencing a previous life event. Traumatic life events such as war, physical or sexual abuse, natural disasters, or murder may lead to a sense of helplessness and reexperiencing of the traumatic event. In the aftermath of the terrorist attack of September 11, 2001, the incidence of PTSD has increased considerably.

14.2 Regions of the Brain Responsible for Anxiety and Wakefulness

Neural systems associated with anxiety and restlessness include the limbic system and the reticular activating system. These are illustrated in Figure 14.1.

The limbic system is an area in the middle of the brain responsible for emotional expression, learning, and memory. Signals routed through the limbic system ultimately connect with the hypothalamus. Emotional states associated with this connection include anxiety, fear, anger, aggression, remorse, depression, sexual drive, and euphoria.

The hypothalamus is an important center responsible for unconscious responses to extreme stress such as high blood pressure, elevated breathing rate, and dilated pupils. These are responses associated with the fight-or-flight

response of the autonomic nervous system as presented in Chapter 13 ⊕ . The many endocrine functions of the hypothalamus are discussed in Chapter 39 ⊕ .

The hypothalamus also connects with the reticular formation, a network of neurons found along the entire length of the brainstem, as shown in Figure 14.1B. Stimulation of the reticular formation causes heightened alertness and arousal; inhibition causes general drowsiness and the induction of sleep.

The larger area in which the reticular formation is found is called the reticular activating system (RAS). This structure projects from the brainstem to the thalamus. The RAS is responsible for sleeping and wakefulness and performs an alerting function for the cerebral cortex. It also helps a person to focus attention on individual tasks by transmitting information to higher brain centers.

If signals are prevented from passing through the RAS, no emotional signals are sent to the brain, resulting in a reduction in general brain activity. If signals coming from the hypothalamus are allowed to proceed, then those signals are further routed through the RAS and on to higher brain centers. This is the neural mechanism thought to be responsible for emotions such as anxiety and fear. It is also the mechanism associated with restlessness and an interrupted sleeping pattern.

14.3 Anxiety Management through Pharmacologic and Nonpharmacologic Strategies

Although stress itself may be incapacitating, it is often only a symptom of an underlying disorder. It is considered more productive to uncover and to address the cause of the anxiety rather than to merely treat the symptoms with medications. Patients should be encouraged to explore and develop nonpharmacologic coping strategies to deal with the underlying causes. Such strategies may include behavioral therapy, biofeedback techniques, meditation, and other complementary therapies. One model for stress management is shown in Figure 14.2.

When anxiety becomes severe enough to significantly interfere with daily activities of life, pharmacotherapy is indicated. In most types of stress, anxiolytics, or drugs having the ability to relieve anxiety, are quite effective. Anxiolytics are usually meant to address generalized anxiety on a short-term basis. Longer term pharmacotherapy for phobias and obsessive-compulsive and posttraumatic stress disorders may include mood disorder drugs (Chapter 16) ⊕ .

INSOMNIA

Insomnia is a condition characterized by a patient's inability to fall asleep or remain asleep. Pharmacotherapy may be indicated if the sleeplessness interferes with normal daily activities.

PHARMFACTS	**Anxiety Disorders**

- About 19 million Americans have anxiety every year.
- Other illnesses that commonly coexist with anxiety include depression, eating disorders, and substance abuse.
- The top five causes of anxiety (as listed in order) occur between the ages of 18 and 54.
  Phobia
  Posttraumatic stress
  Generalized anxiety
  Obsessive-compulsive feelings
  Panic

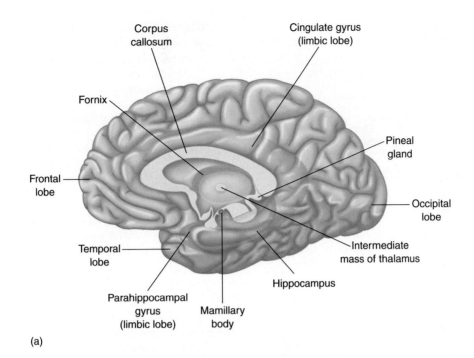

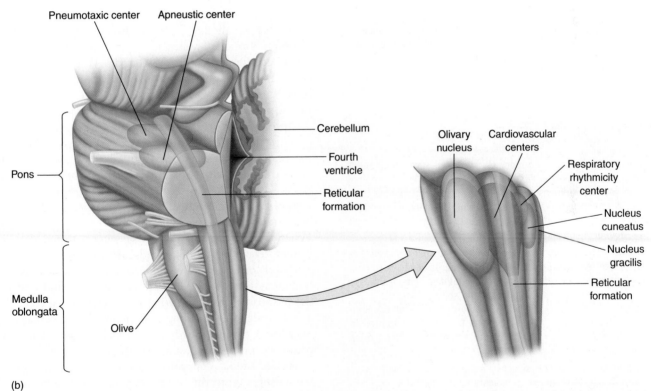

Figure 14.1 | Two regions of the brain are strongly associated with anxiety, expressions of emotion, and a restless state: (a) the limbic system; and (b) the reticular formation, a nucleus where nervous signals ascend to higher centers of the brain; this entire neural network is called the reticular activating system

14.4 Insomnia and Its Link to Anxiety

Why is it that we need sleep? During an average lifetime, about 33% of the time is spent sleeping, or trying to sleep. Although it is well established that sleep is essential for wellness, scientists are unsure of its function or how much is needed. Following are some theories.

- Inactivity during sleep gives the body time to repair itself.
- Sleep is a function that evolved as a protective mechanism. Throughout history, nighttime was the safest time of day.
- Sleep deals with "electrical" charging and discharging of the brain. The brain needs time for processing and filing new information collected throughout the day. When

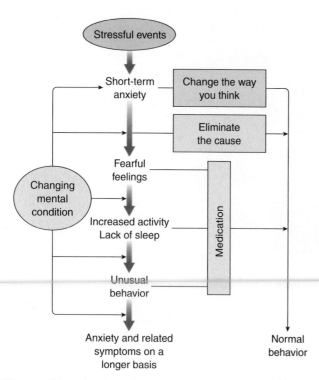

Figure 14.2 A model of anxiety where stressful events or a changing mental condition can produce unfavorable symptoms, some of which may be controlled by medication

NATURAL THERAPIES **Melatonin**

Melatonin is a natural hormone (N-acetyl-5 methoxytryptamine) produced especially at night in the pineal gland. Its secretion is stimulated by darkness and inhibited by light. Tryptophan is converted to serotonin and finally to melatonin. As melatonin production rises, alertness decreases, and body temperature starts to fall, both of which make sleep more inviting.

Melatonin production is also related to age. Children manufacture more melatonin than elderly patients; however, melatonin production begins to drop at puberty. Melatonin is one of only two hormones not regulated by the FDA and sold OTC without a prescription (DHEA, or dehydroepiandrosterone, is the other). Supplemental melatonin, 0.5 to 3.0 mg at bedtime, is purported to decrease the time required to fall asleep and to produce a deep and restful sleep.

Melatonin should not be taken by pregnant or nursing patients, as there is a lack of studies to indicate its safety. Large doses of melatonin have been shown to inhibit ovulation, so women trying to conceive should reconsider taking melatonin.

People with severe allergies, autoimmune diseases, and immune system cancers such as lymphoma and leukemia should not take melatonin, because it could exacerbate such conditions by stimulating the immune system. Patients taking corticosteroids should be advised that melatonin may interfere with the efficacy of these hormones. Melatonin use in some children with seizure disorders may lead to increased seizure activity. Melatonin should not be given to healthy children, as they already produce it in abundance.

this is done without interference from the outside environment, these vast amounts of data can be retrieved through memory.

The acts of sleeping and waking are synchronized to many different bodily functions. Body temperature, blood pressure, hormone levels, and respiration all fluctuate on a cyclic basis throughout the 24-hour day. When this cycle becomes impaired, pharmacologic or other interventions may be needed to readjust it. Increased levels of the neurotransmitter, serotonin, help initiate the various processes of sleep.

Insomnia, or sleeplessness, is a disorder sometimes associated with anxiety. There are several major types of insomnia. Short-term or behavioral insomnia may be attributed to stress caused by a hectic lifestyle or the inability to resolve day-to-day conflicts within the home environment or the workplace. Worries about work, marriage, children, and health are common reasons for short-term loss of sleep. When stress interrupts normal sleeping patterns, patients cannot sleep because their minds are too active.

Foods or beverages containing stimulants such as caffeine may interrupt sleep. Patients may also find that the use of tobacco products makes them restless and edgy. Alcohol, while often enabling a person to fall asleep, may produce vivid dreams and frequent awakening that prevent restful sleep. Ingestion of a large meal, especially one high in protein and fat, consumed close to bedtime can interfere with sleep, due to the increased metabolic rate needed to digest the food. Certain medications cause CNS stimulation, and these should not be taken immediately before bedtime. Stressful conditions such as too much light, uncomfortable room temperature (especially one that is too warm), snoring, sleep apnea, and recurring nightmares also interfere with sleep. Long-term insomnia may be caused by depression, manic disorders, and chronic pain.

Nonpharmacologic means should be attempted prior to initiating drug therapy for sleep disorders. Long-term use of sleep medications is likely to worsen insomnia and may cause physical or psychological dependence. Some patients

PHARMFACTS	Insomnia Linked to Insulin Resistance

- Chronic lack of sleep may make people more prone to developing type 2, or noninsulin-dependent diabetes mellitus (NIDDM).
- Chronic lack of sleep can provide the impetus for the body to acquire a reduced sensitivity to insulin.
- In one study, healthy adults who averaged little more than 5 hours of sleep per night over 8 consecutive nights, secreted 50% more insulin than those who averaged 8 hours of sleep per night for the same period. Those who slept less were 40% less sensitive to insulin than those who got more sleep.
- Sleep deprivation (6.5 hours or less per night) may explain why type 2 diabetes is becoming more prevalent.

experience a phenomenon referred to as rebound insomnia. This occurs when a sedative drug is discontinued abruptly or after it has been taken for a long time; sleeplessness and symptoms of anxiety then become markedly worse.

Older patients are more likely to experience medication-related sleep problems. Drugs may seem to help the insomnia of an elderly patient for a night or two, only to produce generalized brain dysfunction as the medication accumulates in the system. The agitated patient may then be mistakenly overdosed with further medication. Nurses, especially those who work in geriatric settings, are responsible for making accurate observations and reporting patient responses to drugs so the healthcare provider can determine the lowest effective maintenance dose. The need for PRN medication for sleep requires individualized assessment by the nurse, as well as follow-up evaluation and documentation of its effect on the patient.

14.5 Use of the Electroencephalogram to Diagnose Sleep and Seizure Disorders

The electroencephalogram (EEG) is a tool for the diagnosis of sleep disorders, seizure activity, depression, and dementia. Four types of brain waves—alpha, beta, delta, and theta—are identified by their shape, frequencies, and height on a graph. Brain waves give the healthcare provider an idea of how brain activity changes during various stages of sleep and consciousness. For example, alpha waves indicate an awake but drowsy patient. Beta waves indicate an alert patient whose mind is active.

Two distinct types of sleep can be identified on the EEG: nonrapid eye movement (NREM) sleep and rapid eye movement (REM) sleep. There are four progressive stages that advance into REM sleep. After going through the four stages of NREM sleep, the sequence goes into reverse. Under normal circumstances, after returning from the depths of stage IV back to stage I of NREM, a person will still not awaken. Sleep quality begins to change; it is not as deep, and hormone lev-

els and body temperature begin to rise. At that point, REM sleep occurs. REM sleep is often called paradoxical sleep, because this stage has a brain wave pattern similar to when persons are drowsy but awake. This is the stage when dreaming occurs. People with normal sleep patterns move from NREM to REM sleep about every 90 minutes.

Patients who are deprived of stage IV NREM sleep experience depression and a feeling of apathy and fatigue. Stage IV NREM sleep appears to be linked to repair and restoration of the physical body, while REM sleep is associated with learning, memory, and the capacity to adjust to changes in the environment. The body requires the dream state associated with REM sleep to keep the psyche functioning normally. When test subjects are deprived of REM sleep, they experience a sleep debt and become frightened, irritable, paranoid, and even emotionally disturbed. Judgment is impaired and reaction time is slowed. It is speculated that, to make up for their lack of dreaming, they experience far more daydreaming and fantasizing throughout the day. The stages of sleep are shown in Table 14.1.

CENTRAL NERVOUS SYSTEM DEPRESSANTS

CNS depressants are used to slow brain activity in patients experiencing anxiety or sleep disorders. These medications are grouped into three classes: benzodiazepines, barbiturates, and nonbarbiturate/nonbenzodiazepine CNS depressants.

14.6 Treating Anxiety and Insomnia with CNS Depressants

CNS depressants are drugs that slow neuronal activity in the brain. CNS depression should be viewed as a continuum ranging from relaxation, to sedation, to the induction of sleep and anesthesia. Coma and death are the end stages of CNS depression. Some drug classes are capable of producing the full range of CNS depression from calming to anesthesia, whereas others are less efficacious. CNS depressants used for anxiety and sleep disorders are categorized into two major classes, the benzodiazepines and barbiturates. A third class consists of miscellaneous drugs that are chemically unrelated to the benzodiazepines or barbiturates, but have similar therapeutic uses. Other CNS depressants include the opioids (Chapter 19) and ethyl alcohol (Chapter 12) .

Medications that depress the CNS are sometimes called sedatives because of their ability to sedate or relax a patient. At higher doses, some of these drugs are called hypnotics because of their ability to induce sleep. Thus, the term sedative-hypnotic is often used to describe a drug with the ability to produce a calming effect at lower doses while having the ability to induce sleep at higher doses. Tranquilizer is an older term, sometimes used to describe a drug that produces a calm or tranquil feeling.

Many CNS depressants can cause physical and psychological dependence, as discussed in Chapter 12 . The

Table 14.1	Stages of Sleep
Stage	**Description**
NREM stage 1	At the onset of sleep, the patient is in a stage of drowsiness for about 1 to 7 minutes. During this time, the patient can be easily awakened. This stage lasts for about 4% to 5% of total sleep time.
NREM stage 2	Patient can still be easily awakened. Comprises the greatest amount of total sleep time, 45% to 55%.
NREM stage 3	Patient may move into or out of a deeper sleep. Heart rate and blood pressure falls; gastrointestinal activity rises. This stage lasts for about 4% to 6% of total sleep time.
NREM stage 4	The deepest stage of sleep; lasts a little longer than stage 1 or stage 3 sleep, about 12% to 15%. This is the stage during which nightmares occur in children. Sleepwalking is also a common behavior for this stage. Heart rate and blood pressure remain low; gastrointestinal activity remains high.
REM sleep	Characterized by eye movement and a loss of muscle tone. Eye movement occurs in bursts of activity. Dreaming takes place in this stage. The mind is very active and resembles a normal waking state.

withdrawal syndrome for some CNS depressants can cause life-threatening neurologic reactions, including fever, psychosis, and seizures. Other withdrawal symptoms include increased heart rate and lowered blood pressure; loss of appetite; muscle cramps; impairment of memory, concentration, and orientation; abnormal sounds in the ears and blurred vision; and insomnia, agitation, anxiety, and panic. Obvious withdrawal symptoms typically last 2 to 4 weeks. Subtle ones can last months.

Benzodiazepines

The benzodiazepines are one of the most widely prescribed drug classes. The root word *benzo* refers to an aromatic compound, one having a carbon ring structure attached to different atoms or another carbon ring. Two nitrogen atoms incorporated into the ring structure are the reason for the diazepine (*di* = two; *azepine* = nitrogen) portion of the name.

14.7 Treating Anxiety and Insomnia with Benzodiazepines

The benzodiazepines are drugs of choice for various anxiety disorders and for insomnia (see Table 14.2). Since the introduction of the first benzodiazepines—chlordiazepoxide (Librium) and diazepam (Valium)—in the 1960s, the class has become one of the most widely prescribed in medicine. Although about 15 benzodiazepines are available, all have the same actions and adverse effects, and differ primarily in their onset and duration of action. Some, such as midazolam (Versed), have a rapid onset time of 15 to 30 minutes; others, such as halazepam (Paxipam), take 1 to 3 hours to reach peak serum levels. The benzodiazepines are categorized as Schedule IV drugs, although they produce considerably less physical dependence and result in less tolerance than the barbiturates.

Benzodiazepines act by binding to the gamma-aminobutyric acid (GABA) receptor-chloride channel molecule. These drugs intensify the effect of GABA, which is a natural inhibitory neurotransmitter found throughout the brain. Most are metabolized in the liver to active metabolites and excreted primarily in urine. One major advantage of the benzodiazepines is that they do not produce life-threatening respiratory depression or coma if taken in excessive amounts. Death is unlikely, unless the benzodiazepines are taken in large quantities in combination with other CNS depressants, or the patient suffers from sleep apnea.

Most benzodiazepines are given orally. Those that can be given parenterally, such as diazepam (Valium) and lorazepam (Ativan), should be monitored carefully due to their rapid onset of CNS effects, and possible respiratory depression.

The benzodiazepines are drugs of choice for the short-term treatment of insomnia caused by anxiety, having replaced the barbiturates because of their greater margin of safety. Benzodiazepines shorten the length of time it takes to fall asleep and reduce the frequency of interrupted sleep. Although most benzodiazepines increase total sleep time, some reduce stage IV sleep, and some affect REM sleep. In general, the benzodiazepines used to treat short-term insomnia are different from those used to treat generalized anxiety disorder.

Benzodiazepines have a number of other important indications. Diazepam (Valium) is featured as a prototype in Chapter 15 for its use in treating seizure disorders. Other uses include treatment of alcohol withdrawal symptoms, central muscle relaxation (Chapter 45), and as induction agents in general anesthesia (Chapter 20) .

NURSING CONSIDERATIONS

The role of the nurse in benzodiazepine therapy involves careful monitoring of a patient's condition and providing education as it relates to the prescribed drug regimen. The

Table 14.2	Benzodiazepines for Anxiety and Insomnia
Drug	**Route and Adult Dose (max dose where indicated)**
Anxiety Therapy	
alprazolam (Xanax)	For anxiety: PO 0.25–0.5 mg tid For panic attacks: PO 1–2 mg tid
chlordiazepoxide (Librium)	Mild anxiety: PO 5–10 mg tid or qid; IM/IV 50–100 mg 1 hr before a medical procedure Severe anxiety: PO 20–25 mg tid or qid; IM/IV 50–100 mg followed by 25–50 mg tid or qid
clonazepam (Klonopin)	PO; 1–2 mg/day in divided doses (max 4 mg/day)
clorazepate (Tranxene)	PO; 15 mg/day at hs (max 60 mg/day in divided doses)
Pr diazepam (Valium)	PO; 2–10 mg bid; IM/IV 2–10 mg, repeat if needed in 3–4 hr
halazepam (Paxipam)	PO; 20–40 mg tid or qid
Pr lorazepam (Ativan)	PO; 2–6 mg/day in divided doses (max 10 mg/day)
oxazepam (Serax)	PO; 10–30 mg tid or qid
Insomnia Therapy	
estazolam (Prosom)	PO; 1 mg at hs, may increase to 2 mg if necessary
flurazepam (Dalmane)	PO; 15–30 mg at hs
quazepam (Doral)	PO; 7.5–15 mg at hs
temazepam (Restoril)	PO; 7.5–30 mg at hs
triazolam (Halcion)	PO; 0.125–0.25 mg at hs; (max 0.5 mg/day)

nurse should assess patient needs for antianxiety drugs, including intensity and duration of symptoms. The assessment should include identification of factors that precipitate anxiety or insomnia: physical symptoms, excessive CNS stimulation, excessive daytime sleep, or too little exercise or activity. The nurse should obtain a drug history, including hypersensitivity and the use of alcohol and other CNS depressants. The nurse should assess for the likelihood of drug abuse and dependence, and identify coping mechanisms used in managing previous episodes of stress, anxiety, and insomnia. These drugs should be used with caution in patients with a suicidal tendency, as the risk of suicide may be increased. The nurse should assess for the existence of a primary sleep disorder, such as sleep apnea, as benzodiazepines depress respiratory drive.

Alterations in neurotransmitter activity produce changes in intraocular pressure; therefore, benzodiazepines are contraindicated in narrow-angle glaucoma. The presence of any organic brain disease is contraindicated, as these drugs alter the level of consciousness. Liver and kidney function should be monitored in long-term use, and these drugs should be used cautiously in those patients with impaired renal or liver function. Because benzodiazepines cross the placenta and are excreted in breast milk, they are not recommended in pregnant or nursing women (pregnancy category D).

The risk of respiratory depression should be taken into consideration when administering to patients with impaired respiratory function, those taking other CNS depressants, and with intravenous doses. The nurse should assess for common side effects related to CNS depression such as drowsiness and dizziness, as these increase a patient's risk of injury and may indicate a need for dose reduction. Should an overdose occur, flumazenil (Romazicon) is a specific benzodiazepine receptor antagonist that can be administered to reverse CNS depression.

Benzodiazepines are used illegally for recreation, most often by adolescents, young adults, and opioid or cocaine addicts. Nurses should help patients evaluate the social context of their environment, and take any precautions necessary to safeguard the medication supply.

See "Nursing Process Focus: Patients Receiving Benzodiazepine and Nonbenzodiazepine Antianxiety Therapy" for specific teaching points.

Barbiturates

Barbiturates are drugs derived from barbituric acid. They are powerful CNS depressants prescribed for their sedative, hypnotic, and antiseizure effects that have been used in pharmacotherapy since the early 1900s.

PROTOTYPE DRUG | LORAZEPAM (Ativan)

ACTIONS AND USES

Lorazepam is a benzodiazepine that acts by potentiating the effects of GABA, an inhibitory neurotransmitter, in the thalamic, hypothalamic, and limbic levels of the CNS. It is one of the most potent benzodiazepines. It has an extended half-life of 10 to 20 hours that allows for once or twice a day oral dosing. In addition to its use as an anxiolytic, lorazepam is used as a preanesthetic medication to provide sedation, and for the management of status epilepticus.

Administration Alerts

- When administering IV, monitor respirations every 5 to 15 minutes. Have airway and resuscitative equipment accessible.
- Pregnancy category D.

ADVERSE EFFECTS AND INTERACTIONS

The most common side effects of lorazepam are drowsiness and sedation, which may decrease with time. When given in higher doses or by the IV route, more severe effects may be observed, such as amnesia, weakness, disorientation, ataxia, sleep disturbance, blood pressure changes, blurred vision, double vision, nausea, and vomiting.

Lorazepam interacts with multiple drugs. For example, concurrent use of CNS depressants, including alcohol, potentiate sedation effects and increase the risk of respiratory depression and death. Lorazepam may contribute to digoxin toxicity by increasing the serum digoxin level. Symptoms include visual changes, nausea, vomiting, dizziness, and confusion.

Use with caution with herbal supplements. For example, sedation-producing herbs such as kava, valerian, chamomile, or hops may have an additive effect with medication. Stimulant herbs such as gotu-kola and ma huang may reduce the drug's effectiveness.

 See the companion website for a Nursing Process Focus specific to this drug.

14.8 Use of Barbiturates as Sedatives

Until the discovery of the benzodiazepines, barbiturates were the drugs of choice for treating anxiety and insomnia (see Table 14.3). While barbiturates are still indicated for several conditions, they are rarely, if ever, prescribed for treating anxiety or insomnia because of significant side effects and the availability of more effective medications. The risk of psychological and physical dependence is high—several are Schedule II drugs. The withdrawal syndrome from barbiturates is extremely severe and can be fatal. Overdose results in profound respiratory depression, hypotension, and shock. Barbiturates have been used to commit suicide, and death due to overdose is not uncommon.

Barbiturates are capable of depressing CNS function at all levels. Like benzodiazepines, barbiturates act by binding to GABA receptor-chloride channel molecules, intensifying the effect of GABA throughout the brain. At low doses they reduce anxiety and cause drowsiness. At moderate doses they inhibit seizure activity (Chapter 15) and promote sleep, presumably by inhibiting brain impulses traveling through the limbic system and the reticular activating system. At higher doses, some barbiturates can induce anesthesia (Chapter 20) .

When taken for prolonged periods, barbiturates stimulate the microsomal enzymes in the liver that metabolize medications. Thus, barbiturates can stimulate their own metabolism, as well as that of hundreds of other drugs that use these enzymes for their breakdown. With repeated use, tolerance develops to the sedative effects of the drug; this includes cross-tolerance to other CNS depressants such as the opioids. Tolerance does not develop, however, to the respiratory depressant effects (see Chapter 15, page 163, for "Nursing Process Focus: Patients Receiving Barbiturate Therapy for Seizures") .

14.9 Other CNS Depressants for Anxiety and Sleep Disorders

The final group of CNS depressants used for anxiety and sleep disorders consists of miscellaneous agents that are chemically unrelated to either benzodiazepines or barbiturates (see Table 14.4). Some of these, such as paraldehyde (Paracetaldehyde), chloral hydrate (Noctec), meprobamate (Equanil), and glutethimide (Doriglute) have only historical interest, because they are so rarely prescribed. Several, however, such as buspirone (BuSpar) and zolpidem (Ambien), are relatively new agents, and are commonly prescribed for their anxiolytic and hypnotic effects.

The mechanism of action for buspirone (BuSpar) is unclear, but appears to be related to D_2 dopamine receptors in the brain. The drug has agonist effects on presynaptic dopamine receptors and a high affinity for serotonin receptors. Buspirone is less likely than benzodiazepines to affect cognitive and motor performance and rarely interacts with other CNS depressants. Common side effects include dizziness, headache, and drowsiness. Dependence and withdrawal problems are less of a concern with buspirone. Therapy may take several weeks to achieve optimal results.

Zolpidem (Ambien) is a Schedule IV controlled substance limited to the short-term treatment of insomnia. It preserves deep sleep. As with other CNS depressants it should be used cautiously in patients with respiratory impairment,

Table 14.3	Barbiturates for Sedation and Insomnia
Drug	**Route and Adult Dose (max dose where indicated)**
Short acting	
pentobarbital sodium (Nembutal)	Sedative: PO; 20–30 mg bid or qid Hypnotic: PO; 120–200 mg, 150–200 mg IM
secobarbital (Seconal)	Sedative: PO; 100–300 mg/day in three divided doses Hypnotic: PO/IM; 100–200 mg
Intermediate acting	
amobarbital (Amytal)	Sedative: PO; 30–50 mg bid or tid Hypnotic: PO/IM; 65–200 mg (max 500 mg)
aprobarbital (Alurate)	Sedative: PO; 40 mg tid Hypnotic: PO; 40–160 mg
butabarbital sodium (Butisol)	Sedative: PO; 15–30 mg tid or qid Hypnotic: PO; 50–100 mg at hs
Long acting	
mephobarbital (Mebaral) phenobarbital (Luminal) (see page 162 for the Prototype Drug box)	Sedative: PO; 32–100 mg tid or qid Sedative: PO; 30–120 mg/day IV/IM; 100–200 mg/day

Table 14.4	Nonbenzodiazepine, Nonbarbiturate CNS Depressants
Drug	**Route and Adult Dose (max dose where indicated)**
buspirone (BuSpar)	PO; 7.5–15 mg in divided doses; may increase by 5 mg/day every 2–3 days if needed (max 60 mg/day)
chloral hydrate (Noctec)	Sedative: PO or by suppositories; 250 mg tid after meals Hypnotic: PO; 500 mg–1 g 15–30 min before hs
dexmedetomidine HCl (Precedex)	IV; Loading dose 1 μg/kg over 10 min, Maintenance dose 0.2–0.7 μg/kg/hr
ethchlorvynol (Placidyl)	Sedative: PO; 200 mg bid or tid Hypnotic: PO; 500 mg–1 g at hs
glutethimide (Doriglute)	Hypnotic: PO 250–500 mg at hs
meprobamate (Equanil)	Sedative: PO; 1.2–1.6 g/day in three to four divided doses (max 2.4 g/day) Hypnotic: PO 400–800 mg
paraldehyde (Paracetaldehyde)	Sedative: PO; 5–10 ml prn Hypnotic: 10–30 ml prn
zolpidem (Ambien)	PO; 5–10 mg at hs

the elderly, and when used concurrently with other CNS depressants. Lower dosages may be necessary. Also, because of the rapid onset of this drug (7 to 27 minutes), it should be taken just prior to expected sleep. Because zolpidem is metabolized in the liver and excreted by the kidneys, impaired liver or kidney function can increase serum drug levels. Zolpidem is in pregnancy category B.

Diphenhydramine (Benadryl) and hydroxyzine (Vistaril) are antihistamines that produce drowsiness and may be beneficial in calming patients. They offer the advantage of not causing dependence, although their use is often limited by anticholinergic side effects. Diphenhydramine is a common component of OTC sleep aides (Chapter 31) .

PROTOTYPE DRUG | ZOLPIDEM (Ambien)

ACTIONS AND USES

Although a nonbenzodiazepine, zolpidem acts in a similar fashion to facilitate GABA-mediated CNS depression in the limbic, thalamic, and hypothalamic regions. It preserves stages III and IV sleep and has only minor effects on REM sleep. The only indication for zolpidem is for short-term insomnia management (7 to 10 days). Zolpidem is pregnancy category B.

Administration Alert

- Because of rapid onset, 7 to 27 minutes, give immediately before bedtime.

ADVERSE EFFECTS AND INTERACTIONS

Side effects include daytime sedation, confusion, amnesia, dizziness, depression, nausea, and vomiting.

Drug interactions with zolpidem include an increase in sedation when used concurrently with other CNS depressants, including alcohol. When taken with food, absorption is slowed significantly and the onset of action may be delayed.

 See the companion website for a Nursing Process Focus specific to this drug.

NURSING PROCESS FOCUS | PATIENTS RECEIVING BENZODIAZEPINE AND NONBENZODIAZEPINE ANTIANXIETY THERAPY

ASSESSMENT

Prior to administration:
- Obtain complete health history (both physical/mental), including allergies and drug history for possible drug interactions.
- Identify factors that precipitate anxiety or insomnia.
- Assess likelihood of drug abuse and dependence.
- Establish baseline vital signs and level of consciousness.

POTENTIAL NURSING DIAGNOSES

- Risk for Injury
- Anxiety
- Deficient Knowledge, related to drug therapy
- Ineffective Individual Coping
- Disturbed Sleep Pattern

PLANNING: PATIENT GOALS AND EXPECTED OUTCOMES

The patient will:
- Experience an increase in psychological comfort
- Report absence of physical and behavioral manifestations of anxiety
- Demonstrate an understanding of the drug's action by accurately describing drug side effects and precautions

IMPLEMENTATION

Interventions and (Rationales)	Patient Education / Discharge Planning
- Monitor vital signs. Observe respiratory patterns, especially during sleep, for evidence of apnea or shallow breathing. (Benzodiazepines can reduce the respiratory drive in susceptible patients.)	Instruct patient: - To consult the healthcare provider before taking this drug if snoring is a problem. Snoring may indicate an obstruction in the upper respiratory tract resulting in hypoxia - Regarding methods to monitor vital signs at home, especially respirations

continued

Nursing Process Focus: **Patients Receiving Benzodiazepine and Nonbenzodiazepine Antianxiety Therapy (continued)**

Interventions and (Rationales)	*Patient Education / Discharge Planning*
■ Monitor neurological status, especially level of consciousness. (Confusion or lack of response may indicate overmedication.)	■ Instruct patient to report extreme lethargy, slurred speech, disorientation, or ataxia.
■ Ensure patient safety. (Drug may cause excessive drowsiness.)	Instruct patient: ■ Do not drive or perform hazardous activities until effects of drug are known ■ To request assistance when getting out of bed and ambulating until effect of medication is known
■ Monitor the patient's intake of stimulants, including caffeine (in beverages such as coffee, tea, cola and other soft drinks, and OTC analgesics such as Excedrin), and nicotine from tobacco products, and nicotine patches. (These products can reduce the drug's effectiveness.)	Instruct patient to: ■ Avoid taking OTC sleep-inducing antihistamines, such as diphenhydramine ■ Consult the healthcare provider before self-medicating with any OTC preparation
■ Monitor affect and emotional status. (Drug may increase risk of mental depression, especially in patients with suicidal tendencies.)	Instruct patient to: ■ Report significant mood changes, especially depression ■ Avoid consuming alcohol or taking other CNS depressants while on benzodiazepines because these increase depressant effect
■ Avoid abrupt discontinuation of therapy. (Withdrawal symptoms, including rebound anxiety and sleeplessness, are possible with abrupt discontinuation after long-term use.)	Instruct patient: ■ To take drug exactly as prescribed ■ To keep all follow-up appointments as directed by healthcare provider to monitor response to medication ■ About nonpharmacologic methods for reestablishing sleep regimen

EVALUATION OF OUTCOME CRITERIA

Evaluate effectiveness of drug therapy by confirming that patient goals and expected outcomes have been met (see "Planning").

See Tables 14.2 and 14.4 for lists of drugs to which these nursing actions apply.

CHAPTER REVIEW

Key Concepts

The numbered key concepts provide a succinct summary of the important points from the corresponding numbered section within the chapter. If any of these points are not clear, refer to the numbered section within the chapter for review. Expanded versions can be found on the companion website.

14.1 Generalized anxiety disorder is the most common type of anxiety; phobias, obsessive-compulsive disorder, panic attacks, and posttraumatic stress disorders are other important categories.

14.2 The limbic system and the reticular activating system are specific regions of the brain responsible for anxiety and wakefulness.

14.3 Anxiety can be managed through pharmacologic and nonpharmacologic strategies.

14.4 Insomnia is a sleep disorder that may be caused by anxiety. Nonpharmacologic means should be attempted prior to initiating pharmacotherapy.

14.5 The electroencephalogram records brain waves and is used to diagnose sleep and seizure disorders.

14.6 CNS depressants, including anxiolytics, sedatives, and hypnotics, are used to treat anxiety and insomnia.

14.7 Benzodiazepines are drugs of choice for generalized anxiety and insomnia.

14.8 Because of their side effects and high potential for dependency, barbiturates are rarely used to treat insomnia.

14.9 Some commonly prescribed CNS depressants used for anxiety and sleep disorders are not related to either benzodiazepines or barbiturates.

Review Questions

1. Compare and contrast each of following terms in relation to anxiety and alertness: CNS depressants, sedatives, hypnotics, and anxiolytics.

2. What is the major drug class used to treat generalized anxiety disorder and panic disorder? Name popular drugs within this class.

3. Why might a patient not be able to enjoy normal sleep? Why is long-term pharmacotherapy for lack of sleep not recommended?

4. Identify the major drug classes used for daytime sedation and insomnia. Why are CNS depressants especially dangerous if administered in high doses?

5. How can the nurse best support a patient who is suffering from anxiety and insomnia?

Critical Thinking Questions

1. A 58-year-old male patient has undergone an emergency coronary artery bypass graft. He suffered complications while in the cardiac intensive care unit and spent 3 days on a ventilator. He is still experiencing a high degree of pain and also states that he cannot fall asleep. The patient has been ordered secobarbital (Seconal) hs for sleep and also has a prescribed opioid analgesic. Should the nurse medicate the patient with both agents?

2. A 42-year-old female patient with ovarian cancer suffered profound nausea and vomiting after her first round of chemotherapy. The oncologist has added lorazepam (Ativan) 2 mg per IV piggyback with ondansetron (Zofran) as part of the prechemotherapy regimen. Consult a drug handbook and discuss the purpose for adding this benzodiazepine.

3. An 82-year-old female patient complains that she "just can't get good rest anymore." She says that she has come to her doctor to get something to help her sleep. What information can the nurse offer this patient regarding the normal changes in sleep patterns associated with aging? What would you recommend for this patient?

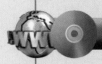 **EXPLORE MEDIALINK**

NCLEX review, case studies, and other interactive resources for this chapter can be found on the companion website at www.prenhall.com/adams. Click on "Chapter 14" to select the activities for this chapter. For animations, more NCLEX review questions, and an audio glossary, access the accompanying CD-ROM in this textbook.

CHAPTER 15

Drugs for Seizures

DRUGS AT A GLANCE

DRUGS THAT POTENTIATE GABA ACTION

Barbiturates

Pr *phenobarbital (Luminal)*

Miscellaneous GABA agents

Pr *valproic acid (Depakene)*

Benzodiazepines

Pr *diazepam (Valium)*

HYDANTOINS AND PHENYTOIN-LIKE DRUGS

Hydantoins

Pr *phenytoin (Dilantin)*

Phenytoin-like Drugs

SUCCINIMIDES

Pr *ethosuximide (Zarontin)*

metabolized and eliminated by the body.
of this process
PHARMACOLOGY
1. The study of medicines; the discipline
pertaining to how drugs improve the heal
of the human body
PHARMACOPOEIA

 MediaLink   www.prenhall.com/adams

CD-ROM

Animation:
   Mechanism in Action: Diazepam (Valium)
Audio Glossary
NCLEX Review

Companion Website

NCLEX Review
Dosage Calculations
Care Plans
Case Study
Expanded Key Concepts

OBJECTIVES

After reading this chapter, the student should be able to:

1. Compare and contrast the terms epilepsy, seizures, and convulsions.
2. Recognize the causes of epilepsy.
3. Relate signs and symptoms to specific types of seizures.
4. Describe the nurse's role in the pharmacologic management of epilepsy.
5. Explain the importance of patient drug compliance in the pharmacotherapy of epilepsy.

6. For each of the drug classes listed in Drugs at a Glance, know representative drug examples and explain their mechanism of drug action, primary actions, and important adverse effects.
7. Categorize drugs used in the treatment of epilepsy based on their classification and mechanism of action.
8. Use the Nursing Process to care for patients receiving drug therapy for epilepsy.

Epilepsy may be defined as any disorder characterized by recurrent seizures. The symptoms of epilepsy depend on the type of seizure and may include blackout, fainting spells, sensory disturbances, jerking body movements, and temporary loss of memory. As the most common neurologic disease, over 2 million Americans have epilepsy. This chapter will examine the pharmacotherapy of the different types of seizures.

SEIZURES

A **seizure** is a disturbance of electrical activity in the brain that may affect consciousness, motor activity, and sensation. The symptoms of seizure are caused by abnormal or uncontrollable neuronal discharges within the brain. These abnormal discharges can be measured using an electroencephalogram (EEG), a valuable tool in diagnosing seizure disorders. Figure 15.1 compares normal and abnormal EEG recordings.

The terms *convulsion* and *seizure* are not synonymous. **Convulsions** specifically refer to involuntary, violent spasms of the large skeletal muscles of the face, neck, arms, and legs. While some types of seizures do indeed involve convulsions, other seizures do not. Thus, it may be stated that all convulsions are seizures, but not all seizures are convulsions. Because of this difference, agents used to treat epilepsy should correctly be called antiseizure medications, rather than anticonvulsants.

15.1 Causes of Seizures

A seizure is considered a symptom of an underlying disorder, rather than a disease in itself. There are many different etiologies of seizure activity. Seizures can result from acute situations or occur on a chronic basis, as with **epilepsy**. In some cases, the exact etiology may not be identified. The following are known causes of seizures.

- *Infectious diseases* Acute infections such as meningitis and encephalitis can cause inflammation in the brain.
- *Trauma* Physical trauma such as direct blows to the skull may increase intracranial pressure; chemical trauma such as the presence of toxic substances or the ingestion of poisons may cause brain injury.
- *Metabolic disorders* Changes in fluid and electrolytes such as hypoglycemia, hyponatremia, and water intoxication may cause seizures by altering electrical impulse transmission at the cellular level.
- *Vascular diseases* Changes in oxygenation such as that caused by respiratory hypoxia and carbon monoxide poisoning, and changes in perfusion such as that caused by hypotension, cerebral vascular accidents, shock, and cardiac dysrhythmias may be causes.
- *Pediatric disorders* Rapid increase in body temperature may result in a febrile seizure.
- *Neoplastic disease* Tumors, especially rapidly growing ones, may occupy space, increase intracranial pressure, and damage brain tissue by disrupting blood flow.

Certain medications for mood disorders, psychoses, and local anesthesia when given in high doses may cause seizures because of increased levels of stimulatory neurotransmitters.

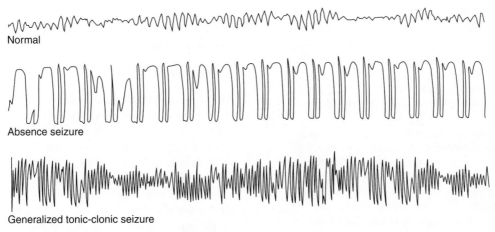

Normal

Absence seizure

Generalized tonic-clonic seizure

Figure 15.1 | EEG recordings showing the differences between normal, absence seizure, and generalized tonic-clonic seizure tracings

Seizures may also occur from drug abuse, as with cocaine, or during withdrawal syndromes from alcohol or sedative-hypnotic drugs.

Pregnancy is a major concern for patients with epilepsy. Additional barrier methods of birth control should be practiced to avoid unintended pregnancy, as some antiseizure medications decrease the effectiveness of oral contraceptives. Most antiseizure drugs are pregnancy category D. Patients should consult with their healthcare provider prior to pregnancy to determine the most appropriate plan of action for seizure control, given their seizure history. As some antiseizure drugs may cause folate deficiency, a condition correlated with increased risk of neural tube defects, vitamin supplements may be necessary. Pregnant women may experience seizures with eclampsia, a pregnancy-induced hypertensive disorder.

In some cases, the etiology of the seizures cannot be found. Patients may have a lower tolerance to environmental triggers and seizures may occur when sleep deprived, exposed to strobe or flickering lights, or when small fluid and electrolyte imbalances occur. Seizures represent the most common serious neurologic problem affecting children, with an overall incidence approaching 2% for febrile seizures and 1% for idiopathic epilepsy. Seizures that result from acute situations generally do not reoccur after the situation has been resolved. If a brain abnormality exists after the acute situation resolves, continuing seizures are likely.

Seizures can have a significant impact on quality of life. They may cause serious injury if they occur while a person is driving a vehicle or performing a dangerous activity. Without pharmacotherapy, epilepsy can severely limit participation in school, employment, and social activities and affect self-esteem. Chronic depression may accompany poorly controlled seizures. Proper treatment, however, can eliminate seizures completely in many patients. Important considerations in nursing care include identifying patients at risk for seizures, documenting the pattern and type of seizure activity, and implementing safety precautions. In collaboration with the patient, healthcare provider, and pharmacist, the nurse is instrumental in achieving positive therapeutic outcomes. Through a combination of pharmacotherapy, patient-family support, and education, effective seizure control can be achieved by the majority of patients.

15.2 Types of Seizures

The differing presentation of seizures relates to the areas of the brain affected by the abnormal electrical activity. Symptoms of a seizure can range from sudden, violent shaking and total loss of consciousness to muscle twitching or slight tremor of a limb. Staring into space, altered vision, and difficult speech are other behaviors a person may exhibit during a seizure. Determining the cause of recurrent seizures is important, to plan appropriate treatment options.

Methods of classifying epilepsy have evolved over time. The terms *grand mal* and *petit mal* epilepsy have, for the

SPECIAL CONSIDERATIONS

Seizure Etiologies Based on Genetics and Age-Related Factors

- The etiologies that trigger the development of childhood epilepsy vary according to age.
- Congenital abnormalities of the CNS, perinatal brain injury, and metabolic imbalances are usually related to seizure activity in neonates, infants, and toddlers.
- Inherited epilepsies, CNS infections, and neurologic degenerative disorders are linked to seizures that have their onset in later childhood.
- Cerebral trauma, cerebrovascular disorders, and neoplastic disease represent the most frequent causes of seizures in the adult population.

most part, been replaced by more descriptive and detailed categorization. Epilepsies are typically identified using the International Classification of Epileptic Seizures nomenclature, as partial (focal), generalized, and special epileptic syndromes. Types of partial or generalized seizures may be recognized based on symptoms observed during a seizure episode. Some symptoms are subtle and reflect the simple nature of neuronal misfiring in specific areas of the brain; others are more complex.

Partial Seizures

Partial (focal) seizures involve a limited portion of the brain. They may start on one side and travel only a short distance before they stop. The area where the abnormal electrical activity starts is known as an abnormal focus (plural = *foci*).

Simple partial seizures have an onset that may begin as a small, limited focus, and subsequently progress to a generalized seizure. Patients with simple partial seizures may feel for a brief moment that their precise location is vague, and they may hear and see things that are not there. Some patients smell and taste things that are not present, or have an upset stomach. Others may become emotional and experience a sense of joy, sorrow, or grief. The arms, legs, or face may twitch.

Complex partial seizures (formerly known as psychomotor or temporal lobe seizures) show sensory, motor, or autonomic symptoms, with some degree of altered or impaired consciousness. Total loss of consciousness may not occur during a complex partial seizure, but a brief period of somnolence or confusion may follow the seizure. Such seizures are often preceded by an aura that is often described as an unpleasant odor or taste. Seizures may start with a blank stare and patients may begin to chew or swallow repetitively. Some patients fumble with clothing; others may try to take off their clothes. Most patients will not pay attention to ver-

bal commands and act as if they are having a psychotic episode. After the seizure, patients do not remember the seizure incident.

Generalized Seizures

As the name suggests, generalized seizures are not localized to one area but travel throughout the entire brain on both sides. The seizure is thought to originate bilaterally and symmetrically within the brain.

Absence seizures (formerly known as petit mal seizures) most often occur in children and last only a few seconds. Absence seizures involve a loss or reduction of normal activity. Staring and transient loss of responsiveness are the most common signs, but there may be slight motor activity with eyelid fluttering or myoclonic jerks. Because these episodes are subtle and only last a few seconds, absence epilepsy may go unrecognized for a long time or be mistaken for daydreaming or attention deficit disorder.

Atonic seizures are sometimes called drop attacks, because patients often stumble and fall for no apparent reason. Episodes are very short, lasting only a matter of seconds.

Tonic-clonic seizures are the most common type of seizure in all age groups. Seizures may be preceded by an aura, a warning that some patients describe as a spiritual feeling, a flash of light, or a special noise. Intense muscle contractions indicate the tonic phase. A hoarse cry may occur at the onset of the seizure due to air being forced out of the lungs and patients may temporarily lose bladder or bowel control. Breathing may become shallow and even stop momentarily. The clonic phase is characterized by alternating contraction and relaxation of muscles. The seizure usually lasts 1 to 2 minutes, after which the patient becomes drowsy, disoriented, and sleeps deeply (known as the postictal state).

Special Epileptic Syndromes

Special epileptic seizures include the febrile seizures of infancy, reflex epilepsies, and other forms of myoclonic epilepsies. Myoclonic epilepsies often go along with other neurologic abnormalities or progressive symptoms.

Febrile seizures typically cause tonic-clonic motor activity lasting 1 or 2 minutes with rapid return of consciousness. They occur in conjunction with a rapid rise in body temperature and usually occur only once during any given illness. Febrile seizures are most likely to occur in the 3-month to 5-year age group, and as many as 5% of all children experience febrile seizures. Preventing the onset of high fever is the best way to control these seizures.

Myoclonic seizures are characterized by large, jerking body movements. Major muscle groups contract quickly, and patients appear unsteady and clumsy. They may fall from a sitting position or drop whatever they are holding. Infantile spasms exemplify a type of generalized, myoclonic seizure distinguished by short-lived muscle spasms involving the trunk and extremities. Such spasms are often not identified as seizures by parents or healthcare providers, because the movements are much like the normal infantile Moro (startle) reflex.

Status epilepticus is a medical emergency that occurs when a seizure is repeated continuously. It could occur with any type of seizure, but usually generalized tonic-clonic seizures are exhibited. When generalized tonic-clonic seizures are prolonged or continuous, the time in which breathing is affected by muscle contraction is lengthened and hypoxia may develop. The continuous muscle contraction also can lead to hypoglycemia, acidosis, and hypothermia due to increased metabolic needs, lactic acid production, and heat loss during contraction. Carbon dioxide retention also leads to acidosis. If not treated, status epilepticus could lead to brain damage and death. Medical treatment involves the IV administration of antiseizure medications. Steps must also be taken to ensure that the airway remains open.

15.3 General Concepts of Epilepsy Pharmacotherapy

The choice of drug for epilepsy pharmacotherapy depends on the type of seizures the patient is experiencing, the patient's previous medical history, diagnostic studies, and the pathologic processes causing the seizures. Once a medication is selected, the patient is placed on a low initial dose. The amount is gradually increased until seizure control is achieved, or the side effects of the drug prevent additional increases in dose. Serum drug levels may be obtained to assist the healthcare provider in determining the most effective drug concentration. If seizure activity continues, a different medication is added in small dose increments while the dose of the first drug is slowly reduced. Because seizures are likely to occur with abrupt withdrawal, antiseizure medication is withdrawn over a period of 6 to 12 weeks.

In most cases, effective seizure management can be obtained using a single drug. In some patients, two antiseizure medications may be necessary to control seizure activity, although additional side effects may become evident. Some antiseizure drug combinations may actually increase the incidence of seizures. The nurse should consult with current drug guides regarding compatibility before a second antiseizure agent is added to the regimen.

Once seizures have been controlled, patients are continued indefinitely on the antiseizure drug. After several years of being seizure free, patients may question the need for their medication. In general, withdrawal of antiseizure drugs should only be attempted after at least 3 years of being seizure free, and only under the close direction of the healthcare provider. Doses of medications are reduced slowly, one at a time, over a period of several months. If seizures recur during the withdrawal process, pharmacotherapy is resumed, usually with the same drug. The nurse must strongly urge patients to maintain compliance with pharmacotherapy and not attempt to discontinue antiseizure drug use without professional guidance. Table 15.1 shows antiseizure drugs, based on the type of seizure.

Holistic medicine, as a treatment philosophy considering the health and well-being of the whole person, does not differ from the standard treatment of epilepsy, according to the Epilepsy Foundation of America. Living a healthy, active life is good therapy for epilepsy, but only as an adjunct to medically prescribed antiseizure drug, not instead of it. With a valid diagnosis of epilepsy, there is no substitute for effective antiseizure pharmacotherapy. There are situations, however, when the medicines cannot be tolerated. Sometimes another medical therapy, such as the ketogenic diet, is used, along with natural remedies.

Antiseizure pharmacotherapy is directed at controlling the movement of electrolytes across neuronal membranes or affecting neurotransmitter balance. In a resting state, neurons are normally surrounded by a higher concentration of sodium, calcium, and chloride ion. Potassium levels are higher inside of the cell. An influx of sodium or calcium into the neuron *enhances* neuronal activity, whereas an influx of chloride ion *suppresses* neuronal activity.

Table 15.1	Drugs Used for the Management of Specific Types of Seizures			
	Partial Seizures	*Generalized Seizures*		
	(Simple or Complex)	(Absence)	(Atonic, Myoclonic)	(Tonic-clonic, Status Epilepticus)
Benzodiazepines				
diazepam (Valium)				✓
lorazepam (Ativan)				✓
Phenytoin-like				
phenytoin (Dilantin)	✓			✓
carbamazepine (Tegretol)	✓			✓
valproic acid (Depakene)	✓	✓	✓	✓
Succinimide				
ethosuximide (Zarontin)		✓	✓	

The goal of antiseizure pharmacotherapy is to suppress neuronal activity just enough to prevent abnormal or repetitive firing. To this end, there are three general mechanisms by which antiseizure drugs act.

- Stimulating an influx of chloride ion, an effect associated with the neurotransmitter, **gamma-aminobutyric acid (GABA)**
- Delaying an influx of sodium
- Delaying an influx of calcium

Within these three *pharmacologic* classes are four major *chemical* classes: benzodiazepines, barbiturates, hydantoins, and succinimides. A fifth category consists of miscellaneous drug types not chemically related to the four major classes.

DRUGS THAT POTENTIATE GABA

Several important antiseizure drugs act by changing the action of GABA, the primary inhibitory neurotransmitter in the brain. These agents mimic the effects of GABA by stimulating an influx of chloride ions that interact with the GABA receptor-chloride channel molecule. A model of this receptor is shown in Figure 15.2. When the receptor is stimulated, chloride ions move into the cell, thus supressing the ability of neurons to fire.

Barbiturates and Miscellaneous GABA Agents

Barbiturates, benzodiazepines, and several miscellaneous drugs reduce seizure activity by intensifying GABA action. The major effect of enhancing GABA activity is CNS depression. These agents are shown in Table 15.2. The antiseizure properties of phenobarbital were discovered in 1912, and the drug is still one of the most commonly prescribed for epilepsy.

15.4 Treating Seizures with Barbiturates and Miscellaneous GABA Agents

As a class, barbiturates have a low margin for safety, cause profound CNS depression, and have a high potential for dependence. Phenobarbital, however, is able to suppress abnormal neuronal discharges without causing sedation. It is inexpensive, long acting, and produces a low incidence of adverse effects. When given orally, several weeks may be necessary to achieve optimum antiseizure activity.

Other barbiturates are occasionally used for epilepsy. Mephobarbital (Mebaral) is converted to phenobarbital in the liver, and offers no significant advantages over phenobarbital. Amobarbital (Amytal) is an intermediate-acting barbiturate that is given IM or IV to terminate status epilepticus. Unlike phenobarbital, which is a Schedule IV drug, amobarbital is a Schedule II drug and has a higher risk for dependence; it is not given orally as an antiseizure drug.

Several nonbenzodiazepine, nonbarbiturate agents act by the GABA mechanism. Examples of these newer drugs, first approved by the FDA in the 1990s, are gabapentin (Neurontin) and tiagabine (Gabitril).

NURSING CONSIDERATIONS

The role of the nurse in barbiturate therapy for seizures involves careful monitoring of a patient's condition and providing education as it relates to the prescribed drug regimen. Of those drugs that mimic or enhance GABA production, barbiturates produce the most pronounced adverse effects, including sedation and respiratory depression.

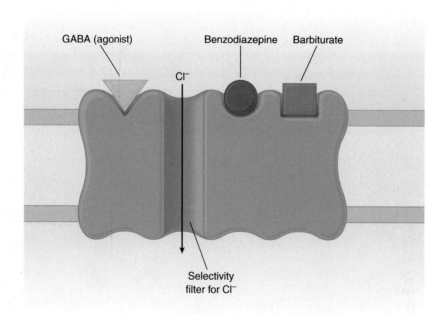

Figure 15.2 | Model of the GABA receptor-chloride channel molecule

Table 15.2	Antiseizure Drugs that Potentiate GABA Action
Drug	**Route and Adult Dose (max dose where indicated)**
Barbiturates	
amobarbital (Amytal)	IV; 65–500 mg, (max 1 g)
pentobarbital (Nembutal)	PO/IM; 150–200 mg in two divided doses IV; 100 mg, may increase to 500 mg if necessary
◉ phenobarbital (Luminal)	For seizures: PO; 100–300 mg day; IV/IM; 200–600 mg up to 20 mg/kg. For status epilepticus: IV; 15–18 mg/kg in single or divided doses (max 20 mg/kg)
secobarbital (Seconal)	IM/IV; 5.5 mg/kg repeated 3–4 hr if necessary (IV infusion at less than 50 mg/15 sec)
Benzodiazepines	
clonazepam (Klonopin)	PO; 1.5 mg/day in three divided doses, increased by 0.5–1.0 mg every 3 days until seizures are controlled
clorazepate (Tranxene)	PO; 7.5 mg tid
◉ diazepam (Valium)	IM/IV; 5–10 mg (repeat as needed at 10–15 min intervals up to 30 mg; repeat again as needed every 2–4 hr); IV push; administer emulsion at 5 mg/min
lorazepam (Ativan) (see p. 150 for the Prototype Drug box) ⊕	IV; 4 mg injected slowly at 2 mg/min; if inadequate response after 10 min, may repeat once
Miscellaneous	
gabapentin (Neurontin)	For additional therapy: PO; start with 300 mg on day 1; 300 mg bid on day 2; 300 mg tid on day 3; continue to increase over 1 week to a dose of 1200 mg/day (400 mg tid); may increase to 1800–2400 mg/day
primidone (Mysoline)	PO; 250 mg/day; increased by 250 mg/week up to max of 2 g in two to four divided doses
tiagabine (Gabitril)	PO; Start with 4 mg/day; may increase by 4–8 mg/day every week up to 56 mg/day in two to four divided doses
topiramate (Topamax)	PO; Start with 50 mg/day; increase by 50 mg/week to effectiveness (max 1600 mg/day)

Barbiturates are metabolized in the liver and excreted primarily in urine. These drugs should be used with caution in patients with impaired hepatic or renal capacity; liver and kidney function must be monitored regularly with long-term usage. Barbiturates cross the placenta and are excreted in breast milk; therefore, they are not recommended for pregnant or nursing women. The nurse should assess women of childbearing age for pregnancy or intent to become pregnant. There is an increased risk of congenital malformations when the drug is taken during the first trimester (pregnancy category D). These drugs may also produce folic acid deficiency, which is associated with an increased risk of neural tube birth defects, including spina bifida and hydrocephalus. Barbiturates may also decrease the effectiveness of oral contraceptives.

Barbiturates produce biochemical changes at the cellular level that result in accelerated metabolism and subsequent depletion of nutrients such as vitamins D and K. Alterations in vitamin synthesis can result in reduced bone density (vitamin D deficiency) and impaired blood coagulability (vitamin K deficiency). Bleeding caused by vitamin K deficiency may present as simple bruising or petechiae, or may manifest as a more serious adverse reaction, such as epistaxis, GI bleeding, menorrhagia, or hematuria. The elderly can be particularly at risk of significant vitamin deficiency caused by barbiturates due to nutritional imbalances that may already exist due to aging. Diminished renal, hepatic, and respiratory function associated with aging also places the elderly at risk of CNS depression. GABA-enhancing drugs may produce an idiosyncratic response in children, resulting in restlessness and psychomotor agitation.

The risk of respiratory depression must be considered when administering barbiturates to patients with impaired respiratory function, those taking other CNS depressants, and with intravenous doses. The nurse should monitor for common side effects such as drowsiness, dizziness, and postural hypotension, which increase a patient's risk of injury. CNS depressants should not be stopped abruptly; abrupt cessation can result in potentially life-threatening rebound seizure activity. Patients should avoid consuming alcohol while taking barbiturates. The use of the herb ginkgo biloba may decrease the antiseizure effect of these drugs. Concurrent use of other antiseizure drugs may also decrease their anticonvulsant effect.

Patients taking gabapentin (Neurontin) and tiagabine (Gabitril) should be monitored for dizziness and drowsiness. Drugs with GABA-intensifying action are not recommended for pregnant or nursing women (pregnancy category C).

See "Nursing Process Focus: Patients Receiving Barbiturate Therapy for Seizures" for specific teaching points.

Benzodiazepines

Like barbiturates, benzodiazepines intensify the effect of GABA in the brain. The benzodiazepines bind to the GABA receptor directly, suppressing abnormal neuronal foci.

15.5 Treating Seizures with Benzodiazepines

Benzodiazepines used in treating epilepsy include clonazepam (Klonopin), clorazepate (Tranxene), lorazepam (Ativan), and diazepam (Valium). Indications include ab-

sence seizures and myoclonic seizures. Parenteral diazepam is used to terminate status epilepticus. Because tolerance may begin to develop after only a few months of therapy with benzodiazepines, seizures may recur unless the dose is periodically adjusted. These agents are generally not used alone in seizure pharmacotherapy, but instead serve as adjuncts to other antiseizure drugs for short-term seizure control.

The benzodiazepines are one of the most widely prescribed classes of drugs, used not only to control seizures but also for anxiety, skeletal muscle spasms, and alcohol withdrawal symptoms.

NURSING CONSIDERATIONS

The following content provides nursing considerations that apply to benzodiazepines when given to treat seizure disorders. For the complete nursing process applied to benzodiazepine therapy, see Chapter 14, page 152, "Nursing Process Focus: Patients Receiving Benzodiazepine and Nonbenzodiazepine Antianxiety Therapy." ∞

The role of the nurse in benzodiazepine therapy for seizures involves careful monitoring of a patient's condition and providing education as it relates to the prescribed drug regimen. The nurse should assess patient needs for seizure medication. The assessment should include identification of factors associated with the seizures such as frequency, symptoms, and previous therapies. A drug history should be obtained, including the use of CNS depressants and OTC drugs. The nurse should assess for the likelihood of drug abuse and dependence, as benzodiazepines are Schedule IV drugs. The nurse should assess women of childbearing age for pregnancy, intent to become pregnant, or lactation status, as these drugs are pregnancy category D, and are secreted into breast milk. Benzodiazepines may also decrease the effectiveness of oral contraceptives.

Pr PROTOTYPE DRUG	PHENOBARBITAL (Luminal)
ACTIONS AND USES	**ADVERSE EFFECTS AND INTERACTIONS**

ACTIONS AND USES

Phenobarbital is a long-acting barbiturate, used for the management of a variety of seizures. It is also used for insomnia. Phenobarbital should not be used for pain relief, as it may increase a patient's sensitivity to pain.

Phenobarbital acts biochemically in the brain by enhancing the action of the neurotransmitter GABA, which is responsible for suppressing abnormal neuronal discharges that can cause epilepsy.

Administration Alerts

- Parenteral phenobarbital is a soft tissue irritant. IM injections may produce local inflammatory reaction. IV administration is rarely used, because extravasation may produce tissue necrosis.
- Pregnancy category D.

ADVERSE EFFECTS AND INTERACTIONS

Phenobarbital is a Schedule IV drug that may cause dependence. Common side effects include drowsiness, vitamin deficiencies (vitamin D, folate: B_9 and B_{12}), and laryngospasms. With overdose, phenobarbital may cause severe respiratory depression, CNS depression, coma, and death.

Phenobarbital interacts with many other drugs. For example, it should not be taken with alcohol or other CNS depressants. These substances potentiate the action of barbiturates, increasing the risk of life-threatening respiratory depression or cardiac arrest. Phenobarbital increases the metabolism of many other drugs, reducing their effectiveness.

 See the companion website for a Nursing Process Focus specific to this drug.

ASSESSMENT	POTENTIAL NURSING DIAGNOSES
Prior to administration: ■ Obtain complete health history including allergies and drug history, to determine possible drug interactions. ■ Assess neurological status, including identification of recent seizure activity.	■ Disturbed Sensory Perception ■ Risk for Injury, related to drug side effect ■ Risk for Imbalanced Nutrition: Less Than Body Requirements ■ Deficient Knowledge, related to drug therapy ■ Disturbed Sleep Pattern

PLANNING: PATIENT GOALS AND EXPECTED OUTCOMES

The patient will:
■ Experience the absence of, or a reduction in, the number or severity of seizures
■ Avoid physical injury related to seizure activity or medication-induced somnolence
■ Demonstrate an understanding of the drug's action by accurately describing drug effects and precautions

IMPLEMENTATION

Interventions and (Rationales)	*Patient Education/Discharge Planning*
■ Monitor vital signs, especially blood pressure and depth and rate of respirations. (These drugs can cause severe respiratory depression.)	■ Instruct patient to withhold medication for any difficulty in breathing or respirations below 12 breaths per minute.
■ Monitor neurological status. Monitor changes in level of consciousness. (Excessive somnolence may occur.) Observe for persistent seizures.	Instruct patient to: ■ Report any significant change in sensorium such as lethargy, stupor, auras, visual changes, and other effects that may indicate an impending seizure ■ Report dizziness, which may indicate hypotension ■ Be aware that drug will cause initial drowsiness, which may diminish with continued therapy ■ Keep a seizure diary to chronicle symptoms
■ Monitor for signs of hepatic or renal toxicity. (Barbiturates are metabolized by the liver and excreted by the kidneys.)	Instruct patient to: ■ Observe for signs of toxicity such as nausea, vomiting, diarrhea, rash, jaundice, abdominal pain, tenderness or distention, or change in color of stool, flank pain, hematuria ■ Adhere to a regular schedule of laboratory testing for liver and kidney function as ordered by the healthcare provider
■ Ensure patient safety. (Barbiturates can cause drowsiness and dizziness.)	Instruct patient to: ■ Request assistance when getting out of bed and ambulating until effect of drug is known ■ Avoid driving and hazardous activities until effect of drug is known
■ Monitor effectiveness of drug therapy. ■ Monitor children for paradoxical response to drug, which may cause hyperactivity.	Instruct patient to: ■ Be aware that full therapeutic effect of oral barbiturate may take 2 to 3 weeks ■ Not discontinue abruptly, or reduce dosage, as increased seizure activity and/or withdrawal symptoms may occur
■ Monitor for signs of vitamin deficiency (vitamin D, vitamin K, folate, and other B vitamins). ■ Obtain consult with dietitian per healthcare provider's order as needed.	Instruct patient: ■ Regarding the role of vitamins and nutrition in maintaining health ■ To immediately report signs of vitamin deficiency: vitamin K—easy bleeding, tarry stools, bruising, pallor; vitamin D—joint pain, bone deformities; vitamin B_6—skin changes, dandruff, peripheral neuropathy, fatigue

EVALUATION OF OUTCOME CRITERIA

Evaluate effectiveness of drug therapy by confirming that patient goals and expected outcomes have been met (see "Planning").

See Table 15.2, "Barbiturates," for a list of drugs to which these nursing actions apply.

Alterations in neurotransmitter activity produce changes in intraocular pressure; therefore, benzodiazepines are contraindicated in narrow-angle glaucoma. Liver and kidney function should be monitored in long-term use and these drugs should be used cautiously in those with impaired renal or liver function.

The risk of respiratory depression should be taken into consideration, especially when administering to patients with impaired respiratory function, those taking other CNS depressants, and with intravenous doses. The nurse should assess for common side effects related to CNS depression such as drowsiness and dizziness. Should an overdose occur, flumazenil (Romazicon) is a specific benzodiazepine receptor antagonist that can be administered to reverse CNS depression.

Intravenous benzodiazepines such as diazepam (Valium) and lorazepam (Ativan) are used in the treatment of status epilepticus or continuous seizures. When administering these drugs IV it is important to have supplemental oxygen and resuscitation equipment available. The nurse should monitor respiratory effort and oxygen saturation. Because the desired action is to terminate seizure activity, severe respiratory depression would be treated with intubation and ventilation rather than by reversing the benzodiazepine effects with flumazenil (Romazicon). Because IV administration may cause hypotension, tachycardia, and muscular weakness, monitoring heart rhythm, heart rate, and blood pressure is necessary. These drugs have a tendency to precipitate from solution and are irritating to veins. They should not be mixed with other drugs or IV fluid additives and should be given in a large vein if possible.

Patient education as it relates to benzodiazepines should include goals, reasons for obtaining baseline data, and possible side effects. Following are the education points the nurse should include regarding benzodiazepines.

- Avoid alcohol and other CNS depressants, including herbal and OTC drugs, unless advised by the healthcare provider.
- Tobacco use, or nicotine patches can decrease benzodiazepine effectiveness.
- Benzodiazepines can potentiate the action of digoxin, thus raising blood levels.
- Do not drive or perform hazardous activities until effects of the drug are known.
- Do not discontinue drug abruptly, as this may result in rebound seizure activity.
- Take with food if GI upset occurs.
- Benzodiazepines are used illegally for recreation; patients should evaluate the social context of their environment, and take any precautions necessary to safeguard their medication supply.

DRUGS THAT SUPPRESS SODIUM INFLUX

This class of drugs dampens CNS activity by delaying an influx of sodium ions across neuronal membranes. Hydantoins and several other related antiseizure drugs act by this mechanism.

Hydantoin and Phenytoin-like Drugs

Sodium channels guide the movement of sodium across neuronal membranes into the intracellular space. Sodium movement is the major factor that determines whether a neuron will undergo an action potential. If these channels are temporarily inactivated, neuronal activity will be suppressed. With hydantoin and phenytoin-like drugs, sodium channels are not blocked; they are just desensitized. If channels are blocked, neuronal activity completely stops, as

---

Pr PROTOTYPE DRUG | **DIAZEPAM (Valium)**

ACTIONS AND USES	ADVERSE EFFECTS AND INTERACTIONS
Diazepam binds to the GABA receptor-chloride channels throughout the CNS. It produces its effects by suppressing neuronal activity in the limbic system and subsequent impulses that might be transmitted to the reticular activating system. Effects of this drug are suppression of abnormal neuronal foci that may cause seizures, calming without strong sedation, and skeletal muscle relaxation. When used orally, maximum therapeutic effects may take from 1 to 2 weeks. Tolerance may develop after about 4 weeks. When given IV, effects occur in minutes and its anticonvulsant effects last about 20 minutes.	Diazepam should not be taken with alcohol or other CNS depressants because of combined sedation effects. Other drug interactions include cimetidine, oral contraceptives, valproic acid, and metoprolol, which potentiate diazepam's action; and levodopa and barbiturates, which decrease diazepam's action. Diazepam increases the levels of phenytoin in the bloodstream, and may cause phenytoin toxicity. When given IV, hypotension, muscular weakness, tachycardia, and respiratory depression are common. Because of tolerance and dependency, use of diazepam is reserved for short-term seizure control, or for status epilepticus.
Administration Alerts	Use with caution with herbal supplements, such as kava and chamomile, which may cause an increased effect.
- When administering IV, monitor respirations every 5 to 15 minutes. Have airway and resuscitative equipment accessible.	
- Pregnancy category D.	

 See the companion website for a Nursing Process Focus specific to this drug.

Table 15.3	Hydantoins and Phenytoin-like Drugs
Drug	**Route and Adult Dose (max dose where indicated)**
Hydantoins	
fosphenytoin (Cerebyx)	IV; Initial dose 15–20 mg PE/kg at 100–150 mg PE/min followed by 4–6 mg PE/kg/d (PE = phenytoin equivalents)
℗ phenytoin (Dilantin)	PO; 15–18 mg/kg of 1 g initial dose; then 300 mg/day in one to three divided doses; may be gradually increased 100 mg/week
Phenytoin-like Agents	
carbamazepine (Tegretol)	PO; 200 mg bid; gradually increased to 800–1200 mg/day in three to four divided doses
felbamate (Felbatol)	Lennox-Gastaut syndrome: start at 15 mg/kg/day PO in three to four divided doses; may increase 15 mg/kg at weekly intervals to max of 45 mg/kg/day Partial seizures: PO; start with 1200 mg/day in three to four divided doses; may increase by 600 mg/day every 2 weeks (max 3600 mg/day)
lamotrigine (Lamictal)	PO; 50 mg/day for 2 weeks, then 50 mg bid for 2 weeks; may increase gradually up to 300–500 mg/day in two divided doses (max 700 mg/day)
valproic acid (Depakene, Depakote)*	PO/IV; 15 mg/kg/day in divided doses when total daily dose is greater than 250 mg; increase 5–10 mg every week until seizures are controlled (max 60 mg/kg/day)
℗ zonisamide (Zonegran)	PO; 100–400 mg/day

*Other formulations of valproic acid include its salts, valproate and divalproex sodium.

occurs with local anesthetic drugs. These agents are shown in Table 15.3.

15.6 Treating Seizures with Hydantoins and Phenytoin-like Drugs

The oldest and most commonly prescribed hydantoin is phenytoin (Dilantin). Approved in the 1930s, phenytoin is a broad-spectrum drug that is useful in treating all types of epilepsy except absence seizures. It is able to provide effective seizure suppression, without the abuse potential or CNS depression associated with barbiturates. Patients vary significantly in their ability to metabolize phenytoin; therefore, dosages are highly individualized. Because of the very narrow range between a therapeutic dose and a toxic dose, patients must be carefully monitored. The other hydantoins are used much less frequently than phenytoin.

Several widely used drugs share a mechanism of action similar to the hydantoins, including carbamazepine (Tegretol) and valproic acid (Depakene, Depakote), which is also available as valproate and divalproex sodium. Carbamazepine is a drug of choice for tonic-clonic and partial seizures, because it produces fewer adverse effects than phenytoin or phenobarbital. Valproic acid is a drug of choice for absence seizures. Both carbamazepine and valproic acid are also used for bipolar disorder (Chapter 16) ⊕. Newer antiseizure drugs having more limited uses include zonisamide (Zonegran), felbamate (Felbatol), and lamotrigine (Lamictal).

NURSING CONSIDERATIONS

The role of the nurse in hydantoin and phenytoin-like drug therapy involves careful monitoring of a patient's condition and providing education as it relates to the prescribed drug regimen. Some of these drugs are monitored via serum drug levels, so regular laboratory testing is required. When serum drugs levels stray outside of the normal range, dosage adjustments are made.

Common signs of hydantoin toxicity include dizziness, ataxia, diplopia, and lethargy. These drugs affect vitamin K metabolism; therefore, blood dyscrasias and bleeding may ensue. Because hydantoins may increase serum glucose levels, a CBC and urinalysis should be obtained. Urinalysis is also important to identify the presence of hematuria; phenytoin may change urine color to pink, red, or brown. These drugs should be used cautiously in patients with hepatic or renal disease.

Recent evidence has discovered several cases of fatal hepatotoxicity in patients taking valproic acid (Depakene, Depakote). The risk is higher for patients taking multiple antiseizure drugs, those with existing liver disease, those with organic brain disease and those under 2 years of age. Extreme caution must be taken when administering this drug to these patients.

Pregnancy tests must be conducted on all women of childbearing age before beginning therapy, as drugs in this class are pregnancy class D (phenytoin, carbamazepine, and valproic acid) or class C (felbamate and lamotrigine). Hydantoins may also decrease the effectiveness of oral contraceptives. Additional contraindications include heart block and seizures due to hypoglycemia.

Patient education as it relates to hydantoin and phenytoin-like drugs should include the goals and reasons for obtaining baseline data, and possible side effects. See "Nursing Process Focus: Patients Receiving Antiseizure Drug Therapy" for specific teaching points.

DRUGS THAT SUPPRESS CALCIUM INFLUX

Succinimides are medications that suppress seizures by delaying calcium influx into neurons. They are generally only effective against absence seizures.

Succinimides

15.7 Treating Seizures with Succinimides

Neurotransmitters, hormones, and some medications bind to neuronal membranes, stimulating the entry of calcium. Without calcium influx, neuronal transmission would not be possible. Succinimides delay entry of calcium into neurons by blocking calcium channels, increasing the electrical threshold and reducing the likelihood that an action potential will be generated. By raising the seizure threshold, suc-

cinimides keep neurons from firing too quickly, thus suppressing abnormal foci. The succinimides are shown in Table 15.4.

Ethosuximide (Zarontin) is the most commonly prescribed drug in this class. It remains a drug of choice for absence seizures, although valproic acid is also effective for these types of seizures. Some of the newer antiseizure agents, such as lamotrigine (Lamictal) and zonisamide (Zonegran), are being investigated for their roles in treating absence seizures.

NURSING CONSIDERATIONS

The role of the nurse in succinimide therapy involves careful monitoring of a patient's education and providing education as it relates to the prescribed drug regimen. The nurse should obtain a medical history confirming the baseline seizure activity. Baseline renal and hepatic function tests should be obtained, because these drugs are metabolized by the liver and excreted by the kidneys. Succinimides should be used cautiously in patients with liver or renal insufficiency. Succinimides are pregnancy category C.

The nurse should review the patient's current drug history to determine if any medications interact with succinimides. Succinimides may alter the effectiveness of other antiseizure drugs. Many drugs that alter CNS activity, such

Pr PROTOTYPE DRUG	PHENYTOIN (Dilantin)
ACTIONS AND USES	**ADVERSE EFFECTS AND INTERACTIONS**

ACTIONS AND USES

Phenytoin acts by desensitizing sodium channels in the CNS responsible for neuronal responsivity. Desensitization prevents the spread of disruptive electrical charges in the brain that produce seizures. It is effective against most types of seizures except absence seizures. Phenytoin has antidysrhythmic activity similar to lidocaine (class IB). An unlabeled use is for digitalis-induced dysrhythmias.

Administration Alerts

- When administering IV, mix with saline only, and infuse at the maximum rate of 50 mg/min. Mixing with other medications or dextrose solutions produces precipitate.
- Always prime or flush IV lines with saline before hanging phenytoin as a piggy-back, since traces of dextrose solution in an existing main IV or piggyback line can cause microscopic precipitate formation, which become emboli if infused. Use an IV line with filter when infusing this drug.
- Phenytoin injectable is a soft tissue irritant that causes local tissue damage following extravasation.
- To reduce the risk of soft tissue damage, do not give IM; inject into a large vein or via central venous catheter.
- Avoid using hand veins to prevent serious local vasoconstrictive response (purple glove syndrome).
- Pregnancy category D.

ADVERSE EFFECTS AND INTERACTIONS

Phenytoin may cause dysrhythmias, such as bradycardia or ventricular fibrillation, severe hypotension and hyperglycemia. Severe CNS reactions include headache, nystagmus, ataxia, confusion and slurred speech, paradoxical nervousness, twitching, and insomnia. Peripheral neuropathy may occur with long-term use. Phenytoin can cause multiple blood dyscrasias, including agranulocytosis and aplastic anemia. It may cause severe skin reactions, such as rashes, including exfoliative dermatitis, and Stevens-Johnson syndrome. Connective tissue reactions include lupus erythematosa, hypertrichosis, hirsutism, and gingival hypertrophy.

Phenytoin interacts with many other drugs, including oral anticoagulants, glucocorticoids, H_2 antagonists, antituberculin agents, and food supplements such as folic acid, calcium, and vitamin D. It impairs the efficacy of drugs such as digitoxin, doxycycline, furosemide, estrogens and oral contraceptives, and theophylline. Phenytoin, when combined with tricyclic antidepressants, can trigger seizures.

Use with caution with herbal supplements, such as herbal laxatives (buckthorn, cascara sagrada, and senna), which may increase potassium loss.

 See the companion website for a Nursing Process Focus specific to this drug.

Pr PROTOTYPE DRUG | VALPROIC ACID (Depakene)

ACTIONS AND USES

The mechanism of action of valproic acid is the same as phenytoin, although effects on GABA and calcium channels may cause some additional actions. It is useful for a wide range of seizure types, including absence seizures and mixed types of seizures. Other uses include prevention of migraine headaches and treatment of bipolar disorder.

Administration Alerts

- Valproic acid is a gastrointestinal irritant. Extended-release tablets must not be chewed, as mouth soreness will occur.
- Valproic acid syrup must not be mixed with carbonated beverages, because they will trigger immediate release of the drug, which causes severe mouth and throat irritation.
- Capsules may be opened and sprinkled on soft foods.
- Pregnancy category D.
- Contraindicated in patients with liver disease

ADVERSE EFFECTS AND INTERACTIONS

Side effects include sedation, drowsiness, GI upset, and prolonged bleeding time. Other effects include visual disturbances, muscle weakness, tremor, psychomotor agitation, bone marrow suppression, weight gain, abdominal cramps, rash, alopecia, pruritus, photosensitivity, erythema multiforme, and fatal hepatotoxicity.

Valproic acid interacts with many drugs. For example, aspirin, cimetidine, chlorpromazine, erythromycin, and felbamate may increase valproic acid toxicity. Concomitant warfarin, aspirin, or alcohol use can cause severe bleeding. Alcohol, benzodiazepines, and other CNS depressants potentiate CNS depressant action. Lamotrigine, phenytoin, and rifampin lower valproic acid levels. Valproic acid increases serum phenobarbital and phenytoin levels. Use of clonazepam concurrently with valproic acid may induce absence seizures.

 See the companion website for a Nursing Process Focus specific to this drug.

NURSING PROCESS FOCUS | PATIENTS RECEIVING ANTISEIZURE DRUG THERAPY

ASSESSMENT

Prior to administration:
- Obtain complete health history including allergies and drug history, to determine possible drug interactions.
- Assess neurological status, including identification of recent seizure activity.
- Assess growth and development.

POTENTIAL NURSING DIAGNOSES

- Risk for Injury, related to drug side effects
- Deficient Knowledge, related to drug therapy
- Noncompliance

PLANNING: PATIENT GOALS AND OUTCOMES

The patient will:
- Experience the absence of, or a reduction in the number or severity of, seizures
- Avoid physical injury related to seizure activity or medication-induced sensory changes
- Demonstrate an understanding of the drug's action by accurately describing drug effects and precautions

IMPLEMENTATION

Interventions and (Rationales)

- Monitor neurological status, especially changes in level of consciousness and/or mental status. (Sedation may indicate impending toxicity.)

- Protect the patient from injury during seizure events until therapeutic effects of drugs are achieved.

Patient Education/Discharge Planning

Instruct the patient to:
- Report any significant change in sensorium, such as slurred speech, confusion, hallucinations, or lethargy
- Report any changes in seizure quality or unexpected involuntary muscle movement, such as twitching, tremor, or unusual eye movement

- Instruct patient to avoid driving and other hazardous activities until effects of the drug are known.

continued

NURSING PROCESS FOCUS: *Patients Receiving Antiseizure Drug Therapy (continued)*

Interventions and (Rationales)	Patient Education/Discharge Planning
■ Monitor effectiveness of drug therapy. Observe for developmental changes, which may indicate a need for dose adjustment.	Instruct patient to: ■ Keep a seizure diary to chronicle symptoms phase, or during dose adjustment ■ Take the medication exactly as ordered, including the same manufacturer's drug each time the prescription is refilled (Switching brands may result in alterations in seizure control.) ■ Take a missed dose as soon as remembered, but do not take double doses (Doubling doses could result in toxic serum level.)
■ Monitor for adverse effects. Observe for hypersensitivity, nephrotoxicity, and hepatotoxicity.	■ Instruct patient to report side effects specific to drug regimen.
■ Monitor oral health. Observe for signs of gingival hypertrophy, bleeding, or inflammation (phenytoin specific).	Instruct patient to: ■ Use a soft toothbrush and oral rinses as prescribed by the dentist ■ Avoid mouthwashes containing alcohol ■ Report changes in oral health such as excessive bleeding or inflammation of the gums ■ Maintain a regular schedule of dental visits
■ Monitor gastrointestinal status. (Valproic acid is a GI irritant and anticoagulant.) ■ Conduct guaiac stool testing for occult blood. (Phenytoin's CNS depressant effects decrease GI motility, producing constipation.)	Instruct patient to: ■ Take drug with food to reduce GI upset ■ Immediately report any severe or persistent heartburn, upper GI pain, nausea, or vomiting ■ Increase exercise, fluid and fiber intake to facilitate stool passage
■ Monitor nutritional status. (Phenytoin's action on electrolytes may cause decreased absorption of folic acid, vitamin D, magnesium, and calcium. Deficiencies in these vitamins and minerals lead to anemia and osteoporosis. Valproic acid may cause an increase in appetite and weight.)	■ Instruct patient in dietary or drug administration techniques specific to prescribed medications. ■ Instruct patient to report significant changes in appetite or weight gain.

EVALUATION OF OUTCOME CRITERIA

Evaluate effectiveness of drug therapy by confirming that patient goals and expected outcomes have been met (see "Planning").

See Tables 15.3 and 15.4 for lists of drugs to which these nursing actions apply.

Table 15.4	Succinimides
Drug	**Route and Adult Dose (max dose where indicated)**
ethosuximide (Zarontin)	PO; 250 mg, bid, increased every 4–7 days (max 1.5 g/day)
methsuximide (Celontin)	PO; 300 mg/day; may increase every 4–7 days (max 1.2 g/day)
phensuximide (Milontin)	PO; 0.5–1.0 g bid or tid

as phenothiazines and antidepressants, lower the seizure threshold and can decrease the effectiveness of succinimides.

The nurse should observe for common adverse reactions during therapy, including drowsiness, headache, fatigue, dizziness, depression or euphoria, nausea and vomiting, diarrhea, weight loss, and abdominal pain. Life-threatening adverse reactions include severe mental depression with overt suicidal intent, Stevens-Johnson syndrome, and blood dyscrasias such as agranulocytosis, pancytopenia, and leukopenia.

Seizure activity should be monitored during therapy, to confirm the drug's efficacy. Symptoms of overdose include CNS depression, stupor, ataxia, and coma. These symptoms may occur when ethosuximide (Zarontin) is given alone or in combination with other anticonvulsants. Combined usage must be monitored carefully, with regular testing for serum levels of each drug.

Patient education as it relates to succinimides should include goals, reasons for obtaining baseline data, and possible side effects. Following are the points the nurse should include when teaching patients about succinimides.

- Immediately report changes in mood, mental depression, or suicidal urges.
- Do not drive or on perform hazardous activities until effect of drug is known.
- Do not discontinue drug abruptly as this may result in rebound seizure activity.
- Take with food if GI upset occurs.
- Immediately report symptoms suggestive of infection (e.g., fever, sore throat, malaise).
- Report weight loss and anorexia.

NATURAL THERAPIES | The Ketogenic Diet

The ketogenic diet is used when seizures cannot be controlled through pharmacotherapy, or there are unacceptable side effects to the medications. Before antiepileptic drugs were developed, this diet was a primary treatment for epilepsy. The ketogenic diet may be used for babies, children, or adults. With adults, however, it is harder to develop the ketones that are necessary for the diet.

The ketogenic diet is a stringently calculated diet that is high in fat and low in carbohydrates and protein. It limits water intake to avoid ketone dilution and carefully controls caloric intake. Each meal has the same ketogenic ratio of 4 g of fat to 1 g of protein and carbohydrate. Extra fat is usually given in the form of cream. Research suggests that the diet produces success rates similar to use of medication, with one-third of the children using it becoming seizure free, one-third having their seizures reduced, and one-third not responding.

The diet appears to be equally effective for every seizure type, though drop attacks (atonic seizures) may be the most rapid responders. It also helps children with Lennox-Gastaut syndrome, and shows promise in babies with infantile spasms. Side effects include hyperlipidemia, constipation, vitamin deficiencies, kidney stones, acidosis, and possibly slower growth rates. Those interested in trying the diet must consult with their healthcare provider; this is not a do-it-yourself diet and may be harmful if not carefully monitored by skilled professionals.

Pr PROTOTYPE DRUG | ETHOSUXIMIDE (Zarontin)

ACTIONS AND USES

Ethosuximide is a drug of choice for absence (petit mal) seizures. It depresses the activity of neurons in the motor cortex by elevating the neuronal threshold. It is usually ineffective against psychomotor or clonic-tonic seizures; however, it may be given in combination with other medications, which better treat these conditions. It is available in tablet and flavored syrup formulations.

Administration Alerts

- Pregnancy category C.
- Abrupt withdrawal of this medication may induce grand mal seizures.

ADVERSE EFFECTS AND INTERACTIONS

Ethosuximide may impair mental and physical abilities. Psychosis or extreme mood swings, including depression with overt suicidal intent, can occur. Behavioral changes are more prominent in patients with a history of psychiatric illness. Central nervous system effects include dizziness, headache, lethargy, fatigue, ataxia, sleep pattern disturbances, attention difficulty, and hiccups. Bone marrow suppression and blood dyscrasias are possible, as is systemic lupus erythematosa.

Other reactions include gingival hypertrophy and tongue swelling. Common side effects are abdominal distress and weight loss.

Drug interactions include ethosuximide, which increases phenytoin serum levels. Valproic acid causes ethosuximide serum levels to fluctuate (increase or decrease).

 See the companion website for a Nursing Process Focus specific to this drug.

CHAPTER REVIEW

Key Concepts

The numbered key concepts provide a succinct summary of the important points from the corresponding numbered section within the chapter. If any of these points are not clear, refer to the numbered section within the chapter for review. Expanded versions can be found on the companion website.

15.1 Seizures are associated with many causes including head trauma, brain infection, fluid and electrolyte imbalance, hypoxia, stroke, brain tumors, and high fever in children.

15.2 The three broad categories of seizures are partial seizures, generalized seizures, and special epileptic syndromes. Each seizure type has a characteristic set of signs, and different drugs are used for different types.

15.3 Antiseizure drugs act by distinct mechanisms: potentiation of GABA, and delaying the influx of sodium or calcium ions into neurons. Pharmacotherapy may continue for many years and withdrawal from these agents must be done gradually to avoid seizure recurrence.

15.4 Barbiturates act by potentiating the effects of GABA. Phenobarbital is used for tonic-clonic and febrile seizures.

15.5 Benzodiazepines reduce seizure activity by intensifying GABA action. Their use is limited to being short-term adjuncts to other more effective agents.

15.6 Hydantoin and phenytoin-like drugs act by delaying sodium influx into neurons. Phenytoin is a broad-spectrum drug used for all types of epilepsy except absence seizures.

15.7 Succinimides act by delaying calcium influx into neurons. Ethosuximide (Zarontin) is a drug of choice for absence seizures.

Review Questions

1. While obtaining a medical history, a new patient claims to have a history of epilepsy but cannot remember the type. What sort of questions should the nurse ask to determine the type of seizures this patient has experienced?

2. Explain the importance of the neurotransmitter GABA in neuronal transmission.

3. A patient has been seizure free for 4 years and wants to be taken off phenytoin. Explain the process by which this withdrawal should be accomplished.

Critical Thinking Questions

1. The nurse practitioner reviews the laboratory results on a 16-year-old patient who presents to the clinic with fatigue and pallor. The patient's hematocrit is 26% and the nurse notes multiple small petechiae and bruises over the arms and legs. This patient has a generalized tonic-clonic seizure disorder that has been managed well on carbamazepine (Tegretol). Relate the drug regimen to this patient's presentation.

2. A 24-year-old woman is brought to the emergency room by her husband. He tells the triage nurse that his wife has been treated for seizure disorder secondary to a head injury she received in an automobile accident. She takes Dilantin 100 mg q8h. He relates a history of increasing drowsiness and lethargy in his wife over the past 24 hours. A Dilantin level is performed and the nurse notes that the results are 24 μg/dl. What is the probable cause of this patient's CNS depression?

3. The nurse is admitting a 17-year-old female patient with a history of seizure disorder. The patient has broken her leg in a car accident, in which she was the driver. The patient states that she hates having to take Dilantin, and that she stopped the drug because she couldn't drive and it was making her ugly. Instead of reassuring the patient, the nurse first considers the possible side effects of long-term phenytoin therapy. Discuss these and how they might impact patient compliance.

EXPLORE MediaLink

NCLEX review, case studies, and other interactive resources for this chapter can be found on the companion website at www.prenhall.com/adams. Click on "Chapter 15" to select the activities for this chapter. For animations, more NCLEX review questions, and an audio glossary, access the accompanying CD-ROM in this textbook.

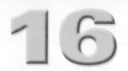

CHAPTER 16

Drugs for Emotional and Mood Disorders

DRUGS AT A GLANCE

ANTIDEPRESSANTS

Tricyclic antidepressants (TCAs)

Pr *imipramine (Tofranil)*

Selective serotonin reuptake inhibitors (SSRIs)

Pr *fluoxetine (Prozac)*

Atypical antidepressants

MAO inhibitors (MAOI)

Pr *phenelzine (Nardil)*

DRUGS FOR BIPOLAR DISORDER: MOOD STABILIZERS

Pr *lithium (Eskalith)*

Miscellaneous drugs

DRUGS FOR ATTENTION DEFICIT–HYPERACTIVITY DISORDER (ADHD)

CNS stimulants

Pr *methylphenidate (Ritalin)*

Nonstimulant drugs for ADHD

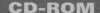

MediaLink **www.prenhall.com/adams**

CD-ROM

Animations:

   Mechanism in Action: Fluoxetine (Prozac)

   Mechanism in Action: Methylphenidate (Ritalin)

Audio Glossary

NCLEX Review

Companion Website

NCLEX Review

Dosage Calculations

Care Plans

Case Study

Expanded Key Concepts

attention deficit–hyperactivity disorder
(**ADHD**) *page 186*

bipolar disorder (manic depression) *page 184*

depression *page 173*

electroconvulsive therapy (**ECT**) *page 174*

mania *page 184*

monoamine oxidase inhibitor (**MAOI**)
page 179

mood disorder *page 173*

mood stabilizer *page 185*

selective serotonin reuptake inhibitor
(**SSRI**) *page 177*

serotonin syndrome (**SES**) *page 178*

tricyclic antidepressant (**TCA**) *page 175*

tyramine *page 180*

OBJECTIVES

After reading this chapter, the student should be able to:

1. Identify the two major categories of mood disorders and their symptoms.
2. Explain the etiology of clinical depression.
3. Discuss the nurse's role in the pharmacologic management of patients with depression, bipolar disorder, or attention deficit–hyperactivity disorder.
4. Identify symptoms of attention deficit–hyperactivity disorder.

5. For each of the drug classes listed in Drugs at a Glance, know representative drug examples, explain their mechanism of action, primary actions, and important adverse effects.
6. Categorize drugs used for mood and emotional disorders based on their classification and drug action.
7. Use the Nursing Process to care for patients receiving drug therapy for mood and emotional disorders.

Inappropriate or unusually intense emotions are among the leading causes of mental health disorders. Although mood changes are a normal part of life, when those changes become severe and result in impaired functioning within the family, work environment, or interpersonal relationships, an individual may be diagnosed as having a mood disorder. The two major categories of mood disorders are depression and bipolar disorder. A third emotional disorder, attention deficit–hyperactivity disorder, is also included in this chapter.

DEPRESSION

Depression is a disorder characterized by a sad or despondent mood. Many symptoms are associated with depression, including lack of energy, sleep disturbances, abnormal eating patterns, and feelings of despair, guilt, and misery.

16.1 Characteristics of Depression

People suffer from depression for a variety of reasons. In some cases, depression may be situational or reactive, meaning that it results from challenging circumstances such as severe physical illness, loss of a job, death of a loved one, divorce, or financial difficulties coupled with inadequate psychosocial support. In other cases, the depression may be biological or organic in origin, associated with dysfunction of neurological processes leading to an imbalance of neurotransmitters. Family history of depression increases the risk for biological depression. Depression is the most common mental health disorder of the elderly, encompassing a variety of physical, emotional, cognitive, and social considerations.

The majority of depressed patients are not found in psychiatric hospitals, but in mainstream everyday settings. The recognition of depression, in order for proper diagnosis and treatment to occur, is a collaborative effort among healthcare providers. Because depressed patients are present in multiple settings and in all areas of practice, every nurse should possess proficiency in the assessment and nursing care of patients afflicted with this disorder. Often times it is the pharmacist, working in a neighborhood pharmacy or supermarket, who may recognize that a person is faced with depression when people are self-medicating with remedies to enhance mood or using OTC sleep aids.

Some women experience intense mood shifts associated with hormonal changes during the menstrual cycle, pregnancy, childbirth, and menopause. For example, up to 80% of women experience depression 2 weeks to 6 months after the birth of a baby. Many women face additional stresses such as responsibilities both at work and home, single parenthood, and caring for children and for aging parents. If mood is severely depressed and persists long enough, many women may benefit from medical treatment, including women with premenstrual distress disorder, postpartum depression, or menopausal distress.

During the dark winter months, some patients experience a type of depression known as seasonal affective disorder (SAD). This type of depression is associated with a reduced release of the brain neurohormone, melatonin. Exposing patients on a regular basis to specific wavelengths of light may relieve SAD depression and prevent future episodes.

16.2 Assessment and Treatment of Depression

The first step to implementing appropriate treatment for depression is a complete health examination. Certain drugs, such as glucocorticoids, levodopa, and oral contraceptives can cause the same symptoms as depression, and the healthcare provider should rule out this possibility. Depression may be mimicked by a variety of medical and neurological disorders, ranging from B-vitamin deficiencies to thyroid gland problems to early Alzheimer's disease. If physical causes for the depression are ruled out, a psychological evaluation is often performed by a psychiatrist or psychologist to confirm the diagnosis.

During the health examination, inquiries should be made about alcohol and drug use, and if the patient has thoughts about death or suicide. Further, a history should include questions about whether other family members have had a depressive illness and, if treated, what therapies they may have received and which were effective.

To determine a course of treatment, healthcare providers and nurses assess for well-accepted symptoms of depression. Patients diagnosed with major depression must show at least five of the following symptoms.

- Difficulty sleeping or sleeping too much
- Extremely tired; without energy

- Abnormal eating patterns (eating too much or not enough)
- Vague physical symptoms (GI pain, joint/muscle pain, or headaches)
- Inability to concentrate or make decisions
- Feelings of despair, lack of self-worth, guiltiness, and misery
- Obsessed with death (expressing a wish to die or to commit suicide)
- Avoiding psychosocial and interpersonal interactions
- Lack of interest in personal appearance or sex
- Delusions or hallucinations

In general, severe depressive illness, particularly that which is recurrent, will require both medication and psychotherapy to achieve the best response. Counseling therapies help patients gain insight into and resolve their problems through verbal "give-and-take" with the therapist. Behavioral therapies help patients learn how to obtain more satisfaction and rewards through their own actions and how to unlearn the behavioral patterns that contribute to or result from their depression.

Short-term psychotherapies that are helpful for some forms of depression are interpersonal and cognitive-behavioral therapies. Interpersonal therapy focuses on the patient's disturbed personal relationships that both cause and exacerbate the depression. Cognitive-behavioral therapies help patients change the negative styles of thought and behavior that are often associated with their depression.

Psychodynamic therapies focus on resolving the patient's internal conflicts. These therapies are often postponed until the depressive symptoms are significantly improved.

In patients with serious and life-threatening mood disorders that are unresponsive to pharmacotherapy, electroconvulsive therapy (ECT) has been the traditional treatment. Although ECT has been found to be safe, there are still deaths (1 in 10,000 patients) and other serious complications related to seizure activity and anesthesia caused by ECT (Janicak, 2002). Recent studies suggest that repetitive transcranial magnetic stimulation (rTMS) is an effective somatic treatment for major depression. In contrast to

PHARMFACTS | **Patients with Depressive Symptoms**

- Major depression, manic depression, and situational depression are some of the most common mental health challenges worldwide.
- Clinical depression affects more than 19 million Americans each year.
- Fewer than half of those suffering from depression actually seek medical treatment.
- Most patients consider depression a weakness rather than an illness.
- There is no common age, sex, or ethnic factor related to depression—it can happen to anyone.

ECT, it has minimal effects on memory, does not require general anesthesia, and produces its effects without a generalized seizure.

Even with the best professional care, the patient with depression may take a long time to recover. Many individuals with major depression have multiple bouts of the illness over the course of a lifetime. This can take its toll on the patient's family, friends, and other caregivers who may sometimes feel burned out, frustrated, or even depressed themselves. They may experience episodes of anger toward the depressed loved one, only to subsequently suffer reactions of guilt over being angry. Although such feelings are common, they can be distressing, and the caregiver may not know where to turn for help, support, or advice. It is often the nurse who is best able to assist the family members of a person suffering from emotional and mood disorders. Family members may need counseling themselves.

ANTIDEPRESSANTS

Drugs for depression are called antidepressants. Antidepressants treat major depression by enhancing mood.

16.3 Mechanism of Action of Antidepressants

Depression is associated with an imbalance of neurotransmitters in certain regions of the brain. Although medication does not completely restore these chemical imbalances, it does help to reduce depressive symptoms while the patient develops effective means of coping.

Antidepressants enhance the action of certain neurotransmitters in the brain, including norepinephrine and serotonin. The two basic mechanisms of action are blocking the enzymatic breakdown of norepinephrine and slowing the reuptake of serotonin. The four primary classes of antidepressant drugs, also shown in Table 16.1, are as follows:

- Tricyclic antidepressants (TCAs)
- Selective serotonin reuptake inhibitors (SSRIs)
- Monoamine oxidase inhibitors (MAOIs)
- Atypical antidepressants

The atypical antidepressants include agents that do not fit into the first three categories. Agents such as bupropion (Wellbutrin) not only inhibit the reuptake of serotonin, but may also affect the activity of norepinephrine and dopamine. Examples of atypical antidepressants are maprotiline (Ludiomil), mirtazapine (Remeron), nefazodone (Serzone), trazodone (Desyrel), and venlafaxine (Effexor).

Tricyclic Antidepressants

Tricyclic antidepressants (TCAs) are drugs named for their three-ring chemical structure. They were the mainstay of depression pharmacotherapy from the early 1960s until the 1980s, and are still widely used.

16.4 Treating Depression with Tricyclic Antidepressants

Tricyclic antidepressants act by inhibiting the reuptake of both norepinephrine and serotonin into presynaptic nerve terminals, as shown in Figure 16.1. TCAs are used mainly for major depression and occasionally for milder situational depression. Clomipramine (Anafranil) is approved for treatment of obsessive-compulsive disorder, and other TCAs are sometimes used as unlabeled treatments for panic attacks. One use for TCAs, not related to psychopharmacology, is treatment of childhood enuresis (bed-wetting).

Shortly after their approval as antidepressants in the 1950s, it was found that the tricyclic antidepressants produced fewer side effects and were less dangerous than MAO inhibitors. However, TCAs have some unpleasant and serious side effects. The most common side effect is orthostatic hypotension, which occurs due to alpha$_1$ blockade on blood vessels. The most serious adverse effect occurs when TCAs accumulate in cardiac tissue. Although rare, cardiac dysrhythmias can occur.

Sedation is a frequently reported complaint at the initiation of therapy, though patients may become tolerant to this effect after several weeks of treatment. Most have a long half-life, which increases the risk of side effects for patients with delayed excretion. Anticholinergic effects, such as dry mouth, constipation, urinary retention, blurred vision, and tachycardia, are common. These effects are less severe if the drug is gradually increased to the therapeutic dose over 2 to 3 weeks. Significant drug interactions can occur with CNS depressants, sympathomimetics, anticholinergics, and MAO inhibitors. With the availability of newer antidepressants that have fewer side effects, TCAs are less likely to be used as first line drugs in the treatment of depression.

NURSING CONSIDERATIONS

The role of the nurse in tricyclic antidepressant therapy involves careful monitoring of a patient's condition and providing education as it relates to the prescribed drug regimen. The therapeutic effects of TCAs may take 2 to 6 weeks to occur. Suicide potential increases as blood levels of a tricyclic increase but have not yet reached their peak therapeutic levels. The nurse needs to monitor the patient closely for symptoms of suicidal ideation throughout treatment. As patients begin to recover from both psychological and physical depression (psychological depression slows all body processes), their energy level rises.

TCAs are contraindicated in patients in the acute recovery phase of an MI, heart block, or history of dysrhythmias because of their effects on cardiac tissue. Because TCAs lower the seizure threshold, patients with epilepsy must be carefully monitored. Patients with urinary retention, narrow-angle glaucoma, or prostatic hypertrophy may not be good candidates for TCAs because of anticholinergic side effects. Annoying anticholinergic effects, coupled with the weight gain effect of TCAs, may lead to

Table 16.1	Antidepressants
Drug	**Route and Adult Dose (max dose where indicated)**
MAO Inhibitors (MAOI)	
isocarboxazid (Marplan)	PO; 10–30 mg/day (max 30 mg/day)
℗ phenelzine (Nardil)	PO; 15 mg tid (max 90 mg/day)
tranylcypromine (Parnate)	PO; 30 mg/day (give 20 mg in A.M. and 10 mg in P.M.); may increase by 10 mg/day at 3-week intervals up to 60 mg/day
Tricyclic Antidepressants (TCAs)	
amitriptyline (Elavil)	Adult: PO; 75–100 mg/day (may gradually increase to 150–300 mg/day) Geriatric: PO; 10–25 mg at hs (may gradually increase to 25–150 mg/day)
amoxapine (Asendin)	Adult: PO; begin with 100 mg/day, may increase on day 3 to 300 mg/day Geriatric: PO; 25 mg at hs; may increase every 3–7 days to 50–150 mg/day (max 300 mg/day)
desipramine (Norpramin)	PO; 75–100 day; may increase to 150–300 mg/day
doxepin (Sinequan)	PO; 30–150 mg/day at hs; may gradually increase to 300 mg/day
℗ imipramine (Tofranil)	PO; 75–100 mg/day (max 300 mg/day)
maprotiline (Ludiomil)	Mild to moderate depression: PO; start at 75 mg/day; gradually increase every 2 weeks to 150 mg/day; Severe depression: PO; start at 100–150 mg/day; gradually increase to 300 mg/day
nortriptyline (Aventyl, Pamelor)	PO; 25 mg tid or qid; may increase 100–150 mg/day
protriptyline (Vivactil)	PO; 15–40 mg/day in three to four divided doses (max 60 mg/day)
trimipramine (Surmontil)	PO; 75–100 mg/day (max 300 mg/day)
Selective Serotonin Reuptake Inhibitors (SSRIs)	
citalopram (Celexa)	PO; Start at 20 mg/day (max 40 mg/day)
escitalopram oxalate (Lexapro)	PO; 10 mg qd; may increase to 20 mg after 1 week
℗ fluoxetine (Prozac)	PO; 20 mg/day in the A.M. (max 80 mg/day)
fluvoxamine (Luvox)	PO; Start with 50 mg/day (max 300 mg/day)
paroxetine (Paxil)	Depression: PO; 10–50 mg/day (max 80 mg/day) Obsessive-compulsive disorder: PO; 20–60 mg/day Panic attacks: PO; 40 mg/day
sertraline (Zoloft)	Adult: PO; start with 50 mg/day; gradually increase every few weeks to a range of 50–200 mg Geriatric: start with 25 mg/day
Atypical Antidepressants	
bupropion (Wellbutrin)	PO; 75–100 mg tid (greater than 450 mg/day increases risk for adverse reactions)
mirtazapine (Remeron)	PO; 15 mg/day in a single dose at hs; may increase every 1–2 weeks (max 45 mg/day)
nefazodone (Serzone)	PO; 50–100 mg bid; may increase up to 300–600 mg/day
trazodone (Desyrel)	PO; 150 mg/day; may increase by 50 mg/day every 3–4 days up to 400–600 mg/day
venlafaxine (Effexor)	PO; 25–125 mg tid

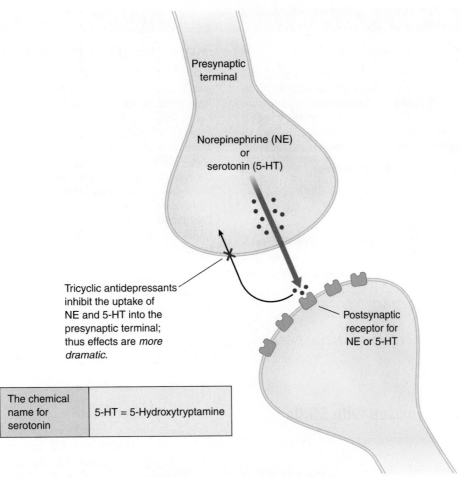

Figure 16.1 | Tricyclic antidepressants produce their effects by inhibiting the reuptake of neurotransmitters into presynaptic nerve terminals. The neurotransmitters particularly affected are norepinephrine and serotonin

noncompliance. Tricyclics must be given with extreme caution to patients with asthma, cardiovascular disorders, gastrointestinal disorders, alcoholism, and other psychiatric disorders including schizophrenia and bipolar disorder. Most TCAs are pregnancy category C or D, so they are only used during pregnancy or lactation when medically necessary. Should a patient desire to become pregnant while taking a TCA, she should discuss her depression medication with her healthcare provider immediately. The TCAs should be withdrawn over several weeks and not discontinued abruptly.

Significant drug interactions may occur with TCAs. Oral contraceptives may decrease the efficacy of tricyclics. Cimetidine (Tagamet) interferes with their metabolism and excretion. Tricyclics affect the efficacy of clonidine (Catapres) and guanethidine (Ismelin). Concurrent use of alcohol and other CNS depressants may result in excessive sedation, and should be avoided.

Patient education as it relates to tricyclic antidepressants should include the goals, reasons for obtaining baseline data such as vital signs and tests for cardiac and renal disorders, and possible side effects. Following are other important points the nurse should include when teaching patients regarding TCAs.

- Be aware that it may take several weeks or more to achieve the full therapeutic effect of the drug.
- Maintain follow-up appointments with the healthcare provider.
- Sweating, along with anticholinergic side effects, may occur.
- Take medication exactly as prescribed and report side effects if they occur.
- Do not take any prescription, OTC drugs, or herbal products without first consulting with the healthcare provider.
- Change position slowly especially when sitting or standing from a lying position.
- Do not drive or engage in hazardous activities until sedative effect is known; it may be taken at bedtime if sedation occurs.

Selective Serotonin Reuptake Inhibitors

Selective serotonin reuptake inhibitors (SSRIs) are drugs that slow the reuptake of serotonin into presynaptic nerve terminals. They have become drugs of choice in the treatment of depression.

Pr PROTOTYPE DRUG | IMIPRAMINE (Tofranil)

ACTIONS AND USES

Imipramine blocks the reuptake of serotonin and norepinephrine into nerve terminals. It is mainly used for clinical depression, although it is occasionally used for the treatment of nocturnal enuresis in children. The nurse may find imipramine prescribed for a number of unlabeled uses including intractable pain, anxiety disorders, and withdrawal syndromes from alcohol and cocaine.

Administration Alerts

- Paradoxical diaphoresis can be a side effect of TCAs; therefore, diaphoresis may not be a reliable indicator of other disease states such as hypoglycemia.
- Imipramine causes anticholinergic effects and may potentiate effects of anticholinergic drugs administered during surgery.
- Do not discontinue abruptly because rebound dysphoria, irritability, or sleeplessness may occur.
- Pregnancy category C.

ADVERSE EFFECTS AND INTERACTIONS

Side effects include sedation, drowsiness, blurred vision, dry mouth, and cardiovascular symptoms such as dysrhythmias, heart block, and extreme hypertension. Agents that mimic the action of norepinephrine or serotonin should be avoided because imipramine inhibits their metabolism and may produce toxicity. Some patients may experience photosensitivity. Concurrent use of other CNS depressants, including alcohol, may cause sedation. Cimetidine (Tagamet) may inhibit the metabolism of imipramine, leading to increased serum levels and possible toxicity. Clonidine may decrease its antihypertensive effects, and increase risk for CNS depression. Use of oral contraceptives may increase or decrease imipramine levels. Disulfiram may lead to delirium and tachycardia.

Use with caution with herbal supplements, such as evening primrose oil or ginkgo, which may lower the seizure threshold. St. John's wort used concurrently may cause serotonin syndrome.

 See the companion website for a Nursing Process Focus specific to this drug.

16.5 Treating Depression with SSRIs

Serotonin is a natural neurotransmitter in the CNS, found in high concentrations in certain neurons in the hypothalamus, limbic system, medulla and spinal cord. It is important to several body activities, including the cycling between NREM and REM sleep, pain perception, and emotional states. Lack of adequate serotonin in the CNS can lead to depression. Serotonin is metabolized to a less active substance by the enzyme monoamine oxidase (MAO). Serotonin is also known by its chemical name, 5-hydroxytryptamine (5-HT).

In the 1970s, it became increasingly clear that serotonin had a more substantial role in depression than once thought. Clinicians knew that the tricyclic antidepressants altered the sensitivity of serotonin to certain receptors in the brain, but they did not know how this was connected with depression. Ongoing efforts to find antidepressants with fewer side effects led to the development of a third category of medications, the selective serotonin reuptake inhibitors (SSRIs).

While the tricyclic class inhibits the reuptake of both norepinephrine and serotonin into presynaptic nerve terminals, the SSRIs are selective for serotonin. Increased levels of serotonin in the synaptic gap induce complex neurotransmitter changes in pre- and postsynaptic neurons in the brain. Presynaptic receptors become less sensitive while postsynaptic receptors become more sensitive. This concept is illustrated in Figure 16.2.

SSRIs have approximately the same efficacy at relieving depression as the MAO inhibitors and the tricyclics. The major advantage of the SSRIs, and the one that makes them drugs of choice, is their greater safety. Sympathomimetic effects (increased heart rate and hypertension) and anticholinergic effects (dry mouth, blurred vision, urinary re-

tention, and constipation) are less common with this drug class. Sedation is also experienced less frequently, and cardiotoxicity is not observed. All drugs in the SSRI class have equal efficacy and similar side effects.

The most common side effects of SSRIs relate to sexual dysfunction. Up to 70% of both men and women can experience decreased libido and lack of ability to reach orgasm. In men, delayed ejaculation and impotence may occur. For patients who are sexually active, these side effects may result in noncompliance with pharmacotherapy. Other common side effects of SSRIs include nausea, headache, anxiety, and insomnia.

Serotonin syndrome (SES) may occur when taking another medication that affects the metabolism, synthesis, or reuptake of serotonin, causing serotonin to accumulate in the body. Symptoms can begin as early as 2 hours after taking the first dose, or as late as several weeks after the initiating pharmacotherapy. SES can be produced by the concurrent administration of a SSRI with a MAOI, a tricyclic antidepressant, lithium, or a number of other medications. Symptoms of SES include mental status changes (confusion, anxiety, restlessness), hypertension, tremors, sweating, hyperpyrexia, or ataxia. Conservative treatment is to discontinue the SSRI and provide supportive care. In severe cases, mechanical ventilation and muscle relaxants may be necessary. If left untreated, death may occur.

NURSING CONSIDERATIONS

The role of the nurse in SSRI therapy involves careful monitoring of a patient's condition and providing education as it relates to the prescribed drug regimen. The nurse should assess the patient's needs for antidepressant drugs, includ-

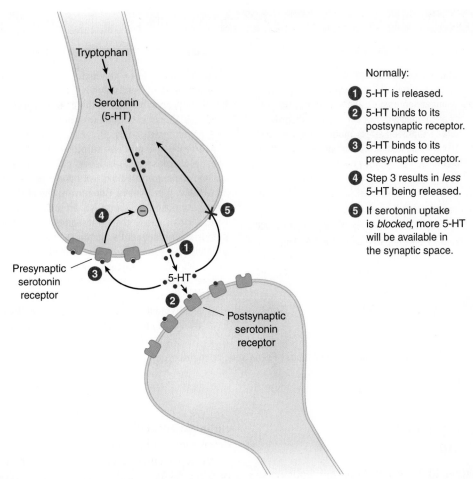

Normally:

1 5-HT is released.

2 5-HT binds to its postsynaptic receptor.

3 5-HT binds to its presynaptic receptor.

4 Step 3 results in *less* 5-HT being released.

5 If serotonin uptake is *blocked*, more 5-HT will be available in the synaptic space.

Figure 16.2 | SSRIs block the reuptake of serotonin into presynaptic nerve terminals. Increased levels of serotonin induce complex changes in pre- and postsynaptic neurons of the brain. Presynaptic receptors become less sensitive while postsynaptic receptors become more sensitive

ing intensity and duration of symptoms. The assessment should include identification of factors that led to depression, such as life events and health changes. The nurse should obtain a careful drug history, including the use of CNS depressants, alcohol and other antidepressants, especially MAOI therapy, as these may interact with SSRIs. The nurse should assess for hypersensitivity to SSRIs. The nurse should assess suicide ideation, because the drugs may take several weeks before full therapeutic benefit is obtained. The medical history should include any disorders of sexual function, as these drugs have a high incidence of side effects of this nature.

Although the SSRIs are safer than other antidepressants, serious adverse effects can still occur. Baseline liver function laboratory tests should be obtained, because SSRIs are metabolized in the liver and hepatic disease can result in higher serum levels. A baseline body weight should be obtained, as SSRIs can cause weight gain.

Patient education as it relates to SSRIs should include goals and reasons for obtaining baseline data such as vital signs and concurrent medications. The nurse should inform the patient that SSRIs take up to 5 weeks to reach their maximum therapeutic effectiveness.

Following are other important points the nurse should include when teaching patients regarding SSRIs.

- Do not take any prescription or OTC drugs or herbal products without first consulting with the healthcare provider.
- Maintain follow-up appointments with healthcare provider.
- Report side effects to healthcare provider as they occur.
- Do not drive or engage in hazardous activities until sedative effect is known; it may be taken at bedtime if sedation occurs.
- Do not discontinue drug abruptly after long-term use.
- Exercise and restrict caloric intake to avoid weight gain.

Monoamine Oxidase Inhibitors

Monoamine oxidase inhibitors (MAOIs) inhibit monoamine oxidase, the enzyme that terminates the actions of neurotransmitters such as dopamine, norepinephrine, epinephrine, and serotonin. Because of their low safety margin, these drugs are reserved for patients who have not responded to TCAs or SSRIs.

PROTOTYPE DRUG | FLUOXETINE (Prozac)

ACTIONS AND USES

Therapeutic actions of fluoxetine can be attributed to its ability to selectively inhibit serotonin reuptake into presynaptic nerve terminals. Its main use is clinical depression, although it may be prescribed for obsessive-compulsive and eating disorders. Therapeutic actions include improved affect, mood enhancement, and increased appetite with maximum effects observed after several days to weeks. Fluoxetine is pregnancy category B.

Administration Alerts

■ Fluoxetine is available in both daily and weekly dose oral formulations. Weekly dose capsules should be dispensed in small quantity or in the healthcare setting to reduce the risk of suicide by overdose.

■ Fluoxetine tends to be eliminated slowly and to accumulate in the body. Active metabolites may persist for weeks.

ADVERSE EFFECTS AND INTERACTIONS

Fluoxetine may cause headaches, nervousness, insomnia, nausea, and diarrhea. Foods high in the amino acid tryptophan should be avoided, as tryptophan is the chemical precursor for serotonin synthesis. Coadministration with selegiline may increase the risk of a hypertensive crisis. Tricyclic antidepressants administered concurrently may produce serotonin syndrome. Symptoms of fluoxetine overdose include fever, confusion, shivering, sweating, and muscle spasms. Fluoxetine cannot be used if the patient took an MAOI within 14 days. Concurrent use of benzodiazepines may cause increased adverse CNS effects. Concurrent use of beta-blockers can cause their decreased elimination, leading to hypotension or bradycardia. Concurrent use of phenytoin, clozapine, or theophylline may lead to decreased elimination of these drugs and toxicity. Concurrent use of warfarin may lead to increased risk of bleeding due to competitive protein binding.

Use with caution with herbal supplements such as St. John's wort or L-tryptophan, which may cause serotonin syndrome, and kava, which may increase the effects of fluoxetine.

 See the companion website for a Nursing Process Focus specific to this drug.

16.6 Treating Depression with MAO Inhibitors

As discussed in Chapter 13, the action of norepinephrine at adrenergic synapses is terminated through two means: reuptake into the presynaptic nerve and enzymatic destruction by the enzyme monoamine oxidase ⊚ . Monoamine oxidase inhibitors inhibit the breakdown of norepinephrine, dopamine, and serotonin in CNS neurons. The higher levels of these neurotransmitters in the brain intensify neurotransmission and alleviate the symptoms of depression. MAO is located within presynaptic nerve terminals as shown in Figure 16.3.

The monoamine oxidase inhibitors were the first drugs approved to treat depression, in the 1950s. They are as effective as TCAs and SSRIs in treating depression. However, because of drug-drug and food-drug interactions, hepatotoxicity, and the development of safer antidepressants, MAOIs are now reserved for patients who are not responsive to other antidepressant classes.

Common side effects of the MAOIs include orthostatic hypotension, headache, insomnia, and diarrhea. A primary concern is that these agents interact with a large number of foods and other medications, sometimes with serious effects. A hypertensive crisis can occur when a MAOI is used concurrently with other antidepressants or sympathomimetic drugs. Combining a MAOI with an SSRI can produce serotonin syndrome. If given with antihypertensives, the patient can experience excessive hypotension. MAOIs also potentiate the hypoglycemic effects of insulin and oral antidiabetic drugs. Hyperpyrexia is known to oc-

cur in patients taking MAOIs with meperidine (Demerol), dextromethorphan (Pedia Care and others), and TCAs.

A hypertensive crisis can also result from an interaction between MAOIs and foods containing tyramine, a form of the amino acid tyrosine. In many respects, tyramine resembles norepinephrine. Tyramine is usually degraded by MAO in the intestines. If a patient is taking MAOIs, however, tyramine enters the bloodstream in high amounts, and displaces norepinephrine in presynaptic nerve terminals. The result is a sudden increase in norepinephrine, causing acute hypertension. Symptoms usually occur within minutes of ingesting the food, and include occipital headache, stiff neck, flushing, palpitations, diaphoresis, and nausea. Calcium channel blockers may be given as an antidote. Examples of foods containing tyramine are shown in Table 16.2.

NURSING CONSIDERATIONS

The role of the nurse in MAOI therapy involves careful monitoring of a patient's condition and providing education as it relates to the prescribed drug regimen. The nurse should assess patient needs for antidepressant drugs, including intensity and duration of symptoms. The assessment should include identification of factors that led to depression, such as life events and health changes. The nurse should assess suicide ideation, because the drugs may take several weeks before full therapeutic benefit is obtained. Cardiovascular status should be assessed, as these agents may affect blood pressure. Phenelzine (Nardil) is contraindicated in cardiovascular disease, heart failure, CVA, hepatic or renal dysfunction and paranoid schizophrenia. A CBC should be

NURSING PROCESS FOCUS | PATIENTS RECEIVING ANTIDEPRESSANT THERAPY

ASSESSMENT

Prior to administration:
- Obtain complete health history including allergies, drug history, and possible drug interactions.
- Obtain history of cardiac (including recent MI), renal, biliary, liver, and mental disorders including EKG and blood studies: CBC, platelets, glucose, BUN, creatinine, electrolytes, liver function tests and enzymes, and urinalysis.
- Assess neurologic status, including seizure activity and identification of recent mood and behavior patterns.

POTENTIAL NURSING DIAGNOSES

- Ineffective Coping
- Powerlessness
- Disturbed Thought Processes, related to side effects of drug, lack of positive coping skills
- Impaired Adjustment
- Deficient Knowledge, related to drug therapy
- Risk for Self-Directed Violence
- Urinary Retention related to anticholinergic side effects of drug

PLANNING: PATIENT GOALS AND EXPECTED OUTCOMES

The patient will:
- Report mood elevation and effectively engage in activities of daily living
- Report an absence of suicidal ideations and improvement in thought processes
- Demonstrate a decrease in anxiety (e.g., ritual behaviors)
- Demonstrate an understanding of the drug's action by accurately describing drug effects and precautions

IMPLEMENTATION

Interventions and (Rationales)	Patient Teaching/Discharge Planning
• Monitor vital signs especially pulse and blood pressure. (Imipramine may cause orthostatic hypotension.)	Instruct patient to: • Report any change in sensorium particularly impending syncope • Avoid abrupt changes in position • Monitor vital signs (especially blood pressure) ensuring proper use of home equipment • Consult the nurse regarding "reportable" blood pressure readings (e.g., lower than 80/50)
• Observe for serotonin syndrome in SSRI use. • If suspected, discontinue drug and initiate supportive care. Respond according to ICU/emergency department protocols.	• Inform patient that overdosage may result in serotonin syndrome, which can be life-threatening.
• Monitor for paradoxical diaphoresis, which must be considered a significant sign, especially serious when coupled with nausea/vomiting or chest pain.	• Instruct patient to seek immediate medical attention for dizziness, headache, tremor, nausea/vomiting, anxiety, disorientation, hyperreflexia, diaphoresis, and fever.
• Monitor cardiovascular status. Observe for hypertension and signs of impending stroke or MI and heart failure.	• Instruct patient to immediately report severe headache, dizziness, paresthesias, bradycardia, chest pain, tachycardia, nausea/vomiting, or diaphoresis.
• Monitor neurologic status. Observe for somnolence and seizures. (TCAs may cause somnolence related to CNS depression. May reduce the seizure threshold.)	Instruct patient to: • Report significant changes in neurological status, such as seizures, extreme lethargy, slurred speech, disorientation, or ataxia and discontinue the drug • Take dose at bedtime to avoid daytime sedation
• Monitor mental and emotional status. Observe for suicidal ideation. (Therapeutic benefits may be delayed. Outpatients should have no more than a 7-day medication supply.) • Monitor for underlying or concomitant psychoses such as schizophrenia or bipolar disorders. (May trigger manic states.)	Instruct patient: • To immediately report dysphoria or suicidal impulses • To commit to a "no-self harm" verbal contract • That it may take 10 to 14 days before improvement is noticed, and about 1 month to achieve full therapeutic effect

continued

NURSING PROCESS FOCUS: *Patients Receiving Antidepressant Therapy (continued)*

Interventions and (Rationales)	*Patient Teaching/Discharge Planning*
■ Monitor sleep-wake cycle. Observe for insomnia and/or daytime somnolence.	Instruct patient to: ■ Take drug very early in the morning if insomnia occurs to promote normal timing of sleep onset ■ Avoid driving or performing hazardous activities until effects of drug are known ■ Take at bedtime if daytime drowsiness persists
■ Monitor renal status and urinary output. (May cause urinary retention due to muscle relaxation in urinary tract. Imipramine is excreted through the kidneys. Fluoxetine is slowly metabolized and excreted, increasing the risk of organ damage. Urinary retention may exacerbate existing symptoms of prostatic hypertrophy.)	Instruct patient to: ■ Monitor fluid intake and output ■ Notify the healthcare provider of edema, dysuria (hesitancy, pain, diminished stream), changes in urine quantity or quality (e.g., cloudy, with sediment) ■ Report fever or flank pain that may be indicative of a urinary tract infection related to urine retention
■ Use cautiously with the elderly or young. (Diminished kidney and liver function related to aging can result in higher serum drug levels, and may require lower doses. Children, due to an immature CNS, respond paradoxically to CNS drugs.)	Instruct patient that: ■ The elderly may be more prone to side effects such as hypertension and dysrhythmias ■ Children on imipramine for nocturnal enuresis may experience mood alterations
■ Monitor gastrointestinal status. Observe for abdominal distention. (Muscarinic blockade reduces tone and motility of intestinal smooth muscle, and may cause paralytic ileus.)	Instruct patient to: ■ Exercise, drink adequate amounts of fluid, and add dietary fiber to promote stool passage ■ Consult the nurse regarding a bulk laxative or stool softener if constipation becomes a problem
■ Monitor liver function. Observe for signs and symptoms of hepatotoxicity. ■ Monitor blood studies including CBC, differential, platelets, PT, PTT, and liver enzymes.	Instruct patient to: ■ Report nausea, vomiting, diarrhea, rash, jaundice, epigastric or abdominal pain, tenderness, or change in color of stool ■ Adhere to laboratory testing regimen for blood tests and urinalysis as directed
■ Monitor hematologic status. Observe for signs of bleeding. (Imipramine may cause blood dyscrasias. Use with warfarin may increase bleeding time.)	■ Instruct patient to report excessive bruising, fatigue, pallor, shortness of breath, frank bleeding, and/or tarry stools. ■ Demonstrate guaiac testing on stool for occult blood.
■ Monitor immune/metabolic status. Use with caution in patients with diabetes mellitus or hyperthyroidism. (If given in hyperthyroidism, can cause agranulocytosis. Imipramine may either increase or decrease serum glucose. Fluoxetine may cause initial anorexia and weight loss, but with prolonged therapy may result in weight gain of up to 20 pounds.)	■ Instruct diabetics to monitor glucose level daily and consult nurse regarding reportable serum glucose levels (e.g., less than 70 and more than 140). ■ Instruct patient that anorexia and weight loss will diminish with continued therapy.
■ Observe for extrapyramidal and anticholinergic effects. In overdosage, 12 hours of anticholinergic activity is followed by CNS depression. ■ Do not treat overdosage with quinidine, procainamide, atropine, or barbiturates. (Quinidine and procainamide can increase the possibility of dysrhythmia, atropine can lead to severe anticholinergic effects, and barbiturates can lead to excess sedation.)	Instruct patient to: ■ Immediately report involuntary muscle movement of the face or upper body (e.g., tongue spasms), fever, anuria, lower abdominal pain, anxiety, hallucinations, psychomotor agitation, visual changes, dry mouth, and difficulty swallowing ■ Relieve dry mouth with (sugar-free) hard candies, chewing gum, and drinking fluids ■ Avoid alcohol-containing mouthwashes which can further dry oral mucous membranes

continued

NURSING PROCESS FOCUS: *Patients Receiving Antidepressant Therapy (continued)*

Interventions and (Rationales)	Patient Teaching/Discharge Planning
■ Monitor visual acuity. Use with caution in narrow-angle glaucoma. (Imipramine may cause an increase in intraocular pressure. Anticholinergic effects may produce blurred vision.)	Instruct patient to: ■ Report visual changes, headache, or eye pain ■ Inform eye care professional of imipramine therapy
■ Ensure patient safety. (Dizziness caused by postural hypotension increases the risk of fall injuries.)	Instruct patient to: ■ Call for assistance before getting out of bed or attempting to ambulate alone ■ Avoid driving or performing hazardous activities until blood pressure is stabilized and effects of the drug are known

EVALUATION OF OUTCOME CRITERIA

Evaluate effectiveness of drug therapy by confirming that patient goals and expected outcomes have been met (see "Planning").

See Table 16.1 for a list of drugs to which these nursing actions apply.

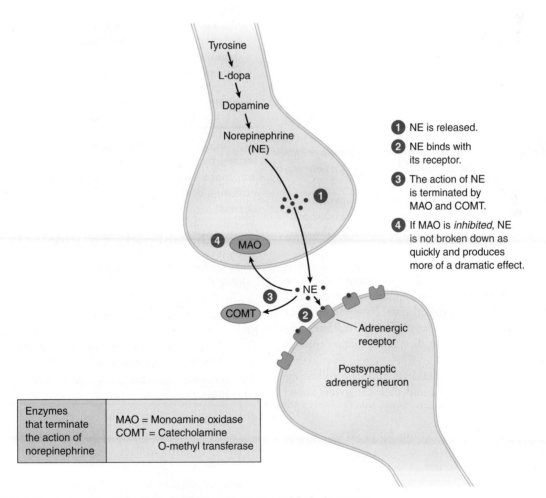

Figure 16.3 | Termination of norepinephrine activity through enzyme activity in the synapse

Table 16.2	**Foods Containing Tyramine**		
Fruits	**Dairy Products**	**Alcohol**	**Meats**
avocados	cheese (cottage cheese is okay);	beer	beef or chicken liver
bananas	sour cream	wines (especially red wines)	pate
raisins	yogurt		meat extracts
papaya products including meat tenderizers			pickled or kippered herring pepperoni
canned figs			salami
			sausage
			bologna/hot dogs
Vegetables	**Sauces**	**Yeast**	**Other foods to avoid**
pods of broad beans (fava beans)	soy sauce	all yeast or yeast extracts	chocolate

obtained, because MAOIs can inhibit platelet function. The nurse should assess for the possibility of pregnancy; these agents are pregnancy category C, and enter breast milk. A patient taking a MAOI must refrain from foods that contain tyramine, which is found in many common foods. MAOIs should be used with caution in epilepsy, as they may lower the seizure threshold.

The nurse should obtain a careful drug history; common drugs that may interact with a MAOI include other MAOIs, insulin, caffeine-containing products, other antidepressants, meperidine (Demerol), and possibly opioids and methyldopa (Dopamet). There must be at least a 14-day interval between the use of MAOIs and these other drugs.

Some patients may not achieve the full therapeutic benefits of a MAOI for 4 to 8 weeks. Because depression continues during this time, patients may discontinue the drug if they do not feel it is helping them.

Because of the serious side effects possible with MAOIs, patient education is vital. The patient's ability to comprehend restrictions and be compliant with them may be impaired in a severely depressed state. Patient education should include goals, reasons for obtaining baseline data such as vital signs, laboratory studies, and a dietary consult for possible side effects.

In addition, the nurse should include the following points when educating patients and their caregivers about MAOIs.

- Strictly observe dietary restrictions for foods containing tyramine.
- Do not take any prescription or OTC drugs or herbal products without first consulting with the healthcare provider.
- Refrain from caffeine intake.
- Wear a medic alert bracelet identifying the MAOI medication.
- Be aware that it may take several weeks or more to obtain the full therapeutic effect of drug.

- Maintain follow-up appointments with healthcare provider.
- Do not drive or engage in hazardous activities until sedative effect is known; it may be taken at bedtime if sedation occurs.
- Observe for and report signs of impending stroke or MI.

BIPOLAR DISORDER

Bipolar disorder, also called **manic depression**, is characterized by extreme and opposite moods, such as euphoria and depression. Patients may oscillate rapidly between both extremes, or there may be prolonged periods where mood is normal.

16.7 Characteristics of Bipolar Disorder

During the depressive stages of bipolar disorder, patients exhibit the symptoms of major depression described earlier in this chapter. Patients with bipolar disorder also display signs of mania, an emotional state characterized by high psychomotor activity and irritability. Patients may shift quickly from emotions of extreme depression to extreme rage and agitation. Symptoms of mania, as shown in the following list, are generally opposite of depressive symptoms.

- Insomnia
- Active for days without appearing tired
- Easily agitated and aggressive
- Feelings of exaggerated confidence
- Making choices without regard for a long-term plan or consequences of action
- Seeking the company or attention of others
- Unusual interest in sex
- May abuse drugs including alcohol, cocaine, or sleeping medication
- Denial that their behavior is a problem

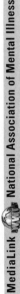

Pr **PROTOTYPE DRUG** | **PHENELZINE** (Nardil)

ACTIONS AND USES

Phenelzine produces its effects by irreversible inhibition of monoamine oxidase; therefore, it intensifies the effects of norepinephrine in adrenergic synapses. It is used to manage symptoms of depression not responsive to other types of pharmacotherapy, and is occasionally used for panic disorder. Drug effects may persist for 2 to 3 weeks after therapy is discontinued.

Administration Alerts

- Wash-out periods of 2 to 3 weeks are required before introducing other drugs.
- Abrupt discontinuation of this drug may cause rebound hypertension.
- Pregnancy category C.

ADVERSE EFFECTS AND INTERACTIONS

Common side effects are constipation, dry mouth, orthostatic hypotension, insomnia, nausea, and loss of appetite. It may increase heart rate and neural activity leading to delirium, mania, anxiety, and convulsions. Severe hypertension may occur when ingesting foods containing tyramine. Seizures, respiratory depression, circulatory collapse, and coma may occur in cases of severe overdose. Many other drugs affect the action of phenelzine. Concurrent use of tricyclic antidepressants and SSRIs should be avoided, since the combination can cause temperature elevation and seizures. Opiates, including meperidine should be avoided due to increased risk of respiratory failure or hypertensive crisis.

Use with caution with herbal supplements, such as ginseng, which could cause headache, tremors, mania, insomnia, irritability, and visual hallucinations. Concurrent use of ephedra could cause hypertensive crisis.

 See the companion website for a Nursing Process Focus specific to this drug.

NATURAL THERAPIES | St. John's Wort for Depression

St. John's wort (*Hypericum perforatum*) is an herb found throughout Britain, Asia, Europe, and North America commonly used as an antidepressant. It gets its name from a legend that red spots once appeared on its leaves on the anniversary of St. John's beheading. The word *wort* is a British term for "plant". Researchers once claimed that it produced its effects the same way MAO inhibitors do, by increasing the levels of serotonin, norepinephrine, and dopamine in the brain. More recent evidence suggests that it may selectively inhibit serotonin reuptake. Some claim that it is just as effective as fluoxetine (Prozac), paroxetine (Paxil), or sertraline (Zoloft) and with fewer side effects. It may also be used as an anti-infective agent for conditions such as *staphylococcus* and *streptococcus*, for nerve pains such as neuralgia and sciatica, and for mental burnout. St. John's wort should not be taken concurrently with antidepressant medications.

An active ingredient in St. John's wort is a photoactive compound that, when exposed to light, produces substances that can damage myelin. Patients have reported feeling stinging pain on the hands after sun exposure while taking the herbal remedy. Advise patients who take this herb to apply sunscreen or to wear protective clothing when outdoors.

MOOD STABILIZERS

Drugs for bipolar disorder are called **mood stabilizers**, because they have the ability to moderate extreme shifts in emotions between mania and depression. Some antiseizure drugs are also used for mood stabilization in bipolar patients.

16.8 Pharmacotherapy of Bipolar Disorder

The mainstay for the treatment of bipolar disorder is lithium (Eskalith), as monotherapy or in combination with other drugs. Lithium was approved in the United States in 1970. Before that time, its benefit in manic-depressive illness had been known; however, its therapeutic safety had not been proven. Other drugs that stabilize mood have multiple uses. For example, carbamazepine (Tegretol) and valproic acid (Depakene) are antiseizure drugs that have adjunct uses in bipolar disease. Table 16.3 shows selected drugs used to treat bipolar disorder.

Lithium has a narrow therapeutic index and is monitored via serum levels every 1 to 3 days when beginning therapy, and every 2 to 3 months thereafter. To ensure therapeutic action, concentrations of lithium in the blood must remain within the range of 0.6 to 1.5 mEq/L. Close monitoring encourages compliance and helps to avoid toxicity. Lithium acts like sodium in the body, so conditions where sodium is lost (e.g., excessive sweating or dehydration) can cause lithium toxicity. Lithium overdose may be treated with hemodialysis and supportive care.

It is not unusual for other drugs to be used in combination with lithium for the control of bipolar disorder. During the depressed stage, a tricyclic antidepressant or bupropion (Wellbutrin) may be necessary. During the manic phases, a benzodiazepine will moderate manic symptoms. In cases of extreme agitation, delusions, or hallucinations, an antipsychotic agent may be indicated. Continued patient compliance is essential to achieve successful pharmacotherapy, because some patients do not perceive their condition as abnormal.

Table 16.3	Drugs for Bipolar Disorder: Mood Stabilizers
Drug	**Route and Adult Dose (max dose where indicated)**
lithium (Eskalith)	PO; Initial: 600 mg tid; maintenance 300 mg tid (max 2.4 g/day)
Antiseizure Drugs	
carbamazepine (Tegretol)	PO; 200 mg bid, gradually increased to 800–1200 mg/day in three to four divided doses
lamotrigine (Lamictal)	PO; 50 mg/day for 2 weeks, then 50 mg bid for 2 weeks; may increase gradually up to 300–500 mg/day in two divided doses (max 700 mg/day)
valproic acid (Depakene) (see page 167 for the Prototype Drug box)	PO; 250 mg tid (max 60 mg/kg/day)

PROTOTYPE DRUG | LITHIUM (Eskalith)

ACTIONS AND USES

Although the exact mechanism of action is not clear, lithium is thought to alter the activity of neurons containing dopamine, norepinephrine, and serotonin by influencing their release, synthesis, and reuptake. Therapeutic actions are stabilization of mood during periods of mania and antidepressant effects during periods of depression. Lithium has neither antimanic nor antidepressant effects in individuals without bipolar disorder. After taking lithium for 2 to 3 weeks, patients are able to better concentrate and function in self-care.

Administration Alerts

- Lithium has a narrow therapeutic/toxic ratio; risk of toxicity is high.
- Acute overdosage may be treated by hemodialysis.
- Pregnancy category D.

ADVERSE EFFECTS AND INTERACTIONS

Lithium may cause dizziness, fatigue, short-term memory loss, increased urination, nausea, vomiting, loss of appetite, abdominal pain, diarrhea, dry mouth, muscular weakness, and slight tremors. Some drugs increase the rate at which the kidneys remove lithium from the bloodstream, including diuretics, sodium bicarbonate, and potassium citrate. Other drugs, such as methyldopa and probenecid, inhibit the rate of lithium excretion. Patients should not have a salt-free diet when taking this drug, because it reduces lithium excretion. Diuretics enhance excretion of sodium and increase the risk of lithium toxicity. Concurrent administration of anticholinergic drugs can cause urinary retention that, coupled with the polyuria effect of lithium, may cause a medical emergency. Alcohol can potentiate drug action.

NURSING CONSIDERATIONS

Lithium (Eskalith) is the only drug in its class. See "Nursing Process Focus: Patients Receiving Lithium" for information on this prototype drug. Refer to chapters on antiseizure drugs (Chapter 15), antipsychotics (Chapter 17), and anxiolytics (Chapter 14) for additional nursing considerations on adjunct medications .

ATTENTION DEFICIT–HYPERACTIVITY DISORDER

Attention deficit–hyperactivity disorder (ADHD) is a condition characterized by poor attention span, behavior control issues, and/or hyperactivity. Although normally diagnosed in childhood, symptoms of ADHD may extend into adulthood.

16.9 Characteristics of ADHD

ADHD affects as many as 5% of all children. Most children diagnosed with this condition are between the ages of 3 and 7 years, and boys are 4 to 8 times more likely to be diagnosed than girls.

ADHD is characterized by developmentally inappropriate behaviors involving difficulty in paying attention or focusing on tasks. ADHD may be diagnosed when the child's hyperactive behaviors significantly interfere with normal play, sleep, or learning activities. Hyperactive children usually have increased motor activity that is manifested by a tendency to be fidgety and impulsive, and to interrupt and talk excessively during their developmental years; therefore, they may not be able to interact with others appropriately at home, school, or on the playground. In boys, the activity levels are usually more overt. Girls show less aggression and impulsiveness but more anxiety, mood

NURSING PROCESS FOCUS	PATIENTS RECEIVING LITHIUM (ESKALITH)

ASSESSMENT

Prior to administration:
- Obtain complete health history including allergies, drug history, and possible drug interactions.
- Assess mental and emotional status, including any recent suicidal ideation.
- Obtain cardiac history (including EKG and vital signs); renal, liver disorders, and blood studies: glucose, BUN, creatinine, electrolytes, and liver enzymes.

POTENTIAL NURSING DIAGNOSES

- Risk for Self-Directed Violence
- Disturbed Thought Processes
- Disturbed Sleep Pattern
- Sleep Deprivation (in mania)
- Risk for Fluid Volume Imbalance
- Self-Care Deficit: Dressing/Grooming

PLANNING: PATIENT GOALS AND EXPECTED OUTCOMES

The patient will:
- Demonstrate stabilization of mood, including absence of mania and suicidal depression
- Engage in normal activities of daily living and report subjective improvement in mood
- Demonstrate understanding of drug action by accurately describing drug effects and precautions

IMPLEMENTATION

Interventions and (Rationales)

- Monitor mental and emotional status. Observe for mania and/or extreme depression. (Lithium should prevent mood swings.)

- Monitor electrolyte balance. (Lithium is a salt affected by dietary intake of other salts such as sodium chloride. Insufficient dietary salt intake causes the kidneys to conserve lithium, increasing serum lithium levels.)

- Monitor fluid balance. (Lithium causes polyuria by blocking effects of antidiuretic hormone.)
- Measure intake and output. Weigh patient daily. (Short-term changes in weight are a good indicator of fluctuations in fluid volume. Excess fluid volume increases the risk of HF; pitting edema may signal HF.)

- Monitor renal status. (Lithium may cause degenerative changes in the kidney which increases drug toxicity.)
- Monitor laboratory tests: CBC, differential, BUN, creatinine, uric acid, and urinalysis. Use with caution in kidney disease.

- Monitor cardiovascular status. (Lithium toxicity may cause muscular irritability resulting in cardiac dysrhythmias or angina.)
- Monitor vital signs including apical pulse.
- Use with caution in patients with a history of CAD or heart disease.

- Monitor gastrointestinal status. (Lithium may cause dyspepsia, diarrhea, or metallic taste.)

- Monitor metabolic status. (Lithium may cause goiter with prolonged use and false-positive results on thyroid tests.)

Patient Education/Discharge Planning

- Instruct patient to keep a symptom log to document response to medication.

Instruct patient to:
- Monitor dietary salt intake; consume sufficient quantities, especially during illness or physical activity
- Avoid activities that cause excessive perspiration

Instruct patient to:
- Increase fluid intake to 1 to 1.5 L per day
- Limit or eliminate caffeine consumption (caffeine has a diuretic effect that can cause lithium sparing by the kidneys)
- Notify healthcare provider of excessive weight gain or loss, or pitting edema

Instruct patient to:
- Immediately report anuria, especially accompanied by lower abdominal tenderness, distention, headache, and diaphoresis
- Inform healthcare provider of nausea, vomiting, diarrhea, flank pain or tenderness, and changes in urinary quantity and quality (e.g., sediment)

Instruct patient to:
- Immediately report palpitations, chest pain, or other symptoms suggestive of myocardial infarction
- Monitor vital signs ensuring proper use of home equipment

- Instruct patient to take drug with food to reduce stomach upset and report distressing GI symptoms.

- Instruct patient to report symptoms of goiter or hypothyroidism: enlarged mass on neck, fatigue, dry skin or edema.

continued

EVALUATION OF OUTCOME CRITERIA

Evaluate effectiveness of drug therapy by confirming that patient goals and expected outcomes have been met (see "Planning").

swings, social withdrawal, and cognitive and language delays. Girls also tend to be older at the time of diagnosis, so problems and setbacks related to the disorder exist for a longer time before treatment interventions are undertaken. Symptoms of ADHD are shown in the following list.

- Easily distracted
- Fail to receive or follow instructions properly
- Cannot focus on one task at a time and jump from one activity to another
- Difficulty remembering
- Frequently lose or misplace personal items
- Talk excessively and interrupt other children in a group
- Have an inability to sit still when asked repeatedly
- Often impulsive
- Sleep disturbance

Most children with ADHD have associated challenges. Many find it difficult to concentrate on tasks assigned in school. Even if they are gifted, their grades may suffer because they have difficulty following a conventional routine; discipline may also be a problem. Teachers are often the first to suggest that a child be examined for ADHD and receive medication when behaviors in the classroom escalate to the point of interfering with learning. A diagnosis is based on psychological and medical evaluations.

The etiology of ADHD is not clear. For many years, scientists described this disorder as mental brain dysfunction and hyperkinetic syndrome, focusing on abnormal brain function and overactivity. A variety of physical and neurologic disorders have been implicated; only a small percentage of those affected have a known cause. Known causes include contact with high levels of lead in childhood and prenatal exposure to alcohol and drugs. Genetic factors may also play a role, although a single gene has not been isolated and a specific mechanism of genetic transmission is not known. The interplay of genetics and environment may be a contributing dynamic. Recent evidence suggests that hyperactivity may be related to a deficit or dysfunction of dopamine, norepinephrine, and serotonin in the reticular activating system of the brain. Although once thought to be the culprits, sugars, chocolate, high carbohydrate foods and beverages, and certain food additives have been disproven as causative or aggravating factors for ADHD.

The nurse is often involved in the screening and the mental health assessment of children with suspected ADHD.

PHARMFACTS | **Attention Deficit–Hyperactivity Disorder**

- ADHD is the major reason why children are referred for mental health treatment.
- About one-half are also diagnosed with oppositional defiant or conduct disorder.
- About one-fourth are also diagnosed with anxiety disorder.
- About one-third are also diagnosed with depression.
- And about one-fifth also have a learning disability.

When a child is referred for testing, it is important to remember that both the child and family must be assessed. The family is screened with, or prior to, the child's evaluation. It is the nurse's responsibility to collect comprehensive data about the character and extent of the child's physical, psychological, and developmental health situation, to formulate the nursing diagnoses and create an individualized plan of care. A relevant nursing care plan can only be created if it is based on appropriate communication that fosters rapport and trust.

Once ADHD is diagnosed, the nurse is instrumental in educating the family regarding coping mechanisms that might be used to manage the demands of a child who is hyperactive. For the school-age child, the nurse often serves as the liaison to parents, teachers, and school administrators. The parents and child need to understand the importance of appropriate expectations and behavioral consequences. The child, from an early age and based on his or her developmental level, must be educated about the disorder and understand that there are consequences to inappropriate behaviors. Self-esteem must be fostered in the child so that ego strengths can develop. It is important for the child to develop a trusting relationship with healthcare providers and learn the importance of medication management and compliance.

One-third to one-half of children diagnosed with ADHD also experience symptoms of attention dysfunction in their adult years. Symptoms of ADHD in adults appear similar to mood disorders. Symptoms include anxiety, mania, restlessness, and depression, which can cause difficulties in interpersonal relationships. Some patients have difficulty holding jobs and may have increased risk for alcohol and drug abuse. Untreated ADHD has been linked to low self-esteem, diminished social success, and criminal or violent behaviors.

AGENTS FOR ATTENTION DEFICIT–HYPERACTIVITY DISORDER

The traditional drugs used to treat ADHD in children have been CNS stimulants. These drugs stimulate specific areas of the central nervous system that heighten alertness and increase focus. Recently, a non-CNS stimulant was approved to treat ADHD. Agents for treating ADHD are shown in Table 16.4.

CNS Stimulants

CNS stimulants are the main course of treatment for ADHD. Stimulants reverse many of the symptoms, helping patients to focus on tasks. The most widely prescribed drug for ADHD is methylphenidate (Ritalin). Other CNS stimulants that are rarely prescribed include d- and l-amphetamine racemic mixture (Adderall), dextroamphetamine (Dexedrine), methamphetamine (Desoxyn), or pemoline (Cylert).

16.10 Pharmacotherapy of ADHD

Patients taking CNS stimulants must be carefully monitored. CNS stimulants used to treat ADHD may create paradoxical hyperactivity. Adverse reactions include insomnia, nervousness, anorexia, and weight loss. Occasionally, a patient may suffer from dizziness, depression, irritability, nausea, or abdominal pain. These are Schedule II controlled substances and pregnancy category C.

Non-CNS stimulants have been tried for ADHD; however, they exhibit less efficacy. Clonidine (Catapres) is sometimes prescribed when patients are extremely aggressive, active, or have difficulty falling asleep. Atypical antidepressants such as bupropion (Wellbutrin) and tricyclics such as desipramine (Norpramine) and imipramine (Tofranil) are

SPECIAL CONSIDERATIONS

Zero Tolerance in Schools

Methylphenidate is an effective drug to treat ADHD and is often promoted by teachers and school counselors as an adjunct to improving academic performance and social adjustment. However, most schools have a "zero drug tolerance" policy which creates a hostile environment for students who must take this drug. Zero tolerance policies generally prohibit the possession of *any* drug and define the school's right to search and seizure and the right to demand that students submit to random drug testing, or screening as a condition of participating in sports and extracurricular activities. Schools maintain the right to suspend or expel students found in violation of such policies. In some districts, possession of scheduled drugs may also result in arrest and prosecution of the student.

Methylphenidate is a Schedule II controlled substance considered to have a high abuse potential. Students who take this drug should be made aware of the academic and social consequences of unauthorized possession of this medication. Most schools have strict guidelines regarding medication administration and require original prescriptions and containers of drug to be supplied to the school health office. Students should carry an official notice from the healthcare provider regarding methylphenidate therapy that may be produced in the event of random drug testing.

Table 16.4	Drugs for Attention Deficit–Hyperactivity Disorder
Drug	**Route and Adult Dose (max dose where indicated)**
CNS Stimulants	
d- and l-amphetamine racemic mixture (Adderall)	>6 years old: PO; 5 mg qd to bid; may increase by 5 mg at weekly intervals (max 40 mg/day). 3–5 years old: PO; 2.5 mg one to two times/day; may increase by 2.5 mg at weekly intervals
dextroamphetamine (Dexedrine)	3–5 years old: PO; 2.5 mg qd to bid; may increase by 2.5 mg at weekly intervals. 6 years old: PO; 5 mg qd to bid; increase by 5 mg at weekly intervals (max 40 mg/day)
methamphetamine (Desoxyn)	≤ 6 years old: PO; 2.5–5 mg qd to bid; may increase by 5 mg at weekly intervals (max 20–25 mg/day)
methylphenidate (Ritalin)	PO; 5–10 mg before breakfast and lunch, with gradual increase of 5–10 mg/week as needed (max 60 mg/day)
pemoline (Cylert)	> 6 years old: PO; 37.5 mg/day; may increase by 18.75 mg at weekly intervals (max 112.5 mg/day)
Nonstimulant for ADD/ADHD	
atomoxetine (Strattera)	PO; Start with 40 mg in A.M.; may increase after 3 days to target dose of 80 mg/day given either once in the morning or divided morning and late afternoon/early evening; may increase to max of 100 mg/day if needed

considered second choice drugs, when CNS stimulants fail to work or are contraindicated.

A recent addition to the treatment of ADHD in children and adults is atomoxetine (Strattera). Although its exact mechanism is not known, it is classified as a norepinephrine reuptake inhibitor. Patients on atomoxetine showed improved ability to focus on tasks and reduced hyperactivity. Efficacy appears to be equivalent to methylphenidate (Ritalin), although the drug is too new for long-term comparisons. Common side effects include headache, insomnia, upper abdominal pain, decreased appetite, and cough. Unlike methylphenidate, it is not a scheduled drug; thus, parents who are hesitant to place their child on stimulants now have a reasonable alternative.

NURSING CONSIDERATIONS

Methylphenidate (Ritalin) is the only drug in its class. See "Nursing Process Focus: Patients Receiving Methylphenidate" for information on this prototype drug.

Pr PROTOTYPE DRUG | METHYLPHENIDATE (Ritalin)

ACTIONS AND USES

Methylphenidate activates the reticular activating system, causing heightened alertness in various regions of the brain, particularly those centers associated with focus and attention. Activation is partially achieved by the release of neurotransmitters such as norepinephrine, dopamine, and serotonin. Impulsiveness, hyperactivity, and disruptive behavior are usually reduced within a few weeks. These changes promote improved psychosocial interactions and academic performance.

Administration Alerts

- Sustained-release tablets must be swallowed whole. Breaking or crushing SR tablets cause immediate release of the entire dose.
- Pregnancy category C.

ADVERSE EFFECTS AND INTERACTIONS

In a non-ADHD patient, methylphenidate causes nervousness and insomnia. All patients are at risk for irregular heart beat, high blood pressure, and liver toxicity. Methylphenidate is a Schedule II drug, indicating its potential to cause dependence when used for extended periods. Periodic drug-free "holidays" are recommended to reduce drug dependence and to assess the patient's condition.

Methylphenidate interacts with many drugs. For example, it may decrease the effectiveness of anticonvulsants, anticoagulants, and guanethidine. Concurrent therapy with clonidine may increase adverse effects. Antihypertensives or other CNS stimulants could potentiate the vasoconstrictive action of methylphenidate. MAOIs may produce hypertensive crisis.

NURSING PROCESS FOCUS | PATIENTS RECEIVING METHYLPHENIDATE (RITALIN) Pr

ASSESSMENT

Prior to administration:
- Obtain complete health history including allergies, drug history, and possible drug interactions.
- Obtain history of neurological, cardiac, renal, biliary, and mental disorders including blood studies: CBC, platelets, liver enzymes.
- Assess neurologic status, including identification of recent behavioral patterns.
- Assess growth and development.

POTENTIAL NURSING DIAGNOSES

- Risk for Delayed Development, related to growth retardation secondary to methylphenidate
- Delayed Growth and Development, related to increased motor activity, growth retardation secondary to methylphenidate, unsuccessful interpersonal relationships
- Imbalanced Nutrition: Less than Body Requirements
- Deficient Knowledge, related to drug therapy
- Disturbed Sleep Pattern

PLANNING: PATIENT GOALS AND EXPECTED OUTCOMES

The patient will:
- Experience subjective improvement in attention/concentration and reduction in impulsivity and/or psychomotor symptoms ("hyperactivity")
- Demonstrate understanding of the drug's action by accurately describing drug effects and precautions

continued

NURSING PROCESS FOCUS: Patients Receiving Methylphenidate (Ritalin) (continued)

IMPLEMENTATION

Interventions and (Rationales)	Patient Education/Discharge Planning
■ Monitor mental status and observe for changes in level of consciousness and adverse effects such as persistent drowsiness, psychomotor agitation or anxiety, dizziness, trembling or seizures.	■ Instruct patient to report any significant increase in motor behavior, changes in sensorium, or feelings of dysphoria.
■ Use with caution in epilepsy. (Drug may lower the seizure threshold.)	■ Instruct patient to discontinue drug immediately if seizures occur and notify healthcare provider.
■ Monitor vital signs. (Stimulation of the CNS induces the release of catecholamines with a subsequent increase in heart rate and blood pressure.)	Instruct patient to: ■ Immediately report rapid heartbeat, palpitations, or dizziness ■ Monitor blood pressure and pulse, ensuring proper use of home equipment
■ Monitor gastrointestinal and nutritional status. (CNS stimulation causes anorexia and elevates BMR, producing weight loss.) Other GI side effects include nausea/vomiting and abdominal pain.	Instruct patient to: ■ Report any distressing GI side effects ■ Take drug with meals to reduce GI upset and counteract anorexia; eat frequent small nutrient and calorie dense snacks ■ Weigh weekly and report significant losses over one pound
■ Monitor laboratory tests such as CBC, differential, and platelet count. (Drug is metabolized in the liver and excreted by the kidneys; impaired organ function can increase serum drug levels. Drug may cause leukopenia and/or anemia.)	Instruct patient to: ■ Report shortness of breath, profound fatigue, pallor, bleeding or excessive bruising (these are signs of blood disorder) ■ Report nausea, vomiting, diarrhea, rash, jaundice, abdominal pain, tenderness, distention, or change in color of stool (these are signs of liver disease) ■ Adhere to laboratory testing regimen for blood tests and urinalysis as directed
■ Monitor effectiveness of drug therapy.	Instruct the patient to: ■ Schedule regular drug holidays ■ Not discontinue abruptly as rebound hyperactivity or withdrawal symptoms may occur; taper the dose prior to starting a drug holiday ■ Keep a behavior diary to chronicle symptoms and response to drug ■ Safeguard medication supply due to abuse potential
■ Monitor growth and development. (Growth rate may stall in response to nutritional deficiency caused by anorexia.)	■ Instruct patient that reductions in growth rate are associated with drug usage. Drug holidays may decrease this effect.
■ Monitor sleep-wake cycle. (CNS stimulation may disrupt normal sleep patterns.)	Instruct the patient that: ■ Insomnia may be adverse reaction ■ Sleeplessness can sometimes be counteracted by taking the last dose no later than 4 P.M. ■ Drug is not intended to treat fatigue; warn the patient that fatigue may accompany wash-out period

EVALUATION OF OUTCOME CRITERIA

Evaluate effectiveness of drug therapy by confirming that patient goals and expected outcomes have been met (see "Planning").

CHAPTER REVIEW

Key Concepts

The numbered key concepts provide a succinct summary of the important points from the corresponding numbered section within the chapter. If any of these points are not clear, refer to the numbered section within the chapter for review. Expanded versions can be found on the companion website.

16.1 Depression has many causes and methods of classification. The identification of depression and its etiology is essential for proper treatment.

16.2 Major depression may be treated with medications, psychotherapeutic techniques, or electroconvulsive therapy.

16.3 Antidepressants act by correcting neurotransmitter imbalances in the brain. The two basic mechanisms of action are blocking the enzymatic breakdown of norepinephrine and slowing the reuptake of serotonin.

16.4 Tricyclic antidepressants are older medications used mainly for the treatment of major depression, obsessive-compulsive disorders, and panic attacks.

16.5 SSRIs act by selectively blocking the reuptake of serotonin in nerve terminals. Because of fewer side effects, SSRIs are drugs of choice in the pharmacotherapy of depression.

16.6 MAOIs are usually prescribed in cases when other antidepressants have not been successful. They have more serious side effects than other antidepressants.

16.7 Patients with bipolar disorder display not only signs of depression, but also mania, a state characterized by expressive psychomotor activity and irritability.

16.8 Mood stabilizers such as lithium (Eskalith) are used to treat both the manic and depressive stages of bipolar disorder.

16.9 Attention deficit–hyperactivity disorder (ADHD) is a common condition occurring primarily in children and is characterized by difficulty paying attention, hyperactivity, and impulsiveness.

16.10 The most efficacious drugs for symptoms of ADHD are the CNS stimulants such as methylphenidate (Ritalin). A newer, nonstimulant drug, atomoxetine (Strattera), has shown promise in patients with ADHD.

Review Questions

1. Identify the classes of drugs used to treat major depression. Which class is the most effective? Which exhibits the fewest side effects?

2. A sexually active man insists upon discontinuing his SSRI due to his inability to achieve erections during intercourse. What are his options for controlling depression?

3. A patient with bipolar disorder becomes physically abusive during manic episodes and denies his behavior is abnormal. What advice would you give, and what treatment options are available?

4. The frustrated parents of a 9-year-old insist that their son be medicated for ADHD. What assessment would be needed? What therapeutic options are available?

Critical Thinking Questions

1. A 10-year-old girl has been diagnosed with ADHD. Her parents have been reluctant to agree with the pediatrician's recommendation for pharmacologic management; however, the child's performance in school has deteriorated. A school nurse notes that the child has been placed on amphetamine (Adderall), not methylphenidate (Ritalin). After reviewing the dosing schedule, the nurse identifies the developmental considerations that might support the use of Adderall. Discuss these.

2. A 66-year-old female patient has been diagnosed with clinical depression following the death of her husband. She says that she has not been able to sleep for weeks and that she is "living on coffee and cigarettes." The healthcare provider prescribes fluoxetine (Prozac). The patient seeks reassurance from the nurse regarding when she should begin feeling "more like myself." How should the nurse respond?

3. A 26-year-old mother of three children comes to the prenatal clinic suspecting a fourth pregnancy. She tells the nurse that she got "real low" after her third baby and that she was prescribed sertraline (Zoloft). She tells the nurse that she is really afraid of "going crazy" if she has to stop taking the drug because of this pregnancy. What concerns should the nurse have?

EXPLORE MediaLink

NCLEX review, case studies, and other interactive resources for this chapter can be found on the companion website at www.prenhall.com/adams. Click on "Chapter 16" to select the activities for this chapter. For animations, more NCLEX review questions, and an audio glossary, access the accompanying CD-ROM in this textbook.

DRUGS AT A GLANCE

metabolized and eliminated by the bod
of this process
PHARMACOLOGY
1. The study of medicines; the disciplin
pertaining to how drugs improve the he
of the human body
PHARMACOPOEIA

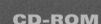

MediaLink www.prenhall.com/adams

CD-ROM
Animation:
   Extrapyramidal Signs (EPS)
Audio Glossary
NCLEX Review

Companion Website
NCLEX Review
Dosage Calculations
Case Study
Care Plans
Expanded Key Concepts

OBJECTIVES

After reading this chapter, the student should be able to:

1. Explain theories for the etiology of schizophrenia.
2. Compare and contrast the positive and negative symptoms of schizophrenia.
3. Discuss the rationale for selecting a specific antipsychotic drug for the treatment of schizophrenia.
4. Explain the importance of patient drug compliance in the pharmacotherapy of schizophrenia.
5. Describe the nurse's role in the pharmacologic management of schizophrenia.

6. Explain the symptoms associated with extrapyramidal side effects of antipsychotic drugs.
7. For each of the drug classes listed in Drugs at a Glance; know representative drug examples, explain their mechanism of action, primary actions, and important adverse effects.
8. Categorize drugs used for psychoses based on their classification and drug action.
9. Use the Nursing Process to care for patients receiving drug therapy for psychoses.

Severe mental illness can be incapacitating for the patient and intensely frustrating for relatives and those dealing with the patient on a regular basis. Before the 1950s, patients with acute mental dysfunction were institutionalized, often for their entire lives. The introduction of chlorpromazine (Thorazine) in the 1950s, and the development of newer agents, revolutionized the treatment of mental illness.

17.1 The Nature of Psychoses

A psychosis is a mental health condition characterized by delusions (firm ideas and beliefs not founded in reality), hallucinations (seeing, hearing, or feeling something that is not there), illusions (distorted perceptions of actual sensory stimuli), disorganized behavior, and a difficulty relating to others. Behavior may range from total inactivity to extreme agitation and combativeness. Some psychotic patients exhibit paranoia, an extreme suspicion and delusion that they are being followed, and that others are trying to harm them. Because they are unable to distinguish what is real from what is illusion, they are often viewed as insane.

Psychoses may be classified as acute or chronic. Acute psychotic episodes occur over hours or days, whereas chronic psychoses develop over months or years. Sometimes a cause may be attributed to the psychosis, such as brain damage, overdoses of certain medications, extreme depression, chronic alcoholism, and drug addiction. Genetic factors are known to play a role in some psychoses. Unfortunately, the vast majority of psychoses have no identifiable cause.

People with psychosis are usually unable to function normally in society without long-term drug therapy. Patients must see their healthcare provider periodically and medication must be taken for life. Family members and social support groups are important sources of help for patients who cannot function without continuous drug therapy.

SCHIZOPHRENIA

Schizophrenia is a type of psychosis characterized by abnormal thoughts and thought processes, disordered communication, withdrawal from other people and the outside environment, and a high risk for suicide. Several subtypes of schizophrenic disorders are based on clinical presentation.

17.2 Signs and Symptoms of Schizophrenia

Schizophrenia is the most common psychotic disorder, affecting 1% to 2% of the population. Symptoms generally begin to appear in early adulthood, with a peak incidence in

MediaLink

men, 15 to 24 years of age; and women, 25 to 34 years of age. Patients experience many different symptoms that may change over time. The following symptoms may appear quickly or take several months or years to develop.

- Hallucinations, delusions, or paranoia
- Strange behavior, such as communicating in rambling statements or made-up words
- Alternating rapidly between extreme hyperactivity and stupor
- Attitude of indifference or detachment toward life activities
- Acting strangely or irrationally
- Deterioration of personal hygiene, and job or academic performance
- Marked withdrawal from social interactions and interpersonal relationships

When observing patients with schizophrenia, nurses should look for both positive and negative symptoms. **Positive symptoms** are those that add on to normal behavior. These include hallucinations, delusions, and a disorganized thought or speech pattern. **Negative symptoms** are those that subtract from normal behavior. These symptoms include a lack of interest, motivation, responsiveness, or pleasure in daily activities. Negative symptoms are characteristic of the indifferent personality exhibited by many schizophrenics. Proper diagnosis of positive and negative symptoms is important for selection of the appropriate antipsychotic drug.

The cause of schizophrenia has not been determined, although several theories have been proposed. There appears to be a genetic component to schizophrenia, since many patients suffering from schizophrenia have family members who have been afflicted with the same disorder. Another theory suggests the disorder is caused by imbalances in neurotransmitters in specific areas of the brain. This theory suggests the possibility of overactive dopaminergic pathways in the basal nuclei, an area of the brain that controls motor activity. The basal ganglia (nuclei), shown in Figure

17.1, are responsible for starting and stopping synchronized motor activity, such as leg and arm motions during walking.

Symptoms of schizophrenia seem to be associated with the **dopamine type 2 (D_2) receptor**. The basal nuclei are particularly rich in D_2 receptors, while the cerebrum contains very few. All antipsychotic drugs act by entering dopaminergic synapses and competing with dopamine for D_2 receptors. By blocking about 65% of the D_2 receptors, antipsychotic drugs reduce the symptoms of schizophrenia. If 80% are blocked, motor abnormalities begin to occur (Seeman & Seeman, 2002). Figure 17.2 illustrates antipsychotic drug action at the dopaminergic receptor.

Schizo-affective disorder is a condition whereby the patient exhibits symptoms of both schizophrenia and mood disorder. For example, an acute schizo-affective reaction may include distorted perceptions, hallucinations, and delusions, followed by extreme depression. Over time, both positive and negative psychotic symptoms will appear. It is challenging to differentiate schizo-affective disorder from bipolar disorder or major depression with psychotic fea-

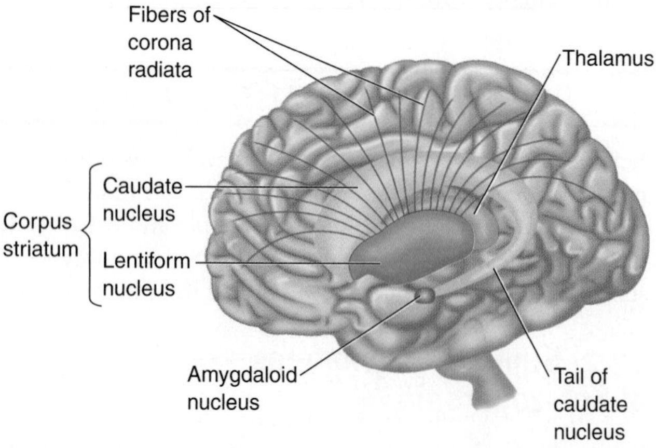

Figure 17.1 | Basal ganglia: overactive dopamine D_2 receptors may be responsible for schizophrenia

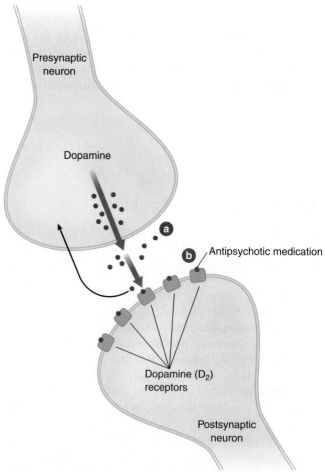

Figure 17.2 | Mechanism of action of antipsychotic drugs: (a) overproduction of dopamine; (b) antipsychotic medication occupies D_2 receptor, preventing dopamine from stimulating the postsynaptic neuron

SPECIAL CONSIDERATIONS

Cultural Views and Treatments of Mental Illness

Some cultures have very different perspectives on the cause of, and treatment for, mental illness. The foundation of many of these mental health treatments involves herbs and spiritual healing methods. American Indians may be treated by the community traditional "medicine man," who may treat mental symptoms with a sweat lodge and herbs. African Americans may be treated by a traditional voodoo priest or other traditional healers, and herbs are frequently used to treat mental symptoms. Hispanics may be treated by a folk healer, called a *curandero*; and herbs such as chamomile, spearmint, and sweet basil are used for mental conditions. Amulets, or charms that are worn on a string or chain, may be used by members of some cultures to protect the wearer from evil spirits that are believed to cause mental illness.

tures, as patients with affective disorders may also experience psychotic episodes.

Many conditions can cause bizarre behavior, and these should be distinguished from schizophrenia. Chronic use of amphetamines or cocaine can create a paranoid syndrome. Certain complex partial seizures (Chapter 15) ⟳ can cause unusual symptoms that are sometimes mistaken for psychoses. Brain neoplasms, infections, or hemorrhage can also cause bizarre, psychoticlike symptoms.

17.3 Pharmacologic Management of Psychoses

Management of severe mental illness is difficult. Many patients do not see themselves as abnormal, and have difficulty understanding the need for medication. When that medication produces undesirable side effects, such as severe twitching or loss of sexual function, compliance diminishes and patients exhibit symptoms of their pretreatment illness. Agitation, distrust, and extreme frustration are common, as patients cannot comprehend why others are unable to think and see the same as them.

From a pharmacologic perspective, therapy has both a positive and a negative side. While many symptoms of psychosis can be controlled with current drugs, adverse effects are common and often severe. The antipsychotic agents do not cure mental illness, and symptoms remain in remission only as long as the patient chooses to take the drug. In terms of efficacy, there is little difference among the various antipsychotic drugs; there is no single drug of choice for schizophrenia. Selection of a specific drug is based on clinician experience, the occurrence of side effects, and the needs of the patient. For example, patients with Parkinson's disease need an antipsychotic with minimal extrapyramidal side effects. Those who operate machinery would need a drug that does not cause sedation. Men who are sexually active may want a drug without negative effects on ejaculation. The experience and skills of the physician and mental health nurse are particularly valuable to achieving successful psychiatric pharmacotherapy.

CONVENTIONAL (TYPICAL) ANTIPSYCHOTIC AGENTS

The two basic categories of drugs for psychoses are conventional antipsychotics and atypical antipsychotics. The conventional antipsychotic agents include the phenothiazines and phenothiazine-like drugs. They are most effective at treating the positive signs of schizophrenia, such as hallucinations and delusions, and have been the treatment of choice for psychoses for 50 years. Antipsychotic drugs are sometimes referred to as **neuroleptics**.

Phenothiazines

17.4 Treating Psychoses with Phenothiazines

The conventional antipsychotics, sometimes called first generation or typical antipsychotics, include the phenothiazine and phenothiazine-like agents (see Table 17.1). Within each category, agents are named by their chemical structure.

The first effective drug used to treat schizophrenia was the low-potency phenothiazine chlorpromazine (Thorazine),

Table 17.1	Conventional Antipsychotic Drugs: Phenothiazines
Drug	**Route and Adult Dose (max dose where indicated)**
chlorpromazine HCl (Thorazine)	PO; 25–100 mg tid or qid (max 1000 mg/day) IM/IV; 25–50 mg (max 600 mg q4–6h)
fluphenazine HCl (Permitil, Prolixin)	PO; 0.5–10 mg/day (max 20 mg/day)
mesoridazine besylate (Serentil)	PO; 10–50 mg bid or tid (max 400 mg/day)
perphenazine (Phenazine, Trilafon)	PO; 4–16 mg bid to qid (max 64 mg/day)
promazine HCl (Prozine, Sparine)	PO/IM; 10–200 mg every 4–6 hours (max 1000 mg/day)
thioridazine HCl (Mellaril)	PO; 50–100 mg tid (max 800 mg/day)
trifluoperazine HCl (Stelazine)	PO; 1–2 mg bid; (max 20 mg/day)

approved by the FDA for this use in 1954. Seven phenothiazines are now available to treat mental illness. All seven are efficacious at blocking the excitement associated with the positive symptoms of schizophrenia, although they differ in their potency and side effect profiles. False perceptions, such as hallucinations and delusions, often begin to diminish within days. Other symptoms, however, may require as long as 7 to 8 weeks of pharmacotherapy to improve. Because of the high rate of recurrence of psychotic episodes, pharmacotherapy should be considered long term, often for the life of the patient. Phenothiazines are thought to act by preventing dopamine and serotonin from occupying their receptor sites in certain regions of the brain. This mechanism is illustrated in Figure 17.2.

Although they revolutionized the treatment of severe mental illness, the phenothiazines exhibit numerous adverse effects that can limit pharmacotherapy. These are listed in Table 17.2. Anticholinergic effects such as dry mouth, postural hypotension, and urinary retention are common. Ejaculation disorders occur in a high percentage of patients taking phenothiazines; delay in achieving orgasm (in both men and women) is a common cause for noncompliance. Menstrual disorders are common. Each phenothiazine has a slightly different side effect spectrum. For example, perphenazine (Phenazine, Trilafon) has a low incidence of anticholinergic effects, whereas mesoridazine (Serentil) has a high incidence of anticholinergic effects. Thioridazine (Mellaril) frequently causes sedation, whereas this side effect is less common with trifluoperazine (Stelazine).

Unlike many other drugs whose primary action is on the CNS (e.g., amphetamines, barbiturates, anxiolytics, alcohol), antipsychotic drugs do not cause dependence. They also have a wide safety margin between a therapeutic and a lethal dose; deaths due to overdoses of antipsychotic drugs are uncommon.

One particularly serious set of adverse reactions to antipsychotic drugs is called extrapyramidal effects. Extrapyramidal side effects (EPS) include acute dystonia, akathisia, Parkinsonism, and tardive dyskinesia. Acute dystonias occur early in the course of pharmacotherapy, and involve severe muscle spasms, particularly of the back, neck, tongue, and face. Akathisia, the most common EPS, is an inability to rest or relax. The patient paces, has trouble sitting or remaining still, and has difficulty sleeping. Symptoms of phenothiazine-induced Parkinsonism include tremor, muscle rigidity, stooped posture, and a shuffling gait. Long-term use of phenothiazines may lead to tardive dyskinesia, which is characterized by unusual tongue and face movements such as lip smacking and wormlike motions of the tongue. If extrapyramidal effects are reported early and the drug is withdrawn or the dosage is reduced, the side effects can be reversible. With higher doses given for prolonged periods, the extrapyramidal symptoms may become permanent. The nurse must be vigilant in observing and reporting EPS, as prevention is the best treatment.

With the conventional antipsychotics, it is not always possible to control the disabling symptoms of schizophrenia without producing some degree of extrapyramidal effects. In these patients, drug therapy may be warranted to treat EPS symptoms. Concurrent pharmacotherapy with an anticholinergic drugs may prevent some of the extrapyramidal signs (Chapter 18) ㊌ . For acute dystonia, benztropine (Cogentin) may be given parenterally. Levodopa (Dopar, Larodopa) is usually avoided, since its ability to increase dopamine function antagonizes the action of the phenothiazines. Beta-adrenergic blockers and benzodiazepines are sometimes given to reduce signs of akathisia.

Table 17.2	Adverse Effects of Conventional Antipsychotic Agents
Effect	**Description**
acute dystonia	severe spasms, particularly the back muscles, tongue, and facial muscles; twitching movements
akathisia	constant pacing with repetitive, compulsive movements
Parkinsonism	tremor, muscle rigidity, stooped posture, and shuffling gait
tardive dyskinesia	bizarre tongue and face movements such as lip smacking and wormlike motions of the tongue; puffing of cheeks, uncontrolled chewing movements
anticholinergic effects	dry mouth, tachycardia, blurred vision
sedation	usually diminishes with continued therapy
hypotension	particularly severe when quickly moving from a recumbent to an upright position
sexual dysfunction	impotence and diminished libido
neuroleptic malignant syndrome	high fever, confusion, muscle rigidity, and high serum creatine kinase; can be fatal

NURSING CONSIDERATIONS

The role of the nurse in phenothiazine therapy involves careful monitoring of a patient's condition and providing education as it relates to the prescribed drug regimen. Assessment information that must be gathered on patients beginning antipsychotic pharmacotherapy includes a complete health history such as any long-term physical problems (e.g., seizure disorders, cardiovascular disease), medication use, allergies, and lifestyle information (e.g., use of alcohol, illegal drugs, caffeine, smoking, herbal preparations). This allows the physician to individualize treatment and minimize the possibility of adverse reactions.

Assessment also includes a complete physical examination, including liver and kidney function tests, vision screening, and mental status to provide a baseline of the patient's health status. If the patient is a child, the nurse should assess for hyperexcitability, dehydration, or gastroenteritis as well as chickenpox or measles, because such conditions increase the chance of EPS. If possible, phenothiazines should not be given to children under 12 years of age. If the patient is elderly, the nurse should also determine whether a lower dose may be indicated due to the slower metabolism in older adults.

Contraindications to the use of phenothiazine and phenothiazine-like drugs include CNS depression, bone marrow suppression, coma, alcohol withdrawal syndrome, lactation, age (children under age 6 months), and presence of Reye's syndrome. This class of drugs must be used with caution in asthma, emphysema, respiratory infections, pregnancy (use only when benefits outweigh risks), and elderly persons or children.

The nurse should monitor the patient for extrapyramidal symptoms. Symptoms include lip smacking; spasms of the face, tongue, or back muscles; facial grimacing; involuntary upward eye movements; jerking motions; extreme restlessness; stooped posture; shuffling gait; and tremors at rest. Observations of EPS symptoms by the nurse should be reported to the physician immediately. These symptoms may be reason to discontinue the drug.

A possible life-threatening side effect of antipsychotic drugs is neuroleptic malignant syndrome (NMS). In this condition, the patient suffers a toxic reaction to therapeutic doses of an antipsychotic drug. The patient exhibits elevated temperature, unstable blood pressure, profuse sweating, dyspnea, muscle rigidity, and incontinence. The nurse should observe for these symptoms and report them immediately to the physician.

In addition, the nurse should assess the patient for drowsiness and sedation, which are both common side effects of this type of medication due to CNS depression. The nurse should evaluate the patient's safety and ability to function.

Patient and family education is an especially important aspect of care for patients with mental illness. Patient education as it relates to phenothiazines should include the goals, reasons for obtaining baseline data, and possible side effects. The nurse should educate the family regarding symptoms indicative of EPS or NMS, instruct them to report such symptoms to the physician immediately. If compliance is a problem, the nurse can supply patients and families with dose calendars and reminder signs. Because these drugs are prescribed for long-term use, the nurse should teach the patient the importance of taking the drug as directed, and to contact their physician immediately if side effects occur, or if symptoms begin to return. See "Nursing Process Focus: Patients Receiving Phenothiazines and Conventional Nonphenothiazine Therapy" for additional specific points that the nurse should include when teaching patients and caregivers regarding these drugs.

Nonphenothiazines

17.5 Treating Psychoses with Conventional Antipsychotics: Nonphenothiazines

The conventional, nonphenothiazine antipsychotic class consists of drugs whose chemical structures are dissimilar to the phenothiazines (see Table 17.3). Introduced shortly after the phenothiazines, initial expectations were that nonphenothiazines would produce fewer side effects. Unfortunately, this appears to not be the case. The spectrum of side effects for the nonphenothiazines is identical to that for the phenothiazines, although the degree to which a particular effect occurs depends on the specific drug. In general, the nonphenothiazine agents cause less sedation and fewer anticholinergic side effects than chlorpromazine (Thorazine), but exhibit an equal or even greater incidence of extrapyramidal signs. Concurrent therapy with other CNS depressants must be carefully monitored due to the potential additive effects.

Drugs in the nonphenothiazine class have the same therapeutic effects and efficacy as the phenothiazines. They are also believed to act by the same mechanism as the phenothiazines, that is, by blocking of postsynaptic D_2 dopamine receptors. As a class, they offer no significant advantages over the phenothiazines in the treatment of schizophrenia.

NURSING CONSIDERATIONS

The role of the nurse in conventional nonphenothiazine therapy involves careful monitoring of a patient's condition and providing education as it relates to the prescribed drug regimen. Assessment data for patients taking a conventional nonphenothiazine antipsychotic includes a complete drug history, including current and past medications to establish any previous allergic reactions or adverse effects from these medications. Elderly patients must be assessed more carefully than younger patients due to the possibility of unusual adverse reactions such as confusion, depression, and hallucinations that are drug induced.

A complete baseline assessment, including physical assessment, mental status (orientation, affect, cognition), vital signs lab studies (CBC, liver and renal function

Pr PROTOTYPE DRUG | CHLORPROMAZINE (Thorazine)

ACTIONS AND USES

Chlorpromazine provides symptomatic relief of positive symptoms of schizophrenia and controls manic symptoms in patients with schizo-affective disorder. Many patients must take chlorpromazine for 7 or 8 weeks before they experience improvement. Extreme agitation may be treated with IM or IV injections, which begin to act within minutes. Chlorpromazine can also control severe nausea and vomiting.

Administration Alerts

- Sustained-release forms should not be crushed or opened.
- When administered IM, give deep IM, only in the upper outer quadrant of the buttocks; patient should remain supine for 30 to 60 minutes after injection, then arise slowly.
- Must be gradually withdrawn over 2 to 3 weeks, and nausea/vomiting, dizziness, tremors, or dyskinesia may occur.
- IV forms should be used only during surgery or for severe hiccups.
- Pregnancy category C (contraindicated during lactation).

ADVERSE EFFECTS AND INTERACTIONS

Strong blockade of alpha-adrenergic receptors and weak blockade of cholinergic receptors explain some of chlorpromazine's adverse effects. Common side effects are dizziness, drowsiness, and orthostatic hypotension.

EPS occur mostly in the elderly, women, and in pediatric patients who are dehydrated. NMS may also occur. Patients taking chlorpromazine and exposed to warmer temperatures should be monitored more closely for symptoms of NMS.

Chlorpromazine interacts with several drugs. For example, concurrent use with sedative medications such as phenobarbital should be avoided. Taking chlorpromazine with tricyclic antidepressants can elevate blood pressure. Concurrent use of chlorpromazine with antiseizure medication can lower the seizure threshold.

Use with caution with herbal supplements, such as kava and St. John's wort, which may increase the risk and severity of dystonia.

See the companion website for a Nursing Process Focus specific to this drug.

Table 17.3	Conventional Antipsychotic Drugs: Nonphenothiazines	
Drug	**Route and Adult Dose (max dose where indicated)**	
chlorprothixene (Taractan)	PO; 75–150 mg/day (max 600 mg/day)	
haloperidol (Haldol)	PO; 0.2–5 mg bid or tid	
loxapine succinate (Loxitane)	PO; Start with 20 mg/day and rapidly increase to 60–100 mg/day in divided doses (max 250 mg/day)	
molindone HCl (Moban)	PO; 50–75 mg/day in three to four divided doses; may increase to 100 mg/day in 3–4 days (max 225 mg/day)	
pimozide (Orap)	PO; 1–2 mg/day in divided doses; gradually increase every other day to 7–16 mg/day (max 10 mg/day)	
thiothixene HCl (Navane)	PO; 2 mg tid; may increase up to 15 mg/day (max 60 mg/day)	

tests), preexisting medical conditions (especially cardiac, kidney, and liver function), and vision screening should be performed. The nurse should also assess the available support system, because many psychiatric clients are unable to self-manage their drug regimen. Contraindications for this class of drugs include Parkinson's disease, CNS depression, alcoholism, seizure disorders, and children under age 3.

When monitoring and teaching about side effects, the nurse should inform the patient and caregivers that sedation is a less severe side effect than with phenothiazines, but there is a greater EPS incidence with nonphenothiazine antipsychotics. A possible life-threatening adverse effect of

antipsychotic drugs is NMS. Refer to information under Nursing Considerations for phenothiazine drugs for information regarding EPS and NMS.

Because of the anticholinergic side effects of these drugs, the nurse should monitor for dry mouth, urinary retention, constipation, and hypotension with resultant tachycardia. Compliance with this classification of drug is equally as important as with the phenothiazines. The nurse should assess for alcohol and illegal drug use, which causes an increased depressant effect when used with antipsychotic drugs. The nurse should also caution the patient that any form of caffeine used with these drugs would likely increase anxiety.

When assessing older patients, the nurse should check for unusual reactions to haloperidol (Haldol). Older adults need smaller doses and more frequent monitoring with a gradual dose increase. There is a great occurrence of tardive dyskinesia in elderly women. This category of drugs is not safe for use with children under 2 years of age.

Patient education as it relates to conventional nonphenothiazines should include the goals, reasons for obtaining baseline data, and possible side effects. The nurse should instruct the family regarding symptoms indicative of EPS or NMS, telling them to report such symptoms to the healthcare provider immediately. See "Nursing Process Focus: Patients Receiving Phenothiazines and Conventional Nonphenothiazine Therapy" for additional teaching points.

ATYPICAL ANTIPSYCHOTIC AGENTS

Atypical antipsychotics treat both positive and negative symptoms of schizophrenia. They have become drugs of choice for treating psychoses.

17.6 Treating Psychoses with Atypical Antipsychotics

The approval of clozapine (Clozaril), the first atypical antipsychotic, marked the first major advance in the pharmacotherapy of psychoses since the discovery of chlorpromazine decades earlier. Clozapine, and the other drugs in this class, are called second generation, or atypical, because they have a broader spectrum of action than the conventional antipsychotics, controlling both the positive and negative symptoms of schizophrenia (see Table 17.4). Furthermore, at therapeutic doses they exhibit their antipsychotic actions without producing the EPS effects of the conventional agents. Some drugs, such as clozapine are especially useful for patients in whom other drugs have proven unsuccessful.

The mechanism of action of the atypical agents is largely unknown, but they are thought to act by blocking several different receptor types in the brain. Like the phenothiazines, the atypical agents block dopamine D_2 receptors. However, the atypicals also block serotonin (5-HT) and alpha-adrenergic receptors, which is thought to account for some of their properties. Because they are only loosely bound to D_2 receptors, fewer extrapyramidal side effects occur than with the conventional antipsychotics.

Although there are fewer side effects with atypical antipsychotics, adverse effects are still significant and patients must be carefully monitored. Although most antipsychotics cause weight gain, the atypical agents are associated with obesity and its risk factors. Risperidone (Risperdal) and some of the other antipsychotic drugs increase prolactin levels, which can lead to menstrual disorders, decreased libido, and osteoporosis in women. In men, high prolactin levels can cause lack of libido and impotence. There is also concern that some atypical agents alter glucose metabolism, which could lead to type 2 diabetes.

Pr PROTOTYPE DRUG | HALOPERIDOL (Haldol)

ACTIONS AND USES

Haloperidol is classified chemically as a butyrophenone. Its primary use is for the management of acute and chronic psychotic disorders. It may be used to treat patients with Tourette's syndrome and children with severe behavior problems such as unprovoked aggressiveness and explosive hyperexcitability. It is approximately 50 times more potent than chlorpromazine, but has equal efficacy in relieving symptoms of schizophrenia. Haldol LA is a long-acting preparation that lasts for approximately 3 weeks following IM or SC administration. This is particularly beneficial for patients who are uncooperative or unable to take oral medications.

Administration Alerts

- Must not be abruptly discontinued, or severe adverse reactions may occur.
- The patient must take medication as ordered for therapeutic results to occur.
- If the patient does not comply with oral therapy, injectable extended-release haloperidol should be considered.
- Pregnancy category C.

ADVERSE EFFECTS AND INTERACTIONS

Haloperidol produces less sedation and hypotension than chlorpromazine, but the incidence of EPS is high. Elderly patients are more likely to experience side effects and often are prescribed half the adult dose until the side effects of therapy can be determined. Although the incidence of NMS is rare, it can occur.

Haloperidol interacts with many drugs. For example, the following drugs decrease the effects/absorption of haloperidol: aluminum- and magnesium-containing antacids, levodopa (also increases chances of levodopa toxicity), lithium (increases chance of a severe neurological toxicity), phenobarbital, phenytoin (also increases chances of phenytoin toxicity), rifampin, and beta-blockers (may increase blood levels of haloperidol thus leading to possible toxicity). Haloperidol inhibits the action of centrally acting antihypertensives.

Use with caution with herbal supplements, such as kava, which may increase the effect of haloperidol.

 See the companion website for a Nursing Process Focus specific to this drug.

NURSING PROCESS FOCUS	PATIENTS RECEIVING PHENOTHIAZINES AND CONVENTIONAL NONPHENOTHIAZINE THERAPY

ASSESSMENT

Prior to administration:
- Obtain complete health history (medical and psychological) including allergies, drug history, and possible drug interactions.
- Obtain baseline lab studies (electrolytes, CBC, BUN, creatinine, WBC, liver enzymes, drug screens).
- Assess for hallucinations, level of consciousness, mental status.
- Assess patient support system(s).

POTENTIAL NURSING DIAGNOSES

- Ineffective Therapeutic Regimen Management, related to noncompliance with medication regimen, presence of side effects, and need for long-term medication use
- Anxiety, related to symptoms of psychosis
- Risk for Injury, related to side effects of medication
- Noncompliance, related to length of time before medication reaches therapeutic levels, desire to use alcohol or illegal drugs
- Deficient Knowledge, related to no previous contact with psychosis or its treatment

PLANNING: PATIENT GOALS AND EXPECTED OUTCOMES

The patient will:
- Report a reduction of psychotic symptoms, including delusions, paranoia, irrational behavior, hallucinations
- Demonstrate an understanding of the drug's action by accurately describing side effects, precautions, and measures to take to decrease any side effects
- Immediately report side effects or adverse reactions
- Adhere to recommended treatment regimen

IMPLEMENTATION

Interventions and (Rationales)

- Monitor for decrease of psychotic symptoms. (If patient continues to exhibit symptoms of psychosis, he or she may not be taking drug as ordered, may be taking an inadequate dose, or may not be affected by the drug; it may need to be discontinued and another antipsychotic begun.)

- Monitor for side effects such as drowsiness, dizziness, lethargy, headaches, blurred vision, skin rash, diaphoresis, nausea/vomiting, anorexia, diarrhea, menstrual irregularities, depression, hypotension, or hypertension.

- Monitor for anticholinergic side effects such as orthostatic hypotension, constipation, anorexia, GU problems, respiratory changes, and visual disturbances.

- Monitor for EPS and NMS. (Presence of EPS may be sufficient reason for patient to discontinue antipsychotic. NMS is life threatening and must be reported and treated immediately.)

Patient Education/Discharge Planning

Instruct patient and caregiver to:
- Notice increases or decreases of symptoms of psychosis, including hallucinations, abnormal sleep patterns, social withdrawal, delusions, or paranoia
- Contact physician if no decrease of symptoms occurs over a 6-week period

- Instruct patient and caregiver to report side effects.
- Inform patient and caregiver that impotence, gynecomastia, amenorrhea, and enuresis may occur.

Instruct patient to:
- Avoid abrupt changes in position
- Not drive or perform hazardous activities until effects of the drug are known
- Report vision changes
- Comply with required laboratory tests
- Increase dietary fiber, fluids, and exercise to prevent constipation
- Relieve symptoms of dry mouth with sugarless hard candy or gum and frequent drinks of water
- Notify physician immediately if urinary retention occurs

Instruct patient and caregiver to:
- Recognize tardive dyskinesia, dystonia, akathisia, pseudoparkinsonism
- Immediately seek treatment for elevated temperature, unstable blood pressure, profuse sweating, dyspnea, muscle rigidity, incontinence

continued

NURSING PROCESS FOCUS: *Patients Receiving Phenothiazines and Conventional Nonphenothiazine Therapy (continued)*

Interventions and (Rationales)	*Patient Education/Discharge Planning*
■ Monitor for alcohol/illegal drug use. (Patient may decide to use alcohol or illegal drugs as a means of coping with symptoms of psychosis, so may stop taking the antipsychotic. Used concurrently, will cause increased CNS depressant effect.)	■ Instruct patient to refrain from alcohol and illegal drug use. Refer patient to community support groups such as AA or NA as appropriate.
■ Monitor caffeine use. (Use of caffeine-containing substances will negate effects of antipsychotics.)	Instruct patient or caregiver of: ■ Common caffeine-containing products ■ Acceptable substitutes, such as decaffeinated coffee and tea, caffeine-free colas
■ Monitor for cardiovascular changes, including hypotension, tachycardia, and EKG changes. (Haloperidol has fewer cardiotoxic effects than other antipsychotics, and may be preferred for patient with existing CV problems.)	■ Instruct patient and caregiver that dizziness and falls, especially upon sudden position changes, may indicate CV changes. Teach safety measures.
■ Monitor for smoking. (Heavy smoking may decrease metabolism of haloperidol, leading to decreased efficacy.)	■ Instruct patient to stop or decrease smoking. Refer to smoking cessation programs, if indicated.
■ Monitor elderly patients closely. (The elderly may need lower doses and a more gradual dosage increase. Elderly women are at greater risk for developing tardive dyskinesia.)	■ Instruct caregiver to observe for unusual reactions such as confusion, depression, and hallucinations, and for symptoms of tardive dyskinesia and to report immediately. ■ Instruct elderly patient or caregiver on ways to counteract anticholinergic effects of medication, while taking into account any other existing medical problems.
■ Monitor lab results, including RBC and WBC counts, and drug levels.	■ Advise patient and caregiver of necessity of having regular lab studies done.
■ Monitor for use of medication. (All antipsychotics must be taken as ordered for therapeutic results to occur.)	■ Instruct patient and caregiver that medication must be continued as ordered, even if no therapeutic benefits are felt, because it may take several months for full therapeutic benefits.
■ Monitor for seizures. (Drug may lower seizure threshold.)	■ Instruct patient and caregiver that seizures may occur and review appropriate safety precautions.
■ Monitor patient's environment. (Drug may cause patient to perceive a brownish discoloration of objects or photophobia. Drug may also interfere with the ability to regulate body temperature.)	Instruct patient and caregiver to: ■ Wear dark glasses to avoid discomfort from photophobia ■ Avoid temperature extremes ■ Be aware that perception of brownish discoloration of objects may appear, but it is not harmful

EVALUATION OF OUTCOME CRITERIA

Evaluate effectiveness of drug therapy by confirming that patient goals and expected outcomes have been met (see "Planning").

See Tables 17.1 and 17.3 for lists of drugs to which these nursing actions apply.

NURSING CONSIDERATIONS

The role of the nurse in atypical antipsychotic therapy involves careful monitoring of a patient's condition and providing education as it relates to the prescribed drug regimen. Assessments of the patient taking atypical antipsychotics include a complete health history, including seizure activity, cardiovascular status, psychological disorders, and neurologic and blood diseases. Baseline lab tests, including CBC, WBC with differential, electrolytes, BUN, creatinine, and liver enzymes, should be obtained. A WBC with differential should be continued every week for the first 6 months, then every 2 weeks for the next 6 months, then every 4 weeks until the drug is

Table 17.4	Atypical Antipsychotic Drugs	
Drug	**Route and Adult Dose (max dose where indicated)**
aripiprazole (Abilify)	PO; 10–15 mg qd (max 30 mg/day)
clozapine (Clozaril)	PO; start at 25–50 mg/day and titrate to a target dose of 50–450 mg/day in 3 days; may increase further (max 900 mg/day)
olanzapine (Zyprexa)	Adult: PO; start with 5–10 mg/day; may increase by 2.5–5 mg every week (range 10–15 mg/day, max 20 mg/day). Geriatric: PO; start with 5 mg/day
quetiapine fumarate (Seroquel)	PO; start with 25 mg bid; may increase to a target dose of 300–400 mg/day in divided doses
risperidone (Risperdal)	PO; 1–6 mg bid; increase by 2 mg daily to an initial target dose of 6 mg/day
ziprasidone (Geodon)	PO; 20 mg bid (max 80 mg bid)

discontinued. The nurse should assess for hallucinations, mental status, dementia, and bipolar disorder, initially and throughout therapy. The nurse should obtain the patient's drug history to determine possible drug interactions and allergies.

Atypical antipsychotics are contraindicated during pregnancy and lactation, as they can cause harm to the developing fetus or to infant. The nurse should instruct female patients to have a negative pregnancy test within 6 weeks of beginning therapy, and to use reliable birth control during treatment. Female patients should also be instructed to notify their physician if they plan to become pregnant. In addition, clozapine (Clozaril) is contraindicated in coma or severe CNS depression, uncontrolled epilepsy, history of clozapine-induced agranulocytosis, and leukopenia (WBC count <3500).

Precautions must be taken when atypical antipsychotics are given to persons with cardiovascular disorders and conditions that predispose the patient to hypotension. Additional precautions include the concurrent use of other CNS depressants, including alcohol, renal or hepatic disorders, exposure to extreme heat, elderly or children, prostatic hypertrophy, glaucoma, and a history of paralytic ileus.

Patient education as it relates to atypical antipsychotic drugs should include the goals, reasons for obtaining baseline data, and possible side effects. The nurse should include the following points when educating patients and their families about atypical antipsychotic medications.

- Avoid abrupt changes in position to decrease dizziness and postural hypotension.
- Take drug strictly as prescribed; do not make any dosage changes or stop taking the medication without approval of the healthcare provider. Medication may take a minimum of 6 weeks before any therapeutic effects are noted.
- Have routine lab studies performed as ordered.
- Call the physician if no improvement in behavior is noted after 6 weeks of therapy.

- Avoid use of alcohol, illegal drugs, caffeine, and tobacco.
- If significant side effects occur, continue taking the medication, but contact the physician immediately.
- Increase intake of fruits, vegetables, and fluids if constipation occurs.

17.7 Treating Psychoses with Dopamine System Stabilizers

Due to side effects caused by conventional and atypical antipsychotic medications, a new drug class was developed to better meet the needs of patients with psychoses (Bailey, 2003). The new class is called dopamine system stabilizers (DSSs) or dopamine partial agonists. Aripiprazole (Abilify) is the first of these agents to receive approval from the FDA. Aripiprazole received approval in November 2002 for the treatment of schizophrenia and schizo-affective disorder.

Aripiprazole-treated patients appear to exhibit fewer extrapyramidal symptoms than patients treated with haloperidol (Haldol). Side effects include headache, nausea/vomiting, fever, constipation, and anxiety.

PHARMFACTS	Psychoses

- Symptoms of psychosis are often associated with other mental health problems including substance abuse, depression, and dementia.
- Psychotic disorders are among the most misunderstood mental health disorders in North America.
- Approximately 3 million Americans have schizophrenia.
- Patients with psychosis often develop symptoms between the age of 13 and the early 20s.
- As many as 50% of homeless people in America have schizophrenia.
- The probability of acquiring schizophrenia is 1 in 100 for the general population; 1 in 10 if one parent has the disorder; and 1 in 4 if both parents are schizophrenic.

Pr PROTOTYPE DRUG | CLOZAPINE (Clozaril)

ACTIONS AND USES

Therapeutic effects of clozapine include remission of a range of psychotic symptoms including delusions, paranoia, and irrational behavior. Of severely ill patients, 25% show improvement within 6 weeks of starting clozapine; 60% show improvement within 6 months. Clozapine acts by interfering with the binding of dopamine to its receptors in the limbic system. Clozapine also binds to alpha-adrenergic, serotonergic, and cholinergic sites throughout the brain. This drug is pregnancy category B.

Administration Alerts

- The patient should be given only a 1-week supply of clozapine at a time, to ensure return for weekly lab studies.
- Dose must be increased gradually.

ADVERSE EFFECTS AND INTERACTIONS

Because seizures and agranulocytosis are associated with clozapine use, a course of therapy with conventional antipsychotics is recommended before starting clozapine therapy. Common side effects are dizziness, drowsiness, headache, constipation, transient fever, salivation, flulike symptoms, and tachycardia. As with the conventional agents, elderly patients exhibit a higher incidence of orthostatic hypotension and anticholinergic side effects. Clozapine may also cause bone marrow suppression, which has proven fatal in some cases.

Clozapine interacts with many drugs. For example, it should not be taken with alcohol, other CNS depressants, or with drugs that suppress bone marrow function, such as anticancer drugs.

Concurrent use with antihypertensives may lead to hypotension. Benzodiazepines taken with clozapine may lead to severe hypotension and a risk for respiratory arrest. Concurrent use of digoxin or warfarin may cause increased levels of those drugs, which could lead to increased cardiac problems or hemorrhage, respectively. If phenytoin is taken concurrently with clozapine, seizure threshold will be decreased.

Use with caution with herbal supplements, such as kava, which may increase CNS depression.

 See the companion website for a Nursing Process Focus specific to this drug.

NURSING PROCESS FOCUS | PATIENTS RECEIVING ATYPICAL ANTIPSYCHOTIC THERAPY

ASSESSMENT

Prior to administration:
- Obtain complete health history (medical and psychological) including allergies, drug history, and possible drug interactions.
- Obtain baseline lab studies, especially RBC and WBC counts.
- Assess for hallucinations, mental status, level of consciousness.
- Assess patient support system(s).

POTENTIAL NURSING DIAGNOSES

- Anxiety related to symptoms of psychosis, side effects of medication
- Injury, Risk for related to side effects of medication, psychosis
- Noncompliance related to lack of understanding or knowledge, desire to use alcohol and caffeine-containing products
- Violence, Risk for, self-directed or directed at others

PLANNING: PATIENT GOALS AND EXPECTED OUTCOMES

The patient will:
- Adhere to recommended treatment regimen
- Report a reduction of psychotic symptoms, including delusions, paranoia, irrational behavior, hallucinations
- Demonstrate an understanding of the drug's actions, by accurately describing side effects, precautions, and measures to take to decrease any side effects

IMPLEMENTATION

Interventions and (Rationales)	Patient Education/Discharge Planning
■ Monitor RBC and WBC counts. (If WBC levels drop <3500, drug will need to be stopped immediately; patient may be developing agranulocytosis, which could be life threatening.)	■ Advise patient and caregiver of importance of having weekly lab studies performed.

continued

NURSING PROCESS FOCUS: *Patients Receiving Atypical Antipsychotic Therapy (continued)*

Interventions and (Rationales)	Patient Education/Discharge Planning
■ Monitor for hematologic side effects. (Neutropenia, leukopenia, agranulocytosis, thrombocytopenia may occur, secondary to possible bone marrow suppression caused by drug.)	■ Instruct patient to report immediately any sore throat, signs of infection, fatigue without apparent cause, bruising.
■ Observe for side effects such as drowsiness, dizziness, depression, anxiety, tachycardia, hypotension, nausea/vomiting, excessive salivation, urinary frequency or urgency, incontinence, weight gain, muscle pain or weakness, rash, fever.	■ Instruct patient and caregiver to report side effects.
■ Monitor for anticholinergic side effects, such as mouth dryness, constipation, or urinary retention. (Severe urinary retention may be corrected only by use of an indwelling catheter.)	Instruct patient and caregiver to: ■ Increase dietary fiber, fluids, and exercise to prevent constipation ■ Relieve symptoms of dry mouth with sugarless hard candy or chewing gum, and frequent drinks of water ■ Notify physician immediately if urinary retention occurs
■ Monitor for decrease of psychotic symptoms. (If patient continues to exhibit symptoms of psychosis, he or she may not be taking medication as ordered, may be taking an inadequate dose, or may not be affected by the drug; it may need to be discontinued and another antipsychotic begun.)	Instruct patient and caregiver to: ■ Notice increases or decreases of symptoms of psychosis, including hallucinations, abnormal sleep patterns, social withdrawal, delusions, or paranoia ■ Contact physician if no decrease of symptoms occurs over a 6-week period
■ Monitor for alcohol or illegal drug use. (Used concurrently, will cause increased CNS depression. Patient may decide to use alcohol or illegal drugs as means of coping with symptoms of psychosis, so may stop taking drug.)	■ Instruct patient to refrain from alcohol or illegal drug use. Refer patient to AA, NA, or other support group as appropriate.
■ Monitor caffeine use. (Use of caffeine-containing substances will inhibit effects of antipsychotics.)	Instruct patient and caregiver of: ■ Common caffeine-containing products ■ Acceptable substitutes, including decaffeinated coffee and tea, caffeine-free soda
■ Monitor for smoking. (Heavy smoking may decrease blood levels of drug.)	■ Instruct patient to stop or decrease smoking. Refer to smoking cessation programs if indicated.
■ Monitor elderly closely. (Older patients may be more sensitive to anticholinergic side effects.)	■ Instruct elderly patients on ways to counteract anticholinergic effects of medication, while taking into account any other existing medical problems.
■ Monitor for EPS and NMS. (Presence of EPS may be sufficient reason for patient to discontinue medication. NMS is life threatening and must be reported and treated immediately.)	Instruct patient and caregiver to: ■ Recognize tardive dyskinesia, dystonia, akathisia, pseudoparkinsonism ■ Seek immediate treatment for elevated temperature, unstable blood pressure, profuse sweating, dyspnea, muscle rigidity, incontinence

EVALUATION OF OUTCOME CRITERIA

Evaluate effectiveness of drug therapy by confirming that patient goals and expected outcomes have been met (see "Planning").

∞ See Table 17.4 for a list of drugs to which these nursing actions apply.

CHAPTER REVIEW

Key Concepts

The numbered key concepts provide a succinct summary of the important points from the corresponding numbered section within the chapter. If any of these points are not clear, refer to the numbered section within the chapter for review. Expanded versions can be found on the companion website.

17.1 Psychoses are severe mental and behavioral disorders characterized by disorganized mental capacity and an inability to recognize reality.

17.2 Schizophrenia is a type of psychosis characterized by abnormal thoughts and thought processes, disordered communication, withdrawal from other people and the outside environment, and a high risk for suicide.

17.3 Pharmacologic management of psychoses is difficult because the adverse effects of the drugs may be severe, and patients often do not understand the need for medication.

17.4 The phenothiazines have been effectively used for the treatment of psychoses for over 50 years; however, they have a high incidence of side effects. Extrapyramidal side effects (EPS) and the neuroleptic malignant syndrome (NMS) are two particularly serious conditions.

17.5 The nonphenothiazine, conventional antipsychotics have the same therapeutic applications and side effects as the phenothiazines.

17.6 Atypical antipsychotics are often preferred because they address both positive and negative symptoms of schizophrenia, and produce less dramatic side effects.

17.7 Dopamine system stabilizers are the newest antipsychotic class. It is hoped that this new class will have equal efficacy to other antipsychotic classes, with fewer serious side effects.

Review Questions

1. What is an extrapyramidal sign? What can the nurse do to limit EPS?

2. What is the major difference between a conventional and an atypical antipsychotic?

3. How does each drug class generally affect positive and negative symptoms of schizophrenia?

4. Explain why the pharmacologic management of severe mental illness is so difficult. What can the nurse do to improve the success of antipsychotic pharmacotherapy?

Critical Thinking Questions

1. A 22-year-old male patient has been on haloperidol (Haldol LA) for 2 weeks for the treatment of schizophrenia. During a follow-up assessment, the nurse notices that the patient keeps rubbing his neck and is complaining of neck spasms. What is the nurse's initial action? What is the potential cause of the sore neck and what would be the potential treatment? What teaching is appropriate for this patient?

2. A 68-year-old patient has been put on olanzapine (Zyprexa) for treatment of acute psychoses. What is a pri-

ority of care for this patient? What teaching is important for this patient?

3. A 20-year-old, newly diagnosed schizophrenic patient has been on chlorpromazine (Thorazine) and is doing well. Today the nurse notices that the patient appears more anxious and is demonstrating increased paranoia. What is the nurse's initial action? What is the potential problem? What patient teaching is important?

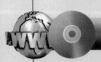 ## EXPLORE MediaLink

NCLEX review, case studies, and other interactive resources for this chapter can be found on the companion website at www.prenhall.com/adams. Click on "Chapter 17" to select the activities for this chapter. For animations, more NCLEX review questions, and an audio glossary, access the accompanying CD-ROM in this textbook.

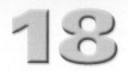
■ DRUGS AT A GLANCE

DRUGS FOR PARKINSON'S DISEASE

Dopaminergic agents

Pr *levodopa (Larodopa)*

Cholinergic blockers (anticholinergics)

Pr *benztropine (Cogentin)*

DRUGS FOR ALZHEIMER'S DISEASE

Acetylcholinesterase inhibitors

Pr *donepezil (Aricept)*

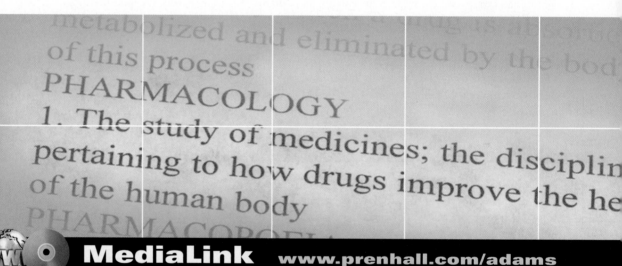

metabolized and eliminated by the bod
of this process
PHARMACOLOGY
1. The study of medicines; the disciplin
pertaining to how drugs improve the he
of the human body

MediaLink www.prenhall.com/adams

CD-ROM

Animation:

   Mechanism in Action: Levodopa (Larodopa)

Audio Glossary

NCLEX Review

Companion Website

NCLEX Review

Dosage Calculations

Case Study

Care Plans

Expanded Key Concepts

OBJECTIVES

After reading this chapter, the student should be able to:

1. Identify the most common degenerative diseases of the CNS.
2. Describe symptoms of Parkinson's disease.
3. Explain the neurochemical basis for Parkinson's disease, focusing on the roles of dopamine and acetylcholine in the brain.
4. Describe the nurse's role in the pharmacologic management of Parkinson's disease and Alzheimer's disease.
5. For each of the drug classes listed in Drugs at a Glance, know representative drug examples, explain their mechanism of action, primary action, and important adverse effects.
6. Describe symptoms of Alzheimer's disease and explain theories about why these symptoms develop.
7. Explain the goals of pharmacotherapy for Alzheimer's disease and the efficacy of existing medications.
8. Categorize drugs used in the treatment of Alzheimer's disease and Parkinson's disease based on their classification and mechanism of action.
9. Use the Nursing Process to care for patients receiving drug therapy for degenerative diseases of the CNS.

Degenerative diseases of the CNS are often difficult to deal with pharmacologically. Medications are unable to stop or reverse the progressive nature of these diseases; they can only offer symptomatic relief. Parkinson's disease and Alzheimer's disease, the two most common debilitating and progressive conditions, are the focus of this chapter.

18.1 Degenerative Diseases of the Central Nervous System

Degenerative diseases of the CNS include a diverse set of disorders differing in their causes and outcomes. Some, such as Huntington's disease, are quite rare, affect younger patients, and are caused by chromosomal defects. Others, such as Alzheimer's disease, affect millions of people, mostly elderly patients, and have a devastating economic and social impact. Table 18.1 lists the major degenerative disorders of the CNS.

The etiology of most neurological degenerative diseases is unknown. Most progress from very subtle signs and symptoms early in the course of the disease, to profound neurologic and cognitive deficits. In their early stages, these disorders may be quite difficult to diagnose. With the exception of Parkinson's disease, pharmacotherapy provides only minimal benefit. Currently, medication is unable to cure any of the degenerative diseases of the CNS.

PARKINSON'S DISEASE

Parkinson's disease is a degenerative disorder of the CNS caused by death of neurons that produce the brain neurotransmitter dopamine. It is the second most common degenerative disease of the nervous system, affecting over 1.5 million Americans. Pharmacotherapy is often successful at reducing some of the distressing symptoms of this disease.

18.2 Characteristics of Parkinson's Disease

Parkinson's disease affects primarily patients older than 50 years of age; however, even teenagers can develop the disorder. Men are affected slightly more than women. The disease is progressive, with the expression of full symptoms

Table 18.1	Degenerative Diseases of the Central Nervous System
Disease	**Description**
Alzheimer's disease	progressive loss of brain function characterized by memory loss, confusion, and dementia
amyotrophic lateral sclerosis	progressive weakness and wasting of muscles caused by destruction of motor neurons
Huntington's chorea	autosomal dominant genetic disorder resulting in progressive dementia and involuntary, spasmodic movements of limb and facial muscles
multiple sclerosis	demyelination of neurons in the CNS resulting in progressive weakness, visual disturbances, mood alterations, and cognitive deficits
Parkinson's disease	progressive loss of dopamine in the CNS causing tremor, muscle rigidity, and abnormal movement and posture

PHARMFACTS **Degenerative Diseases of the Central Nervous System**

- Over 1.5 million Americans have Parkinson's disease.
- Most patients with Parkinson's disease are above the age of 50.
- Greater than 50% of Parkinson's patients who have difficulty with voluntary movement are less than 60 years of age.
- More men than women develop Parkinson's disease.
- Over 4 million Americans have Alzheimer's disease.
- Alzheimer's disease mainly affects patients over the age of 65.
- Of all patients with dementia, 60% to 70% have Alzheimer's disease.
- Over 49,000 American's die annually of Alzheimer's disease. Overall, it is the eighth leading cause of death.

often taking many years. The symptoms of Parkinson's disease, or **Parkinsonism**, are summarized as follows:

- *Tremors*   The hands and head develop a palsy-like motion or shakiness when at rest; pin-rolling is a common behavior in progressive states, in which patients rub the thumb and forefinger together in a circular motion.
- *Muscle rigidity*   Stiffness may resemble symptoms of arthritis; patients often have difficulty bending over or moving limbs. Some patients develop a rigid poker face. These symptoms may be less noticeable at first, but progress to become obvious in later years.
- *Bradykinesia*   The most noticeable of all symptoms, patients may have difficulty chewing, swallowing, or speaking. Patients with Parkinson's disease have difficulties initiating movement and controlling fine muscle movements. Walking often becomes difficult. Patients shuffle their feet without taking normal strides.
- *Postural instability*   Patients may be humped over slightly and easily lose their balance. Stumbling results in frequent falls with associated injuries.

Although Parkinson's disease is a progressive, neurologic disorder primarily affecting muscle movement, other health problems often develop in these patients, including anxiety, depression, sleep disturbances, dementia, and disturbances of the autonomic nervous system such as difficulty urinating and performing sexually. Several theories have been proposed to explain the development of Parkinsonism. Because some patients with Parkinson's symptoms have a family history of this disorder, a genetic link is highly probable. Numerous environmental toxins also have been suggested as a cause, but results have been inconclusive. Potentially harmful agents include carbon monoxide, cyanide, manganese, chlorine, and pesticides. Viral infections, head trauma, and stroke have also been proposed as causes of Parkinsonism.

Symptoms of Parkinsonism develop due to the degeneration and destruction of dopamine-producing neurons found within an area of the brain known as the substantia nigra. Under normal circumstances, neurons in the substantia nigra supply dopamine to the corpus striatum, a region of the brain that controls unconscious muscle movement.

Balance, posture, muscle tone, and involuntary muscle movement depend on the proper balance of the neurotransmitters dopamine (inhibitory) and acetylcholine (stimulatory) in the corpus striatum. If dopamine is absent, acetylcholine has a more dramatic stimulatory effect in this area. For this reason, drug therapy for Parkinsonism focuses not only on restoring dopamine function, but also on blocking the effect of acetylcholine within the corpus striatum. Thus, when the brain experiences a loss of dopamine within the substantia nigra or an overactive cholinergic influence in the corpus striatum, Parkinsonism results.

Extrapyramidal side effects (EPS) develop for the same neurochemical reasons as Parkinson's disease. Recall from Chapter 17 that antipsychotic drugs act through a blockade of dopamine receptors∞. Treatment with certain antipsychotic drugs may induce Parkinsonism-like symptoms, or EPS, by interfering with the same neural pathway and functions affected by the lack of dopamine.

EPS may occur suddenly, and become a medical emergency. With acute EPS, patients' muscles may spasm or become locked up. Fever and confusion are other signs and symptoms of this reaction. If acute EPS occurs in a healthcare facility, short-term medical treatment can be provided by administering diphenhydramine (Benadryl). If recognized outside the healthcare setting, the patient should immediately be taken to the emergency room, as untreated acute episodes of EPS can be fatal.

PARKINSONISM DRUGS

Antiparkinsonism agents are given to restore the balance of dopamine and acetylcholine in specific regions of the brain. These drugs include dopaminergic agents and anticholinergics (cholinergic blockers). Dopaminergic agents are shown in Table 18.2.

Dopaminergics

18.3 Treating Parkinsonism with Dopaminergic Drugs

The goal of pharmacotherapy for Parkinson's disease is to increase the ability of the patient to perform normal daily activities such as eating, walking, dressing, and bathing. Although pharmacotherapy does not cure this disorder, symptoms may be dramatically reduced in some patients.

Drug therapy attempts to restore the functional balance of dopamine and acetylcholine in the corpus striatum of the brain. Dopaminergic drugs are used to increase dopamine levels in this region. The drug of choice for Parkinsonism is levodopa (Larodopa), a dopaminergic drug that has been used more extensively than any other medication for this disorder. As shown in Figure 18.1, levodopa is a precursor of dopamine synthesis. Supplying it directly leads to increased biosynthesis of dopamine within the nerve terminals. Whereas levodopa can cross the blood-brain barrier, dopamine cannot; thus, dopamine itself is not used for therapy. The effectiveness of levodopa can be "boosted" by com-

bining it with carbidopa. This combination, marketed as Sinemet, makes more levodopa available to enter the CNS.

Several additional approaches to enhancing dopamine are used in treating Parkinsonism. Tolcapone (Tasmar), entacapone (Comtan), and selegiline (Carbex, Eldepryl)

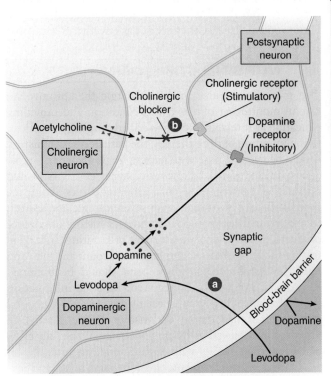

Figure 18.1 | Mechanism of action of antiparkinsonism drugs: (a) levodopa therapy increases dopamine production; (b) cholinergic blocker decreases acetylcholine reaching receptor

Table 18.2	Dopaminergic Drugs Used for Parkinsonism
Drug	**Route and Adult Dose (max dose where indicated)**
amantadine (Symmetrel)	PO; 100 mg qd or bid
bromocriptine (Parlodel)	PO; 1.25–2.5 mg/day up to 100 mg/day in divided doses
carbidopa-levodopa (Sinemet)	PO; 1 tablet containing 10 mg carbidopa/100 mg levodopa or 25 mg carbidopa/100 mg levodopa tid (max 6 tabs/day)
levodopa (L-Dopa, Larodopa)	PO; 500 mg–1 g/day; may be increased by 100–750 mg every 3–7 days
pergolide (Permax)	PO; Start with 0.05 mg daily for 2 days; increase by 0.1 or 0.15 mg/day every 3 days for 12 days; then increase by 0.25 mg every third day (max 5 mg/day)
pramipexole dihydrochloride (Mirapex)	PO; Start with 0.125 mg tid for 1 week; double this dose for the next week; continue to increase by 0.25 mg/dose tid every week to a target dose of 1.5 mg tid
ropinirole hydrochloride (Requip)	PO; Start with 0.25 mg tid; may increase by 0.25 mg/dose tid every week to a target dose of 1 mg tid
selegiline hydrochloride (L-Deprenyl, Eldepryl)	PO; 5 mg/dose bid; doses greater than 10 mg/day are potentially toxic
tolcapone (Tasmar)	PO; 100 mg tid (max 600 mg/day)

inhibit enzymes that normally destroy levodopa and/or dopamine. Bromocriptine (Parlodel), pergolide (Permax), pramipexole (Mirapex), and ropinirole (Requip) directly activate the dopamine receptor and are called dopamine agonists. Amantadine (Symmetrel), an antiviral agent, causes the release of dopamine from its nerve terminals. All of these drugs are considered adjuncts to the pharmacotherapy of Parkinsonism, because they are not as effective as levodopa.

NURSING CONSIDERATIONS

The role of the nurse in dopaminergic therapy involves careful monitoring of a patient's condition and providing education as it relates to the prescribed drug regimen. Prior to the initiation of drug therapy, the patient's health history should be taken. Those with narrow-angle glaucoma, undiagnosed skin lesions, or history of hypersensitivity should not take dopaminergic agents. Dopaminergics should be used cautiously in patients with severe cardiac, renal, liver, or endocrine diseases, mood disorders, a history of seizures or ulcers, or those who are pregnant or lactating. Initial lab testing should include a complete blood count and liver and renal function studies. These tests should be obtained throughout the treatment regimen. Baseline information should include vital signs, especially blood pressure, mental status, and symptoms of Parkinson's disease. Lastly, all other medications taken by the patient should be fully evaluated for compatibility with dopaminergic agonists.

During initial treatment, blood pressure, pulse, and respirations should be closely monitored, because these drugs may cause hypotension and tachycardia. Additional lab testing for diabetes and acromegaly should be done if patient is expected to take the drug long term. The nurse should especially monitor patients for excessive daytime sleepiness, eye twitching, involuntary movements, hand tremors, fatigue, anxiety, mood changes, confusion, agitation, nausea, vomiting, anorexia, dry mouth, and constipation. Muscle twitching and mood changes may indicate toxicity and should be reported at once. The nurse may need to assist patients with drug administration and activities of daily living, including ambulation, at least initially. It is normal for the patient's urine and perspiration to darken in color.

Patient education as it relates to dopaminergic drugs should include goals, reasons for obtaining baseline data, and possible side effects. The nurse should instruct the patient and caregivers as follows:

- Increase fiber and fluid consumption to prevent constipation.
- Avoid foods high in pyridoxine (vitamin B_6) such as beef, liver, ham, pork, egg yolks, sweet potatoes, and oatmeal because they will decrease the effects of these medications.
- Report significant reactions or side effects immediately. It may be several months before the full therapeutic effect of pharmacotherapy is achieved.
- Do not abruptly discontinue taking the drug because Parkinsonian crisis may occur.
- Change positions slowly to prevent dizziness or fainting.

Anticholinergics

18.4 Treating Parkinsonism with Anticholinergics

A second approach to changing the balance between dopamine and acetylcholine in the brain is to give cholinergic blockers, or anticholinergics. By blocking the effect of acetylcholine, anticholinergics inhibit the overactivity of this neurotransmitter in the corpus striatum of the brain. These agents are shown in Table 18.3.

Anticholinergics such as atropine were the first agents used to treat Parkinsonism. The large number of peripheral side effects have limited the uses of this drug class. The anticholinergics now used for Parkinsonism are centrally acting, and produce fewer side effects. Although they act on the CNS, autonomic effects such as dry mouth, blurred vision, tachycardia, urinary retention, and constipation are still troublesome. The centrally acting anticholinergics are not as effective as levodopa at relieving severe symptoms of Parkinsonism. They are used early in the course of the disease when symptoms are less severe, in patients who cannot tolerate levodopa, and in combination therapy with other antiparkinsonism drugs.

NURSING CONSIDERATIONS

The following content provides nursing considerations that apply to anticholinergics when given to treat Parkinsonism. For the complete nursing process applied to anticholinergic therapy, see Chapter 13, page 134, "Nursing Process Focus: Patients Receiving Anticholinergic Therapy".

The role of the nurse in anticholinergic therapy for Parkinsonism involves careful monitoring of a patient's condition and providing education as it relates to the prescribed drug regimen. As with patients taking dopaminergic drugs, the nurse needs to carefully evaluate and monitor patients taking this class of drugs. Before a patient begins treatment, a thorough health history should be obtained. Patients under the age of 3 years, those with known hypersensitivity, narrow-angle glaucoma, myasthenia gravis, or obstruction of the urinary or gastrointestinal tract should not take cholinergic blockers. These drugs should be used carefully in the elderly due to slowed metabolism, and cautiously with patients who have dysrhythmias, BPH, or in pregnant or lactating women. Before treatment begins, the nurse should obtain a history of medications taken and a complete physical to include complete blood count, liver and renal function studies, vital signs, mental status, and progression of Parkinson's disease to establish baseline data. These tests should be repeated throughout the treatment to help determine effectiveness of the drug.

Patient education as it relates to anticholinergics should include goals, reasons for obtaining baseline data, and possible side effects. The following are important points the nurse should include when teaching patients and caregivers about anticholinergics.

- Increase fiber and fluid consumption to prevent constipation.

Pr PROTOTYPE DRUG | LEVODOPA (Larodopa)

ACTIONS AND USES

Levodopa restores the neurotransmitter dopamine in extrapyramidal areas of the brain, thus relieving some Parkinson's symptoms. To increase its effect, levodopa is often combined with other medications, such as carbidopa, which prevent its enzymatic breakdown. As long as 6 months may be needed to achieve maximum therapeutic effects.

Administration Alerts

- The patient may be unable to self-administer medication, and may need assistance.
- Administer exactly as ordered.
- Abrupt withdrawal of drug can result in Parkinsonism crisis or NMS.
- Pregnancy category C.

ADVERSE EFFECTS AND INTERACTIONS

Side effects of levodopa include uncontrolled and purposeless movements such as extending the fingers and shrugging the shoulders, involuntary movements, loss of appetite, nausea, and vomiting. Muscle twitching and spasmodic winking are early signs of toxicity. Orthostatic hypotension is common in some patients. The drug should be discontinued gradually, since abrupt withdrawal can produce acute Parkinsonism.

Levodopa interacts with many drugs. For example, tricyclic antidepressants decrease effects of levodopa, increase postural hypotension, may increase sympathetic activity, with hypertension and sinus tachycardia. Levodopa cannot be used if a MAOI was taken within 14 to 28 days, because concurrent use may precipitate hypertensive crisis. Haloperidol taken concurrently may antagonize therapeutic effects of levodopa. Methyldopa may increase toxicity. Antihypertensives may cause increased hypotensive effects. Anticonvulsants may decrease therapeutic effects of levodopa. Antacids containing magnesium, calcium, or sodium bicarbonate may increase levodopa absorption, which could lead to toxicity. Pyridoxine reverses antiparkinsonian effects of levodopa.

Use with caution with herbal supplements, such as kava, which may worsen symptoms of Parkinson's.

NURSING PROCESS FOCUS | PATIENTS RECEIVING LEVODOPA (LARODOPA) Pr

ASSESSMENT

Prior to administration:
- Obtain complete health history including allergies, drug history, and possible drug interactions.
- Obtain baseline evaluation of severity of Parkinson's disease to determine medication effectiveness.
- Obtain baseline vital signs, especially blood pressure and pulse.

POTENTIAL NURSING DIAGNOSES

- Risk for Falls
- Deficient Knowledge, related to drug therapy
- Impaired Physical Mobility
- Self-Care Deficit: Feeding, Toileting
- Constipation

PLANNING: PATIENT GOALS AND EXPECTED OUTCOMES

The patient will:
- Report increased ease of movement and decreased symptoms of Parkinson's disease
- Demonstrate an understanding of the drug's action by accurately describing drug side effects, precautions, and measures to take to decrease any side effects
- Immediately report side effects and adverse reactions
- Adhere to the medication regimen

IMPLEMENTATION

Interventions and (Rationales)

- Monitor vital signs closely when dose is being adjusted. (Hypotension could occur as a result of dose adjustment. Dysrhythmias can occur in patients predisposed to cardiac problems.)

Patient Education/Discharge Planning

Instruct patient and caregiver to:
- Report signs of hypotension, dizziness, lightheadedness, feelings that heart is racing or skipping beats, or dyspnea
- Have EKGs and vital signs taken periodically

continued

NURSING PROCESS FOCUS: Patients Receiving Levodopa (Larodopa) Therapy (continued)

Interventions and (Rationales)	Patient Education/Discharge Planning
■ Provide for patient safety. (Orthostatic hypotension may occur.)	Instruct patient: ■ To change position slowly and to resume normal activities slowly ■ How to prevent and protect self from falls
■ Monitor for behavior changes. (Drug increases risk of depression or suicidal thoughts, and may cause other mood disturbances such as aggressiveness and confusion.)	Instruct patient and caregiver to: ■ Watch for and report immediately any signs of changes in behavior or mood ■ Seek counseling or a support group to help deal with these feelings; assist patient to find such resources if needed
■ Monitor for symptoms of overdose. (Muscle twitching and blepharospasm are early symptoms.)	■ Instruct patient and caregiver to be aware of newly occurring muscle twitching, including muscles of eyelids and to report immediately.
■ Monitor for improved functional status followed by a loss of therapeutic effects (on-off phenomenon), due to changes in dopamine levels that may last only minutes, or days. (Usually occurs in patients on long-term levodopa therapy.)	■ Instruct patient and caregiver to report rapid, unpredictable changes in motor symptoms to healthcare provider immediately, and that this can be corrected with changes in levodopa dosage schedule.
■ Evaluate diet. (Absorption of levodopa decreases with high protein meals or high consumption of pyridoxine-containing foods.)	Instruct patient to: ■ Take on empty stomach, but food may be eaten 15 minutes after, to decrease GI upset ■ Avoid taking levodopa with high protein meals ■ Avoid high consumption of foods containing vitamin B_6 (pyridoxine) such as bananas, wheat germ, green vegetables, liver, legumes ■ Watch for vitamin B_6 in multivitamins, fortified cereals, and antinauseants, so these products should be avoided
■ Monitor glucose levels in patients with diabetes mellitus. (Loss of glycemic control may occur in the diabetic patient.)	Instruct diabetic patient to: ■ Consistently monitor blood glucose both by self and with periodic lab studies ■ Report symptoms of hypo- or hyperglycemia
■ Monitor for decreased kidney or liver function. (Decrease in these functions may slow metabolism and excretion of drug, possibly leading to overdose or toxicity.)	■ Instruct patient to keep all appointments for liver and kidney function tests during therapy.
■ Monitor for side effects in the elderly. (Elderly patients may experience more rapid and severe side effects, especially those affecting the cardiovascular system.)	■ Instruct elderly patients to report any symptoms involving cardiovascular system: changes in heart rate, dizziness, faintness, edema, palpitations.
■ Monitor for other drug-related changes. (Drug may cause urine and perspiration to darken in color, but it is not a sign of overdose or toxicity.)	■ Inform patient that urine may darken and sweat may be dark colored, but not to be alarmed.

EVALUATION OF OUTCOME CRITERIA

Evaluate effectiveness of drug therapy by confirming that patient goals and expected outcomes have been met (see "Planning").

Table 18.3	Anticholinergic Drugs Used for Parkinsonism
Drug	**Route and Adult Dose (max dose where indicated)**
ⓟ benztropine mesylate (Cogentin)	PO; 0.5–1 mg/day; gradually increase as needed (max 6 mg/day)
biperiden hydrochloride (Akineton)	PO; 2 mg qd to qid
diphenhydramine hydrochloride (Benadryl) (see page 428 for the Prototype Drug box) ⊘	PO; 25–50 mg tid or qid (max 300/day)
procyclidine hydrochloride (Kemadrin)	PO; 2.5 mg tid pc; may be increased to 5 mg tid if tolerated with an additional 5 mg at hs (max 45–60 mg/day)
trihexyphenidyl hydrochloride (Artane)	PO; 1 mg for day 1; double this for day 2; then increase by 2 mg every 3–5 days up to 6–10 mg/day (max 15 mg/day)

- To help relieve dry mouth, take frequent drinks of cool liquids, suck on sugarless hard candy or ice chips, and chew sugarless gum.
- Take with food or milk to prevent GI upset.
- Be evaluated by an eye specialist periodically, as anticholinergics may promote glaucoma development.
- Avoid driving and other hazardous activities because drowsiness may occur.
- Do not abruptly discontinue taking the drug, or withdrawal symptoms such as tremors, insomnia and restlessness may occur.
- Avoid use of alcohol.
- Notify healthcare provider if the following side effects or adverse reactions occur: disorientation, depression, hallucinations, confusion, memory impairment, nervousness, psychoses, vision changes, nausea/vomiting, urinary retention dysuria.
- Wear dark glasses and avoid bright sunlight as necessary.

ALZHEIMER'S DISEASE

Alzheimer's disease is a devastating, progressive, degenerative disease that generally begins after age 60. By age 85, as many as 50% of the population may be affected. Pharmacotherapy has limited success in improving the cognitive function of patients with Alzheimer's disease.

18.5 Characteristics of Alzheimer's Disease

Alzheimer's disease (AD) is responsible for 70% of all dementia. **Dementia** is a degenerative disorder characterized by progressive memory loss, confusion, and inability to think or communicate effectively. Consciousness and perception are usually unaffected. Known causes of dementia include multiple cerebral infarcts, severe infections, and toxins. Although the cause of most dementia is unknown, it is usually associated with cerebral atrophy or other structural changes within the brain. The patient generally lives 5 to 10 years following diagnosis; AD is the fourth leading cause of death.

Despite extensive, ongoing research, the etiology of Alzheimer's disease remains unknown. The early-onset familial form of this disorder, accounting for about 10% of cases, is associated with gene defects on chromosome 1, 14, or 21. Chronic inflammation and excess free radicals may cause neuron damage. Environmental, immunologic, and nutritional factors, as well as viruses, are considered possible sources of brain damage.

Although the cause may be unknown, structural damage in the brain of Alzheimer's patients has been well documented. **Amyloid plaques** and **neurofibrillary tangles**, found within the brain at autopsy, are present in nearly all patients with AD. It is suspected that these structural changes are caused by chronic inflammatory or oxidative cellular damage to the surrounding neurons. There is a loss in both the number and function of neurons.

Alzheimer's patients experience a dramatic loss of ability to perform tasks that require acetylcholine as the neurotransmitter. Because acetylcholine is a major neurotransmitter within the **hippocampus**, an area of the brain responsible for learning and memory, and other parts of the cerebral cortex, neuronal function within these brain areas is especially affected. Thus, an inability to remember and to recall information is among the early symptoms of AD. Symptoms of this disease are as follows:

- Impaired memory and judgment
- Confusion or disorientation
- Inability to recognize family or friends
- Aggressive behavior
- Depression
- Psychoses, including paranoia and delusions
- Anxiety

DRUGS FOR ALZHEIMER'S DISEASE

Drugs are used to slow memory loss and other progressive symptoms of dementia. Some drugs are given to treat associated symptoms such as depression, anxiety, or psychoses. The acetylcholinesterase inhibitors are the most widely used class of drugs for treating AD. These agents are shown in Table 18.4. Memantine (Namenda), the first of a new class of drugs called glutamergic inhibitors, was approved in October 2003.

MediaLink · Alzheimer's Information

PROTOTYPE DRUG | BENZTROPINE (Cogentin)

ACTIONS AND USES

Benztropine acts by blocking excess cholinergic stimulation of neurons in the corpus striatum. It is used for relief of Parkinsonism symptoms and for the treatment of EPS brought on by antipsychotic pharmacotherapy. This medication suppresses tremors but does not affect tardive dyskinesia.

Administration Alerts

- The patient may be unable to self-administer medication, and may need assistance.
- Benztropine may be taken in divided doses, two to four times a day, or the entire day's dose may be taken at bedtime.
- If muscle weakness occurs, dose should be reduced.
- Pregnancy category C.

ADVERSE EFFECTS AND INTERACTIONS

As expected from its autonomic action, benztropine can cause typical anticholinergic side effects such as sedation, dry mouth, constipation, and tachycardia.

Benztropine interacts with many drugs. For example, benztropine should not be taken with alcohol, tricyclic antidepressants, MAO inhibitors, phenothiazines, procainamide, or quinidine because of combined sedative effects. OTC cold medicines and alcohol should be avoided. Other drugs that enhance dopamine release or activation of the dopamine receptor may produce additive effects. Haloperidol will cause decreased effectiveness.

Antihistamines, phenothiazines, tricyclics, disopyramide quinidine may increase anticholinergic effects, and antidiarrheals may decrease absorption.

See the companion website for a Nursing Process Focus specific to this drug.

Table 18.4	Acetylcholinesterase Inhibitors Used for Alzheimer's Disease
Drug	**Route and Adult Dose (max dose where indicated)**
donepezil hydrochloride (Aricept)	PO; 5–10 mg at hs
galantamine (Reminyl)	PO; Initiate with 4 mg bid at least 4 weeks; if tolerated, may increase by 4 mg bid q4wk to target dose of 12 mg bid (max 8–16 mg bid)
rivastigmine tartrate (Exelon)	PO; Start with 1.5 mg bid with food; may increase by 1.5 mg bid q2wk if tolerated; target dose 3–6 mg bid (max 12 mg bid)
tacrine (Cognex)	PO; 10 mg qid; increase in 40 mg/day increments not sooner than every 6 weeks (max 160 mg/day)

Acetylcholinesterase Inhibitors (Parasympathomimetics)

18.6 Treating Alzheimer's Disease with Acetylcholinesterase Inhibitors

The FDA has approved only a few drugs for AD. The most effective of these medications act by intensifying the effect of acetylcholine at the cholinergic receptor, as shown in Figure 18.2. Acetylcholine is naturally degraded in the synapse by the enzyme acetylcholinesterase (AchE). When AchE is inhibited, acetylcholine levels become elevated and produce a more profound effect on the receptor. As described in Chapter 13, the AchE inhibitors are indirect-acting parasympathomimetics .

When treating AD, the goal of pharmacotherapy is to improve function in three domains: activities of daily living, behavior, and cognition. Although the AchE inhibitors improve all three domains, their efficacy is modest, at best. These agents do not cure AD—they only slow its progression. Therapy is begun as soon as the diagnosis of AD is established. These agents are ineffective in treating the severe stages of this disorder, probably because so many neurons have died; increasing the levels of acetylcholine is only effective if there are functioning neurons present. Often, as the disease progresses, the AchE inhibitors are discontinued; their therapeutic benefit is not enough to outweigh their expense or the risks of side effects.

All acetylcholinesterase inhibitors used to treat AD have equal efficacy. Side effects are those expected of drugs that enhance the parasympathetic nervous system (Chapter 13) . The GI system is most affected, with nausea, vomiting, and diarrhea being reported. Of the agents available for AD, tacrine (Cognex) is associated with hepatotoxicity. Rivastigmine (Exelon) is associated with weight loss, a potentially serious side effect in some elderly patients. When discontinuing therapy, doses of the AchE inhibitors should be lowered gradually.

Although acetylcholinesterase inhibitors are the mainstay for the treatment of AD dementia, several other agents are being investigated for their possible benefit in delaying the progression of AD. Because at least some of

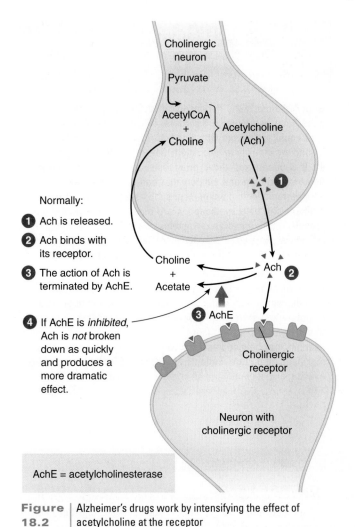

Cholinergic
neuron

Pyruvate

AcetylCoA
+
Choline

Acetylcholine
(Ach)

Normally:

1 Ach is released.

2 Ach binds with
its receptor.

3 The action of Ach is
terminated by AchE.

4 If AchE is *inhibited*,
Ach is *not* broken
down as quickly
and produces a
more dramatic
effect.

1

Choline
+
Acetate

Ach **2**

3 AchE

Cholinergic
receptor

Neuron with
cholinergic receptor

AchE = acetylcholinesterase

Figure 18.2 | Alzheimer's drugs work by intensifying the effect of acetylcholine at the receptor

the neuronal changes in AD are caused by oxidative cellular damage, antioxidants such as vitamin E are being examined for their effects in AD patients. Other agents currently being examined are anti-inflammatory agents, such as the COX-2 inhibitors, estrogen, and ginkgo biloba.

Agitation occurs in the majority of patients with AD. This may be accompanied by delusions, paranoia, hallucinations, or other psychotic symptoms. Atypical antipsychotic agents such as risperidone (Risperdal) and olanzapine (Zyprexa) may be used to control these episodes. Conventional antipsychotics such as haloperidol (Haldol) are occasionally prescribed, though extrapyramidal side effects often limit their use. The pharmacotherapy of psychosis is presented in Chapter 17⟨⟩.

Although not as common as agitation, anxiety and depression may occur in AD patients. Anxiolytics such as buspirone (BuSpar) or some of the benzodiazepines are used to control excessive anxiousness (Chapter 14)⟨⟩. Mood stabilizers such as sertraline (Zoloft), citalopram (Celexa), or fluoxetine (Prozac) are given when major depression interferes with daily activities (Chapter 16)⟨⟩.

NURSING CONSIDERATIONS

The following content provides nursing considerations that apply to acetylcholinesterase inhibitors when given to treat Alzheimer's disease. For the complete Nursing Process applied to acetylcholinesterase inhibitor therapy, see Chapter 13, page 130, "Nursing Process Focus: Patients Receiving Parasympathomimetic Therapy"⟨⟩.

The role of the nurse in AchE inhibitor (parasympathomimetic) therapy involves carefully monitoring the patient's condition and providing education as it relates to the prescribed drug regimen. Prior to the initiation of drug therapy, the patient's health history should be taken. Young children and those with hypersensitivity should not take AchE inhibitors. Patients with narrow-angle glaucoma or undiagnosed skin lesions should not take rivastigmine (Exelon). All AchE inhibitors should be used cautiously in patients with severe cardiac, renal, liver, or respiratory diseases (such as asthma or COPD), a history of seizures, GI bleeding or peptic ulcers, and those who are pregnant or lactating. Lab testing, including a complete blood count and liver and renal function tests, should be done initially and throughout the treatment regimen. Baseline vital signs should be taken. During initial treatment, vital signs should be closely monitored as these medications may cause hypotension. A full assessment of mental status and other signs of Alzheimer's disease should be done to provide a baseline and determine effectiveness of medication. All other medications taken by the patient should be fully evaluated for interactions with AchE inhibitors.

The nurse should monitor patients for side effects or reactions such as changes in mental status, mood changes, dizziness, confusion, insomnia, nausea, vomiting, and anorexia. Additionally, those taking tacrine (Cognex) should be monitored for urinary frequency, hepatotoxicity, and GI bleeding. Patient education as it relates to AchE inhibitors should include goals, reasons for obtaining baseline data, and possible side effects.

Nurses may care for patients with AD in acute or long-term care facilities, or may provide support and education for caregivers in the home. Families and patients who are able to understand must be made aware that currently available medications may slow the progression of the disease but not effect a cure. In addition, the nurse should include the following points when educating patients and caregivers about acetylcholinesterase inhibitors.

- Take with food or milk to decrease GI upset.
- Take drug strictly as prescribed or serious side effects may result.
- Report any changes in mental status or mood.
- Report the following side effects to the healthcare provider: dizziness, confusion, insomnia, constipation, nausea, urinary frequency, GI bleeding, vomiting, seizures, anorexia.
- Make appointments with the healthcare provider on a regular basis.

- To help relieve dry mouth, take frequent drinks of cool liquids, suck on sugarless hard candy, or chew sugarless gum.
- Increase fiber and fluid consumption to prevent constipation.
- Recognize symptoms of overdose: severe nausea/vomiting, sweating, salivation, hypotension, bradycardia, convulsions, increased muscle weakness, including respiratory muscles; if noted, contact healthcare provider immediately.

NATURAL THERAPIES | Ginkgo Biloba for Treatment of Dementia

Ginkgo biloba has been used for many years to improve memory. In Europe, an extract of this herb is already approved for the treatment of dementia. In one of the first U.S. studies, 120 mg of ginkgo taken daily was shown to improve mental functioning and stabilize Alzheimer's disease. In other studies, clinical results were seen between 4 weeks and 6 months of treatment and were found to be relevant. Patients need to speak with their healthcare provider before taking this herb. Although most patients can take ginkgo without problems, those on anticoagulants may have an increased risk for bleeding.

SPECIAL CONSIDERATIONS

Living with Alzheimer's and Parkinson's Diseases

Both Alzheimer's and Parkinson's diseases are progressive, degenerative neurological disorders. While Alzheimer's leads to impairments in memory thinking and reasoning, Parkinson's can lead to the inability to hold small items due to tremors and rigidity. It is because of these progressive symptoms that patients need all the help and support that caregivers can give. While nonpharmacologic management such as providing a safe environment can help, medications are available to slow the progression and minimize symptoms. Caregivers will need to provide assistance with activities of daily living, including making sure that these patients receive their medications.

For patients with Alzheimer's, the side effect of some drugs used to control dementia can disrupt sleep. Additionally, many people with dementia often suffer sleep apnea. In addition to providing a routine and structured environment, new research suggests that as little as a few hours of bright light, especially in the evening, may help people living with Alzheimer's maintain a normal sleeping pattern. Patients who received light therapy in the evening also experienced an improvement in their sleep cycle.

Pr PROTOTYPE DRUG | DONEPEZIL (Aricept)

ACTIONS AND USES

Donepezil is an AchE inhibitor that improves memory in cases of mild to moderate Alzheimer's dementia by enhancing the effects of acetylcholine in neurons in the cerebral cortex that have not yet been damaged. Patients should receive pharmacotherapy for at least 6 months prior to assessing maximum benefits of drug therapy. Improvement in memory may be observed as early as 1 to 4 weeks following medication. The therapeutic effects of donepezil are often short-lived and the degree of improvement is modest, at best. An advantage of donepezil over other drugs in its class is that its long half-life permits it to be given once daily.

Administration Alerts

- Give medication prior to bedtime.
- Medication is most effective when given on a regular schedule.
- Pregnancy category C.

ADVERSE EFFECTS AND INTERACTIONS

Common side effects of donepezil are vomiting, diarrhea, and darkened urine. CNS side effects include insomnia, syncope, depression, headache, and irritability. Musculoskeletal side effects include muscle cramps, arthritis, and bone fractures. Generalized side effects include headache, fatigue, chest pain, increased libido, hot flashes, urinary incontinence, dehydration, and blurred vision. Unlike tacrine, hepatotoxicity has not been observed. Patients with bradycardia, hypotension, asthma, hyperthyroidism, or active peptic ulcer disease should be monitored carefully. Anticholinergics will be less effective. Donepezil interacts with several other drugs. For example, bethanechol causes a synergistic effect. Phenobarbital, phenytoin, dexamethasone, and rifampin may speed elimination of donepezil. Quinidine or ketoconazole may inhibit metabolism of donepezil. Because donepezil acts by increasing cholinergic activity, two parasympathomimetics should not be administered concurrently.

 See the companion website for a Nursing Process Focus specific to this drug.

CHAPTER REVIEW

Key Concepts

The numbered key concepts provide a succinct summary of the important points from the corresponding numbered section within the chapter. If any of these points are not clear, refer to the numbered section within the chapter for review. Expanded versions can be found on the companion website.

18.1 Degenerative diseases of the nervous system such as Parkinson's disease and Alzheimer's disease cause a progressive loss of neuron function.

18.2 Parkinson's disease is characterized by symptoms of tremors, muscle rigidity, and postural instability and ambulation caused by the destruction of dopamine-producing neurons found within the corpus striatum. The underlying biochemical problem is lack of dopamine activity and a related overactivity of acetylcholine.

18.3 The most commonly used medications for Parkinsonism attempt to restore levels of dopamine in the corpus striatum of the brain. Levodopa (Larodopa) is the drug of choice for Parkinson's disease.

18.4 Centrally acting anticholinergic drugs are sometimes used to relieve symptoms of Parkinsonism, although they are less effective than levodopa (Larodopa).

18.5 Alzheimer's disease is a progressive, degenerative disease of older adults. Primary symptoms include disorientation, confusion, and memory loss.

18.6 Acetylcholinesterase inhibitors are used to slow the progression of Alzheimer's disease symptoms. These agents have minimal efficacy, and do not cure the dementia.

Review Questions

1. What is the major pathology of Parkinson's disease? What brain neurotransmitters are affected and how?

2. What major drug category can produce Parkinsonism symptoms with overmedication? What are Parkinson's-like symptoms called?

3. Describe the two basic approaches for restoring neurotransmitter balance in patients with Parkinson's disease.

4. Alzheimer's disease is a dysfunction of which brain neurotransmitters? How do drugs for Alzheimer's disease restore neurotransmitter function and improve Alzheimer's symptoms?

Critical Thinking Questions

1. A 58-year-old Parkinson's patient is placed on levodopa (Larodopa). In obtaining her health history, the nurse notes that the patient takes Mylanta on a regular basis for mild indigestion, takes multivitamins daily (vitamins A, B$_6$, D, and E), and has a history of diabetes mellitus type 2. What should the nurse include in teaching for this patient?

2. A patient is on levodopa and benztropine (Cogentin). During a regular office follow-up, the patient tells the nurse that she is going to Arizona in July to visit her grandchildren. What teaching is important for this patient?

3. A 67-year-old Alzheimer's patient is on donepezil (Aricept) and has a history of congestive heart failure, diabetes mellitus type 2, and hypertension. The patient's wife asks the nurse if this new medicine is appropriate for her husband to take. How should the nurse respond? What teaching should be done?

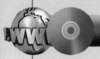 ## EXPLORE MediaLink

NCLEX review, case studies, and other interactive resources for this chapter can be found on the companion website at www.prenhall.com/adams. Click on "Chapter 18" to select the activities for this chapter. For animations, more NCLEX review questions, and an audio glossary, access the accompanying CD-ROM in this textbook.

DRUGS AT A GLANCE

OPIOID (NARCOTIC) ANALGESICS

Opioid agonists

Pr *morphine (Astramorph PF, Duramorph, others)*

Opioids with mixed agonist-antagonist activity

Opioid antagonists

Pr *naloxone (Narcan)*

NONOPIOID ANALGESICS

Acetaminophen

Nonsteroidal anti-inflammatory drugs (NSAIDs)

Aspirin and other salicylates

Pr *aspirin (Acetylsalicylic acid, ASA)*

Ibuprofen and ibuprofen-like drugs

Selective COX-2 inhibitors

Centrally acting agents

ANTIMIGRAINE AGENTS

Triptans

Pr *sumatriptan (Imitrex)*

Ergot alkaloids

Miscellaneous antimigraine agents

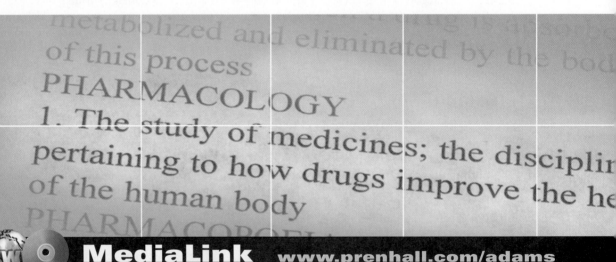

metabolized and eliminated by the bod
of this process
PHARMACOLOGY
1. The study of medicines; the disciplin
pertaining to how drugs improve the he
of the human body

MediaLink www.prenhall.com/adams

CD-ROM

Animation:

Mechanism in Action: Morphine (Astramorph PF)

Audio Glossary

NCLEX Review

Companion Website

NCLEX Review

Dosage Calculations

Case Study

Care Plans

Expanded Key Concepts

Aδ fibers *page 222*

analgesic *page 223*

aura *page 232*

C fibers *page 222*

cyclooxygenase *page 230*

endogenous opioids *page 222*

kappa receptor *page 223*

methadone maintenance *page 229*

migraine *page 232*

mu receptor *page 223*

narcotic *page 223*

neuropathic pain *page 222*

nociceptor *page 222*

nociceptor pain *page 222*

opiate *page 223*

opioid *page 223*

substance P *page 222*

tension headache *page 232*

OBJECTIVES

After reading this chapter, the student should be able to:

1. Relate the importance of pain assessment to effective pharmacotherapy.
2. Explain the neural mechanism for pain at the level of the spinal cord.
3. Explain how pain can be controlled by inhibiting the release of spinal neurotransmitters.
4. Describe the role of nonpharmacologic therapies in pain management.
5. Compare and contrast the types of opioid receptors and their importance to pharmacology.
6. Explain the role of opioid antagonists in the diagnosis and treatment of acute opioid toxicity.
7. Describe the long-term treatment of opioid dependence.
8. Compare the pharmacotherapeutic approaches of preventing migraines to those of aborting migraines.
9. Describe the nurse's role in the pharmacologic management of patients receiving analgesics and antimigraine drugs.
10. For each of the drug classes listed in Drugs at a Glance, know representative drug examples, explain the mechanism of drug action, primary actions, and important adverse effects.
11. Categorize drugs used in the treatment of pain based on their classification and mechanism of action.
12. Use the Nursing Process to care for patients receiving drug therapy for pain.

Pain is a physiological and emotional experience characterized by unpleasant feelings, usually associated with trauma or disease. On a simple level, pain may be viewed as a defense mechanism that helps people to avoid potentially damaging situations and encourages them to seek medical help. Although the neural and chemical mechanisms for pain are straightforward, many psychological and emotional processes can modify this sensation. Anxiety, fatigue, and depression can increase the perception of pain. Positive attitudes and support from caregivers may reduce the perception of pain. Patients are more likely to tolerate their pain if they know the source of the sensation and the medical course of treatment designed to manage the pain. For example, if patients know that the pain is temporary, such as during labor or after surgery, they are more likely to be accepting of the pain.

PHARMFACTS	Pain

Pain is a common symptom:

- Approximately 16 million people experience chronic arthritic pain.
- Over 31 million adults report low back pain, with 19 million people experiencing this on a chronic basis.
- At least 50 million people are fully or partially disabled as a result of pain.
- Over 50% of adults experience muscle pain each year.
- Up to 40% of people with cancer report moderate to severe pain.

19.1 Assessment and Classification of Pain

The psychological reaction to pain is a subjective experience. The same degree and type of pain may be described as excruciating and unbearable by one patient, while not mentioned during physical assessment by another. Several numerical scales and survey instruments are available to help healthcare providers standardize the assessment of pain and measure the progress of subsequent drug therapy. Successful pain management depends on an accurate assessment of both the degree of pain experienced by the patient and the potential underlying disorders that may be causing the

SPECIAL CONSIDERATIONS

Cultural Influences on Pain Expression and Perception

How a person responds to pain and the type of pain management chosen may be culturally determined. Establishment of a therapeutic relationship is of the utmost importance in helping a patient attain pain relief. The nurse should respect the patient's attitudes and beliefs about pain as well as preferred treatment. An assessment of the patient's needs, beliefs, and customs by listening, showing respect, and allowing the patient to help develop and choose treatment options to attain pain relief is the most culturally sensitive approach.

When assessing pain, the nurse must remember that some patients may openly express their feelings and need for pain relief while others believe that the expression of pain symptoms, such as crying, is a sign of weakness. Pain management also varies according to cultural or religious beliefs. Traditional pain medications may or may not be the preferred method for pain control. Asians and Native Americans may prefer to use alternative therapies such as herbs, thermal therapies, acupuncture, massage, and meditation. Prayer plays an important role within African American and Hispanic cultures.

pain. Selection of the correct therapy is dependent on the nature and character of the pain.

Pain can be classified as either acute or chronic. Acute pain is an intense pain occurring over a defined time, usually from injury to recovery. Chronic pain persists longer than 6 months, can interfere with daily activities, and is associated with feelings of helplessness or hopelessness.

Pain can also be classified as to its source. Injury to *tissues* produces **nociceptor pain**. This type of pain may be further subdivided into somatic pain, which produces sharp, localized sensations, or visceral pain, which is described as a generalized dull, throbbing, or aching pain. In contrast, **neuropathic pain** is caused by injury to *nerves* and typically is described as burning, shooting, or numb pain. Whereas nociceptor pain responds quite well to conventional pain relief medications, neuropathic pain has less therapeutic success.

19.2 Nonpharmacologic Techniques for Pain Management

Although drugs are quite effective at relieving pain in most patients, they can have significant side effects. For example, at high doses, aspirin causes gastrointestinal (GI) bleeding, and the opioids cause significant drowsiness and have the potential for dependence. Nonpharmacologic techniques may be used in place of drugs, or as an adjunct to pharmacotherapy to assist patients in obtaining adequate pain relief. When used concurrently with medication, nonpharmacologic techniques may allow for lower doses and possibly fewer drug-related adverse effects. Some techniques used for reducing pain are as follows:

- Acupuncture
- Biofeedback therapy
- Massage
- Heat or cold packs
- Meditation
- Relaxation therapy
- Art or music therapy
- Imagery
- Chiropractic manipulation
- Hypnosis
- Therapeutic touch
- Transcutaneous electrical nerve stimulation (TENS)
- Energy therapies such as Reiki and Qi gong

Patients with intractable cancer pain sometimes require more invasive techniques, as rapidly growing tumors press on vital tissues and nerves. Furthermore, chemotherapy and surgical treatments for cancer can cause severe pain. Radiation therapy may provide pain relief by shrinking solid tumors that may be pressing on nerves. Surgery may be used to reduce pain by removing part of or the entire tumor. Injection of alcohol or another neurotoxic substance into neurons is occasionally performed to cause nerve blocks. Nerve blocks irreversibly stop impulse transmission along the treated nerves, and have the potential to provide total pain relief.

19.3 The Neural Mechanisms of Pain

The process of pain transmission begins when pain receptors are stimulated. These receptors, called **nociceptors**, are free nerve endings strategically located throughout the body. The nerve impulse signaling the pain is sent to the spinal cord along two types of sensory neurons, called Aδ and C fibers. **Aδ fibers** are wrapped in myelin, a lipid substance that speeds nerve transmission. **C fibers** are unmyelinated, thus they carry information more slowly. The Aδ fibers signal sharp, well-defined pain, whereas the C fibers conduct dull, poorly localized pain.

Once pain impulses reach the spinal cord, neurotransmitters are responsible for passing the message along to the next neuron. Here, a neurotransmitter called **substance P** is thought to be responsible for continuing the pain message, although other neurotransmitter candidates have been proposed. Spinal substance P is critical because it controls whether pain signals will continue to the brain. The activity of substance P may be affected by other neurotransmitters released from neurons in the CNS. One group of neurotransmitters called **endogenous opioids** includes endorphins, dynorphins, and enkephalins. Figure 19.1 shows one point of contact where endogenous opioids modify sensory information at the level of the spinal cord. If the pain impulse reaches the brain, it may respond to the sensation with many possible actions, ranging from signaling the skeletal muscles to jerk away from a sharp object, to mental depression caused by thoughts of death or disability in those suffering from chronic pain.

The fact that the pain signal begins at nociceptors located within peripheral tissues and proceeds through the CNS allows several targets for the pharmacologic interven-

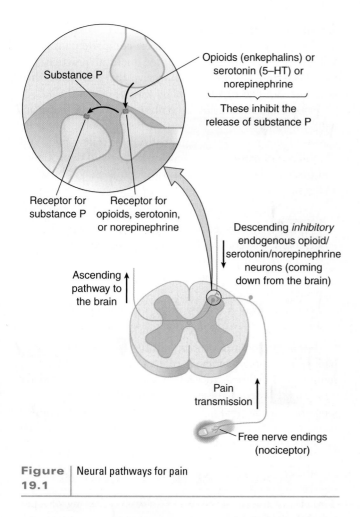

Substance P

Opioids (enkephalins) or
serotonin (5–HT) or
norepinephrine

These inhibit the
release of substance P

Receptor for
substance P

Receptor for
opioids, serotonin,
or norepinephrine

Descending *inhibitory*
endogenous opioid/
serotonin/norepinephrine
neurons (coming
down from the brain)

Ascending
pathway to
the brain

Pain
transmission

Free nerve endings
(nociceptor)

**Figure
19.1** | Neural pathways for pain

tion of pain transmission. In general, the two main classes of pain medications act at different locations: the non-steroidal anti-inflammatory drugs (NSAIDs) act at the peripheral level, whereas the opioids act in the CNS.

OPIOID (NARCOTIC) ANALGESICS

Analgesics are medications used to relieve pain. The two basic categories of analgesics are the opioids and the non-opioids. An opioid analgesic is a natural or synthetic morphine-like substance responsible for reducing severe pain. Opioids are narcotic substances, meaning that they produce numbness or stuporlike symptoms.

19.4 Classification of Opioids

Terminology associated with the narcotic analgesic medications is often confusing. Several of these drugs are obtained from opium, a milky extract from the unripe seeds of the poppy plant, which contains over 20 different chemicals having pharmacologic activity. Opium consists of 9% to 14% morphine and 0.8% to 2.5% codeine. These natural substances are called opiates. In a search for safer analgesics, chemists have created several dozen synthetic drugs with activity similar to that of the opiates. Opioid is a general term referring to any of these substances, natural or synthetic, and is often used interchangeably with the term opiate.

Narcotic is a general term used to describe morphine-like drugs that produce analgesia and CNS depression. Narcotics may be natural, such as morphine, or synthetic such as meperidine (Demerol). In common usage, a narcotic analgesic is the same as an opioid, and the terms are often used interchangeably. In the context of drug enforcement, however, the term narcotic is often used to describe a much broader range of abused illegal drugs such as hallucinogens, heroin, amphetamines, and marijuana. In medical environments, the nurse should restrict use of the term narcotic to specifically refer to opioid substances.

Opioids exert their actions by interacting with at least six types of receptors: mu (types one and two), kappa, sigma, delta, and epsilon. From the perspective of pain management, the mu and kappa receptors are the most important. Drugs that stimulate a particular receptor are called opioid agonists; those that block a receptor are called opioid antagonists. The types of actions produced by activating mu and kappa receptors are shown in Table 19.1.

Some opioid agonists, such as morphine, activate both mu and kappa receptors. Other opioids such as pentazocine (Talwin) exert mixed opioid agonist-antagonist effects by activating the kappa receptor but blocking the mu receptor.

Table 19.1	Responses Produced by Activation of Specific Opioid Receptors	
Response	**Mu Receptor**	**Kappa Receptor**
analgesia	x	x
decreased GI motility	x	x
euphoria	x	
miosis		x
physical dependence	x	
respiratory depression	x	
sedation	x	x

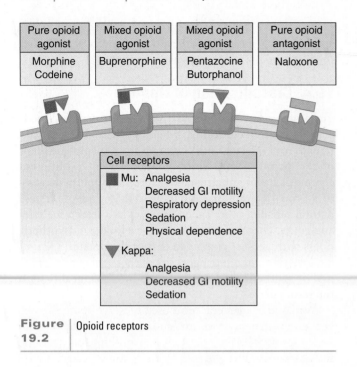

Pure opioid agonist	Mixed opioid agonist	Mixed opioid agonist	Pure opioid antagonist
Morphine Codeine	Buprenorphine	Pentazocine Butorphanol	Naloxone

Cell receptors

■ Mu: Analgesia
Decreased GI motility
Respiratory depression
Sedation
Physical dependence

▼ Kappa:

Analgesia
Decreased GI motility
Sedation

Figure 19.2 | Opioid receptors

Opioid blockers such as naloxone (Narcan) inhibit both the mu and kappa receptors. This is the body's natural way of providing the mechanism for a diverse set of body responses from one substance. Figure 19.2 illustrates opioid actions on the mu and kappa receptors.

19.5 Pharmacotherapy with Opioids

Opioids are drugs of choice for moderate to severe pain that cannot be controlled with other classes of analgesics. Over 20 different opioids are available as medications, which may be classified by similarities in their chemical structures, by their mechanism of action, or by their efficacy (Table 19.2). The most clinically useful method is by efficacy, which places opiates into categories of strong or moderate narcotic activity. Morphine is the prototype drug for severe pain, and the drug to which all other opiates are compared.

Opiates produce many important effects other than analgesia. They are effective at suppressing the cough reflex and at slowing the motility of the GI tract for cases of severe diarrhea. As powerful CNS depressants, opioids can cause sedation, which may be either a therapeutic effect or a side effect, depending on the patient's disease state. Some patients experience euphoria and intense relaxation, which are reasons why opiates are sometimes abused. There are many adverse effects, including respiratory depression, sedation, nausea, and vomiting.

All of the narcotic analgesics have the potential to cause physical and psychological dependence, as discussed in Chapter 12 ⬡. Dependence is more likely to occur when taking high doses for extended periods. Many healthcare providers and nurses are hesitant to administer the proper amount of opioid analgesics for fear of causing patient dependence or of producing serious adverse effects such as se-

dation or respiratory depression. Because of this undermedication, patients may not receive complete pain relief. When used according to accepted medical practice, patients can and indeed should, receive the pain relief they need without fear of addiction or adverse effects.

It is common practice to combine opioids and nonnarcotic analgesics into a single tablet or capsule. The two classes of analgesics work synergistically to relieve pain, and the dose of narcotic can be kept small to avoid dependence and opioid-related side effects. Five common combination analgesics are as follows:

- Vicodin (hydrocodone, 5 mg; acetaminophen, 500 mg)
- Percocet (oxycodone HCl, 5 mg; acetaminophen, 325 mg)
- Percodan (oxycodone HCl, 4.5 mg; oxycodone terephthalate, 0.38 mg; aspirin, 325 mg)
- Darvocet-N 50 (propoxyphene napsylate, 50 mg; acetaminophen, 325 mg)
- Empirin with Codeine No. 2 (codeine phosphate, 15 mg; aspirin, 325 mg)

Some opioids are used primarily for conditions other than pain. For example, alfentanil (Alfenta), fentanyl (Sublimaze), remifentanil (Ultiva), and sufentanil (Sufenta) are used for general anesthesia; these are discussed in Chapter 20. Codeine is most often prescribed as a cough suppressant and is covered in Chapter 24. Opiates used in treating diarrhea are presented in Chapter 25 ⬡.

NURSING CONSIDERATIONS

The role of the nurse involves careful monitoring of a patient's condition and providing education as it relates to the prescribed drug regimen. When providing care for patients taking opioids, the nurse should perform an initial assessment to determine the presence or history of severe respiratory disorders, increased intracranial pressure, seizures, and liver or renal disease. The nurse should obtain an allergy history before administering these drugs. A complete blood count, and liver and renal studies including AST, ALT, amylase, and bilirubin, should be obtained to rule out the presence of disease. The character, duration, location, and intensity of pain should be determined before the administration of these agents. The nurse should obtain history of current medication usage, especially alcohol and other CNS depressants, because these drugs will increase respiratory depression and sedation. Contraindications include hypersensitivity and conditions precluding IV opioid administration such as acute asthma or upper airway obstruction.

Through activation of primarily mu receptors, opioids may cause profound respiratory depression. Vital signs, especially respirations, should be obtained prior to and throughout the treatment regimen. Opioids should not be administered if respirations are below 12 per minute. Narcotic antagonists such as naloxone (Narcan) should be readily available if respirations fall below 10 per minute. The nurse should watch for decreasing level of consciousness and ensure safety by keeping the bed in a low position with

Table 19.2	Opioids for Pain Management
Drug	**Route and Adult Dose (max dose where indicated)**
Opioid Agonists with Moderate Efficacy	
codeine	PO; 15–60 mg qid
hydrocodone bitartrate (Hycodan)	PO; 5–10 mg q4–6h prn (max 15 mg/dose)
oxycodone hydrochloride (OxyContin)	PO; 5–10 mg qid prn
oxycodone terephthalate (Percocet-5, Roxicet, others)	
propoxyphene hydrochloride (Darvon)	PO; 65 mg (HCl form) or 100 mg (napsylate form) q4h
propoxyphene napsylate (Darvon-N)	prn (max 390 HCl/day; max 600 mg napsylate/day)
Opioid Agonists with High Efficacy	
hydromorphone hydrochloride (Dilaudid)	PO; 1–4 mg q4–6h prn
levorphanol tartrate (Levo-Dromoran)	PO; 2–3 mg tid to qid prn
meperidine hydrochloride (Demerol)	PO; 50–150 mg q3–4h prn
methadone hydrochloride (Dolophine)	PO; 2.5–10 mg q3–4h prn
morphine sulfate (Astramorph PF, Duramorph, others)	PO; 10–30 mg q4h prn
oxymorphone hydrochloride (Numorphan)	SC/IM; 1–1.5 mg q4–6h prn PR; 5 mg q4–6h prn
Opioids with Mixed Agonist-Antagonist Effects	
buprenorphine hydrochloride (Buprenex)	IM/IV; 0.3 mg q6h (max 0.6 mg q4h)
butorphanol tartrate (Stadol)	IM; 1–4 mg q3–4h prn (max 4 mg/dose)
dezocine (Dalgan)	IV; 2.5–10 mg (usually 5 mg) q2–4h IM; 5–10 mg (usually 10 mg) q3–4h
nalbuphine hydrochloride (Nubain)	SC/IM/IV; 10–20 mg q3–6h prn (max 160 mg/day)
pentazocine hydrochloride (Talwin)	PO; 50–100 mg q3–4h (max 600 mg/day) SC/IM/IV; 30 mg q3–4h (max 360 mg/day)
Opioid Antagonists	
nalmefene hydrochloride (Revex)	SC/IM/IV; Use 1 mg/ml concentration; nonopioid dependent; 0.5 mg/70 kg; opioid dependent; 0.1 mg/70 kg
naloxone hydrochloride (Narcan)	IV; 0.4–2 mg; may be repeated every 2–3 min up to 10 mg if necessary
naltrexone hydrochloride (Trexan, ReVia)	PO; 25 mg followed by another 25 mg in 1 hour if no withdrawal response (max 800 mg/day)

side rails raised. Assistance may be needed with ambulation and ADLs.

Another severe adverse reaction, increased intracranial pressure (ICP), occurs as an indirect result of the respiratory depression effect. When respiration is suppressed, the CO_2 content of blood is increased, which dilates the cerebral blood vessels and causes ICP to rise. Similarly, orthostatic hypotension may also occur due to the blunting of the baroreceptor reflex and dilation of the peripheral arterioles and veins.

The nurse should continually monitor urinary output for urinary retention. This may occur due to the effect of increasing tone in the bladder sphincter, and through suppression of the bladder stimuli.

Side effects such as constipation, nausea, and vomiting occur due to a combination of actions on the GI tract. By suppressing intestinal contractions, increasing the tone of the anal sphincter, and inhibiting secretion of fluids into the intestine, constipation may occur. Nausea or vomiting may occur due to the direct stimulation of the chemoreceptor trigger zone of the medulla. If this occurs, an antiemetic may be indicated. Opioids may be contraindicated for patients suffering from diarrhea caused by infections, especially following antibiotic therapy (pseudomembranous colitis). Pathogens in the GI tract produce toxins that are shed during diarrhea; constipation causes toxins to build up in the body.

The Influence of Age on Pain Expression and Perception

Pain control in both children and the elderly can be challenging. Knowledge of developmental theories, the aging process, behavioral cues, subtle signs of discomfort, and verbal and nonverbal responses to pain are a must when it comes to effective pain management. Older patients may have a decreased perception of pain or simply ignore pain as a "natural" consequence of aging. Because these patients frequently go undermedicated, a thorough assessment is a necessity. As with adults, it is important that the nurse believe children's self-report when assessing for pain. Developmentally appropriate pain rating tools are available and should be used on a continuous basis. Comfort measures should also be used.

When administering opioids for pain relief, the nurse should always monitor patients closely. Smaller doses are usually indicated and side effects may be heightened. Closely monitor decreased respirations, LOC, and dizziness. Body weight should be taken prior to the start of opioid administration and doses calculated accordingly. Bed/crib rails should be kept raised and the bed in low position at all times to prevent injury from falls. Some opioids, such as meperidine (Demerol), should be used cautiously in children. Many elderly take multiple drugs (polypharmacy); therefore, it is important to obtain a complete list of all medications taken and check for interactions.

Patient education as it relates to opioids should include goals, reasons for obtaining baseline data such as for vital signs, laboratory tests and procedures, and possible side effects. See "Nursing Process Focus: Patients Receiving Opioid Therapy" for important points that the nurse should include when teaching patients regarding this class of drugs.

Opioid Antagonists

19.6 Pharmacotherapy with Opioid Antagonists

Opioid overdose can occur as a result of overly aggressive pain therapy or as a result of substance abuse. Any opioid may be abused for its psychoactive effects; however, morphine, meperidine, and heroin are preferred due to their potency. Although heroin is currently available as a legal analgesic in many countries, it is deemed too dangerous for therapeutic use by the FDA and is a major drug of abuse. Once injected or inhaled, heroin rapidly crosses the blood-brain barrier to enter the brain, where it is metabolized to morphine. Thus, the effects and symptoms of heroin administration are actually caused by the activation of mu and kappa receptors by morphine. The initial effect is an intense euphoria, called a rush, followed by several hours of deep relaxation.

Acute opioid intoxication is a medical emergency, with respiratory depression being the most serious problem. Infusion with the opioid antagonist naloxone (Narcan) may be used to reverse respiratory depression and other acute symptoms. In cases when the patient is unconscious and the healthcare provider is unclear what drug has been taken, opioid antagonists may be given to diagnose the overdose. If the opioid antagonist fails to quickly reverse the acute symptoms, the overdose was likely due to a nonopioid substance.

Pr PROTOTYPE DRUG | **MORPHINE** (Astramorph PF, Duramorph, others)

ACTIONS AND USES

Morphine binds with both mu and kappa receptor sites to produce profound analgesia. It causes euphoria, constriction of the pupils, and stimulation of cardiac muscle. It is used for symptomatic relief of serious acute and chronic pain after nonnarcotic analgesics have failed, as preanesthetic medication, to relieve shortness of breath associated with heart failure and pulmonary edema, and for acute chest pain connected with MI.

Administration Alerts

- Oral solution may be given sublingually.
- Oral solution comes in multiple strengths; carefully observe drug orders and labels before administering.
- Morphine causes peripheral vasodilation, which results in orthostatic hypotension.
- Pregnancy category D in long-term use or with high doses.

ADVERSE EFFECTS AND INTERACTIONS

Morphine may cause dysphoria (restlessness, depression, and anxiety), hallucinations, nausea, constipation, dizziness, and an itching sensation. Overdose may result in severe respiratory depression or cardiac arrest. Tolerance develops to the analgesic, sedative, and euphoric effects of the drug. Cross-tolerance also develops between morphine and other opioids such as heroin, methadone, and meperidine. Physical and psychological dependence develop when high doses are taken for prolonged periods of time. Morphine may intensify or mask the pain of gallbladder disease, due to biliary tract spasms.

Morphine interacts with several drugs. For example, concurrent use of CNS depressants, such as alcohol, other opioids, general anesthetics, sedatives, and antidepressants such as MAO inhibitors and tricyclics, potentiates the action of opiates, increasing the risk of severe respiratory depression and death.

Use with caution with herbal supplements, such as yohimbe, which may potentiate the effect of morphine.

See the companion website for a Nursing Process Focus specific to this drug.

NURSING CONSIDERATIONS

The role of the nurse in opioid antagonist therapy involves careful monitoring of a patient's condition and providing education as it relates to the prescribed drug regimen. The primary indication for use of an opioid antagonist is established or suspected opioid-induced respiratory depression. The primary nursing response is to assess the patient's respiratory status and administer the opioid antagonist if respirations are below 10 breaths per minute. Resuscitative equipment should be immediately accessible. Obtaining key medical information is a priority; the presence/history of cardiovascular disease should be included. Opioids increase cardiac workload, so they must be used with caution in patients with cardiovascular disease. The nurse should assess the social context of the patient's environment for the potential for opioid dependency. Opioid antagonists should be used cautiously in patients who are physically dependent on opioids, because drug-induced withdrawal may be more severe than spontaneous opioid withdrawal. Caution is also advised for pregnant or lactating women, and in children.

The nurse should assess the patient's pain level before administration of these drugs and during therapy. During and immediately after the administration of opioid antagonists, the nurse should check vital signs every 3 to 5 minutes (especially respiratory function and blood pressure), obtain ABGs and EKG, and monitor for the following side effects: drowsiness, tremors, hyperventilation, ventricular tachycardia, and loss of analgesia. If giving these drugs to drug-dependent patients, the nurse should monitor for signs of opioid withdrawal such as cramping, vomiting, hypertension, and anxiety.

Opioid antagonists such as naltrexone (Depade, ReVia, Trexan) are also used for the treatment of opioid addiction. The nurse must monitor for side effects during treatment, many of which reflect the opioid withdrawal syndromes. Symptoms include increased thirst, chills, fever, joint/muscle pain, CNS stimulation, drowsiness, dizziness, confusion, seizures, headache, nausea, vomiting, diarrhea, rash, rapid pulse and respirations, pulmonary edema, and wheezing. Vital signs should be taken every 3 to 5 minutes. Respiratory function should be continually assessed and cardiac status should be monitored for tachycardia and hypertension. As with naloxone (Narcan), resuscitative equipment should always be available.

Patient education regarding opioid antagonists should include goals, reasons for obtaining vital signs, tests and procedures, and possible drug side effects. See "Nursing Process Focus: Patients Receiving Opioid Therapy" for specific teaching points.

19.7 Treatment for Opioid Dependence

Although effective at relieving pain, the opioids have a greater risk for dependence than almost any other class of medications. Tolerance develops relatively quickly to the euphoric effects of opioids, causing users to escalate their doses and take the drugs more frequently. The higher and more frequent doses rapidly cause physical dependence in opioid abusers.

When physically dependent patients attempt to discontinue drug use, they experience extremely uncomfortable symptoms that convince many to continue their drug-taking behavior in order to avoid the suffering. As long as the drug is continued, they feel "normal" and many can continue work or social activities. In cases when the drug is abruptly discontinued, about 7 days of withdrawal symptoms are experienced before the patient overcomes the physical dependence.

Pr PROTOTYPE DRUG	NALOXONE (Narcan)
ACTIONS AND USES	**ADVERSE EFFECTS AND INTERACTIONS**
Naloxone is a pure opioid antagonist, blocking both mu and kappa receptors. It is used for complete or partial reversal of opioid effects in emergency situations when acute opioid overdose is suspected. Given intravenously, it begins to reverse opioid-initiated CNS and respiratory depression within minutes. It will immediately cause opioid withdrawal symptoms in patients physically dependent on opioids. It is also used to treat postoperative opioid depression. It is occasionally given as adjunctive therapy to reverse hypotension caused by septic shock. Naloxone is pregnancy category B.	Naloxone itself has minimal toxicity. However, in reversing the effects of opioids, the patient may experience rapid loss of analgesia, increased blood pressure, tremors, hyperventilation, nausea/vomiting, and drowsiness. It should not be used for respiratory depression caused by nonopioid medications. Drug interactions include a reversal of the analgesic effects of narcotic agonists and angonist-antagonists.
Administration Alert	
■ Administer for respiratory rate of fewer than 10 breaths/ minute. Keep resuscitative equipment accessible.	

 See the companion website for a Nursing Process Focus specific to this drug.

NURSING PROCESS FOCUS | PATIENTS RECEIVING OPIOID THERAPY

ASSSESSMENT

Prior to administration:
- Obtain complete health history including allergies, drug history, and possible drug interactions.
- Assess pain (quality, intensity, location, duration).
- Assess respiratory function.
- Assess level of consciousness before and after administration.
- Obtain vital signs.

POTENTIAL NURSING DIAGNOSES

- Deficient Knowledge, related to drug therapy
- Acute Pain, related to injury; disease; or surgical procedure
- Ineffective Breathing Pattern, related to action of medication
- Constipation
- Disturbed Sleep Pattern, related to surgical pain

PLANNING: PATIENT GOALS AND EXPECTED OUTCOMES

The patient will:
- Report pain relief or a reduction in pain intensity
- Demonstrate an understanding of the drug's action by accurately describing drug side effects and precautions
- Immediately report effects such as untoward or rebound pain, restlessness, anxiety, depression, hallucination, nausea, dizziness, and itching

IMPLEMENTATION

Interventions and (Rationales)	*Patient Education/Discharge Planning*
■ Opioids may be administered PO, SC, IM, IV, or PR. ■ Opioids are Schedule II controlled substances. (Opioids produce both physical and psychological dependence.)	Instruct patient: ■ To take necessary steps to safeguard drug supply; avoid sharing medications with others ■ That oral *capsules* may be opened and mixed with cool foods; extended-release *tablets*, however, may not be chewed, crushed, or broken ■ That oral solution given sublingually may be in a higher concentration than solution for swallowing
■ Monitor liver function via laboratory tests. (Opioids are metabolized in the liver. Hepatic disease can increase blood levels of opioids to toxic levels.)	Instruct patient to: ■ Report nausea, vomiting, diarrhea, rash, jaundice, abdominal pain, tenderness or distention, or change in color of stool ■ Adhere to laboratory testing regimen for liver function as ordered by the healthcare provider
■ Monitor vital signs, especially depth and rate of respirations/pulse oximetry. ■ Withhold the drug if the patient's respiratory rate is below 12, and notify the healthcare provider. ■ Keep resuscitative equipment and a narcotic-antagonist such as naloxone (Narcan) accessible. (Opioid antagonists may be used to reverse respiratory depression, decreased level of consciousness and other symptoms of narcotic overdose.)	Instruct patient or caregiver to: ■ Monitor vital signs regularly, particularly respirations ■ Withhold medication for any difficulty in breathing or respirations below 12 breaths per minute; report symptoms to the healthcare provider
■ Monitor neurological status; perform neurochecks regularly. ■ Monitor changes in level of consciousness. (Decreased LOC and sluggish pupillary response may occur with high doses.) ■ Observe for seizures. (Drug may increase ICP.)	Instruct patient to: ■ Report headache or any significant change in sensorium, such as an aura or other visual affects that may indicate an impending seizure ■ Recognize seizures and methods to ensure personal safety during a seizure ■ Report any seizure activity immediately

continued

NURSING PROCESS FOCUS: *Patients Receiving Opioid Therapy (continued)*

Interventions and (Rationales)	Patient Education/Discharge Planning
■ If ordered prn, administer medication upon patient request or when nursing observations indicate patient expressions of pain.	Instruct patient to: ■ Alert the nurse immediately upon the return or increase of pain ■ Notify the nurse regarding the drug's effectiveness
■ Monitor renal status and urinary output. (May cause urinary retention, which may exacerbate existing symptoms of prostatic hypertrophy.)	Instruct patient or caregiver to: ■ Measure and monitor fluid intake and output ■ Report symptoms of dysuria (hesitancy, pain, diminished stream), changes in urine quality or scanty urine output ■ Report fever or flank pain that may be indicative of a urinary tract infection
■ Monitor for other side effects such as restlessness, dizziness, anxiety, depression, hallucinations, nausea, and vomiting. (Hives or itching may indicate an allergic reaction due to the production of histamine.)	Instruct patient or caregiver to: ■ Recognize side effects and symptoms of an allergic or anaphylactic reaction ■ Immediately report any shortness of breath, tight feeling in the throat, itching, hives or other rash, feelings of dysphoria, nausea, or vomiting ■ Avoid the use of sleep-inducing OTC antihistamines, without first consulting the healthcare provider
■ Monitor for constipation. (Drug slows peristalsis)	Instruct patient to: ■ Maintain an adequate fluid and fiber intake to facilitate stool passage ■ Use a stool softener or laxative as recommended by the healthcare provider
■ Ensure patient safety. ■ Monitor ambulation until response to drug is known. (Drug can cause sedation and dizziness)	Instruct patient to: ■ Request assistance when getting out of bed ■ Avoid driving or performing hazardous activities until effect of drug is known
■ Monitor frequency of requests and stated effectiveness of narcotic administered. (Opioids cause tolerance and dependence)	Instruct patient and caregiver: ■ Regarding cross-tolerance issues ■ To monitor medication supply to observe for hoarding, which may signal an impending suicide attempt ■ When educating patients suffering from terminal illnesses, address the issue of drug dependence from the perspective of reduced life expectancy.

EVALUATION OF OUTCOME CRITERIA

Evaluate effectiveness of drug therapy by confirming that patient goals and expected outcomes have been met (see "Planning").

See Table 19.2 for a list of drugs to which these nursing actions apply.

The intense craving characteristic of psychological dependence may occur for many months, and even years, following discontinuation of opioids. This often results in a return to drug-seeking behavior, unless significant support groups are established.

One common method of treating opioid dependence is to switch the patient from IV and inhalation forms of illegal drugs to methadone (Dolophine). Although an opioid, oral methadone does not cause the euphoria of the injectable opioids. Methadone does not cure the dependence and the patient must continue taking the drug to avoid withdrawal symptoms. This therapy, called methadone maintenance, may continue for many months or years, until the patient decides to enter a total withdrawal treatment program. Methadone maintenance allows patients to return to productive work and social relationships without the physical, emotional, and criminal risks of illegal drug use.

A newer treatment option is to administer buprenorphine (Subutex), a mixed opioid agonist-antagonist, by the sublingual route. Subutex is used early in opioid abuse therapy to prevent opioid withdrawal symptoms. Another combination agent, Suboxone, contains both buprenorphine and naloxone, and is used later in the maintenance of opioid addiction.

NONOPIOID ANALGESICS

The nonopioid analgesics include acetaminophen, the nonsteroidal anti-inflammatory drugs (NSAIDs), and a few centrally acting agents.

Nonsteroidal Antiinflammatory Drugs (NSAIDs)

The NSAIDs inhibit cyclooxygenase, an enzyme responsible for the formation of prostaglandins. When cyclooxygenase is inhibited, inflammation and pain are reduced.

19.8 Pharmacotherapy with NSAIDs

NSAIDs are the drugs of choice for mild to moderate pain, especially for pain associated with inflammation. These drugs have many advantages over the opioids. Aspirin and ibuprofen are available OTC and are inexpensive. They are available in many different formulations, including those designed for children. They are safe and produce adverse effects only at high doses. The NSAIDs have antipyretic and anti-inflammatory activity, as well as analgesic properties. Some of the NSAIDs, such as the selective COX-2 inhibitors, are used primarily for their anti-inflammatory properties. The role of the NSAIDs in the treatment of inflammation and fever is discussed in Chapter 31. Celecoxib (Celebrex) is a featured prototype drug in Chapter 31 ⊙. Table 19.3 highlights the common nonopioid analgesics.

The NSAIDs act by inhibiting pain mediators at the nociceptor level. When tissue is damaged, chemical mediators are released locally, including histamine, potassium ion, hydrogen ion, bradykinin, and prostaglandins. Bradykinin is associated with the sensory impulse of pain. Prostaglandins can induce pain through the formation of free radicals.

Prostaglandins are formed with the help of two enzymes called cyclooxygenase type one (COX-1) and cyclooxygenase type two (COX-2). Aspirin inhibits both COX-1 and COX-2. Because the COX-2 enzyme is more specific for the synthesis of those prostaglandins that cause pain and inflammation, the selective COX-2 inhibitors provide more specific pain relief and produce fewer side effects than aspirin. Figure 19.3 illustrates the mechanisms involved in pain at the nociceptor level.

Several important nonopioid analgesics are not classified as NSAIDs. Acetaminophen is a nonopioid analgesic that has equal efficacy to aspirin and ibuprofen in relieving pain. Acetaminophen is featured as a prototype antipyretic in Chapter 31 ⊙. Clonidine (Catapres) and tramadol (Ultram) are centrally acting analgesics. Tramadol has weak opioid activity, though it is not thought to relieve pain by this mechanism.

NURSING CONSIDERATIONS

The role of the nurse in NSAID therapy involves careful monitoring of a patient's condition and providing education as it relates to prescribed drug regimen. Because NSAIDs are readily available, inexpensive, and taken orally, patients sometimes forget that these medications can have serious side effects. The inhibition of COX-1 by aspirin makes it more likely to cause gastric ulcers and bleeding and acute renal failure. Ibuprofen exerts less of an effect on COX-1 inhibition, so it produces less gastric bleeding than aspirin.

When caring for patients taking high doses of these drugs, a thorough assessment for the presence/history of hypersensitivity, bleeding disorders, gastric ulcers, severe renal/hepatic disease, and pregnancy should be done. NSAIDs are not recommended for patients with these conditions. Renal and liver function studies (BUN, creatinine, AST, ALT, hemoglobin) should be performed before and during pharmacotherapy. An assessment of the location, character, and intensity of pain should be done initially for baseline data and throughout treatment to determine effectiveness. Aspirin has many drug interactions, therefore a complete patient drug list should be obtained (see "Nursing Process Focus: Patients Receiving NSAID Therapy"). Contraindications include hypersensitivity to aspirin or other NSAIDs, bleeding disorders such as hemophilia, von Willebrand's disease, and telangiectasia, and favism (genetic G6PD enzyme deficiency). When taking high doses of these medications, it is important that patients are monitored for nephrotoxicity (dysuria, hematuria, oliguria), blood dyscrasias, hepatitis, and allergic responses (rash and urticaria). The nurse should also monitor patients for the following side effects: nausea, abdominal pain, anorexia, dizziness, and drowsiness. To decrease GI upset, the medication may be taken with food and plenty of fluids. Tablets with enteric coating should not be crushed.

Nurses should exercise extreme caution in administering ASA to children and teenagers. ASA has been implicated in the development of Reye's syndrome in conjunction with flulike illnesses. Febrile, dehydrated children can rapidly develop ASA toxicity. Use ASA with caution in patients who are pregnant or lactating. Pregnancy category C (D in third trimester) denotes potential harm to the fetus.

Patient education for nonopioid analgesics should include goals, reasons for obtaining baseline data such as vital signs, diagnostic procedures and laboratory tests, and possible side effects. See "Nursing Process Focus: Patients Receiving NSAID Therapy" for specific points that the nurse should include when teaching patients regarding this class of drugs.

Table 19.3	Nonopioid Analgesics
Drug	**Route and Adult Dose (max dose where indicated)**
acetaminophen (Tylenol) (see page 425 for the Prototype Drug box)⚬⚬	PO; 325–650 mg q4–6h
NSAIDs	
Selective COX-2 Inhibitors	
celecoxib (Celebrex) (see page 422 for the Prototype Drug box)⚬⚬	PO; 100–200 mg bid or 200 mg qid
rofecoxib (Vioxx)	PO; 12.5–25 mg qd
Ibuprofen and Ibuprofen-like: Nonsalicylates	
diclofenac (Cataflam, Voltaren)	PO; 50 mg bid to qid (max 200 mg/day)
diflunisal (Dolobid)	PO; 1000 mg followed by 500 mg bid to tid
etodolac (Lodine)	PO; 200–400 mg tid to qid
fenoprofen calcium (Nalfon)	PO; 200 mg tid to qid
flurbiprofen (Ansaid)	PO; 50–100 mg tid to qid (max 300 mg/day)
ibuprofen (Advil, Motrin)	PO; 400 mg tid to qid (max 1200 mg/day)
indomethacin (Indocin)	PO; 25–50 mg bid or tid (max 200 mg/day) or 75 mg sustained release one to two times/day
ketoprofen (Actron, Orudis)	PO; 12.5–50 mg tid to qid
ketorolac tromethamine (Toradol)	PO; 10 mg qid prn (max 40 mg/day)
mefanamic acid (Ponstel)	PO; Loading dose 500 mg; maintenance dose 250 mg q6h prn
meloxicam (Mobic)	PO; 7.5 mg qd (max 15 mg/day)
nambumetone (Relafen)	PO; 1000 mg qd (max 2000 mg/day)
naproxen (Naprosyn, Naprolen)	PO; 500 mg followed by 200–250 mg tid to qid (max 1000 mg/day)
naproxen sodium (Aleve, Anaprox, others)	PO; 250–500 mg bid (max 1000 mg/day naproxen); Naprolan is dosed qid
ozaprozin (Daypro)	PO; 600–1200 mg qd (max 1800 mg/day)
piroxicam (Feldene)	PO; 10–20 mg qd to bid (max 20 mg/day)
sulindac (Clinoril)	PO; 150–200 mg bid (max 400 mg/day)
tolmetin (Tolectin)	PO; 400 mg tid (max 2 g/day)
Salicylates	
℗ aspirin (Acetylsalicylic acid, ASA)	PO; 350–650 mg q4h (max 4 g/day)
choline salicylate (Arthropan)	PO; 435–870 mg (2.5–5 ml) q4h
salsalate (Disalcid)	PO; 325–3000 mg qd in divided doses (max 4 g/day)
Centrally Acting Agents	
clonidine (Catapres)	PO; 0.1 mg bid to tid (max 0.8 mg/day)
tramadol (Ultram)	PO; 50–100 mg q4–6h prn (max 400 mg/day); may start with 25 mg/day, and increase by 25 mg every 3 days up to 200 mg/day

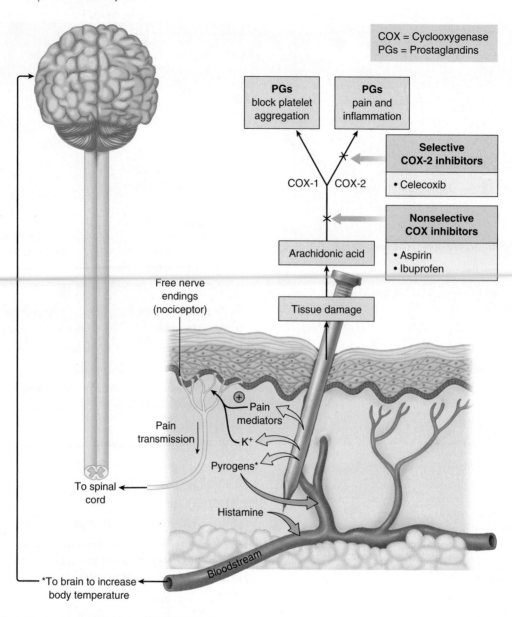

COX = Cyclooxygenase
PGs = Prostaglandins

PGs block platelet aggregation

PGs pain and inflammation

Selective COX-2 inhibitors
• Celecoxib

Nonselective COX inhibitors
• Aspirin
• Ibuprofen

COX-1 COX-2

Arachidonic acid

Tissue damage

Free nerve endings (nociceptor)

Pain transmission

To spinal cord

⊕ Pain mediators

K⁺

Pyrogens*

Histamine

Bloodstream

*To brain to increase body temperature

Figure 19.3 | Mechanisms of pain at the nociceptor level

TENSION HEADACHES AND MIGRAINES

Headaches are some of the most common complaints of patients. Living with headaches can interfere with activities of daily life, thus causing great distress. The pain and inability to focus and concentrate results in work-related absences and the inability to take care of home and family. When the headaches are persistent, or occur as migraines, drug therapy is warranted.

19.9 Classification of Headaches

Of the several varieties of headaches, the most common type is the **tension headache**. This occurs when muscles

of the head and neck become very tight due to stress, causing a steady and lingering pain. Although quite painful, tension headaches are self-limiting and generally considered an annoyance rather than a medical emergency. Tension headaches can usually be effectively treated with OTC analgesics such as aspirin, acetaminophen, or ibuprofen.

The most painful type of headache is the **migraine**, which is characterized by throbbing or pulsating pain, sometimes preceded by an aura. **Auras** are sensory cues that let the patient know that a migraine attack is coming soon. Examples of sensory cues are jagged lines, flashing lights, special smells, tastes, or sounds. Most migraines are accompanied by nausea and vomiting. Triggers for migraines include nitrates, monosodium glutamate (MSG) found in many Asian foods, red wine, perfumes, food additives, caf-

PROTOTYPE DRUG | ASPIRIN (Acetylsalicylic Acid, ASA)

ACTIONS AND USES

Aspirin inhibits prostaglandin synthesis involved in the processes of pain and inflammation and produces mild to moderate relief of fever. It has limited effects on peripheral blood vessels, causing vasodilation and sweating. Aspirin has significant anticoagulant activity and this property is responsible for its ability to reduce the risk of mortality following MI, and to reduce the incidence of strokes. Aspirin has also been found to reduce the risk of colorectal cancer, although the mechanism by which it affords this protective effect is unknown.

Administration Alerts

- Platelet aggregation inhibition caused by ASA is irreversible. Aspirin should be discontinued 1 week prior to elective surgery.
- ASA is excreted in the urine and affects urine testing for glucose and other metabolites, such as vanillylmandelic acid (VMA).
- Pregnancy category D.

ADVERSE EFFECTS AND INTERACTIONS

At high doses, such as those used to treat severe inflammatory disorders, aspirin may cause gastric discomfort and bleeding because of its antiplatelet effects. Enteric-coated tablets and buffered preparations are available for patients who experience GI side effects.

Because aspirin increases bleeding time, it should not be given to patients receiving anticoagulant therapy such as warfarin, heparin, and plicamycin. ASA may potentiate the action of oral hypoglycemic agents. Effects of NSAIDs, uricosuric agents such as probenecid, beta-blockers, spironolactone, and sulfa drugs may be decreased when combined with ASA.

Concurrent use of phenobarbital, antacids, and glucocorticoids may decrease ASA effects. Insulin, methotrexate, phenytoin, sulfonamides, and penicillin may increase effects. When taken with alcohol, pyrazolone derivatives, steroids, or other NSAIDs there is an increased risk for gastric ulcers.

Use with caution with herbal supplements, such as feverfew, which may increase the risk of bleeding.

 See the companion website for a Nursing Process Focus specific to this drug.

feine, chocolate, and aspartame. By avoiding foods containing these substances, some patients can prevent the onset of a migraine attack.

19.10 Drug Therapy for Migraine Headaches

There are two primary goals for the pharmacologic therapy of migraines (see Table 19.4). The first is to stop migraines in progress and the second is to prevent migraines from occurring. For the most part, the drugs used to abort migraines are different than those used for prophylaxis. Drug therapy is most effective if begun before a migraine has reached a severe level.

The two major drug classes used as antimigraine agents, the triptans and the ergot alkaloids, are both serotonin (5-HT) agonists. Serotonergic receptors are found throughout the CNS, and in the cardiovascular and GI systems. At least five receptor subtypes have been identified. In addition to the triptans, other drugs acting at serotonergic receptors include the popular antianxiety agents fluoxetine (Prozac) and buspirone (BuSpar).

Pharmacotherapy of migraine termination generally begins with acetaminophen or NSAIDs. If OTC analgesics are unable to abort the migraine, the drugs of choice are often the triptans. The first of the triptans, sumatriptan (Imitrex), was marketed in the United States in 1993. These agents are selective for the 5-HT$_1$ receptor subtype, and

they are thought to act by constricting certain intracranial vessels. They are effective in aborting migraines with or without auras. Although oral forms of the triptans are most convenient, patients who experience nausea and vomiting during the migraine may require an alternate dosage form. Intranasal formulations and prefilled syringes of triptans are available for patients who are able to self-administer the medication.

For patients who are unresponsive to triptans, the ergot alkaloids may be used to abort migraines. The first purified alkaloid, ergotamine (Ergostat), was isolated from the ergot fungus in 1920, although the actions of the ergot alkaloids had been known for thousands of years. Ergotamine is an inexpensive drug that is available in oral, sublingual, and suppository forms. Modification of the original molecule has produced a number of other pharmacologically useful drugs, such as dihydroergotamine (Migranal). Dihydroergotamine is given parenterally and as a nasal spray. Because the ergot alkaloids interact with adrenergic and dopaminergic receptors, as well as serotonergic receptors, they produce multiple actions and side effects. Many ergot alkaloids are pregnancy category X drugs.

Drugs for migraine prophylaxis include various classes of drugs that are discussed in other chapters of this textbook. These include beta-adrenergic blockers, calcium channel blockers, antidepressants, and antiseizure drugs. Because all of these drugs have the potential to produce side effects, prophylaxis is only initiated if the incidence of

NURSING PROCESS FOCUS — PATIENTS RECEIVING NSAID THERAPY

ASSESSMENT

Prior to administration:
- Obtain complete health history including allergies, drug history, and possible drug interactions.
- Determine pain and analgesic usage patterns.
- Identify infectious agents or other factors responsible for inflammation or pain.

POTENTIAL NURSING DIAGNOSES

- Acute Pain, related to injury or surgical procedure
- Chronic Pain, related to back injury
- Deficient Knowledge, related to drug therapy
- Ineffective Health Maintenance, related to chronic pain

PLANNING: PATIENT GOALS AND EXPECTED OUTCOMES

The patient will:
- Report pain relief or a reduction in pain intensity
- Demonstrate an understanding of the drug's action by accurately describing drug side effects and precautions
- Report ability to manage activities of daily living
- Immediately report effects such as unresolved, untoward, or rebound pain; persistent fever; blurred vision; tinnitus; bleeding; changes in color of stool or urine

IMPLEMENTATION

Interventions and (Rationales)	Patient Education/Discharge Planning
■ NSAIDs may be administered PO. or PR. When using suppositories, monitor integrity of rectum; observe for rectal bleeding.	Inform patient of the following: ■ Enteric-coated tablets must not be cut or crushed. Regular tablets may be broken or pulverized and mixed with food. ■ Administer liquid ASA immediately after mixing because it breaks down rapidly. ■ Different drugs and formulations, such as ibuprofen and naproxen, should not be taken concurrently. Consult the healthcare provider regarding appropriate OTC analgesics for specific types of pain. ■ ASA is an anticoagulant. The body needs time to manufacture new platelets to make clots that promote wound healing. Consult the nurse regarding ASA therapy following surgery. ■ Advise laboratory personnel of aspirin therapy when providing urine samples.
■ Monitor vital signs, especially temperature. (Increased pulse and blood pressure may indicate discomfort; accompanied by pallor and/or dizziness may indicate bleeding.)	Instruct patient to: ■ Report rapid heartbeat, palpitations, dizziness, or pallor ■ Monitor blood pressure and temperature ensuring proper use of home equipment
■ Monitor for signs of GI bleeding or hepatic toxicity. (NSAIDs can be a local irritant to the GI tract with anticoagulant action that is metabolized in the liver.) ■ Monitor gastrointestinal elimination; conduct guaiac stool testing for occult blood. ■ Monitor CBC for signs of anemia related to blood loss.	Instruct patient to: ■ Report any bleeding, abdominal pain, anorexia, heartburn, nausea, vomiting, jaundice, or a change in the color or character of stools ■ Know the proper method of obtaining stool samples and home testing for occult blood ■ Adhere to a regimen of laboratory testing as ordered by the healthcare provider ■ Take NSAIDs with food to reduce stomach upset
■ Assess for character, duration, location, and intensity of pain and the presence of inflammation.	■ Instruct patient to notify nurse if pain and/or inflammation remains unresolved. ■ Advise patient to take only the prescribed amount to decrease the potential for adverse effects.

continued

NURSING PROCESS FOCUS: *Patients Receiving NSAID Therapy (continued)*

Interventions and (Rationales)

- Monitor for hypersensitivity reaction.
- Monitor urinary output and edema in feet/ankles. (Medication is excreted through the kidneys. Long-term use may lead to renal dysfunction.)
- Monitor for sensory changes indicative of drug toxicity: tinnitus, blurred vision.
- Evaluate blood salicylate levels.

Patient Education/Discharge Planning

Advise the patient to:

- Immediately report shortness of breath, wheezing, throat tightness, itching, or hives. If these occur, stop taking ASA immediately and inform the healthcare provider
- Report changes in urination, flank pain or pitting edema immediately
- Return to healthcare provider for prescribed follow-up appointments
- Immediately report any sensory changes in sight or hearing, especially blurred vision or ringing in the ears.

EVALUATION OF OUTCOME CRITERIA

Evaluate effectiveness of drug therapy by confirming that patient goals and expected outcomes have been met (see "Planning").

See Table 19.3 under "NSAIDs" for a list of drugs to which these nursing actions apply.

PHARMFACTS — Headaches and Migraines

- About 28 million Americans suffer from headaches and migraines.
- Of all migraines, 95% are controlled by drug therapy and other measures.
- Before puberty, more boys have migraines than girls.
- After puberty, women have 4 to 8 times more migraines than men.
- Headaches and migraines appear mostly among people in their 20s and 30s.
- Persons with a family history of headache or migraine have a higher chance of developing these disorders.

migraines is high and the patient is unresponsive to the drugs used to abort migraines. Of the various drugs, propranolol (Inderal) is one of the most commonly prescribed. Amitriptyline (Elavil) is preferred for patients who may have a mood disorder or suffer from insomnia in addition to their migraines.

NURSING CONSIDERATIONS

The role of the nurse in antimigraine therapy involves careful monitoring of a patient's condition and providing education as it relates to the prescribed drug regimen. Before starting patients on antimigraine medications, the nurse should gather information about the frequency and intensity of the migraine headaches, the presence/history of an

MI, angina, and hypertension. The nurse should also gather information about the presence/history of renal and liver disease, diabetes, and pregnancy. Lab tests to determine renal and liver disease should be obtained.

The baseline frequency of migraine headaches along with apical pulse, respirations, and blood pressure should be obtained. Because migraines may be stress related, a patient's stress level and coping mechanisms should be investigated. The nurse should always assess for hypersensitivity and the usage of other medications. With triptans, patients should not take MAOIs or SSRIs, which cause an increase in effect.

The nurse should assess the patient's neurological status, including LOC, blurred vision, nausea and vomiting, and tingling in extremities. These signs or symptoms may indicate a migraine is beginning. A quiet, calm environment with decreased noise and subdued lighting should be provided, and care should be organized to limit disruptions and decrease neural stimulation. Cold packs can be applied to help lessen the uncomfortable effects of the migraine. The nurse should monitor for possible side effects, including dizziness, drowsiness, vasoconstriction, warming sensations, tingling, lightheadedness, weakness, and neck stiffness. Use with caution during pregnancy or lactation. Sumatriptan (Imitrex) is excreted in breast milk. Advise the patient that the drug could be harmful to the fetus or infant. Contraindications include hypertension, myocardial ischemia/coronary artery disease (CAD), history of myocardial infarction, dysrhythmia or heart failure, high-risk CAD profile, and diabetes, because of the vasoconstriction action of the drugs.

Table 19.4 Antimigraine Drugs

Drug	Route and Adult Dose (max dose where indicated)
Drugs for Terminating Migraines	
Ergotamine Alkaloids	
dihydroergotamine mesylate (D.H.E. 45, Migranal)	IM; 1 mg; may be repeated at 1 hour intervals to a total of 3 mg (max 6 mg/week)
ergotamine tartrate (Ergostat) ergotamine with caffeine (Cafergot, Ercaf, others)	PO; 1–2 mg followed by 1–2 mg every 30 minutes until headache stops (max of 6 mg/day or 10 mg/week)
Triptans	
almotriptan (Axert)	PO; 6.25–12.5 mg, may repeat in 2 hours if necessary (max 2 tabs/day)
eletriptan (Relpax)	PO; 20–40 mg, may repeat in 2 hours if necessary (max 80 mg/day)
frovatriptan (Frova)	PO; 2.5 mg, may repeat in 2 hours if necessary (max 7.5 mg/day)
naratriptan (Amerge)	PO; 1–2.5 mg; may repeat in 4 hours if necessary (max 5 mg/day)
rizatriptan (Maxalt)	PO; 5–10 mg, may repeat in 2 hours if necessary (max 30 mg/day); 5 mg with concurrent propranolol (max 15 mg/day)
sumatriptan (Imitrex)	PO; 25 mg for 1 dose (max 100 mg)
zolmitriptan (Zomig)	PO; 2.5–5 mg; may repeat in 2 hours if necessary (max 10 mg/day)
Drugs for Preventing Migraines	
almotriptan (Axert)	PO; 6-12.5 mg, may repeat in 2 hours if necessary (max 2 tabs/day)
eletriptan (Relpax)	PO; 20-40 mg, may repeat in 2 hours if necessary (max 80 mg/day)
frovatriptan (Frova)	PO; 2.5 mg, may repeat in 2 hours if necessary (max 7.5 mg/day)
Beta-Adrenergic Blockers	
atenolol (Tenormin) (see page 336 for the Prototype Drug box)	PO; 25–50 mg qd (max 100 mg/day)
metoprolol (Lopressor) (see page 341 for the Prototype Drug box)	PO; 50–100 mg qd-bid (max 450 mg/day)
propranolol hydrochloride (Inderal) (see page 307 for the Prototype Drug box)	PO; 80–240 mg qd in divided doses; may need 160–240 mg/day
timolol (Blocadren)	PO; 10 mg bid; may increase to 60 mg/day in 2 divided doses
Calcium Channel Blockers	
nifedipine (Procardia) (see page 270 for the Prototype Drug box)	PO; 10–20 mg tid (max 180 mg/day)
nimodipine (Nimotop)	PO; 60 mg q4h for 21 days, start therapy within 96 hours of subarachnoid hemorrhage
verapamil hydrochloride (Isoptin) (see page 309 for the Prototype Drug box)	PO; 40–80 mg tid (max 360 mg/day)
Tricyclic Antidepressants	
amitryptyline hydrochloride (Elavil)	PO; 75–100 mg/day
imipramine (Tofranil) (see page 178 for the Prototype Drug box)	PO; 75–100 mg/day (max 300 mg/day)
Miscellaneous Agents	
valproic Acid (Depakene, Depakote) (see page 167 for the Prototype Drug box)	P0; 250 mg bid (max 1000 mg/day)
methysergide (Sansert)	PO; 4–8 mg/day in divided doses
riboflavin (vitamin B_2)	As a supplement: PO 5–10 mg/day; for deficiency: 5–30 mg/day PO in divided doses

Pr PROTOTYPE DRUG | SUMATRIPTAN (Imitrex)

ACTIONS AND USES

Sumatriptan belongs to a relatively new group of antimigraine drugs known as the triptans. The triptans act by causing vasoconstriction of cranial arteries; this vasoconstriction is moderately selective and does not usually affect overall blood pressure. This medication is available in oral, intranasal, and SC forms. SC administration terminates migraine attacks in 10 to 20 minutes; the dose may be repeated 60 minutes after the first injection, to a maximum of two doses per day. If taken orally, sumatriptan should be administered as soon as possible after the migraine is suspected or begun.

Administration Alerts

■ Sumatriptan may produce cardiac ischemia in susceptible persons with no previous cardiac events. Healthcare providers may opt to administer the initial dose of sumatriptan in the healthcare setting.

■ Sumatriptan's systemic vasoconstrictor activity may cause hypertension and may result in dysrhythmias or myocardial infarction. Keep resuscitative equipment accessible.

■ Sumatriptan selectively reduces carotid arterial blood flow. Monitor changes in LOC and observe for seizures.

■ Pregnancy category C.

ADVERSE EFFECTS AND INTERACTIONS

Some dizziness, drowsiness, or a warming sensation may be experienced after taking sumatriptan; however, these effects are not normally severe enough to warrant discontinuation of therapy. Because of its vasoconstricting action, the drug should be used cautiously, if at all, in patients with recent myocardial infarction, or with a history of angina pectoris, hypertension, or diabetes.

Sumatriptan interacts with several drugs. For example, an increase effect may occur when taken with MAOIs and SSRIs. Further vasoconstriction can occur when taken with ergot alkaloids and other triptans.

 See the companion website for a Nursing Process Focus specific to this drug.

The ergot alkaloids promote vasoconstriction, which terminates ongoing migraines. Side effects may include nausea, vomiting, weakness in the legs, myalgia, numbness and tingling in fingers and toes, angina-like pain, and tachycardia. Toxicity may be evidenced by constriction of peripheral arteries: cold, pale, numb extremities and muscle pain. Sumatriptan (Imitrex) is metabolized in the liver and excreted by the kidneys; impaired organ function can increase serum drug levels. The patient should be advised and monitored for constant usage because these medications can cause physical dependence.

Patient education regarding drug therapy for migraines should include goals, reasons for obtaining baseline data such as vital signs, laboratory tests and procedures such as computerized tomography or magnetic resonance images of the brain, lumbar puncture for samples of cerebrospinal fluid, and possible drug side effects. Following are teaching points the nurse should include when educating patients regarding the ergot alkaloids:

■ Take dose immediately after onset of symptoms.
■ Control, avoid, or eliminate factors that trigger a headache or migraine, such as fatigue, anxiety, and alcohol.
■ Report the signs of ergot toxicity, which may include muscle pain, numbness and cold extremities.

■ Do not overuse any of these drugs, as physical dependence may result.

See "Nursing Process Focus: Patients Receiving Triptan Therapy" for specific teaching points about this subclass.

NATURAL THERAPIES | Feverfew for Migraines

Feverfew (*Tanacetum parthenium*) is an herb that originated in southeastern Europe and is now found all over Europe, Australia, and North America. The common name feverfew is derived from its antipyretic properties. The leaves contain the active ingredients, the most prevalent of which is a lactone known as parthenolide. Standardization of this herb is based on the percent parthenolide in the product.

Feverfew has an overall spectrum of action resembling that of aspirin. The herb has been shown to exert anti-inflammatory and antispasmodic effects, as well as to inhibit platelet aggregation. Feverfew extract has also been shown to contain a novel type of mast cell inhibitor, which inhibits anti-IgE-induced histamine release. In clinical trials, feverfew was associated with a reduction in number and severity of migraine attacks, as well as a reduction in vomiting. The most common adverse effect is mouth ulceration, which occurs in about 10% of feverfew users.

NURSING PROCESS FOCUS | PATIENTS RECEIVING TRIPTAN THERAPY

ASSESSMENT

Prior to administration:
- Obtain complete health history including allergies, drug history, and possible drug interactions.
- Determine pain and analgesic usage patterns.
- Identify infectious agents or other factors responsible for inflammation or pain.
- Assess level of consciousness before and after administration.

POTENTIAL NURSING DIAGNOSES

- Acute Pain, related to severe headache
- Deficient Knowledge, related to drug therapy
- Ineffective Coping, related to chronic pain
- Ineffective Health Maintenance, related to inability to manage ADLs

PLANNING: PATIENT GOALS AND EXPECTED OUTCOMES

The patient will:
- Report pain relief or a reduction in pain intensity
- Demonstrate an understanding of the drug's action by accurately describing drug side effects and precautions
- Immediately report effects such as shortness of breath, chest tightness or pressure, jaw pain, untoward or worsened rebound headache, seizures or other neurological changes

IMPLEMENTATION

Interventions and (Rationales)	Patient Education/Discharge Planning
Administer the first dose of the medication under supervision.	Instruct patient that the first dose may need to be given under medical supervision, in the event of cardiac side effects. Reassure patient that this is merely a precautionary measure.
Monitor vital signs, especially blood pressure and pulse. (Triptans have vasoconstrictor action.)	Instruct patient to monitor vital signs, especially blood pressure and pulse, ensuring proper use of home equipment.
Observe for changes in severity, character, or duration of headache. (Sudden severe headaches of "thunderclap" quality can signal subarachnoid hemorrhage. Headaches that differ in quality and are accompanied by such signs as fever, rash, or stiff neck may herald meningitis.)	Instruct patient that changes in the character of migraines could signal other potentially more serious disorders. Provide the patient with written materials on warning signs of stroke; discuss other conditions such as meningitis, which may cause headache.
Monitor neurological status; perform neurochecks regularly	Instruct patient: That feeling dizzy or lightheaded can be the result of the drug's action on the CNS, or coronary ischemia • To report episodes of severe dizziness or impending syncope immediately • To review emergency response and safety measures in the event of a seizure
Monitor for possible side effects: dizziness, drowsiness, warming sensation, tingling, lightheadedness, weakness, or neck stiffness due to vasoconstriction. (Such symptoms can result from decreased blood flow to the brain related to reduced carotid arterial blood supply.)	Advise patient: To immediately report side effects to the healthcare provider • Regarding emergent symptoms suggestive of stroke or MI that may require immediate emergency intervention and transport to a hospital
Monitor dietary intake of foods that contain tyramine. (These foods may trigger an acute migraine.)	Instruct patient to avoid or limit foods containing tyramine such as pickled foods, beer, wine, and aged cheeses. Provide patient with a list of tyramine-containing foods.
Monitor kidney and liver function via laboratory tests.	Instruct patient to: Report nausea, vomiting, diarrhea, rash, jaundice, abdominal pain, tenderness, distention, or change in color of stool • Adhere to laboratory testing regimen for liver function as ordered by healthcare provider

continued

EVALUATION OF OUTCOME CRITERIA

Evaluate effectiveness of drug therapy by confirming that patient goals and expected outcomes have been met (see "Planning").

See Table 19.4 under "Triptans" for a list of drugs to which these nursing actions apply.

CHAPTER REVIEW

Key Concepts

The numbered key concepts provide a succinct summary of the important points from the corresponding numbered section within the chapter. If any of these points are not clear, refer to the numbered section within the chapter for review. Expanded versions can be found on the companion website.

19.1 The ways to assess and classify pain include acute or chronic; nociceptor or neuropathic.

19.2 Nonpharmacologic techniques such as massage, biofeedback therapy, and meditation are often important adjuncts to effective pain management.

19.3 Neural mechanisms include the pain transmission via Aδ or C fibers and the release of substance P.

19.4 Opioids are natural or synthetic substances extracted from the poppy plant that exert their effects through interaction with mu and kappa receptors.

19.5 Opioids are the drugs of choice for severe pain. They also have other important therapeutic effects including dampening of the cough reflex and slowing of the motility of the GI tract.

19.6 Opioid antagonists may be used to reverse the symptoms of opioid toxicity or overdose, such as sedation and respiratory depression.

19.7 Opioid withdrawal can result in severe symptoms, and dependence is often treated with methadone maintenance.

19.8 Nonopioid analgesics, such as aspirin, acetaminophen, and the selective COX-2 inhibitors, are effective in treating mild to moderate pain, inflammation, and fever.

19.9 Headaches are classified as tension headaches or migraines. Migraines may be preceded by auras, and symptoms include nausea and vomiting.

19.10 The goals of pharmacotherapy for migraine headaches are to stop migraines in progress and to prevent them from occurring. Triptans, ergot alkaloids, and a number of drugs from other classes are used for migraines.

Review Questions

1. What questions should the nurse ask during an assessment to identify a patient's type of pain? How would the nurse distinguish between acute pain and chronic pain? Which is the most difficult type of pain to treat?

2. What is a nociceptor? Describe how pain is regulated considering substance P and endogenous opioids.

3. Distinguish between the following terms: *opioid, opiate,* and *narcotic.* Name the classes of opioid receptors and identify those that are connected with analgesia. Under what kinds of conditions should opioid drugs be used?

4. Name three common types of disorders controlled by nonopioid analgesics. Which nonopioid analgesic controls fever only? Which control both fever and inflammation?

Critical Thinking Questions

1. A patient is on a PCA (patient-controlled analgesia) pump to manage postoperative pain related to recent orthopedic surgery. The PCA is set to deliver morphine 6 mg per hour basal rate. The nurse discovers the patient to be unresponsive with a respiratory rate of 8 and oxygen saturation of 84%. What is the nurse's initial response? Subsequent actions?

2. A 64-year-old patient has had a longstanding history of migraine headaches as well as coronary artery disease, diabetes mellitus type 2, and hypertension. Upon review of the medical history, the nurse notes that this patient has recently started on sumatriptan (Imitrex), prescribed by the patient's new neurologist. What intervention and/or teaching should be done for this patient?

3. A 58-year-old patient with history of a recent myocardial infarction is on beta-blocking medications and anticoagulant therapy. The patient also has a history of arthritis and during a recent flare-up began taking aspirin, as this medication has helped in the past. What teaching or recommendation would the nurse have for this patient?

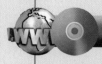

EXPLORE MediaLink

NCLEX review, case studies, and other interactive resources for this chapter can be found on the companion website at www.prenhall.com/adams. Click on "Chapter 19" to select the activities for this chapter. For animations, more NCLEX review questions, and an audio glossary, access the accompanying CD-ROM in this textbook.

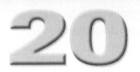
Drugs for Local and General Anesthesia

■ DRUGS AT A GLANCE

LOCAL ANESTHETICS
Amides
Pr *lidocaine (Xylocaine)*
Esters
Miscellaneous agents

GENERAL ANESTHETICS
Inhalation agents
Gasses
Pr *nitrous oxide*
Volatile liquids
Pr *halothane (Fluothane)*

Intravenous agents
Barbiturate and barbiturate-like agents
Pr *thiopental (Pentothal)*
Opioids
Benzodiazepines

ADJUNCTS TO ANESTHESIA
Barbiturate and barbiturate-like agents
Opioids
Neuromuscular blocking agents
Pr *succinylcholine (Anectine)*
Miscellaneous agents

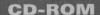

MediaLink www.prenhall.com/adams

CD-ROM
Animation:
   Mechanism in Action: Lidocaine (Xylocaine)
Audio Glossary
NCLEX Review

Companion Website
NCLEX Review
Dosage Calculations
Case Study
Care Plans
Expanded Key Concepts

OBJECTIVES

After reading this chapter, the student should be able to:

1. Compare and contrast the five major clinical techniques for administering local anesthetics.
2. Describe differences between the two major chemical classes of local anesthetics.
3. Explain why epinephrine and sodium hydroxide are sometimes included in local anesthetic cartridges.
4. Identify the actions of general anesthetics on the CNS.
5. Compare and contrast the two primary ways that general anesthesia may be induced.
6. Identify the four stages of general anesthesia.
7. For each of the drug classes listed in Drugs at a Glance, know representative drug examples, explain their mechanism of action, primary actions, and important adverse effects.
8. Categorize drugs used for anesthesia based on their classification and drug action.
9. Use the Nursing Process to care for patients who are receiving anesthesia.

A nesthesia is a medical procedure performed by administering drugs that cause a loss of sensation. Local anesthesia occurs when sensation is lost to a limited part of the body without loss of consciousness. General anesthesia requires differ- ent classes of drugs that cause loss of sensation to the entire body, usually resulting in a loss of consciousness. This chapter will examine drugs used for both local and general anesthesia.

PHARMFACTS | Anesthesia and Anesthetics

- Over 20 million people receive general anesthetics each year in the United States.
- About half of the general anesthetics are administered by a nurse anesthetist.
- The first medical applications of anesthetics were in 1842 with ether and in 1846 with nitrous oxide.
- Herbal products may interact with anesthetics; St. John's wort may intensify or prolong the effects of some opioids and anesthetics.

LOCAL ANESTHESIA

Local anesthesia is loss of sensation to a relatively small part of the body without loss of consciousness to the patient. This technique may be necessary when a relatively brief dental or medical procedure is performed.

20.1 Regional Loss of Sensation Using Local Anesthetics

Although local anesthesia often results in a loss of sensation to a small, limited area, it sometimes affects relatively large portions of the body, such as an entire limb. Because of this, some local anesthetic treatments are more accurately called surface anesthesia or regional anesthesia, depending on how the drugs are administered and their resulting effects.

The five major routes for applying local anesthetics are shown in Figure 20.1. The method employed is dependent upon the location and extent of the desired anesthesia. For example, some local anesthetics are applied topically before a needle stick or minor skin surgery. Others are used to block sensations to large areas such as a limb or the lower abdomen. The different methods of local and regional anesthesia are summarized in Table 20.1.

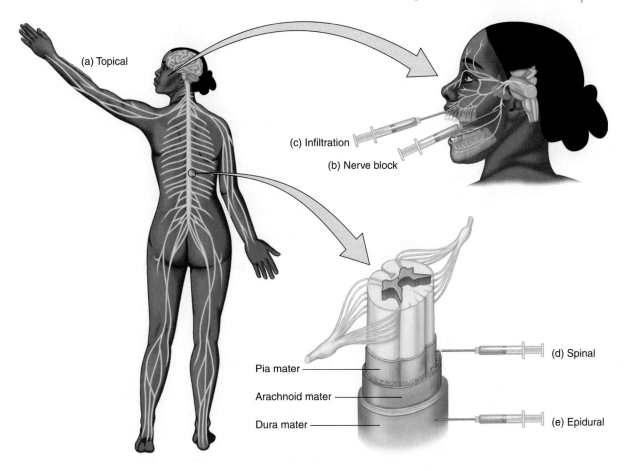

Figure 20.1 | Techniques for applying local anesthesia: (a) topical; (b) nerve block; (c) infiltration; (d) spinal; and (e) epidural

Table 20.1	Methods of Local Anesthetic Administration	
Route	**Formulation/method**	**Description**
topical (surface) anesthesia	creams, sprays, suppositories, drops, and lozenges	applied to mucous membranes including the eyes, lips, gums, nasal membranes, and throat; very safe unless absorbed
infiltration (field block) anesthesia	direct injection into tissue immediate to the surgical site	drug diffuses into tissue to block a specific group of nerves in a small area close to the surgical site
nerve block anesthesia	direct injection into tissue that may be distant from the operation site	drug affects nerve bundles serving the surgical area; used to block sensation in a limb or large area of the face
spinal anesthesia	injection into the cerebral spinal fluid (CSF)	drug affects large, regional area such as the lower abdomen and legs
epidural anesthesia	injection into epidural space of spinal cord	most commonly used in obstetrics during labor and delivery

Local Anesthetics

Local anesthetics are drugs that produce a rapid loss of sensation to a limited part of the body. They produce their therapeutic effect by blocking the entry of sodium ions into neurons.

20.2 Mechanism of Action of Local Anesthetics

The mechanism of action of local anesthetics is well known. Recall that the concentration of sodium ions is normally higher on the outside of neurons than on the inside. A rapid influx of sodium ions into cells is necessary for neurons to fire and conduct an action impulse.

Local anesthetics act by blocking sodium channels, as illustrated in Figure 20.2. Because the blocking of sodium channels is a nonselective process, both sensory and motor impulses are affected. Thus, both sensation and muscle activity will temporarily diminish in the area treated with the local anesthetic. Because of their mechanism of action, local anesthetics are sometimes called sodium channel blockers.

During a medical or surgical procedure, it is essential that the duration of action of the anesthetic last long enough to complete the procedure. Small amounts of epinephrine are sometimes added to the anesthetic solution to constrict blood vessels in the immediate area where the local anesthetic is ap-

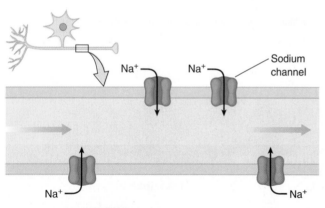

(a) Normal nerve conduction

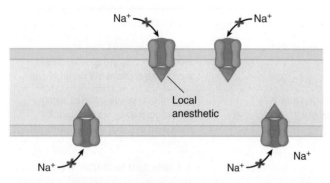

(b) Local anesthetic blocking sodium channels

Figure 20.2 | Mechanism of action of local anesthetics: (a) normal nerve conduction; (b) local anesthetic blocking sodium channels

NATURAL THERAPIES — **Cloves and Anise as Natural Dental Remedies**

One natural remedy for tooth pain is oil of cloves. Extracted from the plant *Eugenia*, eugenol is the chemical extract found in cloves thought to produce its numbing effect. It works especially well for cavities. The herb is applied by soaking a piece of cotton and packing it around the gums close to the painful area. Dentists sometimes recommend it for temporary relief of a toothache. Clove oil has an antiseptic effect that has been reported to kill bacteria, fungi, and helminths.

Another natural remedy is oil of anise, scientific name *Pimpinella*, for jaw pain caused by nerve pressure or gritting of teeth. Anise oil is an antispasmodic agent, which means it relaxes intense muscular pressure around the jaw angle, cheeks, and throat area. It has extra benefits in that it is also a natural expectorant, cough suppressant, and breath freshener. The pharmacologic effects of anise are thought to be due to the chemical anethole, which is similar in structure to natural catecholamines.

plied. This keeps the anesthetic in the area longer, thus extending the duration of action of the drug. The addition of epinephrine to lidocaine (Xylocaine), for example, increases the duration of its local anesthetic effect from 20 minutes to as long as 60 minutes. This is important for dental or surgical procedures that take longer than 20 minutes; otherwise, a second injection of the anesthetic would be necessary.

Sodium hydroxide is sometimes added to anesthetic solutions to increase the effectiveness of the anesthetic in regions that have extensive local infection or abscesses. Bacteria tend to acidify an infected site, and local anesthetics are less effective in an acidic environment. Adding alkaline substances such as sodium hydroxide or sodium bicarbonate neutralizes the region and creates a more favorable environment for the anesthetic.

20.3 Classification of Local Anesthetics

Local anesthetics are classified by their chemical structures; the two major classes are **esters** and **amides** (Table 20.2). The terms ester and amide refer to types of chemical linkages found within the anesthetic molecules, as illustrated in Figure 20.3. Although esters and amides have equal efficacy, important differences exist. A small number of miscellaneous agents are neither esters nor amides.

Cocaine was the first local anesthetic widely used for medical procedures. Cocaine is a natural ester, found in the leaves of the plant *Erythroxylon coca*, native to the Andes Mountains of Peru. As late as the 1880s, cocaine was routinely used for eye surgery, nerve blocks, and spinal anesthesia. Although still available for local anesthesia, cocaine is a Schedule II drug and rarely used therapeutically in the United States. The abuse potential of cocaine is discussed in Chapter 12 ⊝.

Another ester, procaine (Novocain), was the drug of choice for dental procedures from the mid-1900s until the

Table 20.2	Selected Local Anesthetics
Chemical Classification	**Drug**
esters	benzocaine (Americaine, Solarcaine, others)
	chloroprocaine (Nesacaine)
	cocaine
	procaine (Novocain)
	tetracaine (Pontocaine)
amides	articaine (Septodont)
	bupivacaine (Marcaine)
	dibucaine (Nupercaine, Nupercainal)
	etidocaine (Duranest)
	levobupivacaine (Chirocaine)
	lidocaine (Xylocaine)
	mepivacaine (Carbocaine)
	prilocaine (Citanest)
	ropivacaine (Naropin)
miscellaneous agents	dyclonine (Dyclone)
	pramoxine (Tronothane)

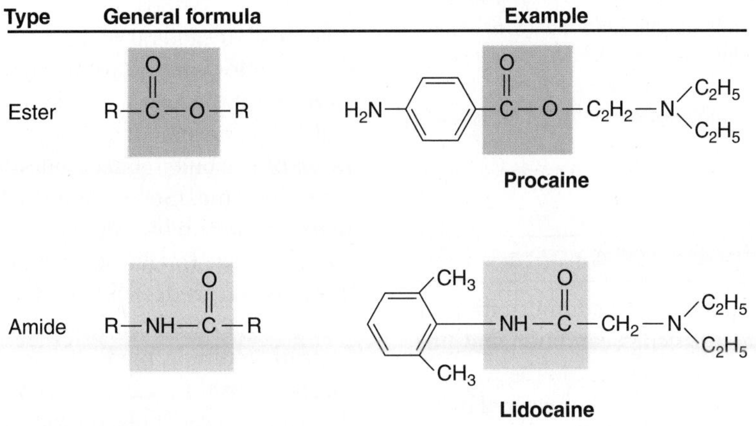

Figure 20.3 | Chemical structures of ester and amide local anesthetics

1960s, until the development of the amide anesthetics led to a significant decline in the use of the drug. One ester, benzocaine (Solarcaine, others) is used as a topical, OTC agent for treating a large number of painful conditions, including sunburn, insect bites, hemorrhoids, sore throat, and minor wounds.

Amides have largely replaced the esters because they produce fewer side effects and generally have a longer duration of action. Lidocaine (Xylocaine) is the most widely used amide for short surgical procedures requiring local anesthesia.

Adverse effects to local anesthetics are uncommon. Allergy is rare. When it does occur, it is often due to sulfites, which are added as preservatives to prolong the shelf life of the anesthetic, or to methylparaben, which may be added to retard bacterial growth in anesthetic solutions. Early signs of adverse effects of local anesthetics include symptoms of CNS stimulation such as restlessness or anxiety. Later effects, such as drowsiness and unresponsiveness, are due to CNS depression. Cardiovascular effects, including hypotension and dysrhythmias, are possible. Patients with a history of cardiovascular disease are often given forms of local anesthetics that contain no epinephrine in order to reduce the potential effects of this sympathomimetic on the heart and blood pressure. CNS and cardiovascular side effects are not expected unless the local anesthetic is absorbed rapidly or is accidentally injected directly into a blood vessel.

SPECIAL CONSIDERATIONS

Effects of Anesthesia on Children and the Elderly

Children are usually more sensitive to anesthesia than adults, because their body systems are not fully developed. Therefore, medication dosages used must be carefully calculated. Some drugs used for anesthesia, such as neuromuscular blockers, are not recommended for use by children under the age of 2 years.

Nurses should also understand that children who are undergoing surgery have fears and concerns about surgery and anesthesia. A child's age and developmental level play a role in his or her thoughts about receiving anesthesia. Children under the age of 1 year are usually not concerned about what will be happening and will easily separate from family members. Fear of needles, the unknown, and being separated from primary caregivers begins to happen during the toddler stage and continues throughout childhood. Children are often perceptive to the anxieties of their parents, therefore it is imperative that caregivers remain calm. Holding the child through induction of anesthesia might help alleviate fears. Local anesthetic creams can be rubbed on the skin to remove the pain of needles.

The elderly are also more affected by anesthesia than younger adults. Because of the changes in drug metabolism that occur with advancing age, these patients are particularly sensitive to the effects of barbiturate and general anesthetics. This increases the chance of side effects, therefore elderly patients should be monitored closely. The elderly are also especially sensitive to the effects of local anesthetics. Sedative-hypnotic drugs used preoperatively may cause increased confusion or excitement in the elderly.

NURSING CONSIDERATIONS

The role of the nurse in local anesthetic administration involves careful monitoring of a patient's condition and providing education as it relates to the prescribed drug regimen. Although these medications are usually administered by the physician to anesthetize an area for medical procedures, the nurse often assists. The nurse's role may include preparing the area to be anesthetized, and monitoring the effectiveness of the medication by assessing pain and comfort levels. The nurse should check for the presence of broken skin, infection, burns, and wounds at the site of anesthetic administration.

Contraindications for these drugs include hypersensitivity to local anesthetics; sepsis and blood dyscrasias; untreated sinus bradycardia; and severe degrees of atrioventricular, sinoatrial, and intraventricular heart block in the absence of a pacemaker. Local anesthetics should be used with caution over large body areas, in patients with extensive surface trauma, and in severe skin disorders because the medication may be absorbed and result in systemic effects. Unless specifically formulated for optic use, local anesthetics should not be used on the eyes.

Although adverse reactions are rare, patients should be monitored for cardiac palpitations and difficulty breathing or swallowing. The nurse should assess vital signs during the procedure and report any changes immediately. The patient should be monitored for reactions such as irritation, rash, and signs of CNS excitation such as restlessness or anxiety.

Patients should be instructed to use benzocaine (Solarcaine, others) cautiously on inflamed skin or mucous membranes as it may increase irritation. Lidocaine viscous is used to anesthetize the throat for some procedures, such as those that require that an endoscope be passed down the throat. After such procedures, the patient should be monitored for return of the gag reflex before drinking water or eating. Advise patients to wait at least 1 hour before eating.

GENERAL ANESTHESIA

General anesthesia is a loss of sensation occurring throughout the entire body, accompanied by a loss of consciousness. General anesthetics are applied when it is necessary for patients to remain still and without pain for a longer period of time than could be achieved with local anesthetics.

20.4 Characteristics of General Anesthesia

The goal of general anesthesia is to provide a rapid and complete loss of sensation. Signs of general anesthesia include total analgesia and loss of consciousness, memory, and body movement. Although these signs are similar to those of sleeping, general anesthesia and sleep are not exactly the same. General anesthetics depress all nervous activity in the brain, whereas sleeping depresses only very specific areas. In fact, some brain activity actually increases during sleep, as described in Chapter 14 ⚭ .

General anesthesia is rarely achieved with a single drug. Instead, multiple medications are used to rapidly induce unconsciousness, cause muscle relaxation, and maintain deep anesthesia. This approach, called balanced anesthesia, allows the dose of inhalation anesthetic to be lower, thus making the procedure safer for the patient.

General anesthesia is a progressive process that occurs in distinct phases. The most efficacious medications can quickly induce all four stages, whereas others are only able to induce stage 1. Stage 3 is where most major surgery occurs; thus it is called surgical anesthesia. When seeking surgical anesthesia, it is desirable to progress through stage 2 as rapidly as possible, as this stage produces distressing symptoms. These stages are shown in Table 20.3 on page 249.

General Anesthetics

General anesthetics are drugs that rapidly produce unconsciousness and total analgesia. These drugs are usually administered by the IV or inhalation routes. To supplement the effects of a general anesthetic, adjunct drugs are given before, during, and after surgery.

PROTOTYPE DRUG | LIDOCAINE (Xylocaine)

ACTIONS AND USES

Lidocaine, the most frequently used injectable local anesthetic, acts by blocking neuronal pain impulses. It is injected as a nerve block, for spinal and epidural anesthesia. Its actions are achieved by blocking sodium channels located within the membranes of neurons.

Lidocaine may be given IV, IM, or SC to treat dysrhythmias, as discussed in Chapter 23 ⊃⊃ . A topical form is also available. Lidocaine is pregnancy category B.

Administration Alerts

■ Solutions of lidocaine containing preservatives or epinephrine are intended for local anesthesia only, and must never be given parenterally for dysrhythmias.

■ Topical lidocaine should not be applied to large skin areas or to broken or abraded areas, as significant absorption may occur. It should also not be allowed to come in contact with the eyes.

■ For spinal or epidural block, use only preparations specifically labeled for IV use.

ADVERSE EFFECTS AND INTERACTIONS

When used for anesthesia, side effects are uncommon. An early symptom of toxicity is CNS excitement, leading to irritability and confusion. Serious adverse effects include convulsions, respiratory depression, and cardiac arrest. Until the effect of the anesthetic diminishes, patients may injure themselves by biting or chewing areas of the mouth that have no sensation following a dental procedure.

Barbiturates may decrease activity of lidocaine. Increased effects of lidocaine occur if taken concurrently with cimetidine, quinidine, and beta blockers. If lidocaine is used on a regular basis, its effectiveness may diminish when used with other medication.

 See the companion website for a Nursing Process Focus specific to this drug.

20.5 Pharmacotherapy with Inhaled General Anesthetics

There are two primary methods of inducing general anesthesia. Intravenous agents are usually administered first because they act within a few seconds. After the patient loses consciousness, inhaled agents are used to maintain the anesthesia. During short surgical procedures or those requiring lower stages of anesthesia, the IV agents may be used alone.

Inhaled general anesthetics, shown in Table 20.4, may be gasses or volatile liquids. These agents produce their effects by preventing the flow of sodium into neurons in the CNS, thus delaying nerve impulses and producing a dramatic reduction in neural activity. The exact mechanism for how this occurs is not exactly known, although it is likely that GABA receptors in the brain are activated. It is not the same mechanism as is known for local anesthetics. There is some evidence suggesting that the mechanism may be related to how some antiseizure drugs work; however, this is still not conclusive. There is not a specific receptor that binds to general anesthetics, and they do not seem to affect neurotransmitter release.

Gaseous General Anesthetics

The only gas used routinely for anesthesia is nitrous oxide, commonly called laughing gas. Nitrous oxide is used for dental procedures and for brief obstetrical and surgical procedures. It may also be used in conjunction with other general anesthetics, making it possible to decrease their dosages with greater effectiveness.

Nitrous oxide should be used cautiously in myasthenia gravis, as it may cause respiratory depression and prolonged hypnotic effects. Patients with cardiovascular disease, especially those with increased intracranial pressure, should be monitored carefully because the hypnotic effects of the drug may be prolonged or potentiated.

NURSING CONSIDERATIONS

Nitrous oxide has a rapid onset and recovery with minimal side effects (e.g., nausea and vomiting). The nurse's responsibilities are to determine knowledge level of the patient and to reassure the patient to alleviate anxiety. Postoperatively, the nurse should monitor the patient's LOC, vital signs, and pain level and give medication to prevent nausea and vomiting. See "Nursing Process Focus: Patients Receiving General Anesthesia" on page 252 for more information, including specific teaching points.

Volatile Liquid General Anesthetics

The volatile anesthetics are liquid at room temperature, but are converted into a vapor and inhaled to produce their anesthetic effects. Commonly administered volatile agents are halothane (Fluothane), enflurane (Ethrane), and isoflurane (Forane). The most potent of these is halothane (Fluothane). Some general anesthetics enhance the sensitivity of the heart to drugs such as epinephrine, norepinephrine, dopamine, and serotonin. Most volatile liquids depress cardiovascular and respiratory function. Because it has less effect on the heart and does not damage the liver,

NURSING PROCESS FOCUS | **PATIENTS RECEIVING LOCAL ANESTHESIA**

ASSESSMENT

Prior to administration:
- Assess for allergies to amide-type local anesthetics.
- Check for the presence of broken skin, infection, burns, and wounds where medication is to be applied.
- Assess for character, duration, location, and intensity of pain where medication is to be applied.

POTENTIAL NURSING DIAGNOSES

- Risk for Aspiration
- Risk for Injury
- Deficient Knowledge, related to drug use

PLANNING: PATIENT GOALS AND EXPECTED OUTCOMES

The patient will:
- Experience no pain during surgical procedure
- Experience no side effects or adverse reactions to anesthesia

IMPLEMENTATION

Interventions and (Rationales)	*Patient Education/Discharge Planning*
Monitor for cardiovascular side effects. (These may occur if anesthetic is absorbed.)	Instruct patient to report any unusual heart palpitations. If using medication on a regular basis, instruct patient to see a healthcare provider regularly.
Monitor skin or mucous membranes for infection or inflammation. (Condition could be worsened by drug.)	Instruct patient to report irritation or increase in discomfort in areas where medication is used.
Monitor for length of effectiveness. (Local anesthetics are effective for 1 to 3 hours.)	Instruct patient to report any discomfort during procedure.
Obtain information and monitor use of other medications.	Instruct patient to report use of any medication to healthcare provider.
Provide for patient safety. (There is a potential for injury related to area being treated having a lack of sensation.)	Inform patient about having no feeling in anesthetized area and taking extra caution to avoid injury, including heat-related injury.
Monitor for gag reflex. (Xylocaine viscous may interfere with swallowing reflex.)	Instruct patient to: - Not eat within 1 hour of administration - Not chew gum while any portion of mouth or throat is anesthetized to prevent biting injuries

EVALUATION OF OUTCOME CRITERIA

Evaluate the effectiveness of drug therapy by confirming that patient goals and expected outcomes have been met (see "Planning").

See Table 20.2 for a list of drugs to which these nursing actions apply.

isoflurane (Forane) has become the most widely used inhalation anesthetic. The volatile liquids are excreted almost entirely by the lungs, through exhalation.

NURSING CONSIDERATIONS

General anesthesia is primarily used for lengthy surgical procedures, and involves significant risks. The patient should be informed that anesthesia will be administered by highly trained personnel, either an anesthesiologist or a nurse anesthetist, and that the nurse will have a major role in monitoring the patient and ensuring patient safety. A comprehensive assessment must be done in each phase of surgical experience. General preoperative information should be obtained such as vital signs, lab tests, health history, level of knowledge concerning procedure, and the presence of anxiety. Preoperatively, the patient should be assessed for the use of alcohol or other CNS

Table 20.3	Stages of General Anesthesia
Stage	**Characteristics**
1	Loss of pain: The patient loses general sensation but may be awake. This stage proceeds until the patient loses consciousness.
2	Excitement and hyperactivity: The patient may be delirious and try to resist treatment. Heart rate and breathing may become irregular and blood pressure can increase. IV agents are administered here to calm the patient.
3	Surgical anesthesia: Skeletal muscles become relaxed and delirium stabilizes. Cardiovascular and breathing activities stabilize. Eye movements slow and the patient becomes still. Surgery begins here and remains until the procedure ends.
4	Paralysis of the medulla region in the brain (responsible for controlling respiratory and cardiovascular activity): If breathing or the heart stops, death could result. This stage is usually avoided during general anesthesia.

Table 20.4	Inhaled General Anesthetics
Type	**Drug**
Volatile liquid	desflurane (Suprane)
	enflurane (Ethrane)
	ⓟ halothane (Fluothane)
	isoflurane (Forane)
	methoxyflurane (Penthrane)
	sevoflurane (Ultane)
Gas	ⓟ nitrous oxide

ⓟ PROTOTYPE DRUG | NITROUS OXIDE

ACTIONS AND USES

The main action of nitrous oxide is analgesia caused by suppression of pain mechanisms in the CNS. This agent has a low potency and does not produce complete loss of consciousness or profound relaxation of skeletal muscle. Because nitrous oxide does not induce surgical anesthesia (stage 3), it is commonly combined with other surgical anesthetic agents. Nitrous oxide is ideal for dental procedures because the patient remains conscious and can follow instructions while experiencing full analgesia.

Administration Alert

Establish an IV if one is not already in place in case emergency medications are needed.

ADVERSE EFFECTS

When used in low to moderate doses, nitrous oxide produces few adverse effects. At higher doses, patients exhibit some adverse signs of stage 2 anesthesia such as anxiety, excitement, and combativeness. Lowering the inhaled dose will quickly reverse these adverse effects. As nitrous oxide is exhaled, the patient may temporarily have some difficulty breathing at the end of a procedure. Nausea and vomiting following the procedure are more common with nitrous oxide than with other inhalation anesthetics. Nitrous oxide has the potential to be abused by users (sometimes medical personnel) who enjoy the relaxed, sedated state that the drug produces.

 See the companion website for a Nursing Process Focus specific to this drug.

depressants within the previous 24 hours, as these products will enhance anesthetic effects. Information concerning the use of other medications should also be obtained.

Use of halothane (Fluothane) is contraindicated in patients who have had this drug within the previous 14 to 21 days, as it can cause halothane hepatitis if used frequently.

Use of halothane is also contraindicated in pregnancy (category D) and in patients with diminished hepatic functioning, as it can be hepatotoxic. Caution should be used in patients with cardiac conditions, especially bradycardia and dysrhythmias, as the medication decreases blood pressure and sensitizes the myocardium to catecholamines, which can lead to serious dysrhythmias.

Pr PROTOTYPE DRUG | HALOTHANE (Fluothane)

ACTIONS AND USES

Halothane produces a potent level of surgical anesthesia that is rapid in onset. Although potent, halothane does not produce as much muscle relaxation or analgesia as other volatile anesthetics. Therefore, halothane is primarily used with other anesthetic agents including muscle relaxants and analgesics. Nitrous oxide is sometimes combined with halothane. Patients recover from anesthesia rapidly after halothane is discontinued.

ADVERSE EFFECTS AND INTERACTIONS

Halothane moderately sensitizes the heart muscle to epinephrine; therefore, dysrhythmias are a concern. This agent lowers blood pressure and the respiration rate. It also abolishes reflex mechanisms that normally keep the contents of the stomach from entering into the lungs. Because of potential hepatotoxicity, use of halothane has declined.

Malignant hyperthermia is rare, but can be a fatal adverse effect triggered by all inhalation anesthetics. It causes muscle rigidity and severe temperature elevation (up to 43°C). This risk is greatest when halothane is used with succinylcholine.

Levodopa taken concurrently increases the level of dopamine in the CNS, and should be discontinued 6 to 8 hours before halothane administration.

Skeletal muscle weakness, respiratory depression, or apnea may occur if halothane is administered concurrently with polymyxins, lincomycin, or aminoglycosides.

 See the companion website for a Nursing Process Focus specific to this drug.

In the immediate postoperative period, the nurse should monitor the patient for side effects of the general anesthesia such as nausea and vomiting, CNS depression, respiratory difficulty, vital sign changes, and complications related to the procedure such as bleeding or impeding shock.

See "Nursing Process Focus: Patients Receiving General Anesthesia" for more details, including patient teaching points.

IV Anesthetics

20.6 Pharmacotherapy with IV Anesthetics

Intravenous anesthetics, shown in Table 20.5, are important supplements to general anesthesia. Although occasionally used alone, they are often administered with inhaled general anesthetics. Concurrent administration of IV and inhaled anesthetics allows the dose of the inhaled agent to be reduced, thus lowering the potential for serious side effects. Furthermore, when combined, they provide additional analgesia and muscle relaxation than could be provided by the inhaled anesthetic alone. When IV anesthetics are administered without other anesthetics, they are generally reserved for medical procedures that take less than 15 minutes.

Drugs employed as IV anesthetics include barbiturates, opioids, and benzodiazepines. Opioids offer the advantage of superior analgesia. Combining the opioid fentanyl (Sublimaze) with the antipsychotic agent droperidol (Inapsine) produces a state known as **neurolept analgesia**. In this state, patients are conscious, though insensitive to pain and unconnected with surroundings. The premixed combination of these two agents is marketed as Innovar. A similar conscious, dissociated state is produced with ketamine (Ketalar).

NURSING CONSIDERATIONS

The role of the nurse in drug therapy with IV anesthetics involves careful monitoring of a patient's condition and providing education as it relates to the anesthetic in use. IV sedation is used to decrease anxiety and fear secondary to confinement of the mask used for inhalation anesthesia. A thorough, complete assessment must be completed prior to selecting an anesthetic or combination of anesthetics. Patients may be given medications other than anesthesia during preoperative, perioperative, or postoperative periods, including antianxiety agents, sedatives, analgesics, opioids, and anticholinergics. The nurse should obtain a complete medical history from the patient. IV anesthetics are contraindicated in patients with drug sensitivity, as allergic reactions can result, ranging from hives to respiratory arrest. Because they are administered intravenously, suitability of an IV access site should be assessed.

Patients with cardiovascular disease should be monitored carefully, as IV anesthetics can cause depression of the myocardium leading to dysrhythmias. Patients with respiratory disorders should also be monitored carefully, because respiratory depression may result in high levels of anesthetic in the blood. Thiopental (Pentothal) should be used with caution in patients with seizure disorders, increased intracranial pressure, neurologic disorders, and myxedema.

The use of general anesthetics brings CNS depression. During the postoperative period, the nurse should monitor the patient for vital sign changes, hallucinations, confusion, and excitability. Other side effects or reactions that should be assessed include respiratory difficulties, shiver-

Table 20.5	Intravenous Anesthetics
Chemical Classification	**Drug**
barbiturate and barbiturate-like agents	etomidate (Amidate)
	methohexital sodium (Brevital)
	propofol (Diprivan)
	Pr thiopental sodium (Pentothal)
benzodiazepines	diazepam (Valium)
	lorazepam (Ativan)
	midazolam hydrochloride (Versed)
opioids	alfentanil hydrochloride (Alfenta)
	fentanyl citrate (Sublimaze, others)
	remifentanil hydrochloride (Ultiva)
	sufentanil citrate (Sufenta)
others	ketamine (Ketalar)

Pr PROTOTYPE DRUG | THIOPENTAL (Pentothal)

ACTIONS AND USES

Thiopental is the oldest IV anesthetic. It is used for brief medical procedures or to rapidly induce unconsciousness prior to administering inhaled anesthetics. It is classified as an ultrashort-acting barbiturate, having an onset time of less than 30 seconds and a duration of only 10 to 30 minutes. Unlike some anesthetic agents, it has very low analgesic properties.

Administration Alert

Pregnancy category C.

ADVERSE EFFECTS AND INTERACTIONS

Like other barbiturates, thiopental can produce severe respiratory depression when used in high doses. It is used with caution in patients with cardiovascular disease because of its ability to depress the myocardium and cause dysrhythmias. Patients may experience emergence delirium postoperatively. This causes hallucinations, confusion, and excitability.

Thiopental interacts with many other drugs. For example, use of CNS depressants potentiate respiratory and CNS depression. Phenothiazines increase the risk of hypotension. Use with caution with herbal supplements, such as kava and valerian, which may potentiate sedation.

 See the companion website for a Nursing Process Focus specific to this drug.

ing and trembling, nausea or vomiting, headache, and somnolence. Preoperative teaching is vital to understanding the anesthetic and the entire surgical experience. It also helps allay fears and anxiety of the patients and caregivers. See "Nursing Process Focus: Patients Receiving General Anesthesia" for specific teaching points.

20.7 Nonanesthetic Drugs as Adjuncts to Surgery

A number of drugs are used either to complement the effects of general anesthetics or to treat anticipated side effects of the anesthesia. These agents, shown in Table 20.6, are called adjuncts to anesthesia. They may be given prior to, during, or after surgery.

The preoperative drugs given to relieve anxiety and to provide mild sedation include barbiturates or benzodiazepines. Opioids such as morphine may be given to counteract pain that the patient will experience after surgery. Anticholinergics such as atropine may be administered to dry secretions and to suppress the bradycardia caused by some anesthetics.

During surgery, the primary adjuncts are the neuromuscular blockers. So that surgical procedures can be carried out safely, it is necessary to administer drugs that cause skeletal muscles to totally relax. Administration of these drugs also allows the amount of anesthetic to be reduced. Neuromuscular blocking agents are classified as depolarizing blockers or nondepolarizing blockers. The only depolarizing blocker is succinylcholine (Anectine), which works by binding to acetylcholine receptors at neuromuscular junctions to cause total skeletal muscle relaxation. Succinylcholine is used in surgery for ease of tracheal intubation. Mivacurium (Mivacron) is the shortest acting of the nondepolarizing blockers, whereas tubocurarine is a longer acting neuromuscular blocking agent. The nondepolarizing

NURSING PROCESS FOCUS | PATIENTS RECEIVING GENERAL ANESTHESIA

ASSESSMENT

Prior to administration:
- Obtain complete health history including allergies, drug history, and possible drug interactions.
- Assess for presence/history of severe respiratory, cardiac, renal, or liver disorders.
- Obtain baseline vital signs.
- Obtain blood work: complete blood count and chemistry panel.
- Assess patient's knowledge of procedure and level of anxiety.

POTENTIAL NURSING DIAGNOSES

- Anxiety, related to surgical procedure
- Impaired Gas Exchange
- Deficient Knowledge, related to drug use
- Nausea, related to drug side effect
- Disturbed Sensory Perception
- Ineffective Breathing Pattern
- Decreased Cardiac Output

PLANNING: PATIENT GOALS AND EXPECTED OUTCOMES

The patient will:
- Experience adequate anesthesia during surgical procedure
- Experience no side effects or adverse reaction to anesthesia
- Demonstrate an understanding of perioperative procedures

IMPLEMENTATION

Interventions and (Rationales)	*Patient Education/Discharge Planning*
■ Preoperatively, assess knowledge level of pre- and postoperative procedures. Ensure that patient has accurate information and questions are answered. (Teaching will reduce patient anxiety.)	■ Give pre- and postoperative instructions. ■ Explain what the patient will see, hear, and feel prior to surgery. ■ Explain the recovery room process. ■ Explain what the patient and family will see and hear postoperatively. ■ Take patient on tour of operative facilities, if possible.
■ Preoperatively, assess emotional state. (Patients who are fearful or extremely anxious may be more difficult to induce and maintain under anesthesia.)	■ Instruct patient about using stress-reduction techniques such as deep breathing, imagery, and distraction.
■ Monitor preoperative status.	Instruct patient to: ■ Remain NPO as ordered prior to surgery to prevent risk of aspiration, nausea, and vomiting ■ Stop taking medications 24 hours prior to surgery as ordered by healthcare provider ■ Refrain from alcohol 24 hours prior to surgery
■ Postoperatively, monitor for respiratory difficulty and adequate O_2-CO_2 exchange. (Anesthetics cause respiratory depression.)	■ Inform patient to report shortness of breath, difficulty breathing, or dizziness.
■ Monitor recovery from anesthesia. Evaluate LOC, nausea, vomiting, and pain.	■ Instruct patient about possible side effects and to report any discomfort immediately.
■ Monitor vital signs. (Respiratory status may be impaired leading to prolonged apnea, respiratory depression, and cyanosis. Blood pressure may drop to shock levels.)	■ Advise patient to report heart palpitations, dizziness, difficulty breathing, or faintness.

EVALUATION OF OUTCOME CRITERIA

Evaluate the effectiveness of drug therapy by confirming that patient goals and expected outcomes have been met (see "Planning").

⊂⊃ See Tables 20.4 and 20.5 for lists of drugs to which these nursing actions apply.

Table 20.6	Selected Adjuncts to Anesthesia
Chemical Classification	**Drug**
barbiturate and barbiturate-like agents	amobarbital (Amytal)
	butabarbital sodium (Butisol)
	pentobarbital (Nembutal)
	secobarbital (Seconal)
opioids	alfentanil hydrochloride (Alfenta)
	fentanyl citrate (Duragesic, Actiq, others)
	fentanyl/droperidol (Innovar)
	remifentanil hydrochloride (Ultiva)
	sufentanil citrate (Sufenta)
miscellaneous agents	bethanechol chloride (Duvoid, Urabeth, Urecholine): anticholinergic
	droperidol (Inapsine): dopamine blocker
	promethazine (Phenazine, Phenergan, others):
	dopamine blocker
	⬦ succinylcholine chloride (Anectine, Quelicin, Sucostrin): neuromuscular blocker
	tubocurarine: neuromuscular blocker

blockers cause muscle paralysis by competing with acetylcholine for cholinergic receptors at neuromuscular junctions. Once on the receptor, the nonpolarizing blockers prevent muscle contraction.

Postoperative drugs include analgesics for pain and antiemetics such as promethazine (Phenergan, others) for the nausea and vomiting that sometimes occur during recovery from the anesthetic. Occasionally a parasympathomimetic such as bethanechol (Urecholine) is administered to stimulate the smooth muscle of the bowel and the urinary tract to begin peristalsis following surgery.

NURSING CONSIDERATIONS

The role of the nurse in neuromusclar blocker therapy involves careful monitoring of a patient's condition and providing education as it relates to the prescribed anesthetic. Neuromuscular blocking agents are used so that the patient experiences complete skeletal muscle relaxation during the surgical procedure. Continuous use is not recommended because of potential side effects. Patients should be aware that these drugs are used only in a controlled acute care setting, usually surgery, by a skilled professional.

In preparation for use of succinylcholine (Anectine), the nurse should assess for the presence/history of hepatic or renal dysfunction, neuromuscular disease, fractures, myasthenia gravis, malignant hyperthermia, glaucoma, and penetrating eye injuries. Use of this drug is contraindicated with these conditions. Use in children under 2 years is contraindicated because it can cause dysrhythmias and malignant hyperthermia.

Mivacurium (Mivacron) is used for intubation and is contraindicated for persons with renal or hepatic disease, fluid and electrolyte imbalances, neuromuscular disorders, respiratory disease, and obesity. It should be used cautiously in the elderly and children. It should not be used during pregnancy or lactation. An anesthesiologist may administer it during cesarean section.

Prior to use of any neuromuscular blocker, the nurse should assess physical status to rule out potential expected problems including vital signs, reflexes, muscle tone and response, pupil size and reactivity, EKG, lung sounds, bowel sounds, affect, and LOC. The nurse should monitor for a decrease in blood pressure, tachycardia, prolonged apnea, bronchospasm, respiratory depression, paralysis, and hypersensitivity.

PROTOTYPE DRUG   SUCCINYLCHOLINE (Anectine)

ACTIONS AND USES

Like the natural neurotransmitter acetylcholine, succinylcholine acts on cholinergic receptor sites at neuromuscular junctions. At first, depolarization occurs and skeletal muscles contract. After repeated contractions, however, the membrane is unable to repolarize as long as the drug stays on the receptor. Effects are first noted as muscle weakness and muscle spasms. Eventually paralysis occurs. Succinylcholine is rapidly broken down by the enzyme pseudocholinesterase; when the IV infusion is stopped, the duration of action is only a few minutes. Use of succinylcholine reduces the amount of general anesthetic needed for procedures.

Administration Alert

Pregnancy category C.

ADVERSE EFFECTS AND INTERACTIONS

Succinylcholine can cause complete paralysis of the diaphragm and intercostal muscles, thus mechanical ventilation is necessary during surgery. Bradycardia and respiratory depression are expected adverse effects. If doses are high, the ganglia are affected causing tachycardia, hypotension, and urinary retention. Patients with certain genetic defects may experience rapid onset of extremely high fever with muscle rigidity may occur—a serious condition known as malignant hyperthermia.

Additive skeletal muscle blockade will occur if succinylcholine is given concurrently with clindamycin, aminoglycosides, furosemide, lithium, quinidine, or lidocaine.

Increased effect of succinylcholine may occur if given concurrently with phenothiazines, oxytocin, promazine, tacrine, or thiazide diuretics. Decreased effect of succinylcholine occurs if given with diazepam.

If this drug is given concurrently with halothane or nitrous oxide, an increased risk of bradycardia, dysrhythmias, sinus arrest, apnea, and malignant hyperthermia exists. If succinylcholine is given concurrently with cardiac glycosides there is increased risk of cardiac dysrhythmias. If narcotics are given concurrently with succinylcholine, there is increased risk of bradycardia and sinus arrest.

 See the companion website for a Nursing Process Focus specific to this drug.

CHAPTER REVIEW

Key Concepts

The numbered key concepts provide a succinct summary of the important points from the corresponding numbered section within the chapter. If any of these points are not clear, refer to the numbered section within the chapter for review. Expanded versions can be found on the companion website.

20.1 Regional loss of sensation is achieved by administering local anesthetics topically or through the infiltration, nerve block, spinal, or epidural routes.

20.2 Local anesthetics act by blocking sodium channels in neurons. Epinephrine is sometimes added to prolong the duration of anesthetic action.

20.3 Local anesthetics are classified as amides or esters. The amides, such as lidocaine (Xylocaine), have generally replaced the esters due to their greater safety.

20.4 General anesthesia produces a complete loss of sensation accompanied by loss of consciousness. This is usually achieved through the use of multiple medications.

20.5 Inhaled general anesthetics are used to maintain surgical anesthesia. Some such as nitrous oxide have low efficacy while others such as halothane (Fluothane) can induce deep anesthesia.

20.6 IV anesthetics are used either alone, for short procedures, or to supplement inhalation anesthetics.

20.7 Numerous nonanesthetic medications, including opioids, antianxiety agents, barbiturates, and neuromuscular blockers, are administered as adjuncts to surgery.

Review Questions

1. What is local anesthesia? Name the five general methods of local and regional anesthesia.

2. How does a local anesthetic work? How does the anesthetic action of lidocaine with epinephrine differ from that of lidocaine without epinephrine?

3. What is the role of IV anesthetics in surgical anesthesia? Why are these drugs not used alone for general anesthesia?

4. What role do adjunct medications serve in anesthesia?

Critical Thinking Questions

1. An elderly patient requires local anesthesia for a 3 cm laceration to the distal fourth metacarpal of the left hand. The healthcare provider requests lidocaine (Xylocaine) 1% with epinephrine. What is the nurse's response?

2. A patient who has a history of heart failure is on digoxin (Lanoxin) and has a history of mild renal failure. The healthcare provider requests the nurse to prepare succinylcholine (Anectine) IV as an anesthetic for this patient who is having an outpatient procedure. What is the nurse's response?

3. The nurse is reviewing the chart of a patient who has recently had abdominal surgery. Which of the following would indicate that this patient may require closer monitoring (and why)? Which is a priority? The patient is 67 years old, has been on digoxin (Lanoxin), ibuprofen, and Maalox daily.

 ## EXPLORE MediaLink

NCLEX review, case studies, and other interactive resources for this chapter can be found on the companion website at www.prenhall.com/adams. Click on "Chapter 20" to select the activities for this chapter. For animations, more NCLEX review questions, and an audio glossary, access the accompanying CD-ROM in this textbook.

UNIT 4

The Cardiovascular and Respiratory Systems

CHAPTER

21

Drugs for Hypertension

◼ DRUGS AT A GLANCE

DIURETICS
Pr *hydrochlorothiazide (HydroDIURIL)*

CALCIUM CHANNEL BLOCKERS
Pr *nifedipine (Procardia)*

DRUGS AFFECTING THE RENIN-ANGIOTENSIN SYSTEM
Angiotensin-converting enzyme (ACE) inhibitors
Pr *enalapril (Vasotec)*

Angiotensin receptor blockers

ADRENERGIC AGENTS
Alpha blockers
Pr *doxazosin (Cardura)*
Beta blockers
Centrally acting agents

DIRECT VASODILATORS
Pr *hydralazine (Apresoline)*

metabolized and eliminated by the bod
of this process
PHARMACOLOGY
1. The study of medicines; the disciplir
pertaining to how drugs improve the he
of the human body

 MediaLink www.prenhall.com/adams

CD-ROM
Animations:
  Mechanism in Action: Nifedipine (Procardia)
  Mechanism in Action: Doxazosin (Cardura)
Audio Glossary
NCLEX Review

Companion Website
NCLEX Review
Dosage Calculations
Case Study
Care Plans
Expanded Key Concepts

OBJECTIVES

After reading this chapter, the student should be able to:

1. Identify the major risk factors associated with hypertension.
2. Summarize the long-term consequences of uncontrolled hypertension.
3. Explain the effects of cardiac output, peripheral resistance, and blood volume on blood pressure.
4. Discuss how the vasomotor center, baroreceptors, chemoreceptors, emotions, and hormones influence blood pressure.
5. Explain how hypertension and prehypertension are defined.

6. Discuss the role of the nurse regarding the nonpharmacologic control of hypertension through patient teaching.
7. Describe the nurse's role in the pharmacologic management of patients receiving drugs for hypertension.
8. For each of the drug classes listed in Drugs at a Glance, know representative drug examples, explain their mechanism of drug action, primary actions, and important adverse effects.
9. Use the Nursing Process to care for patients receiving antihypertensive drugs.

Cardiovascular disease, which includes all conditions affecting the heart and blood vessels, is the most common cause of death in the United States. Hypertension (HTN), or high blood pressure, is the most common of the cardiovascular diseases. According to the American Heart Association, high blood pressure is associated with more than 150,000 deaths in the United States each year. Although mild HTN can often be controlled with lifestyle modifications, moderate to severe HTN requires pharmacotherapy.

Because nurses encounter numerous patients with this disease, having an understanding of the underlying principles of antihypertensive therapy is critical. Healthcare providers play a vital role in teaching the patient safe principles of pharmacotherapy as it relates to hypertension.

21.1 Risk Factors for Hypertension

no cause

Hypertension having no identifiable cause is called primary, idiopathic, or essential. This classification accounts for 90% of all cases. Secondary hypertension, accounting for only 10% of all cases, is caused by identifiable factors such as excessive secretion of epinephrine by the adrenal glands or by narrowing of the renal arteries.

Because chronic hypertension may produce no identifiable symptoms for as long as 10 to 20 years, many people are not aware of their condition. Convincing patients to control their diets, buy costly medications, and take drugs on a regular basis when they are feeling healthy is a difficult task for the nurse. In addition, many patients do not take HTN medications because of their undesirable side effects. Failure to control this condition, however, can result in quite serious consequences. Prolonged or improperly controlled HTN can damage small blood vessels leading to accelerated narrowing of the arteries, resulting in angina, myocardial infarction, and peripheral vascular disease. One of the most serious consequences of chronic hypertension is that the heart must work harder to pump blood to the various organs and tissues. This excessive cardiac workload can cause the heart to fail and the lungs to fill with fluid, a condition

PHARMFACTS | Statistics of Hypertension

- Prehypertension (120–139/80–89) affects approximately 22% of the adult population, or nearly 45 million people.
- High blood pressure affects more than 50 million U.S. adults, or approximately 1 in 4 Americans.
- Hypertension increases with age. It affects approximately:
  - 30% of those over age 50
  - 64% of men over age 65
  - 75% of women over age 75
- Over 13,000 people die of hypertension in the United States each year (8.6 deaths per 100,000 population).
- Diabetics are 2 to 3 times more likely to have hypertension than nondiabetics.
- Hypertension is responsible for over 35 million office visits each year.
- African Americans have the highest rate (33%) of hypertension.
- Among people with HTN, over 32% do not realize they have the disorder.
- Hypertension is the most common complication of pregnancy.
- Approximately 40,000 Americans die of HTN per year; it is a contributing factor in 223,000 additional deaths each year.

known as heart failure (HF). Drug therapy of HF is covered in Chapter 23 ⊕ .

Damage to the vessels that supply blood and oxygen to the brain can result in transient ischemic attacks and cerebral vascular accidents or strokes. Renal damage and retinal damage are also common sequelae of sustained hypertension.

The death rate from cardiovascular-related diseases has dropped significantly over the past 20 years due, in large part, to the recognition and treatment of hypertension, as well as the acceptance of healthier lifestyle habits. Early

treatment is essential, as the long-term cardiovascular damage caused by hypertension may be irreversible if the disease is allowed to progress unchecked.

21.2 Factors Responsible for Blood Pressure

Although many factors can influence blood pressure, the three factors truly responsible for creating the pressure are cardiac output, peripheral resistance, and blood volume. These are shown in Figure 21.1.

The volume of blood pumped per minute is called the **cardiac output**. The higher the cardiac output, the higher the blood pressure. Cardiac output is determined by heart rate and **stroke volume**, the amount of blood pumped by a ventricle in one contraction. This is important to pharmacology, because drugs that change the cardiac output, stroke volume, or heart rate have the potential to influence a patient's blood pressure.

As blood flows at high speeds through the vascular system, it exerts force against the walls of the vessels. Although the inner layer of the blood vessel lining, known as the **endothelium**, is extremely smooth, this friction reduces the velocity of the blood. This turbulence-induced friction in the arteries is called **peripheral resistance**. Arteries have smooth muscle in their walls which, when constricted, will cause the inside diameter or lumen to become smaller, thus creating more resistance and higher pressure. A large number of drugs affect vascular smooth muscle, causing vessels to constrict, thus raising blood pressure. Other drugs cause the smooth muscle to relax, thereby opening the lumen and lowering blood pressure. Chapter 6 presents the role of the auto-

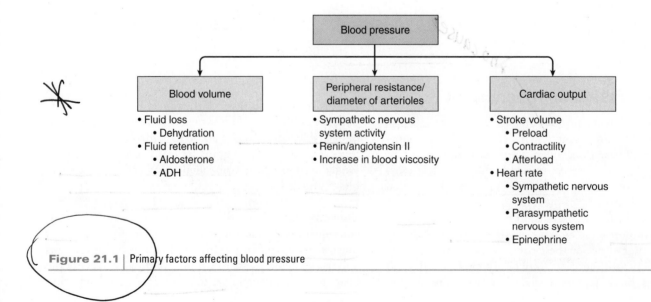

Figure 21.1 | Primary factors affecting blood pressure

nomic nervous system in controlling peripheral resistance⊙ .

The third factor responsible for blood pressure is the total amount of blood in the vascular system, or blood volume. While the average person maintains a relatively constant blood volume of approximately 5 L, this can change due to many regulatory factors and with certain disease states. More blood in the vascular system will exert additional pressure on the walls of the arteries and raise blood pressure. For example, high sodium diets may cause water to be retained by the body, thus increasing blood volume and raising blood pressure. On the other hand, substances known as diuretics can cause fluid loss through urination, thus decreasing blood volume and lowering blood pressure. Loss of blood volume during hemorrhage or shock also lowers blood pressure (Chapter 26)⊙ .

21.3 Normal Regulation of Blood Pressure

It is critical that the body maintains a normal range of blood pressure and that it has the ability to safely and rapidly change pressure as it proceeds through daily activities such as sleep and exercise. Low blood pressure can cause dizziness and lack of adequate urine formation, whereas excessively high pressure can cause vessels to rupture. How the body maintains homeostasis during periods of blood pressure change is shown in Figure 21.2.

Blood pressure is regulated on a minute-to-minute basis by a cluster of neurons in the medulla oblongata called the vasomotor center. Nerves travel from the vasomotor center to the arteries, where the smooth muscle is directed to either constrict (raise blood pressure) or relax (lower blood pressure).

Receptors in the aorta and the internal carotid artery act as sensors to provide the vasomotor center with vital information on conditions in the vascular system. Baroreceptors have the ability to sense pressure within large vessels, whereas chemoreceptors recognize levels of oxygen, carbon dioxide, and the pH in the blood. The vasomotor center reacts to information from baroreceptors and chemoreceptors by raising or lowering blood pressure accordingly.

Emotions can also have a profound effect on blood pressure. Anger and stress can cause blood pressure to rise, whereas mental depression and lethargy may cause it to fall. Strong emotions, if present for a prolonged time period, may become important contributors to chronic hypertension.

A number of hormones and other endogenous agents affect blood pressure on a daily basis. When given as medications, some of these agents may have a profound effect on blood pressure. For example, injection of epinephrine or norepinephrine will immediately raise blood pressure. Antidiuretic hormone (ADH) is a potent vasoconstrictor that can also increase blood pressure by raising blood volume. The renin-angiotensin system is particularly important in the pharmacotherapy of hypertension and is discussed later in this chapter. A summary of the various nervous and hormonal factors influencing blood pressure is shown in Figure 21.3.

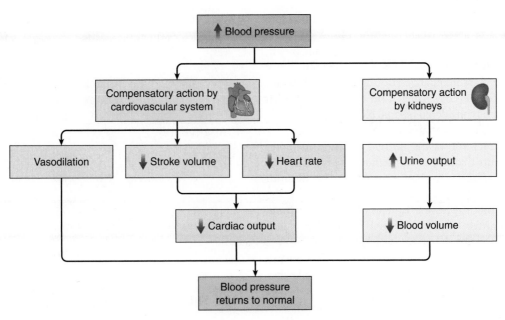

Figure 21.2 | Blood pressure homeostasis

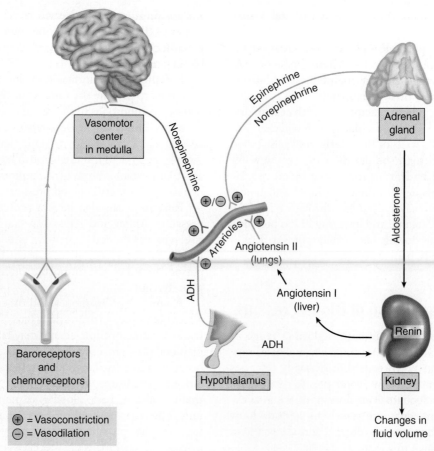

Figure 21.3 | Hormonal and nervous factors influencing blood pressure

21.4 Normal Ranges of Blood Pressure

When the ventricles contract and eject blood, the pressure created in the arteries is called **systolic blood pressure**. When the ventricles relax and the heart is not ejecting blood, pressure in the arteries will fall, and is called **diastolic blood pressure**. Blood pressure changes throughout the lifespan, gradually and continuously rising from childhood through adulthood. What is considered normal blood pressure at one age may be considered abnormal in someone older or younger. Table 21.1 shows the normal variation in blood pressure in patients that occurs throughout the life span.

For many years, blood pressure measuring 120/80 mm Hg had been considered optimal. However, in 2003, the National High Blood Pressure Education Program Coordinating Committee of the National Heart, Lung and Blood Institute, National Institutes of Health, determined the need for new guidelines that addressed the relationship between blood pressure and the risk of cardiovascular disease (CVD). This committee issued the document, *The Seventh Report of the Joint National Committee on Prevention, Detection, Evaluation and Treatment of High Blood Pressure (JNC-7)*, which states the following:

■ The risk of CVD beginning at 115/75 mm Hg *doubles* with each increment of 20/10 mm Hg.

■ Individuals with systolic blood pressure of 120 to 139 mm Hg or a diastolic blood pressure of 80 to 89 mm Hg should be considered as *prehypertensive*. These patients should be strongly encouraged by the nurse to

Table 21.1	Variation in Blood Pressure Throughout the Lifespan	
Age (years)	**Male**	**Female**
1	96/66	95/65
5	92/62	92/62
10	103/69	103/70
20–24	123/76	116/72
30–34	126/79	120/75
40–44	129/81	127/80
50–54	135/83	137/84
60–64	142/85	144/85
70–74	145/82	159/85
80+	145/82	157/83

adopt health-promoting lifestyle modifications to prevent CVD.

- Patients with prehypertension are at increased risk for progression to HTN; those in the 130–139/80–89 mm Hg blood pressure range are at twice the risk to develop hypertension as those with lower values.

The diagnosis of chronic HTN is rarely made on a single blood pressure measurement. A patient having a sustained systolic blood pressure of 140 to 159 or diastolic of 90 to 99 mm Hg, after multiple measurements are made over several clinic visits, is said to have stage 1 hypertension. Pharmacotherapy is indicated at this stage. The recommendations from *JNC-7* are summarized in Table 21.2.

21.5 Nonpharmacologic Therapy for Hypertension

When a patient is first diagnosed with hypertension, a comprehensive medical history is necessary to determine if the disease can be controlled by nonpharmacologic means. In many cases, modifying certain health lifestyle habits, such as changes to nutrition and increased exercise, may eliminate the need for pharmacotherapy. Even if pharmacotherapy is required to manage the hypertension, it is important that the patient continue positive lifestyle changes so that dosages can be minimized, thus lowering the potential for drug side effects. The nurse is key to educating patients about controlling their HTN. Nonpharmacologic methods for controlling hypertension are as follows:

- Limit intake of alcohol.
- Restrict salt consumption.
- Reduce intake of saturated fat and cholesterol.

- Increase aerobic physical activity.
- Discontinue use of all tobacco products.
- Explore measures for dealing with stress.
- Maintain optimum weight.

21.6 Risk Factors and Selection of Antihypertensive Drugs

The goal of antihypertensive therapy is to reduce blood pressure in order to avoid serious, long-term consequences of HTN. Keeping blood pressure within acceptable limits reduces the risk of hypertension-related diseases such as stroke and heart failure. Several strategies that are used to achieve this goal are summarized in Figure 21.4.

The pharmacologic management of hypertension is individualized in regard to the patient's risk factors, concurrent medical conditions, and degree of blood pressure elevation. Once the appropriate drug has been chosen, a low dose is prescribed. Depending on the expected response time of the drug, the patient will be reevaluated, and the dosage may be adjusted. A second drug from a different class may be added if the patient has not responded to the initial medication.

It is common practice for healthcare providers to prescribe two antihypertensives concurrently to manage resistant HTN. The advantage of using two drugs is that lower doses may be used, resulting in fewer side effects and better patient compliance. Unfortunately, compliance decreases when patients need to take more than one drug, or when patients need to take them more often. In an effort to minimize noncompliance, drug manufacturers sometimes combine two drugs into a single pill or capsule. These combination drugs are quite common in the treatment of hypertension. It is important for the patient to receive education on all the

Table 21.2	**Management of Hypertension**		
		Initial Antihypertensive Therapy	
Blood Pressure Classification	**Systolic/Diastolic Blood Pressure (mm Hg)**	**Without Compelling Indication***	**With Compelling Indication***
normal	119/79 or less	No antihypertensive indicated	No antihypertensive indicated
prehypertension	120–139/80–89		
stage 1 hypertension	140–159/90–99	Thiazide diuretic (for most patients)	Other antihypertensives, as needed
stage 2 hypertension	160 or higher/ 100 or higher	Two-drug combination antihypertensive (for most patients)	

* Compelling indications include heart failure, post myocardial infarction, high risk for coronary artery disease, diabetes, chronic kidney disease, and recurrent stroke prevention.

Source: From JNC-7 Express: The Seventh Report of the Joint National Committee on Prevention, Detection, Evaluation and Treatment of High Blood Pressure by National High Blood Pressure Education Program, National Heart, Lung & Blood Institute, 2003, www.nhlbi.nih.gov.

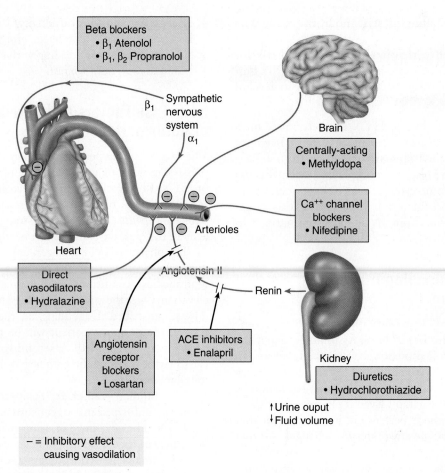

Figure 21.4 | Mechanism of action of antihypertensive drugs

drugs in combination formulas. Selected combination drugs are shown in Table 21.3.

The types of drugs used to treat chronic hypertension generally fall into five primary classes, as follows:

- Diuretics
- Calcium channel blockers
- Agents affecting the renin-angiotensin system
- Adrenergic agents
- Direct-acting vasodilators

DIURETICS

Diuretics act by increasing the volume of urine production. They are widely used in the treatment of hypertension and heart failure. These agents are shown in Table 21.4.

21.7 Treating Hypertension with Diuretics

Diuretics were the first class of drugs used to treat hypertension in the 1950s. Despite many advances in pharmacotherapy, diuretics are still considered first line drugs for this disease because they produce few adverse effects and are very effective at controlling mild to moderate hypertension. Although sometimes used alone, they are frequently pre-

scribed with other antihypertensive drugs to enhance their effectiveness. Diuretics are also used to treat heart failure (Chapter 23) and kidney disorders (Chapter 43)⊖⊙ .

Although many different diuretics are available for hypertension, all produce a similar result: the reduction of blood volume through the urinary excretion of water and electrolytes. **Electrolytes** are ions such as sodium (Na^+), calcium (Ca^{++}), chloride (Cl^-), and potassium (K^+). The mechanism by which diuretics reduce blood volume, specifically where and how the kidney is affected, differs among the various classes of diuretics. Details on the mechanisms of action of the diuretic classes are discussed in Chapter 43⊖⊙ .

When a drug changes urine composition or output, electrolyte depletion is possible; the specific electrolyte lost is dependent upon the mechanism of action of the particular drug. Potassium loss (hypokalemia) is of particular concern for loop and thiazide diuretics. Others such as triamterene (Dyrenium) have less tendency to cause K^+ depletion and for this reason are called potassium-sparing diuretics. Taking potassium supplements with potassium-sparing diuretics may result in dangerously high potassium levels in the blood (hyperkalemia) leading to cardiac conduction abnormalities.

Table 21.3	Combination Drugs Commonly Used to Treat Hypertension				
Trade Name	**Thiazide Diuretic**	**Adrenergic Agent**	**Potassium-Sparing Diuretic**	**ACE Inhibitor or Angiotensin II Blocker**	**Other**
Alazide	hydrochlorothiazide		spironolactone		
Aldactazide	hydrochlorothiazide		spironolactone		
Aldoril	hydrochlorothiazide				methyldopa
Apresazide	hydrochlorothiazide				hydralazine
Capozide	hydrochlorothiazide			captopril	
Combipres	chlorthalidone				clonidine
Diupres	chlorothiazide				reserpine
Dyazide	hydrochlorothiazide		triamterene		
Hydropres	hydrochlorothiazide				reserpine
Hyzaar	hydrochlorothiazide			losartan	
Inderide	hydrochlorothiazide	propranolol			
Lopressor	hydrochlorothiazide	metoprolol			
Lotensin	hydrochlorothiazide			benazepril	
Minizide	polythiazide	prazosin			
Moduretic	hydrochlorothiazide		amiloride		
Tarka				trandolapril	verapamil
Timolide	hydrochlorothiazide	timolol			
Uniretic	hydrochlorothiazide			moexipril	
Vaseretic	hydrochlorothiazide			enalapril	
Zestoretic	hydrochlorothiazide			lisinopril	
Ziac	hydrochlorothiazide	bisoprolol			

NURSING CONSIDERATIONS

The role of the nurse in diuretic therapy for HTN involves careful monitoring of a patient's condition and providing education as it relates to the prescribed drug regimen. Diuretics decrease circulating blood volume, causing the potential development of dehydration and hypovolemia. Orthostatic (postural) hypotension may occur because of the reduced blood volume. The patient may experience dizziness and faintness after rising too quickly from a sitting or lying position.

Because diuretics act by altering the physiological balance of fluid and electrolytes in the body, careful monitoring of laboratory values and body weight are essential. The patient should be weighed daily, and changes reported. The nurse must measure fluid intake and output and assess insensible losses that may occur due to illness, such as high fever, or exercise. The ankles and lower legs should be examined for signs of pitting edema, which signifies fluid retention and may indicate pulmonary edema. The nurse should auscultate breath and heart sounds when taking vital signs; "crackles" and murmurs may indicate impending heart failure. Electrolyte levels, particularly sodium and potassium, should be monitored carefully during diuretic

therapy. Diuretics can reduce the renal excretion of lithium, causing this drug to build up to toxic levels. Most diuretics are contraindicated in patients who are unable to produce urine (anuria).

Because diuretics cause frequent urination, the nurse should assess the patient's ability to safely go to the bathroom or should secure a urinal or bedside commode as needed. Diuretics should be administered early in the day so sleep is not interrupted by frequent urination.

Photosensitivity is also a side effect of many diuretics. Photosensitization occurs when a drug, absorbed into the bloodstream, enters the skin. Sunlight, also absorbed by the skin, chemically changes the drug; the new compound triggers a reaction in the body.

Potassium-Sparing Diuretics

Potassium-sparing diuretics should not be used in patients with renal insufficiency or hyperkalemia, as potassium levels may rise to life-threatening levels. Potassium-sparing diuretics are not normally used for pregnant or lactating women as they range from pregnancy category B (triamterene) to category D (spironolactone). Uric acid levels may increase and patients with a history of gout or kidney stones may not tolerate these diuretics. Complete blood

Table 21.4	Diuretics for Hypertension
Drug	**Route and Adult Dose (max dose where indicated)**
Potassium-sparing Type	
amiloride (Midamor)	PO; 5–20 mg in one to two divided doses (max 20 mg/day)
spironolactone (Aldactone) (see page 647 for the Prototype Drug box) ⌸	PO; 25–100 mg qd (max 200 mg/day)
triamterene (Dyrenium)	PO; 100 mg bid (max 300 mg/day)
Thiazide and Thiazide-like Agents	
benzthiazide (Aquatag, others)	PO; 25–200 mg qd
chlorothiazide (Diuril) (see page 645 for the Prototype Drug box) ⌸	PO; 250–500 mg qd (max 2g/day)
chlorthalidone (Hygroton)	PO; 50–100 mg qd (max 100 mg/day)
hydrochlorothiazide (HydroDIURIL, HCTZ)	PO; 12.5–100 mg qd (max 5 mg/day)
indapamide (Lozol)	PO; 2.5–5.0 mg qd
metolazone (Diulo, others)	PO; 5–20 mg qd
polythiazide (Renese)	PO; 1–4 mg qd
trichlormethiazide (Diurese, others)	PO; 1–4 mg qd
Loop/High Ceiling Type	
bumetanide (Bumex)	PO; 0.5–2.0 mg qd (max 10 mg/day)
furosemide (Lasix) (see page 293 for the Prototype Drug box) ⌸	PO; 20–80 mg qd (max 600 mg/day)
torsemide (Demadex)	PO; 4–20 mg qd

counts should be obtained periodically throughout therapy as agranulocytosis and other hematologic disorders may occur. Because white blood cell levels may be too low to combat infections, patients should report fever, rash, and sore throat. Spironolactone (Aldactone) can cause gynecomastia (breast enlargement) and androgenic effects such as testicular atrophy or accelerated hair growth (hirsutism) in females. Patients should avoid excess potassium in their diet and salt that contain KCl.

Thiazide and Thiazide-Like Diuretics

Because thiazide and thiazide-like diuretics alter blood chemistry, including fluid and electrolyte balance, laboratory values (K^+, Cl^-, Na^+, Ca^{++}, Mg^{++}, CBC, BUN, creatinine, cholesterol, and serum lipids) should be closely monitored. These drugs may cause excess potassium excretion; therefore, patients should increase potassium in their diet. Potassium supplements may be necessary. These diuretics can cause hyperglycemia and decrease the effectiveness of oral antidiabetic drugs. Because uric acid levels may increase, patients should be monitored for signs and symptoms of gout.

Because thiazides may increase blood lipids, these agents should be used cautiously in patients with existing hyperlipidemia. Cautious use is advised during pregnancy (category B) and lactation, and for neonates, as these diuretics cross the placenta and are secreted into breast milk. Thiazides may exacerbate systemic lupus erythematosus (SLE), and therefore are contraindicated in this condition. Elderly patients are at increased risk of electrolyte imbalances due to physiologic changes in the kidneys related to aging. Losses of potassium and magnesium caused by thiazide diuretics increase the risk of digoxin toxicity.

Loop/High Ceiling Diuretics

The efficacious loop or high ceiling group of diuretics is more likely to cause severe potassium loss, hypovolemia, and hypotension, as compared to other diuretic classes. The patient's blood pressure should be monitored frequently, especially with IV administration. Loop diuretics are ototoxic, an effect more likely to occur in patients with renal insufficiency or when high doses are administered. Hearing loss usually reverses when the drug is discontinued. Loop diuretics may also increase glucose and uric acid levels; therefore, these laboratory values should be monitored during therapy.

See "Nursing Process Focus: Patients Receiving Diuretic Therapy" for specific teaching points.

Pr **PROTOTYPE DRUG** | **HYDROCHLOROTHIAZIDE** (HydroDIURIL)

ACTIONS AND USES

Hydrochlorothiazide (HCTZ) is the most widely prescribed diuretic for hypertension, belonging to a large class known as the thiazides. Like many diuretics, it produces few adverse effects and is effective at producing a 10 to 20 mm Hg reduction in blood pressure. Patients with severe HTN, however, may require the addition of a second drug from a different class to control the disease.

Hydrochlorothiazide acts on the kidney tubule to decrease the reabsorption of Na^+. Normally, over 99% of the sodium entering the kidney is reabsorbed by the body so that very little leaves via the urine. When HCTZ blocks this reabsorption, more Na^+ is sent into the urine. When sodium moves across the tubule, water flows with it; thus, blood volume decreases and blood pressure falls. The volume of urine produced is directly proportional to the amount of sodium reabsorption blocked by the diuretic. Hydrochlorothiazide is pregnancy category B.

Administration Alert

Administer the drug early in the day to prevent nocturia.

ADVERSE EFFECTS AND INTERACTIONS

The most common side effects of HCTZ involve potential electrolyte imbalances; K^+ is lost along with the Na^+. Because hypokalemia may cause conduction abnormalities in the heart, patients must closely monitor their dietary potassium and are usually asked to increase their potassium intake as a precaution.

HCTZ potentiates the action of other antihypertensives and increases responsiveness to skeletal muscle relaxants. Thiazides may reduce the effectiveness of anticoagulants, sulfonylureas, antigout drugs, and antidiabetic drugs including insulin. Cholestyramine, colestipol, and NSAIDs reduce the effectiveness of HCTZ.

CNS depressants such as alcohol, barbiturates, and opioids may exacerbate the orthostatic hypotension caused by HCTZ. Steroids or amphotericin B increase potassium loss when given with HCTZ, leading to hypokalemia.

Hydrochlorothiazide increases the risk of serum toxicity of the following drugs: digitalis, lithium, allopurinol, diazoxide, anesthetics, and antineoplastics. HCTZ alters vitamin D metabolism and causes calcium conservation; use of calcium supplements may cause hypercalcemia.

Use with caution with herbal supplements, such as ginkgo biloba, which may produce a paradoxical increase in blood pressure.

 See the companion website for a Nursing Process Focus specific to this drug.

NURSING PROCESS FOCUS | **PATIENTS RECEIVING DIURETIC THERAPY**

ASSESSMENT

Prior to administration:
- Obtain complete health history including allergies, drug history, and possible drug interactions.
- Obtain vital signs; assess in context of patient's baseline values.
- Auscultate chest sounds for rales or rhonchi indicative of pulmonary edema.
- Assess lower limbs for edema; note character/level (e.g., "++ pitting").
- Obtain blood and urine specimens for laboratory analysis.

POTENTIAL NURSING DIAGNOSES

- Excess Fluid Volume, related to excessive diuresis secondary to diuretic use
- Risk for Deficient Fluid Volume
- Impaired Urinary Elimination, related to diuretic use
- Fatigue
- Ineffective Health Maintenance

PLANNING: PATIENT GOALS AND EXPECTED OUTCOMES

The patient will:
- Exhibit a reduction in systolic/diastolic blood pressure
- Demonstrate an understanding of the drug's action by accurately describing drug side effects and precautions
- Maintain normal serum electrolyte levels during drug therapy.

IMPLEMENTATION

Interventions and (Rationales)

- Monitor laboratory values.
  (Diuretic therapy affects the results of laboratory tests.)

Patient Education/Discharge Planning

Instruct patient to:
- Inform laboratory personnel of diuretic therapy when providing blood or urine samples
- Carry a wallet card or wear medical identification jewelry to indicate diuretic therapy

continued

NURSING PROCESS FOCUS: *Patients Receiving Diuretic Therapy (continued)*

Interventions and (Rationales)	*Patient Education/Discharge Planning*
■ Monitor vital signs, especially blood pressure. (Diuretics reduce circulating blood volume, resulting in lowered blood pressure.)	Instruct patient to: ■ Monitor vital signs as specified by the nurse, particularly blood pressure, ensuring proper use of home equipment ■ Withhold medication for severe hypotensive readings as specified by the nurse (e.g., "hold for levels below 88/50")
■ Observe for changes in level of consciousness, dizziness, fatigue, postural hypotension. (Caused by reduction in circulating blood volume.)	Instruct patient to: ■ Report dizziness or lightheadedness ■ Rise slowly from prolonged periods of sitting or lying down ■ Obtain blood pressure readings in sitting, standing, and supine positions to monitor fluctuations in blood pressure
■ Monitor for fluid overload and signs of heart failure. (Increased blood volume causes increased cardiac workload and pulmonary edema.) ■ Measure intake and output, and daily weights.	Instruct patient: ■ To immediately report any severe shortness of breath, frothy sputum, profound fatigue, and edema in extremities ■ To measure and monitor fluid intake and output, and weigh daily ■ To consume enough *plain* water to remain adequately, but not over, hydrated ■ To avoid excessive heat which contributes to excessive sweating and fluid loss ■ That increased urine output and decreased weight indicate that the drug is working
■ Monitor nutritional status. (Electrolyte imbalances may be counteracted by dietary measures.)	For patients taking potassium-wasting diuretics, instruct to: ■ Eat foods high in potassium such as bananas, apricots, kidney beans, sweet potatoes, and peanut butter For patients taking potassium-sparing diuretics, instruct to: ■ Avoid foods high in potassium ■ Consult with nurse before using vitamin/mineral supplements or electrolyte-fortified sports drinks
■ Observe for signs of hyperglycemia. Use with caution in diabetics.	■ Instruct patient to report signs and symptoms of diabetes mellitus to healthcare provider.
■ Monitor liver and kidney function. (Drugs are metabolized by the liver and excreted by the kidneys.)	Instruct patient to: ■ Immediately report symptoms of metabolic imbalances: nausea and vomiting, profound weakness, lethargy, muscle cramps, depression/disorientation, hallucinations, heart spasms, palpitations, numbness or tingling in limbs, extreme thirst, changes in urine output ■ Adhere to laboratory testing regimen as ordered by the healthcare provider
■ Observe for hypersensitivity reaction.	■ Instruct patient to immediately report difficulty breathing, throat tightness, hives or rash, muscle cramps, or tremors.
■ Observe for signs of infection.	■ Instruct patient or caregiver to report any flulike symptoms: shortness of breath, fever, sore throat, malaise, joint pain, or profound fatigue.
■ Monitor hearing and vision. (Loop diuretics such as furosemide are ototoxic. Thiazide diuretics increase serum digitalis levels which may produce visual changes.)	Instruct patient to: ■ Report changes in hearing such as ringing or buzzing in the ears or becoming "hard of hearing" ■ Report dimness of sight, seeing halos or "yellow vision"

continued

NURSING PROCESS FOCUS: *Patients Receiving Diuretic Therapy (continued)*

Interventions and (Rationales)	*Patient Education/Discharge Planning*
■ Monitor for alcohol and caffeine use. (Alcohol potentiates the hypotensive action of some thiazide diuretics. Caffeine is a mild diuretic that could increase diuresis.)	■ Instruct patient to restrict consumption of alcohol and caffeine.
■ Ensure patient safety. Monitor ambulation until effects of drug are known. (Due to postural hypotension caused by drug)	Instruct patient to: ■ Obtain help before getting out of bed or attempting to walk alone ■ Avoid sudden changes of position to prevent dizziness caused by postural hypotension ■ Avoid driving or other activities requiring mental alertness or physical coordination until effects of the drug are known
■ Monitor reactivity to light exposure. (Drug causes photosensitivity.)	Instruct patient to: ■ Limit exposure to the sun ■ Wear dark glasses and light-colored, loose-fitting clothes when outdoors

EVALUATION OF OUTCOME CRITERIA

Evaluate the effectiveness of drug therapy by confirming that patient goals and expected outcomes have been met (see "Planning").

See Table 21.4 for a list of drugs to which these nursing actions apply.

CALCIUM CHANNEL BLOCKERS

Calcium channel blockers exert a number of beneficial effects on the heart and blood vessels by blocking calcium ion channels. They are widely used in the treatment of hypertension and other cardiovascular diseases. These agents are shown in Table 21.5.

21.8 Treating Hypertension with Calcium Channel Blockers

Calcium channel blockers (CCBs) comprise a group of drugs used to treat a number of cardiovascular diseases, including angina pectoris, dysrhythmias, and hypertension. First approved for the treatment of angina in the early

Table 21.5	Calcium Channel Blockers for Hypertension	
Drug	**Route and Adult Dose (max dose where indicated)**
Selective: for Blood Vessels	
amlodipine (Norvasc)	PO; 5–10 mg qd (max 10 mg/day)
felodipine (Plendil)	PO; 5–10 mg qd (max 20 mg/day)
nicardipine (Cardene)	PO; 20–40 mg tid (max 120 mg/day)
nifedipine (Procardia, Adalat)	PO; 10–20 mg tid (max 180 mg/day)
Nonselective: for Both Blood Vessels and Heart	
diltiazem (Cardizem, Dilacor, Tiamate, Triassic) (see page 337 for the Prototype Drug box)	PO; 60–120 mg sustained release bid
isradipine (DynaCirc)	PO; 1.25–10 mg bid (max 20 mg/day)
nisoldipine (Nisocor)	PO; 10–20 mg bid (max 40 mg/day)
verapamil (Calan, Isoptin, Verelan) (see page 309 for the Prototype Drug box)	PO; 80–160 mg tid (max 360 mg/day)

1980s, it was quickly noted that a "side effect" of CCBs was the lowering of blood pressure in hypertensive patients. CCBs have since become a widely prescribed class of drugs for hypertension.

Contraction of muscle is regulated by the amount of calcium ion inside the cell. When calcium enters the cell through channels in the plasma membrane, muscular contraction is initiated. CCBs block these channels and inhibit Ca^{++} from entering the cell, limiting muscular contraction. At low doses, CCBs cause the smooth muscle in arterioles to relax, lowering peripheral resistance and decreasing blood pressure. Some CCBs such as nifedipine (Procardia) are selective for calcium channels in arterioles, while others such as verapamil (Calan) affect channels in both arterioles and the myocardium. CCBs vary in their potency and by the frequency and types of side effects produced. Uses of CCBs in the treatment of dysrhythmias and angina are discussed in Chapters 24 and 25, respectively ∞ .

NURSING CONSIDERATIONS

The role of the nurse in calcium channel blocker therapy for HTN involves careful monitoring of a patient's condition and providing education as it relates to the prescribed drug regimen. CCBs affect the coronary arteries and myocardial conductivity and contractility. EKG, heart rate, and blood pressure should be assessed prior to therapy; vital signs should be monitored regularly thereafter. CCBs are contraindicated in patients with certain types of heart conditions such as sick sinus syndrome or third degree AV blocks without the presence of a pacemaker. Some CCBs reduce myocardial contractility and can worsen heart failure. Due to their potent vasodilating effects, CCBs can cause reflex tachycardia, a condition that occurs when the heart rate increases due to the rapid fall in blood pressure created by the drug. CCBs are pregnancy category C.

Tachycardia and hypotension are most pronounced with IV administration of CCBs. Grapefruit juice increases absorption of these drugs from the GI tract, causing greater than expected effects from the dose. Grapefruit juice taken with a sustained-release CCB could result in rapid toxic overdose which is a medical emergency.

Teaching strategies regarding calcium channel blockers should include the goals for drug therapy, reasons for obtaining baseline data such as vital signs, tests for cardiac and renal disorders including EKG and laboratory values, and possible side effects. See "Nursing Process Focus: Patients Receiving Calcium Channel Blocker Therapy" for specific teaching points.

Pr **PROTOTYPE DRUG** | **NIFEDIPINE** (Procardia)

ACTIONS AND USES

Nifedipine is a CCB generally prescribed for HTN and variant or vasospastic angina. It is occasionally used to treat Raynaud's phenomenon and hypertrophic cardiomyopathy. Nifedipine acts by selectively blocking calcium channels in myocardial and vascular smooth muscle, including that in the coronary arteries. This results in less oxygen utilization by the heart, an increase in cardiac output, and a fall in blood pressure. Nifedipine is as effective as diuretics and beta-adrenergic blockers at reducing blood pressure.

Administration Alerts

- Do not administer immediate-release formulations of nifedipine if an impending MI is suspected, or within 2 weeks following a confirmed MI.
- Administer nifedipine capsules or tablets whole. If capsules or extended-release tablets are chewed, divided, or crushed, the entire dose will be delivered at once.
- Pregnancy category C.

ADVERSE EFFECTS AND INTERACTIONS

Side effects of nifedipine are generally minor and related to vasodilation such as headache, dizziness, and flushing. Fast-acting forms of nifedipine can cause reflex tachycardia. To avoid rebound hypotension, discontinuation of the drug should occur gradually. In rare cases, nifedipine may cause a paradoxical increase in anginal chest pain possibly related to hypotension or heart failure.

Nifedipine may increase serum levels of digitalis, cimetidine, and ranitidine. Nifedipine may potentiate the effects of warfarin, resulting in increased PTT. Potentiation may also occur with fentanyl anesthesia, resulting in severe hypotension and increased fluid volume requirements. Grapefruit juice may cause enhanced absorption of nifedipine. Nifedipine may reduce serum levels of quinidine.

Alcohol potentiates the vasodilating action of nifedipine, and could lead to syncope caused by a severe drop in blood pressure. Nicotine causes vasoconstriction, counteracting the desired effect of nifedipine.

Use with caution with melatonin, which may increase blood pressure and heart rate.

 See the companion website for a Nursing Process Focus specific to this drug.

MediaLink | *Mechanism in Action | Nifedipine*

NURSING PROCESS FOCUS	PATIENTS RECEIVING CALCIUM CHANNEL BLOCKER THERAPY

ASSESSMENT

Prior to administration:
- Obtain complete health history including data on recent cardiac events, allergies, drug history, and possible drug interactions.
- Obtain EKG and vital signs; assess in context of patient's baseline values.
- Assess neurological status and level of consciousness.
- Auscultate chest sounds for rales or rhonchi indicative of pulmonary edema.
- Assess lower limbs for edema; note character/level.

POTENTIAL NURSING DIAGNOSES

- Ineffective Health Maintenance
- Deficient Knowledge, related to drug therapy
- Decreased Cardiac Output
- Altered Tissue Perfusion

PLANNING: PATIENT GOALS AND EXPECTED OUTCOMES

The patient will:
- Exhibit a reduction in systolic/diastolic blood pressure
- Demonstrate an understanding of the drug's action by accurately describing drug side effects and precautions.

IMPLEMENTATION

Interventions and (Rationales)

- Monitor vital signs.
- Monitor EKG during initial therapy.
  (CCBs dilate the arteries, reducing blood pressure.)

- Observe for changes in level of consciousness, dizziness, fatigue, postural hypotension. (Caused by vasodilation)
- Observe for paradoxical increase in chest pain or angina symptoms. (Related to severe hypotension)
- Obtain blood pressure readings in sitting, standing, and supine positions to monitor fluctuations in blood pressure.

- Monitor for signs of heart failure. (CCBs can decrease myocardial contractility, increasing the risk of heart failure.)

- Monitor for fluid accumulation.
- Measure intake and output, and daily weights.
  (Edema is a side effect of some CCBs.)

- Observe for hypersensitivity reaction.

- Monitor liver and kidney function. (CCBs are metabolized in the liver and excreted by the kidneys.)

Patient Education/Discharge Planning

Instruct patient to:
- Monitor vital signs as specified by the nurse, particularly blood pressure, ensuring proper use of home equipment
- Withhold medication for severe hypotensive readings as specified by the nurse (e.g., "hold for levels below 88/50")
- Immediately report palpitations or rapid heartbeat

Instruct patient to:
- Report dizziness or lightheadedeness
- Report chest pain or other angina-like symptoms
- Rise slowly from prolonged periods of sitting or lying down

- Instruct patient to immediately report any severe shortness of breath, frothy sputum, profound fatigue, and swelling. These may be signs of heart failure or fluid accumulation in the lungs.

Instruct patient to:
- Avoid excessive heat, which contributes to excessive sweating and fluid loss
- Measure and monitor fluid intake and output, and weigh daily
- Consume enough *plain* water to remain adequately, but not over, hydrated

- Instruct patient to immediately report difficulty breathing, throat tightness, hives or rash, muscle cramps, or tremors.

Instruct patient to:
- Report signs of liver toxicity: nausea, vomiting, anorexia, bleeding, severe upper or abdominal pain, heartburn, jaundice, or a change in the color or character of stools
- Report signs of renal toxicity: fever, flank pain, changes in urine output, color or character (cloudy, with sediment, etc.)

continued

NURSING PROCESS FOCUS: *Patients Receiving Calcium Channel Blocker Therapy (continued)*

Interventions and (Rationales)	Patient Education/Discharge Planning
	■ Adhere to laboratory testing regimens as ordered by the healthcare provider
■ Observe for constipation. May need to increase dietary fiber or administer laxatives.	Advise patient to: ■ Maintain adequate fluid and fiber intake to facilitate stool passage ■ Use a bulk laxative or stool softener, as recommended by the healthcare provider
■ Ensure patient safety. ■ Monitor ambulation until response to drug are known (due to postural hypotension caused by drug).	■ Instruct patient to avoid driving or other activities requiring mental alertness or physical coordination until effects of the drug is known.

EVALUATION OF OUTCOME CRITERIA

Evaluate the effectiveness of drug therapy by confirming that patient goals and expected outcomes have been met (see "Planning").

See Table 21.5 for a list of drugs to which these nursing actions apply.

Table 21.6	ACE Inhibitors and Angiotensin II Receptor Blockers for Hypertension
Drug	**Route and Adult Dose (max dose where indicated)**
ACE Inhibitors	
benazepril (Lotensin)	PO; 10–40 mg in one to two divided doses (max 40 mg/day)
captopril (Capoten)	PO; 6.25–25 mg tid (max 450 mg/day)
enalapril (Vasotec)	PO; 5–40 mg in one to two divided doses (max 40 mg/day)
fosinopril (Monopril)	PO; 5–40 mg qd (max 80 mg/day)
lisinopril (Prinivil, Zestoretic, Zestril) (see page 292 for the Prototype Drug box)	PO; 10 mg qd (max 80 mg/day)
moexipril (Univasc)	PO; 7.5–30 mg qd (max 30 mg/day)
quinapril (Accupril)	PO; 10–20 mg qd (max 80 mg/day)
ramipril (Altace)	PO; 2.5–5 mg qd (max 20 mg/day)
trandolapril (Mavik)	PO; 1–4 mg qd (max 8 mg/day)
Angiotensin II Receptor Blockers	
candesartan (Atacand)	PO; Start at 16 mg qd (range 8–32 mg divided once or twice daily)
eprosartan (Teveten)	PO; 600 mg qd or 400 mg PO qid-bid (max 800 mg/day)
irbesartan (Avapro)	PO; 150–300 mg qd (max 300 mg/day)
losartan (Cozaar)	PO; 25–50 mg in one to two divided doses (max 100 mg/day)
olmesartan medoxomil (Benicar)	PO; 20–40 mg qd
telmisartan (Micardis)	PO; 40 mg qd; may increase to 80 mg/day
valsartan (Diovan)	PO; 80 mg qd (max 320 mg/day)

DRUGS AFFECTING THE RENIN-ANGIOTENSIN SYSTEM

Drugs that affect the renin-angiotensin pathway decrease blood pressure and increase urine volume. They are widely used in the treatment of hypertension, heart failure, and myocardial infarction. These agents are shown in Table 21.6.

21.9 Pharmacotherapy with ACE Inhibitors and Angiotensin Receptor Blockers

The renin-angiotensin system is a key homeostatic mechanism that controls blood pressure and fluid balance. This mechanism is illustrated in Figure 21.5. Renin is an enzyme secreted by specialized cells in the kidney when blood pressure falls or when there is a decrease in Na^+ flowing through the kidney tubules. Once in the blood, renin converts the inactive liver protein angiotensinogen to angiotensin I. When passing through the lungs, angiotensin I is converted to angiotensin II, one of the most potent natural vasoconstrictors known. The enzyme responsible for the final step in this system is angiotensin-converting enzyme (ACE). The intense vasoconstriction of arterioles caused by angiotensin II raises blood pressure by increasing peripheral resistance.

Angiotensin II also stimulates the secretion of two hormones that markedly affect blood pressure: aldosterone and ADH. Aldosterone, a hormone from the adrenal cortex, increases sodium reabsorption in the kidney. The enhanced sodium reabsorption helps the body retain water, thus increasing blood volume and raising blood pressure. ADH, a hormone from the posterior pituitary, enhances the conservation of water by the kidneys. This raises blood pressure by increasing blood volume. Pharmacotherapy with ADH is discussed in Chapter 39 ∞ .

First detected in the venom of pit vipers in the 1960s, inhibitors of ACE have been approved as drugs for hypertension since the 1980s. Since then, drugs in this class have become key agents in the treatment of hypertension. ACE inhibitors block the effects of angiotensin II, decreasing blood pressure through two mechanisms: lowering peripheral resistance and decreasing blood volume. Some ACE inhibitors have also been approved for the treatment of heart failure and myocardial infarction, as discussed in Chapters 23 and 25, respectively ∞ .

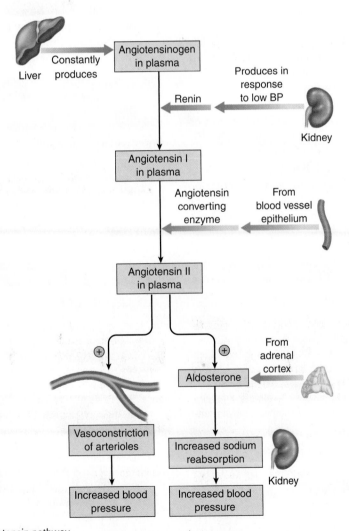

Figure 21.5 | The renin-angiotensin pathway

Side effects of ACE inhibitors are usually minor and include persistent cough and postural hypotension, particularly following the first few doses of the drug. The most serious adverse effect is the development of angioedema, an acute hypersensitivity reaction featuring noninflammatory swelling of the skin, mucous membranes, and other organs. Angioedema may be life threatening; laryngeal swelling can lead to asphyxia and death. The development of angioedema usually occurs within days of taking an ACE inhibitor; however, it can occur as a delayed reaction months or even years into therapy.

A second method of altering the renin-angiotensin pathway is by blocking the action of angiotensin II *after* it is formed. The angiotensin II receptor blockers (ARBs) were the first new class of antihypertensive agents in the United States in more than a decade. The ARBs block receptors for angiotensin II in arteriolar smooth muscle and in the adrenal gland, thus causing blood pressure to fall. Their effects of arteriolar dilation and increased sodium excretion by the kidneys are similar to those of the ACE inhibitors. Angiotensin II receptor blockers have relatively few side effects, most of which are related to hypotension. Drugs in this class are often combined with drugs from other classes in the management of HTN.

Two new methods of altering the renin-angiotensin system show promise for the pharmacotherapy of HTN. Eplerenone (Inspra) is the first aldosterone receptor blocker approved for HTN. This drug prevents aldosterone from reaching its receptors in the kidneys, resulting in less sodium reabsorption and a fall in blood pressure. In addition, several vasopeptidase inhibitors are completing final clinical trials. These new agents have a dual inhibition of both ACE and the enzyme neutral endopeptidase (NEP). Inhibiting NEP leads to a buildup of natriuretic peptides, which causes both vasodilation and diuresis. In clinical trials, vasopeptidase inhibitors appear to be as effective or more effective than conventional antihypertensives. Omapatilat (Vanlev) is the best studied of these agents and the most likely to receive approval.

NURSING CONSIDERATIONS

The role of the nurse in ACE inhibitor therapy for HTN involves careful monitoring of a patient's condition and providing education as it relates to the prescribed drug regimen. ACE inhibitors act on the vasodilator bradykinin, causing a chronic, dry or "tickling" nonproductive cough. Because cough is a significant symptom, it should always be investigated. For example, dry cough may result from vasovagal stimulation related to angina or impending MI. Severe paroxysms of dry cough may indicate laryngeal swelling and the onset of life-threatening angioedema. Suspected angioedema requires immediate discontinuance of ACE inhibitor therapy. Due to the risk of angioedema, resuscitative equipment and oxygen apparatus should remain accessible during initiation of ACE inhibitor therapy, especially during IV administration. Intravenous administration may initiate an immediate, profound hypotensive response, and possible loss of consciousness.

Contraindications to ACE inhibitor therapy include hypersensitivity, any history of angioedema (idiopathic, familial, or drug induced), and patients with heart failure presently taking a potassium-sparing diuretic. ACE inhibitors are also contraindicated in pregnancy (category D), lactation, and in patients with renal insufficiency.

See "Nursing Process Focus: Patients Receiving ACE Inhibitor Therapy" for specific teaching points.

SPECIAL CONSIDERATIONS

Ethnicity and ACE Inhibitor Action

ACE inhibitors can have unique idiosyncratic effects on individuals of particular racial and/or ethnic groups. In particular, African American patients experience reduced efficacy and a higher incidence of angioedema. The nurse should inform patients of African descent of the variations in drug effectiveness and increased risk of angioedema.

 Pr **PROTOTYPE DRUG** | **ENALAPRIL** (Vasotec)

ACTIONS AND USES

Enalapril is one of the most frequently prescribed ACE inhibitors for hypertension. Unlike captopril (Capoten)—the first ACE inhibitor to be marketed—enalapril has a prolonged half-life, which permits administration once or twice daily. Enalapril acts by reducing angiotensin II and aldosterone levels to produce a significant reduction in blood pressure with few side effects. Enalapril may be used by itself, or in combination with other antihypertensives to minimize side effects.

Administration Alerts

- May produce a first dose phenomenon resulting in profound hypotension, which may result in syncope.
- Pregnancy category D.

ADVERSE EFFECTS AND INTERACTIONS

Unlike diuretics, ACE inhibitors such as enalapril have little effect on electrolyte balance; and unlike beta-adrenergic blockers, they cause few cardiac side effects. Enalapril may cause orthostatic hypotension, when moving quickly from a supine to an upright position. A rapid fall in blood pressure may occur following the first dose. Other side effects include headache and dizziness.

ACE inhibitors can cause life-threatening angioedema, neutropenia, or agranulocytosis. Renin-releasing antihypertensives potentiate the action of enalapril and can cause profound hypotension.

Thiazide diuretics increase potassium loss; K^+-sparing diuretics increase the risk of hyperkalemia. Enalapril may induce lithium toxicity by reducing renal clearance of lithium. NSAIDs may reduce the effectiveness of ACE inhibition.

 See the companion website for a Nursing Process Focus specific to this drug.

NURSING PROCESS FOCUS | PATIENTS RECEIVING ACE INHIBITOR THERAPY

ASSESSMENT

Prior to administration:
- Obtain complete health history including data on recent cardiac events and any incidence of angioedema, allergies, drug history, and possible drug interactions.
- Obtain EKG and vital signs; assess in context of patient's baseline values.
- Assess neurological status and level of consciousness.
- Obtain blood and urine specimens for laboratory analysis.

POTENTIAL NURSING DIAGNOSES

- Risk for Injury, related to orthostatic hypotension
- Deficient Knowledge, related to drug therapy
- Ineffective Tissue Perfusion
- Risk for Imbalanced Nutrition: More than Body Requirements, related to hyperkalemia

PLANNING: PATIENT GOALS AND EXPECTED OUTCOMES

The patient will:
- Exhibit a reduction in systolic/diastolic blood pressure
- Maintain normal serum electrolyte levels during drug therapy
- Demonstrate an understanding of the drug's action by accurately describing drug side effects and precautions

IMPLEMENTATION

Interventions and (Rationales)	Patient Education/Discharge Planning
■ Monitor for first dose phenomenon of profound hypotension.	Warn the patient about the first dose phenomenon; reassure that this effect diminishes with continued therapy. Instruct patient: ■ That changes in consciousness may occur due to rapid reduction in blood pressure; immediately report a feelings of faintness ■ That the drug takes effect in approximately 1 hour and peaks in 3 to 4 hours; rest in the supine position beginning 1 hour after administration and for 3 to 4 hours after the first dose ■ Always arise slowly, avoiding sudden posture changes
■ Observe for hypersensitivity reaction, particularly angioedema. (Angioedema may arise at any time during ACE inhibitor therapy, but is generally expected shortly after initiation of therapy.)	Instruct patient: ■ To immediately report difficulty breathing, throat tightness, muscle cramps, hives or rash, or tremors. These symptoms can occur upon the first dose or much later as a delayed reaction ■ That angioedema can be life threatening and to call emergency medical services if severe dyspnea or hoarseness is accompanied by swelling of the face or mouth
■ Monitor for the presence of blood dyscrasia. ■ Observe for signs of infection: fever, sore throat, malaise, joint pain, ecchymoses, profound fatigue, shortness of breath, or pallor. (Bruising is a sign of bleeding which can indicate the presence of a serious blood disorder.)	Instruct patient to: ■ Immediately report any flulike symptoms ■ Observe for bruising and signs of bleeding from the nose, mouth, GI tract ("coffee ground" vomit or tarry stools), menstrual flooding, or bright red rectal bleeding
■ Monitor for changes in level of consciousness, dizziness, drowsiness, or lightheadedness. (Signs of decreased blood flow to the brain are due to the drug's vasodilating hypotensive action. Sudden syncopal collapse is possible.)	Instruct patient to: ■ Report dizziness or fainting which persists beyond the first dose, as well as unusual sensations (e.g., numbness and tingling) or other changes in the face or limbs ■ Contact the healthcare provider, before the next scheduled dose of the drug, if fainting occurs
■ Monitor for persistent dry cough. (This may be triggered by bradykinin's proinflammatory action.) ■ Monitor changes in cough pattern. (This may indicate another disease process.)	Instruct patient to: ■ Expect persistent dry cough ■ Report any change in the character or frequency of cough. Any cough accompanied by shortness of breath, fever, or chest pain should be reported *immediately* because it may indicate MI

continued

NURSING PROCESS FOCUS: *Patients Receiving ACE Inhibitor Therapy (continued)*

Interventions and (Rationales)	*Patient Education/Discharge Planning*
	■ Sleep with head elevated if cough becomes troublesome when in supine position ■ Use nonmedicated sugar-free lozenges or hard candies to relieve cough
■ Monitor for dehydration or fluid overload. (Dehydration causes low circulating blood volume and will exacerbate hypotension. Severe dehydration may trigger syncope and collapse. Pitting edema is a sign of fluid retention can be a sign of heart failure, and may indicate reduced drug efficacy.)	Instruct patient to: ■ Observe for signs of dehydration such as oliguria, dry lips and mucous membranes, or poor skin turgor ■ Report any bodily swelling that leaves sunken marks on the skin when pressed ■ Measure and monitor fluid intake and output, and weigh daily ■ Monitor increased need for fluid caused by vomiting, diarrhea, or excessive sweating ■ Avoid excessive heat which contributes to sweating and fluid loss ■ Consume adequate amounts of *plain* water
■ Monitor for hyperkalemia. (May occur due to reduced aldosterone levels.)	Instruct patient to: ■ Immediately report signs of hyperkalemia: nausea, irregular heartbeat, profound fatigue/muscle weakness, and slow or faint pulse ■ Avoid consuming electrolyte-fortified snacks, or sports drinks that may contain potassium ■ Avoid using salt substitute (KCl) to flavor foods ■ Consult the healthcare provider before taking any nutritional supplements containing potassium
■ Monitor for liver and kidney function. (ACE inhibitors are metabolized by the liver and excreted by the kidneys.)	Instruct patient to: ■ Report signs of liver toxicity: nausea, vomiting, anorexia, diarrhea, rash, jaundice, abdominal pain, tenderness or distention, or change in the color or character of stools ■ Discontinue drug immediately and contact the healthcare provider if jaundice occurs ■ Adhere to laboratory testing regimen as ordered by the healthcare provider
■ Ensure patient safety. (Due to postural hypotension caused by drug) ■ Monitor ambulation until response to the drug is known.	Instruct patient to: ■ Obtain help prior to getting out of bed or attempting to walk alone ■ Avoid driving or other activities that require mental alertness or physical coordination until effects of the drug are known

EVALUATION OF OUTCOME CRITERIA

Evaluate the effectiveness of drug therapy by confirming that patient goals and expected outcomes have been met (see "Planning").

See Table 21.6 under "ACE Inhibitors" for a list of drugs to which these nursing actions apply.

ADRENERGIC AGENTS

The adrenergic receptor has been a site of pharmacologic action in the treatment of hypertension since the first such drugs were developed in the 1950s. Blockade of adrenergic receptors results in a number of beneficial effects on the heart and vessels and these autonomic drugs are used for a wide variety of cardiovascular disorders. Table 21.7 shows the adrenergic agents used for hypertension.

21.10 Pharmacotherapy with Adrenergic Agents

As discussed in Chapter 13, the autonomic nervous system controls involuntary functions of the body such as heart rate,

Table 21.7	Adrenergic Agents for Hypertension
Drug	**Route and Adult Dose (max dose where indicated)**
Beta-blockers	
atenolol (Tenormin): beta$_1$ (see page 336 for the Prototype Drug box) ⬥	PO; 25–50 mg qd (max 100 mg/day)
bisoprolol (Zebeta): beta$_1$	PO; 2.5–5 mg qd (max 20 mg/day)
metoprolol (Toprol, Lopressor): beta$_1$ (see page 341 for the Prototype Drug box) ⬥	PO; 50–100 mg qd-bid (max 450 mg/day)
propranolol (Inderal): Prototype: beta$_1$ and beta$_2$ (see page 307 for the Prototype Drug box) ⬥	PO; 10–30 mg tid or qd (max 320 mg/day) IV; 0.5–3.0 mg every 4 h prn
timolol (Betimol, others): beta$_1$ and beta$_2$ (see page 721 for the prototype Drug box) ⬥	PO; 15–45 mg tid (max 60 mg/day)
Alpha$_1$-blockers	
℗ doxazosin (Cardura)	PO; 1 mg hs; may increase to 16 mg/day in one to two divided doses (max 16 mg/day)
prazosin (Minipress) (see page 138 for the Prototype Drug box) ⬥	PO; 1 mg hs; may increase to 1 mg bid-tid (max 20 mg/day)
terazosin (Hytrin)	PO; 1 mg hs; may increase 1–5 mg/day (max 20 mg/day)
Alpha$_2$-adrenergic Agonists	
clonidine (Catapres)	PO; 0.1 mg bid-tid (max 0.8 mg/day)
guanabenz (Wytensin)	PO; 4 mg bid; may increase by 4–8 mg/day q1–2 weeks (max 32 mg bid)
methyldopa (Aldomet)	PO; 250 mg bid or tid (max 3 g/day)
Alpha$_1$-and Beta-blockers (Centrally Acting)	
carteolol (Cartrol, Ocupress)	PO; 2.5 mg qd; may increase to 5–10 mg if needed (max 10 mg/day)
labetalol (Trandate, Normodyne)	PO; 100 mg bid; may increase to 200–400 mg bid (max 1200–2400 mg/day)
Adrenergic Neuron Blockers (Peripherally Acting)	
guanadrel (Hylorel)	PO; 5 mg bid; may increase to 20–75 mg/day in two to four divided doses
guanethidine (Ismelin)	PO; 10 mg qd; may increase by 10 mg q5–7d up to 300 mg/day (start with 25–50 mg/day in hospitalized patients, increase by 25–50 mg q1–3d)
reserpine (Serpasil)	PO; 1.5 mg qd initially, may reduce to 0.1–0.25 mg/day

pupil size, and smooth muscle contraction, including that in the arterial walls ⬥ . Stimulation of the sympathetic division causes fight-or-flight responses such as faster heart rate, an increase in blood pressure, and bronchodilation. Peripheral blood vessels are innervated only by sympathetic nerves.

Antihypertensive drugs have been developed that affect the sympathetic division through a number of distinct mechanisms, although all have in common the effect of lowering blood pressure. These mechanisms include the following:

- Blockade of alpha$_1$-receptors in the arterioles
- Selective blockade of beta$_1$-receptors in the heart
- Nonselective blockade of both beta$_1$- and beta$_2$-receptors
- Nonselective blockade of both alpha- and beta- receptors

- Stimulation of alpha$_2$-receptors in the brainstem (centrally acting)
- Blockade of peripheral adrenergic neurons

The earliest drugs for hypertension were nonselective agents, blocking nerve transmission at the ganglion or blocking both alpha- and beta-receptors. Although these nonselective agents revolutionized the treatment of hypertension, they produced significant side effects. They are rarely used today, because the selective agents are more efficacious and better tolerated by patients.

The side effects of adrenergic blockers are generally predictable extensions of the fight-or-flight response. The alpha$_1$-adrenergic blockers tend to cause orthostatic hypotension, when moving quickly from a supine to an upright position. Dizziness, nausea, bradycardia, and dry mouth are also common. Less common, though sometimes a major cause for noncompliance, is their adverse effect on male sexual function. These agents can cause decreased libido and erectile dysfunction (impotence). Nonselective beta-blockers will slow the heart rate and cause bronchoconstriction. They should be used with caution in patients with asthma or heart failure. Some beta-blockers are associated with clinical depression.

Some adrenergic agents cause a blood pressure reduction by acting on alpha$_2$-receptors in the central nervous system. Methyldopa (Aldomet) is converted to a "false" neurotransmitter in the brainstem, thus causing a shortage of the "real" neurotransmitter and inhibition of the sympathetic nervous system. Clonidine (Catapres), an alpha$_2$-agonist, affects alpha-adrenergic receptors in the cardiovascular control centers in the brainstem. The centrally acting agents have a tendency to produce sedation and may cause depression. They are not considered first line drugs in the pharmacotherapy of HTN.

NURSING CONSIDERATIONS

The role of the nurse in adrenergic agent therapy for HTN involves careful monitoring of a patient's condition and providing education as it relates to the prescribed drug regimen. Because of their widespread therapeutic applications, discussions of adrenergic antagonists appear in many chapters in this text. Prototypes of adrenergic blockers can be found for carvedilol (Coreg) in Chapter 22, propranolol (Inderal) in Chapter 23, atenolol (Tenormin) and metoprolol (Lopressor) in Chapter 25, and timolol (Timoptic) in Chapter 48 .

Alpha$_1$-Antagonists

Alpha$_1$-antagonists are indicated for hypertension. These drugs are also used to treat benign prostatic hypertrophy (BPH) and urinary obstruction, because they relax smooth muscle in the prostate and bladder neck, thus reducing urethral resistance. The patient may experience hypotension with the first few doses of these medications and orthostatic hypotension may persist throughout treatment. The first dose phenomenon, especially syncope, can occur. Therefore, it remains important to assess blood pressure prior to and routinely during therapy, to maintain patient safety. The nurse should assess for common side effects such weakness, dizziness, headache, and GI complaints such as nausea and vomiting. The elderly are especially prone to the hypotensive and hypothermic effects related to vasodilation caused by these drugs. Drugs in this group range from pregnancy category B (prazosin) to C (terazosin). See Chapter 13, page 139, "Nursing Process Focus: Patients Receiving Adrenergic Antagonist Therapy" .

Alpha$_2$-Agonists

Alpha$_2$-agonists are centrally acting and have multiple side effects. These drugs are usually reserved to treat hypertension uncontrolled by other drugs. The nurse should assess for the presence of common adverse effects such as orthostatic hypotension, sedation, decreased libido, impotence, sodium/water retention and dry mouth. Alpha$_2$-agonists are pregnancy category C; these drugs are distributed into breast milk.

Beta Blockers

Adrenergic antagonists may be cardioselective (beta$_1$) or nonspecific (beta$_1$ and beta$_2$) receptor blockers. Cardioselective beta-blockers decrease heart rate and affect myocardial conduction and contractility. Reduction in myocardial contractility reduces myocardial oxygen demand. Nonspecific beta-blockers produce the same effects, but also act on the respiratory system and the blood vessels, producing vasoconstriction. The nurse should be alert for signs of respiratory distress,

Pr PROTOTYPE DRUG	DOXAZOSIN (Cardura)

ACTIONS AND USES

Doxazosin is a selective alpha$_1$-adrenergic blocker available only in oral form. Because it is selective for blocking alpha$_1$-receptors in vascular smooth muscle, it has few adverse effects on other autonomic organs and is preferred over nonselective beta-blockers. Doxazosin dilates arteries and veins and is capable of causing a rapid, profound fall in blood pressure. Patients who have difficulty urinating due to an enlarged prostate (BPH) sometimes receive this drug to relieve symptoms of dysuria. Doxazosin is pregnancy category B.

Administration Alerts

- May produce a first dose phenomenon resulting in profound hypotension, which may result in syncope.
- The first dose phenomenon can reoccur when medication is resumed after a period of withdrawal and with dosage increases.

ADVERSE EFFECTS AND INTERACTIONS

Upon starting doxazosin therapy, some patients experience orthostatic hypotension, although tolerance normally develops to this side effect after a few doses. Dizziness and headache are also common side effects, although they are rarely severe enough to cause discontinuation of therapy.

Oral cimetidine may cause a mild increase (10%) in the half-life of doxazosin. This increase is not considered to be clinically significant.

 See the companion website for a Nursing Process Focus specific to this drug.

MediaLink | Mechanism in Action | Doxazosin

NURSING PROCESS FOCUS | PATIENTS RECEIVING BETA-ADRENERGIC ANTAGONIST THERAPY

ASSESSMENT

Prior to administration:
- Obtain complete health history including allergies, drug history, and possible drug interactions.
- Assess vital signs, urinary output, and cardiac output (initially and throughout therapy).
- Assess for presence of respiratory disease, including asthma and COPD.

POTENTIAL NURSING DIAGNOSES

- Deficient Knowledge, related to drug therapy
- Decreased Cardiac Output
- Risk for Injury, related to orthostatic hypotension
- Sexual Dysfunction
- Noncompliance, related to therapeutic regimen

PLANNING: PATIENT GOALS AND EXPECTED OUTCOMES

The patient will:
- Exhibit a reduction in systolic/diastolic blood pressure
- Report a decrease in cardiac symptoms such as chest pain and dyspnea on exertion
- Demonstrate an understanding of the drug's action by accurately describing drug side effects and precautions

IMPLEMENTATION

Interventions and (Rationales)	Patient Education/Discharge Planning
■ Monitor vital signs and pulse, observe for signs of bradycardia, heart failure, or pulmonary edema. (Beta blockers affect heart rate.)	■ Instruct patient to monitor vital signs as specified by the nurse, particularly blood pressure, ensuring proper use of home equipment.
■ Monitor for orthostatic hypotension when assisting patient up from a supine position.	Instruct patient to: ■ Withhold medication for severe hypotensive readings as specified by the nurse (e.g., "hold for levels below 88/50") ■ Always arise slowly, avoiding sudden posture changes
■ Observe for additional side effects such as fatigue and weakness.	■ Instruct patient to report side effects such as slow pulse, difficulty in breathing, dizziness, confusion, fatigue, weakness, and impotence.
■ In diabetic patients, monitor for hypoglycemia. (Some beta-adrenergic blockers may lower blood glucose levels.)	■ Instruct the diabetic patient to check blood glucose levels and to report signs of hypoglycemia.
■ Observe for side effects such as drowsiness.	■ Instruct patient to avoid driving or other activities requiring mental alertness or physical coordination until effects of the drug are known.
■ Measure intake and output; measure daily weights.	Instruct patient to: ■ Measure and monitor fluid intake and output and weigh daily ■ Consume enough *plain* water to remain adequately, but not over, hydrated

EVALUATION OF OUTCOME CRITERIA

Evaluate the effectiveness of drug therapy by confirming that patient goals and expected outcomes have been met (see "Planning").

See Table 21.7 under "Beta-Blockers" for a list of drugs to which these nursing actions apply.

including shortness of breath and wheezing, in patients on nonspecific beta-blocking drugs. These side effects tend to occur at high doses and with older drugs. Beta-blockers have several other important therapeutic applications. By decreasing the cardiac workload, beta-blockers can ease the symptoms of angina pectoris (Chapter 25). By slowing conduction through the myocardium, beta-blockers are able to treat certain types of dysrhythmias (Chapter 23). Other therapeutic uses include the treatment of heart failure, myocardial infarction (Chapter 25), and migraines (Chapter 19) .

Because all beta-blockers affect myocardial contractility, the nurse should monitor heart rate, rhythm and sounds, as well as the EKG. Beta-blockers can produce bradycardia and heart block. Reduction in heart rate can also contribute to fatigue and activity intolerance. Beta-blockers cause the heart rate to become less responsive to exertion. Patients should be advised to monitor their pulse as well as blood pressure daily. Diabetics should be warned that symptoms of hypoglycemia (diaphoresis, nervousness, and palpitation) may be less observable while on beta-blocker therapy.

See "Nursing Process Focus: Patients Receiving Beta-Adrenergic Antagonist Therapy" for more information.

DIRECT VASODILATORS

Drugs that directly affect arteriolar smooth muscle are highly effective at lowering blood pressure but produce too many side effects to be drugs of first choice. These agents are shown in Table 21.8.

21.11 Treating Hypertension with Direct Vasodilators

All antihypertensive classes discussed thus far lower blood pressure through indirect means by affecting enzymes (ACE inhibitors), autonomic nerves (alpha- and beta-blockers), or fluid volume (diuretics). It would seem that a more efficient way to reduce blood pressure would be to cause a direct relaxation of arteriolar smooth muscle; unfortunately the direct vasodilator drugs have the potential to produce serious adverse effects. All direct vasodilators can produce reflex tachycardia as a compensatory response to the sudden decrease in blood pressure. Hydralazine (Apresoline) can induce a lupus-like syndrome. Pericardial effusions have been reported with minoxidil (Loniten) use. Because safer drugs are available, the oral direct vasodilators are rarely prescribed.

One direct-acting vasodilator, nitroprusside (Nitropress), is specifically used for those patients who have aggressive, life-threatening hypertension that must be quickly controlled. Nitroprusside (Nitropress), with a half-life of only 2 minutes, has the capability of lowering blood pressure almost instantaneously upon IV administration. It is essential to continuously monitor patients receiving this drug, to avoid hypotension because of overtreatment.

NURSING CONSIDERATIONS

Direct vasodilators are primarily utilized in emergency situations when it is necessary to reduce blood pressure quickly. In the critical care or emergency department setting, the patient

Table 21.8	Direct-acting Vasodilators for Hypertension
Drug	**Route and Adult Dose (max dose where indicated)**
diazoxide (Hyperstat IV)	IV; 1–3 mg/kg push (max 150 mg)
hydralazine (Apresoline)	PO; 10–50 mg qid (max 300 mg/day)
minoxidil (Loniten)	PO; 5–40 mg/day in a single or divided doses (max 100 mg/day)
nitroprusside (Nitropress)	IV; 1.5–10 µg/kg/min

Pr PROTOTYPE DRUG | HYDRALAZINE (Apresoline)

ACTIONS AND USES

Hydralazine was one of the first oral antihypertensive drugs marketed in the United States. It acts through a direct vasodilation of vascular smooth muscle. Although it produces an effective reduction in blood pressure, drugs in other antihypertensive classes have largely replaced hydralazine. The drug is available in both oral and parenteral formulations.

Administration Alerts

- Abrupt withdrawal of drug may cause rebound hypertension and anxiety.
- Pregnancy category C.

ADVERSE EFFECTS AND INTERACTIONS

Hydralazine may produce serious side effects, including severe reflex tachycardia. Patients taking hydralazine sometimes receive a beta-adrenergic blocker to counteract this effect on the heart. The drug may produce a lupus-like syndrome with extended use. Sodium and fluid retention is a potentially serious adverse effect. Because of these side effects, the use of hydralazine is mostly limited to patients whose HTN cannot be controlled with other, safer medications.

MAO inhibitors may potentiate hypotensive action. Other antihypertensive drugs given concomitantly can cause profound hypotension. NSAIDs may decrease the antihypertensive response.

 See the companion website for a Nursing Process Focus specific to this drug.

will likely undergo continuous monitoring of vital signs, EKG, and pulse oximetry. The nurse may also be expected to auscultate blood pressures every 5 to 15 minutes during the drug infusion. The nurse should closely observe monitoring equipment to assess heart rate/EKG for reflex tachycardia.

Contraindications include hypersensitivity, coronary artery disease, rheumatic mitral valve disease, cerebrovascular disease, renal insufficiency, and systemic lupus erythematosus. Direct vasodilators can cause priapism, a sustained, painful penile erection unrelieved by orgasm. Patients may feel embarrassed by priapism, and reluctant to report this side effect. They should be warned that priapism constitutes a medical emergency; if not treated promptly, permanent impotence may result.

There are specific considerations for the various types of direct vasodilators. For minoxidil (Loniten) therapy, the nurse should monitor blood pressure and pulse in both arms while the patient is lying, sitting, and standing to assess for orthostatic hypotension. The patient should be informed these agents may cause elongation, thickening, and increased pigmentation of body hair. This is normal and will stop when the drug is discontinued.

For IV diazoxide (Hyperstat), the nurse should be aware that repeated IV use can result in sodium and water retention; sodium, BUN levels, and the presence of edema and heart failure should be monitored. Diuretics may be used to counteract this effect when used during labor and

NATURAL THERAPIES | Hawthorn for Hypertension

A number of botanicals have been reported to possess antihypertensive activity, including hawthorn, which is sometimes called May bush. Hawthorn (*Crataegus laevigata*) is a thorny shrub or small tree that is widespread in North America, Europe, and Asia. Use of hawthorn dates back to ancient Greece. In some cultures, the shrub is surrounded in magic and religious rites and is thought to ward off evil spirits. The ship *Mayflower* was named after this shrub.

Leaves, flowers, and berries of the plant are dried or extracted in liquid form. Active ingredients are flavonoids and procyanidins. Hawthorn has been purported to lower blood pressure after 4 weeks or longer of therapy, although the effect has been small. The mechanism of action may be inhibition of ACE or reduction of cardiac workload. Patients taking cardiac glycosides should avoid hawthorn, because it has the ability to decrease cardiac output. Patients should be advised not to rely upon any botanical for the treatment of hypertension without frequent measurements of blood pressure to be certain therapy is effective.

NURSING PROCESS FOCUS | PATIENTS RECEIVING DIRECT VASODILATOR THERAPY

ASSESSMENT

Prior to administration:
- Obtain complete health history including allergies, drug history, and possible drug interactions.
- Obtain EKG and vital signs; assess in context of patient's baseline values.
- Auscultate heart and chest sounds.
- Assess neurological status and level of consciousness.
- Obtain blood and urine specimens for laboratory analysis.

POTENTIAL NURSING DIAGNOSES

- Ineffective Tissue Perfusion
- Excess Fluid Volume
- Risk for Injury, related to orthostatic hypotension
- Risk for Impaired Skin Integrity (e.g., IV vasodilators)
- Deficient Knowledge, related to drug therapy

PLANNING: PATIENT GOALS AND EXPECTED OUTCOMES

The patient will:
- Exhibit a reduction in systolic/diastolic blood pressure
- Demonstrate an understanding of the drug's action by accurately describing drug side effects and precautions

IMPLEMENTATION

Interventions and (Rationales)	*Patient Education/Discharge Planning*
■ Observe for signs and symptoms of lupus.	■ Instruct patient to report classic "butterfly rash" over the nose and cheeks, muscle aches, and fatigue when taking hydralazine.
■ Monitor patient vital signs every 5 to 15 minutes and titrate infusion based on prescribed parameters. (These drugs cause rapid hypotension.)	■ Instruct patient to report any burning or stinging pain, swelling, warmth, redness, or tenderness at the IV insertion site which may signal phlebitis or drug seepage into soft tissues.
■ Use with caution with impaired cardiac/cerebral circulation. (The hypotension produced by vasodilators may further compromise individuals who already suffer from ischemia.)	Instruct patient to: ■ Report angina-like symptoms: chest, arm, back and/or neck pain, palpitations

continued

NURSING PROCESS FOCUS: *Patients Receiving Direct Vasodilator Therapy (continued)*

Interventions and (Rationales)	Patient Education/Discharge Planning
	■ Report faintness, dizziness, drowsiness, any sensation of cold, numbness, tingling, pale or dusky look to the hands and feet ■ Report headache or signs of stroke: facial drooping, visual changes, limb weakness, or paralysis ■ Monitor vitals signs (especially blood pressure) daily or as often as advised by the nurse
■ Monitor for dizziness. (This is a sign of hypotension that occurs because the brain is not getting enough blood flow.)	Instruct patient to: ■ Avoid driving or other activities requiring mental alertness or physical coordination until effects of the drug are known ■ Always arise slowly, avoiding sudden posture changes
■ Evaluate for needed lifestyle modifications.	■ Instruct patient to comply with additional interventions for HTN such as weight reduction, modification of sodium intake, smoking cessation, exercise, and stress management.
■ Discontinue medication gradually. (Abrupt withdrawal of drug may cause rebound hypertension and anxiety.)	■ Instruct patient to not stop taking drug suddenly.

EVALUATION OF OUTCOME CRITERIA

Evaluate the effectiveness of drug therapy by confirming that patient goals and expected outcomes have been met (see "Planning").

See Table 21.8 for a list of drugs to which these nursing applications apply.

(side margin: MediaLink — Herbal Therapies for Hypertension)

delivery. However, fetal or neonatal hyperbilirubinemia, thrombocytopenia, or altered carbohydrate metabolism may be complications.

Intravenous nitroprusside is a chemically unstable solution. The only diluent compatible with nitroprusside is 5% dextrose in water (D5W). This drug should never be mixed with any other drugs or diluents. Once dissolved in the vial, nitroprusside solution should be further diluted (in a 250 ml to 1 L bag of D5W) to prevent phlebitis. Reconstituted ni-

troprusside solution is brown and considered stable for up to 24 hours, but the drug is exceptionally light-sensitive. Once reconstituted, the nurse should wrap the IV bag and tubing in an opaque substance (e.g., aluminum foil); labeling should appear on the wrap as well as on the bag itself. The drug solution should be checked periodically and the drug discarded if the color of the solution changes.

See "Nursing Process Focus: Patients Receiving Direct Vasodilator Therapy" for specific teaching points.

CHAPTER REVIEW

Key Concepts

The numbered key concepts provide a succinct summary of the important points from the corresponding numbered section within the chapter. If any of these points are not clear, refer to the numbered section within the chapter for review. Expanded versions can be found on the companion website.

21.1 High blood pressure is classified as essential (primary) or secondary. Uncontrolled hypertension can

lead to chronic and debilitating disorders such as stroke, heart attack, and heart failure.

21.2 The three primary factors controlling blood pressure are cardiac output, peripheral resistance, and blood volume.

21.3 Many factors help to regulate blood pressure, including the vasomotor center, baroreceptors and chemoreceptors in the aorta and internal carotid arteries, and the renin-angiotensin system.

21.4 Hypertension has been recently redefined as a sustained blood pressure of 140/90 mm Hg after multiple measurements made over several clinic visits. A person with sustained blood pressure of 120–139/80–89 mm Hg is said to be prehypertensive, and is at increased risk of developing hypertension.

21.5 Because antihypertensive medications may have uncomfortable side effects, lifestyle changes such as proper diet and exercise should be implemented prior to and during pharmacotherapy to allow lower drug doses.

21.6 Pharmacotherapy of HTN often begins with low doses of a single medication. If ineffective, a second agent from a different class may be added to the regimen.

21.7 Diuretics are often the first line medications for HTN because they have few side effects and can control minor to moderate hypertension.

21.8 Calcium channel blockers block calcium ions from entering cells and cause smooth muscle in arterioles to relax, thus reducing blood pressure. CCBs have emerged as major drugs in the treatment of hypertension.

21.9 Blocking the renin-angiotensin system prevents the intense vasoconstriction caused by angiotensin II. These drugs also decrease blood volume, which enhances their antihypertensive effect.

21.10 Antihypertensive autonomic agents are available which block alpha$_1$-receptors, block beta$_1$- and/or beta$_2$-receptors, or stimulate alpha$_2$- receptors in the brainstem (centrally acting).

21.11 A few medications lower blood pressure by acting directly to relax arteriolar smooth muscle, but these are not widely used due to their numerous side effects.

Review Questions

1. Because hypertension may cause no symptoms, how would the nurse convince a patient to take his or her medication regularly?

2. State the major reasons why a patient should continue lifestyle changes, even though the antihypertensive drug appears to be effective.

3. Why is it important for patients to weigh themselves on a regular basis when taking antihypertensive drugs?

Critical Thinking Questions

1. A 74-year-old patient has a history of hypertension, mild renal failure, and angina. The patient is on a low-sodium, low-protein diet. The most recent BP is 106/84. Should the nurse give the patient benazepril (Lotensin) as scheduled? Why or why not?

2. A patient with diabetes is on atenolol (Tenormin) for hypertension. What teaching should be done for this patient?

3. A patient is having a hypertensive crisis (230/130) and the BP needs to be lowered. The patient has an IV drip of nitroprusside (Nitropress) initiated. How much would the nurse want to lower this patient's BP? Name three nursing factors that are crucial when giving this drip.

 ## EXPLORE MediaLink

NCLEX review, case studies, and other interactive resources for this chapter can be found on the companion website at www.prenhall.com/adams. Click on "Chapter 21" to select the activities for this chapter. For animations, more NCLEX review questions, and an audio glossary, access the accompanying CD-ROM in this textbook.

CHAPTER 22

Drugs for Heart Failure

■ DRUGS AT A GLANCE

CARDIAC GLYCOSIDES
🅿 *digoxin (Lanoxin, Lanoxicaps)*

ANGIOTENSIN-CONVERTING ENZYME (ACE) INHIBITORS
🅿 *lisinopril (Prinivil, Zestril)*

VASODILATORS
🅿 *isosorbide dinitrate (Isordil, Sorbitrate, Dilatrate)*

DIURETICS
Loop or high ceiling
🅿 *furosemide (Lasix)*

Thiazide and thiazide-like agents
Potassium-sparing

PHOSPHODIESTERASE INHIBITORS
🅿 *milrinone (Primacor)*

BETA-ADRENERGIC BLOCKERS (ANTAGONISTS)
🅿 *carvedilol (Coreg)*

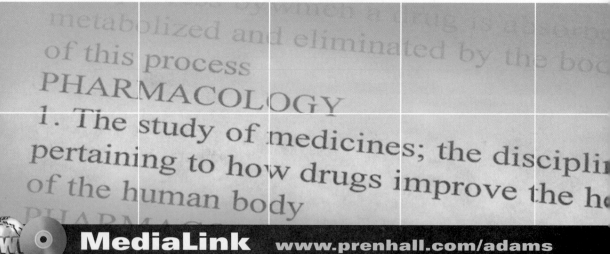

MediaLink www.prenhall.com/adams

CD-ROM
Animations:
 Mechanism in Action: Digoxin (Lanoxin)
 Mechanism in Action: Lisinopril (Prinvil)
 Mechanism in Action: Furosemide (Lasix)
Audio Glossary
NCLEX Review

Companion Website
NCLEX Review
Dosage Calculations
Case Study
Care Plans
Expanded Key Concepts

OBJECTIVES

After reading this chapter, the student should be able to:

1. Identify the major risk factors associated with heart failure.
2. Relate how the classic symptoms associated with heart failure may be caused by weakened heart muscle.
3. Explain how preload and afterload affect cardiac function.
4. Describe the nurse's role in the pharmacologic management of heart failure.
5. For each of the drug classes listed in Drugs at a Glance, know representative drug examples, explain their mechanism of action, primary actions, and important adverse effects.
6. Categorize heart failure drugs based on their classification and mechanism of action.
7. Use the steps of the Nursing Process to care for patients who are receiving drug therapy for heart failure.

Heart failure is one of the most common and fatal of the cardiovascular diseases, and its incidence is expected to increase as the population ages. Despite the dramatic decline in mortality for most cardiovascular diseases that has occurred over the past two decades, the death rate for heart failure has only recently begun to decrease. Although improved treatment of myocardial infarction and hypertension has led to declines in mortality due to heart failure, approximately one in five patients still dies within 1 year of diagnosis of heart failure, and 50% die within 5 years. The incidence of sudden death is as much as 9 times higher in patients with heart failure than in the general population.

PHARMFACTS | Heart Failure

- Heart failure increases with age. It affects:
  2% of those 40 to 50 years old
  5% of those 60 to 69 years old
  10% of those over age 70
- Over 42,000 people die of HF each year.
- Heart failure is responsible for about 3 million office care visits and 1 million hospitalizations each year.
- Heart failure is the most common hospital discharge diagnosis in patients aged 65 or older.
- Blacks have 1.5 to 2 times the incidence of HF as whites.
- Heart failure occurs slightly more frequently in men than women.
- Heart failure is twice as frequent in hypertensive patients and 5 times as frequent in persons who have experienced a heart attack.

THE PATHOPHYSIOLOGY OF HEART FAILURE

22.1 The Etiology of Heart Failure

Heart failure (HF) is the inability of the ventricles to pump enough blood to meet the body's metabolic demands. Though not usually considered a distinct disease, it may be caused or worsened by certain underlying disorders. Indeed, while weakening of cardiac muscle is a natural consequence of aging, the process can be accelerated by the following diseases associated with heart failure.

- Mitral stenosis
- Myocardial infarction
- Chronic hypertension

- Coronary artery disease
- Diabetes mellitus

Since there is no cure for heart failure, the treatment goals are to prevent, treat, or remove the underlying causes when possible, to improve the patient's quality of life. Effective pharmacotherapy can relieve many of the distressing symptoms of heart failure and may prolong patients' lives.

22.2 Cardiovascular Changes in Heart Failure

Although a number of diseases can lead to heart failure, the end result is the same: The heart is unable to pump the volume of blood required to meet the body's metabolic needs. To understand how medications act on the weakened myocardium, it is essential to understand the underlying cardiac physiology.

The right side of the heart receives blood from the venous system and pumps it to the lungs, where the blood receives oxygen and loses its carbon dioxide. The blood returns to the left side of the heart, which pumps it to the rest of the body via the aorta. The amount of blood received by the right side should exactly equal that sent out by the left side. If this does not happen, HF may occur. The amount of blood pumped by each ventricle per minute is the cardiac output. The relationship between cardiac output and blood pressure is explained in Chapter 21 ⬡ .

Although many variables affect cardiac output, the two most important factors are preload and afterload. Just before the chambers of the heart contract (systole), they are filled to their maximum capacity with blood. The degree to which the myocardial fibers are stretched just prior to contraction is called preload. The more these fibers are stretched, the more forceful they will contract, a principle called the Frank-Starling law. This is somewhat similar to a rubber band; the more it is stretched, the more forceful it will snap back. The strength of contraction of the heart is called contractility.

The second important factor affecting cardiac output is afterload. In order for the left ventricle to pump blood out of the heart, it must overcome a fairly substantial pressure in the aorta. Afterload is the pressure in the aorta that must be overcome for blood to be ejected from the left ventricle.

In HF, the myocardium becomes weakened, and the heart cannot eject all the blood it receives. This weakening may occur on the left side, the right side, or on both sides of the heart. If it occurs on the left side, excess blood accumulates in the left ventricle. The wall of the left ventricle may become thicker (hypertrophy) in an attempt to compensate for the extra blood retained in the chamber. Since the left ventricle has limits to its ability to compensate for the increased preload, blood "backs up" into the lungs, resulting in the classic symptoms of cough and shortness of breath, particularly when the patient is lying

down. Left heart failure is sometimes called congestive heart failure (CHF). The pathophysiology of HF is shown in Figure 22.1.

Although left heart failure is more common, the right side of the heart can also become weak, either simultaneously with the left side or independently from the left side. In right heart failure, the blood backs up into the peripheral veins, resulting in peripheral edema and engorgement of organs such as the liver.

22.3 Primary Characteristics of Heart Function

Cardiac physiology is quite complex, particularly when the heart is challenged by a chronic disease such as heart failure. A simplified method for understanding cardiac function and one that is quite useful for pharmacotherapy is to visualize the heart as having the following three fundamental characteristics.

- It contracts with a specific force or strength (contractility).
- It beats at a certain rate (beats per minute).
- It conducts electrical impulses at a particular speed.

Since the fundamental cause of heart failure is a weak myocardium, causing the muscle to beat more forcefully seems to be an ideal solution. The ability to increase the strength of contraction is called a positive inotropic effect and is a fundamental characteristic of the class of drugs known as the cardiac glycosides.

The ability of an agent to change the heart rate is a second characteristic important to pharmacology. A faster heart works harder, but not necessarily more efficiently. A slower heart has a longer time to rest between beats, known as the refractory period. The ability of a drug to change the heart rate is called a chronotropic effect.

A third fundamental characteristic of cardiac physiology, explained in Chapter 23, is the electrical conduction through the heart ⬡ . Some cardiovascular drugs influence the speed of this conduction, known as a dromotropic effect.

DRUGS FOR HEART FAILURE

Drugs can relieve the symptoms of heart failure by a number of different mechanisms, including slowing the heart rate, increasing contractility, and reducing its workload. These mechanisms are illustrated in Figure 22.2.

Cardiac Glycosides

Once used as arrow poisons by African tribes and as medicines by the ancient Egyptians and Romans, the value of the cardiac glycosides in treating heart disorders has been known for over 2,000 years. The chemical classification draws its name from three sugars, or glycosides, which are attached to a steroid nucleus. Information on the cardiac glycosides is provided in Table 22.1.

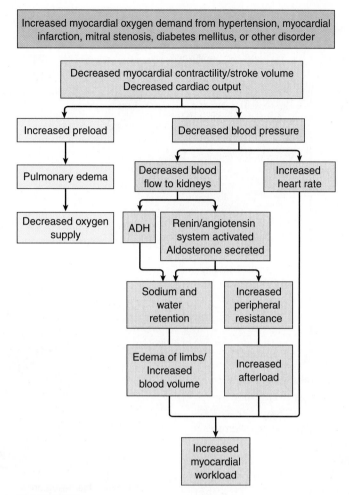

Figure 22.1 | Pathophysiology of heart failure

22.4 Pharmacotherapy with Cardiac Glycosides

Extracted from the beautiful flowering plants, *Digitalis purpurea* (purple foxglove) and *Digitalis lanata* (white foxglove), drugs from this class are also called digitalis glycosides. Until the discovery of ACE inhibitors, cardiac glycosides were the mainstay of HF treatment. Indeed, they are still widely prescribed for this disorder. The cardiac glycosides cause the heart to beat more forcefully and more slowly, improving cardiac output. The two primary cardiac glycosides—digoxin and digitoxin—are quite similar in efficacy; the primary difference is the latter has a more prolonged half-life.

The margin of safety between a therapeutic dose and a toxic dose of digitalis is quite narrow, and severe adverse effects may result from unmonitored treatment. Digitalization refers to a procedure in which the dose of cardiac glycoside is gradually increased until tissues become saturated with the drug, and the symptoms of HF diminish. If the patient is critically ill, digitalization can be accomplished rapidly with IV doses in a controlled clinical environment, where side adverse effects are carefully monitored. As an outpatient, digitalization with digoxin

may occur over a period of 7 days, using oral dosing. In either case, the goal is to determine the proper dose of drug that may be administered, without undue adverse effects.

NURSING CONSIDERATIONS

The role of the nurse in cardiac glycoside therapy involves careful monitoring of a patient's condition and providing education as it relates to the prescribed drug regimen. Prior to beginning therapy with cardiac glycosides, the patient should be evaluated for ventricular dysrhythmias not caused by HF and for any history of hypersensitivity to cardiac glycosides. The patient's renal function should be assessed because the drug is excreted by the kidneys. The nurse should administer these drugs with caution in elderly patients; those with acute myocardial infarction, incomplete heart block, and renal insufficiency; or in pregnant or lactating mothers.

Side effects that the nurse must monitor for when caring for patients taking these drugs include fatigue, drowsiness, dizziness, visual disturbances, anorexia, nausea, and vomiting. The nurse should advise patients to carry or wear identification describing their medical diagnosis and drug regimen. The nurse should instruct patients to eat

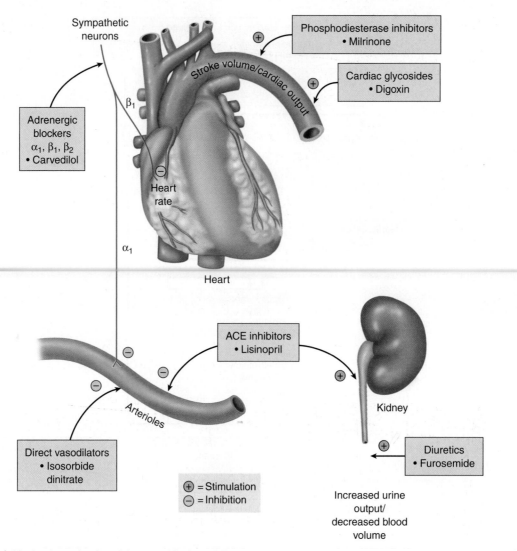

Sympathetic neurons

Phosphodiesterase inhibitors
• Milrinone

Stroke volume/cardiac output

Cardiac glycosides
• Digoxin

Adrenergic blockers
α_1, β_1, β_2
• Carvedilol

β_1

$\ominus$
Heart rate

α_1

Heart

ACE inhibitors
• Lisinopril

Kidney

Arterioles

Direct vasodilators
• Isosorbide dinitrate

$\oplus$ = Stimulation
$\ominus$ = Inhibition

Diuretics
• Furosemide

Increased urine output/ decreased blood volume

Figure 22.2 | Mechanisms of action of drugs used for heart failure

potassium-rich foods, as hypokalemia may predispose the patient to digoxin toxicity. Antacids or antidiarrheal medications should not be taken within 2 hours of cardiac glycoside administration because they decrease the absorption of digoxin.

It is common for dysrhythmias to occur when high doses of digoxin are administered. The nurse should be prepared to administer digoxin immune Fab (Digibind) in the case of life-threatening dysrhythmias. This drug binds and subsequently removes digoxin from the body, and prevents toxic effects of overdose.

See "Nursing Process Focus: Patients Receiving Cardiac Glycoside Therapy" for specific teaching points.

ACE Inhibitors

Drugs affecting the renin-angiotensin system reduce the afterload on the heart and lower blood pressure. They are often drugs of choice in the treatment of heart failure. The ACE inhibitors used for HF are shown in Table 22.1.

22.5 Pharmacotherapy with ACE Inhibitors

Approved for the treatment of hypertension since the 1980s, ACE inhibitors have been shown to slow the progression of heart failure and to reduce mortality from this disease. Due to their relative safety, they have largely replaced digoxin as first line drugs for the treatment of chronic HF.

The primary action of the ACE inhibitors is to lower peripheral resistance and reduce blood volume by enhancing the excretion of sodium and water. The resultant reduction of arterial blood pressure diminishes the afterload required of the heart, thus increasing cardiac output. An additional effect of the ACE inhibitors is dilation of the veins returning blood to the heart. This action, which is probably not directly related to their inhibition of angiotensin, decreases preload and reduces peripheral edema. The combined reductions in preload, afterload, and blood volume substantially decrease the workload on the heart and allow it to work more efficiently for the HF patient. Several ACE inhibitors have been shown to reduce mortality following acute my-

Table 22.1 | Drugs for Heart Failure

Drug	Route and Adult Dose (max dose where indicated)
Cardiac Glycosides	
digitoxin (Crystodigin)	PO; 150 μg qd (max 0.3 mg/day)
℞ digoxin (Lanoxin, Lanoxicaps)	PO; 0.125–0.5 mg qd
ACE Inhibitors	
captopril (Capoten)	PO; 6.25–12.5 mg tid (max 450 mg/day)
enalapril (Vasotec) (see page 274 for the Prototype Drug box) ∞	PO; 2.5 mg qid-bid (max 40 mg/day)
fosinopril (Monopril)	PO; 5–40 mg qd (max 40 mg/day)
℞ lisinopril (Prinivil, Zestoretic, Zestril)	PO; 10 mg qd (max 80 mg/day)
quinapril (Accupril)	PO; 10–20 mg qd (max 40 mg/day)
ramipril (Altace)	PO; 2.5–5.0 mg bid (max 10/day)
Vasodilators	
hydralazine (Apresoline) (see page 280 for the Prototype Drug box) ∞	PO; 10–50 mg qid (max 300 mg/day)
℞ isosorbide dinitrate (Isordil, Sorbitrate, Dilatrate)	PO; 2.5–30 mg qid administer ac and hs (max 160 mg/day)
Diuretics	
Loop or High Ceiling	
bumetanide (Bumex)	PO; 0.5–2.mg qd (max 10 mg/day)
℞ furosemide (Lasix)	PO; 20–80 mg in one or more divided doses (max 600 mg/day)
torsemide (Demadex)	PO; 10–20 mg qd (max 200 mg/day)
Thiazide and Thiazide-like	
chlorothiazide (Diuril) (see page 645 for the Prototype Drug box) ∞	PO; 250 mg–1 g in one to two divided doses (max 2 g/day)
hydrochlorothiazide (HydroDIURIL, HCTZ) (see page 267 for the Prototype Drug box) ∞	PO; 25–200 mg in one to three divided doses (max 200 mg/day)
Potassium-sparing	
spironolactone (Aldactone) (see page 647 for the Prototype Drug box) ∞	PO; 5–200 mg in divided doses (max 200 mg/day)
triamterene (Dyrenium)	PO; 100 mg bid (max 300 mg/day)
Phosphodiesterase Inhibitors	
inamrinone (Inocor)	IV; 0.75 mg/kg bolus given slowly over 2–3 min; then 5–10 μg/kg/min (max 10 mg/kg/day)
℞ milrinone (Primacor)	IV; 50 μkg over 10 min; then 0.375–0.75 μg/kg/min
Beta Adrenergic Blockers	
℞ carvedilol (Coreg)	PO; 3.125 mg bid for 2 wks (max 25 mg bid if <85 kg or 50 mg bid if >85 kg)
metoprolol extended release (Toprol-XL)	PO; 25 mg/day for 2 wks; 12.5 mg/day for severe cases (max 200 mg/day)

ocardial infarction when therapy is started soon after the onset of symptoms (Chapter 25) ∞. More information on ACE inhibitors can be found in Chapter 21 ∞.

NURSING CONSIDERATIONS

The role of the nurse in ACE inhibitor therapy for heart failure involves careful monitoring of a patient's condition and providing education as it relates to the prescribed drug regimen. Prior to beginning therapy, a thorough health history should be taken. These drugs are contraindicated in pregnancy, lactation, and history of angioedema. A complete blood count should be obtained before starting therapy and repeated every month for the first 3 to 6 months of treatment, then at periodic intervals for 1 year. These drugs may cause neutropenia, and should be withheld if the neutrophil

Pr PROTOTYPE DRUG | DIGOXIN (Lanoxin)

ACTIONS AND USES

The primary benefit of digoxin is its ability to increase the contractility or strength of myocardial contraction—a positive inotropic action. Digoxin accomplishes this by inhibiting Na$^+$-K$^+$ ATPase, the critical enzyme responsible for pumping sodium ion out of the myocardial cell in exchange for potassium ion. As sodium accumulates, calcium ions are released from their storage areas in the cell. The release of calcium ion produces a more forceful contraction of the myocardial fibers.

By increasing myocardial contractility, digoxin directly increases cardiac output, thus alleviating symptoms of HF and improving exercise tolerance. The improved cardiac output results in increased urine production and a desirable reduction in blood volume, relieving the distressing symptoms of pulmonary congestion and peripheral edema.

In addition to its positive inotropic effect, digoxin also affects impulse conduction in the heart. Digoxin has the ability to suppress the sinoatrial (SA) node and slow electrical conduction through the atrioventricular (AV) node. Because of these actions, digoxin is sometimes used to treat dysrhythmias, as discussed in Chapter 23 ⊚. Digoxin is pregnancy category A.

Administration Alerts

■ Take the patient's apical pulse for 1 full minute, noting rate, rhythm, and quality before administering. If pulse is below 60 beats per minute, the drug is usually withheld and the healthcare provider notified.

■ Check for recent serum digoxin level results before administering. If level is higher than 1.8, withhold dose and notify healthcare provider.

ADVERSE EFFECTS AND INTERACTIONS

The most dangerous adverse effect of digoxin is its ability to create dysrhythmias, particularly in patients who have low potassium levels in the blood (hypokalemia). Because diuretics can cause hypokalemia and are also often used to treat HF, concurrent use of digoxin and diuretics must be carefully monitored. Other adverse effects of digoxin therapy include nausea, vomiting, anorexia, and visual disturbances such as seeing halos, a yellow/green tinge, or blurring. Periodic serum drug levels should be obtained to determine if the digoxin level is within the therapeutic range, so the dosage may be adjusted based on the laboratory results. Because a small increase in digoxin levels can produce serious adverse effects, the nurse must constantly be on the alert for drug-drug interactions and for changes in renal function.

Digoxin interacts with a number of drugs. Antacids and cholesterol-lowering drugs can decrease absorption of digoxin. If calcium is administered IV together with digoxin, it can increase the risk of dysrhythmias. When the patient is also receiving quinidine, verapamil, or flecainide, digoxin levels will be significantly increased. The digoxin dose should be decreased by 50%.

Use with caution with herbal supplements, such as ginseng, which may increase the risk of digoxin toxicity. Ma-huang and ephedra may induce dysrhythmias. Patients on cardiac glycosides should be strongly advised not to take any other prescription or OTC medication or herbal product without notifying the healthcare provider.

See the companion website for a Nursing Process Focus specific to this drug.

---

count drops below 1,000/mm^3. Additionally, the patient should discontinue diuretics before the nurse initially administers ACE inhibitors, to prevent severe hypotension. Because ACE inhibitors can cause severe hypotension with initial doses, the nurse should monitor the patient closely for several hours. If severe hypotension does occur, the nurse should place the patient in a supine position and notify the healthcare provider. A lower dose is indicated for elderly patients and those with renal insufficiency. These drugs should be used with caution in patients with impaired kidney function, hyperkalemia, and those with autoimmune diseases, especially systemic lupus (SLE).

Patient education as it relates to ACE inhibitors used to treat heart failure should include the goals, reasons for obtaining baseline data such as vital signs and tests for cardiac and renal disorders, and possible side effects. The nurse should instruct the patient on the following:

■ Check with the healthcare provider before taking additional prescription medications or OTC drugs.

■ It may take weeks or months for maximum therapeutic response to be reached.

■ Follow prescribed dietary modifications, including sodium and potassium restrictions, to prevent side effects of hyperkalemia and hyponatremia.

■ Do not take salt or potassium supplements unless ordered by the healthcare provider.

■ Avoid driving until the effect of the drug is known.

Please refer to "Nursing Process Focus: Patients Receiving ACE Inhibitor Therapy," page 275 in Chapter 21, for additional information ⊚.

Vasodilators

Through their hypotensive effects, vasodilators play a minor role in the pharmacotherapy of heart failure. They are also used for hypertension and angina pectoris. Doses for the two vasodilators are given in Table 22.1.

22.6 Pharmacotherapy with Direct Vasodilators

The two drugs in this class act directly to relax blood vessels and lower blood pressure. Hydralazine (Apresoline) acts on arterioles while isosorbide dinitrate (Isordil) acts on veins. Because the two drugs act synergistically, isosorbide dinitrate is usually combined with hydralazine in the treatment of HF. Because of the high incidence of side effects,

NURSING PROCESS FOCUS   PATIENTS RECEIVING CARDIAC GLYCOSIDE THERAPY

ASSESSMENT

Prior to administration:
- Obtain complete health history including allergies, drug history, and possible drug interactions.
- Assess vital signs, urinary output, and cardiac output, initially and throughout therapy.
- Determine the reason the medication is being administered.

POTENTIAL NURSING DIAGNOSES

- Ineffective Tissue Perfusion, related to impaired cardiac status
- Decreased Cardiac Output
- Excess Fluid Volume
- Deficient Knowledge, related to drug therapy

PLANNING: PATIENT GOALS AND EXPECTED OUTCOMES

The patient will:
- Report decreased symptoms of cardiac decompensation related to fluid overload
- Exhibit evidence of improved organ perfusion, including kidney, heart, and brain
- Demonstrate an understanding of the drug's action by accurately describing drug side effects and precautions
- Immediately report side effects such as nausea, vomiting, diarrhea, heart rate below 60, and vision changes

IMPLEMENTATION

Interventions and (Rationales)	*Patient Education/Discharge Planning*
Monitor ECG for rate and rhythm changes during initial digitalization therapy. (Drug has a strong positive inotropic effect)	Instruct patient to: • Count pulse for 1 full minute and record pulse with every dose • Contact healthcare provider if pulse rate is less than 60 or greater than 100
Observe for side effects such as nausea, vomiting, diarrhea, anorexia, shortness of breath, vision changes, and leg muscle cramps.	Instruct patient to report side effects immediately to prevent toxicity.
Weigh patient daily.	Instruct patient to report weight gain of 2 lb or more per day.
Administer precise ordered dose at same time each day. (Overdose may cause serious toxicity.)	Instruct patient to: • Take as directed; do not double dose • Not discontinue drug without advice of healthcare provider
Monitor serum drug level (to determine therapeutic concentration and toxicity). Report serum drug levels greater than 1.8 ng/ml to healthcare provider.	Instruct patient to report to laboratory as scheduled by healthcare provider for ongoing drug level determinations.
Monitor levels of potassium, magnesium, calcium, BUN, and creatinine. (Hypokalemia predisposes the patient to digoxin toxicity.)	Instruct patient to consume foods high in potassium such as bananas, apricots, kidney beans, sweet potatoes, and peanut butter.
Monitor for signs and symptoms of digoxin toxicity.	Instruct patient to immediately report visual changes, mental depression, palpitations, weakness, loss of appetite, vomiting, and diarrhea.

EVALUATION OF OUTCOME CRITERIA

Evaluate the effectiveness of drug therapy by confirming that patient goals and expected outcomes have been met (see "Planning").

See Table 22.1, under "Cardiac Glycosides," for a list of drugs to which these nursing actions apply.

PROTOTYPE DRUG | **LISINOPRIL** (Prinivil, Zestril)

ACTIONS AND USES

Due to its value in the treatment of both HF and hypertension, lisinopril has become one of the most commonly prescribed drugs. Like other ACE inhibitors, doses of lisinopril may require 2 to 3 weeks of adjustment to reach maximum efficacy, and several months of therapy may be needed for a patient's cardiac function to return to normal. Because of their synergistic hypotensive action, combined therapy with lisinopril and diuretics should be carefully monitored.

Administration Alerts

- Measure blood pressure just prior to administering lisinopril to be certain that effects are lasting for 24 hours and to determine if the patient's blood pressure is within acceptable range.
- Pregnancy category D.

ADVERSE EFFECTS AND INTERACTIONS

Although lisinopril causes few side effects, hyperkalemia may occur during therapy; thus, electrolyte levels are usually monitored periodically. Other side effects include cough, taste disturbances, headache, dizziness, chest pain, nausea, vomiting, diarrhea, and hypotension.

Lisinopril interacts with indomethacin and other NSAIDs causing decreased antihypertensive activity. When taken concurrently with potassium-sparing diuretics, hyperkalemia may result. Lisinopril may increase lithium levels and toxicity.

 See the companion website for a Nursing Process Focus specific to this drug.

they are generally reserved for patients who cannot tolerate ACE inhibitors.

NURSING CONSIDERATIONS

The role of the nurse in the care of patients receiving drug therapy with hydralazine for the treatment of hypertension is discussed in Chapter 21 (see "Nursing Considerations," page 280, and "Nursing Process Focus: Patients Receiving Direct Vasodilator Therapy," page 281).

The use of isosorbide dinitrate for therapy of angina pectoris is presented in Chapter 25 (see "Nursing Considerations," page 331).

Diuretics

Diuretics increase urine flow, thereby reducing blood volume and cardiac workload. They are widely used in the treatment of cardiovascular disease. Selected diuretics are shown in Table 22.1.

 PROTOTYPE DRUG | **ISOSORBIDE DINITRATE** (Isordil)

ACTIONS AND USES

Isosorbide dinitrate acts directly and selectively on veins to cause venodilation. This reduces venous return (preload), thus decreasing cardiac workload. The resultant improvement in cardiac output reduces pulmonary congestion and peripheral edema and improves exercise tolerance. Isosorbide dinitrate also dilates the coronary arteries to bring more oxygen to the myocardium. Isosorbide dinitrate belongs to a class of drugs called organic nitrates that are widely used in the treatment of angina.

Administration Alerts

- Do not confuse this drug with isosorbide (Ismotic), an oral osmotic diuretic.
- If administered sublingually, advise patient not to eat, drink, talk, or smoke while tablet is dissolving.
- Pregnancy category C.

ADVERSE EFFECTS AND INTERACTIONS

Common side effects of isosorbide dinitrate include headache and reflex tachycardia. Orthostatic hypotension can cause dizziness and falling, particularly in older adults. Use is contraindicated if the patient is also taking sildenafil (Viagra), as serious hypotension may result.

See the companion website for a Nursing Process Focus specific to this drug.

22.7 Pharmacotherapy with Diuretics

Diuretics are common drugs for the treatment of patients with heart failure, because they produce few adverse effects and are effective at reducing blood volume, edema, and pulmonary congestion. As diuretics reduce fluid volume and lower blood pressure, the workload on the heart is reduced, and cardiac output increases. Diuretics are rarely used alone, but are prescribed in combination with ACE inhibitors or other HF drugs.

The mechanism by which diuretics reduce blood volume, specifically where and how the nephron is affected, differs among the various drugs. Differences in mechanisms among the classes of diuretics are discussed in Chapter 43 ∞ . The role of the thiazide diuretics in the treatment of hypertension is discussed in Chapter 21 ∞ .

NURSING CONSIDERATIONS

The role of the nurse in diuretic therapy for heart failure involves careful monitoring of a patient's condition and providing education as it relates to the prescribed drug regimen. Prior to initiation of diuretic therapy, the patient should be questioned about past history of kidney disease. Diuretics are contraindicated in patients with renal dysfunction, fluid and electrolyte depletion, hepatic coma, pregnancy, and lactation. Diuretics should be used cautiously in patients with hepatic cirrhosis and nephritic syndrome—in infants and in older adults.

Potassium levels should be monitored closely, as non-potassium-sparing diuretics cause hypokalemia with diuresis. The nurse should closely observe elderly patients for weakness, hypotension, and confusion. The nurse should monitor for electrolyte imbalance, elevated BUN, hyperglycemia, and anemia, which can all be side effects of diuretics. The nurse should monitor vital signs as well as intake and output carefully to establish effectiveness of the medication. Rapid and excessive diuresis can result in dehydration, hypovolemia, and circulatory collapse.

Patient education as it relates to diuretics should include the goals, reasons for obtaining baseline data such as vital signs and tests for renal disorders, and possible side effects. Following are important points the nurse should include when teaching patients regarding diuretics.

- Monitor total sodium intake daily. The recommended daily intake should be no more than 4,000 mg per day.
- Report weight loss of more than 2 pounds a week.
- Report fatigue and muscle cramping.
- Make position changes slowly because diuretics in combination with other drugs can cause dizziness.

See "Nursing Process Focus: Patients Receiving Diuretic Therapy," page 267 in Chapter 21, for additional information ∞ .

Phosphodiesterase Inhibitors

Phosphodiesterase inhibitors have a brief half-life and are used for the short-term control of acute heart failure. The doses of these agents are shown in Table 22.1.

22.8 Pharmacotherapy with Phosphodiesterase Inhibitors

In the 1980s, two drugs became available which block the enzyme phosphodiesterase in cardiac and smooth muscle. Blocking phosphodiesterase has the effect of increasing the amount of calcium available for myocardial contraction. The inhibition results in two main actions that benefit patients with HF: a positive inotropic response and

Pr PROTOTYPE DRUG	FUROSEMIDE (Lasix)
ACTIONS AND USES	**ADVERSE EFFECTS AND INTERACTIONS**

ACTIONS AND USES

Furosemide is often used in the treatment of acute HF because it has the ability to remove large amounts of edema fluid from the patient in a short period of time. When given IV, diuresis begins within 5 minutes. Patients often receive quick relief from their distressing symptoms. Furosemide acts by preventing the reabsorption of sodium and chloride, primarily in the loop of Henle region of the nephron. Compared to other diuretics, furosemide is particularly beneficial when cardiac output and renal flow are severely diminished.

Administration Alerts

- Check patient's serum potassium levels before administering drug. If potassium levels are falling or are below normal, notify physician before administering.
- Pregnancy category C.

ADVERSE EFFECTS AND INTERACTIONS

Side effects of furosemide, like those of most diuretics, involve potential electrolyte imbalances, the most important of which is hypokalemia. Because hypokalemia may cause dysrhythmias in patients taking cardiac glycosides, combination therapy with furosemide and digoxin must be carefully monitored. Because furosemide is so efficacious, fluid loss must be carefully monitored to avoid possible dehydration and hypotension.

When furosemide is given with corticosteroids and amphotericin B, it can potentiate hypokalemia. When given with lithium, elimination of lithium is decreased, causing higher risk of toxicity. When given with sulfonylureas and insulin, furosemide may diminish their hypoglycemic effects.

 See the companion website for a Nursing Process Focus specific to this drug.

MediaLink

Mechanism in Action Furosemide

vasodilation. Cardiac output is increased due to the increase in contractility and the decrease in left ventricular afterload. Due to their toxicity, phosphodiesterase inhibitors are normally reserved for patients who have not responded to ACE inhibitors or cardiac glycosides, and they are generally used only for 2 to 3 days.

In 2000, the name of amrinone (Icar) was changed to inamrinone. This was done because practitioners reported confusing amrinone with the drug amiodarone.

NURSING CONSIDERATIONS

The role of the nurse in drug therapy with phosphodiesterase inhibitors involves careful monitoring of a patient's condition and providing education as it relates to the prescribed drug regimen. Prior to administration of phosphodiesterase inhibitors, the nurse should assess potassium levels. If hypokalemia is present, it should be corrected before administering these drugs. The nurse should evaluate the patient for history of renal impairment and dysrhythmias. Baseline vital signs should be obtained, especially blood pressure, because these drugs can cause hypotension. During IV administration, the patient should be continuously monitored for ventricular dysrhythmias such as ectopic beats, supraventricular dysrhythmias, PVCs, ventricular tachycardia, and ventricular fibrillation. If ordered for elderly, pregnant, or pediatric patients, the healthcare provider should be consulted, as safety has not been established in these populations or conditions.

Patient education as it relates to phosphodiesterase inhibitors should include the goals, reasons for obtaining baseline data such as vital signs and tests for cardiac and renal disorders, and possible side effects. Following are the important points the nurse should include when teaching patients about phosphodiesterase inhibitors.

- Report immediately: irregular, fast heartbeat, pain or swelling at infusion site, and fever of 101° F or higher.
- Report immediately any increase in chest pain that might indicate angina.

Beta-Adrenergic Blockers (Antagonists)

Only two beta-blockers are approved for the treatment of heart failure, carvedilol (Coreg) and metoprolol extended release form (Toprol-XL). The doses of these agents are shown in Table 22.1. They reduce the cardiac workload by decreasing afterload.

22.9 Pharmacotherapy with Beta-Adrenergic Blockers

As has been seen with the cardiac glycosides, ACE inhibitors, and phosphodiesterase inhibitors, drugs that produce a positive inotropic effect play important roles in reversing the diminished contractility that is the hallmark of HF. It may seem somewhat unusual, then, to find drugs that

exhibit a negative inotropic effect prescribed for this disease. Yet such is the case with the beta-adrenergic blockers.

Beta-blockers can improve the symptoms of HF by slowing the heart and reducing blood pressure. The decreased afterload reduces the workload on the heart. They are rarely used alone for this disease, but have some value when combined with other agents.

The basic pharmacology of the beta-blockers is presented in Chapter 13 ☞ . Other uses of the beta-adrenergic blockers are discussed elsewhere in this text: hypertension in Chapter 21, dysrhythmias in Chapter 23, and angina/myocardial infarction in Chapter 25 ☞ .

NURSING CONSIDERATIONS

The role of the nurse in beta-adrenergic blocker therapy involves careful monitoring of a patient's condition and providing education as it relates to the prescribed drug regimen. Beta-adrenergic blockers are contraindicated in patients with decompensated heart failure, chronic obstructive pulmonary disease (COPD), bradycardia, or heart block. Beta-blockers are also contraindicated in pregnant or lactating patients. These medications should be used with caution in patients with diabetes, peripheral vascular disease, and hepatic impairment. Caution is needed with elderly patients, as they may need a reduced dose.

The nurse should monitor for worsening signs and symptoms of HF and for signs of hepatic toxicity. Liver function tests should be performed periodically. The nurse should notify the physician if signs or symptoms of liver impairment become apparent.

Patient education as it relates to beta-adrenergic blockers should include the goals, reasons for obtaining baseline data, and possible side effects. Following are the important points the nurse should include when teaching patients regarding beta-adrenergic blockers.

- Monitor blood pressure and pulse. Notify the healthcare provider if pulse rate is less than 50 beats/minute.
- Report immediately signs and symptoms of worsening heart failure, such as shortness of breath, edema of feet and ankles, and chest pain.
- Do not stop taking the drug abruptly without consulting with the healthcare provider.
- Diabetics may experience changes in blood sugar levels while taking medications in this class.
- Report significant side effects such as fainting, difficulty breathing, weight gain, and slow, irregular heart rate.

See "Nursing Process Focus: Patients Receiving Beta-Adrenergic Antagonist Therapy" on page 279 in Chapter 21 for additional information ☞ .

22.10 New Agents for Heart Failure

In 2001, the first new medication for HF in over 10 years was approved. Nesiritide (Natrecor) is a small peptide hormone, produced through recombinant DNA technology,

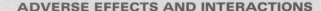

Pr PROTOTYPE DRUG | MILRINONE (Primacor)

ACTIONS AND USES

Of the two phosphodiesterase inhibitors available, milrinone is generally preferred because it has a shorter half-life and fewer side effects. It is only given intravenously and is primarily used for the short-term support of advanced HF. Peak effects occur in 2 minutes. Immediate effects of milrinone include an increased force of myocardial contraction and an increase in cardiac output.

Administration Alerts

- When administering this medication IV, a microdrip set and an infusion pump should be used.
- Pregnancy category C.

 See the companion website for a Nursing Process Focus specific to this drug.

ADVERSE EFFECTS AND INTERACTIONS

The most serious side effect of milrinone is ventricular dysrhythmia, which may occur in at least 1 of every 10 patients taking the drug. The patient's ECG is usually monitored continuously during the infusion of the drug. Milrinone interacts with disopyramide, causing excessive hypotension.

SPECIAL CONSIDERATIONS

Psychosocial Issues and Compliance in Patients with CHF

Patients with depression and lack of social support who have congestive heart failure (CHF) have been shown to be less adherent to their drug therapy regimen. Patients are also less likely to adhere to lifestyle modifications when depressed. The nurse should assess these issues in all patients with CHF and intervene appropriately when warranted. Patients may be referred to cardiac rehabilitation programs, which have been shown to increase compliance.

NATURAL THERAPIES | Carnitine and Heart Disease

L-carnitine supplements have been shown to improve exercise tolerance in patients with angina. The use of L-carnitine may prevent the occurrence of dysrhythmias in the early stages of heart disease. L-carnitine has also been shown to decrease triglyceride levels while increasing HDL serum levels, thus helping to minimize one of the major risk factors associated with heart disease.

Carnitine is a natural substance structurally similar to amino acids. Its primary function in metabolism is to move fatty acids from the bloodstream into cells, where carnitine assists in the breakdown of lipids in the mitochondria. This breakdown produces energy and increases the availability of oxygen, particularly in muscle cells. A congenital deficiency of carnitine leads to severe brain, liver, and heart damage.

Although a normal diet supplies 300 mg per day, certain patients may need additional amounts. Vegetarians are at risk to carnitine depletion, because plant protein supplies little or no carnitine. Endurance athletes and body-builders sometimes use carnitine supplements to build muscle mass. Carnitine is available as a supplement in several forms, including L-carnitine; D, L-carnitine; and acetyl L-carnitine; The best food sources of carnitine are organ meat, fish, muscle meats, and milk products.

Carnitine has a number of additional purported effects including improvement of brain function in patients with Alzheimer's disease. Because of its role in fatty acid metabolism, some claim it assists in treating obesity, although this has not been medically demonstrated.

that is structurally identical to endogenous human beta-type natriuretic peptide (hBNP).

In healthy individuals, the atria secrete atrial natriuretic peptide (ANP), in response to increasing blood pressure. As a natural component of homeostasis, ANP is a hormone that acts on the kidney to increase the excretion of sodium and water and return pressure to normal levels. When heart failure occurs, the ventricles begin to secrete hBNP, in response to the increased stretch on the ventricular walls. hBNP has the same action as ANP: diuresis and renal excretion of sodium. In therapeutic doses, hBNP also causes vasodilation, with also contributes to reduced preload. By reducing preload and afterload, hBNP compensates for diminished cardiac function.

Nesiritide (Natrecor) has limited uses due to its ability to cause severe hypotension. The drug must be given by IV infusion, and patients require continuous monitoring. It is approved for patients with acutely decompensated heart failure.

Pr PROTOTYPE DRUG | CARVEDILOL (Coreg)

ACTIONS AND USES

Carvedilol is the first beta-adrenergic blocker approved for the treatment of HF. It has been found to reduce symptoms, slow the progression of the disease, and increase exercise tolerance when combined with other heart failure drugs such as the ACE inhibitors. Unlike many drugs in this class, carvedilol blocks $beta_1$ and $beta_2$ as well as $alpha_1$- adrenergic receptors. The primary therapeutic effects relevant to HF are a reduction in heart rate and a drop in blood pressure. The lower blood pressure decreases afterload and reduces the workload on the heart.

Administration Alerts

■ To minimize the risk of orthostatic hypotension, give with food to slow absorption.

■ Pregnancy category C.

ADVERSE EFFECTS AND INTERACTIONS

The ability of carvedilol to decrease the heart rate combined with its ability to reduce contractility has the potential to worsen heart failure; thus, dosage must be carefully monitored. Because of the potential for adverse cardiac effects, beta-adrenergic blockers such as carvedilol are not considered first line drugs in the treatment of HF.

Carvedilol interacts with many drugs. For example, levels of carvedilol are significantly increased when taken currently with rifampin. MAO inhibitors, clonidine, and reserpine can cause hypotension or bradycardia when given with carvedilol. When given with digoxin, carvedilol may increase digoxin levels. It may also enhance the hypoglycemic effects of insulin and oral hypoglycemic agents.

 See the companion website for a Nursing Process Focus specific to this drug.

CHAPTER REVIEW

Key Concepts

The numbered key concepts provide a succinct summary of the important points from the corresponding numbered section within the chapter. If any of these points are not clear, refer to the numbered section within the chapter for review. Expanded versions can be found on the companion website.

22.1 Heart failure is not a distinct disease, but is closely associated with chronic hypertension, diabetes, mitral stenosis, and coronary artery disease.

22.2 The central cause of heart failure is weakened heart muscle. Diminished contractility reduces cardiac output.

22.3 The three primary characteristics of heart function are force of contraction, heart rate, and speed of impulse conduction.

22.4 Cardiac glycosides increase the force of myocardial contraction and are the traditional drugs of choice for heart failure. Due to a low safety margin, their use has declined.

22.5 ACE inhibitors improve heart failure by reducing peripheral edema and increasing cardiac output. They are first line drugs for the treatment of HF.

22.6 Vasodilators can help reduce symptoms of heart failure by reducing preload and decreasing the oxygen demand on the heart.

22.7 Diuretics relieve symptoms of heart failure by reducing fluid volume and decreasing blood pressure.

22.8 Phosphodiesterase inhibitors increase the force of contraction and cause vasodilation. They are highly toxic and reserved for acute situations.

22.9 Beta-adrenergic blockers play a role in the treatment of heart failure by slowing the heart rate and decreasing blood pressure. They are not considered first line drugs for HF.

22.10 Human beta natriuretic peptide (hBNP) is a natural hormone secreted by the ventricles of patients with HF. Through recombinant DNA technology, this hormone is now available as nesiritide (Natrecor) for the treatment of acute HF.

Review Questions

1. How can the Frank-Starling law be used to explain the beneficial effects of the cardiac glycosides in treating heart failure?

2. Why are the ACE inhibitors preferred over both the nitrates and the diuretics in the treatment of heart failure?

3. What is the most dangerous adverse effect of digoxin?

Critical Thinking Questions

1. A patient is newly diagnosed with mild congestive heart failure. The patient has been started on digoxin (Lanoxin). What objective evidence would indicate that this drug has been effective?

2. A 69-year-old patient has a sudden onset of acute pulmonary edema. The patient has no past cardiac history, is allergic to sulfa antibiotics, and routinely takes no medica-

tions. The healthcare provider orders furosemide (Lasix) to relieve the pulmonary congestion. What interventions are essential in the care of this patient?

3. A patient who is diabetic and hypertensive is started on carvedilol (Coreg) for mild heart failure. What teaching is important for this patient?

 EXPLORE MediaLink

NCLEX review, case studies, and other interactive resources for this chapter can be found on the companion website at www.prenhall.com/adams. Click on "Chapter 22" to select the activities for this chapter. For animations, more NCLEX review questions, and an audio glossary, access the accompanying CD-ROM in this textbook.

■ DRUGS AT A GLANCE

SODIUM CHANNEL BLOCKERS
Pr *quinidine (Quinidex)*

BETA-ADRENERGIC BLOCKERS
Pr *propranolol (Inderal)*

POTASSIUM CHANNEL BLOCKERS
Pr *amiodarone (Cordarone)*

CALCIUM CHANNEL BLOCKERS
Pr *verapamil (Calan)*

MISCELLANEOUS DRUGS

metabolized and eliminated by the bod
of this process
PHARMACOLOGY
1. The study of medicines; the disciplir
pertaining to how drugs improve the he
of the human body

MediaLink   www.prenhall.com/adams

CD-ROM
Animations:
   Mechanism in Action: Propranolol (Inderal)
   Mechanism in Action: Amiodarone (Cordarone)
Audio Glossary
NCLEX Review

Companion Website
NCLEX Review
Dosage Calculations
Case Study
Care Plans
Expanded Key Concepts

OBJECTIVES

After reading this chapter, the student should be able to:

1. Relate how rhythm abnormalities can affect cardiac function.
2. Illustrate the flow of electrical impulses through the normal heart.
3. Classify dysrhythmias based on their location and type of rhythm abnormality.
4. Explain how an action potential is controlled by the flow of sodium, potassium, and calcium ions across the myocardial membrane.
5. Identify the importance of nonpharmacologic therapies in the treatment of dysrhythmias.

6. Identify the primary mechanisms by which antidysrhythmic drugs act.
7. Describe the nurse's role in the pharmacologic management of patients with dysrhythmias.
8. Know representative drug examples for each of the drug classes listed in Drugs at a Glance, explain their mechanism of action, primary actions, and important adverse effects.
9. Categorize antidysrhythmic drugs based on their classification and mechanism of action.
10. Use the Nursing Process to care for patients receiving drug therapy for dysrhythmias.

D ysrhythmias are abnormalities of electrical conduction that may result in disturbances in heart rate or cardiac rhythm. Sometimes called arrhythmias, they encompass a number of different disorders that range from harmless to life threatening. Diagnosis is often difficult because patients usually must be connected to an electrocardiograph (ECG) and be experiencing symptoms in order to determine the exact type of rhythm disorder. Proper diagnosis and optimum pharmacologic treatment can significantly affect the frequency of dysrhythmias and their consequences.

PHARMFACTS | Dysrhythmias

- Dysrhythmias are responsible for over 44,000 deaths each year.
- Atrial dysrhythmias occur more commonly in men than in women.
- The incidence of atrial dysrhythmias increases with age. They affect:
  <0.5% of those aged 25 to 35
  1.5% of those up to age 60
  9% of those over age 75
- About 15% of strokes occur in patients with atrial dysrhythmias.
- A large majority of sudden cardiac deaths are thought to be caused by ventricular dysrhythmias.
- Sudden cardiac death occurs 3 to 4 times more frequently in blacks.
- Atrial fibrillation affects 1.5 to 2.2 million people in the United States.

23.1 Frequency of Dysrhythmias in the Population

While some dysrhythmias produce no symptoms and have negligible effects on cardiac function, others are life threatening and require immediate treatment. Typical symptoms include dizziness, weakness, decreased exercise tolerance, shortness of breath, and fainting. Many patients report palpitations or a sensation that their heart has skipped a beat. Persistent dysrhythmias are associated with increased risk of stroke and heart failure. Severe dysrhythmias may result in sudden death. Since asymptomatic patients may not seek medical attention, it is difficult to estimate the frequency of the disease, although it is likely that dysrhythmias are quite common in the population.

23.2 Classification of Dysrhythmias

Dysrhythmias are classified by a number of different methods. The simplest method is to name dysrhythmias

MediaLink Childhood Dysrhythmias

Table 23.1	Types of Dysrhythmias
Name of Dysrhythmia	**Description**
premature atrial or premature ventricular contractions (PVCs)	an extra beat often originating from a source other than the SA node; not normally serious unless it occurs in high frequency
atrial or ventricular tachycardia	rapid heart beat greater than 150 bpm; ventricular is more serious than atrial
atrial or ventricular flutter and/or fibrillation	very rapid, uncoordinated beats; atrial may require treatment but is not usually fatal; ventricular requires immediate treatment
sinus bradycardia	slow heart beat, less than 50 beats per minute; may require a pacemaker
heart block	area of nonconduction in the myocardium; may be partial or complete; classified as first, second, or third degree

according to the *type* of rhythm abnormality produced and its *location*. Dysrhythmias that originate in the atria are sometimes referred to as supraventricular. Those that originate in the ventricles are generally more serious, as they more often interfere with the normal function of the heart. Atrial **fibrillation**, a complete disorganization of rhythm, is thought to be the most common type of dysrhythmia. A summary of common dysrhythmias and a brief description of each abnormality is given in Table 23.1. Although obtaining a correct diagnosis of the type of dysrhythmia is sometimes difficult, it is essential for effective treatment.

While the actual cause of most dysrhythmias is elusive, dysrhythmias are associated with certain conditions, primarily heart disease and myocardial infarction. The following are diseases and conditions associated with dysrhythmias.

- Hypertension
- Cardiac valve disease such as mitral stenosis
- Coronary artery disease
- Medications such as digitalis
- Low potassium levels in the blood
- Myocardial infarction
- Stroke
- Diabetes mellitus
- Congestive heart failure

23.3 Conduction Pathways in the Myocardium

Although there are many types of dysrhythmias, all have in common a defect in the generation or conduction of electrical impulses across the myocardium. These electrical impulses, or **action potentials**, carry the signal for the cardiac muscle cells to contract and must be coordinated precisely for the chambers to beat in a synchronized manner. For the heart to function properly, the atria must contract simultaneously, sending their blood into the ventricles. Following atrial contraction, the right and left ventricles then must contract simultaneously. Lack of synchronization of the

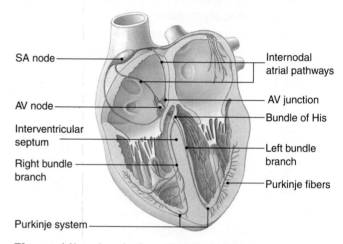

Figure 23.1 | Normal conduction pathway in the heart *Source: Pearson Education/PH College.*

atria and ventricles or of the right and left sides of the heart may have profound consequences. The total time for the electrical impulse to travel across the heart is about 0.22 second. The normal conduction pathway in the heart is illustrated in Figure 23.1.

Normal control of this synchronization begins in a small area of tissue in the wall of the right atrium known as the **sinoatrial (SA) node**. The SA node or pacemaker of the heart has a property called **automaticity**, the ability to spontaneously generate an action potential, without direction from the nervous system. The SA node generates a new action potential approximately 75 times per minute under resting conditions. This is referred to as the normal **sinus rhythm**.

Upon leaving the SA node, the action potential travels quickly across both atria and then to the **atrioventricular (AV) node**. The AV node also has the property of automaticity, although less so than the SA node. Should the SA node malfunction, the AV node has the ability to spontaneously generate action potentials and continue the heart's contraction at a rate of 40 to 60 beats per minute. Compared to other areas in the heart, impulse conduction through the AV node is slow. This allows the atrial contraction to completely empty blood into the ventricles, thereby optimizing cardiac output.

As the action potential leaves the AV node it travels rapidly to the **atrioventricular bundle**, or bundle of His. The impulse is then conducted down the right and left **bundle branches** to the **Purkinje fibers**, which carry the action potential to all regions of the ventricles almost simultaneously. Should the SA and AV nodes become nonfunctional, cells in the AV bundle and Purkinje fibers can continue to generate myocardial contractions at a rate of about 30 beats per minute.

Although action potentials normally begin at the SA node and spread across the myocardium in a coordinated manner, other regions of the heart may begin to initiate beats. These areas, known as **ectopic foci** or **ectopic pacemakers**, may begin to send impulses across the myocardium that compete with those from the normal conduction pathway, thereby affecting the normal flow of impulses. Ectopic foci have the potential to cause many of the types of dysrhythmias noted in Table 23.1.

It is important to understand that the underlying purpose of this conduction system is to keep the heart beating in a regular, synchronized manner so that cardiac output can be maintained. Some dysrhythmias occur sporadically, elicit no symptoms, and do not affect cardiac output. Others, however, profoundly affect cardiac output, result in patient symptoms, and have the potential to produce serious if not mortal consequences. It is these types of dysrhythmias that require pharmacologic treatment.

23.4 The Electrocardiograph

The wave of electrical activity across the myocardium can be measured using the electrocardiograph. The graphic recording from this device, or **electrocardiogram (ECG)**, is useful in diagnosing many types of heart conditions, including dysrhythmias.

Three distinct waves are produced by a normal ECG: the P wave, the QRS complex, and the T wave. Changes to the wave patterns or in their timing can reveal certain pathologies. For example, an exaggerated R wave suggests enlargement of the ventricles and a flat T wave indicates ischemia to the myocardium. A normal ECG and its relationship to impulse conduction in the heart are shown in Figure 23.2.

23.5 Sodium, Potassium, and the Myocardial Action Potential

Because most antidysrhythmic drugs act by interfering with myocardial action potentials, a firm grasp of this phenomenon is necessary for understanding drug mechanisms. Action potentials occur in both nervous and cardiac muscle cells due to the changes in specific ions found inside and outside the cell. Under resting conditions, Na^+ and Ca^{++} are found in higher concentrations *outside* of myocardial cells, while K^+ is found in higher concentration *within* these cells.

These imbalances are, in part, responsible for the inside of a myocardial cell membrane having a slight negative charge (80 to 90 mV), relative to the outside of the membrane. A cell having this negative membrane potential is said to be **polarized**.

An action potential begins when **sodium ion channels** located in the plasma membrane open and Na^+ rushes into the cell producing a rapid **depolarization**, or loss of membrane potential. During this period, Ca^{++} also enters the cell through **calcium ion channels**, although the influx is slower than that of sodium. The entry of Ca^{++} into the cells is a signal for the release of additional calcium that had been held in storage inside the sarcoplasmic reticulum. It is this large increase in intracellular Ca^{++} that is responsible for the contraction of cardiac muscle.

During depolarization, the inside of the cell membrane temporarily reverses its charge, becoming positive. The cell returns to its polarized state by the removal of K^+ through **potassium ion channels**. In cells located in the SA and AV nodes, it is the influx of Ca^{++}, rather than Na^+, which generates the rapid depolarization of the membrane. Blocking potassium, sodium, or calcium ion channels is a pharmacologic strategy used to terminate or prevent dysrhythmias. Figure 23.3 illustrates the ion flows occurring during the action potential.

During depolarization and most of repolarization, the cell cannot initiate another action potential. This time, known as the **refractory period**, ensures that the action potential finishes and the muscle cell contracts before a second action potential begins. The therapeutic effect of some antidysrhythmic agents is due to their prolongation of the refractory period.

23.6 Nonpharmacologic Therapy of Dysrhythmias

The therapeutic goals of antidysrhythmic pharmacotherapy are to terminate existing dysrhythmias or to prevent abnormal rhythms to reduce the risks of sudden death, stroke, or other complications resulting from the disease. Because of their potential to cause serious side effects, antidysrhythmic drugs are normally reserved for those patients experiencing overt symptoms or for those whose condition cannot be controlled by other means. There is little or no benefit to the patient in treating asymptomatic dysrhythmias with medications. Healthcare providers use several nonpharmacologic strategies to eliminate dysrhythmias.

The more serious types of dysrhythmias are corrected through electrical shock of the heart, a treatment called **cardioversion**, or **defibrillation**. The electrical shock momentarily stops all electrical impulses in the heart, both normal and abnormal. Under ideal conditions, the temporary cessation of electrical activity will allow the SA node to automatically return conduction to a normal sinus rhythm.

Other types of nonpharmacologic treatment include identification and destruction of the myocardial cells responsible for the abnormal conduction through a surgical

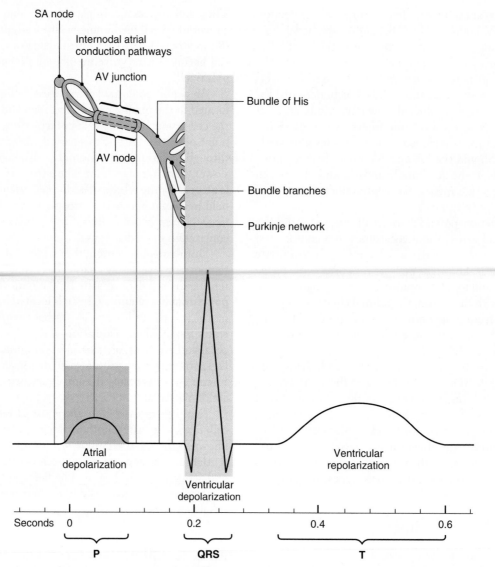

Figure 23.2 | Relationship of the electrocardiogram to electrical conduction in the heart *Source: Pearson Education/PH College.*

procedure called catheter ablation. Cardiac pacemakers are sometimes inserted to correct the types of dysrhythmias that cause the heart to beat too slowly. Implantable cardioverter defibrillators (ICDs) are placed in patients to restore normal rhythm by either pacing the heart or giving it an electric shock when dysrhythmias occur. In addition, the ICD is capable of storing information regarding the heart rhythm for the healthcare provider to evaluate.

23.7 Mechanisms and Classification of Antidysrhythmic Drugs

Antidysrhythmic drugs act by altering electrophysiologic properties of the heart. They do this through two basic mechanisms: blocking flow through ion channels or altering autonomic activity.

Antidysrhythmic drugs are grouped according to the stage in which they affect the action potential. These drugs fall into four primary classes, referred to as classes I, II, III,

and IV, and a fifth group that includes miscellaneous drugs not acting by one of the first four mechanisms. A typical action potential and the phases at which antidysrhythmic drugs act are shown in Figure 23.3. Categories of antidysrhythmics include the following.

- Sodium channel blockers (class I)
- Beta-adrenergic blockers (class II)
- Potassium channel blockers (class III)
- Calcium channel blockers (class IV)
- Miscellaneous antidysrhythmic drugs

Drugs that affect cardiac electrophysiology have a narrow margin between a therapeutic effect and a toxic effect. They not only have the ability to correct dysrhythmias, but also to worsen or even create new dysrhythmias. The nurse must carefully monitor patients taking antidysrhythmic drugs. Often, the patient is hospitalized during the initial stages of therapy so that the optimum dose can be accurately determined.

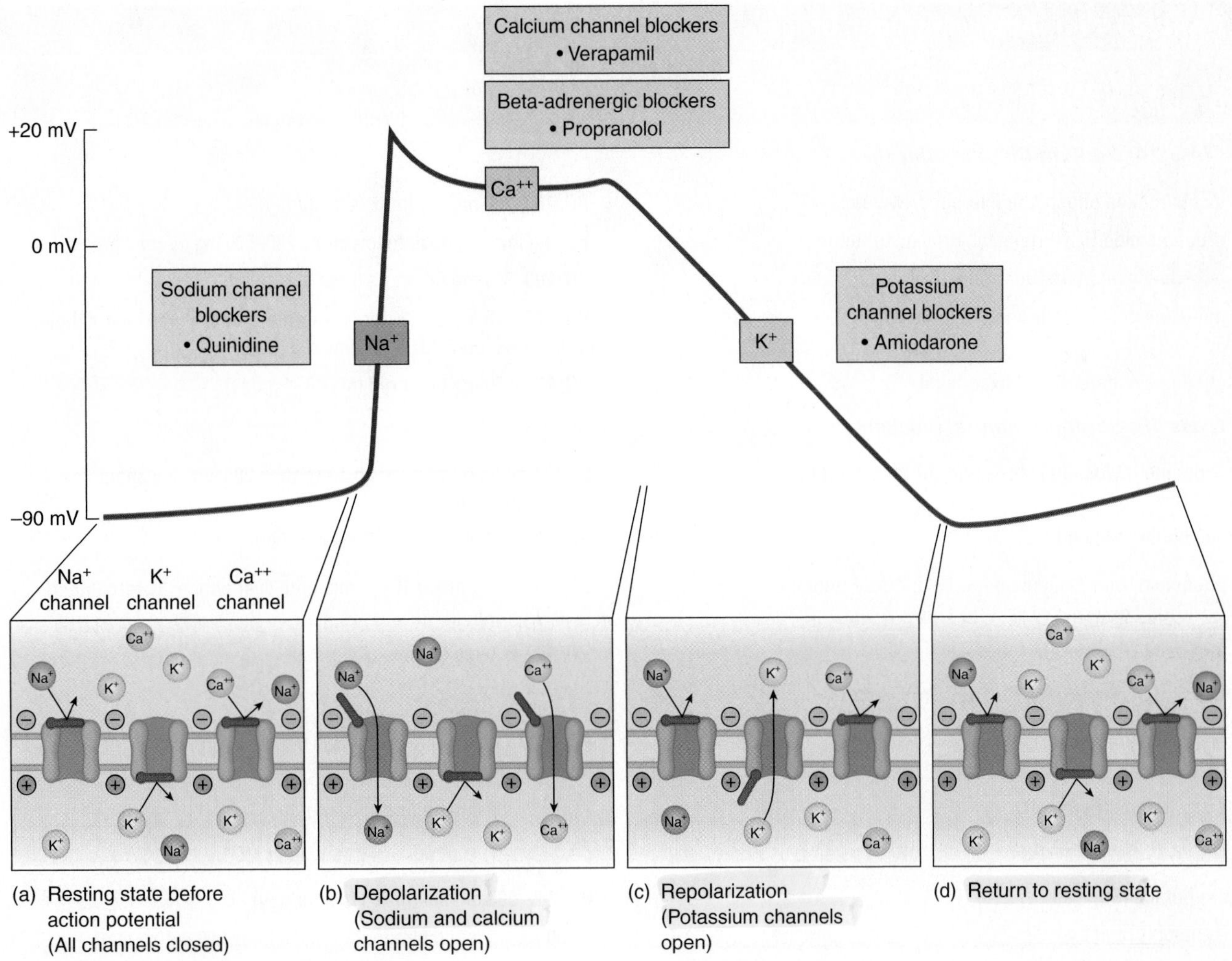

Figure 23.3 | Ion channels in myocardial cells

Sodium Channel Blockers (Class I)

The first medical uses of the sodium channel blockers were recorded in the 18th century. This is the largest class of antidysrhythmics and many are still widely prescribed. The sodium channel blockers are shown in Table 23.2.

23.8 Treating Dysrhythmias with Sodium Channel Blockers

Sodium channel blockers, the class I drugs, are divided into three subgroups, IA, IB, and IC, based on subtle differences in their mechanism of action. Since progression of the action potential is dependent upon the opening of sodium ion channels, a blockade of these channels will prevent depolarization. The spread of the action potential across the myocardium will slow, and areas of ectopic pacemaker activity will be suppressed.

NURSING CONSIDERATIONS

The role of the nurse in sodium channel blocker therapy is included in the "Nursing Process Focus: Patients Receiving Antidysrhythmic Therapies." Additional nursing consider-

ations will vary depending on the drug used. The nurse should be aware of the specific mechanism of action, side effects, administration requirements, and patient teaching for each drug being prescribed.

Because Class I antidysrhythmics have profound effects on the heart, a complete health history and physical examination should be obtained before initiating therapy, including baseline ECG, vital signs, hepatic and urinary function tests, and electrolyte values. The nurse should assess for heart failure, hypotension, myasthenia gravis, and renal or hepatic impairment, as these are contraindicated in Class I antidysrhythmic therapy. A thorough drug history should be obtained because these agents interact with a large number of other drugs, including cardiac glycosides, cimetidine, anticonvulsants, nifedipine, and warfarin.

During pharmacotherapy, the nurse should monitor the patient for changes in the EKG such as an increase in PR and QT intervals and widening of QRS complex. Blood pressure should be monitored frequently, as some agents can cause hypotension. Some drugs in this class can cause arterial embolism. This adverse effect is related to the formation of small blood clots in the atrium that occur while the patient is being treated for atrial fibrillation. Nurses should

Table 23.2	Antidysrhythmic Drugs
Drug	**Route and Adult Dose (max dose where indicated)**
Class 1A: Sodium Channel Blockers	
disopyramide phosphate (Norpace, Napamide)	PO; 100–200 mg qid (max 800 mg/day)
procainamide HCl (Pronestyl, Procan, others)	PO; 1 g loading dose followed by 250–500 mg every 3 hours
quinidine gluconate (Duraquin, Quinaglute)	PO; 200–600 mg tid or qid (max 3–4 g/day)
quinidine polygalacturonate (Cardioquin)	PO; 275–825 mg q3–4h for four or more doses until dysrhythmia terminates, then 137.5–275 mg bid or tid
quinidine sulfate (Quinidex, others)	PO; 200–600 mg tid or qid (max 3–4 g/day)
Class 1B: Sodium Channel Blockers	
lidocaine (Xylocaine) (see page 247 for the Prototype Drug box)	IV; 1–4 mg/min infusion; no more than 200–300 mg should be infused in a 1-hour period
mexiletine (Mexitil)	PO; 200–300 mg tid (max 1200 mg/day)
phenytoin (Dilantin) (see page 166 for the Prototype Drug box)	IV; 50–100 mg every 10–15 min until dysrhythmia is terminated (max 1 g/day)
tocainide (Tonocard)	PO; 400–600 mg tid (max 2.4 g/day)
Class 1C: Sodium Channel Blockers	
flecainide (Tambocor)	PO; 100 mg bid; increase by 500 mg bid every 4 days (max 400 mg/day)
propafanone (Rythmol)	PO; 150–300 mg tid (max 900 mg/day)
Class II: Beta-blockers	
acebutolol (Sectral)	PO; 200–600 mg bid (max 1200 mg/day)
esmolol (Brevibloc)	IV; 50 μg/kg/min maintenance dose (max 200 μg/kg/min)
propranolol (Inderal)	PO; 10–30 mg tid or qid (max 320 mg/day); 0.5–3.1 mg IV every 4h or prn
Class III: Potassium Channel Blockers	
amiodarone (Cordarone, Pacerone)	PO; 400–600 mg/day in one to two divided doses (max 1600 mg/day as loading dose)
dofetilide (Tikosyn)	PO; 125–500 μg bid based on creatinine clearance
sotalol (Betapace)	PO; 80 mg bid (max 320 mg/day)
Class IV: Calcium Channel Blockers	
diltiazem (Cardizem, others) (see page 337 for the Prototype Drug box)	IV; 5–10 mg/hr continuous infusion (max 15 mg/hour) for a maximum of 24h
verapamil (Calan, others)	PO; 240–480 mg/d in divided doses; 5–10 mg IV direct, may repeat in 15–30 min if needed
Miscellaneous Antidysrhythmics	
adenosine (Adenocard, Adenoscan)	IV; 6–12 mg given as a bolus injection
digoxin (Lanoxin) (see page 290 for the Prototype Drug box)	PO; 0.125–0.5 mg qid
ibutilide (Corvert)	IV; 1 mg infused over 10 min

monitor the patient for changes in level of consciousness and respiratory status and report to physician immediately.

The nurse should monitor drug plasma levels during therapy. Also, the patient should be monitored for diarrhea, which occurs in approximately 1/3 of patients on quinidine. This adverse effect is due to the fact that quinidine is chemically related to quinine in structure and action. Diarrhea may be intense, and the nurse should implement appropriate interventions related to the diarrhea to maintain fluid and electrolyte balance.

Patient education as it relates to sodium channel blockers should include the goals, reasons for obtaining baseline data such as vital signs and tests for cardiac and renal disorders, and possible side effects. The nurse should also include the following points when teaching patients regarding sodium channel blockers.

- Do not skip doses of the medications, even if feeling well. Do not take two doses at a time, if the first dose is missed.
- Avoid the use of alcohol, caffeine, and tobacco.
- Comply with monitoring of lab tests as ordered.
- Report the following symptoms immediately: shortness of breath, signs of bleeding, excessive bruising, fever, nausea, persistent headache, changes to vision or hearing, diarrhea, or dizziness.

Beta-Adrenergic Blockers (Class II)

Beta-adrenergic blockers are widely used for cardiovascular disorders. Their ability to slow the heart rate and conduction velocity can suppress several types of dysrhythmias. The beta-blockers are shown in Table 23.2.

23.9 Treating Dysrhythmias with Beta-Adrenergic Blockers

Beta-blockers are used to treat a large number of cardiovascular diseases, including hypertension, MI, heart failure, and dysrhythmias. Because of potentially serious side effects, however, only a few beta-blockers are approved to treat dysrhythmias. Beta-blockers slow the heart rate (negative chronotropic effect), and decrease conduction velocity through the AV node. Myocardial automaticity is reduced and many types of dysrhythmias are stabilized. The main value of beta-blockers as antidysrhythmic agents is to treat atrial dysrhythmias associated with heart failure. Abrupt discontinuation of beta-blockers can lead to dysrhythmias and hypertension. The basic pharmacology of beta-adrenergic blockers is explained in Chapter 13 ⊕.

NURSING CONSIDERATIONS

The role of the nurse caring for patients receiving beta-adrenergic antagonists for dysrhythmias is included in the "Nursing Process Focus: Patients Receiving Antidysrhythmic Therapies". For additional nursing considerations, refer to "Nursing Process Focus: Patients Receiving Beta-Adrenergic Antagonist Therapy" on page 279 in Chapter 21 ⊕.

All drugs in this class are contraindicated in patients with heart block, severe bradycardia, AV block, and asthma. The action of beta-blockers is to decrease the contractions of the myocardium and to lessen the speed of conduction through the AV node. This action predisposes patients with certain existing heart problems to experience a significant decrease in heart rate that may not be well tolerated. The most common adverse reaction to these drugs is hypotension.

The nurse should monitor elderly patients for cognitive dysfunction and depression, as well as hallucinations and psychosis, which are more likely with higher doses. These reactions appear to be related to the lipid solubility of this medication and its ability to cross the blood-brain barrier. The nurse should also monitor for hypoglycemia. There is an increased incidence of hypoglycemia in patients with type 1 diabetes mellitus because beta blockers may inhibit glycogenolysis.

Pr PROTOTYPE DRUG | QUINIDINE SULFATE (Quinidex)

ACTIONS AND USES

Quinidine, the oldest antidysrhythmic drug, was originally obtained as a natural substance from the bark of the South American *Cinchona* tree. Like other drugs in this class, quinidine blocks sodium ion channels in myocardial cells, thus reducing automaticity and slowing conduction of the action potential across the myocardium. This slight delay in conduction velocity prolongs the refractory period and can suppress dysrhythmias. Quinidine is referred to as a broad-spectrum drug because it has the ability to correct many different types of atrial and ventricular dysrhythmias.

Administration Alerts

- The supine position should be used during IV administration because severe hypotension may occur.
- Pregnancy category C.

ADVERSE EFFECTS AND INTERACTIONS

Diarrhea is the most common side effect of quinidine therapy, occurring in up to 50% of all patients. A potentially serious interaction can occur when quinidine is given concurrently with digoxin. Because quinidine has the potential to double digoxin levels in the blood, the dose of digoxin must be reduced accordingly and carefully monitored. Like all antidysrhythmic drugs, quinidine has the ability to produce new dysrhythmias or worsen existing ones, thus patients should be frequently assessed for changes in cardiac status.

Quinidine sulfate interacts with many other drugs. For example, it may increase digoxin levels by 50%. Amiodarone may increase quinidine levels, thus increasing the risk of heart block. Phenothiazines add to cardiac depressant effects.

Use with caution with herbal supplements. For example, aloe and buckthorn, due to their laxative effects, may cause a potassium deficiency and increased antidysrhythmic action.

 See the companion website for a Nursing Process Focus specific to this drug.

NURSING PROCESS FOCUS	PATIENTS RECEIVING ANTIDYSRHYTHMIC THERAPIES

ASSESSMENT

Prior to administration:
- Obtain complete health history including allergies, drug history, and possible drug interactions.
- Assess to determine if cardiac alteration is producing a symptomatic effect on cardiac output including vital signs, level of consciousness, urinary output, skin temperature, and peripheral pulses.
- Obtain baseline ECG to compare throughout therapy.

POTENTIAL NURSING DIAGNOSES

- Ineffective Tissue Perfusion, related to cardiac conduction abnormality
- Deficient Knowledge, related to drug therapy
- Risk for Injury, related to adverse effects of drug

PLANNING: PATIENT GOALS AND EXPECTED OUTCOMES

The patient will:
- Exhibit improved cardiac output as evidenced by stabilization of heart rate, heart rhythm, sensorium, urinary output, and vital signs
- State expected outcomes of drug therapy
- Demonstrate an understanding of the drug's action by accurately describing drug side effects and precautions

IMPLEMENTATION

Interventions and (Rationales)	*Patient Education/Discharge Planning*
■ Monitor cardiac rate and rhythm continuously if administering drug IV. (IV route is used when rapid therapeutic effects are needed. Constant monitoring is needed to detect any potential serious dysrhythmias.)	■ Explain the need for continuous ECG monitoring when administering the medication intravenously.
■ Monitor IV site. Administer all parenteral medication via infusion pump.	■ Instruct patient to report any burning or stinging pain, swelling, warmth, redness, or tenderness at the IV insertion site.
■ Investigate possible causes of the dysrhythmia such as electrolyte imbalances, hypoxia, pain, anxiety, caffeine ingestion, and tobacco use.	Instruct the patient to: ■ Maintain a diet low in sodium and fat with sufficient potassium ■ Report illness such as flu, vomiting, diarrhea, and dehydration to healthcare provider to avoid adverse effects ■ Restrict use of caffeine and tobacco products
■ Observe for side effects specific to the antidysrhythmic used.	Instruct patient to: ■ Report adverse effects specific to prescribed antidysrhythmic ■ Report palpitations, chest pain, dyspnea, unusual fatigue, weakness, and visual disturbances
■ Monitor for proper use of medication.	Instruct patient to: ■ Never discontinue the drug abruptly ■ Take the drug exactly as prescribed, even if feeling well ■ Take pulse prior to taking the drug. (Instruct patient regarding the normal range and rhythm of pulse; instruct to consult the healthcare provider regarding "reportable" pulse.)

EVALUATION OF OUTCOME CRITERIA

Evaluate the effectiveness of drug therapy by confirming that patient goals and expected outcomes have been met (see "Planning").

See Table 23.2 for a list of drugs (Class I–IV) to which these nursing actions apply.

Patient education as it relates to beta-adrenergic blockers should include the goals, reasons for obtaining baseline data such as vital signs and tests for cardiac and renal disorders, and possible side effects. The nurse should provide the following information when teaching patients about beta-adrenergic blockers.

- Take pulse prior to drug administration. Report pulse rate less than 50 to the healthcare provider.
- Rise from a sitting or lying position slowly to avoid dizziness.
- Report the following symptoms immediately: shortness of breath, feeling of skipping a heartbeat, painful or difficult urination, frequent nighttime urination, weight gain of 2 pounds or more, dizziness, insomnia, drowsiness, or confusion.

SPECIAL CONSIDERATIONS

Asian Patients' Sensitivity to Propranolol

Studies have shown that, due to a lack of specific drug metabolizing enzyme (mephenytoin hydroxylase), Asians metabolize propranolol more quickly than Caucasians. Because of this sensitivity to propranolol, the drug has a significantly greater effect on heart rate. The nurse should assess this population for possible overdosage, and monitor for possible adverse reactions due to high drug levels.

Potassium Channel Blockers (Class III)

Although a small class of drugs, the potassium channel blockers have important applications to the treatment of dysrhythmias. These drugs prolong the resting stage of contraction, the refractory period, which stabilizes certain types of dysrhythmias. The potassium channel blockers are shown in Table 23.2.

23.10 Treating Dysrhythmias with Potassium Channel Blockers

The drugs in class III exert their actions by blocking potassium ion channels in myocardial cells. After the action potential has passed and the myocardial cell is in a depolarized state, repolarization depends upon removal of potassium from the cell. The class III medications delay repolarization of the myocardial cells, and lengthen the refractory period, which tends to stabilize dysrhythmias. In addition to blocking potassium channels, sotalol (Betapace) is also a beta-adrenergic blocker.

Drugs in this class generally have restricted uses due to potentially serious side effects. Pharmacologists have been showing considerable interest in class III drugs; in 1999, dofetilide (Tikosyn) was the first new antidysrhythmic drug approved in 10 years and several others are in clinical trials.

NURSING CONSIDERATIONS

The role of the nurse caring for patients receiving potassium channel blockers for dysrhythmias is included in the

---

| Pr PROTOTYPE DRUG | PROPRANOLOL (Inderal) |

ACTIONS AND USES

Until 1978, propranolol was the only beta-blocker approved to treat dysrhythmias. Propranolol is a nonselective beta-adrenergic blocker, affecting beta$_1$-receptors in the heart, and beta$_2$-receptors in pulmonary and vascular smooth muscle. Propranolol reduces heart rate, slows conduction velocity, and lowers blood pressure. Propranolol is most effective against tachycardia caused by excessive sympathetic stimulation. This medication is often combined with other drugs such as digoxin or quinidine in the treatment of cardiovascular disease. It is approved to treat a wide variety of diseases, including hypertension, angina, migraine headaches, and prevention of myocardial infarction.

Administration Alerts

- Abrupt discontinuation may cause myocardial infarction, severe hypertension, and ventricular dysrhythmias because of a potential rebound effect.
- If pulse is less than 60 beats per minute, notify the physician.
- Pregnancy category C.

ADVERSE EFFECTS AND INTERACTIONS

Common side effects of propranolol include fatigue, hypotension, and bradycardia. Because of its ability to slow the heart rate, patients with other cardiac disorders such as heart failure must be carefully monitored. Side effects such as diminished libido and impotence may result in noncompliance in male patients.

Propranolol interacts with many other drugs, including phenothiazines, which have additive hypotensive effects. Propranolol should not be given within 2 weeks of a MAO inhibitor. Beta-adrenergic agonists such as albuterol antagonize the actions of propanolol.

 See the companion website for a Nursing Process Focus specific to this drug.

MediaLink | Mechanism in Action | Propranolol

"Nursing Process Focus: Patients Receiving Antidysrhythmic Therapies". Additional nursing considerations will vary depending on the drug used. The nurse should be aware of the specific mechanism of action, side effects, administration requirements, and patient teaching on each drug prescribed. These drugs are not recommended for use during pregnancy (category C) or lactation.

Patient education should include the goals, reasons for obtaining baseline data such as vital signs and cardiac, renal disorders, and possible side effects. The nurse should instruct the patient with the following information.

- Have regular eye exams, due to possible vision changes.
- Avoid prolonged sun exposure and use sunscreen.
- Take medication with food, or a small snack.
- Report the following symptoms immediately: shortness of breath, feeling that the heart has skipped a beat, cough, vision changes, yellow eyes and skin color (jaundice), right upper abdominal pain, and dizziness.

Calcium Channel Blockers (Class IV)

Like the beta-blockers, the calcium channel blockers are widely prescribed for various cardiovascular disorders. By slowing conduction velocity, they are able to stabilize certain dysrhythmias. The antidysrhythmic calcium channel blockers are shown in Table 23.2.

23.11 Treating Dysrhythmias with Calcium Channel Blockers

Although about 10 calcium channel blockers (CCBs) are available to treat cardiovascular diseases, only a limited number have been approved for dysrhythmias. A few CCBs such as diltiazem (Cardizem) and verapamil (Calan)

block calcium ion channels in the heart; the remainder are specific to calcium channels in vascular smooth muscle. The basic pharmacology of this drug class is presented in Chapter 21 ⊕.

Blockade of calcium ion channels has a number of effects on the heart, most of which are similar to those of beta-adrenergic blockers. Effects include reduced automaticity in the SA node and slowed impulse conduction through the AV node. This prolongs the refractory period and stabilizes many types of dysrhythmias. Calcium channel blockers are only effective against supraventricular dysrhythmias.

NURSING CONSIDERATIONS

The role of the nurse caring for patients receiving calcium channel blockers for dysrhythmias is included in the "Nursing Process Focus: Patients Receiving Antidysrhythmic Therapies". For additional nursing considerations, refer to "Nursing Process Focus: Patients Receiving Calcium Channel Blocker Therapy" on 271 in Chapter 21 ⊕.

Calcium channel blocker therapy should never be initiated in patients with sick sinus syndrome, heart block, severe hypotension, cardiogenic shock, and severe congestive heart failure. The desired action of this class of drugs is to decrease oxygen demand, reduce cardiac workload, and increase oxygen to the myocardium. These therapeutic actions may cause patients with existing heart abnormalities to experience adverse effects to the heart. This class of drugs may produce lethal ventricular arrhythmias.

Because CCBs cause vasodilation of peripheral arterioles and decrease total peripheral vascular resistance, some patients, especially the elderly, may not be able to tolerate these changes in blood pressure. The nurse should instruct patients to move slowly when rising from a sitting or lying position.

Pr PROTOTYPE DRUG | AMIODARONE (Cordarone)

ACTIONS AND USES

Amiodarone is a structural analog of thyroid hormone. It is approved for the treatment of resistant ventricular tachycardia that may prove life threatening, and it has become a drug of choice for the treatment of atrial dysrhythmias in patients with heart failure. In addition to blocking potassium ion channels, some of this drug's actions on the heart relate to its blockade of sodium ion channels. Its onset of action may take several weeks when given orally. Its effects, however, can last 4 to 8 weeks after the drug is discontinued since it has an extended half-life that may exceed 100 days.

Administration Alerts

- Hypokalemia and hypomagnesemia should be corrected prior to initiating therapy.
- Pregnancy category D.

ADVERSE EFFECTS AND INTERACTIONS

The most serious adverse effect from amiodarone occurs in the lung, with the drug causing a pneumonia-like syndrome. The drug also causes blurred vision, rashes, photosensitivity, nausea, vomiting, anorexia, fatigue, dizziness, and hypotension. This medication is concentrated by certain tissues; thus, adverse effects may be slow to resolve. As with other antidysrhythmics, patients must be closely monitored to avoid serious toxicity. Amiodarone interacts with many other drugs. For example, it increases digoxin levels in the blood and enhances the actions of anticoagulants. Use with beta-adrenergic blockers may potentiate sinus bradycardia, sinus arrest, or AV block. Amiodarone may increase phenytoin levels two- to threefold.

Use with caution with herbal supplements, such as echinacea, which may cause an increase in hepatotoxicity. Aloe may cause an increased effect of amiodarone.

 See the companion website for a Nursing Process Focus specific to this drug.

(sidebar) **MediaLink** **Mechanism in Action** **Amiodarone**

Because constipation is a common side effect of these drugs, the nurse also should instruct the patient to eat foods high in fiber. These drugs are not recommended for use during pregnancy (category C) or lactation.

Patient education as it relates to calcium channel blockers used to treat dysrhythmias should include the goals, reasons for obtaining baseline data such as vital signs, and possible side effects. The nurse should instruct the patient with the following information.

- Report any feelings that the heart has skipped a beat.
- Take blood pressure frequently and report changes: either low blood pressure or elevated blood pressure.
- Take pulse frequently and notify healthcare provider if it falls below 60 beats per minute.
- Observe for swelling (edema).
- Report any shortness of breath.

23.12 Treating Dysrhythmias with Digoxin and Miscellaneous Drugs

Several other drugs are occasionally used to treat specific dysrhythmias, but do not act by the mechanisms previously described. These miscellaneous agents are shown in Table 23.2. Although digoxin (Lanoxin) is primarily used to treat heart failure, it is also prescribed for certain types of atrial dysrhythmias because of its ability to decrease automaticity of the SA node and slow conduction through the AV node. Because excessive levels of digoxin can produce serious dysrhythmias, and interactions with other medications are common, patients must be carefully monitored during therapy. Additional information on the mechanism of action and the adverse effects of digoxin may be found in Chapter 22 ∞.

Adenosine (Adenocard) and ibutilide (Corvert) are two additional drugs used for specific dysrhythmias. Adenosine is a naturally occurring nucleoside. When given as a 1- to 2-second bolus IV injection, adenosine terminates serious atrial tachycardia by slowing conduction through the AV node and decreasing automaticity of the SA node. Although dyspnea is common, side effects are generally self-limiting because of its 10-second half-life.

Ibutilide (Corvert) is also used as a short-acting IV intervention, infused over 10 minutes to terminate atrial flutter and fibrillation by prolonging the duration of the cardiac action potential. The infusion is stopped as soon as the dysrhythmia is terminated.

NATURAL THERAPIES | **Magnesium for Dysrhythmias**

Magnesium has been shown to be effective in the treatment of certain cardiac dysrhythmias in those who are magnesium deficient. Magnesium deficiency is associated with a number of dysrhythmias, including atrial fibrillation, premature atrial and ventricular beats, ventricular tachycardia, and ventricular fibrillation. The mechanism of magnesium's antidysrhythmic action is not fully understood, but may be related to its role in maintaining intracellular potassium. It may also be related to its role as a natural calcium channel blocker. Magnesium may be administered intravenously or in liquid or capsule form. Foods that are rich in magnesium include unpolished grains, nuts, and green vegetables.

Pr PROTOTYPE DRUG | **VERAPAMIL (Calan)**

ACTIONS AND USES

Verapamil was the first CCB approved by the FDA. It acts by inhibiting the flow of Ca^{++} into both myocardial cells and in vascular smooth muscle. In the heart, this action slows conduction velocity and stabilizes dysrhythmias. In the vessels, calcium ion channel inhibition lowers blood pressure which reduces cardiac workload. Verapamil also dilates the coronary arteries, an action that is important when the drug is used to treat angina (Chapter 25) ∞.

Administration Alerts

- Capsule contents should not be dissolved or chewed.
- For IV administration, inspect drug preparation to make sure solution is clear and colorless.
- Pregnancy category C.

ADVERSE EFFECTS AND INTERACTIONS

Side effects are generally minor and may include headache, constipation, and hypotension. Because verapamil can cause bradycardia, patients with heart failure should be carefully monitored. Patients should notify their healthcare provider if their heart rate falls below 60 beats per minute or if systolic blood pressure falls below 90 mm Hg. Like many other antidysrhythmics, verapamil has the ability to elevate blood levels of digoxin. Since both digoxin and verapamil have the effect of slowing conduction through the AV node, their concurrent use must be carefully monitored.

Grapefruit juice may increase verapamil levels. Use with caution with herbal supplements, such as hawthorn, which may have additive hypotensive effects.

 See the companion website for a Nursing Process Focus specific to this drug.

CHAPTER REVIEW

Key Concepts

The numbered key concepts provide a succinct summary of the important points from the corresponding numbered section within the chapter. If any of these points are not clear, refer to the numbered section within the chapter for review. Expanded versions can be found on the companion website.

23.1 The frequency of dysrhythmias in the population is difficult to predict because many patients experience no symptoms. Persistent or severe dysrhythmias may be lethal.

23.2 Dysrhythmias are classified by the location (atrial or ventricular) or type (flutter, fibrillation, block) of rhythm abnormality produced.

23.3 The electrical conduction pathway from the SA node, to the AV node, to the bundle branches and Purkinje fibers, keeps the heart beating in a synchronized manner. Some myocardial cells in these regions have the property of automaticity.

23.4 The electrophysiologic events in the heart can be measured with an electrocardiograph.

23.5 Changes in sodium and potassium levels generate the action potential in myocardial cells. Depolarization occurs when sodium (and calcium) rushes in; repolarization occurs when potassium is removed.

23.6 Nonpharmacologic therapy of dysrhythmias, including cardioversion, ablation, and implantable cardioverter defibrillators, are often the treatments of choice.

23.7 Antidysrhythmic drugs are classified by their mechanism of action, namely, classes I through IV.

23.8 Sodium channel blockers are the largest group of antidysrhythmics, and act by slowing the rate of impulse conduction across the heart.

23.9 Beta-adrenergic blockers act by reducing automaticity as well as slowing conduction velocity across the myocardium.

23.10 Potassium channel blockers act by prolonging the refractory period of the heart.

23.11 Calcium channel blockers act by reducing automaticity and by slowing myocardial conduction velocity. Their actions and effects are similar to the beta-blockers.

23.12 Digoxin, adenosine, and ibutilide are used for specific dysrhythmias but do not act by blocking ion channels.

Review Questions

1. Trace the flow of electrical conduction through the heart. What would happen if the impulse never reached the AV node?

2. Why does slowing the speed of the electrical impulse across the myocardium sometimes correct a dysrhythmia?

3. Why are selective alpha-adrenergic blockers such as doxazosin (Cardura) of no value in treating dysrhythmias?

4. Remembering the effects of digoxin on the heart from Chapter 22, explain why most antidysrhythmic drugs have the potential to cause serious side effects in patients taking cardiac glycosides ∞ .

Critical Thinking Questions

1. A patient with a history of COPD and tachycardia has recently been placed on propranolol (Inderal) to control the tachydysrhythmia. What is a priority for the nurse in monitoring this patient?

2. A patient is started on amiodarone (Cordarone) for cardiac dysrhythmias. This patient is also on digoxin (Lanoxin),

warfarin (Coumadin), and insulin. What is a priority teaching for this patient?

3. A patient is on verapamil (Calan) and digoxin (Lanoxin). What is a priority that this patient needs to be monitored for?

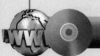

EXPLORE MediaLink

NCLEX review, case studies, and other interactive resources for this chapter can be found on the companion website at www.prenhall.com/adams. Click on "Chapter 23" to select the activities for this chapter. For animations, more NCLEX review questions, and an audio glossary, access the accompanying CD-ROM in this textbook.

CHAPTER 24

Drugs for Coagulation Disorders

DRUGS AT A GLANCE

ANTICOAGULANTS

Parenteral anticoagulants

Pr *heparin (Heplock)*

Oral anticoagulants

Pr *warfarin (Coumadin)*

ANTIPLATELET AGENTS

ADP receptor blockers

Glycoprotein IIb/IIIa blockers

Pr *abciximab (ReoPro)*

ANTICOAGULANT ANTAGONISTS

THROMBOLYTICS

Pr *alteplase (Activase)*

ANTIFIBRINOLYTICS

Pr *aminocaproic acid (Amicar)*

metabolized and eliminated by the bod
of this process
PHARMACOLOGY
1. The study of medicines; the disciplin
pertaining to how drugs improve the he
of the human body

MediaLink www.prenhall.com/adams

CD-ROM

Animation:
   Mechanism in Action: Warfarin (Coumadin)
Audio Glossary
NCLEX Review

Companion Website

NCLEX Review
Dosage Calculations
Case Study
Care Plans
Expanded Key Concepts

OBJECTIVES

After reading this chapter, the student should be able to:

1. Construct a flow chart diagramming the important steps of hemostasis and fibrinolysis.
2. Describe thromboembolic disorders that are indications for coagulation modifiers.
3. Identify the primary mechanisms by which coagulation-modifier drugs act.
4. Explain how laboratory testing of coagulation parameters is used to monitor anticoagulant pharmacotherapy.
5. Describe the nurse's role in the pharmacologic management of coagulation disorders.
6. For each of the classes listed in Drugs at a Glance, explain the mechanism of drug action, primary actions, and important adverse effects.
7. Categorize coagulation-modifying drugs based on their classification and mechanism of action.
8. Use the Nursing Process to care for patients receiving drug therapy for coagulation disorders.

The process of hemostasis, or the stopping of blood flow, is an essential mechanism protecting the body from both external and internal injury. Without efficient hemostasis, bleeding from wounds or internal injuries would lead to shock and perhaps death. Too much clotting, however, can be just as dangerous. The physiological processes of hemostasis must maintain a delicate balance between fluidity and coagulation.

A number of diseases and conditions can affect hemostasis, including myocardial infarction, cerebrovascular accident, venous thrombus, valvular heart disease, and indwelling catheters. Because these disorders are so prevalent, nurses will have frequent occasions to administer and monitor coagulation-modifying drugs.

PHARMFACTS Clotting Disorders

- Von Willebrand's disease (vWD) is the most common hereditary bleeding disorder, caused by a deficiency of von Willebrand factor (vWF), which plays a role in platelet aggregation and acts as a carrier for factor VIII.
- Hemophilia A is a hereditary lack of clotting factor VIII; it accounts for 80% of all hemophilia cases.
- Hemophilia B is a hereditary lack of clotting factor IX.
- More than 15,000 people in the United States have hemophilia A or B.
- Liver disease is a common cause of coagulation disorders, as this organ supplies many of the clotting factors.

24.1 The Process of Hemostasis

The process of hemostasis is complex, involving a number of substances called clotting factors. Hemostasis occurs in a series of sequential steps, sometimes referred to as a cascade. Drugs can be used to modify several of these steps.

When a blood vessel is injured, a series of events initiate the clotting process. The vessel spasms, causing constriction, which limits blood flow to the injured area. Platelets have an affinity for the damaged vessel. They become sticky, adhering to each other and to the injured area. Aggregation is facilitated by adenosine diphosphate (ADP), the enzyme thrombin, and thromboxane A₂,

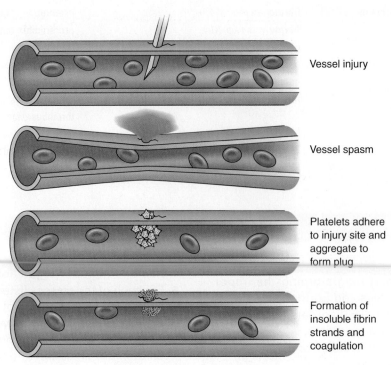

Vessel injury

Vessel spasm

Platelets adhere
to injury site and
aggregate to
form plug

Formation of
insoluble fibrin
strands and
coagulation

Figure 24.1 | Basic steps in hemostasis

while adhesion is made possible by platelet receptor sites and von Willebrand's factor. As the bound platelets break down, they release substances that attract more platelets to the area. Blood flow is further slowed, thus allowing the process of **coagulation**, the formation of an insoluble clot, to occur. The basic steps of hemostasis are shown in Figure 24.1.

When collagen is exposed at the site of injury, the damaged cells initiate a series of complex reactions called the **coagulation cascade**. Coagulation occurs when fibrin threads form to create a meshwork that fortifies the blood constituents so that they develop the clot. During the cascade, various plasma proteins that are circulating in an inactive state, are converted to their active forms. Two separate pathways, along with numerous biochemical processes, lead to coagulation. The intrinsic pathway is activated in response to injury. The extrinsic pathway is activated when blood leaks out of a vessel and enters tissue spaces. There are common steps between the two pathways and the outcome is the same—the formation of the fibrin clot. The steps in each coagulation cascade are shown in Figure 24.2.

Near the end of the common pathway, a chemical called **prothrombin activator** or prothrombinase is formed. Prothrombin activator converts the clotting factor **prothrombin** to an enzyme called **thrombin**. Thrombin then converts **fibrinogen**, a plasma protein, to long strands of **fibrin**. The fibrin strands provide a framework for the structure of the clot. Thus, two of the factors essential to clotting, thrombin and fibrin, are only formed after injury to the vessels. The fibrin strands form an insoluble web over the injured area to

stop blood loss. Normal blood clotting occurs in approximately 6 minutes.

It is important to note that several clotting factors, including thromboplastin and fibrinogen, are proteins made by the liver, which are constantly circulating through the blood in an inactive form. Vitamin K, which is made by bacteria residing in the large intestine, is required for the liver to make four of the clotting factors. Because of the crucial importance of the liver in creating these clotting factors, patients with serious liver disorders often have abnormal coagulation.

24.2 Removal of Blood Clots

The goal of hemostasis has been achieved once a blood clot is formed, protecting the body from excessive hemorrhage. The clot, however, stops most or all of the blood flow to the affected area; circulation must eventually be restored so that the tissue can resume normal activities. The process of clot removal is called **fibrinolysis**. It is initiated within 24 to 48 hours of clot formation and continues until the clot is dissolved.

Fibrinolysis also involves several cascading steps. When the fibrin clot is formed, nearby blood vessel cells secrete the enzyme **tissue plasminogen activator (t-PA)**. t-PA converts the inactive protein **plasminogen**, which is present in the fibrin clot, to its active enzymatic form called **plasmin**. Plasmin then digests the fibrin strands to remove the clot. The body normally regulates fibrinolysis such that unwanted fibrin clots are removed, while fibrin present in wounds is left to maintain hemostasis. The steps of fibrinolysis are shown in Figure 24.3.

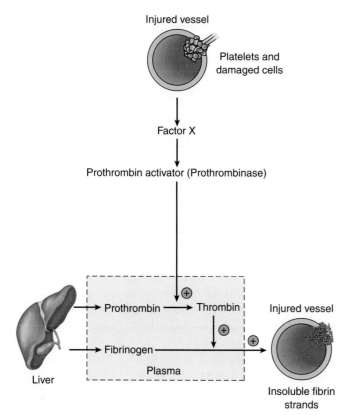

Figure 24.2 | Major steps in the coagulation cascade: Common pathway

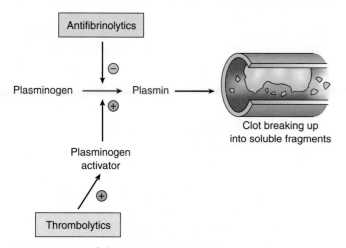

Figure 24.3 | Primary steps in fibrinolysis

24.3 Diseases of Hemostasis

To diagnose bleeding disorders, a thorough health history and physical examination is necessary. Laboratory tests measuring coagulation must be obtained. These usually include a whole blood clotting time, prothrombin time (PT), thrombin time, activated partial thromboplastin time (aPTT), liver function tests, and in some instances a bleeding time. Platelet count is also of interest in assessing

bleeding disorders. Additional tests may be indicated, based on the results of these laboratory analyses.

Thromboembolic disorders are those in which the body forms undesirable clots. Once a stationary clot, called a thrombus, forms in a vessel it often grows larger as more fibrin is added. Arterial thrombi are particularly problematic as they deprive an area of blood flow. Cessation of blood flow results in an infarction and tissue death will result. This is the case in myocardial infarctions and many cerebral vascular accidents (CVAs).

Pieces of a thrombus may break off and travel in the bloodstream to affect other vessels. A traveling clot is called an embolus. Thrombi in the venous system usually form in the veins of the legs in susceptible patients, a condition called deep vein thrombosis (DVT). Thrombi can form in the atria during atrial fibrillation. An embolus from the right atrium will cause pulmonary emboli, whereas an embolus from the left atrium will cause a CVA or an arterial infarction elsewhere in the body. Arterial thrombi and emboli can also result from procedures involving arterial punctures such as angiography. Thromboembolic disorders are the most common indications for pharmacotherapy with anticoagulants.

Bleeding disorders are characterized by abnormal clot formation. The most common bleeding disorder is a deficiency of platelets known as thrombocytopenia, which results from any condition that suppresses bone marrow function. Certain drugs such as immunosuppressants and most drugs used for cancer chemotherapy can cause this condition.

Hemophilias are bleeding disorders caused by genetic deficiencies in certain clotting factors. They are typified by prolonged coagulation times that result in persistent bleeding that can be acute. The classic form, hemophilia A, is caused by a lack of clotting factor VIII and accounts for approximately 80% of all cases. Hemophilia B, or Christmas disease, is caused by a deficiency of factor IX, and makes up about 20% of those afflicted with hemophilia. Hemophilia is treated with the administration of the absent clotting factor and, in acute situations, transfusions of fresh frozen plasma. Of other inherited bleeding disorders, **von Willebrand's disease (vWD)** is the most common. This disorder results in a decrease in quantity or quality of von Willebrand factor (vWF), which has a role in platelet aggregation. This type of bleeding disorder is treated with factor VIII concentrate as well as desmopressin (DDAVP), which promotes the release of stored vWF. For the most severely affected patients, plasma products containing vWF may be required.

24.4 Mechanisms of Coagulation Modification

Drugs can modify hemostasis by four basic mechanisms as summarized in Table 24.1. The most commonly prescribed coagulation modifiers are the **anticoagulants**, which are used to prevent the formation of clots. To accomplish clot prevention, drugs can either inhibit specific clotting factors in the coagulation cascade or diminish the clotting action of platelets. Regardless of the mechanism, all anticoagulant drugs will increase the normal time the body takes to form clots.

Once an abnormal clot has formed in a blood vessel, it may be critical to quickly remove it to restore normal function. This is particularly important for vessels serving the heart, lungs, and brain. A specific class of drugs, the **thrombolytics**, has been developed to dissolve such life-threatening clots.

Occasionally, it is necessary to actually promote the formation of clots. These drugs, called **antifibrinolytics**, inhibit the normal removal of fibrin, thus keeping the clot in place for a longer period of time. Antifibrinolytics are primarily used to speed clot formation, to limit bleeding from a surgical site.

Since hemostasis involves a delicate balance of factors favoring clotting versus those inhibiting clotting, pharmacotherapy with coagulation modifiers is individualized to each patient. Patients will require regular monitoring.

ANTICOAGULANTS

Anticoagulants are drugs used to prolong bleeding time, to prevent blood clots from forming. They are widely used in the treatment of thromboembolic disease.

24.5 Pharmacotherapy with Parenteral and Oral Anticoagulants

Anticoagulants lengthen clotting time and prevent thrombi from forming or growing larger. Thromboembolic disease can be life threatening; thus, therapy is often begun by administering anticoagulants intravenously or subcutaneously to achieve a rapid onset of action. As the disease stabilizes, the patient is switched to oral anticoagulants, with careful monitoring of appropriate coagulation laboratory studies. The most common parenteral anticoagulant is heparin; warfarin (Coumadin) is the most common oral anticoagulant.

Anticoagulants act by a number of different mechanisms, as illustrated in Figure 24.4. These drugs are often referred to as blood thinners, which is actually not the case, because they do not change the viscosity of the blood. Instead, anticoagulants exert a negative charge on the surface of the platelets so the clumping action or aggregation of these cells is inhibited. Heparin acts by enhancing the inhibitory actions of **antithrombin III**. Warfarin (Comuadin) acts by inhibiting the hepatic synthesis of Coagulation factors II, VII, IX and X. Table 24.2 lists the primary anticoagulants.

In recent years, the heparin molecule has been shortened and modified to create a new class of drugs called **low molecular weight heparins (LMWHs)**. The mechanism of action of these agents is similar to that of heparin, except their inhibition is more specific to active factor X (Figure 24.2). LMWHs possess the same degree of anticoagulant activity as heparin but have several advantages. They produce a more stable response than heparin, thus fewer follow-up lab tests are needed, and family members or the patient can be trained to give the necessary SC injections at home. They are less likely to cause thrombocytopenia. LMWHs have become the drugs of choice for a number of clotting disorders, including the prevention of deep vein thrombosis following surgery.

Pentoxifylline (Trental) is a unique agent that has anticoagulation properties, but works by a different mechanism. Pentoxifylline acts on red blood cells to reduce their viscosity and increase their flexibility, thus allowing them

Table 24.1	Mechanisms by which Coagulation Can Be Modified by Drugs	
Type of Modification	**Mechanism**	**Drug Classification**
prevention of clot formation	inhibition of specific clotting factors	anticoagulant
prevention of clot formation	inhibition of platelet actions	anticoagulant/antiplatelet
removal of an existing clot	clot dissolved by the drug	thrombolytic
promotion of clot formation	inhibit the destruction of fibrin	antifibrinolytic

to enter vessels that are partially occluded and prevent thrombi formation. It is given orally to increase the microcirculation in patients with intermittent claudication. Technically, it is classified as a hemorrheologic drug, rather than an anticoagulant.

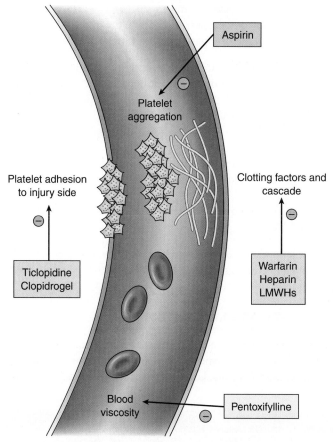

Figure 24.4 | Mechanisms of action of anticoagulants

An experimental oral anticoagulant, exanta (Ximelagatran), is in the final stages of clinical trials. If approved, it would be the first new oral anticoagulant in the last 50 years. It is the first in a new class of anticoagulants, called direct thrombin inhibitors. The primary advantage of this drug is that it is given at a fixed dose with no titrating or coagulation monitoring. Compared to available anticoagulants, it has low potential for food or drug interactions.

NURSING CONSIDERATIONS

The role of the nurse in anticoagulant therapy involves careful monitoring of a patient's condition and providing education as it relates to the prescribed drug regimen. The most serious side effect of anticoagulants is bleeding. The nurse should assess the patient for signs of bleeding, including bruising, nosebleeds, excessive menstrual flow, "coffee-grounds" emesis, tarry stools, tea-colored urine, bright red bleeding from the rectum, dizziness, fatigue, or pale pasty-looking skin. The risk of bleeding is dose dependent: The higher the dose, the higher the risk.

Hypotension accompanied by declining CBC values (RBCs, platelets, hemoglobin, and hematocrit) may signal internal bleeding. Lumbar pain and unilateral abdominal wall bulges or swelling could indicate retroperitoneal hemorrhage. Guaiac tests can be performed on stool to identify occult blood. Use of heparin during breastfeeding can trigger bleeding from the nipples and should be avoided. Use of warfarin (Coumadin) during pregnancy is contraindicated, as it can cause hemorrhage or other abnormalities in the fetus.

Monitoring laboratory values during anticoagulant therapy is essential to patient safety. For heparin, aPTT is measured, with normal values ranging from 25 to 40 seconds. For therapeutic anticoagulation, the aPTT should be 1 to 2 times the patient's baseline. During continuous

Table 24.2	Anticoagulants
Drug	**Route and Adult Dose (max dose where indicated)**
anisindione (Miradon)	PO; 300 mg day 1, 200 mg day 2, then 100 mg qd; adjust dose to maintain desired PT level (dose range 25–250 mg)
heparin (Heplock)	IV; Infusion: 5,000–40,000 units/day
	SC; 15,000–20,000 units bid
pentoxifylline (Trental) *	PO; 400 mg tid
warfarin (Coumadin)	PO; 2–15 mg/day
Low Molecular Weight Heparins (LMWHs)	
ardeparin (Normiflo)	SC; 50 units/kg bid for 14 days
dalteparin (Fragmin)	SC; 2,500–5,000 units/day for 5–10 days
danaparoid (Orgaran)	SC; 750 units bid for 7–10 days
enoxaparin (Lovenox)	SC; 30 mg bid for 7–10 days
tinzaparin (Innohep)	SC; 175 units/kg qd for at least 6 days

* Sometimes classified as a hemorrheologic drug.

intravenous heparin therapy, the aPTT is measured daily and 6 to 8 hours after any changes in dosage.

Prothrombin time (PT) is a laboratory test used to monitor effectiveness of warfarin (Coumadin). The normal PT range is 12 to 15 seconds. During therapeutic anticoagulation, PT should increase to 1 to 2 times the patient's baseline. Because laboratory testing methods for PT vary, prothrombin time is also reported as an international normalized ratio (INR) value; INR values of 2.0 to 3.5 are considered therapeutic. Prothrombin time is measured daily until the therapeutic dose is determined, then the frequency of testing is decreased to weekly or monthly as therapy progresses.

When transitioning from IV heparin to PO warfarin, the two drugs must be administered simultaneously for 2 to 3 days. Heparin has a brief half-life (90 minutes) and warfarin a long one (1 to 3 days). aPTT returns to normal within 2 to 3 hours following discontinuation of heparin, thus concomitant pharmacotherapy is necessary to ensure continuous therapeutic anticoagulation. During this transition, there is increased risk of bleeding, due to the potentiated action of the combined drugs.

LMWHs are given subcutaneously, with dosage calculations based on the patient's weight rather than laboratory values. The nurse should follow manufacturer's recommendations for sites of injection. There is an increased risk of bleeding if injected into muscle. For example, enoxaparin (Lovenox) is given in the subcutaneous tissue of the anterolateral or posterolateral abdominal wall (the "love handles"). To administer safely, the nurse should grasp a skinfold between the thumb and forefinger, insert a 3/8-inch needle fully at a 90-degree angle, and hold the skinfold throughout the injection. For exceptionally lean patients, a longer needle is used and carefully inserted at a 45-degree angle to avoid inadvertent IM injection of the medication. To prevent tissue injury and bruising, an injection site should never be massaged.

Following are important points the nurse should include when teaching patients about heparin and warfarin.

- Immediately report burning, stinging, tightness, tenderness, warmth, or other pain at heparin injection or IV insertion sites; these signs may signal drug seepage into sensitive tissues.
- Notify the nurse of excessive bruising or evidence of swelling at a heparin injection site.
- Take warfarin at the same time each day.
- Balance intake of vitamin K-rich foods when taking warfarin.
- Avoid strenuous or hazardous activities that could result in bleeding injury.

General teaching strategies for anticoagulants can be found in "Nursing Process Focus: Patients Receiving Anticoagulant Therapy."

ANTIPLATELET AGENTS

Antiplatelet drugs cause an anticoagulant effect by interfering with various aspects of platelet function—primarily platelet aggregation. Unlike the anticoagulants, which are

Pr | **PROTOTYPE DRUG** | **HEPARIN** (Heplock)

ACTIONS AND USES

Heparin is a natural substance found in the liver and in the lining of blood vessels. Its normal function is to prolong coagulation time, thereby preventing excessive clotting within blood vessels. As a result, it prevents the enlargement of existing clots and the formation of new ones. The binding of heparin to antithrombin III inactivates several clotting factors and inhibits thrombin activity. The onset of action for IV heparin is immediate, whereas SC heparin may take up to 1 hour for maximum therapeutic effect.

Administration Alerts

- Heparin is poorly absorbed by the GI mucosa because of rapid metabolism by the hepatic enzyme, heparinase. Therefore, it must be given either SC or through IV bolus injection or continuous infusion.
- When administering heparin SC, never draw back the syringe plunger once the needle has entered the skin; never massage the site after injection. Doing either can contribute to bleeding or tissue damage.
- IM administration is contraindicated due to bleeding risk.
- Pregnancy category C.

ADVERSE EFFECTS AND INTERACTIONS

Abnormal bleeding is not uncommon with heparin therapy. Should aPTT become prolonged or toxicity be observed, discontinuation of the drug will result in loss of anticoagulant activity within hours. If serious hemorrhage occurs, a specific antagonist, protamine sulfate, may be administered to neutralize the anticoagulant activity of heparin. Protamine sulfate has an onset of action of 5 minutes and is also an antagonist to the LMWHs.

Oral anticoagulants, including warfarin, potentiate the action of heparin. Drugs that inhibit platelet aggregation, such as ASA, indomethacin, and ibuprofen, may induce bleeding. Nicotine, digitalis, tetracyclines, or antihistamines may inhibit anticoagulation.

Use with caution with herbal supplements, such as arnica, which contains a coumarin component, and may increase the anticoagulant effect.

See the companian website for a Nursing Process Focus specific to this drug.

PROTOTYPE DRUG | **WARFARIN** (Coumadin)

ACTIONS AND USES

Unlike heparin, the anticoagulant activity of warfarin can take several days to reach its maximum effect. This explains why heparin and warfarin therapy are overlapped. Warfarin inhibits the action of vitamin K. Without adequate vitamin K, the synthesis of clotting factors II, VII, IX, and X is diminished. Because these clotting factors are normally circulating in the blood, it takes several days for their plasma levels to fall, and for the anticoagulant effect of warfarin to appear. Another reason for the slow onset is that 99% of the warfarin is bound to plasma proteins and is thus unavailable to produce its effect.

Administration Alerts

■ Should life-threatening bleeding occur during therapy, the anticoagulant effects of warfarin can be reduced in 6 hours through the IM or SC administration of its antagonist, vitamin K_1.
■ Pregnancy category D.

ADVERSE EFFECTS AND INTERACTIONS

The most serious adverse effect of warfarin is abnormal bleeding. Upon discontinuation of therapy, the anticoagulant activity of warfarin may persist for up to 10 days.

Extensive protein binding is responsible for numerous drug-drug interactions, some of which include NSAIDs, diuretics, SSRIs and other antidepressants, steroids, antibiotics and vaccines, and vitamins (e.g., vitamin K). Concurrent use with NSAIDs may increase bleeding risk.

Use with caution with herbal supplements, such as feverfew, garlic, and ginger, which may increase the risk of bleeding; and arnica, which may increase the anticoagulant effect.

See the companion website for a Nursing Process Focus specific to this drug.

used primarily to prevent thrombosis in veins, antiplatelet agents are used to prevent clot formation in arteries. The antiplatelet agents are shown in Table 24.3.

24.6 Inhibition of Platelet Function

Platelets are a central component of the blood hemostasis process and too few platelets or diminished platelet function can profoundly increase bleeding time. Three types of drugs are classified as antiplatelet agents due to their inhibition of platelet function.

 Aspirin
■ Adenosine diphosphate (ADP) receptor blockers
■ Glycoprotein IIb/IIIa receptor blockers

Aspirin deserves special mention as an antiplatelet agent. Because it is available over the counter, patients may not consider aspirin a potent medication; however, its anticoagulant activity is well documented. Aspirin acts by binding irreversibly to the enzyme cyclooxygenase in platelets. This binding inhibits the formation of thromboxane$_2$, a powerful inducer of platelet aggregation. The anticoagulant effect of a single dose of aspirin may persist for as long as a week. Concurrent use of aspirin with other coagulation modifiers should be avoided, unless medically approved. The primary uses of aspirin are described in several places in this textbook: pain relief in Chapter 19, prevention of strokes and myocardial infarction in Chapter 25, and reduction of inflammation in Chapter 31 .

The ADP receptor blockers comprise a small group of drugs that irreversibly alter the plasma membrane of platelets. This alteration changes the platelets so they are unable to receive the chemical signals required for them to aggregate. Both ticlopidine (Ticlid) and clopidogrel (Plavix) are given orally to prevent thrombi formation in patients who have experienced a recent thromboembolic event such as a stroke or MI. Ticlopidine (Ticlid) can cause life-threatening neutropenia and agranulocytosis. Clopidogrel (Plavix) is much safer, having side effects comparable to those of aspirin.

Glycoprotein IIb/IIIa inhibitors are relatively new additions to the treatment of thromboembolic disease. **Glycoprotein IIb/IIIa** is an enzyme necessary for platelet aggregation. Inhibition of this enzyme has the effect of preventing thrombus formation in patients experiencing a recent MI, stroke, or percutaneous transluminal coronary angioplasty (PTCA). Although these drugs are the most efficacious antiplatelet agents, they are very expensive. Another major disadvantage is that they can be given only by the IV route.

NURSING CONSIDERATIONS

The role of the nurse in antiplatelet therapy involves careful monitoring of a patient's condition and providing education as it relates to the prescribed drug regimen. Drugs affecting platelet aggregation increase the risk of bleeding when the patient sustains trauma or undergoes medical procedures or surgery. These drugs are sometimes given in addition to anticoagulants, which further increases bleeding risk. Injection or venipuncture wounds will require prolonged direct pressure over the sites to control bleeding. The nurse should observe for ecchymoses and monitor bleeding time following venipunctures. Bleeding lasting more than 10 minutes may require special medical or nursing interventions, such as suturing or "sand-bagging" a large venipuncture site.

NURSING PROCESS FOCUS | PATIENTS RECEIVING ANTICOAGULANT THERAPY

ASSESSMENT

Prior to administration:
- Obtain complete health history including recent surgeries or trauma, allergies, drug history, and possible drug interactions.
- Obtain vital signs; assess in context of patient's baseline values.

POTENTIAL NURSING DIAGNOSES

- Risk for Injury (bleeding), related to adverse effects of anticoagulant therapy
- Activity Intolerance (Contact Sports)
- Ineffective Tissue Perfusion, related to hemorrhage
- Impaired Tissue Integrity
- Risk for Infection
- Deficient Knowledge, related to drug therapy

PLANNING: PATIENT GOALS AND EXPECTED OUTCOMES

The patient will:
- Experience a decrease in blood coagulability as evidenced by laboratory values ordered by the healthcare provider
- Demonstrate an understanding of the drug's action by accurately describing drug side effects and precautions

IMPLEMENTATION

Interventions and (Rationales)	Patient Education/Discharge Planning
■ Monitor for adverse clotting reaction(s). (Heparin can cause thrombus formation with thrombocytopenia, or "white clot syndrome." Coumadin may cause cholesterol microemboli which result in gangrene, localized vasculitis, or "purple toes syndrome.") ■ Observe for skin necrosis, changes in blue or purple mottling of the feet that blanches with pressure or fades when the legs are elevated. (Patients on anticoagulant therapy remain at risk for developing emboli resulting in CVA or PE.)	Instruct patient to: ■ Immediately report sudden dyspnea, chest pain, temperature or color change in the hands, arms, legs, and feet (Gangrene may occur between day 3 and 8 of warfarin therapy. Purple toes syndrome usually occurs within weeks 3 to 10 or later.) ■ Feel pedal pulses daily to check circulation ■ Protect feet from injury by wearing loose-fitting socks; avoid going barefoot
■ Use with caution in patients with GI, renal and/or liver disease, alcoholism, diabetes, hypertension, hyperlipidemia, and in the elderly and premenopausal women. (Patients with CAD risk factors are at increased risk of developing cholesterol microemboli.)	■ Instruct elderly patients, menstruating women, and those with peptic ulcer disease, alcoholism, or kidney or liver disease that they have an increased risk of bleeding. ■ Diabetics and patients with high blood pressure or cholesterol are at risk of developing microscopic clots, despite anticoagulant therapy.
■ Monitor for signs of bleeding: flulike symptoms, excessive bruising, pallor, epistaxis, hemoptysis, hematemesis, menorrhagia, hematuria, melena, frank rectal bleeding, or excessive bleeding from wounds or in the mouth. (Bleeding is a sign of anticoagulant overdose.)	Advise patient to: ■ Immediately report: flulike symptoms (dizziness, chills, weakness, pale skin); blood coming from a cough, the nose, mouth, or rectum; menstrual "flooding"; "coffee grounds" vomit; tarry stools; excessive bruising; bleeding from wounds that cannot be stopped within 10 minutes; all physical injuries ■ Avoid all contact sports and amusement park rides that cause intense or violent bumping or jostling ■ Use a soft toothbrush and electric shaver ■ Keep a "pad count" during menstrual periods to estimate blood losses
■ Monitor vital signs. (Increase in heart rate accompanied by low blood pressure or subnormal temperature may signal bleeding.)	■ Instruct patient to immediately report palpitations, fatigue, or feeling faint, which may signal low blood pressure related to bleeding.

continued

NURSING PROCESS FOCUS: *Patients Receiving Anticoagulant Therapy (continued)*

Interventions and (Rationales)	*Patient Education/Discharge Planning*
■ Monitor laboratory values: aPTT, PTT for therapeutic values. (Heparin may cause significant elevations of SGOT [S-AST] and SGPT [S-ALT] because the drug is metabolized by the liver.) ■ Monitor CBC, especially in premenopausal women.	Instruct patient to: ■ Always inform laboratory personnel of heparin therapy when providing samples ■ Carry a wallet card or wear medical ID jewelry indicating heparin therapy

EVALUATION OF OUTCOME CRITERIA

Evaluate the effectiveness of drug therapy by confirming that patient goals and expected outcomes have been met (see "Planning").

See Table 24.2 for a list of drugs to which these nursing actions apply.

Table 24.3	**Antiplatelet Agents**
Drug	**Route and Adult Dose (max dose where indicated)**
aspirin (ASA, acetylsalicylic acid) (see page 233 for the Prototype Drug box)	PO; 80 mg qd to 650 mg bid
dipyridamole (Persantine)	PO; 75–100 mg qd
ADP Receptor Blockers	
clopidrogrel (Plavix)	PO; 75 mg qd
ticlopidine (Ticlid)	PO; 250 mg bid
Glycoprotein IIb/IIIa Blockers	
abciximab (ReoPro)	IV; 0.25 mg/kg initial bolus over 5 min then 10 µg/kg/min for 12 hr
eptifibatide (Integrilin)	IV; 180 µg/kg initial bolus over 1–2 min then 2 µg/kg/min for 24–72 hr
tirofiban (Aggrastat)	IV; 0.4 µg/kg/min for 30 min then 0.1 µg/kg/min for 12–24 hr

Aspirin (ASA) may cause gastritis or GI bleeding due to inhibition of prostaglandins in the GI tract (prostaglandins increase bicarbonate and mucous layer production). Aspirin and ticlopidine (Ticlid) may cause nausea and GI upset. Nursing interventions for ASA therapy can be found in "Nursing Process Focus: Patients Receiving NSAID Therapy" in Chapter 19, page 234 .

Patient education as it relates to antiplatelet agents should include the goals, reasons for obtaining baseline data such as vital signs, diagnostic procedures and laboratory tests, and possible side effects. Following are important points the nurse should include when teaching patients regarding antiplatelet agents.

■ Avoid strenuous or hazardous activities that could result in bleeding injury.
■ Do not take OTC products containing aspirin, due to increased risk of bleeding, unless otherwise directed by healthcare provider.
■ If taking antiplatelet agents concurrently with anticoagulants, be aware that the risk of bleeding is greater.

THROMBOLYTICS

Thrombolytics promote fibrinolysis, or clot destruction, by converting plasminogen to plasmin. The enzyme plasmin digests fibrin and breaks down fibrinogen, prothrombin, and other plasma proteins and clotting factors. Unlike the anticoagulants, thrombolytics actually bring about dissolution (lysis) of the insoluble fibrin within intravascular emboli and thrombi. Their therapeutic effect is proportional to the time frame in which they are administered—being more effective when given as soon as possible after clot formation occurs, preferably within 4 hours.

24.7 Pharmacotherapy with Thrombolytics

It is often mistakenly believed that the purpose of anticoagulants such as heparin or warfarin (Coumadin) is to dissolve preexisting clots, but this is not the case. A totally different class of drugs is needed for this purpose. The thrombolytics, shown in Table 24.4, are administered quite

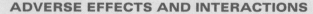

PROTOTYPE DRUG | ABCIXIMAB (ReoPro)

ACTIONS AND USES

Abciximab (ReoPro) is an antibody that binds to the glycoprotein IIb/IIIa receptors of platelets. It is extremely effective, having the ability to reduce platelet function by as much as 90% in just 2 hours. It is of great value with acute coronary syndromes and in conjunction with percutaneous transluminal coronary angioplasty (PTCA), both before and after the procedure. Abciximab is only available by bolus injection and IV infusion.

Administration Alerts

- Give drug as an IV bolus prior to PCTA followed by an infusion for 12 hours after the procedure.
- Do not shake vial, and discard if visible opaque particles are noted.
- Pregnancy category C.

ADVERSE EFFECTS AND INTERACTIONS

Like other drugs having an anticoagulant effect, contraindications for abciximab include active bleeding or recent trauma and the nurse must be observant for bleeding. Abciximab is commonly used with aspirin and heparin, thus increasing the need for careful monitoring. Concurrent use with oral anticoagulants may increase the risk of bleeding.

Use with caution with herbal supplements, such as white willow, which contains salicylates and may create an additive effect with antiplatelet drugs.

See the companion website for a Nursing Process Focus specific to this drug.

Table 24.4	Thrombolytics	
Drug	**Route and Adult Dose (max dose where indicated)**
alteplase (Activase, t-PA)	IV; begin with 60 mg and then infuse 20 mg/h over next 2 h
anistreplase (Eminase)	IV; 30 units over 2–5 min
reteplase (Retavase) (see page 340 for the Prototype Drug box)	IV; 10 units over 2 min; repeat dose in 30 min
streptokinase (Kabikinase)	IV; 250,000–1.5 million units over a short time
urokinase (Abbokinase)	IV; 4,400–6,000 units administered over several minutes to 12 h

differently than the anticoagulants and produce their effects by different mechanisms. Thrombolytics are prescribed for disorders in which an intravascular clot has already formed, such as in acute myocardial infarction, pulmonary embolism, acute ischemic cerebrovascular accident, and deep vein thrombosis (DVT).

Thrombolytics are nonspecific; that is, they will dissolve whatever clots they encounter. Because clotting is a natural and desirable process to prevent excessive bleeding, thrombolytics have a narrow margin of safety between dissolving "normal" and "abnormal" clots. Vital signs must be monitored continuously and any signs of bleeding may call for discontinuation of therapy. Because these drugs are rapidly destroyed in the bloodstream, discontinuation normally results in immediate termination of thrombolytic activity. After the clot is successfully dissolved with the thrombolytic, anticoagulant therapy is generally initiated to prevent the reformation of clots.

Since the discovery of streptokinase, the first thrombolytic, there have been a number of ensuing generations of thrombolytics. The newer drugs such as tenecteplase (TNK t-PA) are more fibrin specific and are reported to have fewer side effects than streptokinase. Tissue plasminogen activator (t-PA), marketed as alteplase (Activase), has replaced urokinase as the drug of choice in clearing thrombosed central intravenous lines. Urokinase was removed from the market due to the possibility of viral contamination, because it is obtained from pooled human donors.

NURSING CONSIDERATIONS

The role of the nurse in thrombolytic therapy involves careful monitoring of a patient's condition and providing education as it relates to the prescribed drug regimen. Thrombolytics are generally administered in the critical care or emergency department setting. The nurse should first identify conditions that exclude the patient from receiving thrombolytics, such as recent trauma, surgery/ biopsies, arterial emboli, recent cerebral embolism, hemorrhage, thrombocytopenia, septic thrombophlebitis, or childbirth (within 10 days). Baseline coagulation tests (aPTT, bleeding time, PT, and/or INR) should be obtained prior to therapy. Baseline Hct, Hgb, and platelet counts should be obtained so they may be compared to later values, to assess for bleeding. Cerebral hemorrhage is a major concern; thus, the nurse should assess for changes in level of consciousness and check neurological status. When given for myocardial infarction, the nurse should observe for dysrhythmias that may occur, as cardiac tissue perfusion is reestablished. IM injections are contraindicated during thrombolytic therapy due to the risk of bleeding.

See "Nursing Process Focus: Patients Receiving Thrombolytic Therapy" for specific teaching points.

The nurse should be aware that these drugs are given in acute situations when time for patient teaching may be limited and the patient may be unable to focus on information related to the stress of the situation.

ANTIFIBRINOLYTICS

Antifibrinolytics have an action opposite to that of anticoagulants: to shorten bleeding time. They are used to prevent excessive bleeding following surgery.

24.8 Pharmacotherapy with Antifibrinolytics

The final class of coagulation modifiers, the antifibrinolytics, is a small group of drugs used to prevent and treat excessive bleeding from surgical sites. All of the antifibrinolytics have very specific indications for use and none are commonly prescribed. Although their mechanisms differ, all drugs in this class prevent fibrin from dissolving, thus enhancing the stability of the clot. Because of their ability to slow blood flow, they are sometimes classified as hemostatic agents.

Desmopressin (DDAVP) differs from the others in being a hormone similar to vasopressin, a hormone naturally present in the body that promotes the renal conservation of water. Unlike the other antifibrinolytics, it has uses beyond hemostasis that include the control of excessive or nocturnal urination (enuresis). The antifibrinolytics are listed in Table 24.5.

NURSING CONSIDERATIONS

The role of the nurse in caring for the patient receiving antifibrinolytic therapy is to assess for clotting. Changes in peripheral pulses, paresthesias, positive Homans' sign, and prominence of superficial veins indicate clotting occurring in peripheral arterial or venous vasculature. Chest pain and shortness of breath may indicate pulmonary thrombus or embolus. Use is contraindicated in patients with disseminated intravascular clotting and severe renal impairment.

Antifibrinolytics are administered intravenously. The nurse should monitor injection sites frequently for thrombophlebitis and extravasation. Antifibrinolytics may affect the muscles, causing wasting and weakness. The nurse should identify and report the presence of myopathy and myoglobinuria, manifesting as reddish-brown urine.

Pr PROTOTYPE DRUG | ALTEPLASE (Activase)

ACTIONS AND USES

Produced through recombinant DNA technology, alteplase is identical to the enzyme human tissue plasminogen activator (t-PA). Like other thrombolytics, the primary action of alteplase is to convert plasminogen to plasmin, which then dissolves fibrin clots. To achieve maximum effect, therapy should begin immediately after the onset of symptoms. Peak effect occurs in 5 to 10 minutes. Alteplase does not exhibit the allergic reactions seen with streptokinase. An unlabeled use is for restoration of patency of IV catheters.

Administration Alerts

- Drug must be given within 6 hours of onset of symptoms of MI and within 3 hours of thrombotic CVA for maximum effectiveness.
- Avoid IM injection, IV punctures, and arterial punctures during infusion to decrease risk of bleeding.
- Pregnancy category C.

ADVERSE EFFECTS AND INTERACTIONS

Thrombolytics such as alteplase are contraindicated in patients with active bleeding or with a history of recent trauma. Trauma may include but is not limited to physical injury, surgery, biopsies, or within the 10-day postpartum period. The nurse must carefully monitor the patient for signs of bleeding every 15 minutes for the first hour of therapy, and every 30 minutes thereafter. Signs of bleeding such as spontaneous ecchymoses, hematomas, or epistaxis should be reported to the healthcare provider immediately.

Use with caution with herbal supplements, such as ginkgo, which may cause an increased thrombolytic effect.

 See the companion website for a Nursing Process Focus specific to this drug.

| NURSING PROCESS FOCUS | PATIENTS RECEIVING THROMBOLYTIC THERAPY |

ASSESSMENT

Prior to administration:
- Obtain complete health history including recent surgeries or trauma, allergies, drug history, and possible drug interactions.
- Obtain vital signs; assess in context of patient's baseline values.
- Assess lab values: aPTT, PT, Hgb, Hct, platelet count.

POTENTIAL NURSING DIAGNOSES

- Risk for Injury (bleeding), related to adverse effects of thrombolytic therapy
- Ineffective Tissue Perfusion, related to increase in size of thrombus due to ineffective thrombolytic therapy
- Deficient Knowledge, related to drug therapy

PLANNING: PATIENT GOALS AND EXPECTED OUTCOMES

The patient will:
- Experience a dissolving of preexisting blood clot(s) as evidenced by laboratory values ordered by the healthcare provider
- Demonstrate an understanding of the drug's action by accurately describing drug side effects and precautions

IMPLEMENTATION

Interventions and (Rationales)

- If necessary, start IV lines, arterial line, or Foley catheter prior to beginning therapy. (This decreases the risk of bleeding from those sites).
- Monitor vital signs every 15 minutes during first hour of infusion, then every 30 minutes during remainder of infusion.
- Patient should be moved as little as possible during the infusion. (This is done to prevent internal injury.)
- If given for thrombotic CVA, monitor neurological status frequently.
- Monitor cardiac response while medication is infusing. (Dysrhythmias may occur with reperfusion of myocardium.)
- Monitor blood tests (Hct, Hgb, platelet counts) during and after therapy for indications of blood loss due to internal bleeding. (Patient has increased risk of bleeding for 2 to 4 days postinfusion.)

Patient Education/Discharge Planning

- Instruct patient about procedures and why they are necessary prior to beginning thrombolytic therapy.

Advise patient:
- Of the need for frequent vital signs
- That activity will be limited during infusion and pressure dressing may be needed to prevent any active bleeding

- Advise patient about assessments and why they are necessary.
- Advise patient that cardiac rhythm will be monitored during therapy.
- Instruct patient of increased risk for bleeding and activity restriction and frequent monitoring during this time.

EVALUATION OF OUTCOME CRITERIA

Evaluate the effectiveness of drug therapy by confirming that patient goals and expected outcomes have been met (see "Planning").

See Table 24.4 for a list of drugs to which these nursing actions apply.

Table 24.5	Antifibrinolytics
Drug	**Route and Adult Dose (max dose where indicated)**
aminocaproic acid (Amicar)	IV; 4–5 g for 1 hour, then 1–1.25 g/h until bleeding is controlled
aprotinin (Trasylol)	IV; 15,000 KIU as a test dose, then give 500,000 KIU during surgery
tranexamic acid (Cyklokapron)	PO; 25 mg/kg qid

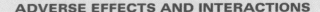

 PROTOTYPE DRUG | **AMINOCAPROIC ACID** (Amicar)

ACTIONS AND USES

Aminocaproic acid acts by inactivating plasminogen, the precursor of the enzyme plasmin that digests the fibrin clot. Aminocaproic acid is prescribed in situations where there is excessive bleeding due to clots being dissolved prematurely. During acute hemorrhages, it can be given IV to reduce bleeding in 1 to 2 hours. It is most commonly prescribed following surgery to reduce postoperative bleeding.

Administration Alerts

- May cause hypotension and bradycardia when given IV. Assess vital signs frequently and place patient on cardiac monitor to assess for dysrhythmias.
- Pregnancy category C.

ADVERSE EFFECTS AND INTERACTIONS

Since aminocaproic acid tends to stabilize clots, it should be used cautiously in patients with a history of thromboembolic disease. Side effects are generally mild.

Drug interactions include hypercoagulation with concurrent use of estrogens and oral contraceptives.

See the companion website for a Nursing Process Focus specific to this drug.

Patient education as it relates to antifibrinolytic agents should include the goals, reasons for obtaining baseline data such as vital signs, diagnostic procedures and laboratory tests, and possible side effects. Following are important points the nurse should include when teaching patients regarding antifibrinolytic agents.

- Report renewed bleeding episodes.
- Avoid the use of aspirin or OTC medications containing aspirin.
- Report the following immediately: excessive bleeding following a medical or dental procedure, altered color vision, decreased amounts of urine, or pain/numbness/tingling in the extremities.

NATURAL THERAPIES | **Garlic for Cardiovascular Health**

Garlic (*Allium sativum*) is one of the best-studied herbs. Purported indications for garlic include arteriosclerosis, common cold, cough/bronchitis, high cholesterol, hypertension, and tendency to infection. It has been proven to be of value in only a few of these disorders.

Several different substances, known as alliaceous oils, have been isolated from garlic and shown to have pharmacologic activity. Dosage forms include eating prepared garlic oil or the fresh bulbs from the plant.

Garlic has been shown to decrease the aggregation or "stickiness" of platelets, thus producing an anticoagulant effect. Platelet aggregation on roughened walls of arteries damaged by atherosclerosis commonly initiates the formation of blood clots that lead to heart attacks and strokes. Claims that garlic can reduce heart disease and the incidence of stroke may be related to this action. Patients taking anticoagulant medications should limit their intake of garlic to avoid bleeding complications.

CHAPTER REVIEW

Key Concepts

The numbered key concepts provide a succinct summary of the important points from the corresponding numbered section within the chapter. If any of these points are not clear, refer to the numbered section within the chapter for review. Expanded versions can be found on the companion website.

24.1 Hemostasis is a complex process involving multiple steps and a large number of enzymes and factors. The final product is a fibrin clot that stops blood loss.

24.2 Fibrinolysis, or removal of a blood clot, is an enzymatic process initiated by the release of t-PA. Plasmin digests the fibrin strands, thus restoring circulation to the injured area.

24.3 Diseases of hemostasis include thromboembolic disorders caused by thrombi and emboli, and bleeding disorders such as hemophilia and von Willebrand's disease.

24.4 The normal coagulation process can be modified by a number of different mechanisms, including inhibiting clotting factors, dissolving fibrin, and influencing platelet function.

24.5 Anticoagulants prevent clot formation. The primary drugs in this category are heparin (parenteral) and warfarin (oral).

24.6 Several drugs prolong bleeding time by interfering with the aggregation of platelets. Antiplatelet agents include aspirin, ADP blockers, and glycoprotein IIb/IIIa receptor blockers.

24.7 Thrombolytics are used to dissolve existing intravascular clots in patients with MI and CVA.

24.8 Antifibrinolytics are used to promote the formation of clots in patients with excessive bleeding from surgical sites.

Review Questions

1. Which clotting factors are always circulating in the blood? Which are only formed after coagulation has been initiated?

2. Both warfarin and heparin are effective anticoagulants. Why would a healthcare provider choose heparin over warfarin?

3. Explain why the commonly used term for anticoagulants, *blood thinners,* is not correct.

4. A patient has begun to hemorrhage while being infused with alteplase (t-PA). What action should be taken?

Critical Thinking Questions

1. The nurse is working on a medical unit where a patient suddenly develops left-sided weakness and garbled speech. The nurse calls the healthcare provider who says that the patient appears to be having a CVA and orders heparin 5,000 units IV and a heparin drip to run at 1,000 units per hour. What should the nurse do?

2. A patient has had an acute myocardial infarction and has received alteplase (Activase) to lyse the clot. What nursing action should have been taken prior to the patient receiving the medication?

3. A patient is receiving Lovenox SQ after being diagnosed with thrombophlebitis. What precautions should be taken when giving this medication?

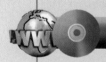

EXPLORE MediaLink

NCLEX review, case studies, and other interactive resources for this chapter can be found on the companion website at www.prenhall.com/adams. Click on "Chapter 24" to select the activities for this chapter. For animations, more NCLEX review questions, and an audio glossary, access the accompanying CD-ROM in this textbook.

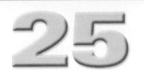

CHAPTER 25

Drugs for Angina Pectoris, Myocardial Infarction, and Cerebrovascular Accident

DRUGS AT A GLANCE

ORGANIC NITRATES
- Pr *nitroglycerin (Nitrostat)*

BETA-ADRENERGIC BLOCKERS
- Pr *atenolol (Tenormin)*
- Pr *metoprolol (Lopressor)*

CALCIUM CHANNEL BLOCKERS
- Pr *diltiazem (Cardizem)*

GLYCOPROTEIN IIB/IIIA INHIBITORS

THROMBOLYTICS
- Pr *reteplase (Retavase)*

ADJUNCT DRUGS FOR MYOCARDIAL INFARCTION AND CEREBROVASCULAR ACCIDENT

metabolized and eliminated by the body.
of this process

PHARMACOLOGY

1. The study of medicines; the discipline pertaining to how drugs improve the heal of the human body

MediaLink   www.prenhall.com/adams

CD-ROM

Animation:
   Mechanism in Action: Reteplase (Retavase)
Audio Glossary
NCLEX Review

Companion Website

NCLEX Review
Dosage Calculations
Case Study
Care Plans
Expanded Key Concepts

OBJECTIVES

After reading this chapter, the student should be able to:

1. Explain the relationship between atherosclerosis and coronary artery disease.

2. Describe the blood supply to the myocardium.

3. Explain the pathophysiology of angina pectoris, myocardial infarction, and cerebrovascular accident.

4. Describe the nurse's role in the pharmacologic management of patients with angina, myocardial infarction, and cerebrovascular accident.

5. For each of the drug classes listed in Drugs at a Glance, know representative drug examples, explain their mechanism of action, primary actions, and important adverse effects.

6. Categorize drugs used in the treatment of angina, myocardial infarction, and cerebrovascular accident based on their classification and mechanism of action.

7. Use the Nursing Process to care for patients who are receiving drug therapy for angina, myocardial infarcation, and cerebrovascular accident.

The tissues and organs of the body are dependent upon the arterial supply of oxygen and other vital nutrients to support life and health. Should the arterial blood supply become compromised, cardiovascular and cerebrovascular functioning may become impaired, resulting in angina pectoris, acute myocardial infarction, or cerebrovascular accident. Such conditions are associated with the development of atherosclerotic plaques or the aggregation of platelets on the intima of blood vessels, with resultant clot formation. Tissues and organs served by the arteries, distal to the site of involvement, become ischemic and suffer varying degrees of damage. This chapter focuses on the pharmacologic and nursing interventions related to these conditions.

25.1 Etiology of Coronary Artery Disease and Myocardial Ischemia

Coronary artery disease (CAD) is one of the leading causes of mortality in the United States. The primary characteristic defining CAD is narrowing or occlusion of the coronary arteries. The narrowing deprives cells of needed oxygen and nutrients, a condition known as myocardial ischemia. If it develops over a long period of time, the heart may compensate for its inadequate blood supply and the patient may experience no symptoms. Indeed, coronary arteries may be occluded as much as 50% or more and cause no symptoms.

As CAD progresses, however, the heart does not receive enough oxygen to meet the metabolic demands of the myocardium. The oxygen deficiency signals the onset of anaerobic metabolism to generate the energy needed to maintain cardiac function. As a result, lactic acid accumulates. As with any muscle, the buildup of lactic acid produces pain and soreness. When lactic acid activates pericardial pain receptors, the body experiences the sensation of chest pain. Persistent myocardial ischemia may lead to heart attack.

The common etiology of CAD in adults is atherosclerosis, the presence of plaque—a fatty, fibrous material within the walls of the coronary arteries. Plaque develops, then builds upon itself, thus producing varying degrees of intravascular narrowing, a situation that results in partial or total blockage of the vessel. In addition, the plaque impairs normal vessel elasticity, and the coronary vessel is unable to dilate properly when the myocardium needs additional blood or oxygen. Plaque accumulation occurs gradually, possibly over periods of 40 to 50 years in some individuals, but actually begins to accrue early in life. As the material collects on the intima (lining) of a vessel, the cardiac muscle distal to the obstruction receives diminished oxygen supply, thus hindering the performance of its metabolic functions. The development of atherosclerosis is illustrated in Figure 25.1.

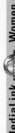

MediaLink   Women and Heart Disease

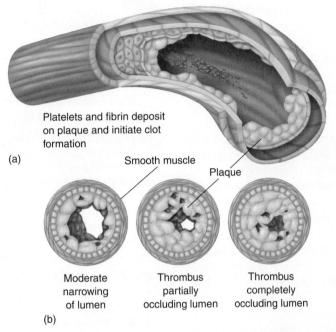

(a)

Platelets and fibrin deposit
on plaque and initiate clot
formation

Smooth muscle

Plaque

Moderate
narrowing
of lumen

Thrombus
partially
occluding lumen

Thrombus
completely
occluding lumen

(b)

Figure 25.1 | Atherosclerosis in the coronary arteries *Source: Pearson Education/PH College.*

25.2 Blood Supply to the Myocardium

The heart, from the moment it begins to function in utero until death, works to distribute oxygen and nutrients via its nonstop pumping action. It is the hardest working organ in the body, functioning continually during both activity and rest. Because the heart itself is a muscle, it needs a steady supply of nourishment to sustain itself and maintain the circulation in a balanced state of equilibrium. Any disturbance in blood flow to the vital organs or the myocardium itself—even for brief episodes—can result in life-threatening consequences.

The myocardium receives its blood via two main arteries that arise within the right and left aortic sinuses at the base of the aorta, called the right and left coronary arteries. These arteries further segregate into smaller branches that encircle the heart, bringing the myocardium a continuous supply of oxygenated nourishment.

The numerous smaller vessels serve as natural communication networks among the coronary arteries and are known as **anastomoses**. In the event that one of the vessels becomes restricted or blocked, blood flow to the myocardium may remain relatively uncompromised as a result of these channels functioning to bypass the block.

ANGINA PECTORIS

25.3 Pathogenesis of Angina Pectoris

Angina pectoris is acute chest pain caused by insufficient oxygen reaching a portion of the myocardium. Over 6 million

Americans have angina pectoris, with over 350,000 new cases each year. It is more prevalent in those over 55 years of age.

The classic presentation of angina pectoris is steady, intense pain, sometimes with a crushing or constricting sensation in the substernal region. Typically, the discomfort radiates to the left shoulder and proceeds down the left arm. It may also extend to the thoracic region of the back or move upward to the jaw. In some patients, the pain is experienced in the midepigastrium or abdominal area. Accompanying the discomfort is severe emotional distress—a feeling of panic with fear of impending death. There is usually pallor, dyspnea with cyanosis, diaphoresis, tachycardia, and elevated blood pressure.

Anginal pain is usually precipitated by physical exertion or emotional excitement—events associated with increased cardiorespiratory oxygen demand. Narrowed coronary arteries containing atherosclerotic deposits block the distribution of oxygen and nutrients to the stressed myocardium. Angina pectoris episodes are usually of short duration. With physical rest and stress reduction, the discomfort subsides within 10 to 15 minutes.

There are three basic types of angina. When anginal occurrences are fairly predictable, as to frequency, intensity, and duration, the condition is described as classic or **stable angina**. The second type of angina, known as atypical or **variant angina** (Prinzmetal's angina), occurs when the decreased myocardial blood flow is caused by spasms of the coronary arteries. It often occurs at the same time each night, during rest or sleep. When episodes of angina arise more frequently, have added intensity, and occur during periods of rest, the condition is termed **unstable angina**. This condition requires more aggressive medical intervention and may be considered a medical emergency, as it is associated with an increased risk for myocardial infarction (MI).

Angina pain closely parallels the signs and symptomatology of a heart attack. It is extremely important that the nurse knows the characteristics that differentiate the two conditions, because the pharmacologic interventions related to angina differ considerably from those of myocardial infarction. Angina, while painful and distressing, rarely leads to a fatal outcome and the chest pain is usually immediately relieved by nitroglycerin. Myocardial infarction, however, carries with it a high mortality rate if appropriate treatment is delayed. Pharmacologic intervention must be immediately initiated and systematically maintained in the event of myocardial infarction.

The nurse should understand that any number of diverse situations—several unrelated to cardiac pathology—may cause chest pain. These include gallstones, peptic ulcer disease, pneumonia, musculoskeletal injuries, and certain cancers. The foremost objective for the healthcare provider, when a person presents with chest pain, is to quickly determine the cause of the pain so that proper, effective interventions can be delivered. This incorporates a detailed individual and family history, a complete physical examination, and laboratory and other diagnostic tests. All healthcare providers work collaboratively to quickly determine the cause of chest pain.

25.4 Nonpharmacologic Management of Angina

A combination of variables influences the development and progression of angina, including dietary patterns and lifestyle circumstances. The nurse is instrumental in assisting patients to control the rate of recurrence of anginal episodes. Such support includes the formulation of a comprehensive plan of care that incorporates psychosocial support and an individualized teaching plan. The patient needs to understand the causes of angina, identify the conditions and situations that trigger it, and develop the motivation to modify behaviors associated with the disease.

In addition to drugs, treatment of angina includes therapies for conditions that worsen coronary artery disease such as diabetes and hypertension. The practice of healthy lifestyle habits can prevent CAD in many individuals, and

---

PHARMFACTS | **Angina Pectoris, Myocardial Infarction, and Cerebrovascular Accident**

Angina
- The incidence of angina peaks in the 75 to 84 age group. Other incidences include:
  4% of those 65 to 74 years old
  6% of those 75 to 84 years old
  4% of those over age 85

Myocardial Infarction
- Over 1.1 million Americans experience a new or recurrent MI each year.
- About one-third of the patients experiencing MIs will die from them.
- About 60% of the patients who died suddenly of MI had no previous symptoms of the disease.
- More than 20% of men and 40% of women will die from MI within 1 year after being diagnosed.

Cerebrovascular Accident
- Stroke is the third leading cause of death, behind heart disease and cancer.
- Of those who suffer stroke, 30% will die within 1 year.
- The incidence of brain attack increases with age (per 1,000 population), although 25% of all strokes occur under age 65.
- Approximately 600,000 new strokes occur each year in the United States.

---

slow the progress of the disease in those who have plaque buildup. The following factors have been shown to reduce the incidence of CAD.

- Limit or abstain from alcohol consumption.
- Eliminate foods high in cholesterol or saturated fats.
- If blood lipids are high (hyperlipidemia), have the condition treated.
- If blood pressure is high, have it treated.
- Exercise regularly and maintain optimum weight.
- Do not use tobacco.

When the coronary arteries are significantly obstructed, the two most common interventions are **percutaneous transluminal coronary angioplasty (PTCA)**, with stent insertion, and **coronary artery bypass graft (CABG) surgery**. PTCA is a procedure whereby the area of narrowing is opened using either a balloon catheter or a laser. The basic concept is to place a catheter, with a small inflatable balloon on the end, within the narrowed section of the artery. Inflation of the balloon catheter causes the balloon to push outward against the narrowed wall of the artery. The stenosis is reduced until it no longer interferes with blood flow. Stenting is done in conjunction with a balloon angioplasty and/or atherectomy, a procedure in which plaque is removed from an artery. Angioplasty with stenting typically leaves less than 10% of the original blockage in the artery.

SPECIAL CONSIDERATIONS

The Influence of Gender and Ethnicity on Angina

Angina occurs more frequently in females than in males. Among racial-ethnic groups, the incidence of angina is highest among African Americans, intermediate in Mexican Americans, and lowest in non-Hispanic Caucasians. African American females have twice the risk of angina as their male counterparts.

Coronary bypass surgery is reserved for severe cases of coronary blockage that cannot be dealt with by any other treatment modality. A portion of a small blood vessel from the leg or chest is used to create a "bypass artery". One end of the graft is sewn to the aorta and the other end to the coronary artery beyond the narrowed area. Blood from the aorta then flows through the new grafted vessel to the heart muscle, "bypassing" or avoiding the blockage in the coronary artery. The result is increased blood flow to the heart muscle, which reduces angina and the risk of heart attack.

25.5 Pharmacologic Goals for the Treatment of Angina

The pharmacologic goals for a patient with angina are twofold: to reduce the frequency of angina episodes and to terminate an incident of acute anginal pain once it is in progress. It is important to remember that interventions are directed toward symptomatic relief and management, as there is no drug treatment available to cure the underlying disorder. The primary means by which antianginal drugs accomplish these goals is to reduce the myocardial demand for oxygen. This can be accomplished by at least four different mechanisms.

- Slowing the heart rate
- Dilating veins so the heart receives less blood (reduced preload)
- Causing the heart to contract with less force (reduced contractility)
- Dilating arterioles to lower blood pressure, thus giving the heart less resistance when ejecting blood from its chambers (reduced afterload)

The pharmacotherapy of angina uses three classes of drugs: organic nitrates, beta-adrenergic blockers, and calcium channel blockers. For stable angina, the first line of pharmacotherapy is with the rapid-acting organic nitrates that are administered during the anginal episode. If episodes become more frequent or severe, prophylactic treatment is initiated using oral or transdermal organic nitrates, beta-adrenergic blockers, or calcium channel blockers. Persistent angina sometimes requires drugs from two or more classes, such as a beta-blocker combined with a long-acting nitrate or calcium channel blocker. Figure 25.2 illustrates the mechanisms of action of drugs used to prevent and treat coronary artery disease.

Organic Nitrates

25.6 Treating Angina with Organic Nitrates

Since their medicinal properties were discovered in 1857, organic nitrates have remained the mainstay for the treatment of angina. Their mechanism of action, and ultimate response, is the end product of a cascade of events. The primary therapeutic action of the organic nitrates is their ability to relax both arterial and venous smooth muscle. With venous vasodilation, the amount of blood returning to the heart (preload) is reduced, and the chambers contain a smaller volume. With less blood for the ventricles to pump, cardiac output is reduced and the workload on the heart is decreased, thereby lowering myocardial oxygen demand. The therapeutic outcome is that chest pain is alleviated and episodes of angina become less frequent. The organic nitrates are shown in Table 25.1.

Organic nitrates also have the ability to dilate coronary arteries, which was once thought to be their primary mechanism of action. It seems logical that dilating a partially occluded coronary vessel would allow more oxygen to get to the ischemic tissue. While this effect does indeed occur, it is no longer considered the primary mechanism of nitrate action in stable angina. This action, however, is important in treating variant angina, in which the chest pain is caused by coronary artery spasm. The organic nitrates can relax these spasms and terminate the pain.

Organic nitrates are of two types, short acting and long acting. The short-acting nitrates, such as nitroglycerin, are taken sublingually to quickly terminate an acute angina attack in progress. Longer acting nitrates, such as isosorbide dinitrate (Isordil, others), are taken orally or delivered through a transdermal patch to decrease the frequency and severity of angina episodes.

Tolerance is a common problem with prolonged use of the longer acting organic nitrates. The magnitude of the tolerance depends on the dosage and the frequency of drug administration. Patients are often instructed to remove the transdermal patch for 6 to 12 hours each day or withhold the nighttime dose of the oral medications to delay the development of tolerance.

Long-acting organic nitrates such as isosorbide dinitrate (Isordil) are also useful in reducing the symptoms of heart failure. Their role in the treatment of this disease is discussed in Chapter 22 ⊙ .

NURSING CONSIDERATIONS

The role of the nurse in nitrate therapy for angina involves careful monitoring of a patient's condition and providing education as it relates to the prescribed drug regimen. Because the main action of nitrates is vasodilation, it is vital for the nurse to assess blood pressure prior to administration. IV nitrates have the greatest risk of causing severe hypotension. These drugs are contraindicated in pericardial tamponade and constrictive pericarditis, because the heart cannot increase cardiac output to maintain blood pressure as vasodilation occurs. In cases when increased vasodilation would be detrimental to the patient (hypotension, shock, head injury with increased intracranial pressure), nitrates are contraindicated, as they worsen the conditions. Sustained-release forms of these drugs should not be given to patients with glaucoma. Nitrates should be used with caution in patients with severe liver or kidney disease or in early MI.

Assessment should include the patient's use of alcohol as this agent can produce an additive vasodilation effect

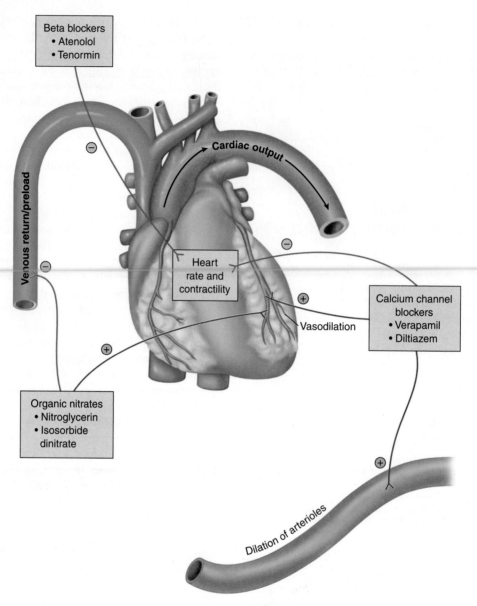

Figure 25.2 | Mechanisms of action of drugs used to treat angina

when taken concurrently with nitrates. Taking isosorbide dinitrate (Isordil, others) or isosorbide mononitrate (Imdur, others) with alcohol may cause severe hypotension and cardiovascular collapse.

With long-acting nitrates, the nurse should monitor for orthostatic hypotension and patients should be advised to change positions gradually. With short-acting forms, the nurse should ensure that patients are sitting or supine during administration and that blood pressure is taken after each dose. If hypotension occurs, the nurse should withhold nitrates and remove topical forms until blood pressure has returned to normal. Frequent blood pressure measurements are done during therapy to monitor for hypotensive effects. Infusions of nitrates are frequently titrated to obtain pain relief for the patient or a specific blood pressure level. The nurse should hold other

forms of nitrates and remove topical forms during the infusion.

Patient education as it relates to nitrates should include the goals, reasons for obtaining baseline data such as vital signs and tests for cardiac and renal disorders, and possible side effects. Following are the important points the nurse should include when teaching patients regarding nitrates.

- Refrain from alcohol use; some patients experience flushing, weakness, and fainting.
- If using transdermal patches, rotate the application site and wash skin thoroughly after patch is removed.
- If using sublingual dosage forms, allow the tablet to dissolve under the tongue; do not chew or swallow the tablet.
- If chest pain is not relieved after three doses of nitroglycerin, call EMS.

Table 25.1	Drugs for Angina, Myocardial Infarction, and Cerebrovascular Accidents
Drug	**Route and Adult Dose (max dose where indicated)**
Organic Nitrates	
amyl nitrite	Inhalation; 1 ampule (0.18–0.3 ml) PRN
isosorbide dinitrate (Iso-Bid, Isordil, Sorbitrate, Dilatrate) (see page 292 for the Prototype Drug box)	PO; 2.5–30 mg qid
isosorbide mononitrate (Imdur, Ismo, Monoket)	PO; 20 mg qid
nitroglycerin (Nitrostat, Nitro-Dur, Nitro-Bid, others)	SL; 1 tablet (0.3–0.6 mg) or 1 spray (0.4–0.8 mg) q3–5min (max three doses in 15 min)
pentaerythritol tetranitrate (Duotrate, Pentylan, Peritrate, others)	PO; 10–20 mg tid or qid
Beta-adrenergic Blockers	
atenolol (Tenormin)	PO; 25–50 mg qd (max 100 mg/day)
metoprolol (Lopressor, Toprol XL)	PO; 100 mg bid (max 400 mg/day)
propranolol (Inderal, Inderal LA) (see page 307 for the Prototype Drug box)	PO; 10–20 mg bid-tid (max 320 mg/day)
timolol maleate (Betimol, Blocadren, Timoptic, Timoptic XE) (see page 721 for the Prototype Drug box)	PO; 15–45 mg tid (max 60 mg/day)
Calcium Channel Blockers	
amlodipine (Norvasc)	PO; 5–10 mg qd (max 10 mg/day)
bepridil (Vascor)	PO; 200 mg qd (max 360 mg/day)
diltiazem (Cardizem, Dilacor XR, Tiamate, Tiazac)	PO; 30 mg qid (max 360 mg/day)
nicardipine (Cardene)	PO; 20–40 mg tid or 30–60 mg SR bid (max 120 mg/day)
nifedipine (Adalat, Procardia) (see page 270 for the Prototype Drug box)	PO; 10–20 mg tid (max 180 mg/day)
verapamil (Calan, Covera-HS, Isoptin, Verelan) (see page 309 for the Prototype Drug box)	PO; 80 mg tid-qid (max 480 mg/day)
Glycoprotein IIb/IIIa Inhibitors	
abciximab (ReoPro) (see page 322 for the Prototype Drug box)	IV; 0.25 mg/kg initial bolus over 5 min then 10 μg/min for 12 hr
eptifibatide (Integrilin)	IV; 18g/kg initial bolus over 1–2 min then 2 μg/kg/min for 24–72 hr
tirofiban HCL (Aggrastat)	IV; 0.4 μg/kg/min for 30 min then 0.1 μg/kg/min for 12–24 hr

- Contact the healthcare provider immediately if blurred vision, dry mouth, or severe headaches occur, which may be signs of overdose.
- Keep medication readily available in its original container, away from excess heat, light, or moisture. Prescription should be replaced every 6 months.

Beta-Adrenergic Blockers

25.7 Treating Angina with Beta-Blockers

Because of their ability to reduce the workload of the heart by slowing heart rate (negative chronotropic effect) and reducing contractility (negative inotropic effect), several beta-blockers are used to decrease the frequency and severity of anginal attacks caused by exertion. They are sometimes considered first line drugs in the pharmacotherapy of chronic angina. Patients should be advised against abruptly stopping beta-blocker therapy, as this may result in a sudden increase in cardiac workload and worsen angina. The beta-blockers used for angina are shown in Table 25.1. The beta-blockers are widely used in medicine, and additional details may be found in Chapters 13, 21, 22, and 23 .

NURSING CONSIDERATIONS

The role of the nurse in beta-blocker therapy for angina involves careful monitoring of a patient's condition and providing education as it relates to the prescribed drug regimen. Before administering beta-blockers, the nurse should assess the patient's apical pulse, especially if the patient is also taking

PROTOTYPE DRUG | NITROGLYCERIN (Nitrostat, Nitro-Bid, Nitro-Dur, others)

ACTIONS AND USES

Nitroglycerin, the oldest and most widely used of the organic nitrates, can be delivered by a number of different routes: sublingual, oral, translingual, IV, transmucosal, transdermal, topical, and extended-release forms. It may be taken while an acute anginal episode is in progress or just prior to physical activity. When given sublingually, it reaches peak plasma levels in approximately 4 minutes, thus terminating angina pain rapidly. Chest pain that does not respond to two or three doses of sublingual nitroglycerin may indicate myocardial infarction.

Administration Alerts

- For IV administration, use glass IV bottle and special IV tubing, because plastic absorbs nitrates significantly, thus reducing patient dose.
- Cover IV bottle to reduce degradation of nitrates due to light exposure.
- Use gloves when applying nitroglycerin paste or ointment to prevent self-administration.
- Pregnancy category C.

ADVERSE EFFECTS AND INTERACTIONS

The side effects of nitroglycerin are usually cardiovascular in nature and are rarely life threatening. Because nitroglycerin can dilate cerebral vessels, headache is a common side effect and may be severe. Occasionally the venodilation created by nitroglycerin causes reflex tachycardia. Some healthcare providers prescribe a beta-adrenergic blocker to diminish this undesirable heart rate increase. The side effects of nitroglycerin often diminish after a few doses.

Concurrent use with sildenafil (Viagra) may cause life-threatening hypotension and cardiovascular collapse. Nitrates should not be taken within 24 hours before or after taking Viagra.

digoxin (Lanoxin), since both drugs slow AV conduction. Because beta-blockers lower blood pressure, vital signs should be monitored periodically. The nurse should monitor the patient for shortness of breath and respiratory distress. These side effects usually occur when nonselective beta-blockers are prescribed at high dosages.

Because beta-blockers slow heart rate and conduction velocity, they are contraindicated in bradycardia and greater than first degree heart block. The nurse should assess heart rate and ECG readings before administering these drugs. They are also contraindicated in cardiogenic shock and overt cardiac failure. Beta-blockers should be used with caution in patients taking digitalis and diuretics for HF, in asthma and COPD, and in patients with impaired renal function. Diabetic patients should be aware that initial symptoms of hypoglycemia, such as palpitations, diaphoresis, nervousness, may not be evident with beta-blockade. Blood glucose levels should be monitored frequently in patients with diabetes mellitus, because insulin doses may need to be decreased when using beta-blockers.

These drugs should never be abruptly discontinued. With long-term use, the heart becomes more sensitive to catecholamines blocked by these drugs. When they are withdrawn abruptly, a rebound excitation occurs and adrenergic receptors are stimulated. This can exacerbate angina, and precipitate tachycardia or even an MI in patients with coronary artery disease. One side effect of beta-blockers is fatigue during exercise, because these drugs prevent the heart rate from increasing with activity.

Patient education as it relates to beta-blockers should include the goals, reasons for obtaining baseline data such as vital signs and tests for cardiac and renal disorders, and possible side effects. Following are important teaching points the nurse should include regarding beta-blockers.

- Change positions slowly; report dizziness or light-headedness.
- Do not take OTC medications or herbal products without discussing with the healthcare provider.
- Do not discontinue medication abruptly.
- If pulse falls below 60, notify healthcare provider.
- Alternate periods of activity with periods of rest in order to avoid fatigue.

See also "Nursing Process Focus: Patients Receiving Sympathomimetic Therapy" page 137 in Chapter 13, for the complete Nursing Process applied to caring for patients receiving beta-adrenergic agonists.

Calcium Channel Blockers

25.8 Treating Angina with Calcium Channel Blockers

Like beta-blockers, the value of calcium channel blockers (CCBs) has been presented in several chapters, including hypertension (Chapter 21) and dysrhythmias (Chapter 23). The first approved use of CCBs was for the treatment of angina. Blockade of calcium channels has a number of effects on the heart, most of which are similar to those of

NURSING PROCESS FOCUS   PATIENTS RECEIVING NITROGLYCERIN

ASSESSMENT

Prior to administration:
- Obtain complete health history including allergies, drug history, and possible drug interactions.
- Assess vital signs, ECG, frequency and severity of angina, and alcohol use.
- Obtain history of cardiac disorders and blood testing including cardiac enzymes, CBC, BUN, creatinine, and liver function tests.
- Assess if patient has taken sildenafil (Viagra) within last 24 hours.

POTENTIAL NURSING DIAGNOSES

- Risk for Ineffective Tissue Perfusion, related to hypotension from drug
- Risk for Injury (dizziness or fainting), related to hypotension from drug
- Acute Pain (headache), related to adverse effects of drug
- Deficient Knowledge, related to drug therapy

PLANNING: PATIENT GOALS AND EXPECTED OUTCOMES

The patient will:
- Experience relief or prevention of chest pain
- Report immediately any chest pain unrelieved by nitroglycerin
- Demonstrate an understanding of the drug's action by accurately describing drug side effects and precautions

IMPLEMENTATION

Interventions and (Rationales)	*Patient Education/Discharge Planning*
■ Ask patient to describe and rate pain prior to drug administration for description/documentation of anginal episode. ■ Obtain 12-lead ECG, to differentiate between angina and infarction. (Pharmacotherapy depends upon which disorder is presenting.)	Instruct patient to: ■ Take one tablet every 5 min until pain is relieved or for up to three doses during an acute anginal attack ■ Call EMS if chest pain is not relieved after three doses ■ Place SL tablet under tongue or spray under tongue; do not inhale spray
■ Monitor blood pressure and pulse. Do not administer drug if patient is hypotensive. (Drug will further reduce blood pressure.)	■ Instruct patient to sit or lie down before taking medication and to avoid abrupt changes in position.
■ Monitor alcohol use. (Extremely low blood pressure may result, which could cause death.)	■ Emphasize the importance of avoiding alcohol while taking nitroglycerin.
■ Monitor for headache in response to use of nitrates.	Instruct patient that: ■ Headache is a common side effect, that usually decreases over time ■ OTC medicines usually relieve the headache
■ Monitor for use of sildenafil (Viagra) concurrently with nitrates, because cardiovascular disease is a major cause of erectile dysfunction in men. (Life-threatening hypotension may result with concurrent use of sildenafil.)	Instruct patient to: ■ Not take Viagra within 24 hours after taking nitrates ■ Wait at least 24 hours after taking Viagra to resume nitrate therapy
■ Monitor need for prophylactic nitrates.	■ Advise patient to take medication prior to a stressful event or physical activity to prevent angina.

EVALUATION OF OUTCOME CRITERIA

Evaluate the effectiveness of drug therapy by confirming that patient goals and expected outcomes have been met (see "Planning").

Pr PROTOTYPE DRUG | ATENOLOL (Tenormin)

ACTIONS AND USES

Atenolol selectively blocks β_1-adrenergic receptors in the heart. Its effectiveness in angina is attributed to its ability to slow heart rate and reduce contractility, both of which lower myocardial oxygen demand. It is also used in the treatment of hypertension and in the prevention of MI. Because of its 7- to 9-hour half-life, it may be taken once a day.

Administration Alerts

- During IV administration, monitor ECG continuously; blood pressure and pulse should be assessed before, during, and after dose is administered.
- Assess pulse and blood pressure before oral administration. Hold if pulse is below 60 bpm or if patient is hypotensive.
- Atenolol may precipitate bronchospasm in susceptible patients with initial doses.
- Pregnancy category C.

ADVERSE EFFECTS AND INTERACTIONS

Being a cardioselective β_1-blocker, atenolol has few adverse effects on the lung. Like other beta-blockers, therapy generally begins with low doses, which are gradually increased until the therapeutic effect is achieved. The most common side effects of atenolol include fatigue, weakness, and hypotension. Anticholinergics may cause decreased absorption from the GI tract.

Concurrent use with calcium channel blockers may cause excessive cardiac suppression. Concurrent use with digitalis may cause slowed AV conduction leading to heart block. Patients should avoid concurrent use of this drug with nicotine or caffeine due to their vasoconstricting effects.

 See the companion website for a Nursing Process Focus specific to this drug.

---

beta-blockers. The calcium channel blockers used for angina are shown in Table 25.1.

CCBs cause arteriolar smooth muscle to relax, thus lowering peripheral resistance and reducing blood pressure. This reduction in afterload decreases the myocardial oxygen demand, thus reducing the frequency of anginal pain.

Some CCBs are selective for arterioles. Others such as verapamil (Calan, Isoptin) and diltiazem (Cardizem) not only affect the arterioles but also have the beneficial effect of slowing the heart rate (negative chronotropic effect). Verapamil and diltiazem produce less reflex tachycardia than the other approved CCBs. Because they relax arterial smooth muscle, the CCBs are useful in treating the acute vasospams of variant angina; they are considered drugs of choice for this type of angina.

NURSING CONSIDERATIONS

The role of the nurse in CCB therapy for angina involves careful monitoring of a patient's condition and providing education as it relates to the prescribed drug regimen. Because of their effects on blood pressure and heart rate, vital signs should be assessed before administering these medications. The nurse should take blood pressure in both arms while the patient is lying, sitting, and standing, to monitor for orthostatic hyoptension. Because CCBs, especially when administered IV, can affect myocardial conduction, they are not used in patients with sick sinus syndrome or third degree AV blocks without the presence of a pacemaker. The ECG should be assessed prior to initiating therapy for any indications of conduction disturbances.

Some CCBs reduce myocardial contractility and can worsen heart failure (HF). The nurse should monitor patient for signs and symptoms of worsening HF such as peripheral edema, shortness of breath, and lung congestion. The nurse should also monitor the patient's weight for a sudden increase indicating fluid retention. Bowel function should be assessed, as some CCBs cause constipation. Extended-release tablets or capsules should not be crushed or split, as this can result in a large dose being released and thus serious hypotension.

Patient education as it relates to calcium channel blockers should include the goals, reasons for obtaining baseline data such as vital signs and tests for cardiac and renal disorders, and possible side effects. Following are important points the nurse should include when teaching patients regarding calcium channel blockers.

- Take blood pressure and pulse before self-administering medication. Withhold drug if either pulse or blood pressure is below established parameters and notify healthcare provider.
- Keep a record of frequency and severity of each anginal attack.
- Change positions slowly and be cautious performing hazardous activities until effects of the drug are known.
- Notify healthcare provider of any symptoms of HF such as shortness of breath, weight gain, or slow heart beat.
- Do not crush or break extended-release capsules or tablets.
- Avoid grapefruit juice, as it can cause CCBs to rise to toxic levels.

See also "Nursing Process Focus: Patients Receiving Calcium Channel Blocker Therapy," page 271 in Chapter 21, for the complete Nursing Process applied to patients receiving calcium channel blockers ∞.

Pr PROTOTYPE DRUG | DILTIAZEM (Cardizem)

ACTIONS AND USES	ADVERSE EFFECTS AND INTERACTIONS
Like other calcium channel blockers, diltiazem inhibits the transport of calcium into myocardial cells. It has the ability to relax both coronary and peripheral blood vessels. It is useful in the treatment of atrial dysrhythmias and hypertension, as well as angina. When given as extended-release capsules, it can be administered once daily.	Side effects of diltiazem are generally not serious and are related to vasodilation: headache, dizziness, and edema of the ankles and feet. Although diltiazem produces few adverse effects on the heart or vessels, it should be used with caution in patients taking other cardiovascular drugs, particularly digoxin or beta-adrenergic blockers. The combined effects of these drugs may cause partial or complete heart block, heart failure, or dysrhythmias.

Administration Alerts

- During IV administration, the patient must be continuously monitored and cardioversion equipment must be available.
- Extended-release version tablets and capsule contents should not be crushed or split.
- Pregnancy category C.

This drug may increase digoxin or quinidine levels when taken concurrently.

Use with caution with herbal supplements, such as dong quai and ginger, as these products interfere with blood clotting.

 See the companion website for a Nursing Process Focus specific to this drug.

Glycoprotein IIb/IIIa Inhibitors

25.9 Treating Myocardial Ischemia with Glycoprotein IIb/IIIa Inhibitors

Glycoprotein IIb/IIIa is a receptor found on the surface of platelets. These receptors bind fibrinogen and von Willebrand's factor to begin the process of platelet aggregation that is essential for blood coagulation.

Several drugs have been developed that occupy the glycoprotein IIb/IIIa receptor and inhibit clot formation. These drugs, sometimes referred to as antiplatelet agents, have a mechanism of action distinct from that of aspirin. The glycoprotein IIb/IIIa inhibitors used for myocardial ischemia are shown in Table 25.1.

Glycoprotein IIb/IIIa inhibitors are sometimes indicated for angina pectoris or myocardial infarction, or for those undergoing PTCA. As with other drugs having an anticoagulant effect, glycoprotein IIb/IIIa inhibitors are contraindicated in the presence of active bleeding, recent surgery, or trauma. They are sometimes used concurrently with aspirin and heparin, thus increasing the need for careful monitoring for bleeding. Additional information on glycoprotein IIb/IIIa inhibitors and a prototype feature for abciximab (ReoPro) are found in Chapter 24 ⌘ .

MYOCARDIAL INFARCTION

25.10 Early Diagnosis of Myocardial Infarction

Heart attacks or myocardial infarctions (MIs) are responsible for a substantial number of deaths each year. Some patients die before reaching a medical facility for treatment and many others die within 1 to 2 days following the initial MI. Clearly, MI is a serious and frightening disease and one responsible for a large percentage of sudden deaths.

The primary cause of myocardial infarction is advanced coronary artery disease. Plaque buildup can severely narrow one or more branches of the coronary arteries. Pieces of plaque can break off and lodge in a small vessel serving a portion of the myocardium. Deprived of its oxygen supply, this area of myocardium becomes ischemic and the tissue can die unless its blood supply is quickly restored. Figure 25.3 illustrates the pathogenesis and treatment of MI.

Goals for the pharmacologic treatment of acute MI are as follows:

- Restore blood supply (perfusion) to the damaged myocardium as quickly as possible through the use of thrombolytics.
- Reduce myocardial oxygen demand with organic nitrates and beta-blockers, to prevent further MIs.
- Control or prevent associated dysrhythmias with beta-blockers or other antidysrhythmics.
- Reduce post-MI mortality with aspirin and ACE inhibitors.
- Control MI pain and associated anxiety with narcotic analgesics.

Laboratory test results are used to aid in diagnosis and monitor progress after an MI. Table 25.2 describes important laboratory values.

Thrombolytics

25.11 Treating Myocardial Infarction with Thrombolytics

In the treatment of MI, the goal of thrombolytic therapy is to dissolve clots obstructing the coronary arteries, thus restoring circulation to the myocardium. Quick restoration of cardiac circulation has been found to reduce mortality caused by acute MI. After the clot is successfully dissolved, anticoagulant therapy is initiated to prevent the formation

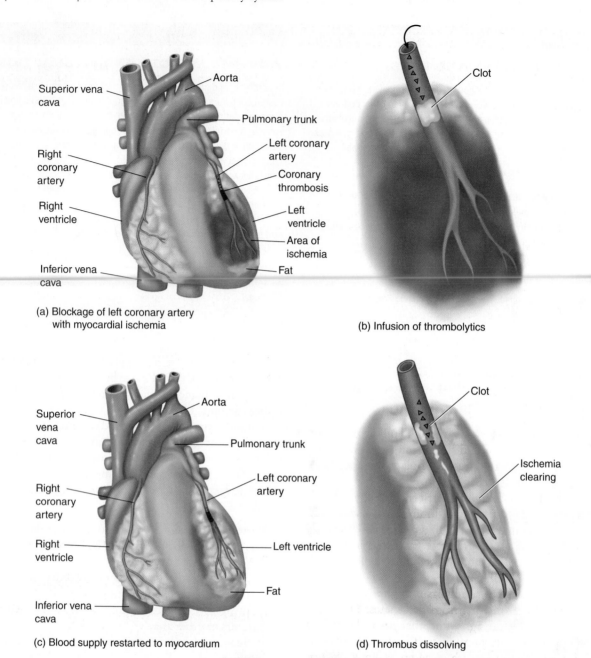

(a) Blockage of left coronary artery with myocardial ischemia

(b) Infusion of thrombolytics

(c) Blood supply restarted to myocardium

(d) Thrombus dissolving

Figure 25.3 | Blockage and reperfusion following myocardial infarction: (a) blockage of left coronary artery with myocardial ischemia; (b) infusion of thrombolytics; (c) blood supply returning to myocardium; (D) thrombus dissolving and ischemia clearing
Source: Figures (a) and (c) Pearson Education/PH College.

of additional clots. Dosages and descriptions of the various thrombolytics are given in Chapter 24 ☉.

Thrombolytics have a narrow margin of safety between dissolving "normal" and "abnormal" clots. It must be understood that once infused in the blood, the drugs travel to all vessels and may cause adverse effects anywhere in the body. The primary risk of thrombolytics is excessive bleeding from interference in the normal clotting process. Vital signs must be monitored continuously and any signs of bleeding generally call for discontinuation of therapy. Because these drugs are rapidly destroyed in the blood, discontinuation of the drug normally results in the rapid termination of adverse effects.

NURSING CONSIDERATIONS

The role of the nurse in thrombolytic therapy for MI involves careful monitoring of a patient's condition and providing education as it relates to the prescribed drug regimen. The nurse should assess for conditions that would be contraindicated including recent trauma or surgery/biopsies, GI bleeding, postpartum (within 10 days), cerebral hemorrhage, bleeding disorders, or thrombocytopenia, because thrombolytics would place the patient at risk for increased bleeding. In septic thrombophlebitis, a favorable clot is in place that would be dissolved by thrombolytics, resulting in

Table 25.2	Changes in Blood Test Values with Acute MI			
Blood Test	**Initial Elevation after MI**	**Peak Elevation after MI**	**Duration of Elevation**	**Normal Range**
Cholesterol			≥4 weeks, during stress response	< 200 mg/dL
CK = creatine kinase/CPK = creatinine phosphokinase	3–8 h	12–24 h	2–4 d	Males: 12–80 U/L Females: 10–70 U/L
	4–8 h	8–24 h	2–3 d	0%–3% of CK
ESR	First week		Several weeks	
Glucose			Duration of stress response	Fasting: 80–120
LDH, LDH1 = lactase dehydrogenase	8–72 h	3–6 d	8–14 d	45–90 U/L
Myoglobin	1–3 h	4–6 h	1–2 d	0–85 ng/mL
Troponin I	2–4 h	24–36 h	7–10 d	< 3.1 μg/L
Troponin T	2–4 h	24–36 h	10–14 d	< 0.2 μg/L
WBC	Few hours		3–7 d	4.8–10.8 × 10^3 μL

patient injury, so they are contraindicated in this condition. These drugs should be used with caution in any condition where bleeding could be a significant hazard, such as severe renal or liver disease.

The nurse should start IV lines, an arterial line, or insert a Foley catheter prior to beginning therapy to decrease the chance of bleeding from those sites. The nurse should monitor for vital signs, and changes in lab values (Hgb, Hct, platelets, coagulation studies) that are indicative of bleeding. Because cerebral hemorrhage is a major concern, changes in level of consciousness should be carefully monitored and neurological status assessed. The nurse should monitor for dysrhythmias that may occur as cardiac tissue is reperfused after myocardial infarction.

The nurse must monitor lab work such as the CBC during and after therapy for indications of blood loss due to internal bleeding. The patient has increased risk of bleeding for 2 to 4 days posttherapy.

Patient education as it relates to thrombolytics should include the goals, reasons for obtaining baseline data such as vital signs and tests for cardiac and renal disorders, and possible side effects. Following are the important points the nurse should include when teaching patients regarding thrombolytics.

- Keep movement of IV sites to a minimum to prevent oozing of blood from site.
- Move as little as possible during the infusion.

- Report any bleeding from gums, rectum, or vagina immediately.
- Continue observing for bleeding for at least 4 days following completion of the infusion.

See also "Nursing Process Focus: Patients Receiving Thrombolytic Therapy" page 324 in Chapter 24, for the complete Nursing Process applied to caring for patients receiving thrombolytics ∞ .

Beta-Adrenergic Blockers

25.12 Treating Myocardial Infarction with Beta Blockers

The use of the beta-adrenergic blockers in the treatment of cardiovascular disease has been discussed in a number of chapters in this textbook. This section will focus on their use in the treatment of MI. The beta-blockers used for MI are shown in Table 25.1.

Beta-blockers have the ability to slow heart rate, decrease contractility, and reduce blood pressure. These three factors reduce myocardial oxygen demand, which is beneficial for patients experiencing a recent MI. In addition, they slow impulse conduction through the heart, which tends to suppress dysrhythmias, which are serious and sometimes fatal complications following an MI. Beta-blockers have been shown to reduce mortality when given within 8 hours of MI onset.

Pr PROTOTYPE DRUG | RETEPLASE (Retavase)

ACTIONS AND USES

Reteplase acts as a catalyst in the cleavage of plasminogen to plasmin, a substance responsible for degrading the fibrin matrix of a clot. Reteplase is one of the newer thrombolytics. Like other drugs in this class, reteplase should be given as soon as possible after the onset of MI symptoms. It usually acts within 20 minutes, and restoration of circulation to the ischemic site may be faster than with other thrombolytics. After the clot has been dissolved, heparin therapy is often started to prevent additional clots from forming.

Administration Alerts

- Must be reconstituted just prior to use with diluent provided by manufacturer; swirl to mix—do not shake.
- Do not give any other drug simultaneously through the same IV line.
- Must be administered within 6 hours of onset of symptoms of MI and within 3 hours of thrombotic CVA to be effective.
- Pregnancy category C.

ADVERSE EFFECTS AND INTERACTIONS

Reteplase is contraindicated in patients with active bleeding. The healthcare provider must be vigilant in recognizing and responding to abnormal bleeding during therapy.

Drug interactions with anticoagulants and platelet aggregation inhibitors will produce an additive effect and increase the risk of bleeding.

 See the companion website for a Nursing Process Focus specific to this drug.

NURSING CONSIDERATIONS

See Nursing Considerations for beta-blockers in Section 25.7.

25.13 Drugs for Symptoms and Complications of Acute Myocardial Infarction

Several additional drugs have proven useful in treating the patient presenting with an acute MI. Unless contraindicated, 180 to 325 mg of aspirin is given as soon as an MI is suspected. Aspirin use in the weeks following an acute MI reduces mortality dramatically. Additional actions of aspirin may be found in Chapters 19 and 31 ∞.

Two ACE inhibitors, captopril (Capoten) and lisinopril (Prinivil, Zestril), also have been determined to improve survival following acute MI. These drugs are most effective when therapy is started within 1 to 2 days following the onset of symptoms. Oral doses are normally begun after thrombolytic therapy is completed and the patient's condition has stabilized. Additional indications for ACE inhibitors may be found in Chapters 21 and 22 ∞.

Pain control is essential following acute MI, to ensure patient comfort and reduce stress. Narcotic analgesics such as morphine sulfate or meperidine (Demerol) are sometimes given to ease extreme pain associated with acute MI and to sedate the anxious patient. The pharmacology of the analgesics is presented in Chapter 19 ∞.

CEREBROVASCULAR ACCIDENT

25.14 Pathogenesis of Cerebrovascular Accident

Cerebrovascular accident (CVA), also called stroke or brain attack, is a major cause of permanent disability. It is the third leading cause of death in the United States, following heart disease and cancer. The majority of CVAs are thrombotic strokes, caused by a thrombus in a vessel serving the brain. Tissues distal to the clot lose their oxygen supply, and neural tissue will die unless circulation is quickly restored. A smaller percentage of CVAs, about 20%, are caused by rupture of a cerebral vessel with associated bleeding into neural tissue, known as a hemorrhagic stroke. Symptoms are the same for the two types of strokes. Mortality from CVA is very high: As many as 40% of the patients die within the first year following the CVA. Most of the risk factors associated with CVA are the same as for other cardiovascular diseases such as hypertension and coronary artery disease.

The signs and symptoms of a CVA depend on a number of factors, the most important of which are the location of the obstruction and how much brain tissue is affected. A stroke affecting one side of the brain will result in neurologic deficits on the opposite side of the body. For example, if the stroke occurs in the right side of the brain, the left side of the body will be affected. Common signs of stroke include the following:

- Paralysis or weakness on one side of the body
- Vision problems

PROTOTYPE DRUG | **METOPROLOL (Lopressor)**

ACTIONS AND USES

Metoprolol is a selective ß₁ antagonist available in tablet, sustained-release tablet, and IV forms. At high doses, it may also affect ß₂-receptors in bronchial smooth muscle. When given IV, it quickly acts to reduce myocardial oxygen demand. Following an acute MI, metoprolol is infused slowly until a target heart rate is reached, usually between 60 and 90 bpm. Upon hospital discharge, patients can be switched to oral forms of the drug. Metoprolol is also approved for angina, hypertension, and myocardial infarction.

Administration Alerts

- During IV administration, monitor EKG, blood pressure, and pulse frequently.
- Assess pulse and blood pressure before oral administration. Hold if pulse is below 60 bpm or if patient is hypotensive.
- Do not crush or chew sustained-release tablets.
- Pregnancy category C.

ADVERSE EFFECTS AND INTERACTIONS

Because it is selective for blocking ß₁-receptors in the heart, metoprolol has few adverse effects on other autonomic targets and thus is preferred over nonselective beta-blockers such as propranolol for patients with lung disorders. Side effects are generally minor and relate to its autonomic activity, such as slowing of the heart rate and hypotension. Because of its multiple effects on the heart, patients with heart failure should be carefully monitored. This agent is contraindicated in cardiogenic shock, sinus bradycardia, and heart block greater than first degree. Concurrent use with digoxin may result in bradycardia. Oral contraceptives may cause increased metoprolol effects.

 See the companion website for a Nursing Process Focus specific to this drug.

- Memory loss
- Speech/language problems
- Difficulty swallowing

25.15 Pharmacotherapy of Thrombotic CVA

Drug therapy for thrombotic CVA focuses on two main goals:

- Prevention of CVAs through the use of anticoagulants and antihypertensive agents
- Restoration of blood supply to the affected neurons as quickly as possible after an acute brain attack through the use of thrombolytics

Sustained, chronic hypertension is closely associated with CVA. Antihypertensive drugs such as the beta-adrenergic blockers, calcium channel blockers, diuretics, and ACE inhibitors can help control blood pressure and reduce the probability of CVA. Diet and lifestyle factors that reduce blood pressure should be implemented concurrently with antihypertensive pharmacotherapy.

Aspirin, through its anticoagulant properties, reduces the incidence of stroke. When given in very low doses, aspirin discourages the formation of clots by inhibiting platelets. Patients are often placed on a daily regimen of low dose aspirin therapy following transient ischemic attacks (TIAs) or following their first CVA. Many healthcare

SPECIAL CONSIDERATIONS

Cultural, Gender, and Age Considerations in Stroke

The American Stroke Association data show that overall, the incidence and prevalence of stroke are about equal for men and women. At all ages, however, more women than men die of stroke. The chance of stroke is greater in people who have a family history of stroke. African Americans have a much higher risk of disability and death from a stroke than Caucasians, in part because blacks have a greater incidence of high blood pressure—a major stroke risk factor.

NATURAL THERAPIES | Ginseng

Ginseng is one of the oldest known herbal remedies, with at least six species being reported to have medicinal properties. *Panax ginseng* is distributed throughout China, Korea, and Siberia, whereas *Panax quinquefolius* is native to Canada and the United States. The plant's popularity has led to its extinction from certain regions, and much of the available ginseng is now grown commercially.

Standardization of ginseng focuses on a group of chemicals called ginsenosides, although there are many other chemicals in the root, which is the harvested portion of the plant. The German E monographs recommend a dose of 20 to 30 mg ginsenosides. This is sometimes reported as a percent, with 5% being the recommended standard of ginsenosides.

There are differences in chemical composition among the various species of ginseng; American ginseng is not considered equivalent to Siberian ginseng. Ginseng is reported to be a calcium channel antagonist. By increasing the conversion of L-arginine to nitric oxide, ginseng improves blood flow to the heart in times of low oxygen supply, such as with myocardial ischemia. The Chinese have found that nitric oxide is a potent antioxidant that combats free radical injury to the heart muscle. The nurse should caution patients who take ginseng, because herb-drug interactions are possible with coumadin and loop diuretics.

MediaLink ⬤ Support For CVA Victims

providers recommend low dose aspirin therapy as a pro-phylactic measure for the prevention of MI and CVA. Ticlopidine (Ticlid) is an antiplatelet drug that may be used to provide anticoagulation in patients who cannot tol-erate aspirin. Other anticoagulants, such as warfarin (Coumadin), may be given to prevent CVAs in high-risk individuals, such as those with prosthetic heart valves. More detailed information on anticoagulants can be found in Chapter 24 ⊂⊃ .

The single most important breakthrough in the phar-macotherapy of CVA was the development of the throm-bolytic drugs called "clot busters". Prior to the advent of these drugs, the treatment of CVA was largely a passive, wait-and-see strategy. Care was directed at habilation or rehabilitation, after the fact. Stroke is now aggressively treated with thrombolytics as soon as the patient arrives at the hospital. Such agents are most effective if administered within 3 hours of the attack. The use of aggressive throm-bolytic therapy can completely restore brain function in a significant number of stroke victims. As a result, a CVA is now considered a condition that mandates immediate treatment. The disease is often referred to by its newer ti-tle, brain attack, which reflects the need for urgent treat-ment.

CHAPTER REVIEW

Key Concepts

The numbered key concepts provide a succinct summary of the important points from the corresponding numbered sec-tion within the chapter. If any of these points are not clear, re-fer to the numbered section within the chapter for review. Expanded versions can be found on the companion website.

25.1 Coronary artery disease includes both angina and myo-cardial infarction. It is caused by narrowing of the arte-rial lumen due to atherosclerotic plaque.

25.2 The myocardium requires a continuous supply of oxy-gen from the coronary arteries in order to function properly.

25.3 Angina pectoris is the narrowing of a coronary artery, resulting in a lack of sufficient oxygen to the heart muscle. Chest pain, upon emotional or physical exer-tion, is the most characteristic symptom.

25.4 Angina management may include nonpharmacologic therapies such as diet and lifestyle modifications, treat-ment of underlying disorders, angioplasty, or surgery.

25.5 The pharmacologic goals for the treatment of angina are to terminate acute attacks and prevent future episodes. This is usually achieved by reducing cardiac workload.

25.6 The organic nitrates relieve angina by dilating veins and coronary arteries. They are drugs of choice for sta-ble angina.

25.7 Beta-adrenergic blockers relieve angina by decreasing the oxygen demands on the heart. They are sometimes considered first line drugs for chronic angina.

25.8 Calcium channel blockers relieve angina by dilating the coronary vessels and reducing the workload on the heart. They are drugs of first choice for treating variant angina.

25.9 Glycoprotein IIb/IIIa inhibitors are antiplatelet agents for the treatment of myocardial ischemia.

25.10 The early diagnosis of myocardial infarction increases chances of survival. Early pharmacotherapy may in-clude thrombolytics, aspirin, beta-blockers, and anti-dysrhythmics.

25.11 If given within hours after the onset of MI, throm-bolytic agents can dissolve clots and restore perfusion to affected regions of the myocardium.

25.12 When given within 24 hours after the onset of my-ocardial infarction, beta-adrenergic blockers can im-prove survival.

25.13 A number of additional drugs are used to treat the symptoms and complications of acute MI. These in-clude analgesics, anticoagulants (including aspirin), and ACE inhibitors.

25.14 CVA is a major cause of death and disability. CVAs may be caused by a clot or by rupture of a cerebral vessel.

25.15 Aggressive treatment of thrombotic CVA with throm-bolytics, to restore perfusion, and anticoagulants, to prevent additional clots from forming, can increase survival.

Review Questions

1. What are the distinguishing characteristics that differentiate stable, variant, and unstable angina?

2. Why does decreasing the cardiac workload result in the reduction of anginal pain?

3. Describe how medication administration with transdermal nitrates can be altered to prevent or delay tolerance in patients with angina pectoris.

4. Why is it important to treat an MI within the first 24 hours after symptoms have begun?

5. What role does aspirin play in the pharmacotherapy of myocardial infarction and CVA?

Critical Thinking Questions

1. A patient on the medical unit is complaining of chest pain (4/10), has a history of angina, and is requesting his PRN nitroglycerin spray. The patient's BP is 96/60 at present. What should the nurse do?

2. A patient is recovering from an acute MI and has been put on atenolol (Tenormin). What teaching should the patient receive prior to discharge from the hospital?

3. A patient with chest pain has been given the calcium channel blocker diltiazem (Cardizem) IV for a heart rate of 118. Blood pressure at this time is 100/60. What precautions should the nurse take?

EXPLORE MediaLink

NCLEX review, case studies, and other interactive resources for this chapter can be found on the companion website at www.prenhall.com/adams. Click on "Chapter 25" to select the activities for this chapter. For animations, more NCLEX review questions, and an audio glossary, access the accompanying CD-ROM in this textbook.

CHAPTER 26

Drugs for Shock

DRUGS AT A GLANCE

FLUID REPLACEMENT AGENTS
Blood and blood products
Crystalloid solutions
Colloid solutions
(Pr) *normal serum albumin (Albuminar, Albutein)*

VASOCONSTRICTORS
(Pr) *norepinephrine (Levarterenol)*

CARDIOTONIC AGENTS
(Pr) *dopamine (Dopastat, Inotropin)*

metabolized and eliminated by the bod
of this process
PHARMACOLOGY
1. The study of medicines; the disciplin
pertaining to how drugs improve the he
of the human body
PHARMACOPEIA

MediaLink   www.prenhall.com/adams

CD-ROM
Animation:
    Mechanism in Action: Dopamine (Dopastat)
Audio Glossary
NCLEX Review

Companion Website
NCLEX Review
Dosage Calculations
Case Study
Care Plans
Expanded Key Concepts

albumin *page 349*

anaphylactic shock *page 346*

cardiogenic shock *page 346*

colloids *page 346*

crystalloids *page 347*

hypovolemic shock *page 346*

inotropic agent *page 351*

neurogenic shock *page 346*

oncotic pressure *page 346*

septic shock *page 346*

shock *page 345*

OBJECTIVES

After reading this chapter, the student should be able to:

1. Compare and contrast the different types of shock.
2. Relate the general symptoms of shock to their physiologic causes.
3. Explain the initial treatment for a patient who is in shock.
4. Compare and contrast the use of colloids and crystalloids in fluid replacement therapy.
5. For each of the classes shown in Drugs at a Glance, know representative drug examples, explain their mechanism of action, primary actions, and important adverse effects.
6. Categorize drugs used in the treatment of shock based on their classification and mechanism of action.
7. Use the steps of the Nursing Process to care for patients who are receiving drug therapy for shock.

Shock is a condition in which vital tissues are not receiving enough blood to function properly. Without adequate oxygen and other nutrients, cells cannot carry out normal metabolic processes. Shock is considered a medical emergency; failure to reverse the causes and symptoms of shock may lead to irreversible organ damage and death. This chapter examines how drugs are used to aid in the treatment of different types of shock.

PHARMFACTS	Shock

- Cardiogenic shock, because it responds poorly to treatment, is the most lethal form of shock and has an 80% to 100% mortality rate.
- Hypovolemic shock carries a 10% to 31% mortality rate.
- With anaphylactic or distributive shock, death can ensue within minutes if treatment is not available to treat the condition.
- Septic or "warm" shock, usually caused by gram negative bacteria, has a mortality rate of 40% to 70% but can be as high as 90%, depending on the causative organism.

26.1 Characteristics of Shock

Shock is a collection of signs and symptoms, many of which are nonspecific. Although symptoms vary somewhat among the different kinds of shock, some similarities exist. The patient appears pale and may claim to feel sick or weak without reporting specific complaints. Behavioral changes are often some of the earliest symptoms and may include restlessness, anxiety, confusion, depression, and apathy. Lack of sufficient blood flow to the brain may result in fainting. Thirst is a common complaint. The skin may feel cold or clammy. Without immediate treatment, multiple body systems will be affected and respiratory failure or renal failure may result. Figure 26.1 shows common symptoms of a patient in shock.

The central problem in most types of shock is the inability of the cardiovascular system to send sufficient blood to the vital organs, with the heart and brain being affected early in the progression of the disease. Assessing the patient's cardiovascular status will often give important indications for a diagnosis of shock. Blood pressure is usually low and cardiac output diminished. Heart rate may be rapid with a weak pulse. Breathing is usually rapid and shallow. Figure 26.2 illustrates the physiologic changes that occur during circulatory shock.

26.2 Causes of Shock

Shock is often classified by naming the underlying pathological process or organ system causing the disease. Table 26.1 lists the different types of shock and their primary causes.

Diagnosis of shock is rarely based on nonspecific symptoms. A careful medical history, however, may give the nurse valuable clues as to what type of shock may be present. For example, obvious trauma or bleeding would

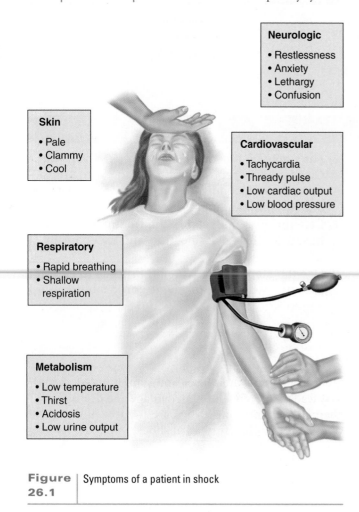

Neurologic
- Restlessness
- Anxiety
- Lethargy
- Confusion

Skin
- Pale
- Clammy
- Cool

Cardiovascular
- Tachycardia
- Thready pulse
- Low cardiac output
- Low blood pressure

Respiratory
- Rapid breathing
- Shallow respiration

Metabolism
- Low temperature
- Thirst
- Acidosis
- Low urine output

Figure 26.1 | Symptoms of a patient in shock

suggest **hypovolemic shock**, related to volume depletion. If trauma to the brain or spinal cord is evident, **neurogenic shock**, a type of distributive shock caused by a sudden loss of nerve impulse communication, may be suspected. A history of heart disease would suggest **cardiogenic shock**, which is caused by a loss of adequate cardiac output due to pump failure. A recent infection may indicate **septic shock**, a type of distributive shock caused by the presence of bacteria and toxins in the blood. A history of allergy with a sudden onset of symptoms following food or drug intake may suggest **anaphylactic shock**, the most severe type I allergic response.

FLUID REPLACEMENT AGENTS

Certain agents are used to replace blood or other fluids lost during hypovolemic shock. Fluid replacement therapy includes blood, blood products, colloids, and crystalloids, as shown in Table 26.2.

26.3 Treatment Priorities for Shock

Shock is treated as a medical emergency and the first goal is to maintain basic life support. Rapid identification of the underlying cause, followed by aggressive treatment, is es-

sential, since the patient's condition may deteriorate rapidly without specific, emergency measures. The initial nursing interventions consist of keeping the patient quiet and warm and offering psychological support and reassurance. Maintaining the ABCs of life support—airway, breathing, and circulation—to sustain normal blood pressure is critical. The patient is immediately connected to a cardiac monitor and a pulse oximeter is applied. Blood pressure readings are taken on the opposite arm of the pulse oximeter, as peripheral vasoconstriction with the inflation of the BP cuff will alter oximetry readings. Unless contraindicated, oxygen is administered at 15 L/min via a nonrebreather mask. Neurologic status and level of consciousness are monitored.

Hypovolemic shock can be triggered by a number of conditions, including hemorrhage, extensive burns, severe dehydration, persistent vomiting or diarrhea, and intensive diuretic therapy. If the patient has lost significant blood or other body fluids, immediate maintenance of blood volume through the administration of fluid and electrolytes or blood products is essential.

Blood and blood products may be administered, depending on the clinical situation. Whole blood is indicated for the treatment of acute, massive blood loss (depletion of more than 30% of the total volume) when there is the need to replace plasma volume and supply red blood cells to increase the oxygen-carrying capacity. The administration of whole blood has been largely replaced with the use of blood components. A unit of whole blood can be separated into its specific constituents (red and white blood cells, platelets, plasma proteins, fresh frozen plasma, and globulins) which can be used to treat more than one patient. The supply of blood products depends on human donors and requires careful crossmatching to ensure compatibility between the donor and the recipient. Whole blood, while carefully screened, has the potential to transmit serious infections such as hepatitis or HIV.

Crystalloids and Colloids

26.4 Treating Shock with Crystalloids and Colloids

Because it is safer to administer only the needed components, rather than whole blood, other products are used to provide volume expansion and to sustain blood pressure. These are of two basic types: colloids and crystalloids. Colloid and crystalloid infusions are often used when up to one-third of an adult's blood volume has been lost.

Colloids are proteins or other large molecules that stay suspended in the blood for a long period, because they are too large to cross membranes. While circulating, they draw water molecules from the cells and tissues into the blood vessels through their ability to increase **oncotic pressure**. Blood product colloids include normal human serum albumin, plasma protein fraction, and serum globulins. The nonblood product colloids are dextran (40, 70, and high molecular weight) and hetastarch (Hespan). These agents are indicated to provide life-sustaining support following massive hemorrhage, for plasma exchange, and to treat

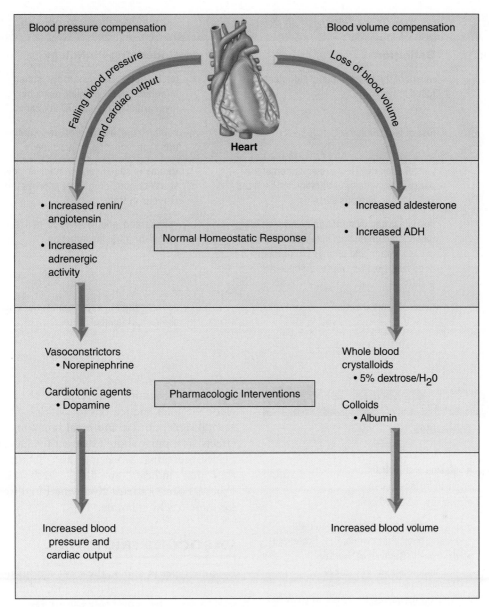

Figure 26.2 | Physiologic changes during circulatory shock: pharmacological intervention

shock as well as for the treatment of burns, acute liver failure, and neonatal hemolytic disease.

Crystalloids are IV solutions that contain electrolytes in concentrations resembling those of plasma. Unlike colloids, crystalloid solutions can readily leave the blood and enter cells. They are used to replace fluids that have been lost and to promote urine output. Common crystalloids include normal saline, lactated Ringer's, Plasmalyte, hypertonic saline, and 5% dextrose in water (D5W).

NURSING CONSIDERATIONS

The role of the nurse in crystalloid and colloid therapy for shock involves careful monitoring of a patient's condition and providing education as it relates to the prescribed drug regimen. Because of the ability of all colloids to pull fluid into the vascular space, circulatory overload is a serious adverse outcome. Monitoring for blood pressure changes is essential; pressure may increase with a healthy heart, or decrease if the heart fails with fluid overload. Lung sounds must also be monitored; crackles will be heard with pulmonary congestion. Pulse oximetry can be utilized to monitor for changes in oxygenation that may become evident before lung sounds change. Monitoring intake, output, and body weight will assist in assessing fluid retention or loss. These products are used with caution in lactation and pregnancy (category C).

Anaphylactic reactions may occur with the use of plasma protein fraction (Plasmanate), dextran 75 (Gentran 75), dextran 70 (Macrodex), and hetastarch (Hespan). Signs and symptoms of an allergic response may include periorbital edema, urticaria, wheezing, and difficulty breathing. The use

Table 26.1	Common Types of Shock	
Type of Shock	**Definition**	**Underlying Pathology**
cardiogenic	failure of the heart to pump sufficient blood to tissues	left heart failure, myocardial ischemia, myocardial infarction, dysrhythmias, pulmonary embolism, myocardial or pericardial infection
hypovolemic	loss of blood volume	hemorrhage, burns, profuse sweating, excessive urination, vomiting, or diarrhea
neurogenic	vasodilation due to overstimulation of the parasympathetic or understimulation of the sympathetic nervous systems	trauma to spinal cord or medulla, severe emotional stress or pain, drugs that depress the central nervous system
septic	multiple organ dysfunction as a result of pathogenic organisms in the blood resulting in vasodilation and changes in permeability of capillaries; often a precursor to ARDS and DIC	widespread inflammatory response to bacterial, fungal, or parasitic infection
anaphylactic	acute allergic reaction	severe reaction to allergen such as penicillin, nuts, shellfish, or animal proteins

Table 26.2	Fluid Replacement Agents
Agent	**Examples**
blood products	• whole blood • plasma protein fraction • fresh frozen plasma • packed red blood cells
colloids	• plasma protein fraction (Plasmanate, Plasma-Plex, Plasmatein, PPF, Protenate) • dextran 40 (Gentran 40, Hyskon, Rheomacrodex) or dextran 70 (Macrodex) • hetastarch (Hespan) • normal serum albumin, human (Albuminar, Albutein, Buminate, Plasbumin)
crystalloids	• normal saline (0.9% sodium chloride) • lactated Ringer's • Plasmalyte • hypertonic saline (3% sodium chloride) • 5% dextrose in water (D5W)

of dextran, a high molecular weight polysaccharide, is further limited because it can interfere with coagulation and platelet adhesion. Hetastarch, a synthetic starch resembling human glycogen, can increase the PT, PTT, and bleeding time when given in large doses, thus limiting its use in conditions where normal clotting is essential. Patients with renal failure exhibiting anuria or oliguria are at great risk for fluid overload because of the fluid shift that will occur and their inability to rid the body of excess fluid through urination.

Patient education as it relates to these drugs should include the goals and reasons for obtaining baseline data such as vital signs, cardiac and renal function, and possible side effects. The nurse should instruct the patient to report difficulty breathing, wheezing, and itching immediately as they may indicate an allergic response. See "Nursing Process Focus: Patients Receiving Fluid Replacer Therapy" for more teaching points.

VASOCONSTRICTORS

In some types of shock, the most serious medical challenge facing the patient is hypotension, which may become so profound as to cause collapse of the circulatory system. Vasoconstrictors are drugs for maintaining blood pressure, when fluid replacement agents have proven ineffective. These agents are shown in Table 26.3.

26.5 Treating Shock with Vasoconstrictors

In the early stages of shock, the body compensates for the fall in blood pressure by increasing the activity of the sympathetic nervous system. This sympathetic activity results in vasoconstriction, thus raising blood pressure and increasing the rate and force of myocardial contraction. The purpose of these compensatory measures is to maintain blood flow to vital organs such as the heart and brain, and to decrease flow to other organs, including the kidneys and liver.

The body's ability to compensate is limited, however, and profound hypotension may develop as shock progresses. In severe cases, fluid replacement agents alone are not effective at raising blood pressure and other medications are indicated. Historically, sympathomimetic vasoconstrictors have been used to stabilize blood pressure in shock patients. When

PROTOTYPE DRUG NORMAL SERUM ALBUMIN (Albuminar, Albutein, Buminate, Plasbumin)

ACTIONS AND USES

Normal serum albumin is a protein extracted from whole blood, plasma, or placental human plasma that contains 96% albumin and 4% globulins and other proteins. Albumin naturally comprises about 60% of all blood proteins. Its normal functions are to maintain plasma osmotic pressure and to shuttle certain substances through the blood, including a substantial number of drug molecules. After extraction from blood or plasma, it is sterilized to remove possible contamination by the hepatitis viruses or HIV.

Administered IV, albumin increases the osmotic pressure of the blood and moves fluid from the tissues to the general circulation. It is used to restore plasma volume in hypovolemic shock, or to restore blood proteins in patients with hypoproteinemia. It has an immediate onset of action and is available in concentrations of 5% and 25%.

Administration Alerts

- Higher concentrations must be infused more slowly because the risk of a large, rapid fluid shift is greater.
- Use large gauge (16–20 gauge) IV cannula for administration of drug.
- Pregnancy category C.

ADVERSE EFFECTS AND INTERACTIONS

Because albumin is a natural blood product, allergic reactions are possible. However, coagulation factors, antibodies, and most other blood proteins have been removed; therefore, the incidence of allergic reactions from albumin is not high. Signs of allergy include fever, chills, rash, dyspnea, and possibly hypotension. Protein overload may occur if excessive albumin is infused.

There have been no clinically significant drug interactions established.

 See the companion website for a Nursing Process Focus specific to this drug.

given intravenously, these drugs will immediately raise blood pressure. Because of side effects and potential organ damage due to the rapid and extreme vasoconstriction, these drugs are used as a last resort. These emergency drugs are considered critical care agents. Sympathomimetics used for shock include norepinephrine (Levarterenol, Levophed), isoproterenol (Isuprel), methoxamine (Vasoxyl), phenylephrine (Neo-Synephrine), and mephentermine (Wyamine). The basic pharmacology of the sympathomimetics, or beta-adrenergic agonists, is presented in Chapter 13 .

NURSING CONSIDERATIONS

The role of the nurse in vasoconstrictor therapy for shock involves careful monitoring of a patient's condition and providing education as it relates to the prescribed drug regimen. Prior to administration, the nurse should assess for the patient's history of narrow angle glaucoma and cardiovascular disease, and obtain an EKG reading. Vasoconstrictors are contraindicated in patients with severe cardiovascular disease and narrow angle glaucoma as they may worsen these conditions. The nurse should assess blood pressure, pulse, and urine output.

In addition to many of the adverse effects described in the Prototype Drug box on page 351 for norepinephrine,

the nurse should be aware that other drugs in this class could cause additional side effects. Phenylephrine (Neo-Synephrine) will cause necrosis of tissue if extravasation occurs. The nurse should ensure IV patency prior to beginning the infusion and observe the IV site during the entire infusion. The nurse should monitor blood pressure and titrate drip if blood pressure is elevated. Urine output should be monitored because extreme vasoconstriction may lead to decreased renal perfusion.

The nurse should monitor the patient for chest pain and ECG changes. Dosages are usually reduced if the heart rate exceeds 110 bpm. The nurse should monitor mental status, skin temperature of extremities, and color of ear lobes, nail beds, and lips.

Patient education as it relates to these drugs should include the goals and reasons for obtaining baseline data such as vital signs, cardiac disorders, and possible side effects. The nurse should explain the use of medication and the rationale for frequent monitoring. The nurse should instruct the patient to report any pain or burning at the IV site immediately. See "Nursing Process Focus: Patients Receiving Sympathomimetic Therapy" page 137 in Chapter 13, for the complete Nursing Process applied to caring for patients receiving sympathomimetics (beta-adrenergic agonists) .

NURSING PROCESS FOCUS	PATIENTS RECEIVING FLUID REPLACER THERAPY

ASSESSMENT

Prior to administration:
- Obtain complete health history, including allergies, drug history, and possible drug interactions.
- Assess lung sounds.
- Obtain vital signs.
- Assess level of consciousness.
- Assess renal function (BUN and creatinine).

POTENTIAL NURSING DIAGNOSES

- Risk for Injury, related to allergic reaction to drug
- Ineffective Tissue Perfusion, related to adverse effects of drug
- Excess Fluid Volume, related to increased intravascular volume
- Deficient Knowledge, related to drug therapy

PLANNING: PATIENT GOALS AND EXPECTED OUTCOMES

The patient will:
- Immediately report difficulty breathing
- Report itching, flushing
- Maintain urinary output at least 50 ml/h
- Demonstrate an understanding of the drug's action by accurately describing drug side effects and precautions

IMPLEMENTATION

Interventions and (Rationales)	*Patient Education/Discharge Planning*
- Monitor respiratory status. (Effects of drugs and rapid infusion may result in fluid overload.)	Instruct patient to: - Report any signs of respiratory distress - Report changes in sensorium such as lightheadedness, drowsiness, or dizziness
- Monitor intake and output for changes in renal function.	- Instruct patient concerning rationale for Foley catheter insertion.
- Monitor electrolytes. (Crystalloid drugs may cause hypernatremia and resulting fluid retention.)	- Instruct patient to report any evidence of edema.
- Observe patient for signs of allergic reactions. (Administration of blood and blood products could cause allergic reactions.)	Instruct patient: - To report itching, rash, chills, and difficulty breathing - That frequent blood draws are necessary to monitor possible complications of drug administration
- Observe urine for changes in color. (Adverse reaction to blood could cause hematuria.)	- Instruct patient to notify the healthcare provider if changes in urine color occur.

EVALUATION OF OUTCOME CRITERIA

Evaluate the effectiveness of drug therapy by confirming that patient goals and expected outcomes have been met (see "Planning").

 See Table 26.2 for a list of the drugs to which these nursing actions apply.

CARDIOTONIC AGENTS

Cardiotonic drugs increase the force of contraction of the heart. In the treatment of shock, they are used to increase the cardiac output. The cardiotonic agents are shown in Table 26.4.

26.6 Treating Shock with Cardiotonic Agents

As shock progresses, the heart may begin to fail; cardiac output decreases, lowering the amount of blood reaching vital tissues and deepening the degree of shock. Car-

Table 26.3	Vasoconstrictors for Shock
Drug	**Route and Adult Dose (max dose where indicated)**
Non-specific Alpha- and Beta-adrenergic Agonists	
mephentermine (Wyamine)	IV; 20–60 mg as an infusion (1.2 mg/ml of D5W)
norepinephrine (Levarterenol, Levophed)	IV; 8–12 μg/min until pressure stabilizes, then 2–4 μg/min for maintenance
Specific Alpha-adrenergic Agonists	
methoxamine (Vasoxyl)	IV; 3–5 mg over 5–10 min
phenylephrine (Neo-Synephrine, others)	IV; 0.1–0.18 mg/min until pressure stabilizes, then 0.04–0.06 mg/min for maintenance

Pr PROTOTYPE DRUG NOREPINEPHRINE (Levarterenol, Levophed)

ACTIONS AND USES

Norepinephrine is a sympathomimetic that acts directly on alpha-adrenergic receptors in vascular smooth muscle to immediately raise blood pressure. It also stimulates beta$_1$-receptors in the heart, thus producing a positive inotropic response that increases cardiac output. The primary indications for norepinephrine are acute shock and cardiac arrest. It is given by the IV route and has a duration of only 1 to 2 minutes after the infusion is terminated.

Administration Alerts

- Drug given as continuous infusion only.
- Infusion should be started only after patency of IV is ensured. The flow rate should be monitored continuously.
- Phentolamine should be available in case of extravasation.
- Do not abruptly discontinue infusion.
- Pregnancy category D.

ADVERSE EFFECTS AND INTERACTIONS

Norepinephrine is a powerful vasoconstrictor; thus, continuous monitoring of the patient's blood pressure is required to avoid hypertension. When first administered, a reflex bradycardia is sometimes experienced. It also has the ability to produce various types of dysrhythmias. Blurred vision and photophobia are signs of overdose.

Norepinephrine interacts with many drugs, including alpha- and beta-blockers, which may antagonize the drug's pressor effects. Conversely, ergot alkaloids and tricyclic antidepressants may potentiate pressor effects. Halothane and cyclopropane may increase the risk of dysrhythmias.

See the companion website for a Nursing Process Focus specific to this drug.

Table 26.4	Cardiotonic Drugs for Shock
Drug	**Route and Adult Dose (max dose where indicated)**
digoxin (Lanoxin, Lanoxicaps) (see page 290 for the Prototype Drug box) ⌐⊃	IV; Digitalizing dose 2.5–5 μg q6 h for 24 h; maintenance dose 0.125–0.5 mg qd
dobutamine (Dobutrex)	IV; Infused at a rate of 2.5–40 μg/kg/min for a max of 72 h
dopamine hydrochloride (Dopastat, Inotropin)	IV; 1.5 μg/kg/min initial dose; may be increased to 30 μg/kg/min

diotonic drugs, also known as **inotropic agents,** have the potential to reverse the cardiac symptoms of shock by increasing the strength of myocardial contraction. Digoxin (Lanoxin) increases myocardial contractility and cardiac output, thus quickly bringing critical tissues their essential oxygen. Chapter 22 should be reviewed, because digoxin and other medications prescribed for heart failure are sometimes used for the treatment of shock ⌐⊃.

Dobutamine (Dobutrex) is a beta$_1$-adrenergic agonist that has value in the short-term treatment of certain types of shock, due to its ability to cause the heart to beat more forcefully. Dobutamine is especially beneficial in cases when the primary cause of shock is related to heart failure, not hypovolemia. The resulting increase in cardiac output assists in maintaining blood flow to vital organs. Dobutamine has a half-life of only 2 minutes, and is only given as an IV infusion.

Dopamine (Dopastat; Inotropin) is both a beta and alpha agonist. Dopamine is utilized at different dosage levels and will have different effects based on what receptors are most affected. It is primarily used in shock conditions to increase blood pressure by causing peripheral vasoconstriction (alpha$_1$ stimulation) and increasing force of myocardial contraction (beta$_1$ stimulation). Dopamine has the potential to cause dysrhythmias, and is only given as an IV infusion.

NURSING CONSIDERATIONS

The role of the nurse in cardiotonic pharmacotherapy for shock involves careful monitoring of a patient's condition and providing education as it relates to the prescribed drug regimen. Prior to administration, the nurse should assess for history of cardiovascular disease, and obtain an ECG. Blood pressure, pulse, urine output, and body weight should also be assessed.

Cardiotonic agents are contraindicated in patients with ventricular tachycardia because they will worsen dysrhythmia, and in hypertrophic idiopathic subaortic stenosis because increasing contractility will precipitate heart failure. Safe use during pregnancy and lactation has not been established (category C). They should be used cautiously with patients who are hypertensive, as they increase blood pressure. With atrial fibrillation, a rapid ventricular response may increase heart rate excessively. Hypovolemia should be corrected with whole blood or plasma prior to the start of dopamine infusion.

Cardiotonic medications may be used separately or concurrently with other antishock agents. They are only given as a continuous infusion, and dosage is based on micrograms/kilogram/minute. Careful calculations must be done to arrive at the appropriate milliliters per hour to set the IV pump to deliver the correct dosage. IV pump technology is such that some will automate calculations, and most have the ability to deliver dosages to a tenth of a milliliter. The IV rate can be found by multiplying the ordered dose times the patient's weight in kilograms times 60 (to get micrograms per hour), then dividing this amount by the concentration of the infusion (micrograms/milliliter). The result will be the milliliters/hour the patient should receive. The nurse should weigh the patient each morning. The patient's dose is recalculated each day, based on that weight.

Patients should be connected to a cardiac monitor prior to and during the infusion of cardiotonic drugs. The nurse should monitor the patient's blood pressure frequently. If a pressure monitoring catheter is in place, pulmonary wedge pressure and cardiac output should be assessed to keep these parameters within normal ranges. The nurse should initiate the IV in a large vein; a central line is preferable. Extravasation of dopamine (Dopastat, Inotropin) can cause severe, localized vasoconstriction resulting in sloughing of tissue and tissue necrosis if not reversed with phentolamine (Regitine) injections at the site of the infiltration. If extravasation occurs, the nurse should discontinue the IV, restart it in another site, and administer the antidote. If infiltration occurs, dobutamine (Dobutrex) can be irritating to the vein and surrounding tissues, although it causes less severe vasoconstriction than dopamine (Dopastat, Inotropin).

Pr PROTOTYPE DRUG	DOPAMINE (Dopastat, Inotropin)
ACTIONS AND USES	**ADVERSE EFFECTS AND INTERACTIONS**
Dopamine is the immediate metabolic precursor to norepinephrine. While classified as a sympathomimetic, dopamine's mechanism of action is dependent upon the dose. At low doses, the drug selectively stimulates dopaminergic receptors, especially in the kidneys, leading to vasodilation and an increased blood flow through the kidneys. This makes dopamine of particular value in treating hypovolemic and cardiogenic shock. At higher doses, dopamine stimulates beta$_1$-adrenergic receptors, causing the heart to beat more forcefully and increasing cardiac output. Another beneficial effect of dopamine when given in higher doses is its ability to stimulate alpha-adrenergic receptors, thus causing vasoconstriction and raising blood pressure.	Because of its profound effects on the cardiovascular system, the nurse must continuously monitor patients receiving dopamine for signs of dysrhythmias and hypotension. Side effects are normally self-limiting because of the short half-life of the drug. Dopamine is a vesicant drug that can cause severe, irreversible damage if the drug escapes from the vein into the surrounding tissues. Dopamine interacts with many other drugs. For example, concurrent administration with MAO inhibitors and ergot alkaloids increase alpha-adrenergic effects. Phenytoin may decrease dopamine action. Beta-blockers may antagonize cardiac effects. Alpha-blockers antagonize peripheral vasoconstriction. Halothane increases the risk of hypertension and ventricular dysrhythmias.

Administration Alerts

- Drug is given as a continuous infusion only.
- Ensure patency of IV prior to beginning infusion.
- Phentolamine is the antidote for extravasation of drug and should be readily available.
- Pregnancy category C.

See the companion website for a Nursing Process Focus specific to this drug.

MediaLink Mechanism in Action Dopamine

The nurse should monitor renal function closely, including urine output, BUN, and creatinine levels. With improved cardiac output, renal function should improve and urine output increase. Low doses of dopamine increase renal perfusion and should enhance urine output. Foley catheters are frequently employed to ensure accurate measurement of urine output.

Patient education as it relates to these drugs should include the goals and reasons for obtaining baseline data such as vital signs, cardiac and renal disorders, and possible side effects. The nurse should explain frequent monitoring and Foley catheter placement. The nurse should advise the patient that continuous cardiac monitoring will occur while receiving the medication.

Following are additional points the nurse should include when teaching patients regarding inotropic agents.

- Report chest pain, difficulty breathing, palpitations, or headache.
- Immediately report burning or pain at IV site.
- Immediately report numbness or tingling in the extremities, or chest pain.

See "Nursing Process Focus: Patients Receiving Sympathomimetic," Therapy page 137 in Chapter 13, for the complete Nursing Process applied to caring for patients receiving beta-adrenergic agonists ∞ .

CHAPTER REVIEW

Key Concepts

The numbered key concepts provide a succinct summary of the important points from the corresponding numbered section within the chapter. If any of these points are not clear, refer to the numbered section within the chapter for review. Expanded versions can be found on the companion website.

26.1 Shock is a clinical syndrome characterized by the inability of the cardiovascular system to pump enough blood to meet the metabolic needs of the tissues.

26.2 Shock is often classified by the underlying pathologic process or by the organ system that is primarily affected, including cardiogenic, hypovolemic, neurogenic, septic, and anaphylactic shock.

26.3 The initial treatment of shock involves administration of basic life support and replacement of lost fluid. Whole blood may be indicated in cases of massive hemorrhage.

26.4 During hypovolemic shock, crystalloids replace lost fluids and electrolytes; colloids expand plasma volume and maintain blood pressure.

26.5 Vasoconstrictors are critical care drugs sometimes needed during severe shock to maintain blood pressure.

26.6 Cardiotonic drugs are useful in reversing the decreased cardiac output resulting from shock.

Review Questions

1. How would an emergency room nurse who is treating a victim of a motorcycle accident determine the cause of the patient's shock?

2. How can cardiotonic drugs reduce the symptoms of shock without causing vasoconstriction?

3. Should the intravenous infusion of dopamine (Inotropin) infiltrate, what nursing intervention is immediately necessary, and why?

Critical Thinking Questions

1. A patient is on a norepinephrine (Levophed) drip for cardiogenic shock with a blood pressure of 84/40. Why is this patient on this medication? When and how should the norepinephrine drip be discontinued?

2. The healthcare provider orders 3 L of 0.9% normal saline (NS) for a 22-year-old patient with vomiting and diarrhea, and a heart rate of 122 and blood pressure of 102/54. Is this an appropriate IV solution for this patient? Why or why not?

3. A patient with a severe head injury has been put on an IV drip of dextrose 5% water running at 150 ml/h. The nurse receives this transfer patient and is reviewing the health-care provider's orders. Is the IV solution appropriate for this patient? Why or why not?

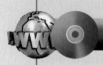

EXPLORE MediaLink

NCLEX review, case studies, and other interactive resources for this chapter can be found on the companion website at www.prenhall.com/adams. Click on "Chapter 26" to select the activities for this chapter. For animations, more NCLEX review questions, and an audio glossary, access the accompanying CD-ROM in this textbook.

CHAPTER 27

Drugs for Lipid Disorders

▪ DRUGS AT A GLANCE

HMG-CoA REDUCTASE INHIBITORS
Ⓟ *atorvastatin (Lipitor)*

BILE ACID RESINS
Ⓟ *cholestyramine (Questran)*

NICOTINIC ACID

FIBRIC ACID AGENTS
Ⓟ *gemfibrozil (Lopid)*

metabolized and eliminated by the body.
of this process
PHARMACOLOGY
1. The study of medicines; the discipline
pertaining to how drugs improve the heal
of the human body
PHARMACOPE

 MediaLink www.prenhall.com/adams

CD-ROM
Animation:
  Mechanism in Action: Atorvastatin (Lipitor)
Audio Glossary
NCLEX Review

Companion Website
NCLEX Review
Dosage Calculations
Case Study
Care Plans
Expanded Key Concepts

OBJECTIVES

After reading this chapter, the student should be able to:

1. Summarize the link between high blood cholesterol, LDL levels, and cardiovascular disease.
2. Compare and contrast the different types of lipids.
3. Illustrate how lipids are transported through the blood.
4. Compare and contrast the different types of lipoproteins.
5. Give examples of how cholesterol and LDL levels can be controlled through nonpharmacologic means.
6. For each of the drug classes listed in Drugs at a Glance, know representative drug examples, explain their mechanism of action, primary actions, and important adverse effects.
7. Categorize antilipidemic drugs based on their classification and mechanism of action.
8. Explain the nurse's role in the pharmacologic management of lipid disorders.
9. Use the Nursing Process to care for patients receiving drug therapy for lipid disorders.

Research during the 1960s and 1970s brought about a nutritional revolution as new knowledge about lipids and their relationship to obesity and cardiovascular disease allowed people to make more intelligent lifestyle choices. Since then, advances in the diagnosis of lipid disorders have helped to identify those patients at greatest risk for cardiovascular disease and those most likely to benefit from pharmacologic intervention. Research in pharmacology has led to safe, effective drugs for lowering lipid levels, thus decreasing the risk of cardiovascular-related diseases. As a result of this knowledge and from advancements in pharmacology, the incidence of death due to most cardiovascular diseases has been declining, although cardiovascular disease remains the leading cause of death in the United States.

PHARMFACTS | **High Blood Cholesterol**

- The incidence of high blood cholesterol increases until age 65.
- Over 100 million Americans are estimated to have total blood cholesterol levels of 200 mg/dl or above. This is 40% to 50% of the adult population.
- Moderate alcohol intake does not reduce LDL-cholesterol, but it does increase HDL-cholesterol.
- Prior to menopause, high blood cholesterol occurs more frequently in men, but after age 50 the condition is more common in women.
- To lower blood cholesterol, both dietary cholesterol and saturated fats must be reduced.
- Familial hypercholesterolemia affects 1 in 500 people and is a genetic disease that predisposes people to high cholesterol levels.

27.1 Types of Lipids

The three types of lipids important to humans are illustrated in Figure 27.1. The most common are the triglycerides, or neutral fats, which form a large family of different lipids all having three fatty acids attached to a chemical backbone of glycerol. Triglycerides are the major storage form of fat in the body and the only type of lipid that serves as an important energy source. They account for 90% of total lipids in the body.

A second class, the phospholipids, is formed when a phosphorous group replaces one of the fatty acids in a triglyceride. This class of lipids is essential to building plasma membranes. The best-known phospholipids are lecithins, which are found in high concentration in egg yolks and soybeans. Once promoted as a natural treatment for high cholesterol levels, controlled studies have not

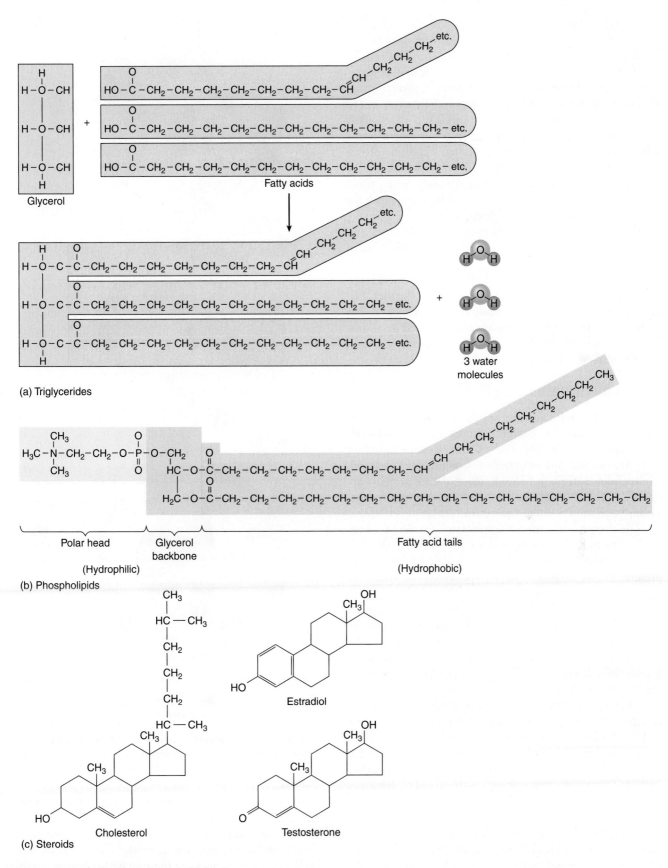

(a) Triglycerides

(b) Phospholipids

(c) Steroids

Figure 27.1 | Chemical structure of lipids

shown lecithin to be of any benefit for this disorder. Likewise, lecithin has been proposed as a remedy for nervous system diseases such as Alzheimer's disease and bipolar disorder, but there is no definite evidence to support these claims.

The third class of lipids is the **steroids**, a diverse group of substances having a common chemical structure called the **sterol nucleus**, or ring. Cholesterol is the most widely known of the steroids, and its role in promoting **atherosclerosis** has been clearly demonstrated. Cholesterol is a natural and vital component of plasma membranes. Unlike the triglycerides that provide fuel for the body during times of energy need, cholesterol serves as the building block for a number of essential biochemicals, including vitamin D, bile acids, cortisol, estrogen, and testosterone. While clearly essential for life, the body only needs minute amounts of cholesterol. The liver, however, is able to synthesize adequate amounts of cholesterol from other chemicals; it is not necessary to provide additional cholesterol in the diet. Dietary cholesterol is obtained solely from animal products; humans do not metabolize the sterols produced by plants. The American Heart Association recommends less than 300 mg of dietary cholesterol per day.

27.2 Lipoproteins

Because lipid molecules are not soluble in plasma, they must be specially packaged for transport through the blood. To accomplish this, the body forms complexes called **lipoproteins** that consist of various amounts of cholesterol, triglycerides, and phospholipids, along with a protein carrier. The protein component is called an **apoprotein** (*apo-* means "separated from or derived from").

The three most common lipoproteins are classified according to their composition, size, and weight or density, which comes primarily from the amount of apoprotein present in the complex. Each type varies in lipid and apoprotein makeup and serves a different function in transporting lipids from sites of synthesis and absorption to sites of utilization. For example, **high-density lipoprotein (HDL)** contains the most apoprotein, up to 50% by weight. The highest amount of cholesterol is carried by **low-density lipoprotein (LDL)**. Figure 27.2 illustrates the three basic lipoproteins and their compositions.

To understand the pharmacotherapy of lipid disorders, it is important to learn the functions of the major lipoproteins and their roles in transporting cholesterol. LDL transports cholesterol from the liver to the tissues and organs, where it is used to build plasma membranes or to synthesize other steroids. Once in the tissues it can also be stored for later use. Storage of cholesterol in the lining of blood vessels, however, is not desirable because it contributes to plaque buildup and atherosclerosis. LDL is often called "bad" cholesterol, because this lipoprotein contributes significantly to plaque deposits and coronary artery disease. **Very low–density lipoprotein (VLDL)** is the primary carrier of triglycerides in the blood. Through a series of steps, VLDL is reduced in size to become LDL. Lowering LDL levels in the blood has been shown to decrease the incidence of coronary artery disease.

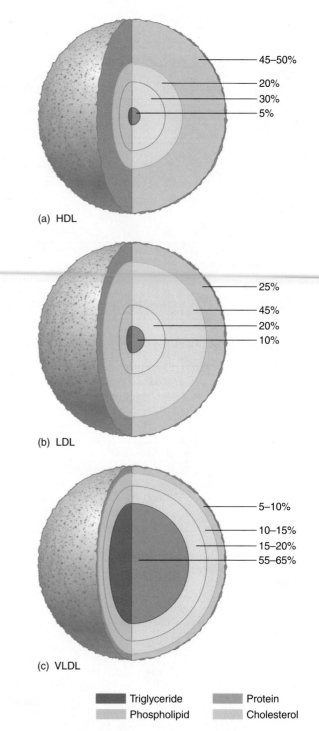

(a) HDL

45–50%
20%
30%
5%

(b) LDL

25%
45%
20%
10%

(c) VLDL

5–10%
10–15%
15–20%
55–65%

■ Triglyceride ■ Protein
■ Phospholipid ■ Cholesterol

Figure 27.2 | Composition of lipoproteins: (a) HDL; (b) LDL; (c) VLDL

HDL is manufactured in the liver and small intestine and assists in the transport of cholesterol away from the body tissues and back to the liver in a process called **reverse cholesterol transport**. The cholesterol component of the HDL is then broken down to unite with bile that is subsequently excreted in the feces. Excretion via bile is the only route the body uses to remove cholesterol. Because HDL transports cholesterol for destruction and removes it from the body, it is considered "good" cholesterol.

Hyperlipidemia, the general term meaning "high levels of lipids in the blood," is a major risk factor for cardiovascular disease. Elevated blood cholesterol, or hypercholesterolemia, is the type of hyperlipidemia that is most familiar to the general public. Dyslipidemia is the term that refers to abnormal (excess or deficient) levels of lipoproteins. The etiology may be inherited and/or acquired.

27.3 LDL and HDL as Predictors of Cardiovascular Disease

Although high serum cholesterol is associated with cardiovascular disease, it is not adequate to simply measure total cholesterol in the blood. Because some cholesterol is being transported for destruction, a more accurate profile is obtained by measuring LDL and HDL. The goal in maintaining normal cholesterol levels is to maximize the HDL and minimize the LDL. This is sometimes stated as a ratio of LDL to HDL. If the ratio is greater than 5.0 (5 times more LDL than HDL), the male patient is considered at risk for cardiovascular disease. The normal ratio in women is slightly lower, at 4.5.

Scientists have further divided LDL into subclasses of lipoproteins. For example, one variety found in LDL, called lipoprotein (a), has been strongly associated with plaque formation and heart disease. It is likely that further research will discover other varieties, with the expectation that drugs will be designed to be more selective toward the "bad" lipoproteins. Table 27.1 gives the desirable, borderline, and high laboratory values for each of the major lipids and lipoproteins.

Establishing treatment guidelines for dyslipidemia has been difficult, as the condition has no symptoms and the progression to cardiovascular disease may take decades. Based on years of research, the National Cholesterol Education Program (NCEP), an expert panel of the National

Heart, Lung and Blood Institute, recently revised the recommended treatment guidelines for dyslipidemia. The new guidelines are based on accumulated evidence that reducing "borderline" high cholesterol levels can result in fewer heart attacks and fewer deaths. Optimal levels of LDL-cholesterol have been lowered from 130 mg/dl to 100 mg/dl. HDL-cholesterol should now be at least 40 mg/dl, compared to the previous 35 mg/dl. In addition, the NCEP guidelines recommend that high cholesterol levels be treated more aggressively in diabetics, and that hormone replacement therapy

SPECIAL CONSIDERATIONS
Pediatric Dyslipidemias

Most people consider dyslipidemia as a condition that occurs with advancing age. Dyslipidemias, however, are also a concern for some pediatric patients. Children at risk include those with a family history of premature coronary artery disease or dyslipidemia, and those who have hypertension, diabetes, or are obese. Lipid levels fluctuate in children, and tend to be higher in girls. Nutritional intervention, regular physical activity, and risk factor management are warranted when the LDL level reaches 110 to 129 mg/dl. More aggressive dietary therapy and pharmacotherapy may be warranted in pediatric patients with LDL levels above 130 mg/dl. The long-term effects of lipid-lowering drugs in children have not been clearly established; therefore, drug therapy is not recommended below 10 years of age. Cholestyramine (Questran) and colestipol (Colestid) are the only approved drugs for hypercholesterolemia in children, although side effects sometimes result in poor compliance. Research into the use of niacin and low dose statin pharmacotherapy in children is continuing.

Table 27.1	Standard Laboratory Lipid Profiles	
Type of Lipid	**Laboratory Value (mg/dl)**	**Standard**
total cholesterol	<200 200–239 >239	desirable borderline high high
LDL-cholesterol	<130 130–159 >159	desirable borderline high high
HDL-cholesterol	Men: 37–70 Women: 40–85 >35 mg/dl	desirable desirable high
LDL-HDL ratio	Men: 1.0 Women: 1.47 Men: >5.0 Women: >4.5	desirable desirable high high
triglycerides	<200 mg/dl 200–400 400–1,000 >1000	desirable borderline high high very high

not be considered as an alternative to cholesterol-lowering medications. The new guidelines will likely lead to more widespread use of medications to treat dyslipidemia.

27.4 Controlling Lipid Levels through Lifestyle Changes

Lifestyle changes should always be included in any treatment plan for reducing blood lipid levels. Many patients with borderline laboratory values can control their dyslipidemia entirely through nonpharmacologic means. It is important to note that all the lifestyle factors for reducing blood lipid levels also apply to cardiovascular disease in general. Because many patients taking lipid-lowering drugs also have underlying cardiovascular disease, these lifestyle changes are particularly important. Following are the most important lipid-reduction interventions.

- Monitor blood lipid levels regularly, as recommended by the healthcare provider.
- Maintain weight at an optimum level.
- Implement a medically supervised exercise plan.
- Reduce dietary saturated fats and cholesterol.
- Increase soluble fiber in the diet, as found in oat bran, apples, beans, grapefruit, and broccoli.
- Reduce or eliminate tobacco use.

Nutritionists recommend that the intake of dietary fat be less than 30% of the total caloric intake. Cholesterol intake should be reduced as much as possible but not exceed 300 mg/day. It is interesting to note that restriction of dietary cholesterol alone will not result in a significant reduction in blood cholesterol levels. This is because the liver reacts to a low cholesterol diet by making more cholesterol and by inhibiting its excretion when saturated fats are present. Thus, the patient must reduce saturated fat in the diet, as well as cholesterol, to control the amount made by the liver and to ultimately lower blood cholesterol levels.

The use of plant sterols and stanols are now recommended by the NCEP to reduce blood cholesterol levels. These plant lipids have a similar structure to cholesterol, and therefore compete with that substance for absorption in the digestive tract. When the body absorbs the plant sterols, cholesterol is excreted from the body. When less cholesterol is delivered to the liver, LDL uptake increases, thereby decreasing serum LDL (the "bad" cholesterol) level. Plant sterols and stanols may be obtained from a variety of sources including wheat, corn, rye, oats, and rice, as well as in nuts and olive oil. Commercially they are available in products fortified with Reducol, found in margarines, salad dressings, certain cereals, and some fruit juices. According to the AHA, the recommended daily intake of plant sterols or stanols is 2 to 3 g.

HMG-CoA Reductase Inhibitors/Statins

The statin class of antihyperlipidemics interferes with a critical enzyme in the synthesis of cholesterol. These agents, shown in Table 27.2, are first line drugs in the treatment of lipid disorders.

27.5 Pharmacotherapy with Statins

In the late 1970s, compounds isolated from various species of fungi were found to inhibit cholesterol production in human cells in the laboratory. This class of drugs, known as the statins, has since revolutionized the treatment of lipid disorders. Statins can produce a dramatic 20% to 40% reduction in LDL-cholesterol levels. In addition to dropping the LDL-cholesterol level in the blood, statins can also lower triglyceride and VLDL levels, and raise the level of "good" HDL-cholesterol.

Cholesterol is manufactured in the liver by a series of more than 25 metabolic steps, beginning with acetyl CoA, a two-carbon unit that is produced from the breakdown of fatty acids. Of the many enzymes involved in this complex pathway, HMG-CoA reductase (3-hydroxy-3-methylglutaryl coenzyme A reductase) serves as the primary regulatory site for cholesterol biosynthesis. Under normal conditions, this enzyme is controlled through negative feedback: High levels of LDL-cholesterol in the blood will shut down production of HMG-CoA reductase, thus turning off the cholesterol pathway. Figure 27.3 illustrates selected steps in cholesterol biosynthesis and the importance of HMG-CoA reductase.

The statins act by inhibiting HMG-CoA reductase, which results in less cholesterol biosynthesis. As the liver makes less cholesterol, it responds by making more LDL receptors on the surface of liver cells. The greater number of LDL receptors in liver cells results in increased removal of LDL from the blood. Blood levels of both LDL and cholesterol are reduced. The drop in lipid levels is not permanent, however, so patients need to remain on these drugs during the remainder of their lives or until their hyperlipidemia can be controlled through dietary or lifestyle changes. Statins have been shown to slow the progression of coronary artery disease and to reduce mortality from cardiovascular disease. The mechanism of actions of the statins and other drugs for dyslipidemia are illustrated in Figure 27.4.

All the statins are given orally and are tolerated well by most patients. Many of them should be administered in the evening, since cholesterol biosynthesis in the body is higher at night. Atorvastatin (Lipitor) is effective regardless of the time of day it is taken.

Much research is ongoing to determine other therapeutic effects of drugs in the statin class. For example, statins block the vasoconstrictive effect of the A-beta protein, a significant protein involved in Alzheimer's disease. Cholesterol and A-beta protein have similar effects on blood vessels, causing them to constrict. Preliminary research suggests that the statins may protect against dementia by inhibiting the protein and thus slowing dementia caused by blood vessel constriction.

Table 27.2	Drugs for Dyslipidemias
Drug	**Route and Adult Dose (max dose where indicated)**
HMG-CoA Reductase Inhibitors	
atorvastatin (Lipitor)	PO; 10–80 mg qd
fluvastatin (Lescol)	PO; 20 mg qd (max 80 mg/day)
lovastatin (Mevacor)	PO; 20–40 mg qd-bid
pravastatin (Pravachol)	PO; 10–40 mg qd
rosuvastatin (Crestor)	PO; 5–40 mg qd
simvastatin (Zocor)	PO; 5–40 mg qd
Bile Acid-binding Agents	
cholestyramine (Questran)	PO; 4–8 g bid-qid ac and hs
colesevelam (Welchol)	PO; 1,350 mg/day
colestipol (Colestid)	PO; 5–15 g bid-qid ac and hs
fenofibrate (Tricor)	PO; 67 mg qd (max 201 mg/d)
Fibric Acid Agents	
clofibrate (Atromid-S)	PO; 2 g/day in two to four divided doses
fenofibrate (Tricor)	PO; 54 mg qd (max 160 mg/day)
gemfibrozil (Lopid)	PO; 600 mg bid (max 1,500 mg/day)
Other Agents	
ezetimibe (Zetia)	Hyperlipidemia: PO; 1.5–3.0 g/day in divided doses (maximum 6 g/day) PO; 10mg/day
niacin (Niac, Nicobid, others)	Niacin deficiency: PO; 10–20 mg/day

NURSING CONSIDERATIONS

The role of the nurse in statin therapy involves careful monitoring of a patient's condition and providing education as it relates to the prescribed drug regimen. Although statin drugs are effective in reducing blood lipid levels, there can be serious adverse effects in some patients. Statins are pregnancy category X, and should not be used in patients who may become pregnant, or are pregnant or breastfeeding. Women taking statin drugs should utilize effective birth control and stop taking the medication if they suspect pregnancy.

Because liver dysfunction may occur with use of statin drugs, the nurse should monitor liver function tests before and during therapy. Statin drugs should not be used in patients with active liver disease, or unexplained elevations in liver function tests. This drug class should be used cautiously in patients who drink large quantities of alcohol; and alcohol use should be restricted or discontinued while on medication. Because myopathy has been reported by some patients, the nurse should assess the patient for muscle pain, tenderness, and weakness. CPK levels should be obtained if myopathy is suspected and, if elevated, statin therapy should be discontinued. The drug may be discontinued if muscle weakness persists even without CPK elevation.

Nausea, vomiting, heartburn, dyspepsia, abdominal cramping, and diarrhea are common, though less serious, side effects. The statins can be taken with the evening meal to help alleviate GI upset.

Patient education as it relates to these drugs should include the goals and reasons for obtaining baseline data such as vital signs, cardiac and hepatic disorders, and possible side effects. Following are the important points the nurse should include when teaching patients regarding HMG-CoA reductase inhibitors.

- Keep all scheduled laboratory visits for liver function tests.
- Do not take other prescription drugs and OTC medications, herbal remedies, or vitamins/minerals without notifying the healthcare provider.
- Practice reliable contraception and notify the healthcare provider if pregnancy is planned or suspected.
- Immediately report unexplained muscle pain, tenderness, or weakness, especially if accompanied by malaise or fever.
- Immediately report unexplained numbness, tingling, weakness, or pain in feet or hands.
- Take with the evening meal to prevent GI disturbances.

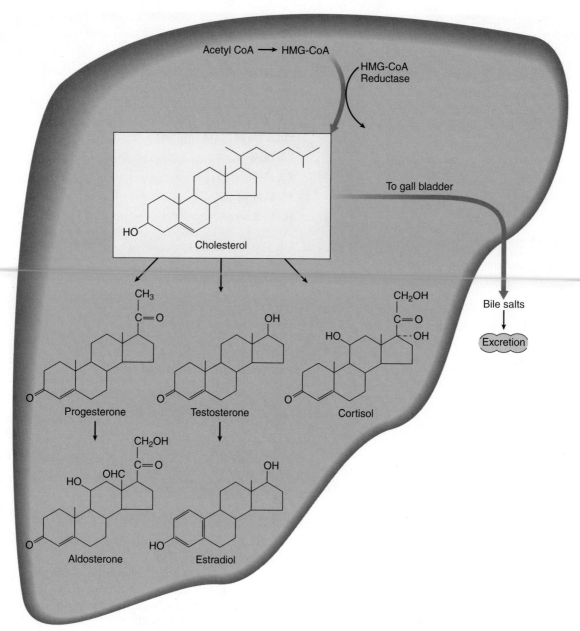

Figure 27.3 | Cholesterol biosynthesis and excretion

Bile Acid Resins

Bile acid resins bind bile acids, thus increasing the excretion of cholesterol. They are sometimes used in combination with the statins. These agents are shown in Table 27.2.

27.6 Bile Acid Resins for Reducing Cholesterol and LDL Levels

Prior to the discovery of the statins, the primary means of lowering blood cholesterol was through use of bile acid-binding drugs. These drugs, called bile acid resins or seques-

trants, bind bile acids, which contain a high concentration of cholesterol. Because of their large size, resins are not absorbed from the small intestine and the bound bile acids and cholesterol are eliminated in the feces. The liver responds to the loss of cholesterol by making more LDL receptors, which removes even more cholesterol from the blood in a mechanism similar to that of the statin drugs.

Although effective at producing a 20% drop in LDL-cholesterol, the bile acid sequestrants tend to cause more frequent side effects than statins. Because of this, they are no longer considered first line drugs for dyslipidemia. A new bile acid-binding agent, colesevelam (Welchol), was recently approved.

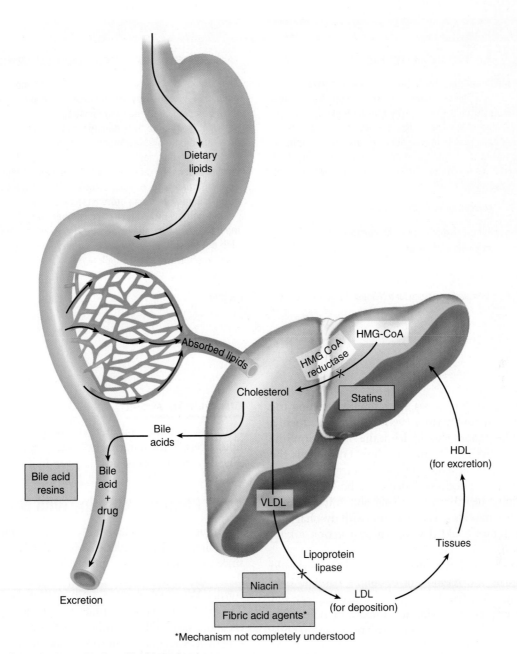

Figure 27.4 | Mechanisms of action of lipid-lowering drugs

NURSING CONSIDERATIONS

The role of the nurse in bile acid-resin therapy involves careful monitoring of a patient's condition and providing education as it relates to the prescribed drug regimen. Because bile acid sequestrants act in the GI tract and are not absorbed, they have no systemic side effects. They can, however, cause significant GI effects such as constipation, abdominal pain, bloating, nausea, vomiting, diarrhea, and steatorrhea. The nurse should assess bowel sounds and the presence of GI disturbance. Bile acid resins should be used cautiously in patients with GI disorders such as peptic ulcer disease, hemorrhoids, inflammatory bowel disease, or chronic constipation as they may worsen or aggravate these conditions. These drugs are generally not used during pregnancy or lactation (pregnancy category C).

Bile acid resins decrease the absorption of vitamins and minerals; deficiencies may occur with extended use. Other medications should be taken more than 1 hour before or 4 hours after taking a bile acid sequestrant because of decreased absorption. Cholestyramine (Questran) powder should be mixed with 60 to 180 ml water, noncarbonated beverages, highly liquid soups, or pulpy fruits (applesauce, crushed pineapple) to prevent esophageal irritation. The nurse should place the contents of the packet of resin on the surface of fluid, allow it to stand,

MediaLink Mechanism in Action Atorvastatin

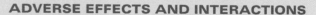

Pr PROTOTYPE DRUG | ATORVASTATIN (Lipitor)

ACTIONS AND USES

The primary indication for atorvastatin is hypercholesterolemia. The statins act by inhibiting HMG-CoA reductase. As the liver makes less cholesterol, it responds by making more LDL receptors on the surface of liver cells. The greater number of LDL receptors in liver cells results in increased removal of LDL from the blood. Blood levels of both LDL and cholesterol are reduced, although at least 2 weeks of therapy are required before these effects are realized.

Administration Alerts

- Administer with food to decrease GI discomfort.
- May be taken at anytime of the day
- Pregnancy category X.

ADVERSE EFFECTS AND INTERACTIONS

Side effects of atorvastatin are rarely severe enough to cause discontinuation of therapy and include GI complaints such as intestinal cramping, diarrhea, and constipation. A small percentage of patients experience liver damage, thus hepatic function is monitored during the first few months of therapy.

Atorvastatin interacts with many other drugs. For example, it may increase digoxin levels by 20%, as well as increase levels of norethindrone and ethinyl estradiol (oral contraceptives). Erythromycin may increase atorvastatin levels 40%.

Grapefruit juice inhibits the metabolism of statins, allowing them to reach toxic levels. Since HMG-CoA reductase inhibitors also decrease the synthesis of coenzyme Q10 (CoQ10), patients may benefit from CoQ10 supplements.

See the companion website for a Nursing Process Focus specific to this drug.

MediaLink Psyllium: A Natural Bile Acid Binder

without stirring, for 2 minutes, occasionally twirling the glass and then stir slowly (to prevent foaming) to form a suspension. The patient should drink the medication immediately after stirring. The patient should not inhale the powder as it may irritate mucous membranes.

Constipation may occur with decreased bowel function. Nausea, vomiting, heartburn, dyspepsia, abdominal cramping, and diarrhea may also occur. Patients with dysphagia or esophageal stricture could develop an obstruction taking this medication.

Patient education as it relates to bile acid resins should include the goals and reasons for obtaining baseline data such as vital signs; cardiac, hepatic, and renal disorders; and possible side effects. Following are important points the nurse should include when teaching patients regarding bile acid resins.

- Take medication before meals.
- Take other medication 1 hour before or 4 hours after taking bile acid resins, to avoid interference with absorption of other drugs.
- A high bulk diet and adequate fluid intake will help to decrease constipation and bloating.
- Take vitamin supplements to replace folic acid, fat-soluble vitamins, and vitamin K.
- Do not take other prescription drugs and OTC medications, herbal remedies, or vitamins/minerals without notifying the healthcare provider.
- Report the following immediately: yellowing of skin or whites of eyes, severe constipation, flatulence, nausea, heartburn, straining with passing of stools, tarry stools, or abnormal bleeding.

Nicotinic Acid

Nicotinic acid is a vitamin that is occasionally used to lower lipid levels. It has a number of side effects that limit its use. The dose for nicotinic acid is given in Table 27.2.

27.7 Pharmacotherapy with Nicotinic Acid

Nicotinic acid, or niacin, is a B complex vitamin. Its ability to lower lipid levels, however, is unrelated to its role as a vitamin, since much higher doses are needed to produce its antilipidemic effects. For lowering cholesterol, the usual dose is 2 to 3 g/day. When taken as a vitamin, the dose is only 25 mg/day. The primary effect of nicotinic acid is to decrease VLDL levels and, since LDL is synthesized from VLDL, the patient experiences a reduction in LDL-cholesterol levels. It also has the desirable effects of reducing triglycerides and increasing HDL levels. As with other lipid-lowering drugs, maximum therapeutic effects may take a month or longer to achieve.

Although effective at reducing LDL-cholesterol by as much as 20%, nicotinic acid produces more side effects than the statins. Flushing and hot flashes occur in almost every patient. In addition, a variety of uncomfortable intestinal effects such as nausea, excess gas, and diarrhea are commonly reported. More serious side effects such as hepatotoxicity and gout are possible. Niacin is not usually prescribed for patients with diabetes mellitus because severe hyperglycemia may result. Because of these adverse effects, nicotinic acid is most often used in lower doses in combination with a statin or bile acid-binding agent, since the beneficial effects of these drugs are additive.

Because niacin is available without a prescription, patients should be instructed not to attempt self-medication

NURSING PROCESS FOCUS — PATIENTS RECEIVING HMG-CoA REDUCTASE INHIBITOR THERAPY

ASSESSMENT

Prior to administration:
- Obtain a complete health history including allergies, drug history, and possible drug interactions.
- Obtain baseline liver function tests, lipid studies, and a pregnancy test in women of childbearing age.

POTENTIAL NURSING DIAGNOSES

- Deficient Knowledge, related to need for altered lifestyle
- Noncompliance, related to dietary and drug regimen
- Chronic Pain, related to drug-induced myopathy
- Impaired Health Maintenance, related to insufficient knowledge of actions and effects of prescribed drug therapy

PLANNING: PATIENT GOALS AND EXPECTED OUTCOMES

The patient will:
- Immediately report skeletal muscle pain, unexplained muscle soreness, or weakness
- Demonstrate compliance with appropriate lifestyle changes
- Demonstrate an understanding of the drug's action by accurately describing drug side effects and precautions

IMPLEMENTATION

Interventions and (Rationales)	Patient Education/Discharge Planning
■ Monitor blood cholesterol and triglyceride levels at intervals during therapy (to determine effectiveness of therapy).	■ Advise patient of the importance of keeping appointments for laboratory testing.
■ Monitor patient compliance with dietary regimen. (Maintenance of controlled saturated fat diet is essential to effectiveness of medications.)	■ Provide patient with information needed to maintain low saturated fat, low cholesterol diet.
■ Monitor patient for alcohol abuse. (Excessive alcohol intake may result in liver damage and interfere with drug effectiveness.)	■ Instruct patient to avoid or limit alcohol use.
■ Monitor CPK level. (Elevated CPK may be indicative of impending myopathy.)	■ Instruct patient to report symptoms of leg or muscle pain to the healthcare provider.
■ Obtain patient's smoking history. (Smoking increases risk of cardiovascular disease and may decrease HDL levels.)	■ Encourage smoking cessation if appropriate.

EVALUATION OF OUTCOME CRITERIA

Evaluate the effectiveness of drug therapy by confirming that patient goals and expected outcomes have been met (see "Planning").

See Table 27.2 for a list of drugs to which these nursing actions apply.

with this drug. One form of niacin available OTC as a vitamin supplement called nicotinamide has no lipid-lowering effects. Patients should be informed that if nicotinic acid is to be used to lower cholesterol, it should be done under medical supervision.

NURSING CONSIDERATIONS

The role of the nurse in nicotinic acid therapy involves careful monitoring of a patient's condition and providing education as it relates to the prescribed drug regimen. Because there is a risk of liver toxicity, niacin therapy must be carefully monitored. This is particularly important with sustained-release versions, which have the highest risk of hepatotoxicity. The nurse should assess liver function prior to and during therapy. Patients with elevated liver enzymes, history of liver disease, or peptic ulcers should not take niacin to lower lipids, as this medication can worsen these conditions. In patients predisposed to gout, nicotinic acid may increase uric acid levels and precipitate acute gout.

Patients are most likely to discontinue nicotinic acid therapy due to the intense flushing and pruritus that occurs 1 to 2 hours after taking the medication. This response may be caused by prostaglandin release; taking one aspirin 30

Pr PROTOTYPE DRUG | CHOLESTYRAMINE (Questran)

ACTIONS AND USES

Cholestyramine is a powder that is mixed with fluid before being taken once or twice daily. It is not absorbed or metabolized once it enters the intestine, thus it does not produce any systemic effects. It may take 30 days or longer to produce its maximum effect. Questran lowers LDL cholesterol levels by increasing LDL receptors on hepatocytes. The resultant increase in LDL intake from plasma decreases circulating LDL levels.

Administration Alerts

- Mix thoroughly with liquid and have the patient drink it immediately to avoid potential irritation or obstruction in the GI tract.
- Other drugs should be taken more than 1 hour before or 4 hours after taking cholestyramine.
- Pregnancy category C.

ADVERSE EFFECTS AND INTERACTIONS

Although cholestyramine rarely produces serious side effects, patients may experience constipation, bloating, gas, and nausea that sometimes limit its use. Because cholestyramine can bind to other drugs and interfere with their absorption, it should not be taken at the same time as other medications. Cholestyramine is sometimes combined with other cholesterol-lowering drugs such as the statins or nicotinic acid, to produce additive effects.

 See the companion website for a Nursing Process Focus specific to this drug.

minutes prior to the nicotinic acid dose will help decrease this effect. The flushing effect decreases with time. Nicotinic acid may affect glycemic control in noninsulin-dependent diabetic patients. Diabetic patients should monitor their blood sugar levels more frequently until the effect of nicotinic acid is known. GI distress is a common side effect that may be decreased by taking the drug with food.

Patient education as it relates to nicotinic acid should include the goals and reasons for obtaining baseline data such as vital signs; cardiac, hepatic, and renal disorders; and possible side effects. Following are important points the nurse should include when teaching patients regarding nicotinic acid.

- Do not take megadoses of niacin due to risk for serious toxic effects.
- Take niacin with cold water, as hot beverages increase flushing.
- Take with or after meals to prevent GI upset.
- Do not take other prescription drugs and OTC medications, herbal remedies, or vitamins/minerals without notifying the healthcare provider.
- Report the following immediately: flank, joint, or stomach pain; skin color changes (advise patient to stay out of the sun if skin changes occur); and yellowing of the whites of eyes.

Fibric Acid Agents

Once widely used to lower lipid levels, the fibric acid agents have been largely replaced by the statins. They are sometimes used in combination with the statins. The fibric acid agents are shown in Table 27.2.

NATURAL THERAPIES | Coenzyme Q10 and Cardiovascular Disease

Coenzyme Q10 (CoQ10) is a vitamin-like substance found in most animal cells. It is an essential component in the cell's mitochondria for producing energy or ATP. Because the heart requires high levels of ATP, a sufficient level of CoQ10 is essential to that organ. Supplementation with CoQ10 is especially important to patients taking the HMG-CoA reductase inhibitors, as these drugs significantly lower blood levels of CoQ10. Coenzyme Q10 and cholesterol share the same metabolic pathways. Inhibition of the enzyme HMG-CoA reductase concurrently decreases CoQ10 levels.

Foods richest in this substance are pork, sardines, beef heart, salmon, broccoli, spinach, and nuts. The elderly appear to have an increased need for CoQ10. Although CoQ10 can be synthesized by the body, many amino acids and other substances are required, thus patients having nutritional deficiencies may be in need of supplementation.

In 1978, a Nobel Prize was awarded for research proving the importance of CoQ10 in energy transfer, but it was not until the 1990s that the substance became the top-selling supplement in health food stores. CoQ10 has been purported to aid a wide range of conditions, including heart failure, hypertension, dysrhythmias, angina, diabetes, neurologic disorders, cancer, and aging. A considerable body of research has begun to accumulate, particularly regarding the role of CoQ10 in heart disease. Some data have found below-normal levels of CoQ10 in patients with heart failure. Studies suggest that the frequency of preventricular contractions may be reduced in some patients by supplementation with CoQ10. Although most studies have demonstrated positive results, CoQ10 has not been widely accepted in the conventional medical community.

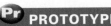 **PROTOTYPE DRUG** | **GEMFIBROZIL** (Lopid)

ACTIONS AND USES

Effects of gemfibrozil include up to a 50% reduction in VLDL with an increase in HDL. The mechanism of achieving this action is unknown. It is less effective than the statins at lowering LDL, thus it is not a drug of first choice for reducing LDL-cholesterol levels. Gemfibrozil is taken orally at 600 to 1,200 mg/day.

Administrative Alert

- Administer with meals to decrease GI distress.
- Pregnancy category B.

ADVERSE EFFECTS AND INTERACTIONS

Gemfibrozil produces few serious adverse effects but it may increase the likelihood of gallstones and occasionally affect liver function. The most common side effects are GI related: diarrhea, nausea, and cramping.

Drug interactions with gemfibrozil include oral anticoagulants; concurrent use with gemfibrozil may potentiate anticoagulant effects. Lovastatin increases the risk of myopathy and rhabdomyolysis.

 See the companion website for a Nursing Process Focus specific to this drug.

27.8 Pharmacotherapy with Fibric Acid Agents

The first fibric acid agent, clofibrate (Atromid-S) was widely prescribed until a 1978 study determined that it did not reduce mortality from cardiovascular disease. Although clofibrate is now rarely prescribed, two other fibric acid agents, fenofibrate (Tricor) and gemfibrozil (Lopid), are sometimes indicated for patients with excessive triglyceride (VLDL) levels. The mechanism of action of the fibric acid agents is largely unknown.

NURSING CONSIDERATIONS

The role of the nurse in fibric acid therapy involves careful monitoring of a patient's condition and providing education as it relates to the prescribed drug regimen. Prior to administering fibric acid, the nurse should assess the patient for abdominal pain, nausea, and vomiting, the most common adverse effects. Taking the medication with meals usually decreases GI distress. The nurse should obtain an accurate pharmacologic history. The use of fibric acid agents with statin drugs increases the risk of myositis. If a patient is taking warfarin (Coumadin), lower dosages will be needed because of competitive protein binding. More frequent monitoring of PT/INR may be necessary until stabilization occurs. Fibric acid is generally not used in lactation or pregnancy (category B). Clofibrate has a tendency to concentrate bile and cause gallbladder disease. This increase in gallbladder disease has not been seen with other fibric acid agents, but drugs in this class are generally not used in patients with preexisting gallbladder or biliary disease.

Patient education as it relates to these drugs should include the goals and reasons for obtaining baseline data such as vital signs, cardiac and renal disorders, and possible side effects. Following are the important points the nurse should include when teaching patients regarding fibric acids.

- Keep appointments for medical follow-up and laboratory tests.
- Report the following immediately: unusual bruising or bleeding, RUQ pain, changes in stool color, or muscle cramping.

CHAPTER REVIEW

Key Concepts

The numbered key concepts provide a succinct summary of the important points from the corresponding numbered section within the chapter. If any of these points are not clear, refer to the numbered section within the chapter for review. Expanded versions can be found on the companion website.

27.1 Lipids can be classified into three types, based on their chemical structures: triglycerides, phospholipids, and sterols. Triglycerides and cholesterol are blood lipids that can lead to atherosclerotic plaque.

27.2 Lipids are carried through the blood as lipoproteins; VLDL and LDL are associated with an increased incidence of cardiovascular disease, whereas HDL exerts a protective effect.

27.3 Blood lipid profiles are important diagnostic tools in guiding the therapy of dyslipidemias.

27.4 Before starting pharmacotherapy for hyperlipidemia, patients should seek to control the condition through lifestyle changes such as restriction of dietary saturated fats and cholesterol, increased exercise, and smoking cessation.

27.5 Statins, which inhibit HMG-CoA reductase, a critical enzyme in the biosynthesis of cholesterol, are drugs of first choice in reducing blood lipid levels.

27.6 The bile acid resins bind bile/cholesterol and accelerate their excretion. These agents can reduce cholesterol and LDL levels but are not drugs of choice due to their side effects.

27.7 Nicotinic acid, or niacin, can reduce LDL levels, but side effects limit its usefulness.

27.8 Fibric acid agents lower triglyceride levels but have little effect on LDL. They are not drugs of choice due to their potential side effects.

Review Questions

1. Why is the cholesterol in high-density lipoproteins considered to be "good" cholesterol?

2. How does the mechanism of action of the statins differ from that of nicotinic acid?

3. During the assessment of a new patient, what kinds of information would guide the healthcare provider in determining the need for pharmacotherapy of a dyslipidemia?

Critical Thinking Questions

1. A patient has been on atorvastatin (Lipitor) for 3 months with no side effects. The patient is moving to Florida and asks about any changes in his medication regimen once he moves. How does the nurse respond?

2. A patient is put on cholestyramine (Questran) for elevated lipids. What teaching is important for this patient?

3. A male diabetic patient presents to the emergency room with complaints of being very red (flushed) and having "hot flashes." The patient admits to self-medicating with niacin for elevated lipids. What is the nurse's response?

EXPLORE MediaLink

NCLEX review, case studies, and other interactive resources for this chapter can be found on the companion website at www.prenhall.com/adams. Click on "Chapter 27" to select the activities for this chapter. For animations, more NCLEX review questions, and an audio glossary, access the accompanying CD-ROM in this textbook.

CHAPTER 28

Drugs for Hematopoietic Disorders

■ DRUGS AT A GLANCE

HEMATOPOIETIC GROWTH FACTORS

Erythropoietin

℗ *epoetin alfa (Epogen, Procrit)*

Colony-stimulating factors

℗ *filgrastim (Neupogen)*

Platelet enhancers

ANTIANEMIC AGENTS

℗ *cyanocobalamin (Cyanabin, others): vitamin B_{12}*

Folic acid (Folvite)

Iron salts

℗ *ferrous sulfate (Ferralyn, others)*

metabolized and eliminated by the body.
of this process
PHARMACOLOGY
1. The study of medicines; the discipline
pertaining to how drugs improve the heal
of the human body
PHARMACOPEIA

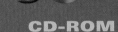 **MediaLink** www.prenhall.com/adams

CD-ROM
Audio Glossary
NCLEX Review

Companion Website
NCLEX Review
Dosage Calculations
Case Study
Care Plans
Expanded Key Concepts

OBJECTIVES

After reading this chapter, the student should be able to:

1. Describe the process of hematopoiesis.
2. Explain how hematopoiesis is regulated.
3. Explain why hematopoietic agents are often administered to patients following chemotherapy or organ transplant.
4. Identify the method by which colony-stimulating factors are named.
5. Classify types of anemia based on their causes.
6. Identify the role of intrinsic factor in the absorption of vitamin B_{12}.
7. Compare and contrast anemias caused by vitamin B_{12} and folate deficiency.

8. Describe the metabolism, storage, and transfer of iron in the body.
9. Describe the nurse's role in the pharmacologic management of hematopoietic disorders.
10. For each of the drug classes listed in Drugs at a Glance, know representative drugs, explain their mechanism of drug action, primary actions, and important adverse effects.
11. Categorize drugs used in the treatment of hematopoietic disorders based on their classification and mechanism of action.
12. Use the Nursing Process to care for patients who are receiving drug therapy for hematopoietic disorders.

The blood serves all other cells in the body and is the only fluid tissue. Because of its diverse functions, diseases affecting blood constituents have widespread effects on the body. Correspondingly, drugs for treating blood disorders will affect cells in many different tissues. Pharmacology of the hematopoietic system is a small, though emerging, branch of medicine.

28.1 Hematopoiesis

Blood is a highly dynamic tissue; over 200 billion new blood cells are formed every day. The process of blood cell formation is called hematopoiesis, or hemopoiesis. Hematopoiesis occurs primarily in red bone marrow and requires B vitamins, vitamin C, copper, iron, and other nutrients.

Hematopoiesis is responsive to the demands of the body. For example, the production of white blood cells can increase to 10 times the normal number in response to infection. The number of red blood cells can also increase as much as 5 times normal, in response to anemia or hypoxia. Homeostatic control of hematopoiesis is influenced by a number of hormones and growth factors, which allow for points of pharmacologic intervention. The process of hematopoiesis is illustrated in Figure 28.1.

The process of hematopoiesis begins with a hematopoietic stem cell, which is capable of maturing into any type of blood cell. The specific path taken by the stem cell, whether it becomes an erythrocyte, leukocyte, or platelet, depends on the internal needs of the body. Regulation of hematopoiesis occurs through messages from cer-

tain hormones such as erythropoietin, chemicals secreted by leukocytes known as colony-stimulating factors, and other circulating substances. Through recombinant DNA technology, some of these growth agents are now available in sufficient quantity to be used as medications.

HEMATOPOIETIC GROWTH FACTORS

Natural hormones that promote some aspect of blood formation are called hematopoietic growth factors. Several growth factors, shown in Table 28.1, are used pharmacologically to stimulate erythrocyte, leukocyte, or platelet production.

Human Erythropoietin and Related Drugs

28.2 Pharmacotherapy with Erythropoietin

The process of red blood cell formation, or erythropoiesis, is primarily regulated by the hormone erythropoietin. Secreted by the kidney, erythropoietin travels to the bone

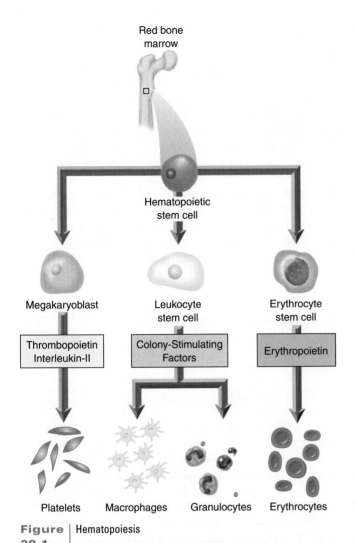

Red bone
marrow

Hematopoietic
stem cell

Megakaryoblast

Leukocyte
stem cell

Erythrocyte
stem cell

Thrombopoietin
Interleukin-II

Colony-Stimulating
Factors

Erythropoietin

Platelets   Macrophages   Granulocytes   Erythrocytes

**Figure
28.1** | Hematopoiesis

marrow where it interacts with receptors on hematopoietic stem cells with the message to increase erythrocyte production. The primary signal for the increased secretion of erythropoietin is a reduction in oxygen reaching the kidney. Serum levels of erythropoietin may increase as much as 1,000-fold in response to severe hypoxia. Hemorrhage, chronic obstructive pulmonary disease, anemia, or high altitudes may cause this hypoxia. Human erythropoietin is marketed as epoetin alfa (Epogen, Procrit)

PHARMFACTS | **Hematopoietic Disorders**

- A pregnant woman's body produces 45% more blood because it contains nutrients and oxygen for the growing fetus. The greatest increase in blood production occurs around week 20 of pregnancy when the need for iron is greatest. Many pregnant women feel tired and short of breath around this time.
- A deficiency of vitamin B_{12}, folate, or vitamin B_6 may increase the blood level of homocysteine, an amino acid normally found in the blood. An elevated blood level of homocysteine is a risk factor for heart disease and stroke.
- Vitamin B_{12} is only present in animal products. Vegetarians who do not eat meats, fish, eggs, milk or milk products, or B_{12}-fortified foods consume no vitamin B_{12} and thus are at high risk of developing a deficiency. Vegetarians may find adequate amounts in fortified cereals, nutritional supplements, or yeast.
- Administration of folic acid during pregnancy has been found to reduce birth defects in the nervous system of the baby.
- Heavy menstrual periods may result in considerable iron loss.

Table 28.1	**Hematopoietic Growth Factors**
Drug	**Route and Adult Dose (max dose where indicated)**
epoetin alfa (Epogen): erythropoietin	SC/IV; 3–500 U/kg/dose three times/wk, usually starting with 50–100 U/kg/dose until target Hct range of 30%–33% (max: 36%) is reached. Hct should not increase by more than 4 points in any 2-wk period. May increase dose if Hct has not increased 5–6 points after 8 wk of therapy, reduce dose after target range is reached, or the Hct increases by greater than 4 points in any 2-wk period, dose usually increased or decreased by 25 U/kg increments
Darbepoietin alfa (Aranesp)	SC/IV; 0.45 μg/kg once per week
Colony-stimulating Factors	
filgrastim (Neupogen): granulocyte-CSF	IV; 5 μg/kg/d by 30 min infusion, may increase by 5 μg/kg/d (max: 30 μg/kg/d); 5 μg/kg/d SC as single dose, may increase by 5 μg/kg/d (max: 20 μg/kg/d)
sargramostim (Leukine): granulocyte-macrophage-CSF	IV; 250 μg/m²/d infused over 2 h for 21 d, begin 2–4 h after bone marrow transfusion and not less than 24 h after last dose of chemotherapy or 12 h after last radiation therapy
Platelet Enhancer	
oprelvekin (Neumega)	SC; 50 μg/kg once daily starting 6–24 h after completing chemotherapy

Darbepoietin alfa (Aranesp) is a recently approved agent that is closely related to erythropoietin and epoetin alfa. It has the same pharmacologic action, efficacy, and safety profile as these other agents; however, it has an extended duration of action that allows it to be administered once weekly. Darbepoietin alfa is only approved for the treatment of anemia associated with chronic renal failure, although it is likely that other indications will be approved as additional clinical trials are completed.

NURSING CONSIDERATIONS

The role of the nurse in hematopoietic growth factor therapy involves careful monitoring of a patient's condition and providing education as it relates to the prescribed drug regimen. Since its development, epoetin alfa (Epogen, Procrit) has significantly improved the quality of life for patients with cancer, AIDS, and chronic renal failure. Although this drug does not cure the primary disease condition, it helps reduce the anemia that dramatically affects the patient's ability to perform daily activities. The nurse should assess for food or drug allergies because epoetin alfa is contraindicated in individuals who are hypersensitive to many protein-based products. The nurse should also assess for a history of uncontrolled hypertension, as the drug can raise blood pressure to dangerous levels. Baseline laboratory tests, especially a CBC, and vital signs should be obtained. Hematocrit and hemoglobin levels provide a reference for evaluating the drug's effectiveness. Epoetin alfa should be used with caution in pregnant and lactating patients (pregnancy category C).

Because this drug increases the risk of thromboembolic disease, the patients should be monitored for early signs of stroke or heart attack. Patients on dialysis are at higher risk for TIA, stroke, and MI and may need increased doses of heparin while receiving epoetin alfa. The nurse should also monitor for side effects such as nausea and vomiting, constipation, medication site reaction and headache.

See "Nursing Process Focus: Patients Receiving Epoetin Alfa" for specific teaching points.

Colony-Stimulating Factors

28.3 Pharmacotherapy with Colony-Stimulating Factors

Control of white blood cell production, or leukopoiesis, is more complicated than erythropoiesis due to the many different types of leukocytes in the blood. The two basic categories of growth factors are interleukins and colony-stimulating factors (CSFs). Because the primary action of the interleukins is to modulate the immune system rather than enhance leukopoiesis, they are presented in Chapter 31 ⊙⊃. One interleukin stimulates the production of platelets and is discussed in Section 28.4.

The leukopoietic growth factors are active at very low concentrations. It is believed that each stem cell stimulated by these growth factors is capable of producing as many as 1,000 mature leukocytes. The growth factors not only increase the production of leukocytes, but also activate existing white blood cells. Examples of enhanced functions include increased migration of leukocytes to antigens, increased antibody toxicity, and increased phagocytosis.

CSFs are named according to the types of blood cells that they stimulate. For example, granulocyte colony-stimulating factor (G-CSF) increases the production of neutrophils, the most common type of granulocyte. Granulocyte/macrophage colony-stimulating factor (GM-CSF) stimulates both neutrophil and macrophage production. The process of identifying the many endogenous CSFs, determining their normal functions, and discovering their potential value as therapeutic agents is an emerging area of pharmacology. Made through recombinant DNA technology, the two CSFs available as medications are filgrastim (Neupogen) and sargramostim (Leukine). Filgrastim is primarily used for chronic neutropenia or neutropenia secondary to chemotherapy. Sargramostim is used specifically to treat non-Hodgkins lymphoma, acute lymphoblastic leukemia, and Hodgkin's disease patients who are having autologous bone marrow transplantation.

NURSING CONSIDERATIONS

The role of the nurse in CSF therapy involves careful monitoring of a patient's condition and providing education as it relates to the prescribed drug regimen. Prior to administration of filgrastim (Neupogen), the nurse should assess for hypersensitivity to certain foreign proteins, specifically those in *E. coli*. Due to its structural components, the drug is contraindicated in patients with this type of hypersensitivity. The nurse should obtain a health history, especially checking for myeloid cancers such as leukemia, because filgrastim may stimulate proliferation of these malignant cells. This drug should not be administered simultaneously with chemotherapy. A baseline CBC with differential and platelet count should be obtained for baseline data to evaluate drug effectiveness. Usage of filgrastim (Neupogen) may cause dysrhythmias and tachycardia; therefore, a thorough initial and ongoing cardiac assessment should be performed throughout the treatment regimen.

The nurse should assess for both hypertension and skeletal pain, which are adverse effects of filgrastim therapy. The ECG readings should be monitored for abnormal ST segment depression, which is also a side effect of the drug. See "Nursing Process Focus: Patients Receiving Filgrastim" for further details on this drug.

With sargramostim (Leukine), the nurse should obtain a CBC prior to administration, because this drug is contraindicated when excessive leukemic myeloid blasts are present in blood or bone marrow. The nurse should also obtain a health history, specifically for any known hypersensitivity to GM-CSF or yeast products. Sargramostim should be used cautiously in patients with cardiac disease such as dysrhythmias or HF, because this agent may cause supraventricular dysrhythmias. This is usually a temporary side effect that disap-

Pr PROTOTYPE DRUG | **EPOETIN ALFA (Epogen, Procrit)**

ACTIONS AND USES

Epoetin alfa is made through recombinant DNA technology and is functionally identical to human erythropoietin. Because of its ability to stimulate erythropoiesis, epoetin alfa is effective in treating specific disorders caused by a deficiency in red blood cell formation. Patients with chronic renal failure often cannot secrete enough endogenous erythropoietin, and thus will benefit from epoetin administration. Epoetin is sometimes given to patients undergoing cancer chemotherapy, to counteract the anemia caused by antineoplastic agents. It is occasionally prescribed for patients prior to blood transfusions or surgery and to treat anemia in HIV-infected patients. Epoetin alfa is usually administered three times per week until a therapeutic response is achieved.

Administration Alerts

- The SC route is generally preferred over IV since lower doses are needed and absorption is slower.
- Premature infants must be given the preservative-free formulation to prevent "fetal gasping" syndrome, because infants are especially sensitive to benzyl alcohol which may be present in epoetin alfa.
- Do not shake vial because this may deactivate the drug. Visibly inspect solution for particulate matter.
- Pregnancy category C.

ADVERSE EFFECTS AND INTERACTIONS

The most common adverse effect of epoetin alfa is hypertension, which may occur in as many as 30% of patients receiving the drug. Blood pressure should be monitored during therapy, and an antihypertensive drug may be indicated. The risk of thromboembolic events is increased.

Patients who are on dialysis may require increased doses of heparin. Transient ischemic attacks (TIAs), heart attacks, and strokes have occurred in chronic renal failure patients on dialysis who are also being treated with epoetin alfa.

The effectiveness of epoetin alfa will be greatly reduced in patients with iron deficiency or other vitamin depleted states, since erythropoiesis cannot be enhanced without these vital nutrients.

There are no clinically significant drug interactions with epoetin alfa.

---

pears when the drug is discontinued. It should also be used with caution in patients with kidney and liver impairment.

It is often difficult to assess the adverse effects of CSF medications because the symptoms may also be attributed to the chemotherapy or the disease itself. A serious side effect of sargramostim is respiratory distress that occurs during the IV infusion, which develops because granulocytes become trapped in the pulmonary circulation. If this occurs, it is recommended that the nurse decrease the infusion rate. Occasionally patients will develop a syndrome that occurs the first time the drug is administered. The patient develops difficulty breathing, tachycardia, low blood pressure, and lightheadedness. This also appears to be related to the trapping of granulocytes in the pulmonary circulation. If these symptoms occur during the first infusion, the nurse should restart the infusion at half the rate after all symptoms have resolved.

Patient education is an important aspect in nursing care. Following are the general patient education points the nurse should include regarding colony-stimulating factors.

- Wash hands frequently and avoid people with infections such as colds and flu.
- Immediately report symptoms such as chest pain or palpitations, respiratory difficulty, nausea, vomiting, fever, chills, and malaise.
- Keep all physician and laboratory appointments.

Platelet Enhancers

28.4 Pharmacotherapy with Platelet Enhancers

The production of platelets, or thrombocytopoiesis, begins when megakaryocytes in the bone marrow start shedding membrane-bound packets. These packets enter the bloodstream and become platelets. A single megakaryocyte can produce thousands of platelets.

Megakaryocyte activity is controlled by the hormone thrombopoietin, which is produced by the kidneys. Thrombopoietin is not available as a medication, although it is currently undergoing clinical trials.

Oprelvekin (Neumega) is a drug, produced through recombinant DNA technology, which stimulates the production of megakaryocytes and thrombopoietin. Although it differs slightly from endogenous interleukin-11, the two are considered functionally equivalent. Oprelvekin is used to stimulate the production of platelets in patients who are at risk for thrombocytopenia caused by cancer chemotherapy. The onset of action is 5 to 9 days, and platelet counts will remain elevated for about 7 days after the last dose. Oprelvekin is only given by the SC route.

NURSING PROCESS FOCUS   PATIENTS RECEIVING EPOETIN ALFA **Pr**

ASSESSMENT

Prior to administration:
- Obtain complete health history including allergies, drug history, and possible drug reactions.
- Assess reason for drug administration such as presence/history of anemia secondary to chronic renal failure, malignancy, chemotherapy, autologous blood donation, and HIV-infected patients treated with zidovudine.
- Assess vital signs, especially blood pressure.
- Assess complete blood count, specifically hematocrit and hemoglobin levels, to establish baseline values.

POTENTIAL NURSING DIAGNOSES

- Ineffective Tissue Perfusion, related to ineffective response to drug
- Risk for Injury (weakness, dizziness, syncope), related to anemia
- Risk for Injury, related to seizure activity secondary to drug
- Activity Intolerance, related to RBC deficiency
- Deficient Knowledge, related to drug therapy

PLANNING: PATIENT GOALS AND EXPECTED OUTCOMES

The patient will:
- Exhibit an increase in hematocrit level and improvement in anemia-related symptoms
- Immediately report effects such as severe headache, chest pain, confusion, numbness, or loss of movement in an extremity
- Demonstrate an understanding of the drug's action by accurately describing drug side effects and precautions

IMPLEMENTATION

Interventions and (Rationales)	*Patient Education/Discharge Planning*
Monitor vital signs, especially blood pressure. (The rate of hypertension is directly related to the rate of rise of the hematocrit. Patients who have existing hypertension are at higher risk for stroke and seizures. Hypertension is also much more likely in patients with chronic renal failure.)	Instruct patient: • In the importance of periodic blood pressure monitoring and on the proper use of home blood pressure monitoring equipment • Of "reportable" blood pressure ranges ("Call healthcare provider when blood pressure is greater than. . . ")
Monitor for side effects, especially symptoms of neurologic or cardiovascular events.	• Instruct patient to report side effects such as nausea, vomiting, constipation, redness/pain at injection site, confusion, numbness, chest pain, and difficulty breathing.
Monitor patient's ability to self-administer medication.	Instruct patient: • In the technique for SC injection if patient is to self-administer the medication • On proper disposal of needles and syringes
Monitor laboratory values such as hematocrit and hemoglobin to evaluate effectiveness of treatment. (Increases in hematocrit and hemoglobin values indicate increased RBC production.)	Instruct patient: • On the need for initial and continuing laboratory blood monitoring • To keep all laboratory appointments • Of latest hematocrit value so that physical activities may be adjusted accordingly
Monitor patient for signs of seizure activity. (Seizures result in a rapid rise in the hematocrit—especially during first 90 days of treatment.)	• Instruct patient to not drive or perform hazardous activities until the effects of the drug are known.
Monitor patient for signs of thrombus such as swelling, warmth, and pain in an extremity. (As hematocrit rises, there is an increased chance of thrombus formation particularly for patients with chronic renal failure.)	Instruct patient: • To report any increase in size, pain, and/or warmth in an extremity • On signs and symptoms of blood clots • Not to rub or massage calves and to report leg discomfort

continued

NURSING PROCESS FOCUS: *Patients Receiving Epoetin Alfa (continued)*

Interventions and (Rationales)	Patient Education/Discharge Planning
■ Monitor dietary intake. Ensure adequate intake of all essential nutrients. (Response to this medication is minimal if blood levels of iron, folic acid, and vitamin B$_{12}$ are deficient.)	Instruct patient to: ■ Maintain adequate dietary intake of essential vitamins and nutrients ■ Continue to follow necessary dietary restrictions if receiving renal dialysis

EVALUATION OF OUTCOME CRITERIA

Evaluate the effectiveness of drug therapy by confirming that patient goals and expected outcomes have been met (see "Planning").

Pr **PROTOTYPE DRUG** | **FILGRASTIM** (Neupogen)

ACTIONS AND USES

Filgrastim is human G-CSF produced through recombinant DNA technology. Its two primary actions are to increase neutrophil production in the bone marrow and to enhance the phagocytic and cytotoxic functions of existing neutrophils. This is particularly important for patients with neutropenia, a reduction in circulating neutrophils that often results in severe bacterial and fungal infections. Administration of filgrastim will shorten the length of neutropenia in cancer patients whose bone marrow has been suppressed by antineoplastic agents or in patients following organ transplants. It may also be used in patients with AIDS-related immunosuppression. It is administered SC or by slow IV infusion.

Administration Alerts

- Do not administer within 24 hours before or after chemotherapy with cytotoxic agents as this will greatly decrease the effectiveness of filgrastim.
- Pregnancy category C.

ADVERSE EFFECTS AND INTERACTIONS

Bone pain is a common side effect of high dose filgrastim therapy. A small percentage of patients may develop an allergic reaction. Frequent laboratory tests are conducted to ensure that excessive numbers of neutrophils, or leukocytosis, does not occur. Because the antineoplastic drugs and colony-stimulating factors produce opposite effects, filgrastim is not administered until at least 24 hours after a chemotherapy session.

NURSING CONSIDERATIONS

The role of the nurse in platelet enhancer therapy involves careful monitoring of a patient's condition and providing education as it relates to the prescribed drug regimen. Oprelvekin should not be given to patients with hypersensitivity to this drug. It is used with caution in patients with cardiac disease, especially HF, dysrhythmias, and left ventricular dysfunction since fluid retention is a common side effect.

As with the colony-stimulating factors, oprelvekin should not be used within 24 hours of chemotherapy, because the cytotoxic effects of the antineoplastic agents decrease the effectiveness of the drug. Adverse effects are related to fluid retention and may be severe, and include pleural effusion and papilledema. Patients should be advised to report edema to the nurse and to avoid activities that could cause bleeding until the platelet count has returned to normal.

Oprelvekin should be withheld for 12 hours before or after radiation therapy, because the breakdown of cells after radiation will decrease the effectiveness of the medication. The nurse should monitor patients with history of edema, as this drug aggravates fluid retention and oprelvekin may cause pleural effusion or congestive heart failure.

See "Nursing Process Focus: Patients Receiving Filgrastim" for additional teaching points.

ANEMIAS

Anemia is a condition in which red blood cells have a diminished capacity to carry oxygen. Although there are many different causes of anemia, they fall into one of the following categories.

- Blood loss due to hemorrhage

NURSING PROCESS FOCUS | PATIENTS RECEIVING FILGRASTIM (NEUPOGEN) **Pr**

ASSESSMENT

Prior to administration:
- Obtain complete health history including allergies, drug history, and possible drug reactions.
- Assess reason for drug administration such as presence/history of severe bacterial or fungal infections, chemotherapy-induced neutropenia, or AIDS-related immunosuppression.
- Assess vital signs.
- Assess complete blood count, specifically WBCs with differential, to establish baseline values.

POTENTIAL NURSING DIAGNOSES

- Risk for Infection, related to impaired immune defense (low WBC)
- Risk for Injury, related to side effects of drug therapy
- Deficient Knowledge, related to drug therapy

PLANNING: PATIENT GOALS AND EXPECTED OUTCOMES

The patient will:
- Exhibit an increase in leukocyte levels and experience a decrease in the incidence of infection
- Demonstrate an understanding of the drug's action by accurately describing drug side effects and precautions
- Immediately report significant adverse effects from the medication such as nausea, vomiting, fever, chills, malaise, and skeletal pain, and allergic type responses such as rash, urticaria, wheezing, and dyspnea

IMPLEMENTATION

Interventions and (Rationales)	*Patient Education/Discharge Planning*
■ Monitor vital signs. (Myocardial infarction and dysrhythmias have occurred in a small number of patients because the drug has been known to cause abnormal ST segment depression.)	■ Instruct patient to report any chest pain or palpitations.
■ Monitor for signs and symptoms of infection. ■ Limit the patient's exposure to pathogenic microorganisms. (Patients are more susceptible to infection until WBC response is achieved)	Instruct the patient to: ■ Wash hands frequently ■ Avoid crowds and people with colds, flu, and infections ■ Cook all foods completely and thoroughly ■ Clean surfaces touched by raw foods ■ Avoid fresh fruits, vegetables, and plants until WBC level is within normal limits ■ Limit exposure to children and animals ■ Increase fluid intake and empty bladder frequently ■ Cough and deep breathe several times per day
■ Monitor complete blood count with differential until WBC count is at an acceptable level.	■ Inform patients of WBC status during the course of the treatment so they may take necessary precautions to avoid infection.
■ Monitor hepatic status during pharmacotherapy. (Filgrastim may cause an elevation in liver enzymes.)	Instruct patient: ■ On the need for initial and continuing laboratory blood monitoring ■ To keep all laboratory appointments
■ Assess for bone pain. (Drug works by stimulating bone marrow cells.)	■ Instruct patient to report any pain not relieved by OTC analgesics
■ Monitor for significant side effects and allergic type reactions. (Patient may be hypersensitive to *E.coli*.)	Instruct patient to immediately report: ■ Side effects such as nausea, vomiting, fever, chills, and malaise ■ Symptoms of allergic reaction such as rash, urticaria, wheezing, and dyspnea

continued

NURSING PROCESS FOCUS: *Patients Receiving Filgrastim (Neupogen) (continued)*

Interventions and (Rationales)	*Patient Education/Discharge Planning*
■ Monitor patient's ability to self-administer medication.	Instruct patient about: ■ Self-injection technique ■ Proper disposal of needles and syringes

EVALUATION OF OUTCOME CRITERIA

Evaluate the effectiveness of drug therapy by confirming that patient goals and expected outcomes have been met (see "Planning").

■ Excessive erythrocyte destruction
■ Diminished erythrocyte synthesis due to a deficiency in a substance needed for erythropoiesis

28.5 Classification of Anemias

Classification of anemia is generally based on a description of the erythrocyte's size and color. Sizes are described as normal (normocytic), small (microcytic), or large (macrocytic). Color is based on the amount of hemoglobin present and is described as normal red (normochromic) or light red (hypochromic). This classification is shown in Table 28.2.

Each type of anemia has specific characteristics, but all have common signs and symptoms. The patient often exhibits pallor, a paleness of the skin and mucous membranes due to hemoglobin deficiency. Decreased exercise tolerance, fatigue, and lethargy occur because of insufficient oxygen reaching muscles. Dizziness and fainting are common as the brain needs more oxygen to properly function. The cardiovascular system attempts to compensate for the oxygen depletion by increasing respiration rate and heart rate. Long-standing or severe disease can result in heart failure.

ANTIANEMIC AGENTS

Several vitamins and minerals are given to enhance the oxygen-carrying capacity of blood in patients with certain anemias. The two most common agents are cyanocobalamin (Cyanabin, others), a purified form of vitamin B_{12}, and ferrous sulfate (Ferralyn, others), an iron supplement. These agents are shown in Table 28.3.

Vitamin B_{12} and Folic Acid

28.6 Pharmacotherapy with Vitamin B_{12} and Folic Acid

Vitamin B_{12} and folic acid are dietary nutrients essential for rapidly dividing cells. Because erythropoiesis is occurring at a continuously high rate throughout the lifespan, deficiencies in these nutrients often manifest as anemias.

Vitamin B_{12} is an essential component of two coenzymes that are required for normal cell growth and replication. Vitamin B_{12} is not synthesized by either plants or animals; only bacteria serve this function. Because only miniscule amounts of vitamin B_{12} are required (3 mcg/day), deficiency of this vitamin is usually not due to insufficient dietary intake. Instead, the most common cause of vitamin B_{12} deficiency is lack of intrinsic factor, a protein secreted by stomach cells. Intrinsic factor is required for vitamin B_{12} to be absorbed from the intestine. Figure 28.2 illustrates the metabolism of vitamin B_{12}. Inflammatory diseases of the stomach or surgical removal of the stomach may result in deficiency of intrinsic factor. Inflammatory diseases of the small intestine that affect food and nutrient absorption may also cause vitamin B_{12} deficiency.

The most profound consequence of B_{12} deficiency is a condition called pernicious or megaloblastic anemia which affects both the hematologic and nervous systems. The stem cells produce abnormally large erythrocytes that do not fully mature. Red blood cells are most affected, though lack of maturation of all blood cell types may occur in severe disease. Nervous system symptoms may include

Table 28.2	Classification of Anemia	
Morphology	**Description**	**Examples**
normocytic-normochromic	loss of normal erythroblasts or mature erythrocytes	aplastic anemia hemorrhagic anemia sickle cell anemia hemolytic anemia
macrocytic-normochromic	large, abnormally shaped erythrocytes with normal hemoglobin	pernicious anemia folate deficiency anemia
microcytic-hypochromic	small, abnormally shaped erythrocytes with diminished hemoglobin	iron deficiency anemia thalassemia

Table 28.3	Antianemic Agents	
Drug	**Route and Adult Dose (max dose where indicated)**
ⓟcyanocobalamin (Cyanabin, others): vitamin B_{12}	IM/deep SC; 30 μg/d for 5–10 d, then 100–200 μg/mo
folic acid (Folvite)	PO/IM/SC/IV; <1 mg/d
Iron Salts	
ferrous fumarate (Feostat, others)	PO; 200 mg tid or qid
ferrous gluconate (Fergon)	PO; 325–600 mg qid, may be gradually increased to 650 mg qid as needed and tolerated
ⓟferrous sulfate (Ferralyn, others)	PO; 750–1500 mg/d in one to three divided doses

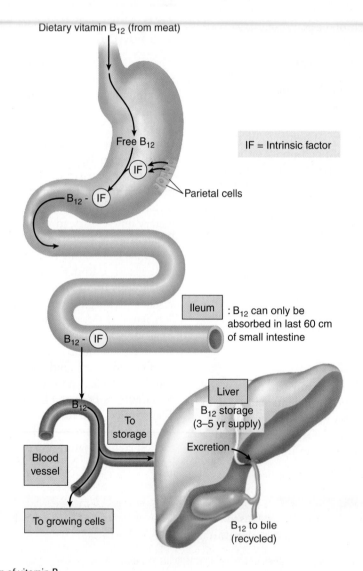

Figure 28.2 | Metabolism of vitamin B_{12}

memory loss, confusion, unsteadiness, tingling or numbness in the limbs, delusions, mood disturbances, and even hallucinations in severe deficiencies. Permanent nervous system damage may result if the disease remains untreated.

Folic acid, or folate, is another vitamin essential for normal DNA and RNA synthesis. Like B_{12} deficiency,

insufficient folic acid can manifest itself as anemia. In fact, the metabolism of vitamin B_{12} and folic acid are intricately linked; a B_{12} deficiency will create a lack of activated folic acid.

Unlike vitamin B_{12}, folic acid does not require intrinsic factor for intestinal absorption, and the most common cause of folate deficiency is insufficient dietary intake. This is most commonly observed in chronic alcoholism, although other absorption diseases of the small intestine can result in folate anemia. Hematopoietic signs of folate deficiency are the same as those for B_{12} deficiency; however, no neurologic signs are present. Folate deficiency during pregnancy has been linked to neural birth defects such as spina bifida; thus, the nurse should take special care to advise pregnant patients and those planning to become pregnant to take adequate amounts of this vitamin. Treatment is often accomplished by increasing the dietary intake of folic acid through fresh green vegetables and wheat products. In cases when adequate dietary intake cannot be achieved, therapy with folate sodium (Folvite) or folic acid is warranted. Folic acid is discussed further in Chapter 38 .

NURSING CONSIDERATIONS

The role of the nurse in antianemic agent therapy involves careful monitoring of a patient's condition and providing education as it relates to the prescribed drug regimen. Although most vitamin B_{12} deficiencies are caused by a lack of intrinsic factor, the nurse should investigate the possibility of inadequate dietary intake of the vitamin. Prior to administration the nurse should assess for other causes of anemia including GI dysfunction, GI surgery, tapeworm infestation, and gluten enteropathy.

Prior to and at regular intervals during treatment, a complete blood count is needed to evaluate the effectiveness of vitamin B_{12} therapy. This drug is not an effective treatment for iron deficiency anemias. Cyanocobalamin (Cyanabin, others) is contraindicated in patients with severe pulmonary disease and is used cautiously in patients with heart disease.

Potassium levels should be monitored during pharmacotherapy because hypokalemia is a possible side effect of this drug. The nurse should also assess patients for additional side effects such as itching, rash, or flushing. Patients taking this drug may develop pulmonary edema and heart failure, so cardiovascular status must be monitored.

See "Nursing Process Focus: Patients Receiving Cyanocobalamin" for specific teaching points.

Iron

Iron is a mineral essential to the function of several biological molecules, the most significant of which is hemoglobin. Of all iron in the body, 60% to 80% is associated with the hemoglobin in erythrocytes. Iron is also essential for a number of mitochondrial enzymes involved in metabolism and energy production in the cell. Because free iron is toxic, the body binds the mineral to the protein complexes ferritin, hemosiderin, and transferrin. Ferritin and hemosiderin maintain iron stores *inside* cells, whereas transferrin *transports* iron to sites in the body where it is needed.

28.7 Pharmacotherapy with Iron

The most common cause of nutritional anemia is iron deficiency. A primary cause of iron deficiency anemia is blood loss, such as may occur from peptic ulcer disease. Certain individuals have an increased demand for iron, including those who are pregnant, experiencing heavy menstruation, or undergoing intensive athletic training. These conditions may require more than the recommended daily allowance (RDA) of iron (Chapter 38). The most significant effect of iron deficiency is a reduction in erythropoiesis, resulting in symptoms of anemia .

Pr **PROTOTYPE DRUG**	**CYANOCOBALAMIN** (Cyanabin, others)
ACTIONS AND USES	**ADVERSE EFFECTS AND INTERACTIONS**
Cyanocobalamin is a purified form of vitamin B_{12} that is administered in deficiency states. Treatment of vitamin B_{12} deficiency is most often by weekly, biweekly, or monthly IM or SC injections. Although oral B_{12} supplements are available, they are only effective in patients having sufficient intrinsic factor and normal absorption in the small intestine. Parenteral administration rapidly reverses most signs and symptoms of B_{12} deficiency. If the disease has been prolonged, symptoms may take longer to resolve, and some neurologic damage may be permanent. In most cases, treatment must often be maintained for the remainder of the patient's life.	Side effects from cyanocobalamin are uncommon. Hypokalemia is possible, thus serum potassium levels are monitored periodically. A small percentage of patients receiving B_{12} exhibit rashes, itching, or other signs of allergy. Anaphylaxis is possible, though rare. Drug interactions with cyanocobalamin include a decrease in absorption when given concurrently with alcohol, aminosalicylic acid, neomycin, and colchicine. Chloramphenicol may interfere with therapeutic response to cyanocobalamin.

Administration Alerts

- With PO preparations, if mixed with fruit juices, administer quickly because ascorbic acid affects the stability of vitamin B_{12}.
- Pregnancy category C when used parenterally.

NURSING PROCESS FOCUS | PATIENTS RECEIVING CYANOCOBALAMIN (CYANABIN)

ASSESSMENT

Prior to administration:
- Obtain complete health history including allergies, drug history, and possible drug reactions.
- Assess vital signs.
- Assess for other causes of anemia.

POTENTIAL NURSING DIAGNOSES

- Risk for Injury (weakness, dizziness, syncope), related to anemia
- Ineffective Tissue Perfusion, related to adverse effects of drug therapy
- Deficient Knowledge, related to drug therapy

PLANNING: PATIENT GOALS AND EXPECTED OUTCOMES

The patient will
- Report a decrease in symptoms of vitamin B_{12} deficiency
- Immediately report significant side effects such as dyspnea, palpitations, fatigue, muscle weakness, and dysrhythmias
- Demonstrate an understanding of the drug's action by accurately describing drug side effects and precautions

IMPLEMENTATION

Interventions and (Rationales)	Patient Education/Discharge Planning
■ Monitor vital signs. (Altered potassium levels and overexertion may produce cardiovascular complications, especially irregular rhythm.)	■ Instruct patient to monitor pulse rate and report irregularities and changes in rhythm.
■ Monitor potassium levels during first 48 hours of therapy. (Conversion to normal red blood cell production increases the need for potassium.)	■ Instruct patient on the need for initial and continuing laboratory blood monitoring, and to keep all laboratory appointments.
■ Monitor respiratory pattern. (Pulmonary edema may occur early in therapy related to a possible sensitivity to the drug. Reactions may take up to 8 days to occur.)	■ Instruct patient to immediately report any respiratory difficulty.
■ Monitor serum vitamin B_{12}, RBCs, and hemoglobin levels to determine effectiveness of drug. (Initial doses of B_{12} stimulate rapid RBC regeneration and should return to near normal within 2 weeks.)	■ Advise patient that treatment for pernicious anemia (usually IM injection) must be continued throughout life to prevent neurologic damage.
■ Assist patient to plan activities and allow for periods of rest to conserve energy.	■ Instruct patient to rest when they begin to feel tired and avoid strenuous activities.
■ Encourage patient to maintain adequate dietary intake of essential nutrients and vitamins.	Instruct patient: ■ That dietary control, by itself, is not possible in treating pernicious anemia ■ To consume adequate dietary intake of essential nutrients and vitamins
■ Monitor for side effects such as palpitations, fatigue, muscle weakness, and dysrhythmias.	■ Teach patient to immediately report side effects to their healthcare provider.

EVALUATION OF OUTCOME CRITERIA

Evaluate the effectiveness of drug therapy by confirming that patient goals and expected outcomes have been met (see "Planning").

After erythrocytes die, nearly all of the iron in their hemoglobin is incorporated into transferrin and recycled for later use. Because of this efficient recycling, only about 1 mg of iron is excreted from the body per day, making daily dietary iron requirements in most individuals quite small. However, the amount of iron lost by some women during menstruation may be significant enough to produce anemic symptoms. Ferrous sulfate (Feosol, others),

SPECIAL CONSIDERATIONS

Iron Deficiency in Children

Iron deficiency and iron deficiency anemia have been identified as significant problems among children 1 to 2 years of age. Inadequate iron intake and storage is the main reason for this condition. Extremely low levels of iron can cause permanent mental and psychomotor impairment; therefore, prevention is of utmost importance. Primary prevention of iron deficiency can be accomplished by daily supplementation of 10 mg of elemental iron with iron-fortified vitamins, iron drops, or an iron-fortified nutritional drink. Accidental overdosing due to products containing iron is one of the leading causes of fatal poisoning in children. It is extremely important that iron be kept out of the reach of children. If overdosing occurs, caregivers should call the healthcare provider or poison control center.

ferrous gluconate (Fertinic, others), and ferrous fumarate (Feostat, others) are the most commonly used oral iron preparations.

NURSING CONSIDERATIONS

The role of the nurse in iron pharmacotherapy involves careful monitoring of a patient's condition and providing education as it relates to the prescribed drug regimen. All iron preparations have essentially the same nursing considerations. Before initiating therapy with these medicines, the nurse should obtain vital signs and a CBC, including hemoglobin and hematocrit levels, to establish baseline values. The nurse should obtain a health history, assessing for peptic ulcer, regional enteritis, ulcerative colitis, and cirrhosis of the liver, because these drugs are contraindicated in such disorders.

Iron dextran can be given as an IM injection or as an IV infusion and is often used for patients who cannot tolerate oral iron preparations. Prior to administering an infusion, the patient must receive a test dose to determine possible allergic reaction, which may cause respiratory arrest and circulatory collapse. Vital signs must be monitored during this initial infusion.

Possible GI reactions such as nausea, vomiting, constipation, and diarrhea are common with the oral iron preparations. The nurse should inform the patient that these effects will diminish over time, and that iron will turn stools a harmless dark green or black color. Taking oral iron with food reduces GI distress but also greatly reduces absorption. Common adverse reactions of iron dextran are headache and muscle and joint pain; these are more severe when given IV. These symptoms are lessened when the drug is given IM. Iron dextran appears to increase bone density in the joints, which is the probable cause of the muscle and joint pain.

See "Nursing Process Focus: Patients Receiving Ferrous Sulfate" for specific teaching points.

Pr PROTOTYPE DRUG | FERROUS SULFATE (Ferralyn, others)

ACTIONS AND USES

Ferrous sulfate is an iron supplement containing about 30% elemental iron. It is available in a wide variety of dosage forms to prevent or rapidly reverse symptoms of iron deficiency anemia. Other forms of iron include ferrous fumarate (Feostat, others), which contains 33% elemental iron, and ferrous gluconate (Fergon), which contains 12% elemental iron. The doses of these various preparations are based on their iron content.

Laboratory evaluation of hemoglobin or hematocrit values is conducted regularly, as excess iron is toxic. Although a positive therapeutic response may be achieved in 48 hours, therapy may continue for several months.

Ferrous sulfate is pregnancy category A.

Administration Alerts

- When administering IV, be careful to prevent infiltration as iron is highly irritating to tissues.
- Use the Z-track method (deep muscle) when giving IM.
- Do not crush tablet or empty contents of capsule when administering.
- Do not give tablets or capsules within 1 hour of bedtime.

ADVERSE EFFECTS AND INTERACTIONS

The most common side effect of ferrous sulfate is GI upset. Taking the drug with food will diminish GI upset but can decrease the absorption of iron by as much as 70%. In addition, antacids should not be taken with ferrous sulfate because they also reduce absorption of the mineral. Ideally, iron preparations should be administered 1 hour before or 2 hours after a meal. Patients should be advised that iron preparations may darken stools, but this is a harmless side effect. Constipation is also a common side effect. Excessive doses of iron are very toxic, and the nurse should advise patients to take their medication exactly as directed.

Drug interactions with ferrous sulfate include reduced absorption when given concurrently with antacids. Also, iron decreases the absorption of tetracyclines, thyroid hormone, levodopa, and methyldopa. It is advisable to take iron supplements *at least* 1 hour before or after other medications.

ASSESSMENT

Prior to administration:
- Obtain complete health history including allergies, drug history, and possible drug reactions.
- Assess reason for drug administration such as presence/history of anemia, or prophylaxis during infancy, childhood, and pregnancy.
- Assess complete blood count specifically hematocrit and hemoglobin levels, to establish baseline values.
- Assess vital signs.

POTENTIAL NURSING DIAGNOSES

- Risk for Imbalanced Nutrition, related to inadequate iron intake
- Risk for Impaired Gas Exchange, related to low RBC count resulting in decreased oxygenation
- Risk for Injury (weakness, dizziness, syncope), related to anemia
- Deficient Knowledge, related to drug therapy

PLANNING: PATIENT GOALS AND EXPECTED OUTCOMES

The patient will:
- Exhibit an increase in hematocrit level and improvement in anemia-related symptoms
- Demonstrate an understanding of the drug's action by accurately describing drug side effects and precautions
- Immediately report significant side effects such as gastrointestinal distress

IMPLEMENTATION

Interventions and (Rationales)

- Monitor vital signs especially pulse.
  (Increased pulse is an indicator of decreased oxygen content in the blood.)

- Monitor complete blood count to evaluate effectiveness of treatment.
  (Increases in hematocrit and hemoglobin values indicate increased RBC production.)

- Monitor changes in stool.
  (May cause constipation, change stool color, and cause false positives when stool tested for occult blood.)

- Plan activities and allow for periods of rest to help patient conserve energy.
  (Diminished iron levels result in decreased formation of hemoglobin leading to weakness.)

- Administer medication on an empty stomach (if tolerated) at least 1 hour before bedtime.
  (Maximizes absorption; taking closer to bedtime may increase the chance of GI distress.)

- Administer liquid iron preparations through a straw or place on the back of the tongue (to avoid staining the teeth).

- Monitor dietary intake to ensure adequate intake of foods high in iron.

- Monitor for potential for child access to medication.
  (Iron poisoning can be fatal to young children.)

Patient Education/Discharge Planning

- Instruct patient to monitor pulse rate and report irregularities and changes in rhythm.

Instruct patient:
- On the need for initial and continuing laboratory blood monitoring
- To keep all laboratory appointments

Instruct patient:
- That stool color may change and this is not a cause for alarm
- On measures to relieve constipation, such as including fruits and fruit juices in diet and increasing fluid intake and exercise

Instruct patient to:
- Rest when they are feeling tired and not to overexert
- Plan activities to avoid fatigue

Instruct patient:
- Not to crush or chew sustained-release preparations
- That medication may cause GI upset
- To take medication with food if GI upset becomes a problem
- To take at least 1 hour before bedtime

Instruct patient to
- Dilute liquid medication before using and to use a straw to take medication
- Rinse the mouth after swallowing to decrease the chance of staining the teeth

- Instruct patient to increase intake of iron-rich foods such as liver, egg yolks, brewer's yeast, wheat germ, and muscle meats.

- Advise parents to store iron-containing vitamins out of reach of children and in childproof containers.

EVALUATION OF OUTCOME CRITERIA

Evaluate the effectiveness of drug therapy by confirming that patient goals and expected outcomes have been met (see "Planning").

CHAPTER REVIEW

Key Concepts

The numbered key concepts provide a succinct summary of the important points from the corresponding numbered section within the chapter. If any of these points are not clear, refer to the numbered section within the chapter for review. Expanded versions can be found on the companion website.

28.1 Hematopoiesis is the process of erythrocyte production that begins with primitive stem cells that reside in bone marrow. Homeostatic control of erythropoiesis is through hematopoietic growth factors.

28.2 Erythropoietin is a hormone that stimulates the production of red blood cells and is used, as epoetin alfa, to treat specific anemias.

28.3 Colony-stimulating factors (CSFs) are growth factors that stimulate the production of leukocytes and are used following chemotherapy or organ transplants.

28.4 Platelet enhancers stimulate the activity of megakaryocytes and thrombopoietin, and increase the production of platelets.

28.5 Anemias are disorders in which blood has a reduced capacity to carry oxygen, due to hemorrhage, excessive erythrocyte destruction, or insufficient erythrocyte synthesis.

28.6 Deficiencies in either vitamin B_{12} or folic acid can lead to pernicious anemia. Treatment with cyanocobalamin or folate can reverse these anemias in many patients.

28.7 Iron deficiency is the most common cause of nutritional anemia and can be successfully treated with iron supplements.

Review Questions

1. Colony-stimulating factors are used for various disorders affecting leukocytes. Identify the usage and action for each drug in this class.

2. Although deficiencies of both vitamin B_{12} and folic acid produce megaloblastic anemias, distinct differences exist. Compare and contrast the pharmacotherapy of the two anemias.

3. Explain why iron supplements are not an effective pharmacologic treatment for anemias caused by a deficiency of intrinsic factor.

Critical Thinking Questions

1. A newly diagnosed renal failure patient asks the nurse why he must be on injections of epoetin alfa (Epogen, Procrit). How would the nurse respond?

2. A patient is receiving filgrastim (Neupogen). The healthcare provider orders vital signs to be done every shift. Is this an appropriate order? Why or why not?

3. A patient is taking ferrous sulfate (Ferralyn, others). What teaching should the nurse provide to this patient?

EXPLORE MediaLink

NCLEX review, case studies, and other interactive resources for this chapter can be found on the companion website at www.prenhall.com/adams. Click on "Chapter 28" to select the activities for this chapter. For animations, more NCLEX review questions, and an audio glossary, access the accompanying CD-ROM in this textbook.

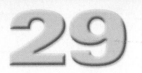

CHAPTER 29

Drugs for Pulmonary Disorders

◼ DRUGS AT A GLANCE

BRONCHODILATORS

Beta-adrenergic agonists

Pr *salmeterol (Serevent)*

Methylxanthines

Anticholinergics

Pr *ipratropium (Atrovent)*

ANTI-INFLAMMATORY AGENTS

Glucocorticoids

Pr *beclomethasone (Beclovent, Beconase, Vancenase, Vanceril)*

Mast cell stabilizers

Leukotriene modifiers

COMMON COLD AGENTS

Antitussives

Pr *dextromethorphan (Benylin)*

Expectorants

Mucolytics

of this process
metabolized and eliminated by the bod
PHARMACOLOGY
1. The study of medicines; the disciplin
pertaining to how drugs improve the he
of the human body

◎ MediaLink   www.prenhall.com/adams

CD-ROM

Animations:

   Mechanism in Action: Salmeterol (Serevent)

   Small Volume Nebulizer

   Metered Dose Inhaler (MDI)

   Dry Powder Inhaler (DPI)

Audio Glossary

NCLEX Review

Companion Website

NCLEX Review

Dosage Calculations

Care Plans

Expanded Key Concepts

aerosol *page 386*

antitussive *page 395*

asthma *page 387*

bronchospasm *page 386*

chronic bronchitis *page 397*

chronic obstructive pulmonary disease (COPD) *page 397*

dry powder inhaler (DPI) *page 387*

emphysema *page 398*

expectorants *page 397*

leukotrienes *page 395*

metered dose inhaler (MDI) *page 387*

methylxanthine *page 390*

mucolytics *page 397*

nebulizer *page 387*

perfusion *page 385*

respiration *page 385*

ventilation *page 385*

OBJECTIVES

After reading this chapter, the student should be able to:

1. Identify anatomical structures associated with the respiratory system.
2. Explain how the autonomic nervous system controls airflow in the bronchial tree, and how this can be modified with drugs.
3. Compare the advantages and disadvantages of using the inhalation route of drug administration for pulmonary drugs.
4. Describe the types of devices used to deliver aerosol therapies via the inhalation route.
5. Describe some common causes and symptoms of asthma, chronic bronchitis, and emphysema.
6. Describe the nurse's role in the pharmacologic treatment of pulmonary disorders.
7. For each of the classes listed in Drugs at a Glance, know representative drugs, explain their mechanism of drug action, primary actions on the respiratory system, and important adverse effects.
8. Categorize drugs used in the treatment of pulmonary disorders based on their classification and mechanisms of action.
9. Use the Nursing Process to care for patients who are receiving pharmacotherapy for respiratory disorders.

MediaLink Canadian Lung Association

The respiratory system is one of the most important organ systems; a mere 5 to 6 minutes without breathing may result in death. When functioning properly, the respiratory system provides the body with the oxygen critical for all cells to carry on normal activities. Measurement of respiration rate and depth and listening to chest sounds with a stethoscope provide the nurse with valuable clues as to what may be happening internally. The respiratory system also provides a means by which the body can rid itself of excess acids and bases, a topic that is covered in Chapter 44 ⌘ . This chapter examines drugs used in the pharmacotherapy of asthma, the common cold, and chronic obstructive pulmonary disease.

29.1 Physiology of the Respiratory System

The primary function of the respiratory system is to bring oxygen into the body and to remove carbon dioxide. The process by which gasses are exchanged is called respiration. The basic structures of the respiratory system are shown in Figure 29.1.

Ventilation is the process of moving air into and out of the lungs. As the diaphragm contracts and lowers in position, it creates a negative pressure that draws air into the lungs, and inspiration occurs. During expiration, the diaphragm relaxes and air leaves the lung passively, with no energy expenditure required. Ventilation is a purely mechanical process that occurs approximately 12 to 18 times per minute in adults, a rate determined by neurons in the brainstem.

This rate may be modified by a number of factors, including emotions, fever, stress, and the pH of the blood.

Air entering the respiratory system travels through the nose, pharynx, and trachea into the bronchi, which divide into progressively smaller passages called bronchioles. The bronchial tree ends in dilated sacs called alveoli which have no smooth muscle, but are abundantly rich in capillaries. An extremely thin membrane in the alveoli separates the airway from the pulmonary capillaries, allowing gasses to readily move between the internal environment of the blood and the inspired air. As oxygen crosses this membrane, it is exchanged for carbon dioxide, a cellular waste product that travels from the blood to the air. The lung is richly supplied with blood. Blood flow through the lung is called perfusion. The process of gas exchange is shown in Figure 29.1.

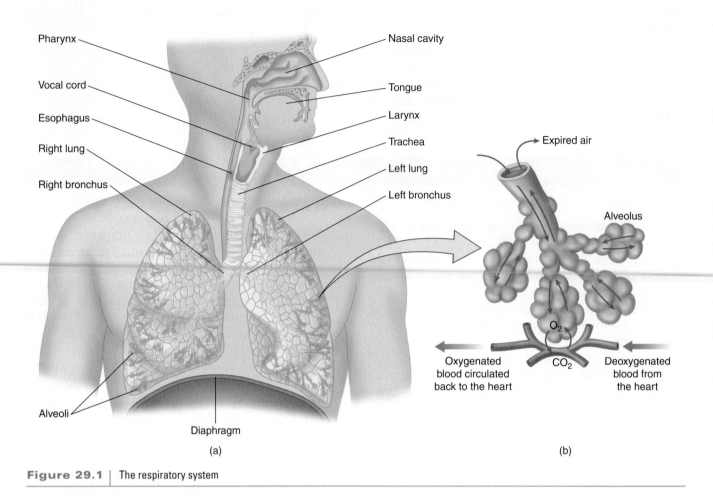

Pharynx

Vocal cord

Esophagus

Right lung

Right bronchus

Alveoli

Diaphragm

(a)

Nasal cavity

Tongue

Larynx

Trachea

Left lung

Left bronchus

Expired air

Alveolus

O_2

CO_2

Oxygenated
blood circulated
back to the heart

Deoxygenated
blood from
the heart

(b)

Figure 29.1 | The respiratory system

29.2 Bronchiolar Smooth Muscle

Bronchioles are muscular, elastic structures whose diameter, or lumen, varies with the specific needs of the body. Changes in the diameter of the bronchiolar lumen are made possible by smooth muscle controlled by the autonomic nervous system. During the fight-or-flight response, beta$_2$-adrenergic receptors of the sympathetic nervous system are stimulated, the bronchiolar smooth muscle relaxes, and bronchodilation occurs. This allows more air to enter the alveoli, thus increasing the oxygen supply to the body during periods of stress or exercise. Sympathetic nervous system activation also increases the rate and depth of breathing. Drugs that stimulate beta$_2$-adrenergic receptors to cause bronchodilation are some of the most common drugs for treating pulmonary disorders.

When nerves from the parasympathetic nervous system are activated, bronchiolar smooth muscle contracts and the airway diameter narrows, resulting in bronchoconstriction. Bronchoconstriction increases airway resistance, causing breathing to be more labored and the patient to become short of breath. Parasympathetic stimulation also has the effect of slowing the rate and depth of respiration.

29.3 Administration of Pulmonary Drugs via Inhalation

The respiratory system offers a rapid and efficient mechanism for delivering drugs. The enormous surface area of the bronchioles and alveoli, and the rich blood supply to these areas, results in an almost instantaneous onset of action for inhaled substances.

Pulmonary drugs are delivered to the respiratory system by aerosol therapy. An **aerosol** is a suspension of minute liquid droplets or fine solid particles suspended in a gas. Aerosol therapy can give immediate relief for **bronchospasm**, a condition during which the bronchiolar smooth muscle contracts, leaving the patient gasping for breath. Drugs may also be given to loosen viscous mucus in the bronchial tree. The major advantage of aerosol therapy is that it delivers the drugs to their immediate site of action, thus reducing systemic side effects. To produce the same therapeutic action, an oral drug would have to be given at higher doses, and be distributed to all body tissues.

It should be clearly understood that agents delivered by inhalation can produce systemic effects due to absorption. For example, anesthetics such as nitrous oxide and halothane (Fluothane) are delivered via the inhalation route

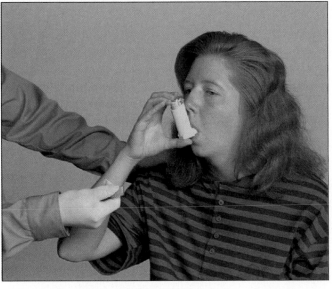

(a) Metered dose inhaler

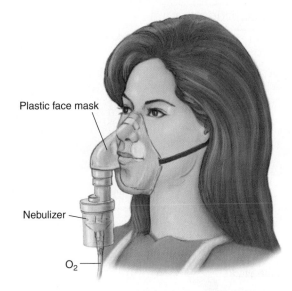

Plastic face mask

Nebulizer

O₂

(b) Nebulizer with attached face mask

Figure 29.2 | Devices used to deliver respiratory drugs *Source: Pearson Education/PH College.*

and are rapidly distributed to cause CNS depression (Chapter 20). Solvents such as paint thinners and glues are sometimes intentionally inhaled and can cause serious adverse effects on the nervous system and even death. The nurse must always monitor for systemic effects from inhalation drugs.

Several devices are used to deliver drugs via the inhalation route. Nebulizers are small machines that vaporize a liquid medication into a fine mist that can be inhaled, using a facemask or handheld device. If the drug is a solid, it may be administered using a dry powder inhaler (DPI). A DPI is a small device that is activated by the process of inhalation to deliver a fine powder directly to the bronchial tree. Turbohalers and rotahalers are types of DPIs. Metered dose inhalers (MDIs) are a third type of device commonly used to deliver respiratory drugs. MDIs use a propellant to deliver a measured dose of drugs to the lungs during each breath. The patient times the inhalation to the puffs of drug emitted from the MDI.

There are disadvantages to administering aerosol therapy. The precise dose received by the patient is difficult to measure because it depends on the patient's breathing pattern and the correct use of the aerosol device. Even under optimal conditions, only 10% to 50% of the drug actually reaches the bronchial tree. The nurse must carefully instruct patients on the correct use of these devices. To reduce the oral absorption of inhaled medicines, patients should rinse their mouth thoroughly following drug use. Two devices used to deliver respiratory drugs are shown in Figure 29.2.

ASTHMA

Asthma is a chronic disease with both inflammatory and bronchospasm components. Drugs may be given to de-

NATURAL THERAPIES | **Horehound for Respiratory Disorders**

Horehound has been used as an herbal remedy since the ancient Egyptians and was popular with American Indians. In folklore, horehound was reported to aid in a number of respiratory disorders, including asthma, bronchitis, whooping cough, and infections such as tuberculosis. Nonrespiratory uses include bowel disorders, jaundice, and wound healing.

Active ingredients of horehound are found throughout the flowering plant. The chief constituent is a bitter substance called marrubium that stimulates secretions. Formulations include tea, dried or fresh leaves, and liquid extracts. Horehound has an expectorant action when treating colds and is also available as cough drops. It is purported to restore normal secretions to the lung and other organs.

crease the frequency of asthmatic attacks or to terminate attacks in progress.

29.4 Pathophysiology of Asthma

Asthma is one of the most common chronic conditions in the United States, affecting almost 15 million Americans. The disease is characterized by acute bronchospasm, causing intense breathlessness, coughing, and gasping for air. Along with bronchoconstriction, the acute inflammatory response is initiated, stimulating mucous secretion and edema in the airways. These conditions are illustrated in Figure 29.3. Status asthmaticus is a severe, prolonged form of asthma unresponsive to drug treatment that may lead to respiratory failure. Typical causes of asthmatic attacks are shown in Table 29.1.

MediaLink Small Volume Nebulizer Animation

MediaLink DPI Animation

MediaLink MDI Animation

NORMAL BRONCHIOLE

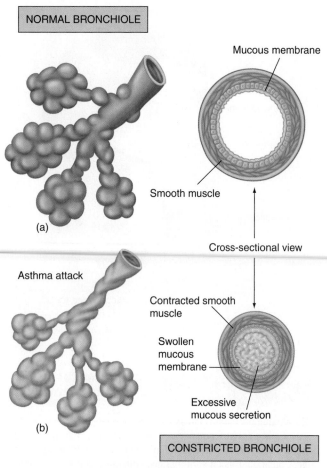

Mucous membrane

Smooth muscle

(a)

Cross-sectional view

Asthma attack

Contracted smooth muscle

Swollen mucous membrane

Excessive mucous secretion

(b)

CONSTRICTED BRONCHIOLE

Figure 29.3 Changes in bronchioles during an asthma attack: (a) normal bronchiole; and (b) in asthma attack.

Table 29.1	Common Causes of Asthma
Cause	**Sources**
air pollutants	tobacco smoke ozone nitrous and sulfur oxides fumes from cleaning fluids or solvents burning leaves
allergens	pollen from trees, grasses, and weeds animal dander household dust mold
chemicals and food	drugs, including aspirin, ibuprofen, and beta-blockers sulfite preservatives food and condiments, including nuts, monosodium glutamate (MSG), shellfish, and dairy products
respiratory infections	bacterial, fungal, and viral
stress	emotional stress/anxiety exercise in dry, cold climates

Although the exact etiology of asthma is unknown, it is believed to be the result of chronic airway inflammation. Because asthma has both a bronchoconstriction component and an inflammation component, pharmacotherapy of the disease focuses on one or both of these mechanisms. The goals of drug therapy are twofold: to terminate acute bronchospasms in progress and to reduce the frequency of acute asthma attacks. Different medications are usually needed to achieve each of these goals. A summary of the various classes of drugs used to treat respiratory diseases is illustrated in Figure 29.4.

Beta-Adrenergic Agonists

Selective beta$_2$ agonists are effective at relieving acute bronchospasm. They are some of the most frequently prescribed agents for the pharmacotherapy of asthma and other pulmonary diseases. These drugs are shown in Table 29.2.

29.5 Treating Asthma with Beta-Adrenergic Agonists

Beta-adrenergic agonists, or sympathomimetics, are drugs of choice in the treatment of acute bronchoconstriction. Sympathomimetics selective for beta$_2$-receptors in the lung have largely replaced the older, nonselective agents such as epinephrine, because they produce fewer cardiac side effects. Sympathomimetics act by relaxing bronchial smooth muscle; the resulting bronchodilation lowers airway resistance and makes breathing easier for the patient.

A practical method for classifying beta-adrenergic agonists for asthma is by their duration of action. The ultrashort-acting drugs, including isoproterenol (Isuprel) and isoetharine (Bronkosol), produce bronchodilation immediately, but their effects only last 2 to 3 hours. Short-acting agents such as metaproterenol (Metaprel), terbutaline (Brethine), and pirbuterol (Maxair), also act quickly, but last 5 to 6 hours. Intermediate-acting sympathomimetics such as albuterol (Proventil), levalbuterol (Xopenex), and bitolterol (Tornalate) last about 8 hours. The longest acting agent, salmeterol (Serevent), has effects lasting as long as 12 hours. The ultrashort-, short-, and intermediate-acting drugs act quickly enough to terminate acute asthmatic episodes. The onset of action for salmeterol is too long for it to be indicated for asthma termination. Formoterol (Foradil) is the newest beta$_2$-adrenergic agonist which combines a very rapid onset of action (1–3 minutes) with a 12 hour duration.

Inhaled beta-adrenergic agonists produce little systemic toxicity because only small amounts of the drugs are absorbed. When given orally, a longer duration of action is achieved, but systemic side effects such as tachycardia are more frequently experienced; they are sometimes contraindicated for patients with dysrhythmias. Tolerance may develop to the therapeutic effects of the beta agonists; therefore, the patient must be instructed to seek medical attention should the drugs become less effective with continued use.

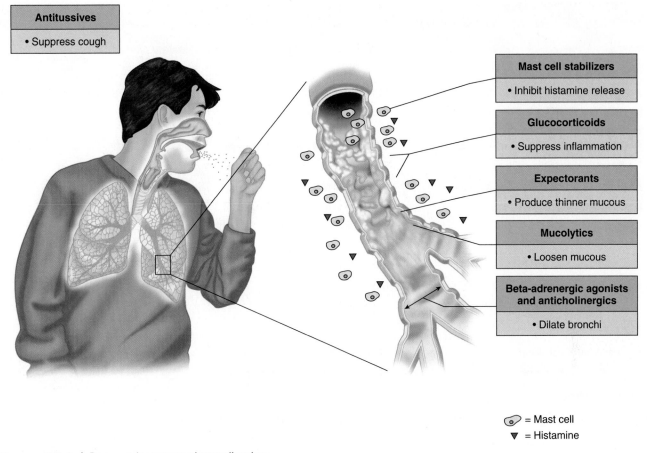

Figure 29.4 | Drugs used to treat respiratory disorders

PHARMFACTS | **Asthma**

- Over 15 million people have asthma.
- Asthma is responsible for over 1.5 million emergency room visits and over 500,000 hospitalizations each year.
- Over 5,500 patients die of asthma each year.
- Estimated direct and indirect costs for asthma total more than $12 billion each year.
- The incidence of asthma has been dramatically increasing each year since 1980 in all age, sex, and ethnic groups. The highest rate of increase has been among blacks.
- The highest incidence of asthma is in patients under the age of 18; from 7% to 10% of children have the disease.
- In adults, asthma is slightly more common in females than in males. In children, however, the disease affects twice as many boys as girls.

NURSING CONSIDERATIONS

The role of the nurse in asthma therapy with beta-adrenergic agonists involves careful monitoring of a patient's condition and providing education as it relates to the prescribed drug regimen. Experiencing breathing difficulties can be distressing and greatly impact a patient's quality of life. Controlling asthma is vital to a person's ability to perform normal activities of daily living. When beta-adrenergic agonists are used as bronchodilators, they help to reduce respiratory distress.

The nurse should assess the patient's adherence to medication and the presence of side effects. The nurse should also assess for the presence/history of bradycardia, dysrhythmias, myocardial infarction, hypothyroidism, decreased renal function, diabetes mellitus, glaucoma, benign prostatic hyperplasia, and tuberculosis. Beta-adrenergic agonists should not be used if the patient has a history of dysrhythmia or myocardial infarction. Drugs in this class may cause many undesirable side effects. For patients using isoproterenol (Isuprel), rebound bronchospasm may occur when effects of the drug wear off.

The nurse should instruct the patient on the use of the inhaler, and observe its use. The patient should hold his or her breath for 10 seconds after inhaling the medication, and wait 2 full minutes before the second inhalation. Saliva and sputum may appear pink after inhalation.

Patient education as it relates to beta-adrenergic agonists should include the goals, reasons for obtaining baseline data such as vital signs and tests for cardiac and renal disorders, and possible side effects. Following are important points the nurse should include when teaching patients regarding beta-adrenergic agonists.

- Limit the use of products that contain caffeine.
- Immediately report difficulty breathing, heart palpitations, tremor, vomiting, nervousness, or vision changes.

Table 29.2	Bronchodilators Used for Asthma
Drug	**Route and Adult Dose (max dose where indicated)**
Beta Agonists/Sympathomimetics	
albuterol (Proventil, Salbutamol, others)	PO; 2–4 mg tid-qid
bitolterol mesylate (Tornalate)	MDI; Two inhalations tid-qid
epinephrine (Adrenalin, Bronkaid, Primatene) (see page 435 for the Prototype Drug box) ∞	SC; 0.1–0.5 ml of 1:1000 q 20 min–4h
formoterol fumarate (Foradil)	DPI; 12 μg inhalation capsule q12h
isoetharine HCl (Bronkosol, Bronkometer)	MDI; One to two inhalations q4h up to 5 days
isoproterenol (Isuprel, Medihaler-Iso)	MDI; One to two inhalations q4h qid
levalbuterol HCl (Xopenex)	Nebulizer; 0.63 mg tid-qid
metaproterenol sulfate (Alupent, Metaprel)	MDI; Two to three inhalations q3–4h (max 12 inhalations/day)
pirbuterol acetate (Maxair)	MDI; Two inhalations qid (max 12 inhalations/day)
Pr salmeterol (Serevent)	MDI; Two inhalations bid
terbutaline sulfate (Brethaire, Brethine)	PO; 2.5–5 mg tid
Methylxanthines	
aminophylline (Truphylline)	PO; 0.25–0.75 mg/kg/hr divided qid
theophylline (Theo-Dur, others)	PO; 0.4–0.6 mg/kg/hr divided tid-qid
Anticholinergic	
Pr ipratropium bromide (Atrovent, Combivent)	MDI; Two inhalations qid (max 12 inhalations/day)

See "Nursing Process Focus: Patients Receiving Sympathomimetic Therapy," page 137 in Chapter 13, for the complete Nursing Process applied to caring for patients receiving beta-adrenergic agonists (sympathomimetics) ∞ .

Methylxanthines and Anticholinergics

Although beta agonists are drugs of choice for treating acute bronchospasm, drugs in the methylxanthine and anticholinergic classes are alternatives in the treatment of asthma. The methylxanthines are older, established drugs. Only one anticholinergic is in widespread use. These agents are shown in Table 29.2.

29.6 Treating Asthma with Methylxanthines and Anticholinergics

The methylxanthines comprise a group of bronchodilators chemically related to caffeine. Theophylline (Theo-Dur, others) and aminophylline (Somophyllin) were considered drugs of choice for bronchoconstriction 20 years ago. Theophylline, however, has a narrow margin of safety and interacts with a large number of other drugs. Side effects such as nausea, vomiting, and CNS stimulation are relatively common and dysrhythmias may be observed at high doses. Because of their chemical similarities, patients should avoid caffeine-containing foods and beverages when taking methylxanthines. These agents are given by the PO or IV routes. Having been largely replaced by safer and more effective drugs, the current use of theophylline is primarily for the long-term oral prophylaxis of persistent asthma.

Blocking the parasympathetic nervous system produces similar effects to stimulation of the sympathetic nervous system. It is predictable, then, that anticholinergic drugs would cause bronchodilation and have potential use in the pharmacotherapy of asthma and other pulmonary diseases. Despite its many side effects, atropine was once widely used in asthma pharmacotherapy prior to the discovery of the inhaled beta agonists. A newer anticholinergic, ipratropium (Atrovent), is the only anticholinergic commonly used for asthma pharmacotherapy. Combivent is a combination of ipratropium and albuterol in a single MDI canister.

NURSING CONSIDERATIONS

The role of the nurse in asthma therapy with methylxanthines and anticholinergics involves careful monitoring of a patient's condition and providing education as it relates to the prescribed drug regimen. The nurse should carefully assess respiration rate before and after the first dose of a metered dose inhaler because the first dose may precipitate bronchospasm. The nurse should monitor vital signs and intake and output throughout therapy, as these drugs cause diuresis. Elderly patients using methylxanthines should be carefully monitored for toxicity as these patients may exhibit increased sensitivity due to decreased hepatic metabolism.

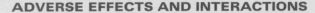

Pr PROTOTYPE DRUG | SALMETEROL (Serevent)

ACTIONS AND USES

Salmeterol acts by selectively binding to beta$_2$-adrenergic receptors in bronchial smooth muscle to cause bronchodilation. When taken 30 to 60 minutes prior to physical activity, it has been shown to prevent exercise-induced bronchospasm. Its 12-hour duration of action is longer than many other bronchodilators, thus making it ideal for asthma maintenance therapy. Because salmeterol takes 15 to 25 minutes to act, it is not indicated for the termination of acute bronchospasm.

Administration Alerts

- Proper use of the metered dose inhaler is important to effective delivery of drug. Observe and instruct patient in proper use.
- Pregnancy category C.

ADVERSE EFFECTS AND INTERACTIONS

Serious adverse effects from salmeterol are uncommon. Like other beta agonists, some patients experience headaches, nervousness, and restlessness. Because of its potential to cause tachycardia, patients with heart disease should be monitored regularly.

Concurrent use of beta-blockers will antagonize the effects of salmeterol.

 See the companion website for a Nursing Process Focus specific to this drug.

Pr PROTOTYPE DRUG | IPRATROPIUM BROMIDE (Atrovent, Combivent)

ACTIONS AND USES

Ipratropium is an anticholinergic muscarinic antagonist that causes bronchodilation by blocking cholinergic receptors in bronchial smooth muscle. It is taken via inhalation and can relieve acute bronchospasm within minutes after administration. Effects may continue for up to 6 hours. Ipratropium is less effective than the beta$_2$ agonists but is sometimes combined with beta-agonists or glucocorticoids for their synergistic effects. It is also prescribed for chronic bronchitis and for the symptomatic relief of nasal congestion. Ipratropium is pregnancy category B.

Administration Alerts

- Proper use of the metered dose inhaler is important to effective delivery of drug. Observe and instruct patient in proper use.
- Avoid contact with eyes.

ADVERSE EFFECTS AND INTERACTIONS

Because it is not readily absorbed from the lungs, ipratropium produces few systemic side effects. Irritation of the upper respiratory tract may result in cough, drying of the nasal mucosa, or hoarseness. It produces a bitter taste, which may be relieved by rinsing the mouth after use.

 See the companion website for a Nursing Process Focus specific to this drug.

Methylxanthines may cause dysrhythmias, nausea, vomiting, and irritation of the upper respiratory tract, which may result in cough, drying of mucus membranes, and a bitter taste. To help with dry mouth and bitterness, patients can rinse their mouths frequently, or use sugarless, hard candy.

Anticholinergic bronchodilators should be used cautiously in elderly men with benign prostatic hypertrophy and in all patients with glaucoma. The complete Nursing Process applied to patients receiving anticholinergics is presented in "Nursing Process Focus: Patients Receiving Anticholinergic Therapy," on page 134 in Chapter 13. ∞

Patient education as it relates to methylxanthines should include the goals, reasons for obtaining baseline data such as vital signs and tests for cardiac and renal disorders, and possible side effects. The nurse should instruct the patient to report the following immediately: inability to urinate or have a bowel movement, severe headache, heart palpitations, difficulty breathing, changes in vision, or eye pain.

For additional nursing considerations, please refer to "Nursing Process Focus: Patients Receiving Bronchodilators".

Glucocorticoids

Inhaled glucocorticoids are used for the long-term prevention of asthmatic attacks. Oral glucocorticoids may be used for the short-term management of acute asthma. The glucocorticoids are shown in Table 29.3.

NURSING PROCESS FOCUS — PATIENTS RECEIVING BRONCHODILATORS

ASSESSMENT

Prior to administration:
- Obtain complete health history including allergies, drug history, and possible drug reactions.
- Assess for symptoms related to respiratory deficiency such as dyspnea, orthopnea, cyanosis, nasal flaring, wheezing, and weakness.
- Obtain vital signs.
- Auscultate bilateral breath sounds for air movement and adventitious sounds (rales, rhonchi, wheezes).
- Assess pulmonary function with pulse oximeter, peak expiratory flow meter, and/or arterial blood gasses to establish baseline.

POTENTIAL NURSING DIAGNOSES

- Impaired Gas Exchange, related to bronchial constriction
- Activity Intolerance, related to ineffective drug therapy
- Deficient Knowledge, related to drug therapy
- Anxiety, related to difficulty in breathing
- Disturbed Sleep Pattern, related to side effects of drugs
- Ineffective Tissue Perfusion, related to adverse effects of drugs

PLANNING: PATIENT GOALS AND EXPECTED OUTCOMES

The patient will:
- Exhibit adequate oxygenation as evidenced by improved lung sounds and pulmonary function values
- Report a reduction in subjective symptoms of respiratory deficiency
- Demonstrate an understanding of the drug's action by accurately describing drug side effects and precautions
- Report at least 6 hours of uninterrupted sleep

IMPLEMENTATION

Interventions and (Rationales)	Patient Education/Discharge Planning
■ Monitor vital signs including pulse, blood pressure, and respiratory rate.	Instruct patient to: ■ Use medication as directed even if asymptomatic ■ Report difficulty with breathing
■ Monitor pulmonary function with pulse oximeter, peak expiratory flow meter, and/or arterial blood gasses. (Monitoring is necessary to assess drug effectiveness.)	■ Instruct patient to report symptoms of deteriorating respiratory status such as increased dyspnea, breathlessness with speech, and/or orthopnea.
■ Monitor the patient's ability to use inhaler. (Proper use ensures correct dosage.)	Instruct patient: ■ In proper use of metered dose inhaler ■ To strictly use the medication as prescribed; do not "double up" on doses ■ To rinse mouth thoroughly following use
■ Observe for side effects specific to the medication used.	■ Instruct patient regarding side effects and to report specific drug side effects.
■ Maintain environment free of respiratory contaminants such as dust, dry air, flowers, and smoke. (These substances may exacerbate bronchial constriction.)	Instruct patient to: ■ Avoid respiratory irritants ■ Maintain "clean air environment" ■ Stop smoking and avoid second-hand smoke, if applicable
■ Maintain dietary intake adequate in essential nutrients and vitamins. (Dyspnea interferes with proper nutrition.) ■ Ensure patient maintains adequate hydration of 3 to 4 L/day (to liquefy pulmonary secretions).	Instruct patient to: ■ Maintain nutrition with foods high in essential nutrients ■ Consume small frequent meals to prevent fatigue ■ Consume 3 to 4 L of fluid/day if not contraindicated ■ Avoid caffeine (increases CNS irritability)
■ Provide emotional and psychosocial support during periods of shortness of breath.	■ Instruct patient in relaxation techniques and controlled breathing techniques.
■ Monitor patient compliance. (Maintaining therapeutic drug levels is essential to effective therapy.)	■ Inform the patient of the importance of ongoing medication compliance and follow-up.

continued

EVALUATION OF OUTCOME CRITERIA

Evaluate the effectiveness of drug therapy by confirming that patient goals and expected outcomes have been met (see "Planning").

See Table 29.2 for a list of drugs to which these nursing actions apply.

29.7 Pharmacotherapy of Asthma with Glucocorticoids

Glucocorticoids are the most effective drugs available for the prevention of acute asthmatic episodes. When inhaled on a daily schedule, these hormones suppress inflammation without major side effects. Patients should be informed that inhaled glucocorticoids must be taken daily to produce their therapeutic effect and that these drugs are not effective at terminating episodes in progress. For some patients, a beta-adrenergic agonist may be prescribed along with an inhaled glucocorticoid, since this permits the dose of the glucocorticoid to be reduced as much as 50%.

For severe, persistent asthma that is unresponsive to other treatments, oral glucocorticoids may be prescribed. If taken for longer than 10 days, oral glucocorticoids can produce significant adverse effects, including adrenal gland atrophy, peptic ulcers, and hyperglycemia. Other uses and adverse effects of glucocorticoids are presented in Chapters 31 and 39.

NURSING CONSIDERATIONS

The role of the nurse in asthma pharmacotherapy with glucocorticoids involves careful monitoring of a patient's condition and providing education as it relates to the prescribed drug regimen. The nurse should assess the patient for presence/history of asthma, seasonal rhinitis, hypertension, heart disease, and blood clots. The nurse should also monitor the patient's vital signs and body weight, and assess for signs and symptoms of infection. The steroid inhalers should be used cautiously in patients with hypertension, GI disease, congestive heart failure, and thromboembolic disease.

Since the primary purpose of inhaled glucocorticoids is to *prevent* respiratory distress, the patient should be advised that this medication should not be used during an acute asthma attack. Additionally, the patient should be alerted to watch for signs and symptoms of simple infections, as glucocorticoids inhibit the inflammatory response and can mask the signs of infection. The patient should be advised to rinse the mouth after using steroid inhalers because the drugs may promote fungal infections of the mouth and throat. Glucocorticoids also increase blood glucose levels and should be closely monitored in individuals with diabetes mellitus.

Patient education as it relates to glucocorticoids should include the goals, reasons for obtaining baseline data such as vital signs and tests for cardiac and renal disorders, and possible side effects. Following are the important points the nurse should include when teaching patients regarding corticosteroids.

- Monitor temperature and blood pressure daily and report elevation to the healthcare provider.
- If diabetic, monitor blood glucose level closely and report unexplained or consistent elevations.
- Report occurrence of tarry stools, edema, dizziness, or difficulty breathing.
- Do not use these medications to terminate acute asthma attacks. Discuss with healthcare provider the appropriate medication to stop attacks.

See "Nursing Process Focus: Patients Receiving Systemic Glucocorticoid Therapy" 584 in Chapter 39, for the complete Nursing Process applied to caring for patients receiving glucocorticoids.

Mast Cell Stabilizers

Two mast cell stabilizers serve limited though important roles in the prophylaxis of asthma. The mast cell stabilizers act by inhibiting the release of histamine from mast cells. These drugs are shown in Table 29.3 (page 394).

29.8 Treating Asthma with Mast Cell Stabilizers

Cromolyn (Intal) and nedocromil (Tilade) are classified as mast cell stabilizers, because their action serves to inhibit mast cells from releasing histamine and other chemical mediators of inflammation. By reducing inflammation they are able to prevent asthma attacks. As with the glucocorticoids, patients must be informed that these agents should be taken on a daily basis and that they are not effective at terminating acute attacks. Maximum therapeutic benefit may take several weeks. Both cromolyn and nedocromil are pregnancy category B.

Cromolyn (Intal) was the first mast stabilizer discovered. When administered via an MDI or a nebulizer, this drug is a safe alternative to glucocorticoids. An intranasal form of cromolyn (Nasalcrom) is used in the treatment of seasonal allergies. Side effects include stinging or burning of the nasal mucosa, irritation of the throat, and nasal congestion. Although not common, bronchospasm and anaphylaxis have been reported. Because of its short half-life (80 minutes), it must be inhaled four to six times per day.

Nedocromil (Tilade) is a newer mast cell stabilizer that has actions and uses similar to cromolyn. Administered with an MDI, the drug produces side effects similar to cromolyn although its longer half-life of 2.3 hours allows less frequent dosing. Patients often experience a bitter, unpleasant taste.

Leukotriene Modifiers

The leukotriene modifiers are newer drugs, approved in the 1990s, used to reduce inflammation and ease bronchoconstriction. They modify the action of leukotrienes, which are mediators of the inflammatory response in asthmatic patients. These drugs are shown in Table 29.3.

Table 29.3	Anti-inflammatory Drugs Used for Asthma
Drug	**Route and Adult Dose (max dose where indicated)**
Glucocorticoids	
beclomethasone (Beclovent, Vanceril, others)	MDI; One to two inhalations tid or qid (max 20 inhalations/day)
budesonide (Pulmicort Turbuhaler)	DPI; One to two inhalations (200 μg/inhalation) qid (max 800 μg/day)
flunisolide (AeroBid)	MDI; Two to three inhalations bid or tid (max 12 inhalations/day)
fluticasone (Flovent) (see page 432 for the Prototype Drug box)	MDI (44 mcg); Two inhalations bid (max 10 inhalations/day)
methylprednisolone (Depo-Medrol, others)	PO; 4–48 mg qd
prednisone (Deltasone, Meticorten, others) (see page 423 for the Prototype Drug box)	PO; 5–60 mg qd
triamcinolone (Azmacort)	MDI; Two inhalations tid or qid (max 16 inhalations/day)
Mast Cell Stabilizers	
cromolyn (Intal)	MDI; One inhalation qid
nedocromil sodium (Tilade)	MDI; Two inhalations qid
Leukotriene Modifiers	
montelukast (Singulair)	PO; 10 mg qd in evening
zafirlukast (Accolate)	PO; 20 mg bid 1 h before or 2 h after meals
zileuton (Zyflo)	PO; 600 mg qid

Pr PROTOTYPE DRUG | BECLOMETHASONE (Beclovent, Beconase, Vancenase, Vanceril)

ACTIONS AND USES

Beclomethasone is a glucocorticoid available through aerosol inhalation (MDI) for asthma or as a nasal spray for allergic rhinitis. For asthma, two inhalations, two to three times per day, usually provide adequate prophylaxis. Beclomethasone acts by reducing inflammation, thus decreasing the frequency of asthma attacks. It is not a bronchodilator and should not be used to terminate asthma attacks in progress.

Administration Alerts

■ Do not use if the patient is experiencing an acute asthma attack.
■ Oral inhalation products and nasal spray products are not to be used interchangeably.
■ Pregnancy category C.

ADVERSE EFFECTS AND INTERACTIONS

Inhaled beclomethasone produces few systemic side effects. Because small amounts may be swallowed with each dose, the patient should be observed for signs of glucocorticoid toxicity when taking the drug for prolonged periods. Local effects may include hoarseness in the voice. Like all glucocorticoids, the anti-inflammatory properties of beclomethasone can mask signs of infections and the drug is contraindicated if active infection is present. A large percentage of patients taking beclomethasone on a long-term basis will develop candidiasis, a fungal infection in the throat, due to the constant deposits of drug in the oral cavity.

 See the companion website for a Nursing Process Focus specific to this drug.

29.9 Treating Asthma with Leukotriene Modifiers

Leukotrienes are mediators of the immune response that promote airway edema, inflammation, and bronchoconstriction. Zileuton (Zyflo) acts by blocking lipoxygenase, the enzyme that converts arachidonic acid into leukotrienes. The remaining two agents in this class, zafirlukast (Accolate) and montelukast (Singulair) act by blocking leukotriene receptors.

The leukotriene modifiers are approved for the prophylaxis of chronic asthma. They are not bronchodilators, and are ineffective in terminating acute asthma attacks. They are all given orally. Because zileuton (Zyflo) is taken four times a day, it offers less patient convenience than montelukast (Singulair) or zafirlukast (Accolate), which are taken every 12 hours. Zileuton has a more rapid onset of action (2 hours) than the other two leukotriene modifiers which take as long as 1 week to obtain therapeutic benefit.

Few serious adverse effects are associated with the leukotriene modifiers. Headache, cough, nasal congestion, or GI upset may occur. Patients over age 55 must be monitored carefully for signs of infection, because these patients have been found to experience an increased frequency of infections when taking leukotriene modifiers. These agents may be contraindicated in patients with significant hepatic dysfunction or in chronic alcoholics, because they are extensively metabolized by the liver.

COMMON COLD

The common cold is a viral infection of the upper respiratory tract that produces a characteristic array of annoying symptoms. It is fortunate that the disorder is self-limiting, because there is no cure or effective prevention for colds. Therapies used to relieve symptoms may include the same classes of drugs used for allergic rhinitis (Chapter 31), such as antihistamines, decongestants, and additional drugs such as those that suppress cough and loosen bronchial secretions⊙.

Antitussives

Antitussives are drugs used to dampen the cough reflex. They are of value in treating coughs due to allergies or the common cold.

29.10 Pharmacotherapy with Antitussives

Cough is a natural reflex mechanism that serves to forcibly remove excess secretions and foreign material from the respiratory system. In diseases such as emphysema and bronchitis, or when liquids have been aspirated into the bronchi, it is not desirable to suppress the normal cough reflex. Dry, hacking, nonproductive cough, however, can be quite irritating to the membranes of the throat and can deprive a patient of much needed rest. It is these types of conditions in which therapy with medications that control cough, known as antitussives, may be warranted. Antitussives are classified as opioids or nonopioids and are shown in Table 29.4.

Opioids, the most efficacious antitussives, act by raising the cough threshold in the CNS. Codeine and hydrocodone are the most frequently used opioid antitussives. Doses needed to suppress the cough reflex are very low; thus, there is minimal potential for dependence. Most opioid cough mixtures are classified as Schedule III, IV, or V drugs, and are reserved for more serious cough conditions. Though not common, overdose from opioid cough remedies may result in significant respiratory depression. Care must be taken when using these medications in patients with asthma or allergies, since bronchoconstriction may occur. Opioids may be combined with other agents such as antihistamines, decongestants, and nonopioid antitussives

Table 29.4	Agents for the Common Cold and Removal of Excessive Bronchial Mucus
Drug	**Route and Adult Dose (max dose where indicated)**
Antitussives: Opioids	
codeine	PO; 10–20 mg q4–6h PRN (max 120 mg/24 h)
hydrocodone bitartrate (Hycodan, others)	PO; 5–10 mg q4–6h PRN (max 15 mg/dose)
Antitussives: Nonopioids	
benzonatate (Tessalon)	PO; 100 mg tid PRN up to 600 mg/d
dextromethorphan (Pedia Care, others)	PO; 10–20 mg q4h or 30 mg q6–8h (max 120 mg/d)
Expectorant	
guaifenesin (Robitussin, others)	PO; 200–400 mg q4h (max 2.4 g/d)
Mucolytic	
acetylcysteine (Mucomyst)	MDI; Inhalation 1–10 ml of 20% solution q4–6h or 2–20 ml of 10% solution q4–6h

Table 29.5	Opioid Combination Drugs for Severe Cold Symptoms	
Trade Name	**Opioid**	**Nonopioid Ingredients**
Ambenyl Cough Syrup	codeine	bromodiphenhydramine
Calcidrine Syrup	codeine	calcium iodide
Codamine Syrup	hydrocodone	phenylpropanolamine
Codiclear DH Syrup	hydrocodone	guaifenesin
Codimal DH	hydrocodone	phenylephrine, pyrilamine
Hycodan	hydrocodone	homatropine
Hycomine Compound	hydrocodone	phenylephrine, chlorpheniramine, acetaminophen
Hycotuss Expectorant	hydrocodone	guaifenesin
Novahistine DH	codeine	pseudoephedrine, chlorpheniramine
Phenergan with Codeine	codeine	promethazine
Robitussin A-C	codeine	guaifenesin
Tega-Tussin Syrup	hydrocodone	phenylephrine, chlorpheniramine
Triaminic Expectorant DH	hydrocodone	phenylpropanolamine, pyrilamine, pheniramine, guaifenesin
Tussionex	hydrocodone	chlorpheniramine

in the therapy of severe cold or flu symptoms. Some of these combinations are shown in Table 29.5.

The most frequently used nonopioid antitussive is dextromethorphan. At low doses, this drug is available in OTC cold and flu medications. Higher doses are available by prescription to treat more severe cough. Dextromethorphan is chemically similar to the opioids, and also acts in the CNS to raise the cough threshold. Though not as efficacious as codeine, there is no risk of dependence with dextromethorphan.

Benzonatate (Tessalon) is a nonopioid antitussive that acts by a different mechanism. Chemically related to the local anesthetic tetracaine (Pontocaine), benzonatate suppresses the cough reflex by anesthetizing stretch receptors in the lungs. If chewed, the drug can cause the side effect of numbing the mouth and pharynx. Side effects are uncommon, but may include sedation, nausea, headache, and dizziness.

NURSING CONSIDERATIONS

The role of the nurse in antitussive therapy involves careful monitoring of a patient's condition and providing education as it relates to the prescribed drug regimen. The nursing care related to patients receiving antitussive drugs is dependent on the agent used. For all antitussive drugs, the nurse should assess for presence/history of persistent nonproductive cough, respiratory distress, shortness of breath, and/or productive cough.

When codeine or other opioids are prescribed, the patient should be monitored for drowsiness. Since cough is a protective mechanism used to cleanse the lungs of microbes, antitussive drugs should be used in moderation and only to treat cough when it interferes with activities of daily living, rest, or sleep. Extreme caution should be used in administering antitussive drugs to individuals with chronic lung conditions, as normal respiratory function is already impaired. Because cough may be a symptom of other serious pulmonary conditions, antitussive drugs should only be used for 3 days, unless otherwise approved by the healthcare provider.

Patient education as it relates to antitussives includes the goals, reasons for obtaining baseline data such as vital signs and tests for cardiac and renal disorders, and possible side effects. Following are the specific points the nurse should include when teaching patients regarding antitussives.

- Avoid driving or performing hazardous activities while taking opioid antitussives.
- Avoid use of alcohol, which can cause increased CNS depression.
- Immediately report the following: coughing up green-or yellow-tinged secretions, difficulty breathing, excessive drowsiness, constipation, nausea/vomiting.
- Store opioid antitussives away from children.

Expectorants and Mucolytics

Certain drugs are available to control excess mucus production. Expectorants increase bronchial secretions and mucolytics help loosen thick bronchial secretions. These agents are shown in Table 29.4.

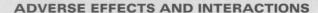

Pr **PROTOTYPE DRUG** | **DEXTROMETHORPHAN** (Benylin)

ACTIONS AND USES

Dextromethorphan is a drug included in most severe cold and flu preparations. It is available in a large variety of formulations, including tablets, liquid-filled capsules, lozenges, and liquids. It has a rapid onset of action, usually within 15 to 30 minutes. Like codeine, it acts in the medulla, though it lacks the analgesic and euphoric effects of the opioids and does not produce dependence. Patients whose cough is not relieved by dextromethorphan after several days of therapy should see their healthcare provider.

Administration Alerts

- Avoid pulmonary irritants, such as smoking or other fumes, as these agents may decrease drug effectiveness.
- Pregnancy category C.

ADVERSE EFFECTS AND INTERACTIONS

Side effects due to dextromethorphan are rare. Dizziness, drowsiness, and GI upset occur in some patients.

Drug interactions with dextromethorphan include a high risk of excitation, hypotension, and hyperpyrexia when used concurrently with MAO inhibitors. Concurrent use with alcohol may result in increased CNS depression.

 See the companion website for a Nursing Process Focus specific to this drug.

29.11 Pharmacotherapy with Expectorants and Mucolytics

Expectorants are drugs that increase bronchial secretions. They act by reducing the thickness or viscosity of bronchial secretions, thus increasing mucus flow that can then be re-

moved more easily by coughing. The most effective OTC expectorant is guaifenesin (Resyl, others). Like dextromethorphan, guaifenesin produces few adverse effects and is a common ingredient in many OTC cold and flu preparations. Higher doses of guaifenesin are available by prescription.

Acetylcysteine (Mucomyst) is one of the few drugs available to directly loosen thick, viscous bronchial secretions. Drugs of this type, **mucolytics**, break down the chemical structure of mucus molecules. The mucus becomes thinner, and more able to be removed by coughing. Acetylcysteine is delivered by the inhalation route and is not available OTC. It is used in patients who have cystic fibrosis, chronic bronchitis, or other diseases that produce large amounts of thick bronchial secretions. A second mucolytic, dornase alfa (Pulmozyme), was approved in 1994 for maintenance therapy in the management of thick bronchial secretions. Dornase alfa breaks down DNA molecules in the mucus, causing it to become less viscous.

CHRONIC OBSTRUCTIVE PULMONARY DISEASE

Chronic obstructive pulmonay disease (COPD) is a generic term used to describe several pulmonary conditions characterized by cough, mucus production, and impaired gas exchange. Drugs may be used to bring symptomatic relief but they do not cure the disorders.

29.12 Pharmacotherapy of COPDs

COPD is a major cause of death and disability. The three specific COPD conditions are asthma, chronic bronchitis, and emphysema. Chronic bronchitis and emphysema are strongly associated with smoking tobacco products and, secondarily, breathing air pollutants. In chronic bronchitis,

SPECIAL CONSIDERATIONS

Respiratory Distress Syndrome

Respiratory distress syndrome (RDS) is a condition, primarily occurring in premature babies, in which the lungs are not producing surfactant. Surfactant forms a thin layer on the inner surface of the alveoli to raise the surface tension. This prevents the alveolus from collapsing during expiration. If birth occurs before the pneumocytes in the lung are mature enough to secrete surfactant, the alveoli collapse and RDS results.

Surfactant medications can be delivered to the newborn, either as prophylactic therapy or as rescue therapy, after symptoms develop. The two surfactant agents used for RDS are colfosceril (Exosurf) and beractant (Survanta). These drugs are administered intratracheally every 4 to 6 hours, until the patient's condition improves.

excess mucus is produced in the bronchial tree due to the inflammation and irritation from cigarette smoke or pollutants. The airway becomes partially obstructed with mucus, thus resulting in the classic signs of dyspnea and coughing. An early sign of bronchitis is often a productive cough that occurs upon awakening. Wheezing and decreased exercise tolerance are additional clinical signs. Because microbes enjoy the mucus-rich environment, pulmonary infections are common. Gas exchange may be impaired.

COPD is progressive, with the terminal stage being emphysema. After years of chronic inflammation, the bronchioles lose their elasticity and the alveoli dilate to maximum size, to allow more air into the lungs. The patient suffers extreme dyspnea from even the slightest physical activity.

Patients with COPD may receive a number of pulmonary drugs for symptomatic relief. The goals of pharmacotherapy are to treat infections, control cough, and relieve bronchospasm. Most patients receive bronchodilators such as ipratropium (Atrovent), beta$_2$ agonists, or inhaled glucocorticoids. Mucolytics and expectorants are sometimes used to reduce the viscosity of the bronchial mucus and to aid in its removal. Oxygen therapy assists breathing in emphysema patients. Antibiotics may be prescribed for patients who experience multiple bouts of pulmonary infections.

Patients should be taught to avoid taking any drugs that have beta-antagonist activity or otherwise cause bronchoconstriction. Respiratory depressants such as opioids and barbiturates should be avoided. It is important to note that none of the pharmacotherapies offer a cure for COPD; they only treat the symptoms of a progressively worsening disease. The most important teaching point for the nurse is to strongly encourage smoking cessation in these patients.

CHAPTER REVIEW

Key Concepts

The numbered key concepts provide a succinct summary of the important points from the corresponding numbered section within the chapter. If any of these points are not clear, refer to the numbered section within the chapter for review. Expanded versions can be found on the companion website.

29.1 The physiology of the respiratory system involves two main processes. Ventilation moves air into and out of the lungs and perfusion allows for gas exchange across capillaries.

29.2 Bronchioles are lined with smooth muscle that controls the amount of air entering the lungs. Dilation and constriction of the airways are controlled by the autonomic nervous system.

29.3 Inhalation is a common route of administration for pulmonary drugs because it delivers drugs directly to the sites of action. Nebulizers, MDIs, and DPIs are devices used for aerosol therapies.

29.4 Asthma is a chronic disease that has both inflammation and bronchospasm components.

29.5 Beta-adrenergic agonists are the most effective drugs for relieving acute bronchospasm. These agents act by activating beta$_2$-receptors in bronchial smooth muscle to cause bronchodilation.

29.6 Methylxanthines and anticholinergics are bronchodilators occasionally used as alternatives to the beta agonists in asthma therapy.

29.7 Glucocorticoids are effective for the long-term prophylaxis of asthma. Both oral and inhaled products are available.

29.8 Cromolyn (Intal), a mast cell stabilizer, is a safe drug used for the prophylaxis of asthma, but is ineffective at relieving acute bronchospasm.

29.9 The leukotriene modifiers, whose primary use is in asthma prophylaxis, act by reducing the inflammatory component of asthma.

29.10 Antitussives are effective at relieving cough due to the common cold. Opioids are used for severe cough. Nonopioids such as dextromethorphan are used for mild or moderate cough.

29.11 Expectorants promote mucous secretion, making it thinner and easier to remove by cough. Mucolytics are agents used to break down thick bronchial secretions.

29.12 Chronic obstructive pulmonary disease (COPD) is a progressive disorder treated with multiple pulmonary drugs. Bronchodilators, expectorants, mucolytics, antibiotics, and oxygen may offer symptomatic relief.

Review Questions

1. What is the difference between ventilation and perfusion?

2. Name the three types of devices used to deliver drugs by the inhalation route. What are the differences between them?

3. Distinguish between the classes of drugs that prevent asthma attacks and those that can terminate an attack in progress. Name at least one drug in each class.

4. What is the difference in the mechanism of action between an antitussive and an expectorant?

Critical Thinking Questions

1. A 72-year-old male patient has recently been started on an ipratropium (Atrovent) inhaler. What teaching is important for the nurse to provide?

2. A 65-year-old patient has bronchitis and has been coughing for several days. Which is the antitussive of choice for this patient, dextromethorphan or codeine? Why?

3. A 45-year-old chronic asthmatic is on glucocorticoids. What must be monitored on this patient?

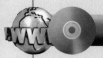

EXPLORE MediaLink

NCLEX review, case studies, and other interactive resources for this chapter can be found on the companion website at www.prenhall.com/adams. Click on "Chapter 29" to select the activities for this chapter. For animations, more NCLEX review questions, and an audio glossary, access the accompanying CD-ROM in this textbook.

specific to antigen
have recollection

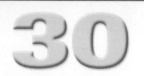

CHAPTER 30

Drugs for Immune System Modulation

DRUGS AT A GLANCE

IMMUNIZATION AGENTS
Vaccines
Immune globulin preparations

IMMUNOSTIMULANTS
Interferons
interferon alfa (Roferon-A, Intron A)
Interleukins
Other agents

IMMUNOSUPPRESSANTS
Antibodies
Antimetabolites and cytotoxic agents
Calcineurin inhibitors
cyclosporine (Neoral, Sandimmune)
Glucocorticoids

MediaLink   www.prenhall.com/adams

CD-ROM
Audio Glossary
NCLEX Review

Companion Website
NCLEX Review
Dosage Calculations
Case Study
Care Plans
Expanded Key Concepts

OBJECTIVES

After reading this chapter, the student should be able to:

1. Identify the components of the lymphatic system and their functions.
2. Compare and contrast specific and nonspecific body defenses.
3. Compare and contrast the humoral and cell-mediated immune responses.
4. Explain why immunosuppressant medications are necessary following organ transplants.
5. Identify the types of agents used as immunosuppressants.
6. Compare and contrast active immunity and passive immunity.
7. Describe the nurse's role in the pharmacologic management of immune disorders.
8. For each of the drug classes listed in Drugs at a Glance, know representative drugs, explain their mechanism of drug action, primary actions related to the immune system, and important adverse effects.
9. Categorize drugs used in the treatment of immune disorders based on their classification and mechanism of action.
10. For each of the major vaccines, give the recommended dosage schedule.
11. Use the Nursing Process to care for patients receiving drug therapy for immune disorders.

The body comes under continuous attack from a host of foreign agents that include viruses, bacteria, fungi, and even single-celled animals. Our extensive body defenses are capable of mounting a rapid and effective response against many of these pathogens. In some cases, pharmacotherapy can be used to stimulate body defenses so that microbes can be more readily attacked and disease prevented. On other occasions, it is desirable to dampen the immune response to allow a transplanted organ to survive. The purpose of this chapter is to examine the pharmacotherapy of agents affecting the body's response to disease.

PHARMFACTS | Vaccines and Organ Transplants

- Vaccines have eradicated smallpox from the world and the poliovirus from the Western Hemisphere.
- Vaccines lowered the number of diphtheria cases in the United States from 175,000 in 1922 to 1 in 1998.
- Vaccines lowered the number of measles cases in the United States from over 503,000 in 1962 to 89 in 1998.
- Over 79,000 patients are waiting for organ transplants, with 3,000 added to the list every month.
- Because of lack of available transplants, many patients die every year. This includes approximately 2,000 kidney patients, 1,300 liver patients, 450 heart patients, and 361 lung patients.
- The most common transplanted organs are kidney, liver, and heart.

30.1 Nonspecific Body Defenses and the Immune Response

The lymphatic system consists of lymphoid cells, tissues, and organs such as the spleen, thymus, tonsils, and lymph nodes. The overall purpose of the lymphatic system is to protect the body from pathogens.

The first line of protection from pathogens involves **nonspecific defenses**, those that protect the body from invasion by general hazards. Nonspecific defenses include physical barriers such as the epithelial lining of the skin and the respiratory and gastrointestinal mucous membranes that are potential entry points for pathogens. Other nonspecific defenses are phagocytes, natural killer (NK) cells, the complement system, fever, and interferons. From a pharmacologic perspective, one of the most important nonspecific defenses is inflammation. Because of its significance, inflammation is discussed separately, in Chapter 31 ⊝.

The body also has the capability to mount a second line of defense that is specific to certain pathogens. This defense is known as the **immune response**. Foreign agents that elicit an immune response are called **antigens**. Foreign proteins, such as those present on the surfaces of pollen grains, bacteria, nonhuman cells, and viruses, are the strongest antigens. The primary cell of the immune response that interacts with antigens is the lymphocyte.

The immune response is extremely complex. Steps involve recognition of the antigen, communication and coordination with other defense cells, and destruction or suppression of the antigen. A large number of chemical messengers and interactions are involved in the immune response, many of which have yet to be discovered. The two basic divisions of the immune response are antibody-mediated (humoral) immunity and cell-mediated immunity. These are shown in Figure 30.1.

30.2 Humoral Immunity and Antibodies

Humoral immunity is initiated when an antigen encounters a type of lymphocyte known as a **B cell**. The activated B cell divides rapidly to form clones of itself. Most cells in this clone

are called **plasma cells** whose primary function is to secrete **antibodies** which are specific to the antigen that initiated the challenge. Circulating through the body, antibodies, also known as immunoglobulins, physically interact with the antigen to neutralize it or mark the foreign agent for destruction by other cells of the immune response. Peak production of antibodies occurs about 10 days after an antigen challenge. The important functions of antibodies are illustrated in Figure 30.2

Some B cells, called memory B cells, remember the initial antigen interaction. Should the body be exposed to the same antigen in the future, the immune system will be able to manufacture even higher levels of antibodies in a shorter period, approximately 2 to 3 days. For some antigens, memory can be retained for an entire lifetime. Vaccines are sometimes administered to produce these memory cells in advance of exposure to the antigen, so that when the body is exposed to the actual organism it can mount a fast, effective response.

VACCINES

Vaccines are biological agents used to stimulate the immune system. The goal of vaccine administration is to prevent serious infections by life-threatening pathogens.

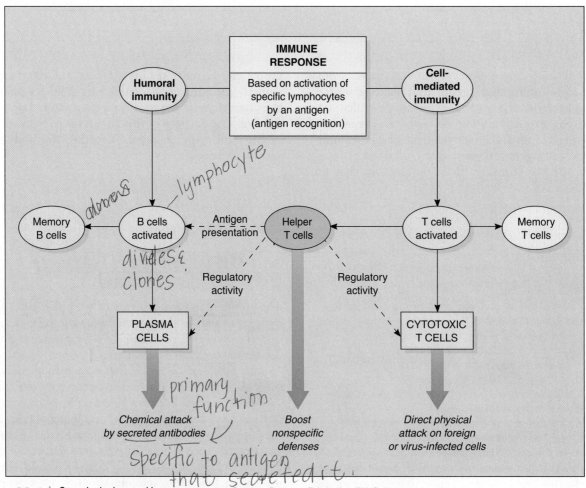

Figure 30.1 | Steps in the humoral immune response *Source: Pearson Education/PH College.*

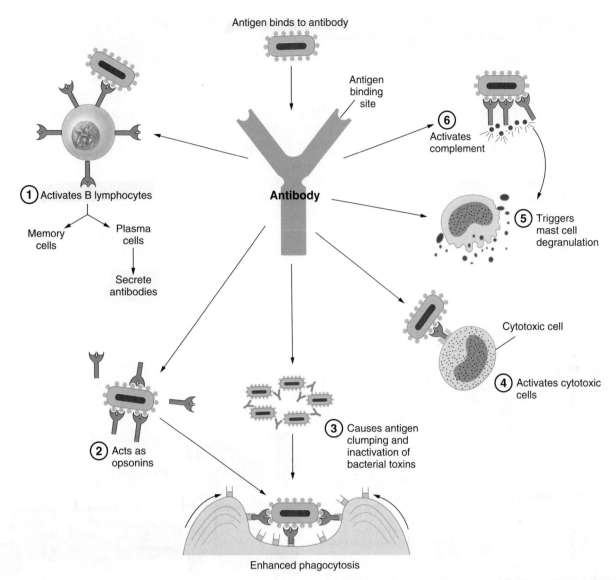

Figure 30.2 | Functions of antibodies

30.3 Administration of Vaccines

Lymphocytes attack antigens by recognizing certain foreign proteins on their surface. Sometimes they recognize a toxin or secretion produced by the organism. Pharmacologists have used this knowledge to create biological products that prevent disease, called **vaccines** which consist of suspensions of one of the following:

- Microbes that have been killed
- Microbes that are alive but weakened (attenuated) so they are unable to produce disease
- Bacterial toxins, called **toxoids**, that have been modified to remove their hazardous properties

Vaccination, or **immunization**, is performed to expose the patient to the modified, harmless microorganism or its toxoid so that an immune response occurs in the following weeks or months. As a result of the vaccination, memory B cells are formed. When later exposed to the actual infectious organism, these cells will react quickly by producing large quantities of antibodies. While some immunizations are only needed once, most require follow-up vaccinations, called boosters, to provide continuous protection. The effectiveness of most vaccines can be assessed by measuring the amount of antibody produced after the vaccine has been administered, a quantity called **titer**.

The type of immunity achieved through the administration of a vaccine is called **active immunity**. In active immunity, the patient's immune system is stimulated to produce antibodies due to exposure to the antigen (vaccine). **Passive immunity** may be obtained by directly administering antibodies to a patient. Examples of agents used to provide passive immunity include infusion of gamma globulin following exposure to hepatitis, antivenoms used for snakebites, and sera used to treat botulism, tetanus, and rabies. Because these drugs do not stimulate the patient's immune system, their protective effects last only 2 to 3 weeks. Table 30.1 lists selected immune

Table 30.1	Immune Globulin Preparations
Drug	**Route and Adult Dose (max dose where indicated)**
cytomegalovirus immune globulin (CytoGam)	IV; 150 mg/kg within 72 h of transplantation, then 100 mg/kg for 2, 4, 6, and 8 wk post-transplant, then 50 mg/kg for 12 and 16 wk post-transplant
hepatitis B immune globulin (BayHep B, HyperHep, H-BIG)	IM; 0.06 ml/kg as soon as possible after exposure, preferably within 24 h, but no later then 7 d, repeat 28–30 d after exposure
immune globulin intramuscular (Gamastan)	IM; 0.02–0.06 ml/kg as soon as possible after exposure if H-BIG is unavailable
immune globulin intravenous (Gamimune N, Gammagard, Gammar-P, IGIV, Iveegam, Sandoglobulin, Venoglobulin-S)	IV; 100–200 mg/kg/mo IM; 1.2 ml/kg followed by 0.6 ml/kg q2–4wk
rabies immune globulin (Bayrab, Imogam Rabis-HT, Hyperab)	IM; (gluteal) 20 IU/kg
Rh$_o$(D) immune globulin (BayRho-D, WinRho SDF, MICRhoGAM, RhoGAM)	IM/IV; One vial or 300 μg at approximately 28 wk; followed by one vial of minidose or 120 μg within 72 h of delivery if infant is Rh-positive
tetanus immune globulin (BayTet, HyperTet)	IM; 250 units

globulin preparations. Figure 30.3 illustrates the development of immunity through vaccines or the administration of antibodies.

Most vaccines are administered with the goal of preventing illness, and include vaccines used to prevent patients from acquiring measles, polio, whooping cough, tetanus, and hepatitis B. In the case of HIV infection, however, experimental HIV vaccines are given after infection has occurred for the purpose of enhancing the immune system, rather than preventing the disease. Unlike other vaccines, experimental vaccines for HIV have thus far been unable to prevent AIDS. Pharmacotherapy of HIV is discussed in Chapter 34 ⊙ .

Vaccines are not without adverse effects. Common side effects include redness and discomfort at the site of injection and fever. Although severe reactions are uncommon, anaphylaxis is possible. Vaccinations are contraindicated for patients who have a weak immune system or who are currently experiencing symptoms such as diarrhea, vomiting, or fever.

Effective vaccines have been produced for a number of debilitating diseases and their widespread use has prevented serious illness in millions of patients, particularly children. One disease, smallpox, has been completely eliminated from the planet through immunization, and others such as polio have diminished to extremely low levels. Table 30.2 gives some common childhood vaccines and their recommended schedules.

Although vaccinations have proved a resounding success in children, many adults die of diseases that could be prevented by vaccination. Most mortality from vaccine-preventable disease in adults is from influenza and pneumococcal disease. Recent studies have shown that, in adults over age 65, only 67% had received influenza vaccine in the past 12 months and only 56% had ever received pneumococcal vaccine. In 2002, the CDC published an adult immunization schedule that contained both age-based and risk-based recommendations (see www.cdc.gov). Risk-based considerations include pregnancy, diabetes, heart disease,

renal failure, and various other serious and debilitating conditions.

30.4 Cell-Mediated Immunity and Cytokines

A second branch of the immune response involves lymphocytes called T cells. Two major types of T cells are called helper T cells and cytotoxic T cells. These cells are sometimes named after a protein receptor on their plasma membrane; the helper T cells have a CD4 receptor and the cytotoxic T cells have a CD8 receptor. The helper T cells are particularly important because they are responsible for activating most other immune cells, including B cells. Cytotoxic T cells travel throughout the body and can directly kill certain bacteria, parasites, virus-infected cells, and cancer cells.

Activated or sensitized T cells rapidly form clones after they encounter their specific antigen. Unlike B cells, however, T cells do not produce antibodies. Instead, activated T cells produce huge amounts of cytokines: hormonelike proteins that regulate the intensity and duration of the immune response and mediate cell-to-cell communication. Some cytokines kill foreign organisms directly, while others induce inflammation or enhance the killing power of macrophages. Specific cytokines released by activated T cells include interleukins, gamma interferon, and perforin. Some cytokines are used therapeutically to stimulate the immune system, as discussed in Section 30.5.

As with B cells, some sensitized T cells become memory cells. Should the body encounter the same antigen in the future, the memory T cells will assist in mounting a more rapid immune response.

IMMUNOSTIMULANTS

Despite attempts over many decades to develop effective drugs that stimulate the immune system to fight disease,

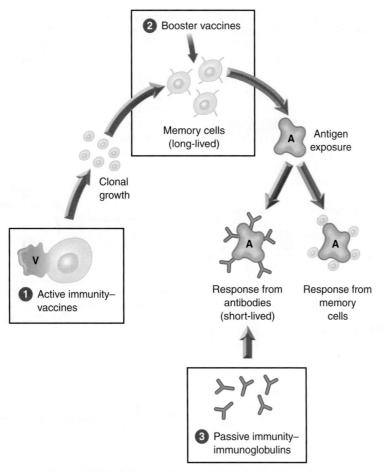

Figure 30.3 | Active and passive immunity: (1) administration of vaccine gives long-lasting active immunity; (2) booster vaccines maintain enough memory cells to give quick response; (3) administration of immunoglobulins gives short-lived passive immunity

Table 30.2	Common Childhood Vaccines and Their Schedules
Vaccine	**Schedule and Age**
diphtheria, tetanus, and pertussis (Tri-Immunol, Tripedia, Acel-Imune, Infanrix, Certiva)	first: 2 months second: 4 months third: 6 months fourth: 15–18 months fifth: 4–6 years
haemophilus influenza (HibTITER, OmniHIB, PedvaxHIB, Comvax)	first: 2 months second: 4 months third: 6 months fourth: 12–15 months
hepatitis B (Recombivax HB, Energix-B)	first: birth–2 months second: 1–4 months third: 6–18 months
measles, mumps, and rubella (MMR II)	first: 12–15 months second: 4–6 years
poliovirus, oral (Orimune)	first: 2 months second: 4 months third: 6–18 months fourth: 4–6 years
varicella zoster/chickenpox (Varivax)	one dose: 12–18 months

Childhood immunizations have proven to be some of the most effective means of preventing and controlling the spread of infectious and communicable diseases, although thousands of preschool children are not being immunized. In general, immunization levels are lower among African American, Hispanic and American Indian/Alaska Native children. According to recent CDC statistics: 76% of white 2-year-olds compared to 68% for African American and Hispanics 2-year-olds were fully vaccinated according to the immunization schedule. Children are not the only ones affected. In 1999, Hispanics and African Americans aged 65 years and older were less likely than whites to report having received influenza and pneumococcal vaccines. Limited access to preventative services, parental skepticism, attitudes, and cultural beliefs about healthcare may contribute to these statistics.

Community outreach programs have proven effective at reaching underserved ethnic groups. Healthy People 2010, a set of health objectives for the nation to achieve in the first decade of the 21st century, has as one of its goals eliminating racial and ethnic disparities in health. Racial and Ethnic Approaches to Community Health (REACH) 2010 serves as one of CDC's efforts to eliminate the disparities. Launched in 1999, REACH funds community coalitions designed to implement unique community-driven strategies. Government-funded health programs, such as Children's Health Initiative Program (CHIP), were also initiated in the 1990s to promote preventative healthcare for America's children.

Echinacea purpurea or purple coneflower is a popular medicinal botanical. Native to the midwestern United States and central Canada, the flowers, leaves, and stems of this plant are harvested and dried. Preparations include dried powder, tincture, fluid extracts, and teas. No single ingredient seems to be responsible for the herb's activity; a large number of active chemicals have been identified from the extracts.

Echinacea was used by Native Americans to treat various wounds and injuries. Echinacea is purported to boost the immune system by increasing phagocytosis and inhibiting the bacterial enzyme hyaluronidase. Some substances in Echinacea appear to have antiviral activity; thus, the herb is sometimes taken to treat the common cold and influenza—an indication for which it has received official approval in Germany. In general, it is used as a supportive treatment for any disease involving inflammation and to enhance the immune system. Side effects are rare; however, it may interfere with drugs that have immunosuppressant effects.

only a few such drugs have been approved. These agents include interferons and interleukins produced by recombinant DNA technology. Immunostimulants are shown in Table 30.3.

Biologic Response Modifiers

30.5 Pharmacotherapy with Biologic Response Modifiers

When challenged by specific antigens, certain macrophages, B and T lymphocytes, mast cells, endothelial cells, and stromal cells of the spleen, thymus, and bone marrow secrete cytokines that help defend against the invading organism. These natural cytokines have been identified and, through recombinant DNA technology, enough quantity has been made available to treat certain disorders. A handful of immunostimulants, sometimes called **biologic response modifiers**, have been approved to boost certain functions of the immune system.

Interferons are cytokines secreted by lymphocytes and macrophages that have been infected with a virus. After secretion, interferons attach to uninfected cells and signal them to secrete antiviral proteins. Part of the nonspecific defense system, interferons slow the spread of viral infections and enhance the activity of existing leukocytes. The actions of interferons include modulation of immune func-

tions such as increasing phagocytosis and enhancing the cytotoxic activity of T cells. The two major classes of interferons having clinical utility are alpha and beta. The alpha class has the widest therapeutic application (when used as medications, the spelling is changed to alfa). Indications for interferon alpha therapy include hairy cell leukemia, AIDS-related Kaposi's sarcoma, chronic myelogenous leukemia (alfa-2a), and chronic hepatitis B or C (alfa-2b). Interferon beta is primarily reserved for the treatment of severe multiple sclerosis.

Interleukins are another class of cytokines synthesized by lymphocytes, monocytes, macrophages, and certain other cells, that enhance the capabilities of the immune system. At least 20 different interleukins have been identified, though only a few are available as medications. The interleukins have widespread effects on immune function including stimulation of T-cell function, stimulation of B-cell and plasma cell production, and promotion of inflammation. Interleukin-2, derived from T helper lymphocytes, causes proliferation of T lymphocytes and activated B lymphocytes. It is available as aldesleukin (Proleukin), which is approved for the treatment of metastatic renal carcinoma. Interleukin-11, derived from bone marrow cells, is a growth factor with multiple hematopoietic effects. It is marketed as oprelvekin (Neumega) for its ability to stimulate platelet production in immunosuppressed patients (Chapter 28) ∞.

In addition to interferons and interleukins, a few additional biologic response modifiers are available to enhance the immune system. Levamisole (Ergamisole) is used to stimulate B cells, T cells, and macrophages in patients with colon cancer. Bacillus Calmette-Guérin (BCG) vaccine (Tice, TheraCys) is an attenuated strain of *Mycobacterium bovis* used for the pharmacotherapy of certain types of bladder cancer.

Table 30.3	Immunostimulants
Drug	**Route and Adult Dose (max dose where indicated)**
aldesleukin (Proleukin): interleukin-2	IV; 600,000 IU/kg (0.037 mg/kg) q8h by a 15-min IV infusion for a total of 14 doses
bacilles Calmette-Guérin (BCG) vaccine (Tice, TheraCys)	interdermal; 0.1 ml
interferon alfa-2 (Roferon-A, Intron A)	IM/SC; 2 million U/m² three times/wk
interferon beta-1a (Avonex, Rebif)	IM; 30 μg qwk
interferon beta-1b (Betaseron)	SC; 0.25 mg (8 million IU) qod
levamisole (Ergamisol)	Initial: 50 mg q8h for 3 days; maintenance: 50 mg q8h for 3 days q 2 weeks for 1 year
oprelvekin (Neumega): interleukin-11	SC; 50 μg/kg once daily starting 6–24 h after completing chemotherapy and continuing until platelet count is ≥50,000 cells/mcL or up to 21 d
peginterferon alfa-2a (Pegasys)	SC; 180 μg once weekly for 48 weeks

Pr PROTOTYPE DRUG | INTERFERON ALFA-2 (Roferon-A, Intron A)

ACTIONS AND USES

Interferon alfa-2 is a biologic response modifier that consists of two similar drugs, interferon alfa-2a (Roferon-A) and interferon alfa-2b (Intron A). Interferon 2b is a natural protein that is produced by human lymphocytes 4 to 6 hours after viral stimulation. Indications include hairy cell leukemia, hepatitis C, and malignant melanoma. An unlabeled use is for AIDS-related Kaposi's sarcoma. Interferon 2b affects cancer cells by two mechanisms. First, it enhances or stimulates the immune system to remove antigens. Secondly, the drug suppresses the growth of cancer cells. As expected from its origin, interferon alfa-2 also has antiviral activity.

Administration Alerts

- Should be administered under the careful guidance of a qualified healthcare provider.
- SC administration is recommended for patients at risk for bleeding.
- Pregnancy category C.

ADVERSE EFFECTS AND INTERACTIONS

Like many immunostimulants, the most common side effect is a flu-like syndrome of fever, chills, dizziness, and fatigue that usually diminishes as therapy progresses. Nausea, vomiting, diarrhea, and anorexia are relatively common. With prolonged therapy, more serious toxicity such as immunosuppression, hepatotoxicity, and neurotoxicity may be observed.

Interferon alfa-2 interacts with many drugs; for example, it may increase theophylline levels. There is additive myelosuppression with antineoplastics. Zidovudine may increase hematologic toxicity.

 See the companion website for a Nursing Process Focus specific to this drug.

NURSING CONSIDERATIONS

The role of the nurse in immunostimulant therapy involves careful monitoring of a patient's condition and providing education as it relates to the prescribed drug regimen. Immunostimulants are powerful drugs that not only affect target cells, but may also seriously impact other body systems. Prior to starting a patient on these drugs, a thorough assessment including a complete health history and present signs and symptoms should be performed, because these drugs have serious side effects. The nurse should assess for the presence and/or history of the following diseases or disorders: chronic hepatitis, hairy cell leukemia, malignant melanoma, condylomata acuminata,

AIDS-related Kaposi's sarcoma, and renal disorders including cancer. Assessment of infections and cancer verifies the need for these drugs. Immunostimulants are contraindicated for patients with renal or liver disease and pregnancy. Also before beginning therapy, lab tests including a complete blood count, electrolytes, renal function, and liver enzymes should be obtained to provide baseline data. Vital signs and body weight should be measured at the initial assessment and throughout the treatment regimen to monitor progress. As with any drug, the nurse should check for allergies and drug interactions.

Interferon alfa-2b (Intron A) should be used with caution in patients with hepatitis other than hepatitis C, leukopenia, and pulmonary disease. Interferon alfa-2a

(Roferon-A) should be used with caution in cardiac disease, herpes zoster, and recent exposure to chickenpox.

The patient should be kept well hydrated during pharmacotherapy. Use of immunostimulants can lead to the development of encephalopathy; therefore, the nurse should assess for changes in mental status. The nurse should be especially vigilant for signs and symptoms of depression and suicidal ideation. Additional nursing interventions may be needed depending on the medication given. When interferon alfa-2b (Intron A) is administered, it may promote development of leukemia because of bone marrow suppression. Periodic blood tests should be obtained to exclude the possibility of leukemia development.

Assessment of a patient's pregnancy status prior to beginning interferon beta-1b (Betaseron) therapy and throughout therapy should be done as this drug may cause spontaneous abortion. The nurse should instruct the patient to use reliable birth control while taking this drug. During the use of interleukin-2 (aldesleukin [Proleukin]), the patient should be instructed not to use corticosteroids, because these hormones reduce the drug's antitumor effectiveness. Liver, endocrine, or neurologic adverse effects that occur during therapy may be permanent.

Unlike most immunostimulants, levamisole (Ergamisol) restores depressed immune function rather than stimulating the body's immune system above normal levels. While taking this drug, patients should be advised not to consume alcohol because it may induce a disulfiram (Antabuse) reaction. The patient should be monitored for depression. Concurrent use of phenytoin (Dilantin) also may produce a possible drug reaction; thus, the nurse will need to monitor phenytoin levels closely.

Because immunosuppressants act on fast-growing cells such as on the lining of the stomach, nausea and stomatitis are common side effects. The nurse should provide small, frequent feedings and use nonalcohol-based mouthwash to treat mouth ulcers. Patients taking immunostimulants should immediately report any of the following side effects: hematuria, petechiae, tarry stools, bruising, fever, sore throat, jaundice, dark-colored urine, clay-colored stools, feelings of sadness, and nervousness.

See "Nursing Process Focus: Patients Receiving Immunostimulant Therapy" for specific teaching points.

IMMUNOSUPPRESSANTS

Drugs used to inhibit the immune response are called immunosuppressants. They are used for patients who are receiving transplanted tissues or organs. These agents are shown in Table 30.4 (page 412).

30.6 Immunosuppressants to Prevent Transplant Rejection

The immune response is normally viewed as a life saver, protecting individuals from a host of pathogens in the environment. For those receiving organ or tissue transplants, however, the immune response is the enemy. Transplanted organs always contain some antigens that trigger the immune response. This response, called **transplant rejection**, is often acute; antibodies sometimes destroy the transplanted tissue within a few days. The cell-mediated system responds more slowly to the transplant, attacking it about 2 weeks following surgery. Even if the organ survives these attacks, chronic rejection of the transplant may occur months or even years after surgery.

Immunosuppressants are drugs given to dampen the immune response. Transplantation would be impossible without the use of effective immunosuppressant drugs. In addition, these agents may be prescribed for severe cases of rheumatoid arthritis or other inflammatory diseases. Although the mechanisms of action of the immunosuppressant drugs differ, most are toxic to bone marrow and produce significant adverse effects. Due to the suppressed immune system, infections are common and the patient must be protected from situations in which exposure to pathogens is likely. Certain tumors such as lymphomas occur more frequently in transplant recipients than in the general population.

Drugs used to dampen the immune response include glucocorticoids, antimetabolites, antibodies, and calcineurin inhibitors. The glucocorticoids are potent inhibitors of inflammation that are discussed in detail in Chapters 31 and 39 ⊙. Antimetabolites such as sirolimus (Rapamune) and azathioprine (Imuran) inhibit aspects of lymphocyte replication. Monoclonal and polyclonal antibodies such as basiliximab (Simulect) and muromonab-CD3 (Orthoclone OKT3) interact with specific antigens on the surface of lymphocytes to destroy them. By binding to the intracellular messenger **calcineurin**, cyclosporine (Sandimmune, Neoral) and tacrolimus (Prograf) disrupt T-cell function. Because the primary indication for some of these immunosuppressants is to treat specific cancers, the student should also refer to Chapter 35 ⊙.

NURSING CONSIDERATIONS

The role of the nurse in immunosuppressant therapy involves careful monitoring of a patient's condition and providing education as it relates to the prescribed drug regimen. When providing care for patients taking immunosuppressants, an assessment should be done to determine the presence or history of organ transplant or grafting and to verify need for these drugs. A patient with leukemia, metastatic cancer, active infection, renal or liver disease, or pregnancy could be made worse by taking immunosuppressants, so they are contraindicated. These drugs should be used with caution in patients who have pancreatic or bowel dysfunction, hyperkalemia, hypertension, and infection. The nurse should obtain vital signs and lab testing, including a complete blood count, electrolytes, and liver profile to provide baseline data and reveal any abnormalities.

Many immunosuppressants act on T lymphocytes, suppressing the normal cell-mediated immune reaction. Due

NURSING PROCESS FOCUS | PATIENTS RECEIVING IMMUNOSTIMULANT THERAPY

ASSESSMENT

- Obtain health history including allergies, drug history, and possible drug interactions.
- Assess history of cytomegalovirus and any malignancies for verification of need.
- Obtain laboratory work: complete blood count, electrolytes, and liver enzymes.
- Obtain weight and vital signs, especially blood pressure.
- Assess mental alertness.

POTENTIAL NURSING DIAGNOSES

- Risk for Injury, related to side effects of drug
- Risk for Imbalanced Nutrition, related to gastrointestinal upset secondary to drug
- Risk for Infection, related to bone marrow suppression secondary to drug

PLANNING: PATIENT GOALS AND EXPECTED OUTCOMES

The patient will:
- Experience increased immune system function
- Demonstrate an understanding of the drug's action by accurately describing drug side effects and precautions
- Immediately report effects such as fever, chills, sore throat, unusual bleeding, chest pain, palpitations, dizziness, and change in mental status
- Demonstrate the ability to self-administer IM or SC injection

IMPLEMENTATION

Interventions and (Rationales)	Patient Education/Discharge Planning
■ Monitor for leukopenia, neutropenia, thrombocytopenia, anemia, increased liver enzymes (due to possible bone marrow suppression and liver damage).	Instruct patient to: ■ Comply with all ordered laboratory tests ■ Immediately report any unusual bleeding or jaundice ■ Avoid crowds and people with infections ■ Avoid activities that can cause bleeding or impairment of skin integrity
■ Ensure drug is properly administered.	■ Instruct patient in proper technique for self-administration of IM or SC injection.
■ Monitor vital signs. (Loss of vascular tone leading to extravasation of plasma proteins and fluids into extravascular spaces may cause hypotension and dysrhythmias.)	Instruct patient to: ■ Monitor blood pressure and pulse every day and report any reading outside normal limits ■ Report any palpitations immediately
■ Monitor for common side effects such as muscle aches, fever, weight loss, anorexia, nausea and vomiting, and arthralgia (due to high doses of medications).	Instruct patient to: ■ Take medication at bedtime to reduce side effects ■ Use frequent mouth care and small frequent feedings to reduce gastrointestinal disturbances ■ Take acetaminophen for flulike symptoms
■ Monitor blood glucose levels. (Blood glucose may increase in patients with pancreatitis.)	■ Instruct patient to have blood glucose checked at regular intervals.
■ Monitor for changes in mental status. May cause depression, confusion, fatigue, visual disturbances, and numbness. (Alpha interferons cause or aggravate neuropsychiatric disorders.)	■ Patient should report any mental changes, particularly depression or thoughts of suicide.

EVALUATION OF OUTCOME CRITERIA

Evaluate the effectiveness of drug therapy by confirming that patient goals and expected outcomes have been met (see "planning").

See Table 30.3 for a list of drugs to which these nursing actions apply.

Table 30.4	Immunosuppressants
Drug	**Route and Adult Dose (max dose where indicated)**
Antibodies	
alemtuzumab (Campath)	IV; 3–30 mg/day
basiliximab (Simulect)	IV; 20 mg times two doses (first dose 2 h before surgery, second dose 4 d after transplant)
daclizumab (Zenapax)	IV; 1 mg/kg start first dose no more than 24 h prior to transplant, then repeat q14d for four more doses
infliximab (Remicade)	IV; 3 mg/kg infused over at least 2 h, followed by 2 mg/kg on weeks 2 and 6, then 2 mg/kg q8wk
lymphocyte immune globulin (Antithymocyte Globulin)	IV; 10–30 mg/kg/d
muromonab-CD3 (Orthoclone OKT3)	IV; 5 mg/d administered in <1 min for 10–14d
rituximab (Rituxan)	IV; 375 mg/m^2 infused at 50 mg/h, may increase infusion rate q30min (max: 400 mg/h if tolerated), repeat dose on days 8, 15, and 22
Antimetabolites and Cytotoxic Agents	
azathioprine (Imuran)	PO; 3–5 mg/kg/d initially, may be able to reduce to 1–3 mg/kg/d; IV; 3–5 mg/kg/d initially, may be able to reduce to 1–3 mg/kg/d
cyclophosphamide (Cytoxan) (see page 506 for the Prototype Drug box) ⌧	PO Initial; 1–5 mg/kg/d; maintenance: 1–5 mg/kg q7–10d IV; Initial: 40–50 mg/kg in divided doses over 2–5 d up to 100 mg/kg; maintenance: 10–15 mg/kg q7–10d or 3–5 mg twice weekly
methotrexate (Amethopterin, Folex, Rheumatrex) (see page 506 for the Prototype Drug box) ⌧	PO; 15–30 mg/d for 5 d, repeat q12wk for three courses IM/IV; 15–30 mg/d for 5 d, repeat q12wk for three to five courses
mycophenolate mofetil (CellCept)	PO/IV; Start within 24 h of transplant, 1 g bid in combination with corticosteroids and cyclosporine
sirolimus (Rapamune)	PO; 6 mg loading dose immediately after transplant, then 2 mg/d
thalidomide (Thalomid)	PO; 100–300 mg qd (max: 400 mg/d) times at least 2 wk
Calcineurin Inhibitors	
cyclosporine (Sandimmune, Neoral)	PO; 250 mg q12h for 2 wk, may increase to 500 mg q12h (max 1g/d)
tacrolimus (Prograf)	PO; 0.15–0.3 mg/kg/d in two divided doses q12h, start no sooner than 6 h after transplant; give first oral dose 8–12 h after discontinuing IV therapy
	IV; 0.05–0.1 mg/kg/d as continuous infusion, start no sooner than 6 h after transplant and continue until patient can take oral therapy
Glucocorticoids (see Chapter 39 for individual doses) ⌧	

to their effect on the immune system, a superimposed infection may occur causing an increase in white blood cell count. The nurse needs to monitor vital signs, especially temperature, and blood testing for indications of infection. The degree of bone marrow suppression (thrombocytopenia and leukopenia) must be carefully monitored, as these adverse effects may be life threatening.

It is important that patients immediately report the following signs and symptoms: alopecia, increased pigmentation, arthralgia, respiratory distress, edema, nausea, vomiting, paresthesia, fever, blood in the urine, black stools, and feelings of sadness. Patients taking azathioprine (Imuran) should be informed and monitored for the development of secondary malignancies.

See "Nursing Process Focus: Patients Receiving Immunosuppressant Therapy" for specific teaching points.

Pr PROTOTYPE DRUG | CYCLOSPORINE (Neoral, Sandimmune)

ACTIONS AND USES

Cyclosporine is a complex chemical obtained from a soil fungus. Its primary mechanism of action is to inhibit helper T cells. Unlike some of the more cytotoxic immunosuppressants, it is less toxic to bone marrow cells. When prescribed for transplant recipients, it is primarily used in combination with high doses of a glucocorticoid such as prednisone.

Administration Alerts

■ Neoral (microemulsion) and Sandimmune are not bioequivalent, and cannot be used interchangeably without healthcare provider supervision.
■ Pregnancy category C.

ADVERSE EFFECTS AND INTERACTIONS

The primary adverse effect of cyclosporine occurs in the kidney, with up to 75% of patients experiencing reduction in urine flow. Other common side effects are tremor, hypertension, and elevated hepatic enzymes. Although infections are common during cyclosporine therapy, they are fewer than with some of the other immunosuppressants. Periodic blood counts are necessary to be certain that WBCs do not fall below 4,000 or platelets below 75,000.

Drugs that decrease cyclosporine levels include phenytoin, phenobarbital, carbamazepine, and rifampin. Drugs that increase cyclosporine levels include antifungal drugs and macrolide antibiotics. Grapefruit juice can raise cyclosporine levels by 50% to 200%.

Use with caution with herbal supplements; for example, the immune-stimulating effects of astragalus and echinacea may interfere with immunosuppressants.

 See the companion website for a Nursing Process Focus specific to this drug.

NURSING PROCESS FOCUS | PATIENTS RECEIVING IMMUNOSUPPRESSANT THERAPY

ASSESSMENT

■ Obtain health history including allergies, drug history, and possible drug interactions.
■ Assess for presence of metastatic cancer, active infection, renal or liver disease, and pregnancy.
■ Assess for skin integrity; specifically look for lesions and skin color.
■ Obtain laboratory work: complete blood count, electrolytes, and liver enzymes.
■ Obtain vital signs especially temperature and blood pressure.

POTENTIAL NURSING DIAGNOSES

■ Risk for Infection, related to depressed immune response secondary to drug
■ Risk for Injury, related to thrombocytopenia secondary to drug

PLANNING: PATIENT GOALS AND EXPECTED OUTCOMES

The patient will:
■ Experience no symptoms of organ or allograft rejection
■ Immediately report elevated temperature, unusual bleeding, sore throat, mouth ulcers, and fatigue to healthcare provider
■ Demonstrate an understanding of the drug's action by accurately describing drug side effects and precautions

IMPLEMENTATION

Interventions and (Rationales)	Patient Education/Discharge Planning
■ Assess renal function. (Drugs cause nephrotoxicity in many patients due to physiological changes in the kidneys such as microcalcifications and interstitial fibrosis.)	Advise patient to: ■ Keep accurate record of urine output ■ Report significant reduction in urine flow
■ Monitor liver function. (There is an increased risk for liver toxicity.)	■ Instruct patient as to the importance of regular laboratory testing.
■ Watch for signs and symptoms of infection, including elevated temperature. (There is an increased risk of infection due to immune suppression.)	Instruct patient to: ■ Use thorough, frequent handwashing ■ Avoid crowds and people with infection

continued

NURSING PROCESS FOCUS: *Patients Receiving Immunosuppressent Therapy (continued)*

Interventions and (Rationales)	*Patient Education/Discharge Planning*
■ Monitor vital signs, especially temperature and blood pressure. (Drugs may cause hypertension, especially in patients with kidney transplants.)	Teach patient to: ■ Monitor blood pressure and temperature ensuring proper use of home equipment ■ Keep all appointments with healthcare provider
■ Monitor for the following possible side effects: hirsutism, leukopenia, gingival hyperplasia, gynecomastia, sinusitis, and hyperkalemia.	Advise patient to: ■ See a dentist on a regular basis ■ Comply with regular laboratory assessments (complete blood count, electrolytes, and hormone levels)
■ Monitor patient for avoidance of drinking grapefruit juice. (This will increase cyclosporine levels 50% to 200%.)	Instruct patient to ■ Completely avoid drinking grapefruit juice ■ Take medication with food to decrease GI upset
■ Assess nutritional status. (Drugs may cause weight gain.)	■ Instruct patient regarding a healthy diet that avoids excessive fats and sugars.

EVALUATION OF OUTCOME CRITERIA

Evaluate the effectiveness of drug therapy by confirming that patient goals and expected outcomes have been met (see "Planning").

See Table 30.4 for a list of drugs to which these nursing actions apply.

CHAPTER REVIEW

Key Concepts

The numbered key concepts provide a succinct summary of the important points from the corresponding numbered section within the chapter. If any of these points are not clear, refer to the numbered section within the chapter for review. Expanded versions can be found on the companion website.

30.1 Protection from pathogens is provided through nonspecific defenses that protect the body from general hazards, and specific body defenses that are activated by specific antigens.

30.2 Humoral immunity involves the production of antibodies by plasma cells, which neutralize the foreign agent or destroy it.

30.3 Vaccines are biological agents used to prevent illness by boosting antibody production. Vaccines are classified as live, attenuated, or toxoid.

30.4 Cell-mediated immunity involves the activation of specific T cells and the secretion of cytokines such as interferons and interleukins that rid the body of the foreign agent.

30.5 Immunostimulants are biologic response modifiers that boost the patient's immune system and are used to treat infections, immunodeficiencies, and cancer.

30.6 Immunosuppressants are used to inhibit the patient's immune system and avoid tissue rejection following organ transplantation.

Review Questions

1. Why are oral glucocorticoids usually used concurrently with immunosuppressant drugs following a transplant operation?

2. Compare and contrast the type and duration of immunity achieved by administering a vaccine versus gamma globulin.

Critical Thinking Questions

1. A patient is taking sirolimus (Rapamune) following a liver transplant. On the most recent CBC, the nurse noted a marked 50% decrease in platelets and leukocytes. As the patient is being examined, what signs and symptoms should the nurse look for, and what are some possible interventions?

2. A patient has been exposed to hepatitis A and has been referred for an injection of gamma globulin. The patient is hesitant to get a "shot" and says that his immune system is fine. How would the nurse respond?

3. A patient has had a renal transplant 6 months ago and is taking cyclosporine (Neoral, Sandimmune) daily. Name three precautions that the nurse should know when caring for this patient.

EXPLORE MediaLink

NCLEX review, case studies, and other interactive resources for this chapter can be found on the companion website at www.prenhall.com/adams. Click on "Chapter 30" to select the activities for this chapter. For animations, more NCLEX review questions, and an audio glossary, access the accompanying CD-ROM in this textbook.

CHAPTER

31

Drugs for Inflammation, Fever, and Allergies

■ DRUGS AT A GLANCE

ANTI-INFLAMMATORY DRUGS

Nonsteroidal anti-inflammatory drugs (NSAIDs)

Pr *celecoxib (Celebrex)*

Systemic glucocorticoids

Pr *prednisone (Meticorten, others)*

ANTIPYRETICS

Pr *acetaminophen (Tylenol)*

ALLERGY DRUGS

H₁ receptor antagonists (antihistamines)

Pr *diphenhydramine (Benadryl, others)*

Pr *fexofenadine (Allegra)*

Intranasal glucocorticoids

Pr *fluticasone (Flonase)*

Sympathomimetics

Pr *oxymetazoline (Afrin, others)*

ANAPHYLAXIS DRUGS

Pr *epinephrine (Adrenalin)*

MediaLink www.prenhall.com/adams

CD-ROM

Animations:

    Mechanism in Action: Diphenhydramine (Benadryl, others)

    Mechanism in Action: Naproxen (Naprosyn, others)

Audio Glossary

NCLEX Review

Companion Website

NCLEX Review

Dosage Calculations

Case Study

Care Plans

Expanded Key Concepts

OBJECTIVES

After reading this chapter, the student should be able to:

1. Identify common signs and symptoms of inflammation.
2. Outline the basic steps in the acute inflammatory response.
3. Differentiate between H_1 and H_2 histamine receptors.
4. Describe common causes and symptoms of allergic rhinitis.
5. Describe the nurse's role in the pharmacologic management of inflammation, fever, and allergies.
6. For each of the classes listed in Drugs at a Glance, know representative drugs, explain their mechanisms of drug action, primary actions related to inflammation, and/or allergies and important adverse effects.
7. Categorize drugs used in the treatment of inflammation, fever, and allergies based on their classification and mechanism of action.
8. Use the Nursing Process to care for patients receiving drug therapy for inflammation, fever, and allergies.

The pain and redness of inflammation following minor abrasions and cuts is something everyone has experienced. Although there is some discomfort from such scrapes, inflammation is a normal and expected part of our body's defense against injury. For some diseases, however, inflammation can become abnormal and rage out of control, producing severe pain, fever, and other distressing symptoms. It is these sorts of conditions in which pharmacotherapy may be warranted.

Similarly, the allergy symptoms of nasal congestion, scratchy throat, and postnasal drip are familiar to millions of patients. Allergy symptoms may range from annoying to life threatening and are common indications for drug therapy.

PHARMFACTS
Inflammatory and Allergic Disorders in the United States

- Arthritis is the leading cause of disability.
- Inflammatory bowel disease affects 300,000 to 500,000 Americans each year.
- About 175 people die from food allergies each year in the United States.
- Of food allergies, 85% are related to milk, eggs, and nuts.
- Incidence of anaphylaxis may be twice as high in women as in men.
- About 3 million Americans (1.1%) are allergic to nuts.
- More than 80 million prescriptions are written for NSAIDs each year, accounting for about 4.5% of all prescriptions written in the United States.
- More than 1% of the U.S. population uses NSAIDs on a daily basis.
- Worldwide, more than 30 million people consume NSAIDs daily, and of these, 40% are more than 60 years of age.

INFLAMMATION

Inflammation is a nonspecific defense system of the body. Through the process of inflammation a large number of potentially damaging chemicals and foreign agents may be neutralized.

31.1 The Function of Inflammation

The human body has developed many complex means to defend against injury and invading organisms. Inflammation is one of these defense mechanisms. Inflammation is a complex process that may occur in response to a large number of different stimuli, including physical injury, exposure to toxic chemicals, extreme heat, invading microorganisms, or death of cells. It is considered a nonspecific defense mechanism because the physiological processes of inflammation proceed in the same manner, regardless of the cause. The specific immune defenses of the body are presented in Chapter 30 🔗 .

The central purpose of inflammation is to contain the injury or destroy the foreign agent. By neutralizing the foreign agent and removing cellular debris and dead cells, repair of the injured area can proceed at a faster pace. Signs of inflammation include swelling, pain, warmth, and redness of the affected area.

Inflammation may be classified as acute or chronic. During acute inflammation, such as that caused by minor physical injury, 8 to 10 days are normally needed for the symptoms to resolve and for repair to begin. If the body cannot contain or neutralize the damaging agent, inflammation may continue for prolonged periods and become chronic. In chronic autoimmune disorders such as lupus and rheumatoid arthritis, inflammation may persist for years, with symptoms becoming progressively worse over time. Other disorders such as seasonal allergy arise at predictable times during each year, and inflammation may produce only minor, annoying symptoms.

The pharmacotherapy of inflammation includes drugs that dampen the natural inflammatory response. Most anti-inflammatory drugs are nonspecific; it does not matter whether the inflammation is caused from injury or allergy, the drug will exhibit the same actions. A few anti-inflammatory drugs are specific to certain diseases, such as those used to treat gout (Chapter 46) 🔗 . Following are diseases that have an inflammatory component and that may benefit from anti-inflammatory drugs.

- Allergic rhinitis
- Anaphylaxis
- Ankylosing spondylitis
- Contact dermatitis
- Crohn's disease
- Glomerulonephritis
- Hashimoto's thyroiditis
- Peptic ulcers
- Rheumatoid arthritis
- Systemic lupus erythematosus
- Ulcerative colitis

31.2 The Role of Histamine in Inflammation

Whether the injury is due to microorganisms, chemicals, or physical trauma, the damaged tissue releases a number of chemical mediators that act as "alarms" to notify the surrounding area of the injury. Chemical mediators of inflammation include histamine, leukotrienes, bradykinin, complement, and prostaglandins. Table 31.1 lists the sources and actions of these mediators.

Histamine is a key chemical mediator of inflammation. It is primarily stored within mast cells located in tissue spaces under epithelial membranes such as the skin, bronchial tree, digestive tract, and along blood vessels. Mast cells detect foreign agents or injury and respond by releasing histamine, which initiates the inflammatory response within seconds. In addition to its role in inflammation, histamine also directly stimulates pain receptors.

When released at an injury site, histamine dilates nearby blood vessels, causing capillaries to become more permeable. Plasma and components such as complement proteins and phagocytes can then enter the area to neutralize foreign agents. The affected area may become congested with blood, a condition called hyperemia, which can lead to significant swelling and pain. Figure 31.1 illustrates the fundamental steps in acute inflammation.

Rapid release of the chemical mediators of inflammation on a larger scale throughout the body is responsible for the distressing symptoms of anaphylaxis, a life-threatening allergic response that may result in shock and death. A number of chemicals, insect stings, foods, and some therapeutic drugs can elicit this widespread release of histamine from mast cells, if the person has an allergy to these substances.

31.3 Histamine Receptors

There are at least two different receptors by which histamine can elicit a response. H_1 receptors are present in the smooth muscle of the vascular system, the bronchial tree, and the digestive tract. Stimulation of these receptors results in itching, pain, edema, vasodilation, and bronchoconstriction. In contrast, H_2 receptors are primarily

Table 31.1	Chemical Mediators of Inflammation
Mediator	**Description**
bradykinin	present in an inactive form in plasma, and also found in mast cells; vasodilator that causes pain; effects are similar to those of histamine
complement	series of at least 20 proteins that combine in a cascade fashion to neutralize or destroy an antigen
histamine	stored and released by mast cells; causes dilation of blood vessels, smooth muscle constriction, tissue swelling, and itching
leukotrienes	stored and released by mast cells; effects are similar to those of histamine
prostaglandins	present in most tissues and stored and released by mast cells; increase capillary permeability, attract white blood cells to site of inflammation, and cause pain

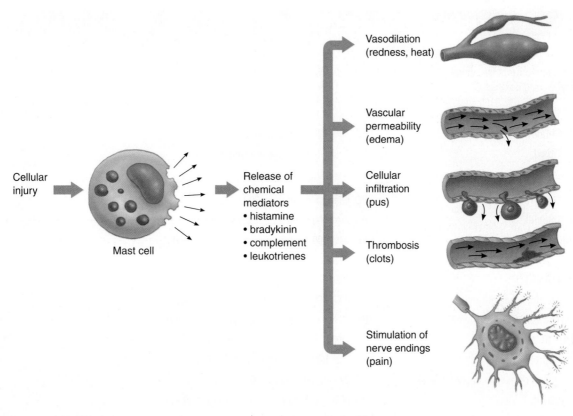

Figure 31.1 | Steps in acute inflammation *Source: Pearson Education/PM College.*

present in the stomach and their stimulation results in the secretion of large amounts of hydrochloric acid.

Drugs that act as specific antagonists for H_1 and H_2 receptors are in widespread therapeutic use. H_1 receptor antagonists, used to treat allergies and inflammation, are discussed later in this chapter. H_2 receptor antagonists are used to treat peptic ulcers and are discussed in Chapter 36 ⊜.

Nonsteroidal Anti-Inflammatory Drugs

Nonsteroidal anti-inflammatory drugs (NSAIDs) such as aspirin and ibuprofen have analgesic, antipyretic, and anti-inflammatory effects. They are drugs of choice in the treatment of mild to moderate inflammation. These agents are shown in Table 31.2.

31.4 Treating Inflammation with NSAIDs

Because of their high safety margin and availability as OTC drugs, the NSAIDs are first line drugs for the treatment of mild to moderate inflammation. The NSAID class includes some of the most widely used drugs in medicine, including aspirin, ibuprofen, and the newer COX-2 inhibitors. All NSAIDs have approximately the same efficacy, although the side effect profiles vary among the different drugs. The NSAIDs also exhibit analgesic and antipyretic actions. Although acetaminophen shares the analgesic and antipyretic properties of these other drugs,

it has no anti-inflammatory action and is not considered an NSAID.

First generation NSAIDs such as aspirin and ibuprofen block the enzymes **cyclooxygenase-1 (COX-1)** and **cyclooxygenase-2 (COX-2)**. This slows the synthesis of both thromboxane and prostaglandin mediators of inflammation. Although inflammation is reduced, the inhibition of COX-1 results in undesirable side effects such as bleeding, gastric upset, and reduced kidney function. Second generation NSAIDs such as celecoxib (Celebrex) and rofecoxib (Vioxx) block the inflammatory pathway selectively, at the level of COX-2. This reduces inflammation without causing most of the serious adverse effects of the older NSAIDs. A comparison of the two forms of the cyclooxygenase enzyme is shown in Table 31.3.

Aspirin binds to both COX-1 and COX-2 enzymes, changing their structures and preventing them from forming inflammatory prostaglandins. This inhibition of cyclooxygenase is particularly prolonged in platelets, where a single dose of aspirin may cause total inhibition for the entire 8- to 11-day lifespan of the platelet. Because it is readily available, inexpensive, and efficacious, aspirin is often a drug of first choice for treating mild inflammation. The fundamental pharmacology and a drug prototype for aspirin are presented in Chapter 19 ⊜.

Unfortunately, large doses of aspirin are necessary to suppress severe inflammation, which results in a greater incidence of side effects than when the drug is used for pain

Table 31.2	Selected Nonsteroidal Anti-Inflammatory Drugs
Drug	**Route and Adult Dose (max dose where indicated)**
aspirin (ASA and others) (see page 233 for the Prototype Drug box) 🔗	PO; 350–650 mg q4h (max 4 g/day)
Selective COX-2 Inhibitors	
celecoxib (Celebrex)	PO; 100–200 mg bid (max 400 mg/day)
rofecoxib (Vioxx)	PO; 12.5–25 mg qd (max 50 mg/day)
Ibuprofen and Similar Agents	
diclofenac (Voltaren, Cataflam)	PO; 50 mg bid-qid (max 200 mg/day)
diflunisal (Dolobid)	PO; 250–500 mg bid (max 1,500 mg/day)
etodolac (Lodine)	PO; 200–400 mg tid-qid (max 1,200 mg/day)
fenoprofen (Nalfon)	PO; 300–600 mg tid-qid (max 3,200 mg/day)
flurbiprofen (Ansaid)	PO; 50–100 mg tid-qid (max 300 mg/day)
ibuprofen (Motrin, Advil, others)	PO; 400–800 mg tid-qid (max 3,200 mg/day)
ketoprofen (Actron, Orudis, Oruvail)	PO; 75 mg tid or 50 mg qid (max 300 mg/day)
nabumetone (Relafen)	PO; 1,000 mg qd (max 2,000 mg/day)
naproxen (Naprosyn, others)	PO; 250–500 mg bid (max 1,000 mg/day)
naproxen sodium (Aleve, Anaprox, others)	PO; 275 mg bid (max 1,100 mg/day)
oxaprozin (Daypro)	PO; 600–1,200 mg qd (max 1,800 mg/day)
piroxicam (Feldene)	PO; 10–20 mg qd-bid (max 20 mg/day)
tolmetin (Tolectin)	PO; 400 mg tid (max 2 g/day)

Table 31.3	Forms of Cyclooxygenase	
	Cyclooxygenase 1	**Cyclooxygenase 2**
Location	present in all tissues	present at sites of tissue injury
Functions	protects gastric mucosa, supports kidney function, promotes platelet aggregation	mediates inflammation, sensitizes pain receptors, mediates fever in the brain
Inhibition by medications	undesirable: increases risk of gastric bleeding and kidney failure	desirable: results in suppression of inflammation

or fever. The most common adverse effects observed during high-dose aspirin therapy relate to the digestive system. By increasing gastric acid secretion and irritating the stomach lining, aspirin may produce epigastric pain, heartburn, and even bleeding due to ulceration. Some aspirin formulations are buffered or given an enteric coating to minimize GI side effects. Because aspirin also has a potent anticoagulant effect, the potential for bleeding must be carefully monitored. High doses may produce salicylism, a syndrome that includes symptoms such as tinnitus (ringing in the ears), dizziness, headache, and sweating.

Ibuprofen and a large number of ibuprofen-like drugs are first generation NSAIDs developed as alternatives to aspirin. Like aspirin, they exhibit their effects through inhibition of both COX-1 and COX-2, although the inhibition by these drugs is reversible. Because they share the same mechanism of action, all drugs in this class have similar pharmacologic properties and a low incidence of adverse effects. The most common side effects of ibuprofen-like NSAIDs are nausea and vomiting. These agents have the potential to cause gastric ulceration and bleeding; however, the incidence is less than that of aspirin. There is some cross-hypersensitivity between aspirin and other first generation NSAIDs.

The newest class of NSAIDs includes celecoxib (Celebrex) and rofecoxib (Vioxx) that selectively inhibit COX-2. Celecoxib is 375 times more selective for COX-2 than traditional NSAIDs; rofecoxib is 1,000 times more selective. Inhibition of COX-2 produces the analgesic, anti-inflammatory, and antipyretic actions typical of NSAIDs without adverse effects on the digestive system. Because they have no GI side effects and do not affect blood coagulation, these drugs are becoming drugs of choice for the treatment of moderate to severe inflammation.

NURSING CONSIDERATIONS

The role of the nurse in NSAID pharmacotherapy involves careful monitoring of the patient's condition and providing education as it relates to the prescribed drug regimen. The nurse should assess for congestive heart failure, fluid retention, hypertension, and renal disease because these drugs are contraindicated in such conditions. Drugs in this class should not be administered to patients with liver dysfunction, because NSAIDs are primarily metabolized in the liver. When the liver is not functioning effectively, toxic levels of metabolites are produced, which may result in hepatic failure. The nurse should assess for sensitivity, as these drugs are contraindicated in patients with a history of NSAID sensitivity.

Pregnant women, children, patients with cardiac, GI, or bleeding disorders, as well as those with diminished kidney or liver function, must be monitored closely while taking NSAIDs. Salicylates (including ASA) are contraindicated for persons under 19 years of age due to an established risk of Reye's syndrome associated with flulike illnesses. Reye's syndrome is a potentially fatal complication of infection characterized by fat accumulation in the brain and liver. NSAIDs promote fluid retention, which may exacerbate hypertension and heart failure. NSAIDs may affect kidney function. Prior to starting on high-dose NSAID pharmacotherapy, baseline kidney and liver function tests and a CBC should be obtained. The nurse should inform the patient that these blood tests will be repeated during therapy, to prevent adverse reactions such as blood dyscrasias.

Despite their selectivity, the COX-2 inhibitors can cause GI bleeding, especially among the elderly, and those who abuse alcohol, smoke cigarettes, or have peptic ulcer disease. NSAIDs may cause fetal abnormalities (pregnancy category C in first trimester, D in second trimester). Patients should not breastfeed while taking COX-2 inhibitors, as they can be transmitted to the baby through breast milk.

Patient education as it relates to nonsteroidal anti-inflammatory drugs should include the goals, reasons for obtaining baseline data such as vital signs and laboratory tests, and possible side effects. The following are important points the nurse should include when teaching patients regarding NSAIDs.

- Reye's syndrome is a life-threatening disorder; do not give drugs containing aspirin to children. Aspirin compounds are ingredients in many OTC drugs such as Excedrin and Pepto-Bismol.
- Take NSAIDs with food or milk to decrease gastric upset.
- Consult a healthcare provider before taking any OTC medications or herbal alternatives while taking NSAIDs.
- Report immediately the following: blood in urine or stool, emesis, heartburn or abdominal pain, unexplained fatigue, headache or dizziness, changes in hearing (especially ringing in the ears), swelling, itching, or skin rash.

NATURAL THERAPIES | Fish Oils for Inflammation

Fish oils, also known as marine oils, are lipids found primarily in coldwater fish. These oils are rich sources of long-chain polyunsaturated fatty acids of the omega-3 type. The two most studied fatty acids found in fish oils are EPA (eicosapentaenoic acid) and DHA (docosahexaenoic acid). These fatty acids are known for their triglyceride-lowering activity and they may also have anti-inflammatory actions.

Several mechanisms are believed to account for the anti-inflammatory activity of EPA and DHA. The two competitively inhibit the conversion of arachidonic acid to the proinflammatory prostaglandins, thus reducing their synthesis.

Interactions may occur between fish oil supplements and aspirin and other NSAIDs. Although rare, such interactions might be manifested by increased susceptibility to bruising, nosebleeds, hemoptysis, hematuria, and blood in the stool.

See "Nursing Process Focus: Patients Receiving NSAID Therapy," page 234 in Chapter 19, for additional teaching points ⊙ .

Systemic Glucocorticoids

Glucocorticoids have wide therapeutic application. One of their most useful properties is a potent anti-inflammatory action that can suppress severe cases of inflammation. Because of potentially serious adverse effects, however, systemic glucocorticoids are reserved for the short-term treatment of severe disease. These agents are shown in Table 31.4.

31.5 Treating Acute or Severe Inflammation with Systemic Glucocorticoids

Glucocorticoids are natural hormones released by the adrenal cortex that have powerful effects on nearly every cell in the body. When used to treat inflammatory disorders, the drug doses are many times higher than those naturally present in the blood. The uses of glucocorticoids include the treatment of neoplasia (Chapter 35), asthma (Chapter 29), arthritis (Chapter 46), and corticosteroid deficiency (Chapter 39) ⊙ .

Glucocorticoids have the ability to suppress histamine release and inhibit the synthesis of prostaglandins by COX-2. In addition, they can inhibit the immune system by suppressing certain functions of phagocytes and lymphocytes. These multiple actions markedly reduce inflammation, making glucocorticoids the most efficacious medications available for the treatment of severe inflammatory disorders.

Unfortunately the glucocorticoid drugs have a number of serious adverse effects that limit their therapeutic utility. These include suppression of the normal functions of the adrenal gland (adrenal insufficiency), hyperglycemia, mood changes, cataracts, peptic ulcers, electrolyte imbalances, and osteoporosis. Because of their effectiveness at reducing the

Pr PROTOTYPE DRUG | CELECOXIB (Celebrex)

ACTIONS AND USES

Approved in 1998, celecoxib is an NSAID that inhibits prostaglandin synthesis through the selective inhibition of COX-2. Its efficacy at relieving pain, fever, and inflammation is similar to that of other NSAIDs. Common indications include musculoskeletal disorders such as rheumatoid and osteoarthritis, acute pain and dysmenorrhea. Unlike many NSAIDs, celecoxib has little effect on blood coagulation, and gastric irritation is minimal. Celecoxib also is used to reduce the number of adenomatous colorectal polyps in adults with familial adenomatous polyposis (FAP). Patients with FAP have an inherited mutation in a gene that results in hundreds of polyps and an almost 100% risk of colon cancer.

Administration Alerts

- Administer 2 hours before or after magnesium- or aluminum-containing antacids.
- Pregnancy category C in first and second trimesters; category D in the third trimester.

ADVERSE EFFECTS AND INTERACTIONS

Side effects of celecoxib are generally mild and include nausea, diarrhea, abdominal pain, flatulence, headache, and insomnia. Celecoxib may cause hypersensitivity in patients allergic to sulfonamides, because this drug contains sulfur.

Drug interactions with celecoxib include a decreased effectiveness of ACE inhibitors. Celecoxib may cause lithium toxicity. Celecoxib may increase INR when used concurrently with warfarin.

See the companion website for a Nursing Process Focus specific to this drug.

Table 31.4	Selected Glucocorticoids for Severe Inflammation
Drug	**Route and Adult Dose (max dose where indicated)**
betamethasone (Celestone, Betacort, others)	PO; 0.6–7.2 mg/day
cortisone (Cortistan, Cortone)	PO; 20–300 mg/day in divided doses
dexamethasone (Decadron, others)	PO; 0.25–4 mg bid-qid
hydrocortisone (Cortef, others) (see page 583 for the Prototype Drug box)	Topical: 0.5% cream applied qd-qid; PO; 10–320 mg tid-qid
methylprednisolone (Depo-Medrol, Medrol, others)	PO; 4–48 mg/day in divided doses
prednisolone (Delta-Cortef, Hydeltrasol, Key-Pred, others)	PO; 5–60 mg qd-qid
prednisone (Medicorten, others)	PO; 5–60 mg qd-qid
triamcinolone (Kenalog, Azmacort, others)	PO; 4–48 mg qd-qid

signs and symptoms of inflammation, glucocorticoids can mask infections that may be present in the patient. This combination of masking signs of infection and suppressing the immune response creates a potential for existing infections to grow rapidly and undetected. An active infection is usually a contraindication for glucocorticoid therapy.

Because the appearance of these adverse effects is a function of the dose and duration of therapy, treatment is often limited to the short-term control of acute disease. When longer therapy is indicated, doses are kept as low as possible and alternate-day therapy is sometimes implemented; the medication is taken every other day to encourage the patient's adrenal gland to function on the days when no drug is given. During long-term therapy, the nurse must be alert for signs of overtreatment, a condition referred to as Cushing's syndrome. Because the body becomes accustomed to high doses of glucocorticoids, patients must dis-

continue glucocorticoids gradually; abrupt withdrawal can result in acute lack of adrenal function.

NURSING CONSIDERATIONS

The role of the nurse in systemic glucocorticoid therapy involves careful monitoring of a patient's condition and providing education as it relates to the prescribed drug regimen. Before beginning therapy, the nurse should screen the patient for existing infection. If infection is discovered prior to or during therapy, antibiotics may be required. Glucocorticoids should be used with great caution in patients with HIV or tuberculosis infections.

Prior to therapy, the nurse must also assess the patient's metabolic status and fluid and electrolyte balance. Baseline laboratory data should be obtained, including CBC, serum glucose, sodium and potassium levels, and body weight.

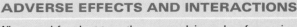

PROTOTYPE DRUG	**PREDNISONE** (Meticorten, others)

ACTIONS AND USES	**ADVERSE EFFECTS AND INTERACTIONS**
Prednisone is a synthetic glucocorticoid. Its actions are the result of being metabolized to an active form, which is also available as a drug called prednisolone (Delta-Cortef, others). When used for inflammation, duration of therapy is commonly 4 to 10 days. Alternate-day dosing is used for longer term therapy. Prednisone is occasionally used to terminate acute bronchospasm in patients with asthma and for patients with certain cancers such as Hodgkin's disease, acute leukemia, and lymphomas.	When used for short-term therapy, prednisone has few serious adverse effects. Long-term therapy may result in Cushing's syndrome, a condition that includes hyperglycemia, fat redistribution to the shoulders and face, muscle weakness, bruising, and bones that easily fracture. Because glucocorticoids can raise blood glucose levels, diabetic patients may require an adjustment in insulin dose. Gastric ulcers may occur with long-term therapy and an antiulcer medication may be prescribed prophylactically.
Administration Alerts	Prednisone interacts with many drugs. For example, barbiturates, phenytoin, and rifampin increase steroid metabolism. Concurrent use with amphotericin B or diuretics increases potassium loss. Prednisone may inhibit antibody response to toxoids and vaccines.
■ IM injections should be administered deep into the muscle mass to avoid atrophy or abscesses. ■ Do not use if a systemic infection is present. ■ Drug should not be discontinued abruptly. ■ Pregnancy category C.	Use with caution with herbal supplements, such as aloe and senna, which may increase potassium loss. Licorice may potentiate the effect of glucocorticoids.

See the companion website for a Nursing Process Focus specific to this drug.

Patients with blood disorders should be observed for possible exacerbation, because glucocorticoids promote red blood cell proliferation. These drugs also suppress osteoblast formation, so they should be administered with caution to patients with osteoporosis or other bone disorders. Patients with diabetes mellitus must be monitored carefully, because glucocorticoids increase serum glucose. Patients with heart failure, hypertension, or renal disease must be monitored closely due to drug-induced sodium and fluid retention. Glucocorticoids can cross the placenta and affect the developing fetus, so they should be used in pregnancy only when benefits outweigh risks (pregnancy category C). Women receiving high-dose glucocorticoid therapy should be warned against breastfeeding.

The nurse should monitor the patient for development of Cushing's syndrome (adrenocortical excess). Signs include bruising and a characteristic pattern of fat deposits in the cheeks (moon face), shoulders (buffalo hump), and abdomen. Patients with existing mental or emotional disorders should be monitored closely; glucocorticoids may trigger mania in bipolar patients. Glucocorticoids may also exacerbate the symptoms of myasthenia gravis, contributing to the risk of respiratory failure.

Glucocorticoids promote the development of gastric ulcers by altering the protective mucous lining of the stomach. Local irritation may be reduced by administering oral doses with food or an antacid. However, the risk of GI bleeding remains, especially with long-term therapy, since changes in the stomach result from *systemic* drug action. Therefore, these drugs should always be administered with caution to patients with a history of peptic ulcer disease. Glucocorticoids also promote capillary fragility; IM injections should be administered deep into the muscle mass to avoid atrophy or abscesses.

Patient education as it relates to glucocorticoids should include the goals, reasons for obtaining baseline data such as blood tests and body weight, and possible side effects. Following are important points the nurse should include when teaching patients regarding glucocorticoids.

■ Take the medication at the same time each day.
■ Never discontinue taking the medication abruptly.
■ Take with food to avoid gastric irritation.
■ Guard against infection: avoid persons with infections and wash hands frequently.
■ Weigh yourself daily and check ankles/legs for signs of swelling.
■ Immediately report the following: difficulty breathing; heartburn; chest, abdominal, or joint/bone pain; nose bleed; bloody cough, vomit, urine or stools; fever; chills; red streaks from wounds or any other sign of infection; increased thirst or urination; fruity breath odor (or significantly elevated daily serum glucose); falls or other accidents (deep lacerations may require antibiotic therapy); and mood swings.

See "Nursing Process Focus: Patients Receiving Systemic Glucocorticoid Therapy," page 584 in Chapter 39 , for additional teaching points.

FEVER

Like inflammation, fever is a natural mechanism in the body's defense system to remove foreign organisms. Many species of bacteria are killed by high fever. The goal of antipyretic therapy is to lower body temperature while treating the underlying cause of the fever, usually an infection. The NSAIDs and acetaminophen are generally safe, effective drugs for reducing fever.

Prolonged, high fever can become quite dangerous, especially in young children in which fever can stimulate febrile seizures. In adults, excessively high fever can break down body tissues, reduce mental acuity, and lead to delirium or coma, particularly among elderly patients. In rare instances, an elevated fever may be fatal. Often, the healthcare provider must determine whether the fever needs to be dealt with aggressively or allowed to run its course. Drugs used to treat fever are called **antipyretics**.

31.6 Treating Fever with Antipyretics

In most patients, fever is more of a discomfort than a life-threatening problem and can be controlled effectively by inexpensive, OTC drugs. Aspirin, ibuprofen, and acetaminophen are all effective antipyretics. Examples of common brand-name drugs taken for fever are Advil, Aleve, Bayer, Cope, Excedrin, Motrin, and Tylenol. Many of these drugs are marketed for different age groups including special, flavored brands for infants and children. For fast delivery and effectiveness, drugs may come in various forms including gels, caplets, enteric-coated tablets, and suspensions. ASA and acetaminophen are also available as suppositories. The antipyretics come in various dosages and concentrations, including extra strength.

Until the 1980s, aspirin was the most common therapy for fever in children; however, aspirin has been implicated in the development of Reye's syndrome. Aspirin and other salicylates are now contraindicated for children and teenagers with fever. Because of the potential for Reye's syndrome, some healthcare providers also advise against administering *any* NSAID to children or teens. Therefore, acetaminophen has become the antipyretic of choice to treat most fevers.

NURSING CONSIDERATIONS

The role of the nurse in antipyretic therapy involves careful monitoring of a patient's condition and providing education as it relates to the prescribed drug regimen. Prior to administering an antipyretic, the nurse should obtain the patient's vital signs, especially temperature. The nurse should assess the patient's developmental status, the origin of the fever, and associated symptoms to determine the appropriate formulation or route for the antipyretic. For example, patients who are vomiting should receive an antipyretic by suppository, and very young children are generally given flavored elixirs.

Baseline laboratory data are necessary to assess the patient's kidney and liver status; antipyretics may cause toxicity in patients with diminished organ function. Acetaminophen is contraindicated in patients with significant liver disease, including viral hepatitis, cirrhosis, and alcoholism, because it is metabolized by the liver and can greatly increase the risk of hepatotoxicity. Acetaminophen also inhibits warfarin (Coumadin) metabolism, and may produce toxic accumulation of this drug and cause serious bleeding. NSAIDs may be contraindicated with warfarin as well, because they also promote bleeding.

SPECIAL CONSIDERATIONS
Ethnic Considerations in Acetaminophen Metabolism

Certain ethnic populations, including Asians, African Americans, and Saudis, have higher rates of an enzyme deficiency that impacts how they metabolize certain drugs. More than 200 million people worldwide are believed to have a hereditary deficiency of this enzyme, glucose-6-phosphate dehydrogenase (G6PD). Patients with G6PD deficiency are at risk for developing hemolysis after ingestion of certain drugs, including acetaminophen. Conflicting data exist on whether therapeutic dosages of acetaminophen can cause hemolysis in these patients. However, because acetaminophen is one of the most common drugs ingested in intentional overdoses, healthcare providers should recommend that patients with G6PD deficiency avoid this drug.

The nurse should advise the patient or caregiver that liquid forms of acetaminophen or ibuprofen come in different strengths; all children's liquid formulations are not the same. Children under 1 year should be given "infant drops" rather than "children's liquid." Patients should be advised to consult the nurse regarding safe dosages. The nurse should inform the patient that acetaminophen overdosage can cause hepatic failure.

See "Nursing Process Focus: Patients Receiving Antipyretic Therapy" for additional teaching points.

ALLERGY

Allergies are caused by a hyperresponse of body defenses. Because histamine is released during an allergic response, many signs and symptoms of allergy are similar to those of inflammation. Allergies also involve mediators of the immune response.

31.7 Pharmacotherapy of Allergic Rhinitis

Allergic rhinitis, or hay fever, is a common disorder afflicting millions of people annually. Symptoms resemble those of the common cold: tearing eyes, sneezing, nasal congestion, postnasal drip, and itching of the throat. The cause of all allergies is exposure to an antigen. An **antigen** may be defined as anything that is recognized as foreign by the body. Certain foods, industrial chemicals, drugs, pollen, animal proteins, and even latex gloves can be antigens. A more detailed discussion of the immune system and the pharmacotherapy of immune disorders is included in Chapter 30 ∞.

The exact cause of a patient's allergic rhinitis is often difficult to pinpoint; however, common causes include pollen from weeds, grasses and trees, molds, dust mites, certain foods, and animal dander. Chemical fumes, tobacco smoke, or air pollutants such as ozone are nonallergenic factors that may worsen symptoms. While some patients expe-

PROTOTYPE DRUG | **ACETAMINOPHEN** (Tylenol)

ACTIONS AND USES

Acetaminophen reduces fever by direct action at the level of the hypothalamus and causes dilation of peripheral blood vessels enabling sweating and dissipation of heat. Acetaminophen and aspirin have equal efficacy in relieving pain and reducing fever.

Acetaminophen has no anti-inflammatory action; therefore, it is not effective in treating arthritis or pain caused by tissue swelling following injury. The primary therapeutic usefulness of acetaminophen is for the treatment of fever in children and for relief of mild to moderate pain when aspirin is contraindicated. Acetaminophen is pregnancy category B.

Administration Alert

- Liquid forms are available in varying concentrations. For administration in children, the appropriate strength product must be used to avoid toxicity.

ADVERSE EFFECTS AND INTERACTIONS

Acetaminophen is quite safe and adverse effects are uncommon at therapeutic doses. Unlike aspirin, acetaminophen has no direct anti-inflammatory effect and does not affect blood coagulation or cause gastric irritation. It is not recommended in patients who are malnourished. In such cases, acute toxicity may result leading to renal failure, which can be fatal. Other signs of acute toxicity include nausea, vomiting, chills, and abdominal discomfort.

Acetaminophen inhibits warfarin metabolism, causing warfarin to accumulate to toxic levels. High-dose or long-term acetaminophen usage may result in elevated warfarin levels and bleeding. Ingestion of this drug with alcohol is not recommended due to the possibility of liver failure from hepatic necrosis.

The patient should avoid taking herbs that have the potential for liver toxicity, including comfrey, coltsfoot, and chaparral.

See the companion website for a Nursing Process Focus specific to this drug.

---

rience symptoms at specific times of the year, when pollen and mold are at high levels in their environment, other patients are afflicted continuously throughout the year.

The fundamental symptomatic problem of allergic rhinitis is inflammation of the mucous membranes in the nose, throat, and airways. Chemical mediators such as histamine are released that initiate the distressing symptoms. The mechanism of allergic rhinitis is illustrated in Figure 31.2.

Drugs used to treat allergic rhinitis may be grouped into two basic categories: preventers and relievers. Preventers are used for prophylaxis and include antihistamines, glucocorticoids, and mast cell stabilizers. Relievers are used to provide immediate, though temporary, relief for acute allergy symptoms once they have occurred. Relievers include the oral and intranasal sympathomimetics that are used as nasal decongestants.

H₁ Receptor Antagonists/ Antihistamines

Antihistamines block the actions of histamine at the H_1 receptor. They are widely used OTC for relief of allergy symptoms, motion sickness, and insomnia. These agents are shown in Table 31.5.

31.8 Treating Allergic Rhinitis with H₁ Receptor Antagonists

H_1 receptor antagonists are commonly called antihistamines. Because the term *antihistamine* is nonspecific and does not indicate which of the two histamine receptors are affected, H_1 receptor antagonist is a more accurate name. Although a large number of H_1 receptor antagonists

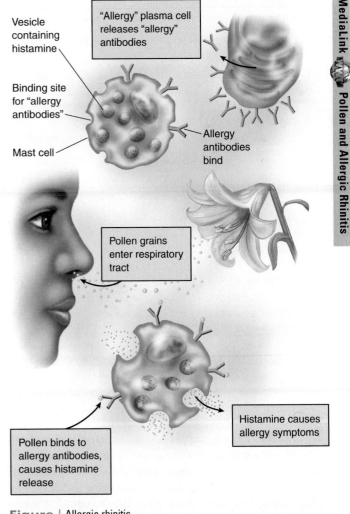

Vesicle containing histamine

Binding site for "allergy antibodies"

Mast cell

"Allergy" plasma cell releases "allergy" antibodies

Allergy antibodies bind

Pollen grains enter respiratory tract

Pollen binds to allergy antibodies, causes histamine release

Histamine causes allergy symptoms

Figure 31.2 | Allergic rhinitis

NURSING PROCESS FOCUS | PATIENTS RECEIVING ANTIPYRETIC THERAPY

ASSESSMENT

Prior to administration:
- Obtain complete health history (mental and physical), including data on origin of fever, recent surgeries, or trauma.
- Obtain vital signs; assess in context of patient's baseline values.
- Obtain patient's complete medication history, including nicotine and alcohol consumption, to determine possible drug allergies and/or interactions.

POTENTIAL NURSING DIAGNOSES

- Pain
- Hyperthermia
- Risk for Injury (hepatic toxicity), related to adverse effects of drug therapy

PLANNING: PATIENT GOALS AND EXPECTED OUTCOMES

The patient will:
- Experience a reduction in body temperature
- Demonstrate an understanding of the drug's action by accurately describing drug side effects and precautions

IMPLEMENTATION

Interventions and (Rationales)	Patient Education/Discharge Planning
Assess for intolerance to ASA for possible cross-hypersensitivity to other NSAIDs or acetaminophen.	Inform patient to immediately report any difficulty breathing, itching, or skin rash.
Monitor hepatic and renal function. (Antipyretics are metabolized in the liver and excreted by the kidneys.)	Instruct patient: ■ To report signs of liver toxicity: nausea, vomiting, anorexia, bleeding, severe upper or lower abdominal pain, heartburn, jaundice, or a change in the color or character of stools ■ To adhere to laboratory testing regimen for serum blood tests as directed
Use with caution in patients with a history of excessive alcohol consumption. (Alcohol increases the risk of liver damage associated with acetaminophen or NSAID administration.)	Advise patient to abstain from alcohol while taking this medication.
Use with caution in diabetics. Observe for signs of hypoglycemia which may occur with acetaminophen usage.	Instruct patient to immediately report: ■ Excessive thirst ■ Large increase or decrease in urine output ■ Advise patients with diabetes mellitus that acetaminophen may cause low blood sugar and require insulin dose adjustments.

EVALUATION OF OUTCOME CRITERIA

Evaluate the effectiveness of drug therapy by confirming that patient goals and expected outcomes have been met (see "Planning").

See Table 31.2 for a list of the drugs to which these nursing actions apply. Acetaminophen is also covered in this Nursing Process Focus chart.

are available for use, their efficacies, therapeutic uses, and side effects are quite similar. These drugs are classified by their generation and their ability to cause sedation, which can be a limiting side effect in some patients. The older, first generation drugs have the potential to cause significant drowsiness, whereas the second generation agents lack this effect in most patients. Care must be taken to avoid alcohol and other CNS depressants when taking antihistamines, because their sedating effects may be additive.

The most common therapeutic use of H_1 receptor antagonists is for the treatment of allergies. These medications provide symptomatic relief from the sneezing, runny nose, and itching of the eyes, nose, and throat which is

Table 31.5	H₁ Receptor Antagonists
Drug	**Route and Adult Dose (max dose where indicated)**
First Generation Agents	
azatadine (Optimine); Trinalin is a combination of azatadine and pseudoephedrine	PO; 1–2 mg bid
azelastine (Astelin)	Intranasal; two sprays per nostril bid
brompheniramine (Dimetapp, others)	PO; 4–8 mg tid-qid (max 40 mg/day)
chlorpheniramine (Chlor-Trimeton, others)	PO; 2–4 mg tid-qid (max 24 mg/day)
clemastine (Tavist)	PO; 1.34 mg bid (max 8.04 mg/day)
cyproheptadine (Periactin)	PO; 4 mg tid or qid (max 0.5 mg/kg/day)
dexbrompheniramine (Drixoral)	PO; 6 mg bid
dexchlorpheniramine (Dexchlor, Poladex, Polargen, Polaramine)	PO; 2 mg q4–6h (max 12 mg/day)
⊕ diphenhydramine (Benadryl, others)	PO; 25–50 mg tid-qid (max 300 mg/day)
promethazine (Phenergan, Anergan, Phenazine, Promacot, others)	PO; 12.5 mg qd (max 150 mg/day)
tripelennamine (PBZ-SR, Pelamine)	PO; 25–50 mg q4–6h (max 600 mg/day)
triprolidine (Actifed, Actidil)	PO; 2.5 mg bid or tid
Second Generation Agents	
cetirizine (Zyrtec)	PO; 5–10 mg qd
desloratidine (Clarinex)	PO; 5 mg qd
⊕ fexofenadine (Allegra)	PO; 60 mg qd-bid (max 120 mg/day)
loratadine (Claritin)	PO; 10 mg qd

Table 31.6	Selected Antihistamine Combinations Available OTC for Allergic Rhinitis		
Brand Name	**Antihistamine**	**Decongestant**	**Analgesic**
Actifed Cold and Allergy tablets	Triprolidine	Pseudoephedrine	-
Actifed Cold and Sinus caplets	Chlorpheniramine	Pseudoephedrine	Acetaminophen
Benadryl Allergy/Cold tablets	Diphenhydramine	Pseudoephedrine	Acetaminophen
Chlor-Trimeton Allergy/ Decongestant tablets	Chlorpheniramine	Pseudoephedrine	-
Dimetapp Cold and Allergy chewable tablets	Brompheniramine	Phenylpropanolamine	-
Drixoral Allergy Sinus Extended Relief tablets	Dexbrompheniramine	Pseudoephedrine	Acetaminophen
Sinutab Sinus Allergy tablets	Chlorpheniramine	Pseudoephedrine	Acetaminophen
Sudafed Cold and Allergy tablets	Chlorpheniramine	Pseudoephedrine	-
Tavist Allergy 12-hour tablets	Clemastine	-	-
Triaminic Cold/Allergy softchews	Chlorpheniramine	Pseudoephedrine	-
Tylenol Allergy Sinus Nighttime caplets	Diphenhydramine	Pseudoephedrine	Acetaminophen

characteristic of allergic rhinitis. H₁ receptor antagonists are used in OTC cold and sinus medicines, often in combination with other drugs such as decongestants and antitussives. Common OTC antihistamine combinations used to treat allergies are shown in Table 31.6.

Antihistamines are most effective when taken prophylactically to prevent allergic symptoms. Their effectiveness may diminish with long-term use. It should be noted that during severe allergic reactions such as anaphylaxis, histamine is just one of several chemical mediators released;

thus, H_1 receptor antagonists alone are not efficacious in treating these acute disorders.

Although most antihistamines are given orally, azelastine (Astelin) was the first to be available by the intranasal route. Azelastine is considered as safe and effective as the oral antihistamines. Although a first generation agent, azelastine causes less drowsiness than others in its class because it is applied locally, and little systemic absorption occurs.

H_1 receptor antagonists are effective in treating a number of other disorders. Motion sickness responds well to these drugs. They are also some of the few drugs available to treat vertigo, a form of dizziness that causes significant nausea. Some of the older antihistamines are marketed as OTC sleep aids, taking advantage of their ability to cause drowsiness.

NURSING CONSIDERATIONS

First Generation H_1 Receptor Antagonists

The role of the nurse in drug therapy with first generation H_1 receptor antagonists involves careful monitoring of a patient's condition and providing education as it relates to the prescribed drug regimen. Before administering a first generation antihistamine, the nurse should obtain baseline vital signs, including ECG in patients with a history of heart disease. First generation H_1 receptor antagonists are contraindicated in patients with a history of dysrhythmias

and heart failure. These drugs can cause vasodilation due to H_1 stimulation.

First generation H_1 receptor antagonists may cause CNS depression, so they may be contraindicated in patients with a history of depression or sleep disorders, such as narcolepsy or apnea. Because the anticholinergic effects of H_1 receptor antagonists can place patients with narrow angle glaucoma at risk for injury, they are contraindicated in these patients. Drugs in this class sometimes cause idiosyncratic CNS stimulation; therefore, they may be contraindicated in patients with seizure disorders. Idiosyncratic CNS stimulation, causing hyperactivity, is more common in children.

Elderly patients should be monitored for profound sedation and altered consciousness, which may contribute to falls or other injuries. Prior to initiation of therapy, the nurse should assess for history of allergy and identify the presence of symptoms, such as urticaria, angioedema, nausea, vomiting, motion sickness, or excess mucous production. The agents should be used with caution during pregnancy (pregnancy category C). H_1 antagonists are secreted in breast milk and should not be used by patients who are breastfeeding.

Patient education as it relates to first generation H_1 receptor antagonists should include goals, reasons for obtaining baseline data such as vital signs, EKG and laboratory blood work, and possible side effects. See "Nursing Process Focus: Patients Receiving Antihistamine Therapy" for specific teaching points.

Pr PROTOTYPE DRUG | DIPHENHYDRAMINE (Benadryl, others)

ACTIONS AND USES

Diphenhydramine is a first generation H_1 receptor antagonist that is a component of some OTC drugs. Its primary use is to treat minor symptoms of allergy and the common cold such as sneezing, runny nose, and tearing of the eyes. OTC preparations may combine diphenhydramine with an analgesic, decongestant, or expectorant. Diphenhydramine is also used as a topical agent to treat rashes, and an IM form is available for severe allergic reactions. Other indications for diphenhydramine include Parkinson's disease, motion sickness, and insomnia.

Administration Alerts

- There is an increased risk of anaphylactic shock when this drug is administered parenterally.
- When administering IV, inject at a rate of 25 mg/min to reduce the risk of shock.
- When administering IM, inject deep into the muscle, to minimize tissue irritation.
- Antihistamines may cause false positive readings for allergy skin tests.
- Pregnancy category C.

ADVERSE EFFECTS AND INTERACTIONS

Older H_1 receptor antagonists such as diphenhydramine cause significant drowsiness, although this usually diminishes with long-term use. Occasionally, a patient will exhibit CNS stimulation and excitability rather than drowsiness. Anticholinergic effects such as dry mouth, tachycardia, and mild hypotension are seen in some patients. Diphenhydramine may cause photosensitivity.

Diphenhydramine interacts with multiple drugs, particularly CNS depressants such as alcohol which enhance sedation. Other OTC cold preparations may increase anticholinergic side effects.

See the companion website for a Nursing Process Focus specific to this drug.

Second Generation H₁ Receptor Antagonists

The role of the nurse in drug therapy with second generation H₁ receptor antagonists involves careful monitoring of a patient's condition and providing education as it relates to the prescribed drug regimen. Prior to initiating therapy, the nurse should assess for the presence/history of allergic rhinitis, conjunctivitis, urticaria, and atopic dermatitis. Baseline vital signs, including ECG in patients with a history of cardiac disease, should be obtained.

Second generation H₁ receptor antagonists are generally contraindicated in patients with dysrhythmias because the drugs prolong the Q-T interval. Due to their anticholinergic effects on the respiratory system, these agents are contraindicated in patients with asthma and in patients who use nicotine. These drugs are metabolized by the liver and excreted by the kidneys; therefore, they are contraindicated in patients with severe liver or renal impairment. Loratadine (Claritin) is most effective when given on an empty stomach.

These drugs should be used with caution in patients with urinary retention due to their anticholinergic effects on the bladder. Anticholinergic activity also affects patients with open angle glaucoma and hypertension; these patients must be monitored closely. Drugs in this classification are contraindicated in pregnant women in their third trimester due to the possibility of fetal malformation. These drugs should be used with caution in young children, because the long-term effects of these drugs on growth and development has not been established.

Patient education as it relates to second generation H₁ receptor antagonists should include goals, reasons for obtaining baseline data such as vital signs, ECG and laboratory blood work, and possible side effects. See "Nursing Process Focus: Patients Receiving Antihistamine Therapy" for specific teaching points.

Intranasal Glucocorticoids

Glucocorticoids may be applied directly to the nasal mucosa to prevent symptoms of allergic rhinitis. They have begun to replace antihistamines as drugs of choice for the treatment of chronic allergic rhinitis. These drugs are shown in Table 31.7.

31.9 Treating Allergic Rhinitis with Intranasal Glucocorticoids

Section 31.5 presents the importance of the glucocorticoids in treating severe inflammation. As systemic drugs, their use is limited by serious side effects. Intranasal glucocorticoids, however, produce none of the potentially serious adverse effects that are observed when these hormones are given orally or parenterally. Because of their effectiveness and safety, the intranasal glucocorticoids have joined antihistamines as first line drugs in the treatment of allergic rhinitis.

Intranasal glucocorticoids are administered with a metered-spray device that delivers a consistent dose of drug per spray. When administered properly, their action is limited to the nasal passages. The most frequently reported side effects are an intense burning sensation in the nose immediately after spraying and drying of the nasal mucosa.

NURSING CONSIDERATIONS

The role of the nurse in drug therapy with intranasal glucocorticoids involves careful monitoring of a patient's condition and providing education as it relates to the prescribed drug regimen. Prior to administering glucocorticoid nasal spray, the nurse should assess the nares for excoriation or bleeding. Broken mucous membranes allow direct access to the bloodstream, increasing the likelihood of systemic effects. The mouth and throat should be examined for signs of infection, because glucocorticoids may slow the healing process and mask infections. Intranasal glucocorticoids are contraindicated in patients who demonstrate hypersensitivity to any of the ingredients, including preservatives, in the nasal spray.

Pr PROTOTYPE DRUG	FEXOFENADINE (Allegra)

ACTIONS AND USES

Fexofenadine is a second generation H₁ receptor antagonist with efficacy equivalent to that of diphenhydramine. Its primary action is to block the effects of histamine at H₁ receptors. When taken prophylactically, it reduces the severity of nasal congestion, sneezing, and tearing of the eyes. Its long half-life of over 14 hours offers the advantage of being administered once or twice daily. Fexofenadine is only available in oral form. Allegra-D combines fexofenadine with pseudoephedrine, a decongestant.

Administration Alert

■ Pregnancy category C.

ADVERSE EFFECTS AND INTERACTIONS

The major advantage of fexofenadine over first generation antihistamines is it causes less drowsiness. Although considered nonsedating, drowsiness can still occur in some patients. Other side effects are usually minor and include headache and upset stomach.

No clinically significant drug interactions have been established. However, concurrent use with other antihistamines or CNS depressants may cause synergistic sedative effects.

 See the companion website for a Nursing Process Focus specific to this drug.

NURSING PROCESS FOCUS **PATIENTS RECEIVING ANTIHISTAMINE THERAPY**

ASSESSMENT

Prior to administration:
- Obtain complete health history including data on anaphylaxis, asthma, or cardiac disease, plus allergies, drug history, and possible drug interactions.
- Obtain EKG and vital signs; assess in context of patient's baseline values.
- Assess respiratory status: breathing pattern.
- Assess neurologic status and level of consciousness.

POTENTIAL NURSING DIAGNOSES

- Ineffective Airway Clearance
- Ineffective Breathing Pattern
- Disturbed Sleep Pattern, related to somnolence or agitation

PLANNING: PATIENT GOALS AND EXPECTED OUTCOMES

The patient will:
- Report relief from allergic symptoms such as congestion, itching, or postnasal drip
- Demonstrate an understanding of the drug's action by accurately describing drug side effects and precautions

IMPLEMENTATION

Interventions and (Rationales)	*Patient Education/Discharge Planning*
■ Auscultate breath sounds before administering. Use with extreme caution in patients with asthma or COPD. Keep resuscitative equipment accessible. (Anticholinergic effects of antihistamines may trigger bronchospasm.)	■ Instruct patient to immediately report wheezing or difficulty breathing. ■ Advise asthmatics to consult the nurse regarding the use of injectable epinephrine in emergency situations.
■ Monitor vital signs (including EKG) before administering. Use with extreme caution in patients with a history of cardiovascular disease. (Anticholinergic effects can increase heart rate and lower blood pressure. Fatal dysrhythmias and cardiovascular collapse have been reported in some patients receiving antihistamines.)	Instruct patient to: ■ Immediately report dizziness, palpitations, headache, or chest, arm, or back pain accompanied by nausea/vomiting and/or sweating ■ Monitor vital signs daily, ensuring proper use of home equipment
■ Monitor thyroid function. Use with caution in patients with a history of hyperthyroidism. (Antihistamines exacerbate CNS-stimulating effects of hyperthyroidism and may trigger thyroid storm.)	■ Instruct patient to immediately report nervousness or restlessness, insomnia, fever, profuse sweating, thirst, and mood changes.
■ Monitor for vision changes. Use with caution in patients with narrow angle glaucoma. ■ (Antihistamines can increase intraocular pressure and cause photosensitivity.)	Instruct patient to: ■ Immediately report head or eye pain and visual changes ■ Wear dark glasses, use sunscreen, and avoid excessive sun exposure
■ Monitor neurologic status, especially LOC. Use with caution in patients with a history of seizure disorder. (Antihistamines lower the seizure threshold. The elderly are at increased risk of serious sedation and other anticholinergic effects.)	Instruct patient to: ■ Immediately report seizure activity, including any changes in character and pattern of seizures ■ Avoid driving or performing hazardous activities until effects of the drug are known
■ Observe for signs of renal toxicity. Measure intake and output. Use with caution in patients with a history of kidney or urinary tract disease. (Antihistamines promote urinary retention.)	■ Instruct patient to immediately report flank pain, difficulty urinating, reduced urine output, and changes in the appearance of urine (cloudy, with sediment, odor, etc.).
■ Use with caution in patients with diabetes mellitus. Monitor serum glucose levels with increased frequency (e.g, from daily to tid, ac). (Antihistamines decrease serum glucose levels.)	Instruct patient to: ■ Immediately report symptoms of hypoglycemia ■ Consult the healthcare provider regarding timing of glucose monitoring and reportable results (e.g., "less than 70 mg/dl")

continued

NURSING PROCESS FOCUS: *Patients Receiving Antihistamine Therapy (continued)*

Interventions and (Rationales)	Patient Education/Discharge Planning
■ Monitor for GI side effects. Use with caution in patients with a history of GI disorders, especially peptic ulcers or liver disease. (Antihistamines block H_1 receptors, altering the mucosal lining of the stomach. These drugs are metabolized in the liver, increasing the risk of hepatotoxicity.)	Instruct patient to: ■ Immediately report nausea, vomiting, anorexia, bleeding, chest or abdominal pain, heartburn, jaundice, or a change in the color or character of stools ■ Avoid substances that irritate the stomach such as spicy foods, alcoholic beverages, and nicotine; take drug with food to avoid stomach upset
■ Monitor for side effects such as dry mouth; observe for signs of anticholinergic crisis.	Instruct patient to: ■ Immediately report fever or flushing accompanied by difficulty swallowing ("cotton mouth"), blurred vision, and confusion ■ Avoid mixing OTC antihistamines; always consult the healthcare provider before taking any OTC drugs or herbal supplements ■ Suck on hard candy to relieve dry mouth and maintain adequate fluid intake

EVALUATION OF OUTCOME CRITERIA

Evaluate the effectiveness of drug therapy by confirming that patient goals and expected outcomes have been met (see "Planning").

See Table 31.6 for a list of drugs to which these nursing actions apply.

Table 31.7	**Intranasal Glucocorticoids**
Drug	**Route and Adult Dose (max dose where indicated)**
beclomethasone (Beconase, Vancenase) (see page 394 for the Prototype Drug box)	Intranasal: one spray bid-qid
budesonide (Rhinocort)	Intranasal: two sprays bid
flunisolide (Nasalide, Nasarel)	Intranasal: two sprays bid; may increase to tid if needed
fluticasone propionate (Flonase)	Intranasal: one spray qd-bid (max qid)
mometasone furoate (Nasonex)	Intranasal: two sprays qd
triamcinolone acetonide (Nasacort AQ)	Intranasal: 2–4 sprays qid

The nurse should monitor the patient for alterations in the nasal and oral mucosa, and for signs of upper respiratory (especially oropharyngeal) infection. Signs and symptoms of GI distress should be monitored, because swallowing large quantities of the drug may contribute to dyspepsia and systemic drug absorption. The nurse should monitor for signs of Cushing's syndrome.

Patient education as it relates to intranasal glucocorticoids should include goals, reasons for obtaining baseline data such as vital signs and laboratory blood work, and possible side effects. The nurse should instruct the patient in the correct use and care of the nasal spray device. Because these medications may take 2 to 4 weeks to be effective, the nurse must advise the patient not to discontinue use prematurely. Patients may expect these drugs to act as quickly and effectively as decongestants. All patients, especially chil-

dren, must be urged not to swallow excess amounts of the drug which is likely to drain down the back of the throat following application. Swallowing large amounts of drug residue increases the risks of systemic side effects. Nasal decongestant sprays are sometimes prescribed with intranasal glucocorticoids for patients with chronic rhinitis. Decongestant sprays should be administered first to clear the nasal passages, allowing for adequate application of the glucocorticoid mist.

Following are other important points the nurse should include when teaching patients regarding intranasal glucocorticoids.

■ Take the medication exactly as prescribed; additional dosing will not speed relief.
■ Shake inhalers thoroughly before spraying.

- Gently clear the nose before spraying. Avoid clearing the nose immediately after spraying.
- Report nosebleeds, nasal burning or irritation that lasts more than a few doses.
- Following administration, spit out the postnasal medication residue.
- Use a humidifier, preservative-free nasal saline spray, or petroleum jelly to ease nasal dryness.

Sympathomimetics

Sympathomimetics stimulate the sympathetic nervous system. They may be administered orally or intranasally to dry the nasal mucosa. The agents used for nasal congestion are shown in Table 31.8.

31.10 Treating Nasal Congestion with Sympathomimetics

As discussed in Chapter 13, sympathomimetics, or adrenergic agonists, are agents that stimulate the sympathetic branch of the autonomic nervous system ⊙. Sympathomimetics with alpha-adrenergic activity are effective at relieving the nasal congestion associated with allergic rhinitis when given by either the oral or intranasal routes. The intranasal preparations such as oxymetazoline (Afrin, others)

are available OTC as sprays or drops, and produce an effective response within minutes. Because of their local action, intranasal sympathomimetics produce few systemic effects. The most serious, limiting side effect of the intranasal preparations is **rebound congestion**. Prolonged use causes hypersecretion of mucous and nasal congestion to worsen, once the drug effects wear off. This sometimes leads to a cycle of increased drug use, as the condition worsens. Because of this rebound congestion, intranasal sympathomimetics should be used for no longer than 3 to 5 days.

When administered orally, sympathomimetics do not produce rebound congestion. Their onset of action by this route, however, is much slower than the intranasal preparations and they are less effective at relieving severe congestion. The possibility of systemic side effects is also greater with the oral drugs. Potential side effects include hypertension and CNS stimulation that may lead to insomnia and anxiety. Pseudoephedrine is the most common sympathomimetic found in oral OTC cold and allergy medicines.

Because the sympathomimetics only relieve nasal congestion, they are often combined with antihistamines to control the sneezing and tearing of allergic rhinitis. It is interesting to note that some OTC drugs having the same basic name (Neo-Synephrine, Afrin, Vicks) may contain different sympathomimetics. For example, Neo-Synephrine preparations with a 12-hour duration contain the drug

Pr PROTOTYPE DRUG	FLUTICASONE (Flonase)
ACTIONS AND USES	**ADVERSE EFFECTS AND INTERACTIONS**
Fluticasone is typical of the intranasal glucocorticoids used to treat seasonal allergic rhinitis. Therapy usually begins with two sprays in each nostril, twice daily, and decreases to one dose per day. Fluticasone acts to decrease local inflammation in the nasal passages thus decreasing nasal stuffiness. ***Administration Alerts*** ■ Directions for use provided by the manufacturer should be carefully followed by the patient. ■ Pregnancy category C.	Side effects to fluticasone are rare. Small amounts of the intranasal glucocorticoids are sometimes swallowed, thus increasing the potential for systemic side effects. Nasal irritation and bleeding occur in a small number of patients. Concomitant use of a local nasal decongestant spray may increase the risk of irritation or bleeding. Use with caution with herbal supplements, such as licorice, which may potentiate the effects of glucocorticoids.

 See the companion website for a Nursing Process Focus specific to this drug.

Table 31.8	**Sympathomimetics for Allergic Rhinitis**
Drug	**Route and Adult Dose (max dose where indicated)**
ephedrine (Pretz-D, Primatene)	Intranasal (0.1%): one to two drops bid
naphazoline (Privine)	Intranasal: two drops q3–6h.
oxymetazoline (Afrin 12 Hour, Neo-synephrine 12 Hour, others)	Intranasal (0.05%): two to three sprays bid for up to 3–5 days
phenylephrine (Afrin 4–6 Hour, Neo-synephrine 4–6 Hour, others)	Intranasal (0.1%): two to three drops or sprays q3–4h, as needed
pseudoephedrine (Actifed, Sudafed, others)	PO; 60 mg 4–6h (max 120 mg/day)
xylometazoline (Otrivin)	Intranasal (0.1%): one to two sprays bid (max three doses/day)

oxymetazoline; Neo-Synephrine preparations that last 4 to 6 hours contain phenylephrine.

NURSING CONSIDERATIONS

The role of the nurse in drug therapy with sympathomimetics for nasal congestion involves careful monitoring of a patient's condition and providing education as it relates to the prescribed drug regimen. The nurse should assess for the presence/history of nasal congestion, and should assess the nares for signs of excoriation or bleeding. Before and during pharmacotherapy, the nurse should assess vital signs, especially pulse and blood pressure. Oral sympathomimetics are contraindicated in patients with hypertension due to vasoconstriction caused by stimulation of alpha-adrenergic receptors on systemic blood vessels.

Alpha-adrenergic agonists should be used with caution in patients with prostatic enlargement, since these drugs increase smooth muscle activity in the prostate gland and may diminish urinary outflow (Chapter 42). Patients with thyroid disorders and diabetes mellitus are at risk because sympathomimetics can increase serum glucose and body metabolism.

These agents should be used with caution for patients with psychiatric disorders due to an increased risk of agitation. The CNS depression effect of these drugs can seriously exacerbate symptoms of clinical depression.

Patient education as it relates to sympathomimetics for nasal congestion should include goals, reasons for obtaining baseline data such as vital signs and tests for cardiac or metabolic disorders, and possible side effects. The following are important points the nurse should include when teaching patients regarding sympathomimetics.

- Limit use of intranasal preparations to 3 to 5 days, to prevent rebound congestion.
- Avoid using other OTC cold or allergy preparations (especially those containing antihistamines) while taking sympathomimetics, because these agents may cause excessive drowsiness.
- Follow the nurse's directions for the use and care of nasal spray dispensers, and proper inhalation technique.
- Report the following immediately: palpitations or chest pain, dizziness or fainting, fever, visual changes, excessively dry mouth and confusion, numbness or tingling in the face or limbs, severe headache, insomnia, restlessness or nervousness, nosebleeds, or persistent intranasal pain or irritation.

See "Nursing Process Focus: Patients Receiving Sympathomimetic Therapy," page 137 in Chapter 13, for more information .

ANAPHYLAXIS

Anaphylaxis is a potentially fatal condition in which body defenses produce a hyperresponse to an antigen. Upon first exposure, the antigen produces no symptoms; however, the body responds by becoming highly sensitized for a subsequent exposure. During anaphylaxis, the body responds quickly, sometimes within minutes after exposure to the antigen, by releasing massive amounts of histamine and other mediators of the inflammatory response. Shortly after exposure to the antigen, the patient may experience itching, hives, and a tightness in the throat or chest. Swelling occurs around the larynx, causing the voice to become hoarse and a nonproductive cough. As anaphylaxis progresses, the patient experiences a rapid fall in blood pressure and difficulty breathing due to bronchoconstriction. The hypotension causes a rebound speeding up of the heart, called reflex tachycardia. Without medical intervention, anaphylaxis leads to a profound shock, which is often fatal. Figure 31.3 illustrates the symptoms of anaphylaxis.

Pr PROTOTYPE DRUG	**OXYMETAZOLINE** (Afrin, others)
ACTIONS AND USES	**ADVERSE EFFECTS AND INTERACTIONS**

ACTIONS AND USES

Oxymetazoline stimulates alpha-adrenergic receptors in the sympathetic nervous system. This causes small arterioles in the nasal passages to constrict, producing a drying of the mucous membranes. Relief from the symptoms of nasal congestion occurs within minutes and lasts for 10 to 12 hours. Oxymetazoline is administered with a metered spray device or by nasal drops.

Administration Alerts

- Wash hands carefully after administration to prevent anisocoria (blurred vision, inequality of pupil size).
- Pregnancy category C.

ADVERSE EFFECTS AND INTERACTIONS

Rebound congestion is common when oxymetazoline is used for longer than 3 to 5 days. Minor stinging and dryness in the nasal mucosa may be experienced. Systemic side effects are unlikely, unless the patient swallows a considerable amount of the medicine. Patients with thyroid disorders, hypertension, diabetes, or heart disease should only use sympathomimetics upon the direction of their healthcare provider.

Oxymetazoline interacts with MAOIs and should not be administered within 2 weeks of MAOI usage.

Use with caution with herbal supplements such as St. John's wort which may have MAOI properties.

 See the companion website for a Nursing Process Focus specific to this drug.

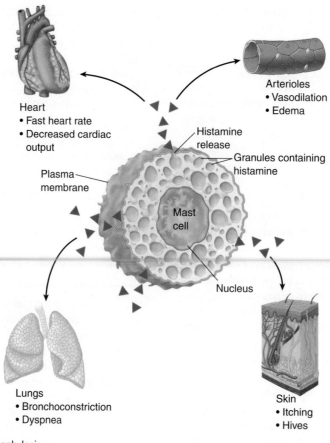

Heart
• Fast heart rate
• Decreased cardiac output

Arterioles
• Vasodilation
• Edema

Histamine release

Granules containing histamine

Plasma membrane

Mast cell

Nucleus

Lungs
• Bronchoconstriction
• Dyspnea

Skin
• Itching
• Hives

Figure 31.3 | Symptoms of anaphylaxis

31.11 Pharmacotherapy of Anaphylaxis

Pharmacotherapy of anaphylaxis is symptomatic and involves supporting the cardiovascular system and preventing further hyperresponse by body defenses. Various medications are used to treat the symptoms of anaphylaxis, depending on the severity of the symptoms. Oxygen is usually administered immediately. Sympathomimetics such as epinephrine can rapidly reverse hypotension. Antihistamines such as diphenhydramine (Benadryl) may be administered IM or IV to prevent stimulation of H_1 receptors. A bronchodilator such as albuterol (Ventolin, Proventil) is sometimes administered by inhalation to relieve the acute shortness of breath caused by histamine. Systemic glucocorticoids such as hydrocortisone may be administered to dampen the inflammatory response. The pharmacotherapy of shock is presented in Chapter 26 ⊙.

NURSING CONSIDERATIONS

The role of the nurse in drug therapy with epinephrine (Adrenalin) involves careful monitoring of a patient's condition and providing education as it relates to the drug. Epinephrine is generally administered as an emergency response to severe allergic reactions. Although epinephrine is contraindicated for patients with known hypersensitivity

to this drug, in life-threatening situations there are no absolute contraindications to its use.

Epinephrine must be administered with caution to patients with cardiac disease or history of cerebral atherosclerosis as it can cause intracranial bleeding, dysrhythmias, or pulmonary edema resulting from a steep rise in blood pressure, and peripheral vascular constriction combined with cardiac stimulation. Epinephrine must also be administered with caution to patients with hyperthyroidism; epinephrine exacerbates tachycardia.

This drug is frequently administered in the emergency department setting; resuscitative equipment must be readily accessible. Parenteral epinephrine is irritating to tissues; thus, IV sites must be closely monitored for signs of extravasation. Vital signs, including EKG, are monitored continuously during epinephrine infusions. The nurse should auscultate the chest before and after epinephrine injection to monitor improvement in bronchoconstriction (wheezing). Patients with a history of closed angle glaucoma should be monitored for visual changes as a result of changes in intraocular pressure.

Patients with a history of recurrent anaphylaxis may be prescribed epinephrine to be self-administered intramuscularly via automatic injectable device (EpiPen). The nurse should instruct these patients regarding safe "pen" storage and disposal and the proper injection technique. Patients

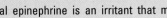 **PROTOTYPE DRUG** | **EPINEPHRINE** (Adrenalin)

ACTIONS AND USES	ADVERSE EFFECTS AND INTERACTIONS
Subcutaneous or intravenous epinephrine is a drug of choice for anaphylaxis because it can reverse many of the distressing symptoms within minutes. Epinephrine is a nonselective adrenergic agonist, stimulating both alpha- and beta-adrenergic receptors. Almost immediately after injection, blood pressure rises due to stimulation of alpha$_1$-receptors. Activation of beta$_2$-receptors in the bronchi opens the airways and relieves the patient's shortness of breath. Cardiac output increases due to stimulation of beta$_1$-receptors in the heart.	When administered parenterally, epinephrine may cause serious adverse effects. Hypertension and dysrhythmias may occur rapidly; therefore, the patient should be monitored continuously following injection. Epinephrine interacts with many drugs. For example, it may increase hypotension with phenothiazines and oxytocin. There may be additive toxicities with other sympathomimetics. MAO inhibitors, tricyclic antidepressants, and alpha- and beta-adrenergic agents inhibit the actions of epinephrine.

Administration Alerts

- Parenteral epinephrine is an irritant that may cause tissue damage if extravasation occurs.
- Pregnancy category C.

 See the companion website for a Nursing Process Focus specific to this drug.

---

should be encouraged to use the medication-free "trainer" auto-inject pen to practice the technique. The nurse should advise the patient to expect some medication to remain in the pen following injection and to report all episodes requiring pen usage to the healthcare provider.

Patient education as it relates to epinephrine should include goals, reasons for obtaining baseline data such as vital signs and EKG, and possible side effects. Following are the important points the nurse should include when teaching patients regarding epinephrine.

- Seek emergency medical attention immediately if a single auto-injection of epinephrine fails to bring relief.

- Report burning, irritation, tenderness, swelling, or hardness at IV or IM injection sites.
- Immediately report changes in level of consciousness, particularly feeling faint.
- Report any of the following: palpitations, chest pain, nausea, vomiting, sweating, weakness, dizziness, confusion, blurred vision, headache, anxiety, or sense of impending doom.

See "Nursing Process Focus: Patients Receiving Sympathomimetic Therapy," page 137 in Chapter 13, for more information.

CHAPTER REVIEW

Key Concepts

The numbered key concepts provide a succinct summary of the important points from the corresponding numbered section within the chapter. If any of these points are not clear, refer to that numbered section within the chapter for review. Expanded versions can be found on the companion website.

31.1 Inflammation is a natural, nonspecific response that limits the spread of invading microorganisms or injury. Acute inflammation occurs over several days, whereas chronic inflammation may continue for months or years.

31.2 Histamine is a key chemical mediator in inflammation. Release of histamine produces vasodilation, allowing capillaries to become leaky thus causing tissue swelling.

31.3 Histamine can produce its effects by interacting with two different receptors. The classic antihistamines used for allergies block H$_1$ histamine receptors in vascular smooth muscle, in the bronchi, and on sensory nerves. The H$_2$ receptor antagonists are used to treat peptic ulcers.

31.4 Nonsteroidal anti-inflammatory drugs (NSAIDs) are the primary drugs for the treatment of simple inflammation. Newer selective COX-2 inhibitors cause less GI distress.

31.5 Systemic glucocorticoids are effective in treating acute or severe inflammation. Overtreatment with these drugs can cause a serious condition called Cushing's syndrome, thus therapy for inflammation is generally short term.

31.6 Acetaminophen and NSAIDs are the primary agents used to treat fever.

31.7 Allergic rhinitis is a disorder characterized by sneezing, watery eyes, and nasal congestion.

31.8 Antihistamines, or H$_1$ receptor antagonists, can provide relief from the symptoms of allergic rhinitis. Newer drugs in this class are nonsedating and offer the advantage of once-a-day dosage.

31.9 Intranasal glucocorticoids have become drugs of choice in treating allergic rhinitis due to their high efficacy and wide margin of safety.

31.10 Oral and intranasal sympathomimetics are used to alleviate the nasal congestion due to allergic rhinitis and the common cold. Intranasal drugs are more efficacious but can only be used for 3 to 5 days due to rebound congestion.

31.11 Anaphylaxis is a serious and often fatal allergic response that is treated with a large number of different drugs, including sympathomimetics, antihistamines, and glucocorticoids.

Review Questions

1. Why are the antihistamines most effective if given *before* inflammation occurs?

2. The sympathomimetics are the most effective drugs for relieving nasal congestion, but healthcare providers often prefer to prescribe antihistamines or intranasal glucocorticoids. Why?

3. Why are oral glucocorticoids primarily used concurrently with the immunosuppressant drugs following a transplant operation?

Critical Thinking Questions

1. A 64-year-old diabetic patient is on prednisone (Meticorten) for rheumatoid arthritis. The patient has recently been admitted to the hospital for stabilization of hyperglycemia. What are the nurse's primary concerns when caring for this patient?

2. A 44-year-old is requesting medication for a painful tendonitis of the elbow. This patient has mild hypertension, a history of alcohol abuse, and nutritional deficits. This patient has a PRN order for acetaminophen (Tylenol), ibuprofen (Motrin), and celecoxib (Celebrex). Which one would the nurse give and why?

3. A 74-year-old male patient informs the nurse that he is taking diphendydramine (Benadryl) to reduce the seasonal allergy symptoms. This patient has a history of an enlarged prostate and mild glaucoma (controlled by medication). What is the nurse's response?

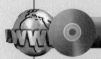 ## EXPLORE MediaLink

NCLEX review, case studies, and other interactive resources for this chapter can be found on the companion website at www.prenhall.com/adams. Click on "Chapter 31" to select the activities for this chapter. For animations, more NCLEX review questions, and an audio glossary, access the accompanying CD-ROM in this textbook.

CHAPTER 32

Drugs for Bacterial Infections

DRUGS AT A GLANCE

PENICILLINS
Pr *penicillin G (Pentids)*

CEPHALOSPORINS
Pr *cefotaxime (Claforan)*

TETRACYCLINES
Pr *tetracycline HCl (Achromycin, others)*

MACROLIDES
Pr *erythromycin (E-Mycin, Erythrocin)*

AMINOGLYCOSIDES
Pr *gentamicin (Garamycin)*

FLUOROQUINOLONES
Pr *ciprofloxacin (Cipro)*

SULFONAMIDES
Pr *trimethoprim-sulfamethoxazole (Bactrim, Septra)*

MISCELLANEOUS ANTIBACTERIALS
Pr *vancomycin (Vancocin)*

ANTITUBERCULAR AGENTS
Pr *isoniazid (INH)*

metabolized and eliminated by the body.
of this process
PHARMACOLOGY
1. The study of medicines; the discipline
pertaining to how drugs improve the heal
of the human body

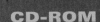 **MediaLink** www.prenhall.com/adams

CD-ROM
Animation:
   Mechanism in Action: Penicillin (Pentids)
Audio Glossary
NCLEX Review

Companion Website
NCLEX Review
Dosage Calculations
Case Study
Care Plans
Expanded Key Concepts

KEY TERMS

acquired resistance *page 440*

aerobic *page 439*

anaerobic *page 439*

antagonism *page 442*

antibiotic *page 439*

anti-infective *page 439*

bacilli *page 439*

bacteriocidal *page 439*

bacteriostatic *page 439*

beta-lactam ring *page 444*

beta-lactamase/penicillinase *page 444*

broad-spectrum antibiotic *page 441*

cocci *page 439*

culture and sensitivity test *page 442*

folic acid *page 455*

gram-positive *page 439*

gram-negative *page 439*

host flora *page 442*

mutations *page 439*

narrow-spectrum antibiotic *page 441*

nosocomial infections *page 441*

pathogen *page 438*

pathogenicity *page 438*

penicillin-binding protein *page 444*

plasmid *page 440*

red-man syndrome *page 458*

spirilla *page 439*

superinfection *page 442*

tubercles *page 459*

virulence *page 438*

OBJECTIVES

After reading this chapter, the student should be able to:

1. Compare and contrast the terms *pathogenicity* and *virulence*.
2. Describe how bacteria are classified.
3. Compare and contrast the terms *bacteriostatic* and *bacteriocidal*.
4. Using a specific example, explain how resistance can develop to an anti-infective drug.
5. Describe the nurse's role in the pharmacologic management of bacterial infections.
6. Explain the importance of culture and sensitivity testing to anti-infective chemotherapy.
7. Identify the mechanism of development and symptoms of superinfections caused by anti-infective therapy.
8. For each of the drug classes listed in Drugs at a Glance, know representative drug examples, explain their mechanism of action, primary actions, and important adverse effects.
9. Categorize antibacterial drugs based on their classification and mechanism of action.
10. Explain how the pharmacotherapy of tuberculosis differs from that of other infections.
11. Use the Nursing Process to care for patients who are receiving drug therapy for bacterial infections.

The human body has adapted quite well to living in a world teeming with microorganisms. In the air, water, food, and soil, microbes are an essential component of life on the planet. In some cases, such as with microorganisms in the colon, microbes play a beneficial role in human health. When in an unnatural environment or when present in unusually high numbers, however, microorganisms can cause a wide variety of ailments ranging from mildly annoying to fatal. The development of the first anti-infective drugs in the mid-1900s was a milestone in the field of medicine. In the last 50 years, pharmacologists have attempted to keep pace with microbes that rapidly become resistant to therapeutic agents. This chapter examines two groups of anti-infectives, the antibacterial agents and the specialized drugs used to treat tuberculosis.

32.1 Pathogenicity and Virulence

A microbe that can cause disease is called a pathogen. Human pathogens include viruses, bacteria, fungi, unicellular organisms, and multicellular animals. To infect humans, pathogens must bypass a number of elaborate body defenses, such as those described in Chapters 30 and 31 . Pathogens may enter through broken skin, or by ingestion, inhalation, or contact with a mucous membrane such as the nasal, urinary, or vaginal mucosa.

The ability of an organism to cause infection is called pathogenicity. Pathogenicity depends on an organism's ability to evade or overcome body defenses. Another common word used to describe a pathogen is virulence. A highly virulent microbe is one that can produce disease when present in minute numbers.

After gaining entry, pathogens generally cause disease by one of two basic mechanisms. Some pathogens grow rapidly and cause disease by their sheer numbers which can overcome immune defenses and disrupt normal cellular function. A second mechanism is the production of toxins that affect human cells. Even very small amounts of some bacterial toxins may disrupt normal cellular activity and, in extreme cases, result in death.

- Infectious diseases are the third most common cause of death in the United States and first in the world.
- Food-borne illness is responsible for 76,000,000 illnesses; 300,000 hospitalizations; and 5,000 deaths each year. About 500 people die of salmonella each year in the United States.
- Urinary tract infection (UTI) is the most common infection acquired in hospitals and nearly all are associated with the insertion of a urinary catheter. Hospital-acquired urinary infections add an average of 3.8 days to a hospital stay and can cost $3,803 per infection.
- Over 2 million nosocomial infections are acquired each year. These infections add 1 day for UTI, 7 to 8 days for surgical site infections, and 6 to 30 days for pneumonia.
- Approximately 200,000 nosocomial infections of the bloodstream occur annually.
- Pneumococcal infections are the most common invasive bacterial infections in children, accounting for 1,400 meningitis; 17,000 bloodstream infections; and 71,000 pneumonia infections under the age of 5 years.
- Up to 30% of all *S. pneumoniae* found in some areas of the United States are resistant to penicillin.
- Nearly all strains of *S. aureus* in the United States are resistant to penicillin.
- About 73,000 cases of *E. coli* poisoning are reported annually in the United States, with the most common source being ground beef.

32.2 Describing and Classifying Bacteria

Because of the enormous number of different bacterial species, several descriptive systems have been developed to simplify their study. It is important for nurses to learn these classification schemes, because drugs that are effective against one organism in a class are likely to be effective against other pathogens in the same class. Common bacterial pathogens with the types of diseases that they cause are shown in Table 32.1.

One of the simplest methods of classifying bacteria is to examine them microscopically after a crystal violet Gram stain is applied. Some bacteria contain a thick cell wall and retain a purple color after staining. These are called **gram-positive** bacteria. Examples of gram-positive bacteria include staphylococci, streptococci, and enterococci. Bacteria that have thinner cell walls will lose the violet stain and are called **gram-negative**. Examples of gram-negative bacteria include bacteroides, *E.coli*, klebsiella, pseudomonas, and salmonella. The distinction between gram-positive and gram-negative bacteria is a profound one that reflects important biochemical and physiological differences between the two groups. Some antibacterial agents are effective only against gram-positive bacteria, whereas others are used to treat gram-negative bacteria.

A second descriptive method is based on cellular shape. Bacteria assume several basic shapes that can be readily determined microscopically. Rod shapes are called **bacilli**, spherical shapes are called **cocci**, and spirals are called **spirilla**.

A third factor used to classify bacteria is their ability to use oxygen. Those that thrive in an oxygen environment are called **aerobic**; those that grow best without oxygen are called **anaerobic**. Some organisms have the ability to change their metabolism and survive in either aerobic or anaerobic conditions, depending on their external environment. Antibacterial drugs differ based on their ability to treat aerobic versus anaerobic bacteria.

32.3 Classification of Anti-infective Drugs

Anti-infective is a general term for any medication that is effective against pathogens. Although **antibiotic** is more frequently used, this term technically refers only to natural substances produced by microorganisms that can kill other microorganisms. In current practice, the terms *antibacterial, anti-infective, antimicrobial,* and *antibiotic* are often used interchangeably, as they are in this textbook.

With over 300 anti-infectives available, it is useful to group these drugs into classes that have similar chemical structures or therapeutic properties. Chemical classes are widely used. Names such as aminoglycoside, fluoroquinolone, and sulfonamide refer to the fundamental chemical structure of a group of anti-infectives. Anti-infectives belonging to the same chemical class share similar antimicrobial properties and side effects.

Another method of classifying anti-infectives is by mechanism of action. Examples include cell wall inhibitors, protein synthesis inhibitors, folic acid inhibitors, and reverse transcriptase inhibitors. These classifications are used in this textbook, where appropriate.

32.4 Actions of Anti-infective Drugs

The primary goal of antimicrobial therapy is to assist in ridding the body of the pathogen. Medications that accomplish this goal by *killing* bacteria are called **bacteriocidal**. Some drugs do not kill the bacteria, but instead slow their growth so that the body's natural defenses can dispose of the microorganisms. These *growth-slowing* drugs are called **bacteriostatic**.

Bacterial cells are quite different from human cells. Bacteria have cell walls and contain certain enzymes and cellular structures that human cells lack. Antibiotics exert selective toxicity on bacterial cells by targeting these unique differences. In that way, bacteria can be killed or their growth severely hampered without major effects on human cells. Of course, there are limits to this selective toxicity, depending on the specific antibiotic and the dose employed and side effects can be expected from all the anti-infectives. The basic mechanisms of action of antimicrobial drugs are shown in Figure 32.1.

32.5 Acquired Resistance

Microorganisms have the ability to replicate extremely rapidly. During this cell division, bacteria make frequent errors duplicating their genetic code. These **mutations** occur

Table 32.1	**Common Bacterial Pathogens and Disorders**	
Name of Organism	**Disease(s)**	**Description**
Borrelia burgdorferi	Lyme disease	from tick bites
Chlamydia trachomatis	venereal disease, endometriosis	most common cause of sexually transmitted diseases in the United States
Escherichia coli	traveler's diarrhea, UTI, bacteremia, endometriosis	part of host flora in GI tract
Haemophilus	pneumonia, meningitis in children, bacteremia, otitis media, sinusitis	some Haemophilus species are host flora in the upper respiratory tract
Klebsiella	pneumonia, UTI	usually infects immunosuppressed patients
Mycobacterium leprae	leprosy	most cases in the United States occur in immigrants from Africa or Asia
Mycobacterium tuberculosis	tuberculosis	incidence very high in HIV-infected patients
Mycoplasma pneumoniae	pneumonia	most common cause of pneumonia in patients age 5–35
Neisseria gonorrhoeae	gonorrhea and other sexually transmitted diseases, endometriosis, neonatal eye infection	some Neisseria species are normal host flora
Neisseria meningitidis	meningitis in children	some Neisseria species are normal host flora
Pneumococci	pneumonia, otitis media, meningitis, bacteremia, endocarditis	part of normal flora in upper respiratory tract
Proteus mirabilis	UTI, skin infections	part of host flora in GI tract
Pseudomonas aeroginosa	UTI, skin infections, septicemia	usually infects immunosuppressed patients
Rickettsia rickettsii	Rocky Mountain spotted fever	from tick bites
Salmonella enteritidis	food poisoning	from infected animal products; raw eggs, undercooked meat or chicken
Salmonella typhi	typhoid fever	from inadequately treated food or water supplies
Staphylococcus aureus	pneumonia, food poisoning, impetigo, abscesses, bacteremia, endocarditis, toxic shock syndrome	some Staphylococcus species are normal host flora
Streptococcus	pharyngitis, pneumonia, skin infections, septicemia, endocarditis	some Streptococcus species are normal host flora
Vibrio cholerae	cholera	from inadequately treated food or water supplies

spontaneously and randomly. Although most mutations are harmful to the organism, mutations occasionally result in a bacterial cell that has reproductive advantages over its neighbors. The mutated bacterium may be able to survive in harsher conditions or perhaps grow faster than other cells. Mutations that are of particular importance to medicine are those that confer drug resistance to a microorganism.

Antibiotics help to promote the appearance of drug-resistant bacterial strains by killing populations of bacteria that are sensitive to the drug. Consequently, the only bacteria remaining are those cells that possess mutations that make them insensitive to the effects of the antibiotic. These

drug-resistant bacteria are then free to grow, unrestrained by their neighbors that were killed by the antibiotic, and the patient develops an infection that is resistant to conventional drug therapy. This phenomenon, acquired resistance, is illustrated in Figure 32.2. Bacteria may pass the resistance gene to other bacteria through conjugation, the transfer of small pieces of circular DNA called plasmids.

It is important to understand that the antibiotic did not create the mutation that caused bacteria to become resistant. The mutation occurred randomly. The role of the antibiotic is to kill the surrounding cells that were susceptible to the drug, leaving the mutated ones plenty of room to di-

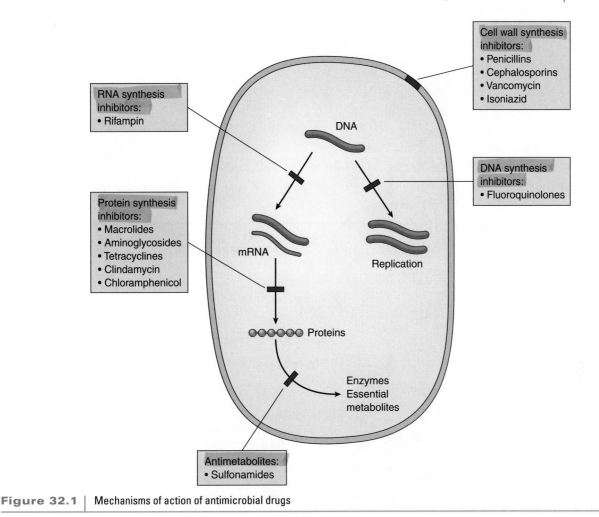

RNA synthesis inhibitors:
• Rifampin

Cell wall synthesis inhibitors:
• Penicillins
• Cephalosporins
• Vancomycin
• Isoniazid

DNA

Protein synthesis inhibitors:
• Macrolides
• Aminoglycosides
• Tetracyclines
• Clindamycin
• Chloramphenicol

DNA synthesis inhibitors:
• Fluoroquinolones

mRNA

Replication

Proteins

Enzymes
Essential metabolites

Antimetabolites:
• Sulfonamides

Figure 32.1 | Mechanisms of action of antimicrobial drugs

vide and infect. It is the bacteria that have become resistant, not the patient. Additionally, an individual with an infection that is resistant to certain antibacterial agents can transmit the resistant bacteria to others.

The widespread and sometimes unwarranted use of antibiotics has led to a large number of resistant bacterial strains. At least 60% of *Staphylococcus aureus* infections are now resistant to penicillin, and resistant strains of *Enterococcus faecalis*, *Enterococcus faecium*, and *Pseudomonas aeruginosa* are becoming major clinical problems. The longer an antibiotic is used in the population and the more often it is prescribed, the larger the percentage of resistant strains. Infections acquired in a hospital or other healthcare setting, called nosocomial infections, are often resistant to common antibiotics. Healthcare providers can play an important role in delaying the emergence of resistance by restricting the use of antibiotics to those conditions deemed medically necessary.

In most cases, antibiotics are given when there is clear evidence of bacterial infection. Some patients, however, receive antibiotics to *prevent* an infection, a practice called prophylactic use, or chemoprophylaxis. Examples of patients who might receive prophylactic antibiotics include those who have a suppressed immune system, those who have experienced deep puncture wounds such as from dog bites, or those patients who have prosthetic heart valves, prior to receiving medical or dental surgery.

It is not uncommon for patients to stop taking an antibiotic once they begin to feel better. Discontinuing an antibiotic before all organisms have been killed promotes the appearance of resistant strains. The nurse should instruct the patient that many organisms still remain, even after the symptoms disappear. The importance of taking the entire drug regimen must be stressed.

32.6 Selection of an Effective Antibiotic

Some antibacterials are effective against a wide variety of different microorganisms. These are called broad-spectrum antibiotics. Narrow-spectrum antibiotics are effective against only one or a restricted group of microorganisms.

The selection of an antibiotic therapy effective against a specific organism is an important task of the healthcare provider. Selecting an incorrect drug will delay proper treatment, thus giving the microorganism more time to infect. Prescribing ineffective antibiotics also promotes the

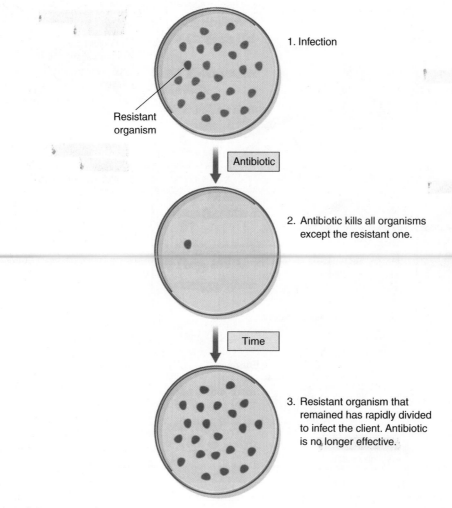

1. Infection

Resistant organism

Antibiotic

2. Antibiotic kills all organisms except the resistant one.

Time

3. Resistant organism that remained has rapidly divided to infect the client. Antibiotic is no longer effective.

Figure 32.2 | Acquired resistance

development of resistance and may cause unnecessary side effects in the patient.

Ideally, laboratory tests should be conducted to identify the organism prior to beginning anti-infective therapy. Lab tests may include examination of body specimens such as urine, sputum, blood, or pus for microorganisms. Organisms isolated from the specimens may be grown in the laboratory and identified. After identification, the laboratory may test several different antibiotics to determine which is most effective against the infecting microorganism. This process of growing the organism and identifying the most effective antibiotic is called **culture and sensitivity testing**.

Proper laboratory testing and identification of bacteria may take several days and, in the case of viruses, several weeks. Some organisms simply cannot be cultured at all. If the infection is severe, the healthcare provider will likely begin therapy immediately with a broad-spectrum antibiotic. After the results of the culture and sensitivity tests are obtained, therapy may be changed to include the antibiotic found to be most effective against the microbe.

In most cases, antibacterial therapy is conducted using a single drug. Combining two antibiotics may actually decrease each drug's efficacy, a phenomenon known as **antagonism**. Use of multiple antibiotics also has the potential to promote resistance. Multidrug therapy may be warranted, however, if several different organisms cause the patient's infection or if the infection is so severe that therapy must be started before laboratory tests have been completed. Multidrug therapy is clearly warranted in the treatment of tuberculosis or in patients infected with HIV.

One common side effect of anti-infective therapy is the appearance of secondary infections, known as **superinfections**, which occur when microorganisms normally present in the body are destroyed. These normal microorganisms, or **host flora**, inhabit the skin and the upper respiratory, genitourinary, and intestinal tracts. Some of these organisms serve a useful purpose by producing antibacterial substances and by competing with pathogenic organisms for space and nutrients. Removal of host flora by an antibiotic gives the remaining microorganisms an opportunity to grow, allowing for overgrowth of pathogenic microbes or nonaffected host flora. Superinfection should be suspected when a new infection appears while the patient is receiving anti-infective therapy. Signs and symptoms of a superinfection may include diarrhea, bladder pain, painful urination, or abnormal vaginal discharges. Broad-spectrum antibiotics are more likely to cause superinfections because they kill so many different species of microorganisms.

32.7 Host Factors

The most important factor in selecting an appropriate antibiotic is to be certain that the microbe is sensitive to the effects of the drug. However, the nurse must also take into account certain host factors that can influence the success of antibacterial chemotherapy.

The primary goal of antibiotic therapy is to kill enough bacteria, or to slow the growth of the infection, such that natural body defenses can overcome the invading agent. Unless an infection is highly localized, the antibiotic alone may not be enough: The patient's immune system and phagocytic cells will be needed to completely rid the body of the infectious agent. Patients with suppressed immune systems may require aggressive antibiotic therapy with bacteriocidal agents. These patients include those with AIDS and those being treated with immunosuppressive or antineoplastic drugs. Since therapy is more successful when the number of microbes is small, antibiotics may be given on a prophylactic basis to patients whose white blood cell count is extremely low.

Local conditions at the infection site should be considered when selecting an antibiotic because factors that hinder the drug from reaching microbes will limit therapeutic success. Infections of the central nervous system are particularly difficult to treat because many drugs cannot cross the blood-brain barrier. Injury or inflammation can cause tissues to become acidic or anaerobic and have poor circulation. Excessive pus formation or hematomas can block drugs from reaching their targets. Although most bacteria are extracellular in nature, pathogens such as *M. tuberculosis*, salmonella, toxoplasma, and listeria may reside intracellularly and thus be resistant to antibacterial action. Consideration of these factors may necessitate a change in the route of drug administration or the selection of a more effective antibiotic specific for the local conditions.

Allergic reactions to antibiotics, while not common, may be fatal. The nurse's assessment must include a thorough drug history; a previous acute allergic incident is highly predictive of future reactions. If severe allergy to a medication is established, it is best to avoid all drugs in the same chemical class. Because the patient may have been exposed to an antibiotic unknowingly, through food products or molds, allergic reactions can occur without previous incident. Penicillins are the class of antibacterials having the highest incidence of allergic reactions; between 0.7% and 4% of all patients who receive the drugs exhibit hypersensitivity.

Other host factors to be considered are age, pregnancy status, and genetics. The very young and very old are often unable to readily metabolize or excrete antibiotics; thus, doses are generally lowered. Some antibiotics cross the placenta. For example, tetracyclines taken by the mother can cause teeth discoloration in the newborn; aminoglycosides can affect the infant's hearing. The benefits of antibiotic use in pregnant or lactating women must be carefully weighed against the potential risks to the fetus and neonate. Lastly, some patients have a genetic absence of certain enzymes used to metabolize antibiotics. For example, patients with a deficiency of the enzyme glucose-6-phosphate dehydrogenase should not receive sulfonamides, chloramphenicol, or nalidixic acid because their erythrocytes may rupture.

ANTIBACTERIAL AGENTS

Antibacterial agents form a large number of chemical classes. Although drugs within a class have similarities in their mechanisms and spectrum of activity, each is slightly different and learning the differences and therapeutic applications among antibacterial agents can be challenging. Basic nursing assessments and interventions apply to all antibiotic therapies; however, the nurse should individualize the plan of care based on the patient's condition, the infection, and the antibacterial agent prescribed.

Penicillins

Although not the first anti-infective discovered, penicillin was the first mass-produced antibiotic. Isolated from the fungus *Penicillium* in 1941, the drug quickly became a miracle product by preventing thousands of deaths from infections. Penicillins are indicated for the treatment of pneumonia; meningitis; skin, bone, joint infections; stomach infections; blood and valve infections; gas gangrene; tetanus; anthrax; and sickle cell anemia in infants. The penicillins are shown in Table 32.2.

Table 32.2	Penicillins	
Drug	**Route and Adult Dose (max dose where indicated)**	
Narrow Spectrum/Pencillinase Sensitive		
penicillin G benzathine (Bicillin)	IM; 1.2 million units as a single dose	
penicillin G procaine (Crysticillin, Wycillin)	IM; 600,000–1.2 million units qd	
penicillin G sodium/potassium (Pentids)	PO; 400,000–800,000 units qd	
penicillin V (Pen-Vee K, Veetids, Betapen)	PO; 125–250 mg qid	
Narrow Spectrum/Pencillinase Resistant		
cloxacillin (Tegopen)	PO; 250–500 mg bid	
dicloxacillin (Dynapen)	PO; 125–500 mg qid	
nafcillin (Nafcil, Unipen)	PO; 250 mg–1 g qid (max 12 g/day)	
oxacillin (Prostaphlin, Bactocill)	PO; 250 mg–1 g qid (max 12 g/day)	
Broad Spectrum (Aminopenicillins)		
amoxicillin (Amoxil, Trimox, Wymox)	PO; 250–500 mg tid	
amoxicillin-clavulanate (Augmentin)	PO; 250 or 500 mg tablet (each with 125 mg clavulanic acid) q8–12h	
ampicillin (Polycillin, Omnipen)	PO; 250–500 mg bid	
bacampicillin (Spectrobid)	PO; 400–800 mg bid	
Extended Spectrum		
carbenicillin (Geocillin, Geopen)	PO; 382–764 mg qid	
mezlocillin (Mezlin)	IM; 1.5–2.0 g qid (max 24 g/day)	
piperacillin sodium (Pipracil)	IM; 2–4 g tid-qid (max 24 g/day)	
piperacillin tazobactam (Zosyn)	IV; 3.375 g qid over 30 min	
ticarcillin (Ticar)	IM; 1–2 g qid (max 40 g/day)	

32.8 Pharmacotherapy with Penicillins

Penicillins kill bacteria by disrupting their cell walls. Many bacterial cell walls contain a substance called **penicillin-binding protein** that serves as a receptor for penicillin. Penicillin weakens the cell wall and allows water to enter, thus killing the organism. Human cells do not contain cell walls, thus the actions of the penicillins are specific to bacterial cells.

The portion of the chemical structure of penicillin that is responsible for its antibacterial activity is called the **beta-lactam ring**. Some bacteria secrete an enzyme, called **beta-lactamase** or **penicillinase**, which splits the beta-lactam ring. This structural change causes these bacteria to become resistant to the effects of most penicillins. Since their discovery, large numbers of resistant bacterial strains have appeared that now limit the therapeutic usefulness of the penicillins. The action of penicillinase is illustrated in Figure 32.3.

Chemical modifications to the original penicillin molecule produced drugs offering several advantages. Oxacillin (Prostaphlin, others) and cloxacillin (Tegopen) are effective against penicillinase-producing bacteria and are called penicillinase-resistant penicillins. The aminopenicillins such as ampicillin (Polycillin, others) and amoxicillin (Amoxil, others) are effective against a wider range of microorganisms and are called broad-spectrum penicillins.

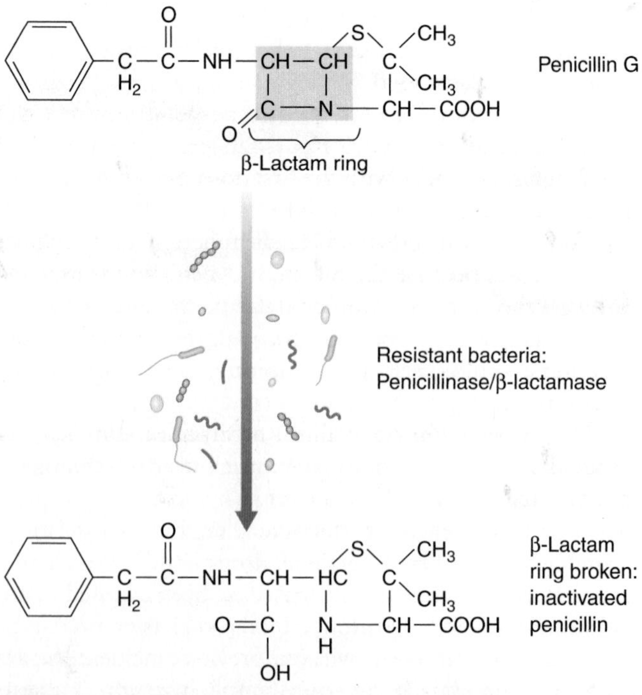

Figure 32.3 Action of penicillinase

The extended-spectrum penicillins, such as carbenicillin (Geocillin, Geopen) and piperacillin (Pipracil), are effective against even more microbes, including pseudomonas, enterobacter, klebsiella, and *Bacteroides fragilis*.

In general, the adverse effects of penicillins are minor; they are one of the safest classes of antibiotics. This has contributed to their widespread use for over 50 years. Allergy to penicillin is the most common adverse effect. Common symptoms of penicillin allergy include rash and fever. Incidence of anaphylaxis ranges from 0.04% to 2%. Allergy to one penicillin increases the risk of allergy to other drugs in the same class.

NURSING CONSIDERATIONS

The role of the nurse in drug therapy with penicillins involves careful monitoring of a patient's condition and providing education as it relates to the prescribed drug regimen. Since allergies occur more frequently with penicillins than with any other antibiotic class, it is essential to assess previous drug reactions to penicillin prior to administration. If the patient has a history of severe penicillin allergic reaction, cephalosporins should also be avoided due to risk of cross sensitization. The nurse should obtain specimens for culture and sensitivity prior to the start of antibiotic therapy.

Vital signs, electrolytes, and renal function tests should be obtained prior to and during therapy. Because some penicillin preparations contain high levels of sodium and potassium salts, the nurse should monitor for hyperkalemia and hypernatremia prior to and during therapy. Cardiac status should be monitored, including EKG changes, due to the possibility of worsening an existing heart failure related to the increased sodium intake. Additionally, the nurse should monitor for indications of response to therapy, including reduced fever, normal white blood cell count, absence of symptoms such as cough, and improved appetite.

After parenteral administration of penicillins, the patient should be observed for possible allergic reactions for 30 minutes, especially with the first dose. Sensitivity may be immediate, accelerated, or delayed.

Patients with impaired renal function may require smaller doses because the majority of penicillin is excreted through the kidneys. Penicillins should be used with caution during lactation because the drug enters breast milk. The nurse should monitor for bleeding in patients on anticoagulant therapy who are receiving high doses of parenteral carbenicillin (Geocillin), piperacillin (Pipracil), or ticarcillin (Ticar), because these drugs may interfere with platelet aggregation.

A small number of patients may develop a serious superinfection called antibiotic-associated pseudomembranous colitis (AAPMC). In this condition, the organism *Clostridium difficile* secretes a toxin that causes severe inflammation of the bowel wall, followed by necrosis. This results in a potentially life-threatening infection. Patients with this condition have two to five semisolid or liquid stools per day. Antidiarrheal drugs should not be adminis-

tered because these agents cause the toxin to be retained in the bowel. When AAPMC occurs, antibiotic therapy should be discontinued and fluid/electrolyte replacement is essential.

As with other antibiotics, penicillins may cause less severe superinfections with symptoms such as abdominal cramping and diarrhea. Replacement of natural colon flora with probiotic supplements or cultured dairy products such as yogurt or buttermilk may help to alleviate symptoms. Superinfections in elderly, debilitated, or immunosuppressed patients may be serious and require immediate interventions.

Patient education as it relates to penicillins should include goals, reasons for obtaining baseline data, and possible side effects. Following are important points the nurse should include when teaching patients regarding penicillins.

- Wear a medical alert bracelet if allergic to penicillins.
- Take Pen V, amoxicillin, and amoxicillin-clavulanate with meals to decrease GI distress. Take all other penicillins with a full glass of water, 1 hour before or 2 hours after meals to increase absorption.
- Oral penicillin G should be taken with water because acidic fruit juice can inactivate the drug's antibacterial activity.
- Do not discontinue the drug regimen before the complete prescription has been taken.
- Avoid use of penicillins while breastfeeding.
- Consult with nurse about taking probiotic supplements and/or cultured dairy products during antibiotic therapy.
- Report significant side effects immediately, including severe abdominal or stomach cramps, abdominal tenderness, convulsions, decreased urine output, and severe watery diarrhea or bloody diarrhea.

See "Nursing Process Focus: Patients Receiving Antibacterial Therapy" on page 457 for the Nursing Process applied to all antibacterials.

Cephalosporins

Isolated shortly after the penicillins, the four generations of cephalosporins comprise the largest antibiotic class. Like the penicillins, the cephalosporins contain a beta-lactam ring that is mostly responsible for their antimicrobial activity. The cephalosporins are bacteriocidal and act by attaching to penicillin-binding protein to inhibit cell wall synthesis. The cephalosporins are shown in Table 32.3.

32.9 Pharmacotherapy with Cephalosporins

Over 20 cephalosporins are available and classified by their "generation." First generation cephalosporins contain a beta-lactam ring; bacteria producing beta-lactamase will usually be resistant to these agents. The second generation cephalosporins are more potent, more resistant to beta-lactamase, and exhibit a broader spectrum than the first generation drugs. The third generation cephalosporins

Pr PROTOTYPE DRUG | PENICILLIN G POTASSIUM (Pentids)

ACTIONS AND USES

Similar to penicillin V, penicillin G is a drug of choice against strep-tococci, pneumococci, and staphylococci organisms that do not produce penicillinase. It is also a medication of choice for gonorrhea and syphilis caused by susceptible strains. Penicillin V is more acid stable; over 70% is absorbed after an oral dose compared to the 15% to 30% from penicillin G. Because of its low oral absorption, penicillin G is often given by the IV or IM routes. Penicillinase-producing organisms inactivate both penicillin G and penicillin V. Penicillin is pregnancy category B.

Administration Alerts

- After parenteral administration, observe for possible allergic reactions for 30 minutes, especially following the first dose.
- Do not mix penicillin and aminoglycosides in the same intravenous solution. Give IV medications 1 hour apart to prevent interactions.

ADVERSE EFFECTS AND INTERACTIONS

Penicillin G has few side effects. Anaphylaxis is the most serious adverse effect.

Diarrhea, nausea, and vomiting are the most common adverse effects and can cause serious complications in certain populations such as children and older adults. Pain at the injection site may occur and superinfections are possible. Since penicillin G is excreted extensively by the kidneys, renal disease can result in excessive accumulation of the drug.

Penicillin G may decrease the efficacy of oral contraceptives. Colestipol taken with this medication will decrease the absorption of penicillin. Potassium-sparing diuretics may cause hyperkalemia when administered with penicillin G potassium.

 See the companion website for a Nursing Process Focus specific to this drug.

---

generally have a longer duration of action, an even broader spectrum, and are resistant to beta-lactamase. Third generation cephalosporins are sometimes the drugs of choice against infections by pseudomonas, klebsiella, neisseria, salmonella, proteus, and *H. influenza*. Newer, fourth generation drugs are more effective against organisms that have developed resistance to earlier cephalosporins. Third and fourth generation agents are capable of entering the cerebrospinal fluid to treat CNS infections. There are not always clear distinctions among the generations.

The primary therapeutic use of the cephalosporins is for gram negative infections and for patients who cannot tolerate the less expensive penicillins. Side effects are similar to those of the penicillins, with allergic reactions being the most common adverse effect. The nurse must be alert that 5% to 10% of the patients who are allergic to penicillin will also be allergic to the cephalosporins. Despite this incidence of cross-sensitivity, the cephalosporins offer a reasonable alternative for patients who are unable to take penicillin. It is common for patients with a mild allergy to penicillin to be given a cephalosporin. Earlier generation cephalosporins exhibited kidney toxicity, but this is diminished with the newer drugs.

NURSING CONSIDERATIONS

The role of the nurse in cephalosporin therapy involves careful monitoring of a patient's condition and providing education as it relates to the prescribed drug regimen. The cephalosporins are generally the treatment of choice for patients with gram negative infections. The nurse should assess for the presence/history of bleeding disorders, because cephalosporins may reduce prothrombin levels through interference with vitamin K metabolism. Renal and hepatic

function should be assessed as most cephalosporins are eliminated by the kidney, and liver function is important in vitamin K production. Culture and sensitivity testing should be performed before and during therapy.

Due to elimination of cephalosporins through the kidneys, it is necessary to monitor intake and output, blood urea nitrogen (BUN), and serum creatinine. If the patient is concurrently taking NSAIDs, the nurse should monitor blood coagulation studies because cephalosporins increase the effect of platelet inhibition.

Cephalosporins should be used with caution in pregnant or lactating patients as they can be transferred to the fetus or infant. Doses should be adjusted appropriately in patients with impaired renal or hepatic function. Certain cephalosporins will cause a disulfiram (Antabuse)–like reaction when alcoholic beverages are consumed. Typical reactions include severe vomiting, weakness, blurred vision, and profound hypotension.

Cephalosporins may predispose patients to pseudomembranous colitis especially if gastrointestinal pathology preexists. Less severe superinfections may also occur. Eating cultured dairy products such as yogurt or kefir may suppress superinfections.

Patient education as it relates to cephalosporins should include goals, reasons for obtaining baseline data, and possible side effects. Following are important points the nurse should include when teaching patients regarding cephalosporins.

- Avoid alcohol use while taking cephalosporins.
- Eat cultured dairy products to help discourage superinfections.
- Report significant side effects, including diarrhea, onset of flulike symptoms, blistering or peeling of skin,

Table 32.3	Cephalosporins
Drug	**Route and Adult Dose (max dose where indicated)**
First Generation	
cefadroxil (Duricef)	PO; 500 mg–1 g qd-bid (max 2 g/day)
cefazolin (Kefzol, others)	IM; 250 mg-2 g tid (max 12 g/day)
cephalexin (Keflex, others)	PO; 250–500 mg qid
cephapirin (Cefadyl)	IM/IV; 500 mg-1 g q4–6h (max 12 g/day)
cephradine (Velosef)	PO; 250–500 mg q6h or 500 mg–1 g q12h (max 4 g/day)
Second Generation	
cefaclor (Ceclor)	PO; 250–500 mg tid
cefamandole (Mandol)	IM; 500 mg–1 g tid-qid (max 12 g/day)
cefmetazole (Zefazone)	IV; 1–2 g q6–12h
cefonicid (Monocid)	IM; 1 g qd (max 2 g/day)
cefotetan (Cefotan)	IV/IM; 1–2 g q12h
cefoxitin (Mefoxin)	IV/IM; 1–2 g q6–8h, (max 12 g/day)
cefprozil (Cefzil)	PO; 250–500 mg qd-bid
cefuroxime (Ceftin, Kefurox, Zinacef)	PO; 250–500 mg bid
loracarbef (Lorabid)	PO; 200–400 mg q12h taken 1 h ac or 2 h pc
Third Generation	
cefdinir (Omnicef)	PO; 300 mg bid
cefditoren pivoxil (Spectracef)	PO; 400 mg bid for 10 d
cefixime (Suprax)	PO; 400 mg qd or 200 mg bid
cefoperazone (Cefobid)	IV/IM; 1–2 g q12h; 16 g/day in two to four divided doses
cefotaxime (Claforan)	IM; 1–2 g bid-tid (max 12 g/day)
cefpodoxime (Vantin)	PO; 200 mg q12h for 10 days
ceftazidime (Fortaz, others)	IV/IM; 1–2 mg q8–12h, up to 2 g q6h
ceftibuten (Cedax)	PO; 400 mg qd for 10 d
ceftizoxime (Cefizox)	IV/IM; 1–2 g q8–12h, up to 2 g q4h
ceftriaxone (Rocephin)	IV/IM; 1–2 g q12–24h (max 4 g/d)
Fourth Generation	
cefepime (Maxipime)	IV/IM; 0.5–1.0 g q12h for 7–10 d

seizures, decreased urine output, hearing loss, skin rash, breathing difficulty, and unusual tiredness or weakness.

See "Nursing Process Focus: Patients Receiving Antibacterial Therapy" on page 457 for the Nursing Process applied to all antibacterials.

Tetracyclines

The first tetracyclines were extracted from *Streptomyces* soil microorganisms in 1948. Tetracyclines exert a bacteriostatic effect by selectively inhibiting bacterial protein synthesis. The six tetracyclines are effective against a large number of different gram negative and gram positive organisms and have one of the broadest spectrums of

any class of antibiotics. The tetracyclines are shown in Table 32.4.

32.10 Pharmacotherapy with Tetracyclines

The widespread use of tetracyclines in the 1950s and 1960s resulted in a large number of resistant bacterial strains that now limit their therapeutic utility. They are drugs of choice for only a few diseases: Rocky Mountain spotted fever, typhus, cholera, Lyme disease, ulcers caused by *Helicobacter pylori*, and chlamydial infections. They are occasionally used for the treatment of acne vulgaris. Because of their ability to bind metal ions such as calcium and iron, tetracyclines should not be taken with

Pr PROTOTYPE DRUG | CEFOTAXIME (Claforan)

ACTIONS AND USES

Cefotaxime is a third generation cephalosporin with a broad spectrum of activity against gram negative organisms. It is effective against many bacteria that have developed resistance to earlier generation cephalosporins and to other classes of anti-infectives. Cefotaxime exhibits bacteriocidal activity by inhibiting cell wall synthesis. It is prescribed for serious infections of the lower respiratory tract, central nervous system, genitourinary system, bones, and joints. It may also be used for blood infections such as bacteremia or septicemia. Like many other cephalosporins, cefotaxime is not absorbed from the GI tract and must be given by the IM or IV route.

Cefotaxime is pregnancy category B.

Administration Alert

- IM injections should be administered deep into a large muscle mass to prevent injury to surrounding tissues.

 See the companion website for a Nursing Process Focus specific to this drug.

ADVERSE EFFECTS AND INTERACTIONS

For most patients, cefotaxime and the other cephalosporins are safe medications. Hypersensitivity is the most common adverse effect, although symptoms may include only a minor rash and itching. Anaphylaxis is possible, thus the nurse should be alert for this reaction. GI-related side effects such as diarrhea, vomiting, and nausea may occur. Some patients experience considerable pain at the injection site.

Cefotaxime interacts with probenecid causing decreased renal elimination of the drug. Alcohol interacts with cefotaxime to produce a disulfiram-like reaction. Cefotaxime interacts with NSAIDs to cause an increase in platelet inhibition.

Table 32.4	Tetracyclines
Drug	**Route and Adult Dose (max dose where indicated)**
demeclocycline (Declomycin)	PO; 150 mg q6h or 300 mg q12h (max 2.4 g/d)
doxycycline (Vibramycin, others)	PO; 100 mg bid on day 1, then 100 mg qd (max 200 mg/day)
methacycline (Rondomycin)	PO; 600 mg/day in 2–4 divided doses
minocycline (Minocin, others)	PO; 200 mg as one dose followed by 100 mg bid
oxytetracycline (Terramycin)	PO; 250–500 mg bid-qid
Pr tetracycline (Achromycin, others)	PO; 250–500 mg bid-qid (max 2 g/day)

milk or iron supplements because the drug's absorption may be decreased by as much as 50%. They may also cause yellow-brown teeth discoloration in young children. Some patients experience photosensitivity during therapy, making their skin particularly susceptible to sunburn. Because of their broad spectrum, the risk for superinfection is relatively high.

NURSING CONSIDERATIONS

The role of the nurse in tetracycline therapy involves careful monitoring of a patient's condition and providing education as it relates to the prescribed drug regimen. The nurse should assess for presence/history of acne vulgaris, actinomycosis, anthrax, malaria, syphilis, urinary tract infection, rickettsial infection, and Lyme disease. This class of antibiotics can treat all of these disorders. Prior to administration, the nurse should assess for a history of hypersensitivity to tetracyclines. If possible, culture and sensitivity results should be obtained before therapy is initiated. Lab tests including CBC and kidney and liver function studies should be done. The nurse should monitor the patient's body temperature, white blood cell count, and culture/sensitivity results to determine the effectiveness of the treatment, as well as observe for superinfections.

Tetracyclines are contraindicated in pregnancy or lactation due to the drug's effect on linear skeletal growth of the fetus and child. They are also contraindicated in children less than 8 years of age due to the drug's ability to cause permanent mottling and discoloration of the teeth. Tetracycline decreases the effectiveness of oral contraceptives, so female patients should use an alternate method of birth control while taking the medication. Tetracyclines should be used with caution in patients with impaired kidney or liver function.

Oral and perineal hygiene care are extremely important to decrease the risk of superinfections due to *Candida*. Tetracyclines cause photosensitivity, which may lead to tingling and burning of the skin, similar to sunburn. Photosensitivity reaction may appear within a few minutes to hours to sun exposure and may persist for several days after pharmacotherapy is completed.

Patient education as it relates to tetracyclines should include goals, reasons for obtaining baseline data such as tests for culture and sensitivity, and possible side effects. Follow-

Pr PROTOTYPE DRUG | TETRACYCLINE HCL (Achromycin, others)

ACTIONS AND USES

Tetracycline is effective against a broad range of gram positive and negative organisms, including chlamydiae, rickettsiae, and mycoplasma. Tetracycline is given orally, though it has a short half-life that may require administration four times per day. Topical and oral preparations are available for treating acne. An IM preparation is available; injections may cause local irritation and be extremely painful.

Administration Alerts

- Administer oral drug with full glass of water to decrease esophageal and GI irritation.
- Administer antacids and tetracycline 1 to 3 hours apart.
- Administer antilipidemic agents at least 2 hours before or after tetracycline.
- Pregnancy category D.

ADVERSE EFFECTS AND INTERACTIONS

Being a broad-spectrum antibiotic, tetracycline has a tendency to affect vaginal, oral, and intestinal flora and cause superinfections. Tetracycline irritates the GI mucosa and may cause nausea, vomiting, epigastric burning, and diarrhea. Diarrhea may be severe enough to cause discontinuation of therapy. Other common side effects include discoloration of the teeth and photosensitivity.

Oral tetracycline interacts with milk products, iron supplements, magnesium-containing laxatives, or antacids. These products reduce the absorption and serum levels of tetracyclines. Tetracyline binds with certain lipid-lowering drugs (colestipol and cholestyramine) thereby decreasing the antibiotic's absorption. This drug decreases the effectiveness of oral contraceptives.

 See the companion website for a Nursing Process Focus specific to this drug.

ing are important points the nurse should include when teaching patients regarding tetracyclines.

- Do not save medication because toxic effects may occur if it is taken past the expiration date.
- Do not take these medications with milk products, iron supplements, magnesium-containing laxatives, or antacids.
- Wait 1 to 3 hours after taking tetracyclines before taking antacids.
- Wait at least 2 hours before or after taking tetracyclines before taking lipid-lowering drugs such as colestipol (Colestid) and cholestyramine (Questran).
- Report significant side effects immediately, including increased photosensitivity of skin to sunlight, abdominal pain, loss of appetite, nausea and vomiting, visual changes, and yellowing of skin.

See "Nursing Process Focus: Patients Receiving Antibacterial Therapy" on page 457 for the Nursing Process applied to all antibacterials.

Macrolides

Erythromycin, the first macrolide antibiotic, was isolated from *Streptomyces* in a soil sample in 1952. The macrolide antibiotics inhibit bacterial protein synthesis and may be either bacteriocidal or bacteriostatic, depending on the dose and the target organism.

32.11 Pharmacotherapy with Macrolides

Macrolides are considered safe alternatives to penicillin, although they are drugs of first choice for relatively few diseases. Common uses of macrolides include the treatment of whooping cough, Legionnaire's disease, and infections by streptococcus, *Haemophilus influenza, Mycoplasma*

pneumoniae, and chlamydia. The macrolides are shown in Table 32.5.

The newer macrolides were synthesized from erythromycin. Although their spectrums are similar, the newer agents have a longer half-life and cause less gastric irritation than erythromycin. For example, azithromycin (Zithromax) has such an extended half-life that it is administered for only 4 days, rather than the 10 days required for most antibiotics. The shorter duration of therapy is thought to increase patient compliance.

NURSING CONSIDERATIONS

The role of the nurse in macrolide therapy involves careful monitoring of a patient's condition and providing education as it relates to the prescribed drug regimen. The nurse should assess for the presence of respiratory infection, GI tract infection, skin and soft tissue infections, otitis media, gonorrhea, nongonococcal urethritis, and *Helicobacter pylori* treatment. Macrolides are indicated for the pharmacologic treatment of these disorders. The patient should be examined for history of cardiac disorders, as macrolides may exacerbate existing heart disease. Due to toxic effects on liver, hepatic enzymes should be monitored with certain macrolides such as erythromycin estolate.

The patient should be assessed for a history of hypersensitivity to macrolides. Rashes or other signs of hypersensitivity should be reported immediately. Culture and sensitivity testing should be performed before initiation of macrolide therapy.

Macrolides are contraindicated in patients with hepatic disease since the liver metabolizes these drugs. These agents should be used with caution in pregnant or breast-feeding women to avoid harm to the fetus or newborn.

Table 32.5	**Macrolides**
Drug	**Route and Adult Dose (max dose where indicated)**
azithromycin (Zithromax)	PO; 500 mg for one dose, then 250 mg qd for 4 days
clarithromycin (Biaxin)	PO; 250–500 mg bid
dirithromycin (Dynabac)	PO; 500 mg qd
erythromycin (E-Mycin, Erythrocin)	PO; 250–500 mg bid or 333 mg tid

---

PROTOTYPE DRUG | ERYTHROMYCIN (E-Mycin, Erythrocin)

ACTIONS AND USES

Erythromycin is inactivated by stomach acid and is thus administered as coated tablets or capsules that are intended to dissolve in the small intestine. Its main application is for patients who are unable to tolerate penicillins or who may have a penicillin-resistant infection. It has a spectrum similar to that of the penicillins and is effective against most gram positive bacteria. It is often a preferred drug for infections by *Bordetella pertussis* (whooping cough) and *Corynebacterium diphtheriae*.

Erythromycin is pregnancy category B.

Administration Alerts

- Administer oral drug on an empty stomach with a full glass of water.
- For suspensions, shake the bottle thoroughly to ensure the drug is well mixed.
- Do not give with or immediately before or after fruit juices.

ADVERSE EFFECTS AND INTERACTIONS

The most common side effects from erythromycin are nausea, abdominal cramping, and vomiting, although these are rarely serious enough to cause discontinuation of therapy. Concurrent administration with food reduces these side effects. The most severe adverse effect is hepatotoxicity caused by the estolate form of the drug.

Anesthetic agents and anticonvulsant drugs may interact to cause serum drug levels to rise and result in toxicity. This drug interacts with cyclosporine increasing the risk for nephrotoxicity. It may increase the effects of warfarin. Erythromycin may interact with medications containing xanthine, to cause an increase in theophylline levels.

 See the companion website for a Nursing Process Focus specific to this drug.

Multiple drug-drug interactions occur with macrolides. Certain anesthetic agents (alfentanil) and anticonvulsant drugs (carbamazepine) may interact with macrolides to cause serum drug levels to rise and result in toxicity. Macrolides should be used cautiously with patients receiving cyclosporine (Sandimmune) and drug levels must be monitored due to the risk for nephrotoxicity. Patients receiving warfarin (Coumadin) need to be monitored closely because macrolides may decrease warfarin metabolism and excretion. Coagulation studies, such as INR, need to be monitored more frequently as dosage adjustments may be required. Clarithromycin (Biaxin) and zidovudine (AZT) must be administered at least 4 hours apart to avoid interaction, which results in a delayed time for peak concentration of AZT.

Patient education as it relates to macrolides should include goals, reasons for obtaining baseline data such as culture and sensitivity tests, and possible side effects. Following are important points the nurse should include when teaching patients regarding macrolides.

- Do not discontinue the medication before the complete prescription has been taken.
- Do not take with or immediately before or after fruit juices.

- Notify the healthcare provider before taking other prescription or OTC medications, or herbal products, because macrolides interact with many substances.
- Report significant side effects immediately, including severe skin rash, itching, or hives; difficulty breathing or swallowing; yellowing of skin or eyes; dark urine; and pale stools.

See "Nursing Process Focus: Patients Receiving Antibacterial Therapy" on page 457 for the Nursing Process applied to all antibacterials.

Aminoglycosides

The first aminoglycoside, streptomycin, was named after *Streptomyces griseus*, the soil organism from which it was isolated in 1942. Once widely used, streptomycin is now usually restricted to the treatment of tuberculosis due to the development of a large number of resistant strains. Although more toxic than other antibiotic classes, aminoglycosides have important therapeutic applications for the treatment of aerobic gram negative bacteria, mycobacteria, and some protozoans. The aminoglycosides are shown in Table 32.6.

Table 32.6	Aminoglycosides
Drug	**Route and Adult Dose (max dose where indicated)**
amikacin (Amikin)	IM; 5.0–7.5 mg/kg as a loading dose, then 7.5 mg/kg bid
gentamicin (Garamycin, others)	IM; 1.5–2.0 mg/kg as a loading dose, then 1–2 mg/kg bid-tid
kanamycin (Kantrex)	IM; 5.0–7.5 mg/kg bid-tid
neomycin (Mycifradin)	IM; 1.3–2.6 mg/kg qid
netilmicin (Netromycin)	IM; 1.3–2.2 mg/kg tid or 2.0–3.25 mg/kg bid
paromomycin (Humatin)	PO; 7.5–12.5 mg/kg tid
streptomycin	IM; 15 mg/kg up to 1 g as a single dose
tobramycin (Nebcin)	IM; 1 mg/kg tid (max 5 mg/kg/day)

32.12 Pharmacotherapy with Aminoglycosides

Aminoglycosides are bacteriocidal and act by inhibiting bacterial protein synthesis and by causing the synthesis of abnormal proteins. They are normally reserved for serious systemic infections caused by aerobic gram negative organisms, including those caused by *E.coli*, serratia, proteus, klebsiella, and pseudomonas. When used for systemic bacterial infections, aminoglycosides are given parenterally, as they are poorly absorbed from the GI tract. They are occasionally given orally to sterilize the bowel prior to intestinal surgery. Neomycin (Mycifradin, others) is available for topical infections of the skin, eyes, and ears. Paromomycin (Humatin) is given orally for the treatment of parasitic infections. The nurse should note the differences in spelling of some drugs, from -mycin to -micin, which reflects the different organisms from which the drugs were originally isolated.

NURSING CONSIDERATIONS

The role of the nurse in aminoglycoside therapy involves careful monitoring of a patient's condition and providing education as it relates to the prescribed drug regimen. The nurse should assess the patient for a history of previous allergic reaction to aminoglycosides. These anti-infectives are most noted for their toxic effects on the kidneys and vestibular apparatus; therefore, the patient should be monitored for ototoxicity and nephrotoxicity during the course of therapy. Baseline audiometry, renal function, and vestibular function need to be assessed prior to the initial administration of aminoglycosides and throughout therapy. Hearing loss may occur after therapy has been completed. Baseline urinalysis is necessary prior to initiation of therapy and throughout therapy as renal impairment may increase the risk of toxicity. With streptomycin therapy, caloric tests are assessed for baseline data and to monitor for vestibular toxicity.

Neuromuscular function may also be impaired in patients receiving aminoglycosides. Patients with neuromuscular diseases, such as myasthenia gravis and Parkinson's disease, may experience greater muscle weakness due to neuromuscular blockade caused by aminoglycosides. These antibiotics also should be used with caution in patients receiving anesthetics due to an interaction causing possible neuromuscular blockade.

These drugs should be used with caution in neonates, infants, and the elderly. Infants may experience neuromuscular blockade from aminoglycosides due to their immature neurologic system. Elderly patients are at a higher risk of nephrotoxicity and ototoxicity because of reduced renal function and may require lower doses. Patients should be instructed to increase fluid intake, unless otherwise contraindicated, to promote excretion of the medications. Superinfection is a side effect of aminoglycoside therapy, and the nurse should monitor carefully for diarrhea, vaginal discharge, stomatitis, and glossitis.

Patient education as it relates to aminoglycosides should include goals, reasons for obtaining baseline data such as vestibular function tests, and possible side effects. Following are important points the nurse should include when teaching patients regarding aminoglycosides.

- Increase fluid intake.
- Report significant side effects immediately, including tinnitus, high-frequency hearing loss, persistent headache, nausea, and vertigo.

See "Nursing Process Focus: Patients Receiving Antibacterial therapy" on page 457 for the Nursing Process applied to all antibacterials.

Fluoroquinolones

In the past decade, the fluoroquinolones have become an increasingly important class of antibiotics. The first drug in this class, nalidixic acid (NegGram) was approved in 1962. Classified as a quinolone, the use of nalidixic acid was restricted to urinary tract infections (UTIs) due to its narrow spectrum of activity and a high incidence of bacterial resistance. The development of fluorinated quinolones with a wider spectrum of activity began in the late 1980s and continues today. Four generations of fluoroquinolones are now available, based on their microbiologic activity. All fluoroquinolones have

PROTOTYPE DRUG | GENTAMICIN (Garamycin)

ACTIONS AND USES

Gentamicin is a broad-spectrum, bacteriocidal antibiotic usually prescribed for serious urinary, respiratory, nervous, or GI infections when less toxic antibiotics are contraindicated. It is often used in combination with other antibiotics or when drugs from other classes have proven ineffective. It is used parenterally, or as drops, for eye infections.

Administration Alerts

- For IM administration, give deep into a large muscle.
- Use only IM and IV drug solutions that are clear and colorless or slightly yellow. Discard discolored solutions or those that contain particulate matter.
- Pregnancy category C.

ADVERSE EFFECTS AND INTERACTIONS

As with other aminoglycosides, adverse effects from gentamicin may be severe. Ototoxicity can produce a loss of hearing or balance, which may become permanent with continued use. Frequent hearing tests should be conducted so that gentamicin may be discontinued if early signs of ototoxicity are detected.

Gentamicin is excreted unchanged, primarily by the kidneys. The nurse must be alert for signs of reduced kidney function, including proteinuria, and elevated BUN and creatinine levels. Nephrotoxicity is of particular concern to patients with preexisting kidney disease, and may limit therapy with gentamicin. Resistance to gentamicin is increasing and some cross-resistance among aminoglycosides has been reported.

The risk of ototoxicity increases if the patient is currently taking amphotericin B, furosemide, aspirin, Bumex, Edecrin, cisplatin, and Humatin.

Concurrent use with amphotericin B, capreomycin, cisplatin, polymyxin B, and vancomycin increases the risk of nephrotoxicity.

 See the companion website for a Nursing Process Focus specific to this drug.

activity against gram negative pathogens; the later generation agents are significantly more effective against gram positive agents. The fluoroquinolones are shown in Table 32.7.

32.13 Pharmacotherapy with Fluoroquinolones

The fluoroquinolones are bacteriocidal and affect DNA synthesis by inhibiting two bacterial enzymes: DNA gyrase and topoisomerase IV. Agents in this class are infrequently first line drugs, although they are extensively used as alternatives to other antibiotics. Clinical applications include infections of the respiratory, gastrointestinal, and gynecologic tracts, and some skin and soft tissue infections. The most widely used drug in this class, ciprofloxacin (Cipro), is an agent of choice for postexposure prophylaxis of *Bacillus anthracis*. Two newer agents, moxifloxacin (Avelox) and trovafloxacin (Trovan), are highly effective against anaerobes. Recent studies suggest that some fluoroquinolones may be effective against *Mycobacterium tuberculosis*.

A major advantage of the fluoroquinolones is that they are well absorbed orally and may be administered either once or twice a day. They have a favorable safety profile with nausea, vomiting, and diarrhea being the most common side effects. Although they may be taken with food, they should not be taken concurrently with multivitamins or mineral supplements, since calcium, magnesium, iron, or zinc ions can reduce absorption of the antibiotic by as much as 90%.

The most serious adverse effects are dysrhythmias (gatifloxacin and moxifloxacin) and liver failure (trovafloxacin). Central nervous system effects such as dizziness, headache, and sleep disturbances affect 1% to 8% of patients. Because an-

imal studies have suggested that fluoroquinolones affect cartilage development, use in children must be monitored carefully. Use in pregnancy or in lactating patients should be avoided.

NURSING CONSIDERATIONS

The role of the nurse in fluoroquinolone therapy involves careful monitoring of a patient's condition and providing education as it relates to the prescribed drug regimen. The nurse should assess for allergic reactions to fluoroquinolones before beginning therapy. Because these agents may decrease leukocytes, the white blood cell count should be carefully monitored. When possible, culture and sensitivity testing should be performed before beginning therapy.

These drugs are contraindicated in patients with a history of hypersensitivity to fluoroquinolones. They should be used with caution in patients with epilepsy, cerebral arteriosclerosis, or alcoholism due to a potential drug interaction that increases the risk of CNS toxicity. Patients with liver and renal dysfunction should be monitored carefully, due to the drug being metabolized by the liver and excreted by the kidneys.

Enoxacin (Penetrex) and norfloxacin (Noroxin) should be taken on an empty stomach. Antacids and ferrous sulfate may decrease the absorption of fluoroquinolones, reducing antibiotic effectiveness. The fluoroquinolones should be administered at least 2 hours before these drugs. Coagulation studies (INR) need to be monitored frequently if these antibiotics are administered concurrently with warfarin (Coumadin) due to interactions leading to increased anticoagulation effects.

The nurse should monitor urinary output and report quantities of less than 1,000 cc in 24 hours to the healthcare provider. The patient should be encouraged to drink eight

Table 32.7	Fluoroquinolones
Drug	**Route and Adult Dose (max dose where indicated)**
First Generation	
cinoxacin (Cinobac)	PO; 250–500 mg bid-qid
nalidixic acid (NeoGram)	PO; Acute therapy: 1 g qid PO; Chronic therapy: 500 mg qid
Second Generation	
ciprofloxacin (Cipro, Septra)	PO; 250–750 mg bid
enoxacin (Penetrex)	PO; 200–400 mg bid
lomefloxacin (Maxaquin)	PO; 400 mg qd
norfloxacin (Noroxin)	PO; 400 mg bid
ofloxacin (Floxin)	PO; 200–400 mg bid
Third Generation	
gatifloxacin (Tequin)	PO; 400 mg tid
levofloxacin (Levaquin)	PO; 250–500 mg/day qd
sparfloxacin (Zagam)	PO; 400 mg on day one then 200 mg qd
Fourth Generation	
gemifloxacin (Factive)	PO; 320 mg qd
moxifloxacin (Avelox)	PO; 400 mg qd
trovafloxacin mesylate (Trovan)	PO; 100–300 mg qd

or more glasses of water per day to decrease the risk of crystalluria, which irritates the kidneys. The nurse should advise the patient to discontinue the drug and notify the healthcare provider if signs of hypersensitivity occur.

The nurse should inform the patient that these drugs may cause dizziness and lightheadedness and to avoid driving or performing hazardous tasks during drug therapy. These agents should be used with caution during pregnancy or breastfeeding due to untoward effects caused by the passage of antimicrobials to the newborn. Safety for use by children under 18 has not been established.

Patients receiving norfloxacin (Noroxin) should be informed that photophobia is possible. Some fluoroquinolones, such as ciprofloxacin (Cipro), may affect tendons especially in children. The patient should refrain from physical exercise if calf, ankle, or Achilles pain occurs.

Patient education as it relates to fluoroquinolones should include goals, reasons for obtaining baseline data such as lab work and culture and sensitivity tests, and possible side effects. Following are important points the nurse should include when teaching patients regarding fluoroquinolones.

- Wear sunglasses; avoid exposure to bright lights and direct sunlight when taking norfloxacin (Noroxin).
- Report the first signs of tendon pain or inflammation.
- Report the following side effects immediately: dizziness, restlessness, stomach distress, diarrhea, psychosis, confusion, and irregular or fast heart rate.

See "Nursing Process Focus: Patients Receiving Antibacterial Therapy" on page 457 for the Nursing Process applied to all antibacterials.

Sulfonamides

The discovery of the sulfonamides in the 1930s heralded a new era in the treatment of infectious disease. With their wide spectrum of activity against both gram positive and gram negative bacteria, the sulfonamides significantly reduced mortality from susceptible microbes and earned its discoverer a Nobel Prize in medicine in 1938. Sulfonamides suppress bacterial growth by inhibiting the essential compound folic acid that is responsible for cellular biosynthesis. Sulfonamides are active against a broad spectrum of microorganisms. The sulfonamides are shown in Table 32.8.

32.14 Pharmacotherapy with Sulfonamides

Several factors have led to a significant decline in the use of sulfonamides. Their widespread use over several decades resulted in a substantial number of resistant strains. The development of the penicillins, cephalosporins, and macrolides gave healthcare providers larger choices of agents, some of which exhibited an improved safety profile over the sulfonamides. Approval of the combination antibiotic sulfamethoxazole-trimethoprim (Bactrim, Septra)

PROTOTYPE DRUG | **CIPROFLOXACIN** (Cipro)

ACTIONS AND USES

Ciprofloxacin, a second generation fluoroquinolone, was approved in 1987 and is the most widely used drug in this class. By inhibiting bacterial DNA gyrase, ciprofloxacin affects bacterial replication and DNA repair. It is more effective against gram negative than gram positive organisms. It is prescribed for respiratory infections, bone and joint infections, GI infections, ophthalmic infections, sinusitis, and prostatitis. The drug is rapidly absorbed after oral administration and is distributed to most body tissues. Oral and intravenous forms are available.

Administration Alerts

- Administer at least 4 hours before antacids and ferrous sulfate.
- Pregnancy category C.

ADVERSE EFFECTS AND INTERACTIONS

GI side effects may occur in as many as 20% of patients. Ciprofloxacin may be administered with food, to diminish adverse GI effects. The patient should not, however, take this drug with antacids or mineral supplements, since drug absorption will be diminished. Some patients report headache and dizziness. Caffeine should be restricted, to avoid excessive nervousness, anxiety, or tachycardia.

Concurrent administration with warfarin may increase anticoagulant effects. This drug may increase theophylline levels 15% to 30%. Antacids, ferrous sulfate, and sucralfate decrease the absorption of ciprofloxacin.

See the companion website for a Nursing Process Focus specific to this drug.

Table 32.8	Sulfonamides
Drug	**Route and Adult Dose (max dose where indicated)**
sulfacetamide (Cetamide, others)	Opthalmic; one to three drops of 10%, 15%, or 30% solution into lower conjunctival sac q2–3h, may increase interval as patient responds or use 1.5–2.5 cm (0.5–1.0 in.) of 10% ointment q6h and at hs
sulfadiazine (Microsulfon)	PO; Loading dose 2–4 g; maintenance dose 2–4 g/d in four to six divided doses
sulfamethizole	PO; 2–4 g initially followed by 1–2 g qid
sulfidoxine-pyrimethamine (Fansidar)	PO; 1 tablet weekly (500 mg sulfidoxine, 25 mg pyrimethamine)
sulfamethoxazole (Gantanol)	PO; 2 g initially followed by 1 g bid-tid
sulfisoxazole (Gantrisin)	PO; 2–4 g initially followed by 1–2 g qid
trimethoprim-sulfamethoxazole (Bactrim, Septa)	PO; 160 mg TMP/800 mg SMZ bid

marked a resurgence in the use of sulfonamides in treating urinary tract infections (UTIs). Agents in this drug class are also given for treatment of *Pneumocystis carini* pneumonia and shigella infections of small bowel.

Sulfonamides are classified by their absorption and excretion characteristics. Some, such as sulfisoxazole (Gantrisin) and sulfamethoxazole (Gantanol), are rapidly absorbed when given orally and excreted rapidly by the kidney. Others such as sulfasalazine (Azulfidine) are poorly absorbed and remain in the alimentary canal to treat intestinal infections. A third group, including sulfadiazine (Microsulfon), is used for topical infections. Sulfadoxine has an exceptionally long half-life and is occasionally prescribed for malarial prophylaxis.

In general, the sulfonamides are safe drugs; however, some adverse effects may be serious. Adverse effects include the formation of crystals in the urine, hypersensitivity reactions, nausea, and vomiting. Although not common, sulfonamides can produce potentially fatal blood abnormalities, such as aplastic anemia, acute hemolytic anemia, and agranulocytosis.

NURSING CONSIDERATIONS

The role of the nurse in sulfonamide therapy involves careful monitoring of a patient's condition and providing education as it relates to the prescribed drug regimen. The nurse should assess for anemia or other hematological disorders, because sulfonamides may cause hemolytic anemia and blood dyscrasias due to a genetically determined deficiency in some patients' red blood cells. The nurse should assess renal function, as sulfonamides may increase the risk for crystalluria. Culture and sensitivity results should be obtained before initiating sulfonamide therapy. CBC and urinalysis should be obtained during therapy.

Sulfonamides are contraindicated during pregnancy and lactation and for infants less than 2 months of age due to the drug's ability to promote jaundice. Agents in this class must be used with caution for patients with renal impairment. Sulfonamides have a low solubility that may cause crystals to form within urine and obstruct the kidneys or ureters. The nurse should encourage fluids to 3,000 cc

PROTOTYPE DRUG | **TRIMETHOPRIM-SULFAMETHOXAZOLE** (Bactrim, Septra)

ACTIONS AND USES

The fixed combination of the sulfonamide sulfamethoxazole (SMZ) with the anti-infective trimethoprim (TMP) is most commonly used in the pharmacotherapy of urinary tract infections. It is also approved for the treatment of *Pneumocystis carinii* pneumonia, shigella infections of the small bowel, and for acute episodes of chronic bronchitis.

Both SMZ and TMP are inhibitors of the bacterial metabolism of folic acid, or folate. Their action is synergistic: a greater bacterial kill is achieved by the fixed combination than would be achieved with either drug used separately. Because humans obtain the precursors of folate in their diets, these medications are selective for bacterial folate metabolism. Another advantage of the combination is that development of resistance is lower than is observed when either of the agents is used alone.

Administration Alerts

■ Administer oral drugs with a full glass of water.
■ Pregnancy category C.

ADVERSE EFFECTS AND INTERACTIONS

The most common side effect of TMP-SMZ involves skin rashes, which are characteristic of sulfonamides. Nausea and vomiting are not uncommon. This medication should be used cautiously in patients with preexisting kidney disease, since crystalluria, oliguria, and renal failure have been reported. Periodic laboratory evaluation of the blood is usually performed to identify early signs of agranulocytosis or thrombocytopenia.

TMP and SMZ may enhance the effects of oral anticoagulants. These drugs may also increase methotrexate toxicity.

See the companion website for a Nursing Process Focus specific to this drug.

---

per day to achieve a urinary output of 1,500 cc/24 hours to decrease the possibility of crystalluria.

Cross-sensitivity exists with diuretics, such as acetazolamide and the thiazides, and with sulfonylurea antidiabetic agents. These agents should be avoided in patients with a history of hypersensitivity to sulfonamides because this can induce a skin abnormality called Stevens-Johnson syndrome. The nurse should instruct the patient to stop taking the drug and contact a healthcare provider if rash occurs.

Patient education as it relates to sulfonamides should include goals, reasons for obtaining baseline data such as lab work and culture and sensitivity tests, and possible side effects. Following are the important points the nurse should include when teaching patients regarding sulfonamides.

■ Avoid exposure to direct sunlight; use sunscreen and protective clothing to decrease effects of photosensitivity.
■ Take oral medications with a full glass of water.
■ Increase fluid intake to 1,500 to 3,000 ml per day unless otherwise contraindicated.
■ Report significant side effects immediately, including abdominal or stomach cramps or pain, blood in urine, confusion, difficulty breathing, and fever.

See "Nursing Process Focus: Patients Receiving Antibacterial Therapy" on page 457 for the Nursing Process applied to all antibacterials.

32.15 Miscellaneous Antibacterials

Some anti-infectives cannot be grouped into classes, or the class is too small to warrant separate discussion. That is not to diminish their importance in medicine, as some of the mis-cellaneous anti-infectives are critical drugs in certain situations. The miscellaneous antibiotics are shown in Table 32.9.

Clindamycin (Cleocin) is effective against gram-positive and gram-negative bacteria. Susceptible bacteria include fusobacterium, and *Clostridium perfringens*. It is sometimes the drug of choice for oral infections caused by bacteroides. It is considered to be appropriate treatment when less toxic alternatives are not effective options. It is contraindicated in patients with a history of hypersensitivity to clindamycin or lincomycin, regional enteritis, or ulcerative colitis. Clindamycin is limited in use because it is associated with pseudomembranous colitis (AAPMC), the most severe adverse effect of this drug. The patient should report significant side effects to the healthcare provider immediately, including diarrhea, rashes, difficulty breathing, itching, and difficulty swallowing.

Quinupristin/dalfopristin (Synercid) is a combination drug that is the first in a new class of antibiotics called streptogamins. This drug is primarily indicated for treatment of vancomycin-resistant *Enterococcus faecium* infections and is contraindicated in patients with hypersensitivity to quinupristin/dalfopristin. It is used cautiously in patients with renal or hepatic dysfunction. Hepatotoxicity is the most serious adverse effect of this drug. The patient should report significant side effects to the healthcare provider immediately, including irritation, pain, or burning at the intravenous infusion site, joint and muscle pain, rash, diarrhea, and vomiting.

Linezolid (Zyvox) is significant in being the first drug in a new class of antibiotics called the oxazolidinones. This drug is as effective as vancomycin against methicillin-resistant *Staphylococcus aureus* (MRSA) infections. Linezolid is administered intravenously or orally. Most patients

MediaLink Emerging Infectious Diseases

Table 32.9	Selected Miscellaneous Antibacterials
Drug	**Route and Adult Dose (max dose where indicated)**
aztreonam (Azactam)	IM; 0.5–2.0 g bid-qid (max 8 g/day)
chloramphenicol (Chlorofair, others)	PO; 12.5 mg/kg qid
clindamycin (Cleocin)	PO; 150–450 mg qid
daptomycin (Cubicin)	IV; 4 mg/kg once every 24h for 7–14 days
fosfomycin (Monurol)	PO; 3 g sachet dissolved in 3–4 oz of water as a single dose
imipenem-cilastatin (Primaxin)	IV; 250–500 mg tid-qid (max 4 g/day)
lincomycin (Lincocin)	PO; 500 mg tid-qid (max 8 g/day)
linezolid (Zyvox)	PO; 600 mg bid
meropenum (Merrem IV)	IV; 1–2 g tid
methenamine (Mandelamine, Hiprex, Urex)	PO; 1 g bid (Hiprex) or qid (Mandelamine)
nitrofurantoin (Furadantin, Macrobid, Macrodantin)	PO; 50–100 mg qid
quinupristin-dalfopristin (Synercid)	IV; 7.5 mg/kg infused over 60 min q8h
spectinomycin (Trobicin)	IM; 2 g as single dose
teicoplanin (Targocid)	IV; 6 mg/kg/day, after two loading doses 12h apart (each 6 mg/kg)
vancomycin (Vancocin, others)	IV; 500 mg qid; 1 g bid

Pr PROTOTYPE DRUG | VANCOMYCIN (Vancocin)

ACTIONS AND USES

Vancomycin is an antibiotic usually reserved for severe infections from gram positive organisms such as *Staphylococcus aureus* and *Streptococcus pneumoniae*. It is often used after bacteria have become resistant to other, safer antibiotics. It is bacteriocidal, inhibiting bacterial cell wall synthesis. Because vancomycin was not used frequently during the first 30 years following its discovery, the incidence of vancomycin-resistant organisms is smaller than with other antibiotics. Vancomycin is the most effective drug for treating methicillin-resistant *S. aureus* infections, which have become a major problem in the United States. Vancomycin resistant strains of *S. aureus*, however, have begun to appear in recent years. Vancomycin is normally given intravenously, as it is not absorbed from the GI tract.

Administration Alerts

- Administer IV slowly at a rate of 10 mg/min over not less than 60 minutes to avoid causing sudden hypotension.
- Pregnancy category C.

ADVERSE EFFECTS AND INTERACTIONS

Frequent, minor side effects include flushing, hypotension, and rash on the upper body, sometimes called the red-man syndrome. More serious adverse effects are possible with higher doses, including nephrotoxicity and ototoxicity. Patients may experience acute allergic reactions, including anaphylaxis.

Vancomycin adds to toxicity of aminoglycosides, amphotericin B, cisplatin, cyclosporine, polymyxin B, and other ototoxic and nephrotoxic medications. It interacts with cholestyramine and colestipol, causing a decrease in absorption of oral vancomycin. It may increase the risk of lactic acidosis when administered with metformin.

 See the companion website for a Nursing Process Focus specific to this drug.

---

can be converted from intravenous to oral routes in about 5 days. Linezolid is contraindicated in patients with hypersensitivity to the drug and in pregnancy and used with caution in patients who have hypertension. Cautious use is also necessary in patients taking MAOI or serotonin reuptake inhibitors because the drugs can interact causing a hypertensive crisis. Linezolid can cause thrombocytopenia. The patient should report significant side effects to the health-

care provider immediately, including bleeding, diarrhea, headache, nausea, vomiting, rash, dizziness, and fever.

Vancomycin (Vancocin) is an antibiotic usually reserved for severe infections from gram positive organisms such as *Staphylococcus aureus* and *Streptococcus pneumoniae*. It is often used after bacteria have become resistant to other, safer antibiotics. Vancomycin is the most effective drug for treating methicillin-resistant *S. aureus* infections. Vancomycin is

NURSING PROCESS FOCUS   PATIENTS RECEIVING ANTIBACTERIAL THERAPY

ASSESSMENT

Prior to administration:
- Obtain complete health history including allergies, drug history, and possible drug interactions.
- Obtain specimens for culture and sensitivity before initiating therapy.
- Perform infection-focused physical examination including vital signs, white blood cell count, and sedimentation rate.

POTENTIAL NURSING DIAGNOSES

- Infection
- Risk for Injury, related to side effects of drug
- Deficient Knowledge, related to disease process, transmission, and drug therapy
- Noncompliance, related to therapeutic regimen

PLANNING: PATIENT GOALS AND EXPECTED OUTCOMES

The patient will:
- Report reduction in symptoms related to the diagnosed infection, and have negative results for laboratory and diagnostic tests for the presenting infection
- Demonstrate an understanding of the drug's action by accurately describing drug side effects and precautions
- Immediately report significant side effects such as shortness of breath, swelling, fever, stomatitis, loose stools, vaginal discharge, or cough
- Complete full course of antibiotic therapy and comply with follow-up care

IMPLEMENTATION

Interventions and (Rationales)	Patient Education/Discharge Planning
■ Monitor vital signs and symptoms of infection to determine antibacterial effectiveness. (Another drug or different dosage may be required.)	■ Instruct patient to notify healthcare provider if symptoms persist or worsen.
■ Monitor for hypersensitivity reaction. (Immediate hypersensitivity reaction may occur within 2 to 30 minutes; accelerated occurs in 1 to 72 hours; and delayed after 72 hours.)	■ Instruct patient to discontinue the medication and inform healthcare provider if symptoms of hypersensitivity reaction develop such as wheezing; shortness of breath; swelling of face, tongue, or hands; and itching or rash.
■ Monitor for severe diarrhea. (The condition may occur due to superinfection or the possible adverse effect of antibiotic associated pseudomembranous colitis, or AAPMC.)	Instruct patient to: ■ Consult healthcare provider before taking antidiarrheal drugs, which could cause retention of harmful bacteria ■ Consume cultured dairy products with live active cultures, such as kefir, yogurt, or buttermilk, to help maintain normal intestinal flora
■ Administer drug around the clock (to maintain effective blood levels).	Instruct patient to: ■ Take medication on schedule ■ Complete the entire prescription even if feeling better, to prevent development of resistant bacteria
■ Monitor for superinfection, especially in elderly, debilitated, or immunosuppressed patients. (Increased risk for superinfections is due to elimination of normal flora.)	■ Instruct patient to report signs and symptoms of superinfection such as fever; black hairy tongue; stomatitis; loose, foul-smelling stools; vaginal discharge; or cough.
■ Monitor intake of OTC products such as antacids, calcium supplements, iron products, and laxatives containing magnesium. (These products interfere with absorption of many antibiotics.)	■ Advise patient to consult with healthcare provider before using OTC medications or herbal products.
■ Monitor for photosensitivity. (Tetracyclines, fluoroquinolones, and sulfonamides can increase patient's sensitivity to ultraviolet light and increase risk of sunburn.)	Encourage patient to: ■ Avoid direct exposure to sunlight during and after therapy ■ Wear protective clothing, sunglasses, and sunscreen when in the sun

TFS

continued

NURSING PROCESS FOCUS: *Patients Receiving Antibacterial Therapy (continued)*

Interventions and (Rationales)	Patient Education/Discharge Planning
■ Determine the interactions of the prescribed antibiotics with various foods and beverages.	■ Instruct patient regarding foods and beverages that should be avoided with specific antibiotic therapies: ■ No acidic fruit juices with penicillins ■ No alcohol intake with cephalosporins ■ No dairy product/calcium products with tetracyclines
■ Monitor IV site for signs and symptoms of tissue irritation, severe pain, and extravasation.	■ Instruct patient to report pain or other symptoms of discomfort immediately during intravenous infusion.
■ Monitor for side effects specific to various antibiotic therapies. (See "Nursing Considerations" for each antibiotic classification in this chapter.)	■ Instruct patient to report side effects specific to antibiotic therapy prescribed.
■ Monitor renal function such as intake and output ratios and urine color and consistency. Monitor lab work including serum creatinine and BUN. (Some antibiotics such as the aminoglycosides are nephrotoxic.)	■ Explain purpose of required laboratory tests and scheduled follow-up with healthcare provider. ■ Instruct patient to increase fluid intake to 2,000 to 3,000 ml/day.
■ Monitor for symptoms of ototoxicity. (Some antibiotics, such as the aminoglycosides and vancomycin, may cause vestibular or auditory nerve damage.)	Instruct patient to notify healthcare provider of: ■ Changes in hearing, ringing in ears, or full feeling in the ears ■ Nausea and vomiting with motion, ataxia, nystagmus, or dizziness
■ Monitor patient for compliance with antibiotic therapy.	Instruct patient in the importance of: ■ Completing the prescription as ordered ■ Follow-up care after antibiotic therapy is completed

EVALUATION OF OUTCOME CRITERIA

Evaluate the effectiveness of drug therapy by confirming that patient goals and expected outcomes have been met (see "Planning").

See Tables 32.2 through 32.9 for lists of drugs to which these nursing actions apply.

contraindicated in patients with known hypersensitivity to the drug, and in patients with hearing loss. Due to ototoxicity, hearing must be evaluated frequently through the course of therapy. It should not be given to pregnant or lactating patients. Vancomycin can also cause nephrotoxicity leading to uremia.

Vancomycin is administered orally and IV, but not IM. A reaction that can occur with rapid IV administration is known as red-man syndrome and includes hypotension with flushing and a red rash on the face and upper body. The patient should report significant side effects to the healthcare provider immediately, including superinfections, generalized tingling after IV administration, chills, fever, skin rash, hives, hearing loss, and nausea.

See "Nursing Process Focus: Patients Receiving Antibacterial Therapy" on page 457 for the Nursing Process applied to all antibacterials.

In September 2003, the first in a new class of antibiotics, the cyclic lipopeptides, was approved. Daptomycin (Cubicin) is approved for the treatment of serious skin and

skin structure infections such as major abscesses, postsurgical skin wound infections, and infected ulcers caused by *Staphylococcus aureus, Streptococcus pyogenes, Streptococcus agalactiae,* and *Enterococcus faecalis.* The most common side effects are GI distress, injection site reactions, fever, headache, dizziness, insomnia, and rash.

TUBERCULOSIS

Tuberculosis is a highly contagious infection caused by *Mycobacterium tuberculosis.* It is treated with multiple antiinfectives for a prolonged period. The antitubercular agents are shown in Table 32.10.

32.16 Pharmacotherapy of Tuberculosis

Tuberculosis (TB) is an infection caused by the organism *M. tuberculosis.* Although the microorganisms typically invade the lung, they may also enter other body systems, par-

Table 32.10	Antituberculosis Drugs
Drug	**Route and Adult Dose (max dose where indicated)**
First Line Agents	
ethambutol (Myambutol)	PO; 15–25 mg/kg qd
isoniazid (INH, others)	PO; 15 mg/kg qd
pyrazinamide (PZA)	PO; 5–15 mg/kg tid-qid (max 2 g/day)
rifampin (Rifadin, Rimactane)	PO; 600 mg qd
rifapentine (Priftin)	PO; 600 mg twice a week for 2 mo, then once a week for 4 mo
rifater: combination of pyrazinamide with isoniazid and rifampin	PO; six tablets qd (for patients weighing 121 lb or more)
streptomycin	IM; 15 mg/kg up to 1.0 g/day as a single dose
Second Line Agents	
amikacin (Amikin)	IM; 5–7.5 mg/kg as a loading dose, then 7.5 mg/kg bid
capreomycin (Capastat Sulfate)	IM; 1 g/d (not to exceed 20 mg/kg/d) for 60–120 d, then 1 g two to three times/wk
ciprofloxacin (Cipro)	PO; 250–750 mg bid
cycloserine (Seromycin)	PO; 250 mg q12h for 2 wk, may increase to 500 mg q12h (max 1 g/day)
ethionamide (Trecator-SC)	PO; 0.5–1.0 g/d divided q8–12h
kanamycin (Kantrex)	IM; 5–7.5 mg/kg bid-tid
ofloxacin (Floxin)	PO; 200–400 mg bid

ticularly bone. *Mycobacteria* activate cells of the immune response, which attempt to isolate the microorganisms by creating a wall around them. The slow-growing *Mycobacteria* usually become dormant, existing inside cavities called tubercles. They may remain dormant during an entire lifetime, or they may become reactivated if the patient's immune system becomes suppressed. When active, tuberculosis can be quite infectious, readily spread by contaminated sputum. With the immune suppression characteristic of AIDS, the incidence of TB has greatly increased; as many as 20% of all AIDS patients develop active tuberculosis infections. Infection by a different species of mycobacterium, *M. leprae*, is responsible for a disease known as leprosy.

Drug therapy of tuberculosis differs from that of most other infections. Mycobacteria have a cell wall that is resistant to penetration by anti-infective drugs. For medications to reach the isolated microorganisms in the tubercles, therapy must continue for 6 to 12 months. Although the patient may not be infectious this entire time and may have no symptoms, it is critical that therapy continue the entire period. Some patients develop multidrug-resistant infections and require therapy for as long as 24 months.

A second difference in the pharmacotherapy of tuberculosis is that at least two, and sometimes four or more, antibiotics are administered concurrently. During the 6- to 24-month treatment period, different combinations of drugs may be used. Multiple drug therapy is necessary because the mycobacteria grow slowly and resistance is common. Using multiple drugs in different combinations during the long treatment period lowers the potential for resistance and increases the success of the therapy. There are two broad categories of antitubercular agents. One class consists of first line drugs, which are safer and generally the most effective. A second group of drugs, more toxic and less effective than the first line agents, are used when resistance develops.

A third difference is that antituberculosis drugs are extensively used for *preventing* the disease in addition to treating it. Chemoprophylaxis is used for close contacts or family members of recently infected tuberculosis patients. Therapy usually begins immediately after a patient receives a positive tuberculin test. Patients with immunosuppression, such as those with AIDS or those receiving immunosuppressant drugs, may receive preventative treatment with antituberculosis drugs. A short-term therapy of 2 months, consisting of a combination treatment with isoniazid (INH) and pyrazinamide (PZA), is approved for tuberculosis prophylaxis in HIV-positive patients.

NURSING CONSIDERATIONS

The role of the nurse in antituberculosis therapy involves careful monitoring of a patient's condition and providing education as it relates to the prescribed drug regimen. Before beginning therapy, the nurse should assess for the presence or history of a positive tuberculin skin test, a positive sputum culture, or a close contact with a person recently infected with TB. These conditions are all indications for the use of antituberculosis drugs. The nurse should also assess the patient for a history of alcohol abuse,

AIDS, liver disease, or kidney disease, because many anti-tuberculosis drugs are contraindicated in those conditions. They are also contraindicated in patients receiving immunosuppressant drugs. A complete physical exam including vital signs should be performed.

Caution must be observed in patients with renal dysfunction, pregnancy and lactation, or a history of convulsive disorders. They are used with caution in patients with chronic liver disease or alcoholism because of the risk for hepatic injury due to the production of toxic levels of drug metabolites. These drugs may cause asymptomatic hyperuricemia because they can inhibit the renal excretion of uric acid, which may lead to gouty arthritis. Ethambutol (Myambutol) is contraindicated in patients with optic neuritis. Some antituberculosis drugs interact with oral contraceptives and decrease their effectiveness, thus female patients should use an alternate form of birth control while using these medications.

See "Nursing Process Focus: Patients Receiving Antituberculosis Agents" for specific teaching points.

NATURAL THERAPIES | The Antibacterial Properties of Goldenseal

Goldenseal (*Hydrastis canadensis*) was once a common plant found in woods in the eastern and midwestern United States. American Indians used the root for a variety of medicinal applications, including wound healing, diuresis, and washes for inflamed eyes. In recent years, the plant has been harvested to near extinction. In particular, goldenseal was reported to mask the appearance of drugs in the urine of patients wanting to hide drug abuse. This claim has since been proven false.

The roots and leaves of goldenseal are dried and available as capsules, tablets, salves, and tinctures. One of the primary active ingredients in goldenseal is hydrastine, which is reported to have antibacterial and antifungal properties. When used topically or locally, it is purported to be of value in treating bacterial and fungal skin infections and oral conditions such as gingivitis and thrush. As an eyewash, it can soothe inflamed eyes. Considered safe for most people, it is contraindicated in pregnancy and hypertension.

Pr PROTOTYPE DRUG | ISONIAZID (INH)

ACTIONS AND USES

Isoniazid has been a drug of choice for the treatment of *M. tuberculosis* for many years. It is bacteriocidal for actively growing organisms but bacteriostatic for dormant mycobacteria. It is selective for *M. tuberculosis*. Isoniazid is used alone for chemoprophylaxis, or in combination with other antituberculosis drugs for treating active disease.

Administration Alerts

- Give on an empty stomach, 1 hour after or 2 hours before meals.
- Give with meals if GI irritation occurs.
- For IM administration, administer deep IM and rotate sites.
- Pregnancy category C.

ADVERSE EFFECTS AND INTERACTIONS

The most common side effects of isoniazid are numbness of the hands and feet, rash, and fever. Although rare, liver toxicity is a serious adverse effect; thus, the nurse should be alert for signs of jaundice, fatigue, elevated hepatic enzymes, or loss of appetite. Liver enzyme tests are usually performed monthly during therapy to identify early hepatotoxicity.

Aluminum-containing antacids decrease the absorption of isoniazid. When disulfiram is taken with INH, lack of coordination or psychotic reactions may result. Drinking alcohol with INH increases the risk of hepatotoxicity.

 See the companion website for a Nursing Process Focus specific to this drug.

NURSING PROCESS FOCUS | PATIENTS RECEIVING ANTITUBERCULOSIS AGENTS

ASSESSMENT

Prior to administration:
- Obtain complete health history including allergies, drug history, and possible drug interactions.
- Perform complete physical examination including vital signs.
- Assess for presence/history of the following:
  - positive tuberculin skin test
  - positive sputum culture or smear
  - close contact with person recently infected with tuberculosis
  - HIV infection or AIDS
  - immunosuppressant drug therapy
  - alcohol abuse
  - liver or kidney disease
- Assess cognitive ability to comply with long-term therapy.

POTENTIAL NURSING DIAGNOSES

- Risk for Infection
- Risk for Injury, related to side effects of medication
- Deficient Knowledge, related to drug therapy
- Noncompliance, related to therapeutic regimen

PLANNING: PATIENT GOALS AND EXPECTED OUTCOMES

The patient will:
- Report reduction in tuberculosis symptoms and have negative results for laboratory and diagnostic tests indicating TB infection
- Demonstrate an understanding of the drug's action by accurately describing drug side effects and precautions
- Immediately report effects such as visual changes, difficulty voiding, changes in hearing, and symptoms of liver or kidney impairment
- Complete full course of antitubercular therapy and comply with follow-up care

IMPLEMENTATION

Interventions and (Rationales)	Patient Education/Discharge Planning
■ Monitor for hepatic side effects. (Antituberculosis agents, such as isoniazid and rifampin, cause hepatic impairment.)	■ Instruct patient to report yellow eyes and skin, loss of appetite, dark urine, and unusual tiredness.
■ Monitor for neurologic side effects such as numbness and tingling of the extremities. (Antituberculosis agents, such as isoniazid, cause peripheral neuropathy and depletion of vitamin B_6.)	Instruct patient to: ■ Report numbness and tingling of extremities ■ Take supplemental vitamin B_6 as ordered to reduce risk of side effects
■ Collect sputum specimens as directed by healthcare provider. (This will determine the effectiveness of the antituberculosis agent.)	■ Instruct the patient in technique needed to collect a quality sputum specimen.
■ Monitor for dietary compliance when patient is taking isoniazid. (Foods high in tyramine can interact with the drug and cause palpitations, flushing, and hypertension.)	■ Advise patients taking isoniazid to avoid foods containing tyramine, such as aged cheese, smoked and pickled fish, beer and red wine, bananas, and chocolate.
■ Monitor for side effects specific to various antituberculosis drugs.	Instruct patient to report side effects specific to antituberculosis therapy prescribed: ■ Blurred vision or changes in color or vision field (ethambutol) ■ Difficulty in voiding (pyrazinamide) ■ Fever, yellowing of skin, weakness, dark urine (isoniazid, rifampin) ■ Gastrointestinal system disturbances (rifampin) ■ Changes in hearing (streptomycin) ■ Numbness and tingling of extremities (isoniazid) ■ Red discoloration of body fluids (rifampin) ■ Dark concentrated urine, weight gain, edema (streptomycin)

continued

NURSING PROCESS FOCUS: Patients Receiving Antituberculosis Agents (continued)

Interventions and (Rationales)	*Patient Education/Discharge Planning*
■ Establish infection control measures based on extent of disease condition, and established protocol.	■ Instruct patient in infectious control measures, such as frequent handwashing, covering the mouth when coughing or sneezing, and proper disposal of soiled tissues.
■ Establish therapeutic environment to ensure adequate rest, nutrition, hydration, and relaxation. (Symptoms of tuberculosis are manifested when the immune system is suppressed.)	■ Teach patient to incorporate health-enhancing activities, such as adequate rest and sleep, intake of essential vitamins and nutrients, and intake of six to eight glasses of water/day.
■ Monitor patient's ability and motivation to comply with therapeutic regimen. (Treatment must continue for the full length of therapy to eliminate all *M. tuberculosis* organisms.)	Explain the importance of complying with the entire therapeutic plan, including: ■ Take all medications as directed by healthcare provider ■ Do not discontinue medication until instructed ■ Wear a medical alert bracelet ■ Keep all appointments for follow-up care

EVALUATION OF OUTCOME CRITERIA

Evaluate the effectiveness of drug therapy by confirming that patient goals and expected outcomes have been met (see "Planning").

See Table 32.10 for a list of drugs to which these nursing actions apply.

CHAPTER REVIEW

Key Concepts

The numbered key concepts provide a succinct summary of the important points from the corresponding numbered section within the chapter. If any of these points are not clear, refer to the numbered section within the chapter for review. Expanded versions can be found on the companion website.

32.1 Pathogens are organisms that cause disease due to their ability to divide rapidly or secrete toxins.

32.2 Bacteria are described by their shape (bacilli, cocci, or spirilla), their ability to utilize oxygen (aerobic or anaerobic), and by their staining characteristics (gram positive or gram negative).

32.3 Anti-infective drugs are classified by their chemical structures (e.g., aminoglycoside, fluoroquinolone) or by their mechanism of action (e.g., cell wall inhibitor, folic acid inhibitor).

32.4 Anti-infective drugs act by affecting the target organism's metabolism or life cycle and may be bacteriocidal or bacteriostatic.

32.5 Acquired resistance causes loss of antibiotic effectiveness and is worsened by the overprescribing of these agents.

32.6 Careful selection of the correct antibiotic, through the use of culture and sensitivity testing, is essential for effective pharmacotherapy and to limit adverse effects.

32.7 Host factors such as immune system status, local conditions at the infection site, allergic reactions, age, and genetics influence the choice of antibiotic.

32.8 Penicillins kill bacteria by disrupting the cell wall. Allergies occur most frequently with the penicillins.

32.9 The cephalosporins are similar in structure and function to the penicillins and are one of the most widely prescribed anti-infective classes. Cross-sensitivity may exist with the penicillins in some patients.

32.10 Tetracyclines have some of the broadest spectrums, but they are drugs of choice for relatively few diseases.

32.11 The macrolides are safe alternatives to penicillin for many diseases.

32.12 The aminoglycosides are narrow-spectrum drugs that have the potential to cause serious adverse effects such as ototoxicity, nephrotoxicity, and neuromuscular blockade.

32.13 The use of fluoroquinolones has expanded far beyond their initial role in treating urinary tract infections.

32.14 Once widely prescribed, resistance has limited the usefulness of sulfonamides to urinary tract infections and a few other specific infections.

32.15 A number of miscellaneous antibacterials have specific indications, distinct antibacterial mechanism, and related nursing care.

32.16 Multiple drug therapies are needed in the treatment of tuberculosis, since the complex microbes are slow growing and commonly develop drug resistance.

Review Questions

1. Why does antibiotic resistance become more of a problem when antibiotics are prescribed too often?

2. If penicillins are inexpensive, why might a healthcare provider prescribe a more expensive cephalosporin or macrolide antibiotic?

3. How does drug therapy of tuberculosis differ from conventional anti-infective chemotherapy? What are the rationales for these differences?

Critical Thinking Questions

1. An 18-year-old female comes to a clinic for prenatal care. She is 8 weeks' pregnant. She is healthy and takes no other medication other than low-dose tetracycline for acne. What is a priority of care for this patient?

2. A 32-year-old patient has a diagnosis of otitis externa and the healthcare provider has ordered erythromycin PO. This patient has a history of hepatitis B, allergies to sulfa and penicillin, and mild hypertension. Should the nurse give the erythromycin?

3. A 66-year-old hospitalized patient has MRSA in a cellulitis of the lower extremity and is on gentamicin IV. What is a priority for the nurse to monitor in this patient?

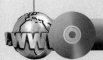 ## EXPLORE MediaLink

NCLEX review, case studies, and other interactive resources for this chapter can be found on the companion website at www.prenhall.com/adams. Click on "Chapter 32" to select the activities for this chapter. For animations, more NCLEX review questions, and an audio glossary, access the accompanying CD-ROM in this textbook.

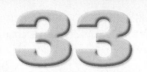

CHAPTER 33

Drugs for Fungal, Protozoan, and Helminth Infections

▪ DRUGS AT A GLANCE

ANTIFUNGAL DRUGS
Agents for systemic infections
- amphotericin B (Fungizone)
- fluconazole (Diflucan)

Agents for topical infections
- nystatin (Mycostatin)

ANTIPROTOZOAN DRUGS
Antimalarial agents
- chloroquine (Aralen)

Nonmalarial antiprotozoan agents
- metronidazole (Flagyl)

Antiparasitic agents

ANTHELMINTIC DRUGS
- mebendazole (Vermox)

metabolized and eliminated by the bod...
of this process
PHARMACOLOGY
1. The study of medicines; the disciplin...
pertaining to how drugs improve the he...
of the human body

MediaLink   www.prenhall.com/adams

CD-ROM
Audio Glossary
NCLEX Review

Companion Website
NCLEX Review
Dosage Calculations
Care Plans
Expanded Key Concepts

OBJECTIVES

After reading this chapter, the student should be able to:

1. Compare and contrast the pharmacotherapy of superficial and systemic fungal infections.
2. Identify the types of patients who are at greatest risk for acquiring serious fungal infections.
3. Identify protozoan and helminth infections that may benefit from pharmacotherapy.
4. Explain how an understanding of the *Plasmodium* life cycle is important to the effective pharmacotherapy of malaria.
5. Describe the nurse's role in the pharmacologic management of fungal, protozoan, and helminth infections.
6. For each of the classes shown in Drugs at a Glance, know representative examples, explain their mechanism of drug action, primary actions, and important adverse effects.
7. Categorize drugs used in the treatment of fungal, protozoan, and helminth infections based on their classification and mechanism of action.
8. Use the Nursing Process to care for patients receiving drug therapy for fungal, protozoan, and helminth infections.

Fungi, protozoans, and multicellular parasites are more complex than bacteria. Because of structural and functional differences, most antibacterial drugs are ineffective against fungi. Although there are fewer drugs to treat these diseases, the available drugs are usually effective.

PHARMFACTS | Fungal, Protozoal, and Helminth Diseases

- Approximately 300 to 500 million cases of malaria occur worldwide each year, with an estimated 2.7 million deaths due to the disease.
- Of the more than 200,000 known species of fungi, fewer than 300 are known to infect humans and 90% of these infections are caused by just a few dozen species.
- Fungi cause 9% of nosocomial infections.
- Of all fungal infections, 86% are caused by candida. The second most common (1.3%) is aspergillosis.
- Chagas' disease, caused by *Trypanosoma cruzi*, is the most significant cause of heart disease in some South American countries. It infects 16 million people annually.
- *Ascaris lumbricoides* is the most common intestinal helminth infection, affecting 1 billion people worldwide.

33.1 Characteristics of Fungi

Fungi are single-celled or multicellular organisms whose primary role on the planet is to serve as decomposers of dead plants and animals, returning their elements to the soil for recycling. Although 100,000 to 200,000 species exist in soil, air, and water, only about 300 are associated with disease in humans. A few species of fungi normally grow on skin and mucosal surfaces, as part of the normal host flora.

Unlike bacteria, which grow rapidly to overwhelm hosts' defenses, fungi grow slowly and infections may progress for many months before symptoms develop. Fungi cause disease by replication; they do not secrete toxins like many bacterial species. With a few exceptions, fungal infections are not readily communicable to those in casual contact with the patient.

The human body is remarkably resistant to infection by these organisms and patients with healthy immune systems experience few serious fungal diseases. Patients who have a suppressed immune system, however, such as those infected with HIV, may experience frequent fungal infections, some of which may require aggressive pharmacotherapy.

The species of pathogenic fungi that attack a host with a healthy immune system are somewhat distinct from those that infect patients who are immunocompromised. Patients with intact immune defenses are afflicted with *community-acquired* infections such as sporotrichosis, blastomycosis, histoplasmosis, and coccidioidomycosis. *Opportunistic* fungal infections acquired in a nosocomial setting are more likely to be candidiasis, aspergillosis, cryptococcosis, and mucormycosis. Table 33.1 lists the most common fungi that cause disease in humans.

33.2 Classification of Mycoses

Fungal diseases are called mycoses. Yeasts, which include the common pathogen *Candida albicans*, are unicellular fungi. A simple and useful method of classifying fungal infections is to consider them as either superficial or systemic. Superficial mycoses affect the scalp, skin, nails, and mucous membranes such as the oral cavity and vagina. Mycoses of this type are often treated with topical drugs, as the incidence of side effects is much lower using this route of administration. Superficial fungal infections are sometimes called dermatophytic.

Systemic mycoses are those affecting internal organs, typically the lungs, brain, and digestive organs. Although less common than superficial mycoses, systemic fungal infections affect multiple body systems and are sometimes fatal to patients with suppressed immune systems. Mycoses of this type often require aggressive oral or parenteral medications that produce more adverse effects than the topical agents.

Historically, the antifungal drugs used for superficial infections were clearly distinct from those prescribed for systemic infections. In recent years, this distinction has become somewhat arbitrary. Many of the newer antifungal agents may be used for either superficial or systemic infections. Furthermore, some superficial infections may be treated either systemically or topically.

33.3 Mechanism of Action of Antifungal Drugs

Biologically, fungi are classified as eukaryotes; their cellular structure and metabolic pathways are more similar to those of humans than to bacteria. Antibiotics that are efficacious against bacteria are ineffective in treating mycoses. Thus, an entirely different set of agents is needed.

One important difference between fungal cells and human cells is the steroid in their plasma membranes. Whereas cholesterol is essential for animal cell membranes, ergosterol is present in fungi. This difference al-

Table 33.1	Fungal Pathogens
Name of Fungus	**Description**
Systemic	
Aspergillus fumigatus, others	aspergillosis: opportunistic, most commonly affects lung but can spread to other organs
Blastomyces dermatitidis	blastomycosis: begins in the lungs and spreads to other organs
Candida albicans, others	candidiasis: most common opportunistic fungal infection; may affect nearly any organ
Coccidioides immitis	coccidioidomycosis: begins in the lungs and spreads to other organs
Cryptococcus neoformans	cryptococcosis: opportunistic, begins in the lungs but is the most common cause of meningitis in AIDS patients
Histoplasma capsulatum	histoplasmosis: begins in the lungs and spreads to other organs
Mucorales (various species)	mucormycosis: opportunistic, affects blood vessels, causes sinus infections, stomach ulcers and others
Pneumocystis carinii	pneumocystis pneumonia: opportunistic, primarily pneumonia of the lung but can spread to other organs
Topical	
Candida albicans, others	candidiasis: affects skin, nails, oral cavity (thrush), vagina
Epidermophyton floccosum	athlete's foot (tinea pedis), jock itch (tinea cruris), and other skin disorders
Microsporum audouini, others	ringworm of scalp (tinea capitis)
Sporothrix schenckii	sporotrichosis: primarily affects skin and superficial lymph nodes
Trichophyton (various species)	affects scalp, skin, and nails

lows antifungal agents such as amphotericin B to be selective for fungal plasma membranes. The largest class of antifungals, the azoles, inhibits ergosterol synthesis, causing the fungal plasma membrane to become porous or leaky.

Some antifungals act by mechanisms that take advantage of enzymatic differences between fungi and humans. For example, in fungi, flucytosine (Ancobon) is converted to the toxic antimetabolite 5-fluorouracil, which inhibits both DNA and RNA synthesis. Humans do not have the enzyme necessary for this conversion. 5-Fluorouracil itself is a common antineoplastic drug (Chapter 35)⬤⬤ .

DRUGS FOR SYSTEMIC ANTIFUNGAL INFECTIONS

Systemic or invasive fungal disease may require intensive pharmacotherapy for extended periods. Amphotericin B (Fungizone) and fluconazole (Diflucan) are drugs of choice. Systemic antifungal drugs are shown in Table 33.2.

33.4 Pharmacotherapy of Systemic Fungal Diseases

Opportunistic fungal disease in AIDS patients spurred the development of several new drugs for systemic fungal infections over the past 20 years. Others who may experience systemic mycoses include those patients receiving prolonged therapy with corticosteroids, experiencing extensive burns, receiving antineoplastic agents, having indwelling vascular catheters, or having recently received organ transplants. Systemic antifungal drugs have little or no antibacterial activity and pharmacotherapy is often extended, lasting several months.

Amphotericin B (Fungizone) has been the drug of choice for systemic fungal infections for many years; however, the newer azole drugs such as ketoconazole (Nizoral) have replaced amphotericin B for the treatment of less severe systemic infections. Although rarely used as a monotherapy, flucytosine (Ancobon) is sometimes used in combination with amphotericin B in the pharmacotherapy of severe candida infections. Flucytosine (Ancobon) can cause immuno-

suppression and liver toxicity, and resistance has become a major problem.

NURSING CONSIDERATIONS

The role of the nurse in systemic antifungal therapy involves careful monitoring of a patient's condition and providing education as it relates to the prescribed drug regimen. Prior to the initiation of therapy, the patient's health history should be taken. This class is contraindicated in patients with hypersensitivity and should be used cautiously in patients with renal impairment or severe bone marrow suppression. The nurse should obtain baseline culture and sensitivity tests prior to the beginning of therapy. Baseline and periodic lab tests including BUN, creatinine, CBC, electrolytes, and liver function tests should be obtained. Vital signs, especially pulse and blood pressure, should be obtained for baseline data, as patients with heart disease may develop fluid overload.

Amphotericin B (Fungizone) causes some degree of kidney damage in 80% of the patients who take it; therefore, the nurse should monitor intake and output, as well as weight. Oliguria, changes in intake and output ratios, hematuria, or abnormal renal function tests should be reported to the physician immediately. Because amphotericin B can cause ototoxicity, the nurse should assess for hearing loss, vertigo, unsteady gait, or tinnitus.

Electrolyte imbalance is a significant side effect due to excretion of the drug in the urine. Hypokalemia is common, so the nurse should monitor for symptoms of low potassium levels, including dysrhythmias. The nurse should also evaluate all other medications taken by the patient for compatibility with systemic antifungal medications. Concurrent therapy with medications that reduce liver or renal function is not recommended.

Patient education as it relates to systemic antifungal medications should include goals, reasons for obtaining baseline data, and possible side effects. The nurse should instruct the patient and caregivers to do the following:

■ Complete the full course of treatment.
■ Avoid drinking alcohol due to its effects on the liver.

Table 33.2	Drugs for Systemic Mycoses
Drug	**Route and Adult Dose (max dose where indicated)**
▣ amphotericin B (Fungizone, Abelcet, Amphotec, AmBisome)	IV; 0.25 mg/kg qd; may increase to 1 mg/kg qd or 1.5 mg/kg qod (max 1.5 mg/kg/day)
caspofungin acetate (Cancidas)	IV; Loading dose 70 mg infused over 1 hr
▣ fluconazole (Diflucan)	PO; 200–400 mg on day 1, then 100–200 mg qd for 2–4 weeks
flucytosine (5-fluorocytosine, Ancobon)	PO; 50–150 mg/kg in divided doses
itraconazole (Sporanox)	PO; 200 mg qd; may increase to 200 mg bid (max 400 mg/day)
ketoconazole (Nizoral)	PO; 200–400 mg qd
terbinafine hydrochloride (Lamisil)	PO; 250 mg qd for 6–13 weeks
voriconazole (Vfend)	IV; 6 mg/kg q12h day 1, then 4 mg/kg q12h; may reduce to 3 mg/kg q12h if not tolerated

Pr PROTOTYPE DRUG	AMPHOTERICIN B (Fungizone)

ACTIONS AND USES

Amphotericin B has a wide spectrum of activity that includes most of the fungi pathogenic to humans; thus, it is a drug of choice for most severe systemic mycoses. It may also be indicated as prophylactic antifungal therapy for patients with severe immunosuppression. It acts by binding to ergosterol in fungal cell membranes, causing them to become permeable or leaky. Because it is not absorbed from the GI tract, it is normally given by IV infusion. Topical preparations are available for superficial mycoses. Treatment may continue for several months. Resistance to amphotericin B is not common.

To reduce toxicity, amphotericin B has been formulated with three lipid preparations: liposomal amphotericin B (AmBisome), amphotericin B lipid complex (Abelcet), and amphotericin B cholesteryl sulfate complex (Amphotec). The principal advantage of the lipid formulations is reduced nephrotoxicity and less infusion-related fever and chills. They are generally used only after therapy with other agents has failed, due to their expense. Amphotericin B is pregnancy category B.

Administration Alerts

- Infuse slowly. Cardiovascular collapse may result when medication is infused too rapidly.
- Administer premedication to help decrease the chance of infusion reactions.
- Withhold drug if BUN exceeds 40 mg/dl or serum creatinine rises above 3 mg/dl.

ADVERSE EFFECTS AND INTERACTIONS

Amphotericin B can cause a number of serious side effects. Many patients develop fever and chills, vomiting, and headache at the beginning of therapy, which subside as treatment continues. Phlebitis is common during IV therapy. Some degree of nephrotoxicity is observed in most patients and kidney function tests are normally performed throughout the treatment period.

Amphotericin B interacts with many drugs. For example, concurrent therapy with aminoglycosides, vancomycin, carboplatin, and furosemide, which reduce renal function, is not recommended. Use with corticosteroids, skeletal muscle relaxants, and thiazole may potentiate hypokalemia. If hypokalemia is present, use with digitalis increases the risk of digitalis toxicity.

- Use effective contraception measures to prevent pregnancy.
- Monitor urinary output and drink plenty of fluids.
- Use caution while performing hazardous activities.

See also "Nursing Process Focus: Patients Receiving Amphotericin B" for specific points the nurse should include when teaching patients regarding this drug.

Azoles

The azole drug class actually consists of two different chemical classes, the imidazoles and the triazoles. Azole antifungal drugs interfere with the biosynthesis of ergosterol, which is essential for fungal cell membranes. By depleting fungal cells of ergosterol, their growth is impaired. Several new azoles are in the final stages of clinical trials, and should become available over the next few years.

33.5 Pharmacotherapy with the Azole Antifungals

Most azoles are given by the topical route, although fluconazole (Diflucan), itraconazole, (Sporanox), and ketoconazole (Nizoral) may be given orally or parenterally for systemic or superficial infections. Ketoconazole is only available orally, and is the most hepatotoxic of the azoles.

Itraconazole has begun to replace ketoconazole in the therapy of systemic mycoses because it has less hepatotoxicity and may be given either orally or intravenously. It also has a broader spectrum of activity than the other systemic azoles. Clotrimazole (Mycelex, others) is a drug of choice for fungal infections of the skin, vagina, and mouth.

The systemic azole drugs have a spectrum of activity similar to that of amphotericin B, are considerably less toxic, and have the major advantage that they can be administered orally. Topical formulations are available for superficial mycoses, although they may also be given by the oral route for these infections. Common side effects of the oral and parenteral azoles include nausea, vomiting, diarrhea, and rash.

NURSING CONSIDERATIONS

The role of the nurse in azole therapy involves careful monitoring of a patient's condition and providing education as it relates to the prescribed drug regimen. Prior to the initiation of pharmacotherapy, the patient's health history should be taken. They are contraindicated in patients with hypersensitivity to azole antifungals, and should be used with caution in patients with renal impairment. Lab tests,

NURSING PROCESS FOCUS | **PATIENTS RECEIVING AMPHOTERICIN B (FUNGIZONE, ABELCET)**

ASSESSMENT

Prior to administration:
- Obtain complete health history including allergies, drug history, and possible drug interactions.
- Obtain a culture and sensitivity of suspected area of infection to determine need for therapy.
- Obtain baseline vital signs, especially pulse and blood pressure.
- Obtain renal function including blood tests (CBC, chemistry panel, BUN, and creatinine).

POTENTIAL NURSING DIAGNOSES

- Risk for Injury, related to adverse effects of drug
- Risk for Infection, related to drug-induced leukopenia
- Deficient Knowledge, related to drug therapy

PLANNING: PATIENT GOALS AND EXPECTED OUTCOMES

The patient will:
- Report fewer symptoms of fungal infection
- Demonstrate an understanding of the drug's action by accurately describing drug side effects and precautions
- Immediately report effects such as fever, chills, fluid retention, dizziness, or decrease in urine output

IMPLEMENTATION

Interventions and (Rationales)	*Patient Education/Discharge Planning*
■ Monitor vital signs, especially pulse and blood pressure, frequently during and after infusion. (Cardiovascular collapse may result when drug is infused too rapidly, which is caused by the drug binding to human cytoplasmic sterols.)	■ Advise patient to report dizziness, shortness of breath, heart palpitations, or faintness immediately.
■ Monitor kidney function, including intake and output, urinalysis, and periodic blood work. (Amphotericin B is nephrotoxic. This medication is excreted in the urine and causes significant electrolyte loss from the kidneys.)	Instruct patient to: ■ Keep all laboratory appointments for blood work (CBC, electrolytes every 2 weeks; BUN, creatinine weekly) ■ Keep an accurate record of intake and output ■ Drink at least 2.5 L of fluids daily ■ Report a decrease in urinary output, change in the appearance of urine, or weight gain or loss
■ Monitor for GI distress.	Instruct patient to: ■ Take an antiemetic prior to drug therapy, if needed ■ Report GI distress such as anorexia, nausea, vomiting, extreme weight loss, and headache
■ Monitor for fluid overload and electrolyte imbalance. (Patients with cardiac disease are at high risk.)	■ Advise patients with any form of cardiac disease to report any palpitations, chest pain, swelling of extremities, and shortness of breath.
■ Monitor for signs/symptoms of toxicity and hypersensitivity.	Instruct patient to report the following: ■ IV: malaise, generalized pain, confusion, depression, hypotension tachycardia, respiratory failure, evidence of ototoxicity such as hearing loss, tinnitus, vertigo, and unsteady gait ■ Topical: irritation, pruritus, dry skin, redness, burning, and itching
■ Monitor IV site frequently for any signs of extravasation. (Medication is irritating to the vein. Use a central line if possible.)	■ Advise patient to report any pain at the IV site.

EVALUATION OF OUTCOME CRITERIA

Evaluate the effectiveness of drug therapy by confirming that patient goals and expected outcomes have been met (see "Planning").

including BUN, creatinine, and liver function tests, should be obtained before therapy begins and through the course of treatment. Ketoconazole (Nizoral) should not be given to patients with chronic alcoholism, because this drug can be toxic to the liver.

Because the azoles can cause GI side effects, the nurse should assess for nausea, vomiting, abdominal pain, or diarrhea. The nurse should also monitor for signs and symptoms of hepatotoxicity, such as pruritus, jaundice, dark urine, and skin rash. Azoles may affect glycemic control in diabetic patients, so blood sugar should be monitored carefully in these patients. The nurse should also evaluate all other medications taken by the patient for compatibility with antifungal drugs. Concurrent therapy with drugs that reduce liver or renal function is not recommended. The nurse should monitor for alcohol use as it increases the risk of side effects such as nausea and vomiting and increases blood pressure.

Patient education as it relates to azole drugs should include goals, reasons for obtaining baseline data, and possible side effects. The nurse should instruct the patient and caregivers to do the following:

- Complete the full course of treatment.
- Report the use of any other prescription or OTC medications.
- Avoid drinking alcohol due to its effects on the liver.
- Use effective contraception measures to prevent pregnancy.
- Monitor urinary output and drink plenty of fluids.
- Use caution while performing hazardous activities.
- Advise diabetic patients to increase blood glucose monitoring and report hypoglycemia.

DRUGS FOR SUPERFICIAL FUNGAL INFECTIONS

Superficial fungal infections are generally not severe. If possible, superficial infections are treated with topical agents because they are safer than their systemic counterparts. Agents used to treat superficial mycoses are shown in Table 33.3.

33.6 Superficial Fungal Infections

Superficial fungal infections of the hair, scalp, nails, and the mucous membranes of the mouth and vagina are rarely medical emergencies. Infections of the nails and skin, for example, may be ongoing for months or even years before a patient seeks treatment. Unlike systemic fungal infections, superficial infections may occur in any patient, not just those who have suppressed immune systems. About 75% of all female patients experience vulvovaginal candidiasis at least once in their lifetime.

Superficial antifungal drugs are much safer than their systemic counterparts because penetration into the deeper layers of the skin is generally poor and only small amounts are absorbed. Many are available as OTC creams, gels, and ointments. If the infection has grown into the deeper skin layers, oral antifungal drugs may be indicated. Extensive superficial mycoses are often treated with oral antifungal drugs along with the topical agents, to be certain that the infection is eliminated.

Selection of a particular antifungal agent is based on the location of the infection and characteristics of the lesion. Griseofulvin (Fulvicin) is an inexpensive, older agent that is indicated for the oral therapy of mycoses of the hair, skin,

Pr PROTOTYPE DRUG	FLUCONAZOLE (Diflucan)
ACTIONS AND USES	**ADVERSE EFFECTS AND INTERACTIONS**
Like other azoles, fluconazole acts by interfering with the synthesis of ergosterol. Fluconazole, however, offers several advantages over other systemic antifungals. It is rapidly and completely absorbed when given orally. Unlike itraconazole (Sporanox) and ketoconazole (Nizoral), it is able to penetrate most body membranes to reach infections in the CNS, bone, eye, urinary tract, and respiratory tract. A major disadvantage of fluconazole is its relatively narrow-spectrum of activity. Although it is effective against *Candida albicans*, it may not be effective against non-*albicans Candida* species, which account for a significant percentage of opportunistic fungal infections. *Administration Alerts* ■ Do not mix IV fluconazole with other drugs. ■ Pregnancy category C.	Fluconazole causes few serious side effects. Nausea, vomiting, and diarrhea are reported at high doses. Because most of the drug is excreted by the kidneys, it should be used cautiously in patients with preexisting kidney disease. Unlike ketoconazole hepatotoxicity with fluconazole is rare. Fluconazole interacts with several drugs. Use with warfarin may cause increased risk for bleeding. Hypoglycemic reaction may be seen with oral sulfonylureas. Fluconazole levels may be decreased with concurrent rifampin or cimetidine use. The effects of fentanyl, alfentanil, or methadone may be prolonged with concurrent administration of fluconazole.

 See the companion website for a Nursing Process Focus specific to this drug.

Table 33.3	Drugs for Superficial Mycoses
Drug	**Route and Adult Dose (max dose where indicated)**
butenafine (Mentax)	Topical: apply qd for 4 wk
butoconazole (Femstat)	Topical: one applicator intravaginally hs for 3 d
ciclopirox olamine (Loprox)	Topical: apply bid for 4 wk
clotrimazole (FemCare, Gyne-Lotrimin, Mycelex, others)	Topical: apply bid for 4 wk; for vaginal mycoses, insert one applicator intravaginally hs for 7 d
econazole (Spectazole)	Topical: apply bid for 4 wk
⊙ fluconazole (Diflucan)	PO; 200–400 mg on day 1, then 100–200 mg qd for 2–4 wk
griseofulvin (Fulvicin)	PO; 500 mg microsize or 330–375 mg ultra microsize qd
haloprogin (Halotex)	Topical: apply bid for 2–3 wk
itraconazole (Sporanox)	PO; 200 mg qd; may increase to 200 mg bid (max 400 mg/day)
ketoconazole (Nizoral)	Topical: apply qd-bid to affected area
miconazole (Micatin, Monistat Cruex, others)	Topical: apply bid for 2–4 wk
naftifine (Naftin)	Topical: apply cream qd or gel bid for 4 wk
⊙ nystatin (Mycostatin, Nilstat, Nystex)	PO; 500,000–1,000,000 units tid, Intravaginal: one to two tablets daily for 2 wk
oxiconazole (Oxistat)	Topical: apply qd in the evening for 2 mo
sulconazole nitrate (Exelderm)	Topical: apply once or twice daily for 2–6 wk
terbinafine (Lamisil)	Topical: apply qd or bid for 7 wk
terconazole (Terazol)	Topical: insert one applicator intravaginally at hs for 3–7 wk
tioconazole (Vagistat)	Topical: insert applicator intravaginally at hs for 1 day
tolnaftate (Aftate, Tinactin)	Topical: apply bid for 4–6 wk
undecylenic acid (Fungi-Nail, Gordochrom, others)	Topical: apply qd-bid

and nails that have not responded to conventional topical preparations. Itraconazole (Sporanox) and terbinafine (Lamisil) are oral preparations that have the advantage of accumulating in nail beds, allowing them to remain active many months after therapy is discontinued.

Although Nystatin (Mycostatin, others) belongs to the same chemical class as amphotericin B (Fungizone), the **polyenes**, nystatin is available in a wider variety of formulations, including cream, ointment, powder, tablet, and lozenge. Too toxic for parenteral administration, it is primarily used topically for candida infections of the vagina, skin, and mouth. When given topically, nystatin produces few adverse effects, other than minor skin irritation. It may also be used orally to treat candidiasis of the intestine, because it travels through the GI tract without being absorbed. When given orally, it may cause diarrhea, nausea, and vomiting.

NURSING CONSIDERATIONS

The role of the nurse in superficial antifungal therapy involves careful monitoring of a patient's condition and providing education as it relates to the prescribed drug regimen. Prior to the initiation of therapy with antifungals, the patient's health history should be obtained. The nurse should

assess for signs of contact dermatitis; if this is present, the drug should be withheld and the physician notified.

Superficial antifungals, such as nystatin (Mycostatin), should not be used vaginally during pregnancy to treat infections caused by *Gardnerella vaginalis* or *Trichomonas* species. They should be used with caution in patients who are lactating.

There are few side effects to antifungals used for superficial mycoses. The medications may be "swished and swallowed" when used to treat oral candidiasis. The nurse should monitor for side effects such as nausea, vomiting, and diarrhea when the patient is taking high doses. If GI side effects are especially disturbing, the patient should be advised to spit out the medication rather than swallowing it. Some orders will be to "swish only" and then to spit out the medication. The nurse should monitor for signs of improvement in the mouth and on the tongue to evaluate the effectiveness of the medication.

Patient education as it relates to superficial antifungal drugs should include goals, reasons for obtaining baseline data, and possible side effects. The nurse should instruct the patient and caregivers to do the following:

- Complete the full course of treatment; some infections require pharmacotherapy for several months.
- If self-treating with OTC preparations, follow the directions carefully and notify the healthcare provider if symptoms do not resolve in 7 to 10 days.

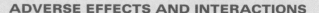

PROTOTYPE DRUG | NYSTATIN (Mycostatin)

ACTIONS AND USES	ADVERSE EFFECTS AND INTERACTIONS
Nystatin binds to sterols in the fungal cell membrane allowing leakage of intracellular contents as the membrane becomes weakened. Although it belongs to the same chemical class as amphotericin B, the polyenes, nystatin is available in a wider variety of formulations, including cream, ointment, powder, tablet, and lozenge. Too toxic for parenteral administration, it is primarily used topically for candida infections of the vagina, skin, and mouth. It may also be used orally to treat candidiasis of the intestine, because it travels through the GI tract without being absorbed.	When given topically, nystatin produces few adverse effects other than minor skin irritation. There is a high incidence of contact dermatitis, related to the preservatives found in many of the formulations. When given orally, it may cause diarrhea, nausea, and vomiting.

Administration Alerts

- Apply with a swab to affected area in infants and children as swishing is difficult or impossible.
- Pregnancy category C.

See the companion website for a Nursing Process Focus specific to this drug.

- Abstain from sexual intercourse during treatment for vaginal infections.
- Teach patients with vaginal candidiasis the correct method for using vaginal suppositories, creams, and ointments.

See also "Nursing Process Focus: Patients Receiving Pharmacotherapy for Superficial Fungal Infections" for specific points the nurse should include when teaching patients regarding this class of drugs.

PROTOZOAN INFECTIONS

Protozoans are single-celled animals. Although only a few of the more than 20,000 species cause disease in humans, they have a significant health impact in Africa, South America, and Asia. Travelers to these continents may acquire these infections overseas and bring them back to the United States and Canada. These parasites often thrive in conditions where sanitation and personal hygiene are poor and population density is high. In addition, protozoan infections often occur in patients who are immunocompromised, such as those in the advanced stages of AIDS. Drugs for malarial infections are shown in Table 33.4.

33.7 Pharmacotherapy of Malaria

Drug therapy of protozoal infections is difficult due to the animals' complicated life cycles. When faced with adverse conditions, protozoans can form cysts that allow the animal to survive in harsh environments, and infect other hosts. When cysts occur inside the host, the parasite is often resistant to pharmacotherapy. With few exceptions, antibiotics, antifungal, and antiviral drugs are ineffective against protozoans.

NATURAL THERAPIES	Remedies for Fungal Infections

Several natural products are reported to have antifungal properties:

- Grape seed extract, which is taken from the seeds of the grape, *Vitis vinifera*; capsules are used internally for 3 to 6 months
- Garlic; in capsule or liquid extract form
- Probiotics; refrigerated supplements that contain *L. acidophilus* and *B. bifidum* are the most potent
- Astragalus root; in capsule and tincture form
- Tea tree oil and thyme oil used externally for fungal infections of the skin; these oils are powerful and should be diluted with another oil such as olive oil

Malaria is caused by four species of the protozoan *Plasmodium*. Although rare in the United States and Canada, malaria is the second most common fatal infectious disease in the world, with 300 to 500 million cases occurring annually.

Malaria begins with a bite from an infected female *Anopheles* mosquito. Once inside the human host, *Plasmodium* multiplies in the liver and transforms into progeny called merozoites. About 14 to 25 days after the initial infection, the merozoites are released into the blood. The merozoites infect red blood cells, which eventually rupture, releasing more merozoites, and causing severe fever and chills. This is called the erythrocytic stage of the infection. *Plasmodium* can remain in body tissues for extended periods and cause relapses months, or even years, after the initial infection. The life cycle of *Plasmodium* is shown in Figure 33.1.

Pharmacotherapy of malaria attempts to interrupt the complex life cycle of *Plasmodium*. Although successful early in the course of the disease, other therapy becomes increasingly difficult as the parasite enters different stages

NURSING PROCESS FOCUS	PATIENTS RECEIVING PHARMACOTHERAPY FOR SUPERFICIAL FUNGAL INFECTIONS

ASSESSMENT

Prior to administration:
- Obtain complete health history including allergies, drug history, and possible drug interactions.
- Obtain a culture and sensitivity of suspected area of infection to determine need for therapy.
- Obtain baseline liver function tests.

POTENTIAL NURSING DIAGNOSES

- Risk for Injury (rash), related to side effect of drug
- Deficient Knowledge, related to drug therapy
- Risk for Impaired Skin Integrity

PLANNING: PATIENT GOALS AND EXPECTED OUTCOMES

The patient will:
- Report healing of fungal infection
- Demonstrate an understanding of the drug's action by accurately describing drug side effects and precautions
- Immediately report effects such as hepatoxicity, GI distress, rash, or decreased urine output

IMPLEMENTATION

Interventions and (Rationales)	Patient Education/Discharge Planning
■ Monitor for possible side effects or hypersensitivity.	Instruct patient to report: ■ Burning, stinging, dryness, itching, erythema, urticaria, angioedema, and local irritation for superficial drugs ■ Symptoms of hepatic toxicity—jaundice, dark urine, light-colored stools, and pruritis ■ Nausea, vomiting, and diarrhea ■ Signs and symptoms of hypo-or hyperglycemia
■ Encourage compliance with instructions when taking oral antifungals. (To increase medication effectiveness.)	Instruct patient to: ■ Swish the oral suspension to coat all mucous membranes, then swallow medication ■ Spit out medication instead of swallowing if GI irritation occurs ■ Allow troche to dissolve completely, rather than chewing or swallowing; it may take 30 minutes for it to completely dissolve ■ Avoid food or drink for 30 minutes following administration ■ Remove dentures prior to using the oral suspension ■ Take ketoconazole with water, fruit juice, coffee, or tea to enhance dissolution and absorption
■ Monitor topical application. ■ Avoid occlusive dressings. (Dressings increase moisture in the infected areas and encourage development of additional yeast infections.)	■ Instruct patient to avoid wearing tight-fitting undergarments if using ointment in the vaginal or groin area.
■ Monitor for contact dermatitis with topical formulations. (This is related to the preservatives found in many of the formulations.)	■ Instruct patient to report any redness or skin rash.
■ Encourage infection control practices. (To prevent the spread of infection.)	Instruct patient to: ■ Clean affected area daily ■ Apply medication with a glove ■ Wash hands properly before and after application ■ Change socks daily if rash is on feet

EVALUATION OF OUTCOME CRITERIA

Evaluate the effectiveness of drug therapy by confirming that patient goals and expected outcomes have been met (see "Planning").

See Table 33.3, as well as the oral and topical systemic drugs in Table 33.2, for a list of drugs to which these nursing actions apply.

Table 33.4	Drugs for Malaria
Drug	**Route and Adult Dose (max dose where indicated)**
atovaquone (Mepron)	PO; 750 mg bid for 21 d
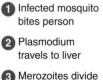 chloroquine hydrochloride (Aralen)	PO; 600 mg initial dose, then 300 mg weekly
halofantrine HCl (Halfan)	PO; 500 mg every 6 hr for three doses; repeat 7 d after the first course
hydroxychloroquine sulfate (Plaquenil) (see page 693 for the Prototype Drug box) ∞	PO; 620 mg initial dose, then 310 mg weekly
mefloquine (Lariam)	PO; Prevention: begin 250 mg once a week for 4 wk, then 250 mg every other week Treatment: 1,250 mg as a single dose
primaquine phosphate	PO; 15 mg qd for 2 wk
proguanil (Paludrine)	PO; 100–200 mg daily taken at least 24 hr before arrival in endemic area, and 6 wk after leaving
pyrimethamine (Daraprim)	PO; 25 mg once per week for 10 wk
quinine (Quinamm)	PO; 260–650 mg tid for 3 d

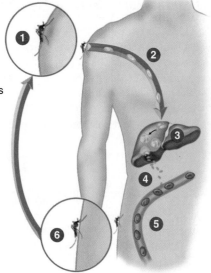

1 Infected mosquito bites person

2 Plasmodium travels to liver

3 Merozoites divide inside hepatocytes

4 Merozoites are released to bloodstream causing fever and chills

5 Merozoites enter red blood cells

6 Mosquito bites person and becomes infected to restart cycle

Figure 33.1 | Life cycle of *Plasmodium*

of its life cycle. Goals of antimalarial therapy include the following:

- *Prevention of the disease* Because of the difficulty in treating malaria once the disease has been acquired, prevention is the best therapeutic option. The Centers for Disease Control (CDC) recommends that travelers to infested areas receive prophylactic antimalarial drugs prior to and during their visit, and for 1 week after leaving. Proguanil (Paludrine) is the prototype antimalarial for prophylaxis.

- *Treatment of acute attacks* Drugs are used to interrupt the erythrocytic stage and eliminate the merozoites from red blood cells. Chloroquine (Aralen) is the classic antimalarial for treating the acute stage.

- *Prevention of relapse* Drugs are given to eliminate the latent forms of *Plasmodium* residing in the liver. Primaquine phosphate is one of the few drugs able to affect a total cure.

NURSING CONSIDERATIONS

The role of the nurse in antimalarial therapy involves careful monitoring of the patient's condition and providing education as it relates to the prescribed drug regimen. Prior to the initiation of drug therapy, the patient's health history should be taken. Those with hematological disorders, severe skin disorders such as psoriasis, or pregnant patients should not take antimalarial drugs. These drugs should be used cautiously in patients with preexisting cardiovascular disease and those who are lactating.

Initial lab work should include a CBC, liver and renal function tests, and a test for G6PD deficiency. Chloroquine (Aralen) may precipitate anemia in those with G6PD deficiency; furthermore, it concentrates in the erythrocytes and leukocytes and may cause bone marrow depression. A baseline EKG should be taken because of potential cardiac complications associated with some antimalarial drugs. Other baseline information should include vital signs, especially temperature and blood pressure, and hearing and vision testing. All other medication taken by the patient also should be fully evaluated for compatibility with antimalarial medications, as drug-drug interactions are common.

During treatment, all vital signs should be closely monitored and periodic EKGs and CBCs should be obtained. The nurse should especially monitor for GI side effects such as vomiting, diarrhea, and abdominal pain; oral antimalarials can be given with food to reduce GI distress. The nurse should assess for signs of allergic reactions, such as flushing, rashes, edema, and pruritus. The nurse should monitor for signs of toxicity, which include ringing in the ears with quinine and severe cardiac complications and/or CNS complications such as seizures and blurred vision with chloroquine (Aralen).

Patient education as it relates to antimalarial drugs should include goals, reasons for obtaining baseline data, and possible side effects. The nurse should instruct the patient and caregivers to do the following:

Pr PROTOTYPE DRUG | CHLOROQUINE (Aralen)

ACTIONS AND USES

Developed to counter the high incidence of malaria among American soldiers in the Pacific Islands during World War II, chloroquine has been the prototype medication for treating malaria for over 60 years. It is effective in treating the erythrocytic stage, but has no activity against latent *Plasmodium*.

Chloroquine concentrates in the food vacuoles of *Plasmodium* residing in red blood cells. Once in the vacuole, it is believed to prevent the metabolism of heme, which then builds to toxic levels within the parasite.

Chloroquine can eliminate the high fever of patients in the acute stage in less than 48 hours. It also is used to prevent malaria by being administered 2 weeks before entering an endemic area and continuing 4 to 6 weeks after leaving. Although chloroquine is a drug of choice, many other agents are available, as resistance to chloroquine is common.

Administration Alerts

- Monitor pediatric dosage closely due to a child's susceptibility to overdose.
- If IM, inject into a deep muscle and aspirate prior to injecting medication because of its irritating effects to the tissues.
- Pregnancy category C.

ADVERSE EFFECTS AND INTERACTIONS

Chloroquine exhibits few serious side effects at low to moderate doses. Nausea and diarrhea may occur. At higher doses, CNS and cardiovascular toxicity may be observed. Symptoms include confusion, convulsions, reduced reflexes, hypotension, and dysrhythmias.

Chloroquine interacts with several drugs. For example, antacids and laxatives containing aluminum and magnesium can decrease chloroquine absorption and they must not be given within 4 hours of each other. Chloroquine may also interfere with the response to rabies vaccine.

 See the companion website for a Nursing Process Focus specific to this drug.

- Complete the full course of treatment.
- Take with food to decrease GI upset.
- Change position slowly to decrease postural hypotension.
- Use effective contraception measures to prevent pregnancy.
- Abstain from alcohol.
- Do not perform hazardous tasks until the effects of the drug are known.
- Report significant side effects such as flushing, rashes, edema, itching, ringing in the ears, blurred vision, or seizures.

33.8 Pharmacotherapy of Nonmalarial Protozoan Infections

Although infection by *Plasmodium* is the most significant protozoan disease worldwide, infections caused by other protozoans affect significant numbers of people in endemic areas. These infections include amebiasis, toxoplasmosis, giardiasis, cryptosporidiosis, trichomoniasis, trypanosomiasis, and leishmaniasis. Like *Plasmodium*, the nonmalarial protozoan infections occur more frequently in areas where public sanitation is poor and population density is high. Several of these infections occur in severely immunocompromised patients. Each of the organisms has unique differences in its distribution pattern and physiology. Descriptions of common nonmalarial protozoal infections are given in Table 33.5.

One such protozoan infection, amebiasis, affects over 50 million people and causes 100,000 deaths worldwide.

Caused by the protozoan *Entamoeba histolytica*, amebiasis is common in Africa, Latin America, and Asia. Although primarily a disease of the large intestine where it causes ulcers, *E. histolytica* can invade the liver and create abscesses. The primary symptom of amebiasis is amebic dysentery, a severe form of diarrhea. Drugs used to treat amebiasis include those that act directly on amebas in the intestine and those that are administered for their systemic effects on the liver and other organs. Drugs for nonmalarial protozoan infections are shown in Table 33.6.

NURSING CONSIDERATIONS

The role of the nurse in nonmalarial, antiprotozoan therapy involves careful monitoring of the patient's condition and providing education as it relates to the prescribed drug regimen. Prior to the initiation of drug therapy, the patient's health history should be taken. Antiprotozoan therapy is contraindicated in patients with blood dyscrasias, active organic disease of the CNS, and during the first month of pregnancy. These drugs are contraindicated in alcoholics; the medication is not administered until more than 24 hours after the patient's last drink of alcohol. It should be used cautiously in patients with peripheral neuropathy or preexisting liver disease. These drugs should be used cautiously in patients who have a history of bone marrow depression because of the possibility of leukopenia. Safety and efficacy have not been established in children.

Table 33.5	Nonmalarial Protozoan Infections
Name of Protozoan	**Description**
Cryptosporidium (various species)	cryptosporidiosis: primarily a disease of the intestines, often seen in immunocompromised patients
Entamoeba histolytica	amebiasis: primarily a disease of the large intestine that may cause liver abscesses; rarely travels to other organs such as the brain, lungs, or kidney
Giardia lamblia	giardiasis: primarily a disease of the intestines that may cause malabsorption, gas, and abdominal distension
Leishmania (various species)	leishmaniasis: affects various body systems including the skin, liver, spleen, or blood depending upon the species
Pneumocystis carinii	pneumocystosis: primarily causes pneumonia in immunocompromised patients
Toxoplasma gondii	toxoplasmosis: causes a fatal encephalitis in immunocompromised patients
Trichomonas vaginalis	trichomoniasis: causes inflammation of the vagina and urethra and is spread through sexual contact
Trypanosoma brucei	trypanosomiasis: the African form, known as sleeping sickness, causes CNS depression in severe infections; the American form, known as Chagas' disease, invades cardiac tissue

Table 33.6	Drugs for Nonmalarial Protozoan Infections
Drug	**Route and Adult Dose (max dose where indicated)**
eflornithine (Ornidyl)	Topical: apply bid for 2 mo
iodoquinol (Yodoxin)	PO; 630–650 mg tid for 20 d (max 2 g/d)
melarsoprol (Arsobal)	IV; 2.0–3.6 mg/kg for 3 days, then repeated on day 7 and days 10–21
ⓟ metronidazole (Flagyl)	PO; 250–750 mg tid
nifurtimox (Lampit)	PO; 2.0–2.5 mg/kg q6h
paromomycin (Humatin)	PO; 25–35 mg/kg divided in three doses for 5–10 days
pentamidine (Pentam 300, Nebupent)	IV; 4 mg/kg qd for 14–21 days; infuse over 60 min
Pentostam (sodium stibogluconate)	IM; 20 mg/kg/day
suramin (Germanin)	IV; 1 g on days 1, 3, 7, 14, and 21
tetracycline (Sumycin) and doxycycline (Vibramycin)	PO; 250–500 mg bid-qid (1–2 g/d) 250 mg IM: qd or 300 mg qd in two to three divided doses
trimetrexate (Neutrexin)	IV; 45 mg/m^2 qd

Initial lab work should include a CBC and thyroid and liver function tests. Baseline vital signs should be obtained. The nurse should evaluate all other drugs taken by the patient for compatibility with antiprotozoan drugs. The nurse should closely monitor vital signs and thyroid function during therapy, because serum iodine may increase and cause thyroid enlargement with iodoquinol (Yodoxin).

The nurse should especially monitor for GI distress; oral medications can be given with food to decrease unpleasant effects. Patients taking metronidazole (Flagyl) may complain of dryness of mouth and a metallic taste. The nurse should monitor for CNS toxicity such as seizures, paresthesia, nausea, and vomiting, and for allergic responses such as urticaria and pruritus.

Patient education as it relates to nonmalarial, antiprotozoan drug therapy should include goals, reasons for obtaining baseline data, and possible side effects. The nurse should instruct the patient and caregivers to do the following:

- Complete the full course of treatment.
- Take with food to decrease GI upset.
- Use effective contraception measures to prevent pregnancy.
- Avoid using hepatotoxic drugs including alcohol—may cause an disulfiram-like reaction.
- Recognize that urine may turn reddish-brown as an effect of the medication.
- Have concurrent treatment of a sexual partner to prevent reinfection.

Pr PROTOTYPE DRUG | METRONIDAZOLE (Flagyl)

ACTIONS AND USES

Metronidazole is the prototype drug for most forms of amebiasis, being effective against both the intestinal and hepatic stages of the disease. Resistant forms of *E. histolytica* have not been a clinical problem with metronidazole. The drug is unique among antiprotozoan drugs in that it also has antibiotic activity against anaerobic bacteria and thus is used to treat a number of respiratory, bone, skin, and CNS infections. Metronidazole is a drug of choice for two other protozoan infections: giardiasis from *Giardia lamblia* and trichomoniasis due to *Trichomonas vaginalis*. Topical forms of this agent are used to treat rosacea, a disease characterized by skin reddening and hyperplasia of the sebaceous glands, particularly around the nose and face. Metronidazole is pregnancy category B.

Administration Alerts

- Extended-release form must be swallowed whole.
- Contraindicated during the first trimester of pregnancy.

ADVERSE EFFECTS AND INTERACTIONS

The most common side effects of metronidazole are anorexia, nausea, diarrhea, dizziness, and headache. Dryness of the mouth and an unpleasant metallic taste may be experienced. Although side effects are relatively common, most are not serious enough to cause discontinuation of therapy.

Metronidazole interacts with several drugs. For example, oral anticoagulants potentiate hypoprothrombinemia. In combination with alcohol, metronidazole may elicit disulfiram reaction. This would include other medications that may contain alcohol. The drug also may elevate lithium levels.

Table 33.7	Drugs for Helminth Infections
Drug	**Route and Adult Dose (max dose where indicated)**
albendazole (Albenza)	PO; 400 mg bid with meals (max 800 mg/day)
bithionol (Bitin)	PO; 10 mg/kg for one dose
diethylcarbamazine (Hetrazan)	PO; 2–3 mg/kg tid
ivermectin (Stromectol)	PO; 150–200 µg/kg for one dose
Pr mebendazole (Vermox)	PO; 100 mg for one dose or 100 mg bid for 3 d
praziquantel (Biltricide)	PO; 5 mg/kg for one dose or 25 mg/kg tid
pyrantel (Antiminth)	PO; 11 mg/kg for one dose (max 1 g)

- Report significant side effects such as seizures, numbness in limbs, nausea, vomiting, hives, or itching.

DRUGS FOR HELMINTHIC INFECTIONS

Helminths consist of various species of parasitic worms which have more complex anatomy, physiology, and life cycles than the protozoans. Diseases due to these pathogens affect more than 2 billion people worldwide, and are quite common in areas lacking high standards of sanitation. Helminth infections in the United States and Canada are neither common nor fatal, although drug therapy may be indicated. Drugs for helminth infections are shown in Table 33.7.

33.9 Pharmacotherapy of Helminthic Infections

Helminths are classified as roundworms (nematodes), flukes (trematodes), or tapeworms (cestodes). The most common helminthic disease worldwide is caused by the roundworm *Ascaris lumbricoides*; however, infection by the pinworm *Ent-* *erobius vermicularis* is more common in the United States. Drugs used to treat these infections are called anthelmintics.

Like protozoans, helminths have several stages in their life cycles, which include immature and mature forms. Typically, the immature forms of helminths enter the body through the skin or the digestive tract. Most attach to the human intestinal tract, although some form cysts in skeletal muscle or in organs such as the liver.

Pharmacotherapy is not indicated for all helminthic infections, because the adult parasites often die without reinfecting the host. When the infestation is severe or complications occur, pharmacotherapy is initiated. Complications caused by extensive infestations may include physical obstruction in the intestine, malabsorption, increased risk for secondary bacterial infections, and severe fatigue. Pharmacotherapy is aimed at eradicating the parasites locally in the intestine and systemically in the tissues and organs they have invaded. Some anthelmintics are effective against multiple organisms, whereas others are specific for a certain species.

NURSING PROCESS FOCUS | **PATIENTS RECEIVING METRONIDAZOLE (FLAGYL)** Pr

ASSESSMENT

Prior to administration:
- Obtain complete health history including allergies, drug history, and possible drug interactions.
- Obtain results from serologic studies, stool samples or cultures of the suspected area of infection to determine the need for therapy.
- Obtain baseline vital signs, especially pulse and blood pressure.
- Obtain complete blood count.

POTENTIAL NURSING DIAGNOSES

- Risk for Injury, related to dizziness secondary to side effect of drug
- Risk for Fluid Volume Imbalance related to nausea and vomiting secondary to side effect of drug

PLANNING: PATIENT GOALS AND EXPECTED OUTCOMES

The patient will:
- Report decreased signs and symptoms amebic or other infection
- Demonstrate an understanding of the drug's action by accurately describing drug side effects and precautions
- Immediately report effects such as seizures, numbness in limbs, nausea, vomiting, hives, or itching

IMPLEMENTATION

Interventions and (Rationales)	*Patient Education/Discharge Planning*
■ Monitor complete blood count periodically. (The drug may cause leukopenia.)	■ Instruct patient to notify the healthcare provider of fever or other signs of infection.
■ Encourage treatment of sexual partner. (Asymptomatic trichomoniasis in the male is a frequent source of reinfection.)	■ Instruct patient that simultaneous treatment of a sexual partner is necessary.
■ Monitor use of alcohol. (Metronidazole interferes with the metabolism of alcohol.)	Instruct patient to: ■ Abstain from alcohol including any OTC medication that contains alcohol (liquid cough and cold products) ■ Report side effects such as cramping, vomiting, flushing, and headache which may result with alcohol use
■ Monitor CNS toxicity. (High doses may cause seizures and peripheral neuropathy possibly related to the medication's distribution into the CSF.)	■ Instruct patient to immediately report seizures, numbness of limbs, nausea, and vomiting.
■ Monitor for allergic reactions.	■ Instruct patient to immediately report hives and itching, rash, flushing, fever, and/or joint pain.
■ Monitor for gastrointestinal distress. (This is the most common adverse effect.)	Instruct patient to: ■ Take medication with food to decrease gastrointestinal distress ■ Recognize that medication may cause a metallic taste in the mouth

EVALUATION OF OUTCOME CRITERIA

Evaluate the effectiveness of drug therapy by confirming that patient goals and expected outcomes have been met (see "Planning").

NURSING CONSIDERATIONS

The role of the nurse in anthelmintic therapy involves careful monitoring of the patient's condition and providing education as it relates to the prescribed drug regimen. Prior to the initiation of drug therapy, the patient's health history should be taken. Anthelmintic therapy should be used cautiously in patients who are pregnant or lactating, have preexisiting liver disease, or are under the age of 2 years.

SPECIAL CONSIDERATIONS

Parasitic Infections in Children

Many parasitic infections are common among children with the national rates highest among children less than 5 years of age. In public health labs, the most commonly diagnosed intestinal parasite is giardiasis. These cases are usually associated with water-related activities such as swimming and possibly the presence of diapers.

Children adopted from Asian countries, central and South America, and Eastern Europe also have a high rate of parasitic infection. Up to 35% of foreign-born adopted children are reported to have *Giardia lamblia*. Environments in which these children have been living, particularly those from orphanages, often provide favorable conditions for infectious disease. The CDC recommends that internationally adopted children undergo examination of at least one stool sample, and three stool samples if GI symptoms are present. Unfortunately, evidence has shown that in communities where helminth infections are common, albeit in the United States or overseas, poor nutritional status, anemia, and impaired growth and learning in children result.

Initial lab tests should include a CBC and liver function studies. A stool specimen is obtained for verification and identification of the parasite and to determine the need for therapy. Other baseline information should include vital signs. The nurse should evaluate all other medications taken by the patient for compatibility with anthelmintic drugs.

The nurse should closely monitor lab results and vital signs during therapy. Cases of leukopenia, thrombocytopenia, and agranulocytosis have been associated with the use of albendazole (Albenza). Assessment of the patient's health habits and living conditions should be done, to locate and treat others that may be exposed to infestation and to identify means to prevent reinfestation.

SPECIAL CONSIDERATIONS

Lifestyle Issues Related to Parasitic Infections

Parasitic infections have long been associated with lifestyle. Sociologic barriers to control these parasites still exist. Conditions such as poverty, poor personal hygiene, and defecation practices contribute to high infection rates, reinfestations, and subsequent problems such as anemia. Medications are available for acute cases; but for long-term control, sanitation and education concerning hygiene practices are important for eradication of these infections. Nurses can help decrease these infections by thoroughly assessing the needs of patients and reinforcing proper hygiene practices.

The nurse should especially monitor for GI symptoms such as abdominal pain and distension, and diarrhea, because these symptoms may occur as worms die. Such side effects are likely to occur more frequently in patients with Crohn's disease and ulcerative colitis because of the inflammatory process in the intestine. The nurse must monitor for CNS side effects such as drowsiness with thiabendazole (Mintezol). Allergic responses include urticaria and pruritus.

Patient education as it relates to anthelmintic drug therapy should include goals, reasons for obtaining baseline data, and possible side effects. The nurse should instruct the patient and caregivers to do the following:

- Complete the full course of treatment.
- Use effective contraception measures to prevent pregnancy during therapy.
- Avoid hazardous activities until the effects of the drug are known.
- Have concurrent treatment of those having close contact with patient to prevent reinfestation.
- Report significant side effects such as itching and hives.

 PROTOTYPE DRUG | **MEBENDAZOLE (Vermox)**

ACTIONS AND USES

Mebendazole is used in the treatment of a wide range of helminth infections, including those caused by roundworm (*Ascaris*) and pinworm (*Enterobiasis*). As a broad-spectrum drug, it is particularly valuable in mixed helminth infections, which are common in areas having poor sanitation. It is effective against both the adult and larval stages of these parasites. It is poorly absorbed after oral administration, which allows it to retain high concentrations in the intestine. For pinworm infections, a single dose is usually sufficient; other infections require 3 days of therapy.

Administration Alerts

- Drug is most effective when chewed and taken with a fatty meal.
- Pregnancy category C.

ADVERSE EFFECTS AND INTERACTIONS

Because so little of the drug is absorbed, mebendazole does not generally cause serious systemic side effects. As the worms die, some abdominal pain, distension, and diarrhea may be experienced.

Carbamazepine and phenytoin can increase the metabolism of mebendazole.

NURSING PROCESS FOCUS | PATIENTS RECEIVING MEBENDAZOLE (VERMOX)

ASSESSMENT

Prior to administration:
- Obtain complete health history including allergies, drug history, and possible drug interactions.
- Obtain a stool specimen for verification of parasite and determine need for therapy.
- Obtain complete blood count.
- Assess the patient's living situation including number of individuals in close contact with the patient.

POTENTIAL NURSING DIAGNOSES

- Pain (abdominal pain), related to side effect of drug
- Risk for Deficient Fluid Volume, related to diarrhea secondary to drug therapy

PLANNING: PATIENT GOALS AND EXPECTED OUTCOMES

The patient will:
- Report decreased signs and symptoms of parasitic infection
- Demonstrate an understanding of the drug's action by accurately describing drug side effects and precautions
- Immediately report effects such as itching, hives, diarrhea, and fever

IMPLEMENTATION

Interventions and (Rationales)	*Patient Education/Discharge Planning*
Monitor stools (to assess effectiveness of drug therapy).	Instruct patient to bring stool sample to lab for testing.
Monitor for side effects.	Instruct patients to report transient abdominal pain, diarrhea, and fever.
Monitor complete blood count. (Thrombocytopenia, reversible neutropenia, and leukopenia may occur during therapy.)	Instruct patient to report any bleeding or signs of infection.
Monitor for pregnancy. (Even one dose of this medication during the first trimester has been shown to cause fetal damage.)	Instruct patient to: - Use effective birth control during drug therapy - Notify healthcare provider of any signs or suspicion of pregnancy
Monitor self-administration of medication, including chewing tablets or crushing and mixing with fatty foods. (Drug is most effective when taken with fatty foods, which increase absorption.)	Instruct patient that tablets can be chewed, swallowed, or crushed and mixed with food, especially fatty foods such as cheese or ice cream.
Evaluate health habits. (Lifestyle changes may be required to prevent the spread of infestation and prevent future infections.)	Instruct patient: - That all family members should be treated at the same time to prevent reinfestation - To wash all fruits and vegetables; cook meat thoroughly - To carefully wash hands with soap and water before and after eating and toileting - To wash toilet seats with disinfectants - To keep nails clean and out of mouth - To wear tight underwear and change daily - To sleep alone and wash bedding - That it is extremely important to complete the entire course of drug therapy

EVALUATION OF OUTCOME CRITERIA

Evaluate the effectiveness of drug therapy by confirming that patient goals and expected outcomes have been met (see "Planning").

CHAPTER REVIEW

Key Concepts

The numbered key concepts provide a succinct summary of the important points from the corresponding numbered section within the chapter. If any of these points are not clear, refer to the numbered section within the chapter for review. Expanded versions can be found on the companion website.

33.1 Fungi are more complex than bacteria and require special classes of drugs because they are unaffected by antibiotics.

33.2 Fungal infections are classified as either superficial, affecting hair, skin, nails, and mucous membranes, or systemic, affecting internal organs.

33.3 Antifungal medications act by disrupting aspects of growth or metabolism that are unique to these organisms.

33.4 Amphotericin B (Fungizone) is a drug of choice for serious fungal infections of internal organs. Systemic mycoses affect the internal organs and may require prolonged and aggressive drug therapy.

33.5 The azole drugs have become widely used in the pharmacotherapy of both systemic and superficial mycoses due to their favorable safety profile.

33.6 Antifungal drugs to treat superficial mycoses may be given topically or orally. They are safe and effective in treating infections of the skin, nails, and mucous membranes.

33.7 Malaria is the most common protozoal disease and requires multidrug therapy due to the complicated life cycle of the parasite.

33.8 Treatment of non-*Plasmodium* protozoan disease generally requires a different set of medications than those used for malaria. Other common protozoal diseases which may be indications for pharmacotherapy include amebiasis, toxoplasmosis, giardiasis, cryptosporidiosis, trichomoniasis, trypanosomiasis, and leishmaniasis.

33.9 Helminths are parasitic worms that cause significant disease in certain regions of the world. The goals of pharmacotherapy are to kill the parasites locally and to disrupt their life cycles.

Review Questions

1. Explain how antibacterial pharmacotherapy differs from antifungal and antiparasitic drug therapy.

2. How do most patients in the United States and Canada acquire protozoan infections?

3. Why is knowledge of a parasite's life cycle important to selecting the proper medication?

Critical Thinking Questions

1. A nurse is caring for a severely immunosuppressed patient who is on IV amphotericin B (Fungizone). The nurse understands that this medication is highly toxic to the patient. What are three priority nursing assessment areas for patients on this medication?

2. A young female patient has been given a prescription for metronidazole (Flagyl) for a vaginal yeast infection. What is a priority of teaching for this patient?

3. A patient is traveling to Africa for 3 months and is requesting a prescription for chloroquine (Aralen) to prevent malaria. What premedication assessment must be done for this patient?

 EXPLORE MediaLink

NCLEX review, case studies, and other interactive resources for this chapter can be found on the companion website at www.prenhall.com/adams. Click on "Chapter 33" to select the activities for this chapter. For animations, more NCLEX review questions, and an audio glossary, access the accompanying CD-ROM in this textbook.

CHAPTER 34

Drugs for Viral Infections

DRUGS AT A GLANCE

AGENTS FOR HIV-AIDS

Nucleoside and nucleotide reverse transcriptase inhibitors

Pr *zidovudine (Retrovir, AZT)*

Nonnucleoside reverse transcriptase inhibitors

Pr *nevirapine (Viramune)*

Protease inhibitors

Pr *saquinavir mesylate (Fortovase, Invirase)*

Fusion inhibitors

AGENTS FOR HERPESVIRUSES

Pr *acyclovir (Zovirax)*

AGENTS FOR INFLUENZA

AGENTS FOR HEPATITIS

Interferons

Noninterferons

metabolized and eliminated by the bod
of this process
PHARMACOLOGY
1. The study of medicines; the discipli
pertaining to how drugs improve the he
of the human body
PHARMACOPELA

MediaLink   www.prenhall.com/adams

CD-ROM

Animation:

   Mechanism in Action: Zidovudine (Retrovir, AZT)

Audio Glossary

NCLEX Review

Companion Website

NCLEX Review

Dosage Calculations

Case Study

Care Plans

Expanded Key Concepts

acquired immune deficiency syndrome (AIDS) *page 484*

antiretroviral *page 484*

capsid *page 483*

CD4 receptor *page 484*

hepatitis *page 493*

highly active antiretroviral therapy (HAART) *page 485*

HIV-AIDS *page 484*

influenza *page 493*

intracellular parasite *page 484*

latent phase (of HIV infection) *page 485*

pegylation *page 495*

protease *page 484*

reverse transcriptase *page 484*

virion *page 483*

virus *page 483*

OBJECTIVES

After reading this chapter, the student should be able to:

1. Describe the structural components of viruses.
2. Identify viral diseases that may benefit from pharmacotherapy.
3. Explain the purpose and expected outcomes of HIV pharmacotherapy.
4. Explain the advantages of HAART in the pharmacotherapy of HIV infection.
5. Describe the nurse's role in the pharmacologic management of patients receiving antiretroviral and antiviral drugs.

6. For each of the classes listed in Drugs at a Glance, know representative drugs, explain the mechanism of drug action, primary actions, and important adverse effects.
7. Categorize drugs used in the treatment of viral infections based on their classification and mechanism of action.
8. Use the Nursing Process to care for patients receiving drug therapy for viral infections.

Viruses are the smallest agents capable of causing infectious disease in humans and other organisms. After infecting an organism, viruses use host enzymes and cellular structures to replicate. Although the number of antiviral drugs has increased dramatically in recent years due to research into the AIDS epidemic, antivirals remain the least effective of all the anti-infective drug classes.

PHARMFACTS   Viral Diseases

- Approximately 85% of adults have serologic evidence of infections by HSV-1.
- About 45 million Americans are infected with genital herpes— 1 of every 5 of the total adolescent and adult population.
- Genital herpes is more common in women than in men, and in blacks over other ethnic groups.
- About 900,000 Americans are currently living with HIV infections, with about 40,000 new infections occurring each year.
- Roughly 70% of new HIV infections occur in men, with the largest risk category being men who have sex with other men.
- Of the new HIV infections in women, 75% are acquired through heterosexual contact.
- Since the beginning of the AIDS epidemic, over 450,000 Americans have died of this disease.

34.1 Characteristics of Viruses

Viruses are nonliving agents that infect bacteria, plants, and animals. Viruses contain none of the cellular organelles necessary for self-survival that are present in living organisms. In fact, the structure of viruses is quite primitive, compared to even the simplest cell. Surrounded by a protein coat or capsid, a virus possesses only a few dozen genes, either in the form of ribonucleic acid (RNA) or deoxyribonucleic acid (DNA), that contain the necessary information needed for viral replication. Some viruses also have a lipid envelope surrounding them. A mature infective particle is called a virion. Figure 34.1 shows the basic structure of the human immunodeficiency virus (HIV).

Although nonliving and structurally simple, viruses are capable of remarkable feats. They infect their host by entering a target cell and then using the machinery inside that

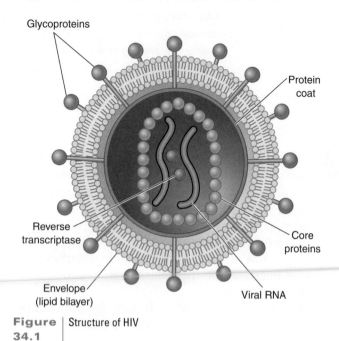

Glycoproteins

Protein coat

Reverse transcriptase

Core proteins

Envelope (lipid bilayer)

Viral RNA

Figure 34.1 | Structure of HIV

cell to replicate. Thus, viruses are intracellular parasites: They must be inside a host cell to cause infection. The viral host is often very specific; it may be a single species of plant, bacteria, or animal or even a single type of cell within that species. Most often viruses infect only one species, although cases have been documented where viruses can mutate and cross species, as is likely the case for HIV.

Many viral infections, such as the rhinoviruses that cause the common cold, are self-limiting and require no medical intervention. Although symptoms may be annoying, the virus disappears in 7 to 10 days and causes no permanent effects, if the patient is otherwise healthy. Others, such as HIV and the hepatitis virus, can result in serious and even fatal consequences and require aggressive drug therapy. Antiviral pharmacotherapy can be extremely challenging due to the rapid mutation rate of viruses, which can quickly render drugs ineffective. Also complicating therapy is the intracellular nature of the virus, which makes it difficult for drugs to find their targets without giving excessively high doses that injure normal cells. Antiviral drugs have narrow spectrums of activity, usually limited to one specific virus.

HIV-AIDS

Acquired immune deficiency syndrome (AIDS) is characterized by profound immunosuppression that leads to opportunistic infections and malignancies not commonly found in patients with functioning immune defenses. Antiretroviral drugs for HIV-AIDS slow the growth of HIV by several different mechanisms. Resistance to these drugs is a major clinical problem and a pharmacologic cure for HIV-AIDS is not yet achievable.

34.2 Replication of HIV

Infection with HIV occurs by exposure to contaminated body fluids, most commonly blood or semen. Transmission may occur through sexual activity (oral, anal, or vaginal) or through contact of infected fluids with broken skin, mucous membranes, or needle sticks. Newborns can receive the virus during birth or from breastfeeding.

Shortly after entry into the body, the virus attaches to its preferred target—the CD4 receptor on T4 (helper) lymphocytes. After entering the host cell, HIV converts its RNA strands to DNA, using the viral enzyme reverse transcriptase. The viral DNA enters the nucleus of the T4 lymphocyte where it becomes incorporated into the host's DNA. It may remain in the host's DNA for many years before it becomes activated to begin producing more viral particles. The new virions eventually bud from the host cell and enter the bloodstream. As a final step, the viral enzyme protease cleaves some of the proteins associated with the HIV DNA, enabling it to infect other T4 lymphocytes. Knowledge of the replication cycle of HIV is critical to understanding the pharmacotherapy of HIV-AIDS, as shown in Figure 34.2.

Only a few viruses such as HIV are able to construct DNA from RNA using reverse transcriptase; no bacteria, plants, or animals are able to perform this unique metabolic function. All living organisms make RNA from DNA. Because of their "backward" or reverse synthesis, these viruses are called retroviruses and drugs used to treat HIV infections are called antiretrovirals.

34.3 General Principles of HIV Pharmacotherapy

The widespread appearance of HIV infection in 1981 created enormous challenges for public health and an unprecedented need for the development of new antiviral drugs. HIV-AIDS is unlike any other infectious disease because it is sexually transmitted, uniformly fatal, and demands a continuous supply of new drugs for patient survival. The challenges of HIV-AIDS have resulted in the development of over 18 new antiretroviral drugs, and many others are in various stages of clinical trials. Unfortunately, the initial hopes of curing HIV-AIDS through antiretroviral therapy or vaccines have not been realized; none of these drugs produce a cure for this disease. HIV mutates extremely rapidly and resistant strains develop so quickly that the creation of novel approaches to antiretroviral drug therapy must remain an ongoing process.

While pharmacotherapy for HIV-AIDS has not produced a cure, it has resulted in a number of therapeutic successes. For example, many patients with HIV infection are able to live symptom-free lives with their disease for a much longer time due to medications. Furthermore, the transmission of the virus from an HIV-infected mother to her newborn has been reduced dramatically due to intensive drug therapy of the mother prior to delivery, and of the baby immediately following birth. These two factors have

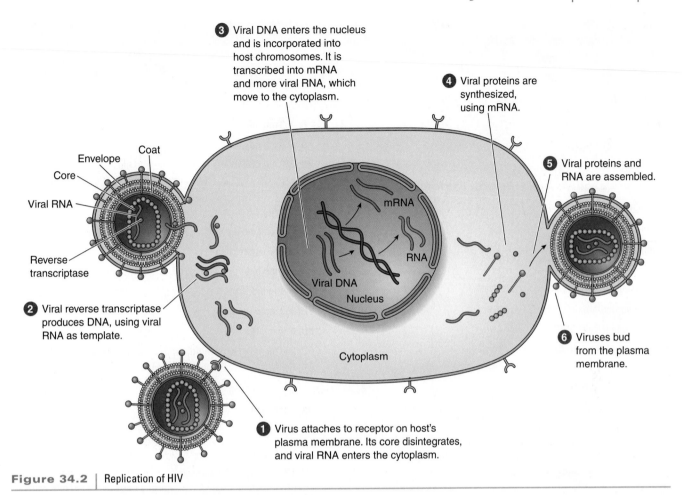

Figure 34.2 | Replication of HIV

resulted in a significant decline in the death rate due to HIV-AIDS in the United States. Unfortunately, this decline has not been observed in African countries, where antiviral drugs are not as readily available, largely due to their high cost.

After HIV incorporates its viral DNA into the nucleus of the T4 lymphocyte, it may remain dormant for several months to many years. During this latent phase, patients are asymptomatic and may not even realize they are infected. Once diagnosis is established, a decision must be made as to when to begin pharmacotherapy. The advantage of beginning during the asymptomatic, chronic stage is that the viral load or burden can be reduced. Presumably, early treatment will delay the onset of acute symptoms and the development of AIDS.

Unfortunately, the decision to begin treatment during the chronic phase has many negative consequences. Drugs for HIV-AIDS are expensive; treatment with some of the newer agents costs more than $20,000 per year. These drugs produce a number of uncomfortable and potentially serious side effects. Therapy over many years promotes viral resistance; when the acute stage eventually develops, the drugs may no longer be effective.

The decision to begin therapy during the acute phase is a much easier decision, because the severe symptoms of

AIDS can rapidly lead to death. Thus, therapy is nearly always initiated during this phase.

The therapeutic goals for the pharmacotherapy of HIV-AIDS include the following:

- Evidence of reduction of HIV in the blood
- Increased lifespan
- Higher quality of life

Two laboratory tests used to guide pharmacotherapy are absolute CD4 lymphocyte count and measurement of the amount of HIV RNA in the plasma. The number of CD4 lymphocytes is an important indicator of immune function and predicts the likelihood of opportunistic disease; however, it does not indicate how rapidly HIV is replicating. HIV RNA counts are a better indicator of viral load. These tests are performed every 3 to 6 months to assess the degree of success of drug therapy.

34.4 Classification of Drugs for HIV-AIDS

Antiretroviral drugs block phases of the HIV replication cycle. The standard pharmacotherapy for HIV-AIDS includes aggressive treatment with as many as four drugs concurrently, a regimen called highly active antiretroviral

Table 34.1 Antiretroviral Drugs for HIV-AIDS

Drug	Route and Adult Dose (max dose where indicated)
Nonnucleoside Reverse Transcriptase Inhibitors	
delavirdine (Rescriptor)	PO; 400 mg tid
efavirenz (Sustiva)	PO; 600 mg qd
Pr nevirapine (Viramune)	PO; 200 mg qd for 14d, then increase to bid
Nucleoside and Nucleotide Reverse Transcriptase Inhibitors	
abacavir (Ziagen)	PO; 300 mg bid
didanosine (Videx, DDI)	PO; 125–300 mg bid
emtricitabine (Emtriva)	PO; 200 mg once daily
lamivudine (Epivir, 3TC)	PO; 150 mg bid
stavudine (Zerit, D4T)	PO; 40 mg bid
tenofovir disoproxil fumarate (Viread)	PO; 300 mg once daily
zalcitabine (Hivid, DDC)	PO; 0.75 mg tid
Pr zidovudine (Retrovir, AZT)	PO; 200 mg q4h (1,200 mg/d), after 1 mo may reduce to 100 mg q4h (600 mg/d); IV; 1–2 mg/kg q4h (1,200 mg/d)
Protease Inhibitors	
amprenavir (Agenerase)	PO; 1,200 mg bid
atazanavir (Reyataz)	PO; 400 mg qd
indinavir (Crixivan)	PO; 800 mg tid
lopinavir/ritonavir (Kaletra)	PO; 400/100 mg (three capsules or 5 ml suspension) bid increase dose to 533/133 mg (four capsules or 6.5 ml) bid, with concurrent efavirenz or nevirapine
nelfinavir (Viracept)	PO; 750 mg tid
ritonavir (Norvir)	PO; 600 mg bid
Pr saquinavir (Invirase, Fortovase)	PO; 600 mg tid
Fusion Inhibitor	
enfuvtiride (Fuzeon)	SC; 90 mg bid

therapy (HAART). The goal of HAART is to reduce the plasma HIV RNA to its lowest possible level. It must be understood, however, that HIV is harbored in locations other than the blood, such as lymph nodes; therefore, elimination of the virus from the blood is not a cure. The simultaneous use of drugs from several classes also reduces the probability that a virus will become resistant to treatment. These drugs are shown in Table 34.1.

HIV-AIDS antiretrovirals are classified into the following five groups, based on their mechanism of activity.

- Nucleoside reverse transcriptase inhibitor (NRTI)
- Nonnucleoside reverse transcriptase inhibitor (NNRTI)
- Protease inhibitor
- Nucleotide reverse transcriptase inhibitor (RTI)
- Fusion inhibitor

The last two classes include recently discovered agents that act by unique mechanisms. Tenofovir (Viread) is a nucleotide reverse transcriptase inhibitor that is structurally similar to adenosine monophosphate (AMP). After metabolism, tenofovir is incorporated into viral DNA in a manner similar to the NRTIs. Enfuvirtide (Fuzeon) blocks the fusion of the HIV virion to the CD4 receptor.

Reverse Transcriptase Inhibitors

Drugs in the reverse transcriptase inhibitor class are comprised of agents which are structurally similar to nucleosides, the building blocks of DNA. This class includes nonnucleoside reverse transcriptase inhibitors, which bind directly to the viral enzyme reverse transcriptase and inhibit its function, and nucleotide reverse transcriptase inhibitors.

34.5 Pharmacotherapy with Reverse Transcriptase Inhibitors

One of the early steps in HIV infection is the synthesis of viral DNA from the viral RNA inside the T4 lymphocyte. The enzyme performing this step is reverse transcriptase. Because reverse transcriptase is a viral enzyme not found in animal cells, selective inhibition of viral replication is possible.

As viral DNA is synthesized, building blocks known as nucleosides are required. The NRTIs chemically resemble naturally occurring nucleosides. As reverse transcriptase uses these NRTIs to build its DNA, however, the viral DNA chain is prevented from lengthening. The prematurely terminated chain prevents the viral DNA from being inserted into the host chromosome.

A second mechanism for inhibiting reverse transcriptase is to affect the enzyme's function. Drugs in the NNRTI class act by binding near the active site of the enzyme, causing a structural change in the enzyme molecule. This causes a direct inhibition of enzyme function.

Although there are differences in their pharmacokinetic and toxicity profiles, no single NRTI or NNRTI offers a significant therapeutic advantage over any other. Choice of agent depends on patient response and the experience of the healthcare provider. Because some of these drugs, such as zidovudine (Retrovir, AZT), have been used consistently for over 15 years, the potential for resistance must be considered when selecting the specific agent. The NRTIs and NNRTIs are nearly always used in multidrug combinations in HAART.

Protease Inhibitors

Drugs in the protease inhibitor class block the viral enzyme protease, which is responsible for the final assembly of the HIV virions.

34.6 Pharmacotherapy with Protease Inhibitors

Near the end of its replication cycle, HIV has assembled all the necessary molecular components for the creation of new virions. Using the metabolic machinery of the host cell, HIV RNA has been synthesized using the viral DNA that was incorporated into the host's genome. The structural and regulatory proteins of HIV have been synthesized, using this viral RNA as a template.

As the newly formed virions bud from the host cell and are released into the surrounding extracellular fluid, one final step remains before the HIV is mature: a long polypeptide chain must be cleaved to produce the final HIV proteins. The enzyme performing this step is HIV protease.

The protease inhibitors attach to the active site of the HIV protease enzyme and prevent the final maturation of the virions. When combined with other antiretroviral drug classes, the protease inhibitors are capable of lowering plasma HIV RNA levels to below the detectable range. The protease inhibitors are metabolized in the liver and have the potential to interact with many different drugs. In general, they are well tolerated, with GI complaints being the most common side effects. Various lipid abnormalities, or lipodystrophies, have been reported including elevated cholesterol and triglyceride levels, and abdominal obesity.

Of the six available protease inhibitors, all have equivalent efficacy and a similar range of adverse effects. Choice of protease inhibitor is generally based on clinical response and the experience of the healthcare provider. Cross-resistance among the various protease inhibitors has been reported.

NURSING CONSIDERATIONS

The following material provides a discussion of NRTIs, NNRTIs, and protease inhibitors. Because antiretrovirals are commonly prescribed for HIV infection, a Nursing Process Focus has been provided for them. See page 491 later in this section.

Although NRTI, NNRTI, and protease inhibitors act by different mechanisms, the associated nursing care is similar. The role of the nurse involves careful monitoring of a patient's condition and providing education as it relates to the prescribed drug regimen. The nurse is instrumental in providing patient education, and psychosocial support will be crucial. Patients will experience tremendous emotional distress at various times during treatment. Denial and anger may be evident in the patient's behavior as they attempt to cope with their diagnosis.

The nurse should assess the patient's understanding of the HIV disease process. Although drug therapies may slow the progression of the virus, they are not a cure. Prior to the administration of antiretroviral drugs, the nurse should assess for symptoms of HIV and for any opportunistic infections. The nurse should also monitor plasma HIV RNA (viral load) assays, CD4 counts, complete blood count, liver and renal profiles, and blood glucose levels.

SPECIAL CONSIDERATIONS

Psychosocial Issues with Antiretroviral Drug Compliance

One key concern for success of an antiretroviral regimen is patient compliance to the prescribed medication plan. Drug compliance is difficult for most people once they feel well; patients may not feel sick while taking the medications and be more prone to skip doses for various reasons. Many factors can enhance the probability that the patient will adhere to treatment. For example, a multidisciplinary assessment can screen patients for depression, alcohol or drug abuse, or negative attitudes with interventions initiated to minimize the impact on compliance. Education at an appropriate level is essential so the patient can understand the disease process as well as the role the medications play in securing a positive outcome. Developing trust and open communication between the patient and healthcare provider is essential to improve the chances of drug compliance and to reach common therapeutic goals.

These diagnostic values will determine the effectiveness as well as the toxicity of the drugs employed.

The nurse should verify the drug combination to determine potential side effects and precautions. All antiretroviral agents are contraindicated during pregnancy and lactation. The list of diseases and conditions that necessitate close observation is quite extensive for the antiretrovirals. Typically, agents classified as NTRI should be used cautiously in patients with pancreatitis, peripheral vascular disease, neuropathy, kidney disorders, liver disorders, cardiac disease, and alcohol abuse. NNTRI agents necessitate judicious use in patients with liver impairment and CNS

diseases. Protease inhibitors are potentially problematic with patients suffering from sensitivity to sulfonamides, liver disorders, and renal insufficiency. It should be understood that in its acute stages, treatment of AIDS may proceed despite relative contraindications.

Some antiretroviral drugs vary in the way in which the drugs should be taken. For example, patients taking an NRTI drug should be instructed to take the medication on an empty stomach. These drugs should always be taken with water only and never with fruit juice, because acidic fruit juices interact with them. On the other hand, nevirapine (Viramune) and saquinavir mesylate (Invirase, Fortovase) should be taken

PROTOTYPE DRUG (NRTI) | ZIDOVUDINE (Retrovir, AZT)

ACTIONS AND USES

Zidovudine was first discovered in the 1960s and its antiviral activity was demonstrated prior to the AIDS epidemic. Structurally, it resembles thymidine, one of the four nucleoside building blocks of DNA. As the reverse transcriptase enzyme begins to synthesize viral DNA, it mistakenly uses zidovudine as one of the nucleosides, thus creating a defective DNA strand. Because of its widespread use since the beginning of the AIDS epidemic, resistant HIV strains are common. It is primarily used in combination with other antiretrovirals.

Administration Alerts

- Administer on an empty stomach, with water only.
- Avoid administering with fruit juice.
- Pregnancy category C.

ADVERSE EFFECTS AND INTERACTIONS

Zidovudine can result in severe toxicity to blood cells at high doses; anemia and neutropenia are common and may limit therapy. Many patients experience anorexia, nausea, and diarrhea. Patients may report fatigue and generalized weakness.

Zidovudine interacts with many drugs. Acetaminophen and ganciclovir may worsen bone marrow suppression. The following drugs may increase the risk of AZT toxicity: atovaquone, amphotericin B, aspirin, doxorubicin, fluconazole, methadone, and valproic acid. Other antiretroviral agents may cause lactic acidosis and severe hepatomegaly with steatosis.

Use with caution with herbal supplements, such as St. John's wort, which may cause a decrease in antiretroviral activity.

See the companion website for a Nursing Process Focus specific to this drug.

PROTOTYPE DRUG (NNRTI) | NEVIRAPINE (Viramune)

ACTIONS AND USES

Nevirapine is an NNRTI that binds directly to reverse transcriptase, disrupting the enzyme's active site. This inhibition prevents viral DNA from being synthesized from HIV RNA. It is readily absorbed following an oral dose. Since resistance develops rapidly when used as monotherapy, nevirapine is nearly always used in combination with other antivirals in treatment using HAART.

Administration Alerts

- Administer with food to minimize gastric distress.
- Pregnancy category C.

ADVERSE EFFECTS AND INTERACTIONS

Nevirapine increases the levels of metabolic enzymes in the liver; thus, it has the potential to interact with drugs handled by this organ. Therapy is sometimes contraindicated in patients with hepatic impairment. GI-related effects such as nausea, diarrhea, and abdominal pain are experienced by some patients. Skin rashes, fever, and fatigue are frequent side effects. Though rare, some patients acquire Stevens-Johnson syndrome, a sometimes fatal skin condition affecting mucous membranes and large areas of the body. Resistance can develop quite rapidly, which may extend to other NNRTIs.

Nevirapine interacts with several other drugs. For example, nevirapine may decrease plasma concentrations of protease inhibitors and oral contraceptives. It may also decrease methadone levels, inducing opiate withdrawal.

Use with caution with herbal supplements, such as St. John's wort, which may cause a decrease in antiretroviral activity.

See the companion website for a Nursing Process Focus specific to this drug.

Pr PROTOTYPE DRUG (Protease Inhibitor) | SAQUINAVIR MESYLATE (Fortovase, Invirase)

ACTIONS AND USES

Saquinavir was the first protease inhibitor approved by the FDA in 1995. By effectively inhibiting HIV protease, the final step in the assembly of an infectious HIV virion is prevented. The first formulation of saquinavir (Invirase) was a hard gelatin capsule that was poorly absorbed. The newer formulation of saquinavir (Fortovase) is a soft gelatin capsule that gives a significantly higher absorption rate, particularly when taken with a high-fat, high-calorie meal. Because of its short half-life, it is usually taken every 8 hours. Saquinavir is pregnancy category B.

Administration Alerts

- Administer with food to minimize gastric distress.
- Invirase and Fortovase are not equivalent and cannot be interchanged.

ADVERSE EFFECTS AND INTERACTIONS

Saquinavir is well tolerated by most patients. The most frequently reported problems are GI related, such as nausea, vomiting, dyspepsia, and diarrhea. General fatigue and headache are possible. Though not common, reductions in platelets and erythrocytes have been reported. Resistance to saquinavir may develop with continued use, and may include cross-resistance with other protease inhibitors.

Saquinavir interacts with several drugs, including rifampin and rifabutin, which significantly decrease saquinavir levels. Phenobarbital, phenytoin, and carbamazepine may also reduce saquinavir levels. Conversely, ketoconazole, and ritonavir may increase saquinavir levels.

Use with caution with herbal supplements such as St. John's wort which may cause a decrease in antiretroviral activity.

 See the companion website for a Nursing Process Focus specific to this drug.

NATURAL THERAPIES | Complementary and Alternative Medicine for HIV

With no cure and the available drugs producing numerous adverse effects, it is not surprising that many patients infected with HIV turn to complementary and alternative medicine (CAM). It is estimated that as many as 70% of HIV-AIDS patients use CAM during the course of their illness. Most patients use CAM in addition to antiretroviral therapy, to control serious side effects, combat weight loss, and boost their immune system. Relieving stress and depression are also common reasons for seeking CAM. The most common herbal products reported by HIV-AIDS patients are garlic, ginseng, Echinacea, and aloe. Unfortunately, few controlled studies have examined the safety or efficacy of CAM in HIV-AIDS patients.

The nurse should provide supportive education regarding the use of CAM. Although the use of these therapies should not be discouraged, patients must be strongly warned not use CAM in place of conventional medical treatment. In addition, some herbs such as St. John's wort can increase the hepatic metabolism of antiretrovirals, resulting in an increased or decreased effect. Garlic coadministered with saquinavir has been shown to greatly reduce plasma levels of the antiretroviral. The nurse should urge the patient to obtain CAM information from reliable sources and to always report the use of CAM therapies to the healthcare provider.

with food to minimize gastric distress. With all antiretroviral drugs it is critical that the patient be instructed to consult with the healthcare provider before taking any OTC medication or herbal supplement to avoid drug interactions.

Many of the side effects of antiretrovirals can dramatically influence activities of daily living. Some of these drugs may cause dizziness or other troublesome CNS effects.

When such side effects occur the patient may be instructed to take the medication just before sleep. The patient should also be advised not to drive or perform hazardous activities until reactions to the medication is known. Specific side effects depend on the drugs used. The nurse must be vigilant in assessing for side effects and assisting patients to manage their therapeutic regimen.

Patient education as it relates to antiretroviral drugs should include the goals, reasons for obtaining baseline data such as vital signs and tests for cardiac and renal disorders, and possible side effects. The nurse should instruct the patient to report adverse effects specific to the antiretroviral agent prescribed. For example, when teaching patients about NRTIs, the nurse should instruct the patient to report fever, skin rash, abdominal pain, nausea, vomiting, numbness, or burning of feet or hands. When teaching patients receiving NNRTIs, the nurse should instruct the patient to report fever, chills, rash, blistering of skin, reddening of the skin, muscle pain, or joint pain to the healthcare provider. Patients taking protease inhibitors should report rash, abdominal pain, headache, insomnia, fever, constipation, cough, fainting, and visual changes.

The role of the nurse in teaching the patient taking antiretroviral agents is critical and may enhance the quality of life of the individual. Because these patients are highly susceptible to infections, it is critical that the nurse describe the symptoms of infections such as fever, chills, sore throat, and cough, and the importance of immediately seeking medical care should these signs develop. Additionally, the patient should be taught methods to minimize exposure to infection. Frequent handwashing, as well as avoiding crowds and people with colds, flu, and other infections, will greatly reduce the patient's likelihood of becoming infected. The patient should also be instructed to take additional measures to reduce microbial infections such as increasing oral fluid intake,

NURSING PROCESS FOCUS   PATIENTS RECEIVING ANTIRETROVIRAL AGENTS

ASSESSMENT	POTENTIAL NURSING DIAGNOSES

Prior to administration:
 ■ Obtain complete health history including allergies, drug history, and possible drug interactions.
 ■ Obtain complete physical examination.
 ■ Assess for the presence/history of HIV infection.
 ■ Obtain the following laboratory studies:
   ■ HIV RNA assay / CD4 count
   ■ Complete blood count (CBC)
   ■ Liver function
   ■ Renal function
   ■ Blood glucose
	■ Risk for Infection, related to compromised immune system
	 ■ Decisional Conflict, related to therapeutic regimen
	 ■ Fear, related to HIV diagnosis
	 ■ Risk for Injury, related to side effects of drugs
	 ■ Deficient Knowledge, related to disease process, transmission, and drug therapy

PLANNING: PATIENT GOALS AND EXPECTED OUTCOMES

The patient will:
- Exhibit a decrease in viral load and an increase in CD4 counts
- Demonstrate knowledge of disease process, transmission, and treatment
- Identify side effects and report to healthcare provider
- Complete full course of therapy and comply with follow-up care

IMPLEMENTATION

Interventions and (Rationales)	Patient Education/Discharge Planning
■ Monitor for symptoms of hypersensitivity reactions. (Zalcitabine may cause anaphylactic reaction.)	■ Instruct patient to discontinue the medication and inform healthcare provider if symptoms of hypersensitivity reaction develop such as wheezing; shortness of breath; swelling of face, tongue, or hands; itching or rash.
■ Monitor vital signs, especially temperature, and for symptoms of infection. Monitor white blood cell count. (Antiretroviral drugs such as delavirdine may cause neutropenia.)	Instruct patient: ■ To report symptoms of infections such as fever, chills, sore throat, and cough ■ On methods to minimize exposure to infection such as frequent handwashing; avoiding crowds and people with colds, flu, and other infections; limiting exposure to children and animals; increasing fluid intake; emptying bladder frequently; and coughing and deep breathing several times per day
■ Monitor patient for signs of stomatitis. (Immunosuppression may result in the proliferation of oral bacteria.)	■ Advise patient to be alert for mouth ulcers and to report their appearance.
■ Monitor blood pressure. (Antiviral agents such as abacavir may cause significant decrease in blood pressure.)	Instruct patient to: ■ Rise slowly from lying or sitting position to minimize effects of postural hypotension. ■ Report changes in blood pressure
■ Monitor HIV RNA assay, CD4 counts, liver function, kidney function, complete blood count, blood glucose, and serum amylase and triglyceride levels. (These will determine effectiveness and toxicity of drug.)	Instruct patient: ■ On the purpose of required laboratory tests and scheduled follow-ups with healthcare provider ■ To monitor weight and presence of swelling ■ To keep all appointments for laboratory tests

NURSING PROCESS FOCUS: *Patients Receiving Antiretroviral Agents (continued)*

Interventions and (Rationales)	*Patient Education/Discharge Planning*
■ Determine potential drug-drug and drug-food interactions. (Antiretroviral medications have multiple drug-drug interactions and must be taken as prescribed.)	Instruct patient: ■ When to take the specific medication in relationship to food intake ■ About foods or beverages to avoid when taking medication some antiretrovirals should not be taken with acidic fruit juice ■ To take medication exactly as directed; do not skip any doses ■ To consult with healthcare provider before taking any OTC medications or herbal supplements
■ Monitor for symptoms of pancreatitis including severe abdominal pain, nausea, vomiting, and abdominal distention. (Antiretroviral agents such as didanosine may cause pancreatitis.)	■ Instruct patient to report the following immediately: Fever, severe abdominal pain, nausea/vomiting and abdominal distention
■ Monitor skin for rash; withhold medication and notify physician at first sign of rash. (Several antiretroviral drugs may cause Stevens-Johnson syndrome which may be fatal.)	■ Advise patient to check skin frequently and notify healthcare provider at first sign of any rash.
■ Establish therapeutic environment to ensure adequate rest, nutrition, hydration, and relaxation. (Support of the immune system is essential in HIV patients to minimize opportunistic infections.)	Teach patient to incorporate the following health-enhancing activities: ■ Adequate rest and sleep ■ Proper nutrition that provides essential vitamins and nutrients ■ Intake of six to eight glasses of water/day
■ Monitor blood glucose levels. (Antiretroviral drugs may cause hyperglycemia, especially in patients with type 1 diabetes.)	■ Instruct patient to report excessive thirst, hunger, and urination to healthcare provider. ■ Instruct diabetic patients to monitor blood glucose levels regularly.
■ Monitor for neurological side effects such as numbness and tingling of the extremities. (Many NRTI agents cause peripheral neuropathy.)	Instruct patient to: ■ Report numbness and tingling of extremities ■ Use caution when in contact with heat and cold due to possible peripheral neuropathy
■ Determine the effect of the prescribed antiretroviral agents on oral contraceptives. (Many agents reduce the effectiveness of oral contraceptives.)	■ Instruct patient to use an alternate form of birth control while taking antiretroviral medications.
■ Provide resources for medical and emotional support.	■ Advise patient on community resources and support groups.
■ Assess patient's knowledge level regarding use and effect of medication.	Advise patient: ■ That medication may decrease the level of HIV infection in the blood but will not prevent transmitting the disease ■ To use barrier protection during sexual activity ■ To avoid sharing needles ■ To not donate blood

EVALUATION OF OUTCOME CRITERIA

Evaluate the effectiveness of drug therapy by confirming that patient goals and expected outcomes have been met (see "Planning").

See Table 34.1 for a list of drugs to which these nursing actions apply.

emptying the bladder frequently, and coughing and deep breathing several times per day to expel invading organisms.

Nurses should also incorporate health promotional teaching to the patient receiving these drugs. Because patients on antiretroviral agents typically have impaired immune systems, the nurse should instruct them to engage in activities that support immune function. These activities include adequate rest and sleep, consuming a diet that provides essential vitamins and minerals, and drinking six to eight glasses of water per day.

Another important factor in health teaching with these patients focuses on disease transmission. The patient should be taught that antiretroviral agents may decrease the level of HIV infection in the blood but will not prevent the risk of transmission of the disease to other individuals. The nurse must discuss sensitive issues with the patient, including abstinence, the use of barrier protection devices such as condoms during sexual activity or the avoidance of sharing needles with other individuals. Open and honest dialogue will occur only if the nurse has developed a therapeutic rapport with the patient based on trust and acceptance. Additional teaching points are discussed in "Nursing Process Focus: Patients Receiving Antiretroviral Agents".

HERPES VIRUSES

Herpes simplex viruses (HSVs) are a family of DNA viruses that cause repeated, blisterlike lesions on the skin, genitals, and other mucosal surfaces. Antiviral drugs can lower the frequency of acute herpes episodes and diminish the intensity of acute disease. These drugs are shown in Table 34.2.

34.7 Pharmacotherapy of Herpesvirus Infections

Herpesviruses are usually acquired through direct physical contact with an infected person. Herpesviruses can also be transmitted from infected mothers to their newborns,

sometimes resulting in severe CNS disease. The herpesvirus family includes the following:

- HSV-type 1 primarily causes infections of the eye, mouth, and lips, although the incidence of genital infections is increasing
- HSV-type 2; genital infections
- cytomegalovirus (CMV); affects multiple body systems in immunosuppressed patients
- varicella-zoster virus (VZV); shingles (zoster) and chickenpox (varicella)
- Epstein-Barr virus (EBV); mononucleosis and a form of cancer known as Burkitt's lymphoma

Pharmacotherapy of initial HSV-1 and HSV-2 infections is usually accomplished through oral antiviral therapy for 7 to 10 days. Topical forms of several antivirals are available for local applications, though they are not as efficacious as the oral forms. In immunocompromised patients, IV acyclovir (Zovirax) may be indicated.

Following its initial entrance into the patient, HSV may remain in a latent, asymptomatic, nonreplicating state in ganglia for many years. Immunosuppression, physical challenges or emotional stress can promote active replication of the virus, and the characteristic lesions to reappear. Although recurrent herpes lesions are usually mild and often require no drug treatment, patients who experience frequent recurrences may benefit from low doses of prophylactic antiviral therapy. It should be noted that the antiviral drugs used to treat herpesviruses do not cure patients; the virus remains in them for their lifetime.

NURSING CONSIDERATIONS

The following material provides a discussion of the nursing considerations for patients receiving antiviral medications not associated with HIV infections.

The role of the nurse in antiviral therapy involves careful monitoring of a patient's condition and providing education as it relates to the prescribed drug regimen. Because

Table 34.2	Drugs for Herpesviruses
Drug	**Route and Adult Dose (max dose where indicated)**
acyclovir (Zovirax)	PO; 400 mg tid
cidofovir (Vistide)	IV; 5 mg/kg q week for 2 wk, then once q week
docosanol (Abreva)	Topical; 10% cream applied to cold sore up to five times/d for 10 d
famciclovir (Famvir)	PO; 500 mg tid for 7 d
foscarnet (Foscavir)	IV; 40–60 mg/kg infused over 1–2 h tid
ganciclovir (Cytovene)	IV; 5 mg/kg infused over 1 h bid
idoxuridine (Herplex)	Topical; one drop in each eye q1h during the day and q2h at night
penciclovir (Denavir)	Topical; apply q2h while awake for 4 d
trifluridine (Viroptic)	Topical; one drop in each eye q2h during waking hours (max nine drops/day)
valacyclovir (Valtrex)	PO; 1.0 g tid
vidarabine (Vira-A)	Topical; 0.5 inch of ointment to each eye q3h not to exceed five applications/d

many of these viral infections are systemic versus localized, the nurse should perform a complete physical assessment prior to drug administration. Once a baseline of assessment findings including vital signs, weight, and laboratory studies (CBC, viral cultures, liver and kidney function) is completed, the nurse should focus on the presenting symptoms of the viral infections. For patients with preexisting renal or hepatic disease, the drugs should be used with extreme caution. Although many antiviral medications are listed as pregnancy categories B or C, their judicious use is still warranted during pregnancy. Viruses that can be treated with antiviral drugs include herpes simplex, CMV infection, Epstein-Barr viral infection, varicella-zoster viral infection, respiratory syncytial viral infections, keratoconjunctivitis, and herpes zoster.

Depending on the specific antiviral drugs, these agents can be administered intravenously, orally, topically, and through inhalation. The nurse should instruct the patient in the proper administration techniques. Additionally, it is important that the nurse emphasize compliance with antiviral therapy such as taking the exact amount around the clock even if sleep is interrupted. Many antiviral drugs cause GI distress and should be taken with food. The nurse should also monitor the patient for side effects throughout the course of the treatment and assist the patient with managing antiviral drug-related problems. For example, because ganciclovir (Cytovene) may cause bone marrow suppression, patients should be monitored for anemia, thrombocytopenia, and neutropenia. Because many antiviral drugs are nephrotoxic and hepatotoxic, the nurse should monitor the patient for dysfunction in the kidneys and liver.

Patient education as it relates to antiviral drugs should include goals, reasons for obtaining baseline data such as vital signs and tests for cardiac and renal disorders, and possible side effects. The nurse should teach the patient modes of transmission and methods to prevent spreading the disease and advise the patient that these drugs do not prevent transmission of the virus to other individuals.

Following are other important points the nurse should include when teaching patients regarding antiviral agents.

- Report the following symptoms immediately. Blood in urine, bruising, yellowing of the skin, fever, chills, confusion, nervousness, dizziness, nausea, and vomiting.
- Take the medications for the full course of therapy and continue taking the medication even if symptoms improve, until the full prescription has been taken.
- Keep all appointments for follow-up care.
- Take necessary safety precautions while taking these drugs, because some antivirals may cause dizziness and drowsiness.
- Do not drive or perform hazardous activities until the effects of the drug are known.
- Consult the healthcare provider before taking any OTC medications or herbal supplements because of potentially toxic drug-drug interactions.
- Apply topical preparations with an applicator or a glove, to prevent the spread of the virus to other areas.
- Do not apply any other types of creams, ointments, or lotions to the infected sites.

INFLUENZA

Influenza is a viral infection characterized by acute symptoms that include sore throat, sneezing, coughing, fever, and chills. The infectious viral particles are easily spread via airborne droplets. In immunosuppressed patients, an influenza infection may be fatal. In 1919, a worldwide outbreak of influenza killed approximately 20 million people. The RNA-containing influenza viruses should not be confused with *Haemophilus influenza*, which is a bacterium that causes respiratory disease.

34.8 Pharmacotherapy of Influenza

The best approach to influenza infection is prevention through annual vaccination. Those who benefit greatly from vaccinations include residents of long-term care facilities, those with chronic cardiopulmonary disease, pregnant women in their second or third trimester during the peak flu season, and healthy adults over age 50. Depending on the stage of the disease, HIV-positive patients usually benefit from vaccination. Adequate immunity is achieved about 2 weeks after vaccination, and lasts for several months up to a year. Additional details on vaccines are presented in Chapter 30 ∞.

Antivirals may be used to prevent influenza or decrease the severity of symptoms. The drug amantadine (Symmetrel) has been available to prevent and treat influenza for many years. Chemoprophylaxis with amantadine or rimantadine (Flumadine) is indicated for unvaccinated individuals, after a confirmed outbreak of influenza type A. Therapy with these antivirals is sometimes started concurrently with vaccination; the antiviral offers protection during the period before therapeutic antibody titers are achieved from the vaccine. These drugs are generally prescribed for patients who are at greatest risk to the severe complications of influenza. Antivirals for influenza are shown in Table 34.3.

A new class of drugs, the neuroaminidase inhibitors, was introduced in 1999 to treat active influenza infections. If given within 48 hours of the onset of symptoms, oseltamivir (Tamiflu) and zanamivir (Relenza) are reported to shorten the normal 7-day duration of influenza symptoms to 5 days. Oseltamivir is given orally, whereas zanamivir is inhaled. Because these agents produce only modest effects on an active infection, prevention through vaccination remains the best alternative.

HEPATITIS

Viral hepatitis is a common infection caused by a number of different viruses. Although each virus has its own unique clinical features, they all cause inflammation and necrosis of liver cells. Symptoms of hepatitis may be acute or chronic. Acute symptoms include fever, chills, fatigue, anorexia, nausea, and

Pr PROTOTYPE DRUG (Antiviral) — ACYCLOVIR (Zovirax)

ACTIONS AND USES

Approved in 1982 as one of the first antiviral drugs, the activity of acyclovir is limited to the herpesviruses, for which it is a drug of choice. It is most effective against HSV-1 and HSV-2 and effective only at high doses against CMV and varicella-zoster. Acyclovir acts by inhibiting the viral enzyme thymidine kinase, thus preventing viral DNA synthesis. Acyclovir decreases the duration and severity of herpes episodes. When given for prophylaxis, it may decrease the frequency of herpes appearance, but it does not cure the patient. It is available in topical form for placement directly on active lesions, in oral form for prophylaxis, and as an IV for particularly severe episodes. Because of its 2.5- to 5-hour half-life, acyclovir is sometimes administered orally up to five times a day.

Administration Alerts

- When given IV, the drug may cause painful inflammation of vessels at the site of infusion.
- Administer around the clock, even if sleep is interrupted.
- Administer with food.
- Pregnancy category C.

ADVERSE EFFECTS AND INTERACTIONS

There are few adverse effects to acyclovir when administered topically or orally. Because nephrotoxicity is possible when the medication is given IV, frequent laboratory tests may be performed to monitor kidney function. Resistance has developed to the drug, particularly in patients with HIV-AIDS.

Acyclovir interacts with several drugs. For example, probenecid decreases acyclovir elimination, and zidovudine may cause increased drowsiness and lethargy.

 See the companion website for a Nursing Process Focus specific to this drug.

Table 34.3	Drugs for Influenza
Drug	**Route and Adult Dose (max dose where indicated)**
Influenza Prophylaxis	
amantadine (Symmetrel)	PO; 100 mg bid
rimantadine (Flumadine)	PO; 100 mg bid
Influenza Treatment: Neuroaminidase Inhibitors	
oseltamivir (Tamiflu)	PO; 75 mg bid for 5 d
zanamivir (Relenza)	Inhalation; two inhalations for 5 d

vomiting. Chronic hepatitis may result in prolonged fatigue, jaundice, liver cirrhosis, and ultimately hepatic failure.

34.9 Pharmacotherapy of Hepatitis

Hepatitis A virus (HAV), sometimes called infectious hepatitis, is caused by an RNA virus. It is spread by the oral-fecal route primarily in regions of the world having poor sanitation. Hepatitis B virus (HBV), known as serum hepatitis, is caused by a DNA virus and is transmitted primarily through exposure to contaminated blood and body fluids. HBV has a much greater incidence of chronic hepatitis and a greater mortality rate than HAV. The hepatitis C, D, and E viruses are sometimes referred to as non A-non B viruses.

The best treatment for viral hepatitis is prevention through immunization, which is available for HAV and HBV. HAV vaccine is indicated for those living in communities or states with high infection rates, or for travelers to countries with high endemic HAV infection rates. Immune globulin, a concentrated solution of antibodies, is sometimes administered to close personal contacts of infected patients to prevent transmission of HAV. The immunoglobulins induce passive protection and provide prophylaxis for about 3 months.

Traditionally, HBV vaccine has been indicated for healthcare workers and others who are routinely exposed to blood and body fluids. Because this vaccination protocol failed to address hepatitis B in early childhood, it is now recommended that universal vaccination of all children be conducted. Postexposure treatment of hepatitis B may include hepatitis B immunoglobulins and an antiviral agent such as interferon alpha-2a (Roferon-A) or lamivudine (Epivir). Adefovir (Hepsera) is a recently approved therapy for chronic hepatitis B infections. Following metabolism, adefovir is incorporated into the growing viral DNA chain, causing it to terminate prematurely.

Most patients recover completely from HAV and HBV infection without drug therapy, though complete recovery may take many months. The overall mortality rate is less than 1%. Neonates and immunocompromised patients are at higher risk to developing chronic hepatitis.

Transmitted primarily through exposure to infected blood or body fluid, hepatitis C virus (HCV) is more common than HBV. Up to 50% of all HIV-AIDS patients are coinfected with HCV. A large percentage of patients infected with HCV proceed to chronic hepatitis; HCV is the most common cause of liver transplants. A specific vaccine is not available for hepatitis C. Current pharmacotherapy for chronic HCV infection includes treatment with Rebetron, a combination agent consisting of interferon alpha-2b (Intron A) and ribavirin (Rebetol). After 24 weeks of treatment with Rebetron, about 30% to 50% of patients will respond with increased liver function. If response is not attained, therapy may continue for as long as 12 to 18 months. Peginterferon alfa-2a (Pegasys) and peginterferon alfa-2b (PEG-Intron) are recently approved therapies for chronic hepatitis C. Pegylation is a process that attaches polyethylene glycol (PEG) to the interferon to extend its pharmacologic activity. This permits the interferon to remain in the body longer and exert prolonged activity. Agents for hepatitis are shown in Table 34.4.

Table 34.4	Drugs for Hepatitis
Drug	**Route and Adult Dose (max dose where indicated)**
Interferons	
interferon alfacon-1 (Infergen)	SC; 9 μg three times/wk for 24 wk
interferon alfa-n1 (Wellferon)	SC/IM; 3 MU three times/wk for 48 wk
interferon alfa-2b (Intron A) (see page 410 for the Prototype Drug box) ∞	IM/SC; 2 million U/m² three times/wk
peginterferon alfa-2a (Pegasys)	SC; 180 μg once weekly for 48 wk
peginterferon alfa-2b (PEG-Intron)	SC; 1 μg/kg/wk for monotherapy; 1.5 g/kg/wk when given with ribavirin
Noninterferons/Combinations	
adefovir dipivoxil (Hepsera)	PO; 10 mg qd
lamivudine (Epivir HBV)	PO; 150 mg bid
ribavirin/interferon alpha-2b (Rebetron/Introl A)	Adults more than 75 kg: Rebeton PO: 3 × 200 mg capsules in the a.m. and 3 × 200 mg capsules in the p.m. Intron A SC: 3 million IU three times/wk

CHAPTER REVIEW

Key Concepts

The numbered key concepts provide a succinct summary of the important points from the corresponding numbered section within the chapter. If any of these points are not clear, refer to the numbered section within the chapter for review. Expanded versions can be found on the companion website.

34.1 Viruses are nonliving intracellular parasites that require host machinery to replicate.

34.2 HIV attacks the T4 lymphocyte, using reverse transcriptase to make viral DNA.

34.3 Antiretroviral drugs used in the treatment of HIV-AIDS do not cure the disease but they do help many patients to live longer. Pharmacotherapy may be initiated in the acute (symptomatic) or chronic (asymptomatic) phase of HIV infection.

34.4 Drugs from five drug classes are combined in the pharmacotherapy of HIV-AIDS. The nucleotide reverse transcriptase inhibitors and the fusion inhibitors have been recently discovered.

34.5 The reverse transcriptase inhibitors block HIV replication at the level of the reverse transcriptase enzyme.

34.6 The protease inhibitors inhibit the final assembly of the HIV virion.

34.7 Pharmacotherapy can lessen the severity of acute herpes simplex infections and prolong the latent period of the disease.

34.8 Drugs are available to prevent and to treat influenza infections. Vaccination is the best choice, as drugs are relatively ineffective once symptoms appear.

34.9 Hepatitis A and B are best treated through immunization. Newer drugs for HBV and HBC have led to therapies for chronic hepatitis.

Review Questions

1. What is the advantage to using combinations of agents to treat HIV infection?

2. Is it better to treat HIV before or after acute symptoms occur? What are the advantages and disadvantages of each?

3. From a pharmacologic perspective, explain why is it better to prevent influenza than to treat it.

4. What are the therapeutic goals for the pharmacotherapy of patients with HAV or HBV?

Critical Thinking Questions

1. The patient is a 72-year-old female who lives in an assisted living community. The home health nurse advises the patient of the necessity to receive an amantadine (Symmetrel) injection. What is the rationale supporting this recommendation? How could the nurse assist the patient to comply with this recommendation?

2. A newly diagnosed HIV-positive patient has been put on zidovudine (Retrovir). What is a priority for the nurse to monitor in this patient?

3. A healthcare provider has ordered acyclovir (Zovirax) as an IV bolus to infuse over 15 minutes. The patient is seriously ill with a systemic herpesvirus infection and the healthcare provider wants the patient to have immediate access to the medication. What is the nurse's response?

 ## EXPLORE MediaLink

NCLEX review, case studies, and other interactive resources for this chapter can be found on the companion website at www.prenhall.com/adams. Click on "Chapter 34" to select the activities for this chapter. For animations, more NCLEX review questions, and an audio glossary, access the accompanying CD-ROM in this textbook.

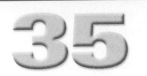

CHAPTER 35

Drugs for Neoplasia

DRUGS AT A GLANCE

ALKYLATING AGENTS
Nitrogen mustards
Pr *cyclophosphamide (Cytoxan)*
Nitrosoureas
Miscellaneous alkylating agents

ANTIMETABOLITES
Folic acid antagonist
Pr *methotrexate (Folex, Mexate, others)*
Pyrimidine analogs
Purine analogs

ANTITUMOR ANTIBIOTICS
Pr *doxorubicin (Adriamycin)*

NATURAL PRODUCTS
Vinca alkaloids
Pr *vincristine (Oncovin)*

Taxoids
Topoisomerase inhibitors

HORMONE AND HORMONE INHIBITORS
Adrenocorticoids
Androgens and androgen antagonists
Estrogens and estrogen antagonists
Pr *Tamoxifen (Nolvadex)*
Progestins
Other hormone agents

MISCELLANEOUS ANTINEOPLASTICS
Biologic response modifiers
Other anticancer drugs

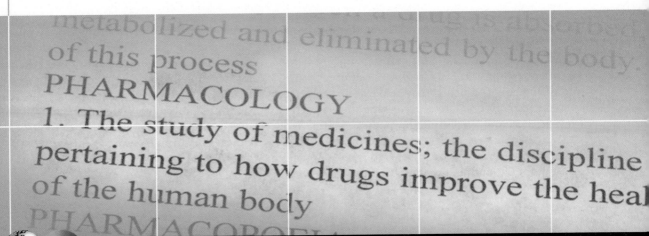

MediaLink www.prenhall.com/adams

CD-ROM
Animation:
Mechanism in Action: Methotrexate (Folex, Mexate, others)
Audio Glossary
NCLEX Review

Companion Website
NCLEX Review
Dosage Calculations
Case Study
Care Plans
Expanded Key Concepts

OBJECTIVES

After reading this chapter, the student should be able to:

1. Explain differences between normal cells and cancer cells.
2. Identify primary causes of cancer.
3. Describe lifestyle factors associated with a reduced risk of acquiring cancer.
4. Identify the three primary therapies for cancer.
5. Explain the significance of growth fraction and the cell cycle to the success of chemotherapy.
6. Describe the nurse's role in the pharmacologic management of cancer.
7. Explain how combination therapy and special dosing protocols increase the effectiveness of chemotherapy.
8. List the general adverse effects of chemotherapeutic agents.
9. For each of the drug classes listed in Drugs at a Glance, know representative drugs, explain their mechanism of drug action, primary actions, and important adverse effects.
10. Categorize anticancer drugs based on their classification and mechanism of action.
11. Use the Nursing Process to care for patients who are receiving antineoplastic medications as part of their treatment of cancer.

ancer is one of the most feared diseases in society for a number of valid reasons. It is often silent, producing no symptoms until it is too far advanced for cure. It sometimes requires painful and disfiguring surgery. It may strike at an early age, even during childhood, to deprive patients of a normal lifespan. Perhaps worst of all, the medical treatment of cancer often cannot offer a cure, and progression to death is sometimes slow, painful, and psychologically difficult for patients and their loved ones.

Despite its feared status, many successes have been made in the diagnosis, understanding, and treatment of cancer. Some types of cancer are now curable and therapies may give the patient a longer, symptom-free life. This chapter examines the role of drugs in the treatment of cancer. Medications used to treat this disease are called anticancer drugs, antineoplastics, or cancer chemotherapeutic agents.

35.1 Characteristics of Cancer: Uncontrolled Cell Growth

Cancer, or carcinoma, is a disease characterized by abnormal, uncontrolled cell division. Cell division is a normal process occurring extensively in most body tissues from conception to late childhood. At some point in time, however, cells stop their rapid division by repressing genes responsible for cell growth. This may result in a total lack of replication, in the case of muscle cells and perhaps brain cells. In other cells, genes controlling replication are turned back on when it becomes necessary to replace worn-out cells, as in the case of blood cells and the mucosa of the digestive tract.

Cancer is thought to result from damage to the genes controlling cell growth. Once damaged, the cell is no longer responsive to normal chemical signals checking its growth. The cancer cells lose their normal functions, divide rapidly, and invade surrounding cells. The abnormal cells often travel to distant sites where they populate new tumors, a process called metastasis. Figure 35.1 illustrates some characteristics of cancer cells.

Tumor is defined as a swelling, abnormal enlargement, or mass. The word neoplasm is often used interchangeably with tumor. Tumors may be solid masses, such as lung or breast cancer, or they may be widely disseminated in the blood, such as leukemia. Tumors are named according to their tissue of origin, generally with the suffix *-oma*. Table 35.1 gives examples of various types of tumors.

35.2 Causes of Cancer

A large number of factors have been found to cause cancer or to be associated with a higher risk for acquiring the disease. These factors are known as carcinogens.

Many chemical carcinogens have been identified. Some of these carcinogens have been associated with a higher incidence of cancer in the workplace, such as asbestos and benzene. Chemicals in tobacco smoke are thought to be responsible for about one-third of all cancer in the United States. In some cases the actual site of the cancer may be distant from the entry location, as with bladder cancer caused by the inhalation of certain industrial chemicals. Some known chemical carcinogens are listed in Table 35.2.

A number of physical factors are also associated with cancer. For example, exposure to large amounts of x-rays is associated with a higher risk of leukemia. Ultraviolet (UV) light from the sun is a known cause of skin cancer.

Viruses are associated with about 15% of all human cancers. Examples include herpes simplex types I and II, Epstein-Barr virus, papillomavirus, cytomegalovirus, and human T-lymphotrophic viruses. Factors that suppress the immune system, such as HIV or drugs given after transplant surgery, may encourage the growth of preexisting cancer cells, as discussed in Chapter 30⬆.

Some cancers have a strong genetic component. The fact that close relatives may acquire the same type of cancer suggests that certain genes, called oncogenes, may predispose close relatives to the condition. These abnormal genes somehow interact with chemical, physical, and biological agents to promote cancer formation. Other genes, called tumor suppressor genes, may inhibit the formation of tumors. If these suppressor genes are damaged, cancer may result. Damage to the suppressor gene known as p53 is associated with cancers of the breast, lung, brain, colon, and bone.

Although the formation of cancer has a genetic component, it also has strong environmental component. Adopting healthy lifestyle habits may reduce the risk of acquiring cancer. Proper nutrition, avoiding chemical and physical risks, and keeping regular health checkups can help prevent cancer from developing into a fatal disease. The following are lifestyle factors regarding cancer prevention or diagnosis that should be used by the nurse when teaching patients about cancer prevention.

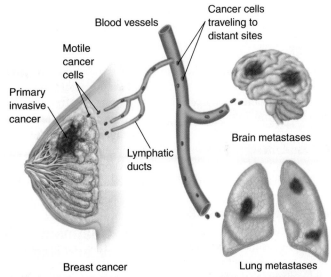

Figure 35.1 | Invasion and metastasis by cancer cells

Table 35.1	Classification and Naming of Tumors	
Name	**Description**	**Examples**
benign tumor	slow growing; do not metastasize and rarely require drug treatment	adenoma, papilloma and lipoma, osteoma, meningioma
malignant tumor	grow rapidly larger; become resistant to treatment and result in death if untreated	
sarcoma	cancer of connective tissue; grow extremely rapidly and metastasize early in the progression of the disease	osteogenic sarcoma, fibrosarcoma, Kaposi's sarcoma, angiosarcoma
carcinoma	cancer of epithelial tissue; most common type of malignant neoplasm; grow rapidly and metastasize	malignant melanoma, renal cell carcinoma, adenocarcinoma, hepatocellular carcinoma
leukemia	cancer of the blood-forming cells in bone marrow; may be acute or chronic	myelocytic leukemia, granulocytic leukemia
lymphoma	cancer of lymphoid tissue	Hodgkin's disease, lymphoblastic lymphoma
glioma	cancer of glial (interstitial) cells in the brain, spinal cord, pineal gland, posterior pituitary gland, or retina	telangiectatic glioma, brainstem glioma

Table 35.2	Agents Associated with an Increased Risk of Cancer
Agent	**Type of Cancer**
alcohol	liver
arsenic	skin and lung
asbestos	lung
benzene	leukemia
nickel	lung and nasal
polycyclic aromatic hydrocarbons	lung and skin
tobacco substances	lung
vinyl chloride	liver

- Eliminate tobacco use and exposure to secondhand smoke.
- Limit or eliminate alcohol beverage use.
- Reduce fat in the diet, particularly that from animal sources.
- Choose most foods from plant sources; increase fiber in the diet.
- Exercise regularly and keep body weight within recommended guidelines.
- Self-examine your body monthly for abnormal lumps and skin lesions.
- When exposed to direct sun, use skin lotions with the highest SPF (sun protection factor) value.
- Have periodic diagnostic testing performed at recommended intervals.
  - Women should have periodic mammograms, as directed by their healthcare provider.
  - Men should have a digital rectal prostate examination and a prostate-specific antigen test annually after age 50.
  - Have a fecal occult blood test (FOBT) and flexible sigmoidoscopy performed at age 50 with FOBT annually following age 50.
  - Women who are sexually active or have reached age 18 should have an annual Pap test and pelvic examination.

35.3 Treatment of Cancer: Chemotherapy, Surgery, and Radiation Therapy

There is a much greater possibility for cure if a cancer is treated in its early stages, when the tumor is small and localized to a single area. Once the cancer has spread to distant sites, cure is much more difficult; thus, it is important to diagnose the disease as early as possible. In an attempt to remove every cancer cell, three treatment approaches are utilized: surgery, radiation therapy, and drug therapy.

Surgery is performed to remove a tumor that is localized to one area, or when the tumor is pressing on nerves, the airways, or other vital tissues. Surgery lowers the number of cancer cells in the body so that radiation and pharmacotherapy can be more successful. Surgery is not an option for tumors of blood cells or when it would not be expected to extend a patient's lifespan or to improve the quality of life.

Radiation therapy is an effective way to kill tumor cells through nonsurgical means; approximately 50% of patients with cancer receive radiation therapy as part of their treatment. High doses of ionizing radiation are aimed directly at the tumor and confined to this area, to the maximum extent possible. Radiation treatments may follow surgery, to kill any cancer cells left behind following the operation. Radiation is sometimes given as palliation for inoperable cancers to shrink the size of a tumor that may be pressing on vital organs, to relieve pain, difficulty breathing, or difficulty swallowing.

Pharmacotherapy of cancer is sometimes called chemotherapy. Because drugs are transported through the blood, they have the potential to reach cancer cells in virtually any location. Some drugs are available to pass across the blood-brain barrier to treat brain tumors. Others are instilled directly into body cavities such as the urinary bladder, to bring the highest dose possible to the cancer cells without producing systemic side effects.

Anticancer drugs are sometimes given, in concert with surgery and radiation, to attempt a total cure or complete eradication of all tumor cells from the body. In other cases, the cancer is too advanced to expect a cure, and antineoplastic agents are given for palliation to reduce the size of the tumor. Palliation eases the severity of pain or discomfort and may extend the patients lifespan or improve quality of life. In a few cases, drugs are given as prophylaxis with

the goal of preventing cancer from occurring in patients at high risk to developing tumors.

35.4 Growth Fraction and Success of Chemotherapy

Although cancers are rapidly growing, not all cells in a tumor are replicating at any given time. Since antineoplastic agents are generally more effective against cells that are replicating, the percentage of tumor cells proliferating at the time of chemotherapy is critical.

Both normal and cancerous cells go through a sequence of events known as the cell cycle which is illustrated in Figure 35.2. Cells spend most of their lifetime in the G_0 phase. Although sometimes called the resting stage, the G_0 phase is when cells conduct their everyday activities such as metabolism, impulse conduction, contraction, or secreting. If the cell receives a signal to divide, it leaves G_0, to enter the G_1 phase, where it synthesizes the RNA, proteins, and other components needed to duplicate its DNA during the S phase. Following duplication of its DNA, it enters the premitotic phase, or G_2. Following mitosis in the M phase, the cell reenters its resting G_0 phase where it may remain for extended periods, depending on the specific tissue and surrounding cellular signals.

The actions of some antineoplastic agents are specific to certain phases of the cell cycle, while others are mostly independent of the cell cycle. For example, mitotic inhibitors such as vincristine (Oncovin) affect the M phase. Antimetabolites such as fluorouracil (Adrucil) are most effective during the S phase. The effects of alkylating agents such as cyclophosphamide (Cytoxan) are generally independent of the phases of the cell cycle. Some of these agents are shown in Figure 35.2.

The growth fraction is a measure of how many cells in a tumor are undergoing mitosis. It is a ratio of the number of replicating cells to the number of resting cells. Solid tumors such as breast and lung cancer generally have a low growth fraction, thus they are less sensitive to antineoplastic agents. Certain leukemias and lymphomas have a higher growth fraction and have a greater antineoplastic success rate. Some normal tissues, such as hair follicles, bone marrow, and the GI epithelium also have a high growth fraction and are sensitive to the effects of these drugs.

35.5 Achieving a Total Cancer Cure

To cure a patient, it is believed that every single cancer cell must be destroyed or removed from the body. Even one malignant cell could potentially produce enough offspring to kill a patient. Unlike anti-infective therapy in which the patient's immune system is an active partner in eliminating massive numbers of microorganisms, the immune system is able to eliminate only a small number of cancer cells.

As an example, consider that a small 1 cm breast tumor may already contain 1 billion cancer cells before it is detected. A drug killing 99% of these cells would be considered a very effective drug, indeed. Yet even with this fantastic achievement, 10 million cancer cells would remain, any one of which

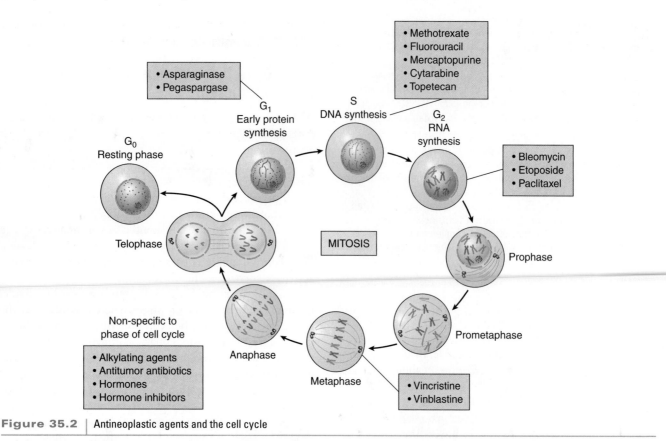

Figure 35.2 | Antineoplastic agents and the cell cycle

could cause the tumor to return and kill the patient. The relationship between cell kill and chemotherapy is shown in Figure 35.3. This example reinforces the need to diagnose and treat tumors at an early stage using several therapies such as drugs, radiation, and surgery when possible.

35.6 Special Pharmacotherapy Protocols and Strategies for Cancer Chemotherapy

While cancer cells are clearly abnormal in many ways, much of their physiology is identical to that of normal cells. It is thus difficult to kill cancer cells selectively without profoundly affecting normal cells. Complicating the chances for a pharmacologic cure is the fact that cancer cells often develop resistance to antineoplastic drugs.

A number of treatment strategies have been found to increase the effectiveness of anticancer drugs. In most cases, multiple drugs from different antineoplastic classes are given during a course of chemotherapy. These multiple drugs affect different stages of the cancer cell's life cycle, attacking the tumor from several mechanisms of action, thus increasing the percentage of cell kill. Combination chemotherapy also allows the dosages of each individual agent to be lower, thus reducing toxicity and slowing the development of resistance. Examples of combination therapies include cyclophosphamide-methotrexate-fluorouracil (CMF) for breast cancer and cyclophosphamide-doxorubicin-vincristine (CDV) for lung cancer.

Specific dosing schedules, or protocols, have been found to increase the effectiveness of the antineoplastic agents. For example, some of the anticancer drugs are given as single doses or perhaps a couple of doses over a few days. Several weeks may pass before the next series of doses begins. This gives normal cells time to recover from the adverse effects of the drugs, and allows tumor cells that may not have been replicating at the time of the first dose to begin dividing and become more sensitive to the next round of chemotherapy.

35.7 Toxicity of Antineoplastic Agents

All anticancer drugs have the potential to cause serious toxicity. These drugs are often pushed to their maximum possible dosages, so that the greatest tumor kill can be obtained. Such high dosages always result in adverse effects in the patient. Table 35.3 provides typical adverse effects of anticancer drugs.

Because these drugs primarily affect rapidly dividing cells, normal cells that are replicating are most susceptible to adverse effects. Hair follicles are damaged resulting in hair loss or **alopecia**. The epithelial lining of the digestive tract is commonly affected, resulting in bleeding or severe diarrhea. The vomiting center in the medulla is triggered by many antineoplastics, resulting in significant nausea and vomiting. Because of this effect, antineoplastics are sometimes classified by their emetic potential. Before starting therapy with the highest emetic potential agents, patients may be pretreated with antiemetic drugs such as prochlorperazine (Compazine), metoclopramide (Reglan, others), or lorazepam (Ativan) (Chapter 37)⊛.

Stem cells in the bone marrow may be destroyed by antineoplastics, causing anemia, leukopenia, and thrombocytopenia. These side effects are the ones that most often cause discontinuation of chemotherapy. Efforts to minimize bone marrow toxicity may include bone marrow transplantation, or therapy with growth factors such as granulocyte colony-stimulating factor (filgrastim [Neupogen]) or granulocyte colony-stimulating factor (sargramostim [Leukine]).

Each antineoplastic drug has a documented **nadir**, the lowest point that the neutrophil count has been depressed by the chemotherapeutic agent. The nurse can calculate the absolute neutrophil count (ANC) by multiplying the white blood cell count times the percentage of neutrophils. This can be obtained by reading the patient's CBC with differential. In general, the drug should not be administered if the patient is immunodeficient.

When possible, antineoplastics are given locally by topical application or through direct instillation into a tumor site to minimize systemic toxicity. Most antineoplastics, however, are given intravenously. Extravasation from an injection site can produce severe tissue and nerve damage, and even loss of a limb. Certain antineoplastics have specific antidotes for extravasation. For example, extravasation of carmustine (BiCNU, Gliadel) is treated with injections of equal parts of sodium bicarbonate and normal saline into the extravasation site. Before administering intravenous antineoplastic agents, the nurse should know the emergency treatment for extravasation.

Drugs used in cancer chemotherapy come from diverse pharmacologic and chemical classes. Antineoplastics have been extracted from plants and bacteria, as well as being created entirely in the laboratory. Some of the drug classes attack vital cellular macromolecules, such as DNA and proteins, while others poison vital metabolic pathways of rapidly growing cells. The common theme among all the antineoplastic agents is that they kill or at least stop the growth of cancer cells.

Classification of the various antineoplastics is quite variable, as some of these drugs kill cancer cells by several different mechanisms and have characteristics from more

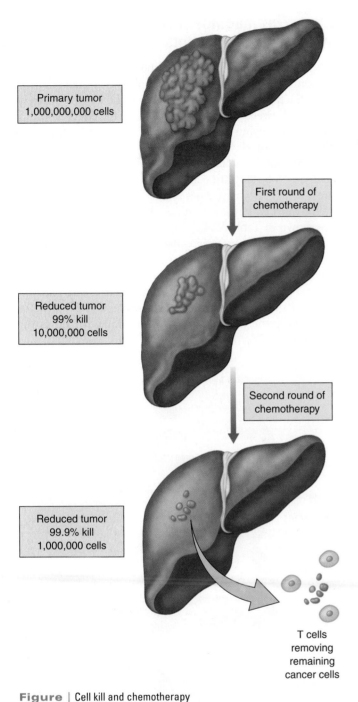

Primary tumor 1,000,000,000 cells

First round of chemotherapy

Reduced tumor 99% kill 10,000,000 cells

Second round of chemotherapy

Reduced tumor 99.9% kill 1,000,000 cells

T cells removing remaining cancer cells

Figure 35.3 | Cell kill and chemotherapy

Table 35.3	**Adverse Effects of Anticancer Drugs**	
Changes to the Blood	**Changes to the GI Tract**	**Other Effects**
anemia (low red blood cells)	anorexia	alopecia
leukopenia or neutropenia (low white blood cells)	bleeding	fatigue
thrombocytopenia (low platelets)	diarrhea	fetal death/birth defects
	extreme nausea and vomiting	opportunistic infections
		ulceration and bleeding of the lips and gums

than one class. Furthermore, the mechanisms by which some antineoplastics act are not completely understood. A simple method of classifying this complex group of drugs includes the following six categories.

- Alkylating agents
- Antimetabolites
- Antitumor antibiotics
- Hormones and hormone antagonists having antineoplastic activity
- Natural products having antineoplastic activity
- Miscellaneous anticancer drugs

Alkylating Agents

The first alkylating agents, the **nitrogen mustards**, were developed in secrecy as chemical warfare agents during World War II. Although the drugs in this class have quite different chemical structures, all share the common characteristic of forming bonds or linkages with DNA, a process called **alkylation**. Figure 35.4 illustrates the process of alkylation.

35.8 Pharmacotherapy with Alkylating Agents

Alkylation changes the shape of the DNA double helix and prevents the nucleic acid from completing normal cell division. Each alkylating agent attaches to DNA in a different manner; however, they collectively have the effect of killing or at least slowing the replication of tumor cells. Although the process of alkylation occurs independently of the cell cycle, the killing action does not occur until the cell begins to divide. The alkylating agents have a broad spectrum, and are used against many types of malignancies. They are some of the most widely used antineoplastic drugs. These agents are shown in Table 35.4.

Blood cells are particularly sensitive to alkylating agents and bone marrow suppression is the most important adverse effect of this class. Within days after administration, declines in erythrocytes, leukocytes, and platelets may be measured. Damaging effects on the epithelial cells lining the GI tract are also common with alkylating agents.

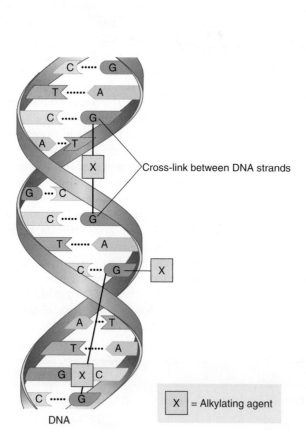

Cross-link between DNA strands

X = Alkylating agent

DNA

(a) Alkylation occuring during G_0 (resting) phase of cell cycle

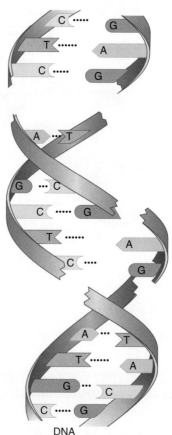

DNA

(b) Strand breaks occuring when DNA replicates during S phase of cell cycle

Figure 35.4 | Mechanism of action of the alkylating agents

Table 35.4	Alkylating Agents
Drug	**Route and Adult Dose (max dose where indicated)**
Nitrogen Mustards	
chlorambucil (Leukeran)	PO; Initial dose 0.1–0.2 mg/kg qd; maintenance dose 4–10 mg/qd
⊙ cyclophosphamide (Cytoxan, Neosar)	PO; Initial dose 1–5 mg/qd; maintenance dose 1–5 mg/kg q 7–10 d
estramustine (Emcyt)	PO; 5 mg/kg tid-qid
ifosfamide (Ifex)	IV; 1.2 g/m^2 qd for 5 consecutive days
mechlorethamine (Mustargen)	IV; 6 mg/m^2 on day 1 and 8 of a 28-day cycle
melphalan (Alkeran)	PO; 6 mg qd for 2–3 wk
Nitrosoureas	
carmustine (BiCNU, Gliadel)	IV; 200 mg/m^2 q 6 wk
lomustine (CeeNU)	PO; 130 mg/m^2 as a single dose
streptozocin (Zanosar)	IV; 500 mg/m^2 for 5 consecutive days
Miscellaneous Alkylating Agents	
busulfan (Myleran)	PO; 4–8 mg qd
carboplatin (Paraplatin)	IV; 360 mg/m^2 once q 4 wk
cisplatin (Platinol)	IV; 20 mg/m^2 qd for 5 d
dacarbazine (DTIC-Dome)	IV; 2–4.5 mg/kg qd for 10 d
oxaliplatin (Eloxatin)	IV; 85 mg/m^2 for 2 hr
temozolomide (Temodar)	PO; 150 mg/m^2 qd for 5 consecutive days

NURSING CONSIDERATIONS

The role of the nurse in alkylating agent therapy involves careful monitoring of a patient's condition and providing education as it relates to the prescribed drug regimen. Before starting any form of chemotherapy, the nurse should assess baseline vital signs, complete blood count, and the patient's overall health status, including renal and liver function, intake and output, and body weight. Alkylating agents must be administered with caution to patients with hepatic or renal impairment, recent steroid therapy, leukopenia, or thrombocytopenia.

Alkylating agents are highly toxic to tissues with a rapid growth rate. Bone marrow depression occurs because these agents kill normal hematopoietic cells. These drugs may cause injury to the GI mucosa and hair follicles. Mustard agents may cause skin eruptions such as blistering. Alkylating agents may depress spermatogenesis and oocyte production, and secondary leukemias are frequently associated with this class of drugs. Platinum compound alkylating agents (e.g., cisplatin) may cause high-frequency hearing loss.

The nurse should remain alert to the possible development of blood dyscrasias by observing the patient for signs and symptoms such as bruising or bleeding, and by closely monitoring the CBC with differential and platelet count. Patients of childbearing age should be informed of the po-

tential adverse impact on fertility. Cyclophosphamide also diminishes sex drive. Patients should be encouraged to frankly discuss sexual issues with the nurse, especially regarding options to preserve fertility.

Alkylating agents range from pregnancy category C (streptozocin, cyclophosphamide) to category X (estramustine). Both females and males should be counseled to abstain from coitus, or to use reliable contraception during therapy and for 4 months thereafter. The nurse can assist the patient in choosing an appropriate method for the patient's cultural background, lifestyle, and health.

Patient education as it relates to alkylating agents should include therapeutic goals; reasons for obtaining baseline data such as vital signs, blood work, tests for cardiac and renal disorders; and possible side effects. Following are important points the nurse should include when teaching patients regarding alkylating agents.

- Sterility and amenorrhea may occur in patients on mechlorethamine (Mustargen) or cyclophosphamide (Cytoxan) therapy, but these are reversible once therapy is discontinued.
- Obtain routine hearing screenings during therapy.
- Report any buzzing, ringing, or tingling sensation in the ears, or decreased hearing.
- Immediately report the following: tachycardia, fever, chills, sore throat, dyspnea, gout, kidney stones, skin rashes.

Please refer to "Nursing Process Focus: Patients Receiving Antineoplastic Therapy" for additional teaching points.

Antimetabolites

Antimetabolites are drugs that are chemically similar to essential building blocks of the cell. They are structurally similar to certain critical cell molecules. They interfere with aspects of the nutrient or nucleic acid metabolism of rapidly growing tumor cells.

35.9 Pharmacotherapy with Antimetabolites

Rapidly growing cancer cells require large quantities of nutrients and other chemicals to construct proteins and nucleic acids. When cancer cells attempt to synthesize proteins, RNA, or DNA, they use the antimetabolites instead of normal precursors. By disrupting metabolic pathways in this manner, antimetabolites can kill cancer cells or slow their growth. These agents are prescribed for leukemias and solid tumors and are shown in Table 35.5.

The purine and pyrimidine analogs resemble the natural precursors to nucleic acid biosynthesis. For example, the pyrimidine analog fluorouracil (Adrucil) is able to block the formation of thymidylate, an essential chemical needed to make DNA, and is used in treating various solid tumors. After becoming activated and incorporated into DNA, cytarabine (Cytosar) blocks DNA synthesis and is an important drug in forcing remission of acute myelocytic leukemia. Figure 35.5 illustrates the structural similarities of some of these antimetabolites to their natural counterparts.

NURSING CONSIDERATIONS

The role of the nurse in antimetabolite therapy involves careful monitoring of a patient's condition and providing education as it relates to the prescribed drug regimen. Before initiating chemotherapy, the nurse should assess baseline vital signs, complete blood count, and the patient's overall health status, including renal and liver function, intake and output, and body weight.

Many antimetabolites are contraindicated in pregnancy; for example, methotrexate (Mexate) is a category X drug and pregnancy should be avoided for at least 6 months following termination of therapy. Further contraindications would include hepatic, cardiac, and renal insufficiency; myelosuppression; and blood dyscrasias. Patients with pep-

---

 PROTOTYPE DRUG | **CYCLOPHOSPHAMIDE** (Cytoxan)

ACTIONS AND USES

Cyclophosphamide is a commonly prescribed nitrogen mustard. It is used alone, or in combination with other drugs, against a wide variety of cancers, including Hodgkin's disease, lymphoma, multiple myeloma, breast cancer, and ovarian cancer. Cyclophosphamide acts by attaching to DNA and disrupting replication, particularly in rapidly dividing cells. It is one of only a few anticancer drugs that are well absorbed when given orally. Because of its potent immunosuppressive properties, it has been used for certain nonneoplastic disorders such as prevention of transplant rejection and severe rheumatoid arthritis.

Administration Alerts

- Dilute prior to IV administration.
- Monitor platelet count prior to IM administration; if low, hold dose.
- To avoid GI upset take with meals or divide doses.
- Pregnancy category C.

ADVERSE EFFECTS AND INTERACTIONS

The powerful immunosuppressant effects of cyclophosphamide peak 1 to 2 days after administration. Leukocyte counts sometimes serve as a guide to dosage adjustments during therapy. Thrombocytopenia is common, though less severe than with many other alkylating agents. Nausea, vomiting, anorexia, and diarrhea are frequently experienced. Cyclophosphamide damages hair follicles to cause alopecia, though this effect is usually reversible. Several metabolites of cyclophosphamide may cause hemorrhagic cystitis if the urine becomes concentrated; patients should be advised to maintain high fluid intake during therapy. Unlike other nitrogen mustards, cyclophosphamide exhibits little neurotoxicity.

Cyclophosphamide interacts with many drugs. For example, immunosuppressant agents used concurrently may increase risk of infections and further development of neoplasms. There is an increased chance of bone marrow toxicity if cyclophosphamide is used concurrently with allopurinol. If anticoagulants are used concurrently, increased anticoagulant effects may occur, leading to hemorrhage.

If used concurrently with digoxin, decreased serum levels of digoxin occur. Concurrent use with insulin may lead to increased hypoglycemia. Phenobarbital, phenytoin, or glucocorticoids used concurrently may lead to an increased rate of cyclophosphamide metabolism by the liver. Thiazide diuretics used concurrently lead to increased possibility of leukopenia.

Use with caution with herbal supplements, such as echinacea, which is an immune stimulator, and may interfere with the drug's immunosuppressant effects.

 See the companion website for a Nursing Process Focus specific to this drug.

Table 35.5	Antimetabolites
Drug	**Route and Adult Dose (max dose where indicated)**
Folic Acid Antagonist	
methotrexate (Folex, Mexate, others)	PO; 10–30 mg/d for 5d
Pyrimidine Analogs	
capecitabine (Xeloda)	PO; 2,500 mg/m^2 qd for 2 wk
cytarabine (Cytosar-U, Tarabine, DepoCyt)	IV; 200 mg/m^2 as a continuous infusion over 24 hr
floxuridine (FUDR)	Intra-arterial: 0.1–0.6 mg/kg qd as a continuous infusion
fluorouracil (5-FU, Adrucil, Efudex, Fluoroplex)	IV; 12 mg/kg qd for 4 consecutive days
gemcitabine (Gemzar)	IV; 1,000 mg/m^2 once weekly for 7 wk
Purine Analogs	
cladribine (Leustatin)	IV; 0.09 mg/m^2 qd as a continuous infusion
fludarabine (Fludara)	IV; 25 mg/m^2 qd for 5 consecutive days
mercaptopurine (Purinethol)	PO; 2.5 mg/kg qd
pentostatin (Nipent)	IV; 4 mg/m^2 q other week
thioguanine (Lanvis)	PO; 2 mg/kg qd

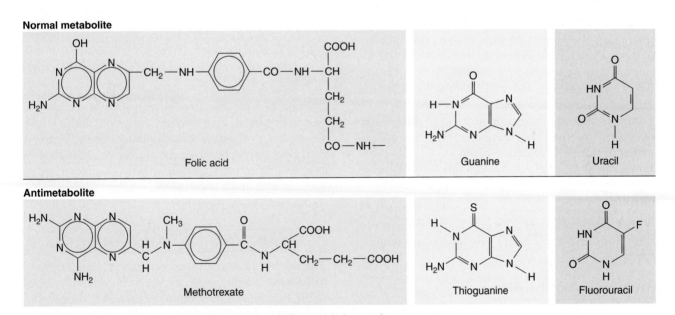

Figure 35.5 | Structural similarities between antimetabolites and their natural counterparts

tic ulcer, ulcerative colitis, or poor nutritional status should be monitored closely. Antimetabolites cause many of the adverse effects common to other antineoplastics, including alopecia, fatigue, nausea, vomiting, diarrhea, bone marrow depression, and blood dyscrasias. These drugs may also cause photosensitivity and idiosyncratic pneumonitis.

The nurse should observe the patient for signs and symptoms of respiratory infection, including shortness of breath, cough, fever, and especially rash or chest pain (pleurisy). Viral infections such as herpes/varicella strains can be especially virulent when experienced during an-

timetabolite therapy. Immunizations, especially attenuated vaccines, should be avoided during this time due to drug-induced impaired immunity. Patients should be encouraged to regularly exercise deep breathing, if necessary, with the aid of an incentive spirometer.

Patient education as it relates to antimetabolites should include goals of therapy; reasons for obtaining baseline data such as vital signs, tests for immune, lung, and renal disorders, and blood work; and possible side effects. Following are important points the nurse should include when teaching patients regarding antimetabolites.

PROTOTYPE DRUG | METHOTREXATE (Folex, Mexate, others)

ACTIONS AND USES

Methotrexate inhibits folic acid (vitamin B_9) metabolism. By blocking the synthesis of folic acid, methotrexate is able to inhibit replication, particularly in rapidly dividing cells. It is prescribed alone or in combination with other drugs for choriocarcinoma, osteogenic sarcoma, leukemias, head and neck cancers, breast carcinoma, and lung carcinoma. It is occasionally used to treat nonneoplastic disorders such as severe psoriasis and rheumatoid arthritis that have not responded to other medications.

Administration Alerts

- Avoid skin exposure to drug. Avoid inhaling drug particles.
- Dilute prior to IV administration.
- Pregnancy category X.

ADVERSE EFFECTS AND INTERACTIONS

The adverse effects of methotrexate appear primarily in rapidly dividing tissues such as the GI epithelium and stem cells in the bone marrow. A potent immunosuppressant, methotrexate can result in fatal bone marrow toxicity at high doses. Leucovorin (Folinic Acid), a reduced form of folic acid, is sometimes administered with methotrexate to "rescue" normal cells, or protect against severe bone marrow damage. Hemorrhage and bruising are often observed due to low platelet counts. Nausea, vomiting, and anorexia are common. Although rare, pulmonary toxicity may develop and be quite serious. Methotrexate interacts with several drugs. Bone marrow suppressants such as chemotherapeutic agents or radiation therapy may cause increased effects; the patient will require a lower dose of methotrexate.

In concurrent use with NSAIDs, methotrexate may lead to severe methotrexate toxicity. Aspirin may interfere with excretion of methotrexate, leading to increased serum levels and toxicity. Concurrent administration with live oral vaccine may result in decreased antibody response and increased adverse reactions to the vaccine.

Use with caution with herbal supplements, such as echinacea, which may interfere with the drug's immunosuppressant effects.

 See the companion website for a Nursing Process Focus specific to this drug.

- Avoid immunizations and people with active infections.
- Regularly practice deep breathing exercises.
- Eliminate or reduce respiratory irritants in the environment such as secondhand tobacco smoke or aerosol cosmetics (e.g., hair spray or deodorants).
- Immediately report the following: shortness of breath, chest pain, cough, fever, rash, dizziness, bruising, or bleeding.

Please refer to "Nursing Process Focus: Patients Receiving Antineoplastic Therapy" for additional teaching points.

Antitumor Antibiotics

The antitumor antibiotics class contains antibiotics, obtained from bacteria, that have the ability to kill cancer cells. They are not widely used, but are very effective against certain tumors.

35.10 Pharmacotherapy with Antitumor Antibiotics

Antitumor properties have been identified in a number of substances isolated from microorganisms. These chemicals are more cytotoxic than the traditional antibiotics, and their use is restricted to treating a few specific types of cancer. For example, the only indication for idarubicin (Idamycin) is acute myelogenous leukemia. Testicular carcinoma is the only indication for plicamycin (Mithramycin). The antitumor antibiotics are shown in Table 35.6.

The antitumor antibiotics bind to DNA and affect its function by a mechanism similar to that of the alkylating agents. Because of this, their general actions and side effects are similar to those of the alkylating agents. Unlike the alkylating agents, however, the antitumor antibiotics must be administered intravenously or through direct instillation via a catheter into a body cavity.

NURSING CONSIDERATIONS

The role of the nurse in antitumor antibiotic therapy involves careful monitoring of a patient's condition and providing education as it relates to the prescribed drug regimen. Before initiating chemotherapy, the nurse should assess the complete blood count and the patient's overall health status, including renal and liver function, intake and output, and body weight. The nurse should interview the patient regarding any history of allergy prior to initiating therapy. Vital signs—including auscultation of heart and chest sounds—and a baseline EKG should be obtained to rule out signs of cardiac abnormality or heart failure. The nurse should also assess for pregnancy and lactation, as antitumor antibiotics range from pregnancy category C (dactinomycin, plicamycin, and valrubicin) to category D (bleomycin, daunorubicin, all others).

Antitumor antibiotics require cautious use in many patients. These drugs produce the same general cytotoxic effects as other antineoplastics, including alopecia, fatigue,

Table 35.6	Antitumor Antibiotics
Drug	**Route and Adult Dose (max dose where indicated)**
bleomycin (Blenoxane)	IV; 0.25–0.5 units/kg q 4–7 d
dactinomycin (Actinomycin-D, Cosmegen)	IV; 500 µg qd for maximum of 5 d
daunorubicin (Cerubidine)	IV; 30–60 mg/m² qd for 3–5 d
daunorubicin liposomal (DaunoXome)	IV; 40 mg/m² q 2 wk
Pr doxorubicin (Adriamycin, Rubex)	IV; 60–75 mg/m² as single dose at 21 d intervals or 30 mg/m² on each of 3 consecutive days (max: total cumulative dose 550 mg/m²)
doxorubicin liposomal (Doxil)	IV; 20 mg/m² q 3 wk
epirubicin (Ellence)	IV; 100–120 mg/m² as a single dose
idarubicin (Idamycin)	IV; 8–12 mg/m² qd for 3 d
mitomycin (Mutamycin)	IV; 2 mg/m² as a single dose
mitoxantrone (Novantrone)	IV; 12 mg/m² qd for 3 d
plicamycin (Mithramycin, Mithracin)	IV; 25–30 µ/kg qd for 8–10 d.
valrubicin (Valstar)	Intrabladder instillation; 800 mg q week for 6 wk

nausea, vomiting, diarrhea, bone marrow supression, and blood dyscrasias. As antibiotics, the risk of hypersensitivity reactions such as life-threatening angioedema exists. Antitumor antibiotics can be damaging to the myocardium; thus, they should be used with extreme caution, if at all, for patients with cardiac disease. Doxorubicin (Adriamycin) should be used cautiously if the patient has received cyclophosphamide, pelvic radiation or radiotherapy to areas surrounding the heart, or has a history of atopic dermatitis. Other effects include hyperpigmentation of the mucosa and nailbeds, particularly among African Americans, and changes in the rectal mucosa. For this reason, suppositories and the taking of rectal temperatures are contraindicated.

The nurse must be extremely cautious when administering antitumor antibiotics. Doxorubicin (Adriamycin) is easily absorbed through the skin and by inhalation, and may cause fetal death or birth defects as well as liver disease. Therefore, the nurse should wear protective clothing (gloves, mask, and apron) when preparing the drug.

Patient education as it relates to antitumor antibiotics should include goals of therapy, reasons for obtaining baseline data such as vital signs, blood work, EKG and other cardiac tests, and possible side effects. Following are important points the nurse should include when teaching patients regarding antitumor antibiotics.

- Proper attention to good oral hygiene is important. Changes in the color of the mucosa can make it difficult to distinguish the degree of tissue oxygenation or the severity of mouth sores. Inform the dentist of antitumor antibiotic therapy.
- Avoid using OTC rectal drugs, such as for hemorrhoids, and taking rectal temperatures.
- Seek emergency medical treatment for signs of severe allergic reaction or possible heart attack, such as shortness of breath, thick tongue, throat tightness or facial swelling, rash, palpitations, chest, arm or back pain.
- Immediately report headache, dizziness, or rectal bleeding.

Please refer to "Nursing Process Focus: Patients Receiving Antineoplastic Therapy" for additional teaching points.

Natural Products (Plant Extracts)

Plants have been a valuable source for antineoplastic agents. These agents act by preventing cell division.

35.11 Pharmacotherapy with Natural Products (Plant Extracts)

Agents with antineoplastic activity have been isolated from a number of plants, including the common periwinkle (*Vinca rosea*), Pacific yew (*Taxus baccata*), mandrake (May apple), and the shrub *Campothecus acuminata*. Although structurally different, medications in this class have the common ability to affect cell division; thus, some of them are called mitotic inhibitors. The plant extracts, or natural products, are shown in Table 35.7

The **vinca alkaloids**, vincristine (Oncovin), and vinblastine (Velban) are older drugs derived from the periwinkle plant. Over 100 alkaloids have been isolated from the periwinkle, and their properties were described in folklore in several regions of the world long before their modern medical uses were discovered. Despite being derived from the same plant, vincristine, vinblastine, and the semisynthetic vinorelbine (Navelbine) exhibit different effects and toxicity profiles.

The **taxoids**, which include paclitaxel (Taxol) and docetaxel (Taxotere), were originally isolated from the bark of the Pacific yew, which is an evergreen found in forests

Pr PROTOTYPE DRUG | DOXORUBICIN (Adriamycin)

ACTIONS AND USES

Doxorubicin attaches to DNA, distorting its double helical structure and preventing DNA synthesis. It is only administered by IV infusion. Doxorubicin is one of the broader-spectrum cytotoxic antibiotics, prescribed for solid tumors of the lung, breast, ovary, and bladder, and for various leukemias and lymphomas. It is structurally similar to daunorubicin (Cerubidine).

A novel delivery method has been developed for both doxorubicin and daunorubicin. The drug is enclosed in small lipid sacs, or vesicles, called **liposomes**. The liposomal vesicle is designed to open and release the antitumor antibiotic when it reaches a cancer cell. The goal is to deliver a higher concentration of drug to the cancer cells, thus sparing normal cells. An additional advantage is that doxorubicin liposomal has a half-life of 50 to 60 hours, which is about twice that of regular doxorubicin. The primary indication for this delivery method is AIDS-related Kaposi's sarcoma.

Administration Alerts

- Extravasation from an injection site can cause severe pain and extensive tissue damage.
- For infants and children, verify concentration and rate of IV infusion with physician.
- Avoid skin contact with drug. If exposure occurs, wash thoroughly with soap and water.
- Pregnancy category D.

ADVERSE EFFECTS AND INTERACTIONS

The most serious concern, which sometimes limits doxorubicin therapy, is cardiotoxicity. Acute effects include dysrhythmias; delayed effects may include irreversible heart failure. Like many of the anticancer drugs, doxorubicin may profoundly lower blood cell counts. Acute nausea and vomiting are common and often require antiemetic therapy. Complete, though reversible, hair loss occurs in most patients. May cause soles of feet, palms of hands, and nail beds to darken.

Doxorubicin interacts with many drugs. For example, if digoxin is taken concurrently, the patient will have decreased serum digoxin levels. Phenobarbital taken concurrently leads to increased plasma clearance of doxorubicin and decreased effectiveness. Concurrent use of phenytoin may lead to decreased phenytoin level, and possible seizure activity. Hepatotoxicity may occur if mercaptopurine is taken concurrently. Concurrent use of verapamil may increase serum doxorubicin levels, leading to doxorubicin toxicity.

Use with caution with herbal supplements. For example, green tea may enhance the antitumor activity of doxorubicin.

 See the companion website for a Nursing Process Focus specific to this drug.

Table 35.7	Plant Extracts with Antineoplastic Activity
Drug	**Route and Adult Dose (max dose where indicated)**
Vinca Alkaloids	
vinblastine sulfate (Velban)	IV; 3.7–18.5 mg/m^2 q week
Pr vincristine sulfate (Oncovin)	IV; 1.4 mg/m^2 q week (max 2 mg/m^2)
vinorelbine tartrate (Navelbine)	IV; 30 mg/m^2 q week
Taxoids	
docetaxel (Taxotere)	IV; 60–100 mg/m^2 q 3 wk
paclitaxel (Taxol)	IV; 135–175 mg/m^2 q 3 wk
Topoisomerase Inhibitors	
etoposide (VePesid)	IV; 50–100 mg/m^2 qd for 5 d
teniposide (Vumon)	IV; 165 mg/m^2 q 3–4 d for 4 wk
irinotecan hydrochloride (Camptosar)	IV; 125 mg/m^2 q week for 4 wk
topotecan hydrochloride (Hycamtin)	IV; 1.5 mg/m^2 qd for 5 d

throughout the western United States. Over 19 different taxane alkaloids have been isolated from the tree and several are being investigated for potential antineoplastic activity. Paclitaxel is approved for metastatic ovarian and breast cancer and for Kaposi's sarcoma. Unlabeled uses include many other cancers. A semisynthetic product of paclitaxel, docetaxel is claimed to have greater antitumor properties, with lower toxicity. Bone marrow toxicity is usually the dose-limiting factor for the taxoids. Like the vinca alkaloids, the taxoids are mitotic inhibitors.

American Indians described uses of the May apple or wild mandrake (*Podophyllum peltatum*) long before pharmacologists isolated podophyllotoxin, the active ingredient in the plant. As a botanical, podophyllum has been used as an antidote for snakebites, a cathartic, and a topical treatment for warts. Teniposide (Vumon) and etoposide (VePesid) are semisynthetic products of podophyllotoxin. These agents act by inhibiting topoisomerase I, an enzyme that helps repair DNA damage. By binding in a complex with topoisomerase and DNA, these antineoplastics cause strand breaks that accumulate and cause permanent damage to the DNA. Etoposide is approved for refractory testicular carcinoma, small oat-cell carcinoma of the lung, and choriocarcinoma. Teniposide is approved only for refractory acute lymphoblastic leukemia in children. Bone marrow toxicity is the primary dose-limiting side effect.

Other recently isolated topoisomerase I inhibitors include topotecan (Hycamtin) and irinotecan (Camptosar). These agents are called camptothecins because they were first isolated from *Camptotheca acuminata*, a tree native to China. The camptothecins are only administered intravenously, and their use is limited. Topotecan is approved for metastatic ovarian cancer and small-cell lung cancer after failure of initial chemotherapy. Irinotecan is indicated for metastatic cancer of the colon or rectum. Like many other cytotoxic natural products, bone marrow suppression is the dose-limiting toxicity for the camptothecins.

NURSING CONSIDERATIONS

The role of the nurse in natural plant extract therapy involves careful monitoring of a patient's condition and providing education as it relates to the prescribed drug regimen. Before initiating chemotherapy, the nurse should assess baseline vital signs, the complete blood count, and the patient's overall health status, including renal and liver function, intake and output, and body weight.

Because natural plant extracts may produce allergic reactions in susceptible individuals, the nurse should interview the patient regarding any allergy to plants or flowers, including herbs or foods, which may provide clues to possible hypersensitivity to these drugs. Infusion hypersensitivity is an adverse reaction, which may be ameliorated by steroid therapy. Vincristine (Oncovin) may produce acute bronchospasm and skin rashes. The nurse should inquire regarding pregnancy and lactation as many of these agents are contraindicated in pregnancy. Vincristine is contraindicated in patients with obstructive jaundice and those with demyelinating forms of Charcot-Marie-Tooth disease.

These drugs produce many of the same cytotoxic effects as other antineoplastics, including alopecia, fatigue, nausea, vomiting, diarrhea, bone marrow suppression, and blood dyscrasias. Natural product antineoplastics should also be used cautiously in many existing conditions, such as seizure disorders; vincristine may lower the seizure threshold. Vincristine should also be used cautiously in patients with leukopenia, neuromuscular disease, and hypertension. Nat-ural products may cause muscle weakness, peripheral neuropathy (including nerve pain), and paralytic ileus. The nurse should emphasize the need to establish a nutritional plan to combat constipation, including high fluid and fiber intake. Natural product antineoplastics can affect blood pressure, causing either hypotension or hypertension. The nurse should observe the patient for symptoms such as headache, dizziness, or syncope. These drugs may produce severe mental depression; thus, the nurse should remain alert to the possibility of suicidal ideation. Referrals for spiritual or emotional care such as a chaplain, mental health nurse, or social worker should be offered.

Patient education as it relates to plant extract antineoplastics should include goals of therapy; reasons for obtaining baseline data such as vital signs, blood work, and renal and liver function tests; and possible side effects. Following are important points the nurse should include when teaching patients regarding this class of drugs.

- Seek emergency medical treatment for signs of severe allergic reaction: shortness of breath, thick tongue, throat tightness or difficulty swallowing, or rash.
- Seek medical treatment for severe convulsions or suicide risk, such as feelings of despair, verbalized suicide plan, or attempt.
- Immediately report the following: muscle weakness; difficulty walking or talking; visual disturbances; stomach, bone, or joint pain; swelling, especially in the legs or ankles; rectal bleeding; or significant changes in bowel habits.
- Avoid using OTC suppositories and taking rectal temperatures.
- Avoid activities requiring physical stamina until effects of the drug are known.
- Obtain assistance with walking if weakness or staggering gait is a problem.
- Maintain good bowel habits including adequate fluid and fiber intake.

Please refer to "Nursing Process Focus: Patients Receiving Antineoplastic Therapy" for additional teaching points.

Antitumor Hormones and Hormone Antagonists

Hormones significantly affect the growth of some tumors. Use of natural or synthetic hormones or their antagonists as antineoplastic agents is a strategy used to slow the growth of hormone-dependent tumors.

35.12 Pharmacotherapy with Antitumor Hormones and Hormone Antagonists

A number of hormones are used in cancer chemotherapy, including glucocorticoids, estrogens, and androgens. In addition, several hormone antagonists have been found to exhibit antitumor activity. The mechanism of hormone antineoplastic activity is largely unknown. It is likely, however, that these antitumor properties are independent of their

Pr PROTOTYPE DRUG | VINCRISTINE (Oncovin)

ACTIONS AND USES

Vincristine is a cell-cycle-specfic agent that affects rapidly growing cells by preventing their ability to complete mitosis. It is thought to exert this action by inhibiting microtubule formation in the mitotic spindle. Although it must be given intravenously, a major advantage of vincristine is that it causes minimal immunosuppression. It has a wider spectrum of clinical activity than vinblastine, and is usually prescribed in combination with other antineoplastics for the treatment of Hodgkin's and non-Hodgkin's lymphomas, leukemias, Kaposi's sarcoma, Wilms' tumor, bladder carcinoma, and breast carcinoma.

Administration Alerts

- Extravasation, could result in serious tissue damage. Stop injection immediately if extravasation occurs. Apply local heat and inject hyaluronidase as ordered. Observe site for sloughing.
- Avoid eye contact which causes severe irritation and corneal changes.
- Pregnancy category D.

ADVERSE EFFECTS AND INTERACTIONS

The most serious limiting adverse effects of vincristine relate to nervous system toxicity. Children are particularly susceptible. Symptoms include numbness and tingling in the limbs, muscular weakness, loss of neural reflexes, and pain. Paralytic ileus may occur in young children. Severe constipation is common. Reversible alopecia occurs in most patients.

Vincristine interacts with many drugs. For example, asparaginase used concurrently with or before vincristine may cause increased neurotoxicity secondary to decreased hepatic clearance of vincristine. Doxorubicin or prednisone may increase bone marrow depression. Calcium channel blockers may increase vincristine accumulation in cells. Concurrent use of digoxin may decrease digoxin levels, so the patient may need increased digoxin dose. When vincristine is given with methotrexate, the patient may need lower doses of methotrexate. Vincristine may decrease serum phenytoin levels, leading to increased seizure activity.

 See the companion website for a Nursing Process Focus specific to this drug.

normal hormone mechanisms, as the doses utilized in cancer chemotherapy are magnitudes larger than the amount normally present in the body. Only the antitumor properties of these hormones are discussed in this section; for other indications and actions, the student should refer to other chapters in this text. The antitumor hormones are shown in Table 35.8.

In general, the hormones and hormone antagonists act by blocking substances needed for tumor growth. Because these agents are not cytotoxic, they produce few of the debilitating side effects seen with other antineoplastics. They can, however, produce significant side effects when given at high doses for prolonged periods. Because they rarely produce cancer cures when used singly, they are normally given for palliation.

The primary adrenocortical hormones used in chemotherapy are dexamethasone and prednisone (Deltasone, others). Because of their natural ability to suppress lymphocytes, the principal value of the glucocorticoids is in the treatment of lymphomas, Hodgkin's disease, and leukemias. They are sometimes given to reduce the nausea, weight loss, and tissue inflammation caused by other antineoplastics. Prolonged use can result in symptoms of Cushing's disease.

The sex hormones are used to treat tumors that contain specific hormone receptors. Two androgens, fluoxymesterone (Halotestin) and testolactone (Teslac), are used for breast cancer in postmenopausal women. The estrogens ethinyl estradiol and diethylstilbestrol (DES) are used to treat metastatic breast cancer and prostate cancer. The progestins medroxyprogesterone and megestrol (Megace) are used to treat endometrial cancer.

Hormone inhibitors include the antiandrogens bicalutamide (Casodex), nilutamide (Nilandron), and flutamide (Eulexin), which are prescribed for advanced prostate cancer. Antiestrogens include tamoxifen (Nolvadex) and anastrozole (Armidex), which are indicated for breast cancer. Anastrozole, letrozole (Femara), and exemestane (Aromasin) are called aromatase inhibitors, because they block the enzyme aromatase, which normally converts adrenal androgen to estradiol. Aromatase inhibitors can reduce plasma estrogen levels by as much as 95%, and are used in postmenopausal women with advanced breast cancer whose disease has progressed beyond tamoxifen therapy.

NURSING CONSIDERATIONS

The role of the nurse in antitumor hormone and hormone antagonist therapy involves careful monitoring of a patient's condition and providing education as it relates to the prescribed drug regimen. Before initiating chemotherapy, the nurse should assess baseline vital signs, the complete blood count, and the patient's overall health status, including renal and liver function, intake and output, and body weight. The nurse should assess for pregnancy and breastfeeding, as both are contraindicated with the antitumor hormones and hormone antagonists.

Therapy using hormones other than tamoxifen (Nolvadex) may be palliative rather than curative; it is important that both patient and family understand this limitation before beginning chemotherapy. They must understand that while the patient may appear to be improving, the cancer is likely continuing to worsen.

Table 35.8	Hormone and Hormone Antagonists Used for Neoplasia
Drug	**Route and Adult Dose (max dose where indicated)**
Hormones	
dexamethasone (Decadron, others)	PO; 0.25 mg bid-qid
diethylstilbestrol (DES, Stilbestrol)	PO; for treatment of prostate cancer, 500 mg tid; for pallation,1–15 mg qd
ethinyl estradiol (Estinyl, others)	PO; for treatment of breast cancer, 1 mg tid for 2–3 months; for palliation of prostate cancer, 0.15–3 mg/day
fluoxymesterone (Halotestin)	PO; 10 mg tid
medroxyprogesterone (Provera, Depo-Provera) (see 618 for the Prototype Drug box) 🔗	IM; 400–1,000 mg q week
megestrol (Megace)	PO; 40–160 mg bid-qid
prednisone (Deltasone, others) (see 423 for the Prototype Drug box) 🔗	PO; 20–100 mg/m^2 qd
testolactone (Teslac)	PO; 250 mg qid
testosterone (Andro, Histerone, Testred, Delatest, others) (see 630 for the Prototype Drug box) 🔗	IM; 200–400 mg q 2–4 weeks
Hormone Antagonists	
aminoglutethimide (Cytadren)	PO; 250 mg bid-qid
anastrozole (Arimidex)	PO; 1 mg qd
bicalutamide (Casodex)	PO; 50 mg qd
exemestane (Aromasin)	PO; 25 mg qd after a meal
flutamide (Eulexin)	PO; 250 mg tid
fulvestrant (Faslodex)	IM; 250 mg once
goserelin (Zoladex)	SC 3.6 mg q 28 days
letrozole (Femara)	PO; 2.5 mg qd
leuprolide (Eligard, Lupron)	SC; 1 mg qd
nilutamide (Nilandron)	PO; 300 mg d for 30 days, then 150 mg qd
PT tamoxifen citrate (Nolvadex)	PO; 10–20 mg 1–2 times/d (morning and evening)
toremifene (Fareston)	PO; 60 mg qd

One of the most common yet distressing side effects of sex hormone therapy is the development of cross-gender secondary sexual characteristics, such as gynecomastia in males and hirsutism in females. Fertility is sometimes affected. The nurse should discuss these effects frankly with the patient and offer support and simple interventions to increase self-esteem. The nurse may discuss clothing options to disguise gynecomastia or methods of facial hair removal, such as waxes or depilatories.

The use of glucocorticoids may increase the risk of sexually transmitted diseases and other infections, by suppressing the immune response. Glucocorticoid therapy may cause swelling, weight gain, redistribution of body fat (Cushing's syndrome), and hyperglycemia. The nurse should discuss body image concerns as well, and nutritional strategies to increase energy and limit weight gain. Weight gain remains a concern for a number of cancer patients—especially in the early phases of the disease. In some cases, cancer patients who are experiencing cachexia may benefit from glucocorticoid-induced weight gain. Glucocorticoids should be administered with caution to patients with diabetes mellitus. The nurse should obtain results of laboratory blood tests, including serum glucose, hormone levels, and electrolytes.

Patient education as it relates to hormone therapy for cancer should include therapeutic goals; reasons for obtaining baseline data such as vital signs and tests for cardiac, renal, and endocrine disorders; and possible side effects. If the patient is diabetic, teach to monitor blood glucose more frequently; the patient may need adjustments in antidiabetic medications. Instruct patient to report serum blood glucose readings as ordered by the healthcare provider (e.g., "less than 60 mg/dl or more than 220 mg/dl").

Following are other important points the nurse should include when teaching patients regarding hormonal therapy for cancer.

PROTOTYPE DRUG | **TAMOXIFEN** (Nolvadex)

ACTIONS AND USES

Tamoxifen is given orally and is a drug of choice for treating metastatic breast cancer. It is sometimes classified as a selective estrogen receptor modulator (SERM). Tamoxifen is effective against breast tumors that require estrogen for their growth. These susceptible cancer cells are known as estrogen receptor (ER) positive cells. While it blocks estrogen receptors on breast cancer cells, tamoxifen actually activates estrogen receptors in other parts of the body. This results in typical estrogen-like effects such as reduced LDL levels and increased mineral density of bone. The drug is unique among antineoplastics, because it is given not only to patients with breast cancer but also to high-risk patients to prevent the disease. Few if any other antineoplastics are given prophylactically, due to their toxicity.

Administration Alerts

- Give with food or fluids to decrease GI irritation.
- Do not crush or chew drug.
- Avoid antacid for 1 to 2 hours following PO dosage of tamoxifen.
- Pregnancy category D.

 See the companion website for a Nursing Process Focus specific to this drug.

ADVERSE EFFECTS AND INTERACTIONS

Other than nausea and vomiting, tamoxifen produces little of the serious toxicity observed with other antineoplastics. Of concern, however, is the association of tamoxifen therapy with an increased risk of endometrial cancer and thromboembolic disease. Hot flashes, fluid retention, and vaginal discharges are relatively common. Patients experiencing abnormal vaginal bleeding or menstrual irregularities during therapy should be evaluated promptly. Tamoxifen causes initial "tumor flare"—an idiosyncratic increase in tumor size, but this is an expected therapeutic event.

Tamoxifen interacts with several other drugs. For example, anticoagulants taken concurrently may increase the risk of of bleeding. Concurrent use with cytotoxic agents may increase the risk of thromboembolism.

- Immediately report the following: shortness of breath, chest pain, difficulty with urination (too much, too little, pain, or irritation), excessive thirst, bleeding or injuries, sore throat, fever, or other signs of infection.
- Avoid persons with active infections.
- Practice excellent oral hygiene and skin care.

Please refer to "Nursing Process Focus: Patients Receiving Antineoplastic Therapy" for additional teaching points.

Biologic Response Modifiers and Miscellaneous Antineoplastics

Biologic response modifiers approach cancer treatment from a different perspective than other chemotherapeutic agents. Rather than being cytotoxic to cancer cells, they stimulate the patient's own immune system to fight the cancer.

35.13 Pharmacotherapy with Biologic Response Modifiers and Miscellaneous Antineoplastics

Certain anticancer drugs act through mechanisms other than those previously described. For example, asparaginase (Elspar) deprives cancer cells of asparagine, an essential amino acid and is used for acute lymphocytic leukemia. Mitotane (Lysodren), similar to the insecticide DDT, poisons cancer cells by forming links to proteins, and is used for advanced adrenocortical cancer. One of the newest antineoplastics, imatinib (Gleevec), inhibits the enzyme tyrosine

SPECIAL CONSIDERATIONS

Chemotherapy in the Elderly

The elderly population has a higher incidence of most types of cancer. This could be a result of a greater accumulation of carcinogenic effects over time and age-related reduction in immune system function.

Due to age-related changes, such as decreasing mobility of the myeloid cells from the bone marrow to bloodstream, elderly patients with cancer are not likely to respond as effectively to stress that would normally trigger hematopoiesis. This in turn results in greater susceptibility to bone marrow suppression. Patient teaching of the elderly and their caregivers should include the following:

- Elderly patients receiving chemotherapy drugs may experience toxic effects from the binding of the drugs to red blood cells at a higher rate due to normal age-related factors of fewer circulating red blood cells. Inform the patient to report and monitor any bleeding or bruising and to avoid all aspirin products.
- For reduction of neutropenia and prevention of infection, instruct the patient in the importance of a daily regimen, including monitoring temperature and avoiding antipyretics to reduce fever before calling healthcare provider. Instruct the patient to avoid crowds and people with respiratory infections. The patient and caregivers should be instructed to use frequent handwashing to prevent the transmission of pathogens.
- Because older adults often have deficient nutritional intake, teach the patient and caregivers regarding healthy food choices and assess for the patient's ability to swallow foods and medications.
- Constipation may occur due to a decrease in elimination pattern. Encourage the patient to obtain adequate fluid intake and to increase dietary fiber by using grains and leafy vegetables.

NURSING PROCESS FOCUS PATIENTS RECEIVING ANTINEOPLASTIC THERAPY

ASSESSMENT

Prior to administration:
- Obtain complete health history including lab values such as platelets, Hct, leukocyte count, liver and kidney function tests, and serum electrolytes.
- Obtain drug history to determine possible drug interactions and allergies.
- Assess neurological status including mood and/or sensory impairment.
- Assess for history or presence of herpes zoster or chickenpox. (Immunosuppressive effects of cyclophosphamide and vincristine can cause life-threatening exacerbations.)

POTENTIAL NURSING DIAGNOSES

- Risk for Infection, related to compromised immune system
- Imbalanced Nutrition, Less than Body Requirements, related to nausea, vomiting, diarrhea, anorexia as a result of drug side effects
- Impaired Skin Integrity, related to extravasation
- Risk for Disturbed Body Image, related to physical changes as a result of drug side effects
- Fatigue, related to side effects of drug

PLANNING: PATIENT GOALS AND EXPECTED OUTCOMES

The patient will:
- Experience a reduction in tumor mass and/or progression of abnormal cell growth
- Demonstrate an understanding of the drug's action by accurately describing drug side effects, precautions, and therapeutic goals

IMPLEMENTATION

Interventions and (Rationales)

- Monitor hematological/immune status.
- Observe for signs and symptoms of myelosuppression. (This could be indicative of overdose.)
- Monitor complete blood count and temperature.
- Collect stool samples for guaiac testing of occult blood. (Antineoplastics may cause anemia.)

Patient Education/Discharge Planning

Instruct patient to:
- Immediately report profound fatigue, fever, sore throat, epigastric pain, coffee-grounds vomit, bruising, tarry stools, or frank bleeding
- Avoid consuming aspirin
- Avoid persons with active infections
- Monitor vital signs (especially temperature) daily, ensuring proper use of home equipment
- Anticipate fatigue and balance daily activities to prevent exhaustion
- Avoid activities requiring mental alertness and physical strength until effects of the drug are known

---

- Monitor cardiorespiratory status.
- Monitor vital signs and chest/heart sounds. (Cyclophosphamide may cause myopericarditis and lung fibrosis. Doxorubicin may cause sinus tachycardia, cardiac depression, and delayed onset CHF.)
- Observe EKG for T-wave flattening, ST depression, or voltage reduction.
- Monitor for shortness of breath and pitting edema.

Instruct patient:
- To immediately report dyspnea; chest, arm, neck, or back pain; tachycardia; cough; frothy sputum; swelling; or activity intolerance
- To maintain a regular schedule of EKGs as advised by the healthcare provider
- That heart changes may be a sign of drug toxicity; HF may not appear for up to 6 months after completion of doxorubicin therapy

---

- Monitor renal status, urinary output, intake and output, and daily weights. (Cyclophosphamide may cause renal toxicity and/or hemorrhagic cystitis. Vincristine and methotrexate increase uric acid levels, contributing to renal calculi and gout. Vincristine may also cause water retention and highly concentrated urine.)

Instruct patient:
- To immediately report the following: changes in thirst; color, quantity, and character of urine (e.g., "cloudy," with odor or sediment); joint, abdominal, flank, or lower back pain; difficult urination; and weight gain
- That doxorubicin will turn urine red-brown for 1 to 2 days after administration; blood in the urine may occur several months after cyclophosphamide has been discontinued
- To consume 3 L of fluid on the day before treatment and daily for 72 hr after (when patient has no prescribed fluid restriction)

continued

NURSING PROCESS FOCUS: *Patients Receiving Antineoplastic Therapy (continued)*

Interventions and (Rationales)	Patient Education/Discharge Planning
■ Monitor GI status and nutrition. Administer antiemetics 30 to 45 minutes prior to antineoplastic administration or at the first sign of nausea. (Profound nausea, dry heaves, and/or vomiting are common with antineoplastic therapy. Dry mouth can also occur.)	Instruct patient to: ■ Report loss of appetite, nausea/vomiting, diarrhea, mouth redness, soreness, or ulcers ■ Consume frequent small meals, drink plenty of cold liquids; avoid strong odors and spicy foods to control nausea ■ Examine mouth daily for changes ■ Use a soft toothbrush; avoid toothpicks
■ Monitor for constipation. (Ileus or constipation and fecal impaction may occur with vincristine use, especially among the elderly.)	Instruct patient to: ■ Report changes in bowel habits ■ Increase activity, fiber, and fluids to reduce constipation
■ Monitor neurological/sensory status. (Antineoplastics may cause peripheral neuropathy and mental depression. Vincristine may cause ataxia and hand/foot drop. Tamoxifen may cause photophobia and decreased vision. Such neurological changes may be irreversible.)	Instruct patient to: ■ Report changes in skin color, vision, hearing, numbness or tingling, staggering gait, or depressed mood; obtain no self-harm contract ■ Limit sun exposure; wear sun screen, sunglasses, and long sleeves when outdoors
■ Monitor genitourinary status. (Antineoplastic agents, including hormones, and especially tamoxifen, may alter menstrual cycles in women and may produce impotence in men. Tamoxifen increases the risk of endometrial cancer.)	Instruct patient to: ■ Report changes in menstruation, sexual functioning and/or vaginal discharge ■ Recognize the risk of endometrial cancer before giving tamoxifen
■ Monitor for hypersensitivity or other adverse reactions.	■ Instruct patient to immediately report chest or throat tightness, difficulty swallowing, swelling (especially facial), abdominal pain, headache or dizziness
■ Monitor hair and skin status. (Alopecia is associated with most chemotherapy and may be a sign of overdosage. Methotrexate can cause a variety of skin eruptions.)	Instruct patient to: ■ Immediately report desquamation of skin on hands and feet, rash, pruritus, acne, or boils ■ Wear a cold gel cap during chemotherapy to minimize hair loss
■ Monitor for conjunctivitis. (Doxorubicin may cause conjunctivitis.)	■ Instruct patient or caregiver to immediately report eye redness, stickiness, or pain or weeping.
■ Monitor liver function tests. (Antineoplastics are metabolized by the liver, increasing the risk of hepatotoxicity.)	Instruct patient to: ■ Report jaundice, abdominal pain, tenderness or bloating, or change in stool color ■ Adhere to laboratory testing regimen for serum blood level tests of liver enzymes as directed
■ Administer with caution to patients with diabetes mellitus. (Hypoglycemia may occur secondary to combination of cyclophosphamide and insulin.)	Instruct patient to: ■ Report signs and symptoms of hypoglycemia (e.g., sudden weakness, tremors) ■ Monitor blood glucose daily; consult the healthcare provider regarding reportable results (e.g., less than 70 mg/dl)

EVALUATION OF OUTCOME CRITERIA

Evaluate the effectiveness of drug therapy by confirming that patient goals and expected outcomes have been met (see "Planning").

⊂⊃ See Tables 35.2 through 35.8 for lists of drugs to which these nursing actions apply.

Table 35.9	Biologic Response Modifiers and Miscellaneous Antineoplastics
Drug	**Route and Adult Dose (max dose where indicated)**
alemtuzumab (Campath)	IV; 3–30 mg qd
altretamine (Hexalen)	PO; 65 mg/m^2 qd
arsenic trioxide (Trisenox)	IV; 0.15 mg/kg qd (max 60 doses)
asparaginase (Elspar)	IV; 200 IU/kg qd
bexarotene (Targretin)	PO; 100–400 mg/m^2 qd; topical; 1% gel applied to lesion qd-qid
bortezomib (Velcade)	IV; 1.3 mg/m^3 as bolus twice weekly for 2 weeks
gefitinib (Iressa)	PO; 250 mg qd
gemtuzumab ozogamicin (Mylotarg)	IV; 9 mg/m^2 for 2 hr
hydroxyurea (Hydrea)	PO; 20–30 mg/kg qd
imatinib mesylate (Gleevec)	PO; 400–600 mg qd
interferon alfa-2 (Roferon-A, Intron A) (see 410 for the Prototype Drug box)	SC/IM; 2–3 million units qd for leukemia; increase to 36 million units qd for Kaposi's sarcoma
levamisole (Ergamisol)	PO; 50 mg tid for 3 d
mitotane (Lysodren)	PO; 3–4 mg tid-qid
pegaspargase (Oncaspar, PEG-L-asparaginase)	IV; 2,500 IU/m^2 q 14 d
procarbazine (Matulane)	PO; 2–4 mg/kg qd
rituximab (Rituxan)	IV; 375 mg/m^2 qd as a continuous infusion
trastuzumab (Herceptin)	IV; 4 mg/kg as a single dose, then 2 mg/kg q wk
tositumomab (Bexxar)	IV; 450 mg over 60 minutes
zoledronic acid (Zometa)	IV; 4 mg over at least 15 minutes

kinase in chronic myeloid leukemia cells and shows promise for treating other cancers. These agents are shown in Table 35.9.

Biologic response modifiers are a relatively new class of medications that do not kill tumor cells directly but instead stimulate the body's immune system. When given concurrently with other antineoplastics, biologic response modifiers help to limit the severe immunosuppressive effects caused by other agents. Refer to Chapter 30 for additional information on the biologic response modifiers, and for a drug prototype for Interferon alfa-2 (Roferon-A, Intron A).

CHAPTER REVIEW

Key Concepts

The numbered key concepts provide a succinct summary of the important points from the corresponding numbered section within the chapter. If any of these points are not clear, refer to the numbered section within the chapter for review. Expanded versions can be found on the companion website.

35.1 Cancer is characterized by rapid, uncontrolled growth of cells that invade normal tissues and eventually metastasize. Benign neoplasms are slow growing and rarely result in death; however, malignant neoplasms are fast growing and often fatal.

35.2 The causes of cancer may be chemical, physical, or biological.

35.3 Cancer may be treated using surgery, radiation therapy, and drugs.

35.4 The growth fraction, the percentage of cancer cells undergoing mitosis at any given time, is a major factor determining success of chemotherapy.

35.5 To achieve a total cure, every malignant cell must be removed or killed through surgery, radiation, drugs, or by the patient's own immune system.

35.6 Use of multiple drugs and special dosing protocols are strategies that allow for lower doses, fewer side effects, and greater success of chemotherapy.

35.7 Serious toxicity, including thrombocytopenia, anemia, leukopenia, alopecia, and severe nausea, vomiting, and diarrhea, limits therapy with most antineoplastic agents.

35.8 Alkylating agents act by changing the structure of DNA in cancer cells. Some have a very broad spectrum of clinical activity.

35.9 Antimetabolites act by disrupting critical pathways in cancer cells, such as folate or DNA metabolism.

35.10 Due to their cytotoxicity, a few antibiotics are used to treat cancer by inhibiting cell growth. They have a narrow spectrum of clinical activity.

35.11 Some plant extracts have been isolated that kill cancer cells by preventing cell division.

35.12 Some hormones and hormone antagonists are noncytotoxic agents that are effective against reproductive-related tumors such as breast, prostate, or uterus. They are less cytotoxic, than other antineoplastics.

35.13 Biologic response modifiers and some additional antineoplastic drugs have been found to be effective against tumors by stimulating the patient's immune system.

Review Questions

1. What is the fundamental feature that makes a cancer cell different from a normal cell?

2. Why is it important to kill or remove 100% of the cancer cells to effect a cure?

3. Why is combination therapy with antineoplastics more successful than monotherapy?

Critical Thinking Questions

1. A patient is newly diagnosed with cancer and is about to start on chemotherapy. What would be the priority teaching for this patient?

2. The chemotherapy medications often cause neutropenia in the cancer patient. What would be a priority for the nurse to teach this patient who is at home receiving outpatient chemotherapy?

3. A nurse is taking chemotherapy IV medication to a patient's room and the IV bag suddenly leaks solution (approximately 50 ml) on the floor. What action should the nurse take?

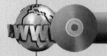

EXPLORE MediaLink

NCLEX review, case studies, and other interactive resources for this chapter can be found on the companion website at www.prenhall.com/adams. Click on "Chapter 35" to select the activities for this chapter. For animations, more NCLEX review questions, and an audio glossary, access the accompanying CD-ROM in this textbook.

The Gastrointestinal System

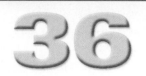

CHAPTER 36

Drugs for Peptic Ulcer Disease

DRUGS AT A GLANCE

H₂-RECEPTOR ANTAGONISTS
ranitidine (Zantac)

PROTON PUMP INHIBITORS
omeprazole (Prilosec)

ANTACIDS
aluminum hydroxide (Amphojel, others)

ANTIBIOTICS

MISCELLANEOUS AGENTS

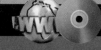

MediaLink www.prenhall.com/adams

CD-ROM

Animation:
   Mechanism in Action: Ranitidine (Zantac)
Audio Glossary
NCLEX Review

Companion Website

NCLEX Review
Dosage Calculations
Case Study
Care Plans
Expanded Key Concepts

OBJECTIVES

After reading this chapter, the student should be able to:

1. Describe the major anatomical structures of the upper gastrointestinal tract.
2. Identify common causes, signs, and symptoms of peptic ulcer disease.
3. Compare and contrast duodenal ulcers and gastric ulcers.
4. Identify the classification of drugs used to treat peptic ulcer disease.
5. Explain why two or more antibiotics are used concurrently in the treatment of *H. pylori*.
6. Describe the nurse's role in the pharmacologic management of patients with peptic ulcer disease.
7. For each of the classes listed in Drugs at a Glance, know representative drugs, explain their mechanism of drug action, describe primary actions, and identify important adverse effects.
8. Categorize drugs used in the treatment of peptic ulcer disease based on their classification and mechanism of action.
9. Use the Nursing Process to care for patients who are receiving drug therapy for peptic ulcer disease.

MediaLink | Digestive Disorders

Very little of the food we eat is directly available to body cells. Food must be broken down, absorbed, and chemically modified before it is in a form useful to cells. The digestive system performs these functions, and more. Some disorders of the digestive system are mechanical in nature, slowing or accelerating the transit of food through the gastrointestinal tract. Others are metabolic, affecting the secretion of digestive fluids or the absorption of essential nutrients. Many signs and symptoms are nonspecific and may be caused by any number of different disorders. This chapter will examine the pharmacotherapy of common diseases of the upper digestive system.

PHARMFACTS | Gastrointestinal Tract Disorders

- Colorectal cancer is the second leading cause of cancer deaths, killing more than 55,000 Americans annually.
- About 140,000 new cases of colorectal cancer occur each year.
- Over 400,000 new cases of peptic ulcer disease are diagnosed each year.
- Ulcers are responsible for about 40,000 surgeries annually.
- About 6,000 people die annually of ulcer-related complications.
- Nonsteriodal anti-inflammatory agents such as Advil and Motrin are commonly used by teenage girls and college-age women to control menstrual cramps. As a result of improper use and failure to control discomfort with lifestyle modification measures, gastroenterology consults are rising to epidemic proportions in this population.

36.1 Normal Digestive Processes

The digestive system consists of two basic anatomical divisions: the alimentary canal and the accessory organs. The **alimentary canal**, or gastrointestinal (GI) tract, is a long, continuous, hollow tube that extends from the mouth to the anus. The accessory organs of digestion include the salivary glands, liver, gallbladder, and pancreas. Major structures of the digestive system are illustrated in Figure 36.1.

Digestion is the process by which ingested food is broken down to small molecules that can be absorbed. The primary functions of the GI tract are to physically transport ingested food and to provide the necessary enzymes and surface area for chemical digestion and absorption.

The inner lining of the alimentary canal is the **mucosa layer**, which provides a surface area for the various acids, bases, mucus, and enzymes to break down food. In many parts of the alimentary canal, the mucosa is folded and contains deep grooves and pits. The small intestine is lined

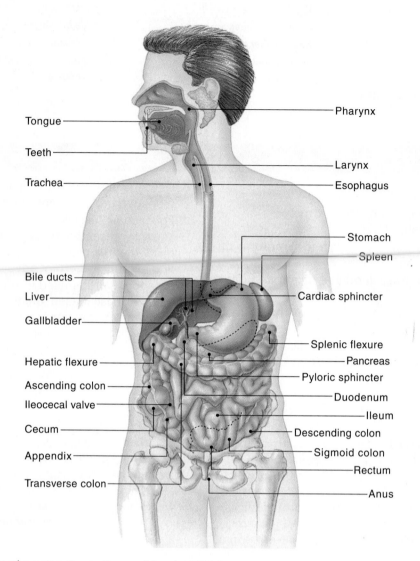

Figure 36.1 | The digestive system *Source: Pearson Education/PH College.*

with tiny projections called villi and microvilli which provide a huge surface area for the absorption of food and medications.

Substances are propelled along the GI tract by **peristalsis**, rhythmic contractions of layers of smooth muscle. The speed at which substances move through the GI tract is critical to the absorption of nutrients and water and for the removal of wastes. If peristalsis is too fast, nutrients and drugs will not have sufficient contact with the mucosa to be absorbed. In addition, the large intestine will not have enough time to absorb water, and diarrhea may result. Abnormally slow transit may result in constipation or even obstructions in the small or large intestine. Disorders of the large intestine are discussed in Chapter 37 ⊙ .

To chemically break down ingested food, a large number of enzymes and other substances are required. Digestive enzymes are secreted by the salivary glands, stomach, small intestine, and pancreas. The liver makes bile, which is stored in the gallbladder, until needed for lipid digestion.

Because these digestive substances are not common targets for drug therapy, their discussion in this chapter is limited, and the student should refer to anatomy and physiology texts for additional information.

36.2 Acid Production by the Stomach

Food passes from the esophagus to the stomach by traveling through the lower esophageal (cardiac) sphincter. This ring of smooth muscle usually prevents the stomach contents from moving backwards, a condition known as **esophageal reflux**. A second ring of smooth muscle, the pyloric sphincter, is located at the entrance to the small intestine. This sphincter regulates the flow of substances leaving the stomach.

The stomach thoroughly mixes ingested food and secretes substances that promote the process of chemical digestion. Gastric glands extending deep into the mucosa of the stomach contain several cell types critical to digestion and the pharmacotherapy of digestive disorders. **Chief cells** secrete pepsinogen, an inactive form of the enzyme pepsin that chemically breaks down proteins. **Parietal cells** secrete 1 to 3 L of hydrochloric acid each day. This strong acid helps to break down food, activates pepsinogen, and kills microbes that may have been ingested. Parietal cells also secrete **intrinsic factor**, which is essential for the absorption of vitamin B_{12} (Chapter 38)⬅⮕.

The combined secretion of the chief cells and parietal cells, gastric juice, is the most acidic fluid in the body, having a pH of 1.5 to 3.5. A number of natural defenses protect the stomach mucosa against this extremely acidic fluid. Certain cells lining the surface of the stomach secrete a thick mucous layer and bicarbonate ion to neutralize acid. These form such an effective protective layer that the pH at the mucosa surface is nearly neutral. Once reaching the duodenum, the stomach contents are further neutralized by bicarbonate from pancreatic and biliary secretions. These natural defenses are shown in Figure 36.2.

36.3 Pathogenesis of Peptic Ulcer Disease

An ulcer is an erosion of the mucosa layer of the GI tract, usually associated with acute inflammation. Although ulcers may occur in any portion of the alimentary canal, the duodenum is the most common site. The term **peptic ulcer** refers to a lesion located in either the stomach (gastric) or small intestine (duodenal). Peptic ulcer disease (PUD) is associated with the following risk factors.

- Close family history of peptic ulcer disease
- Blood group O
- Smoking tobacco
- Beverages and food containing caffeine
- Drugs, particularly glucocorticoids, aspirin, and NSAIDs
- Excessive psychological stress
- Infection with *Helicobacter pylori*

The primary cause of PUD is infection by the gram negative bacterium *Helicobacter pylori*. In noninfected patients, duodenal ulcers are commonly caused by drug therapy with NSAIDs. Secondary factors that contribute to the ulcer and its subsequent inflammation include hypersecretion of gastric acid and hyposecretion of adequate mucous protection. Figure 36.3 illustrates the mechanism of peptic ulcer formation.

The characteristic symptom of duodenal ulcer is a gnawing or burning, upper abdominal pain that occurs 1 to 3 hours after a meal. The pain disappears upon ingestion of food, and nighttime pain, nausea, and vomiting are uncommon. If the erosion progresses deeper into the mucosa, bleeding occurs and may be evident as either bright red blood in vomit or black, tarry stools. Many duodenal ulcers heal spontaneously, although they frequently reoccur after months of remission. Long-term medical follow-up is usually not necessary.

Gastric ulcers are less common than the duodenal type and have different symptoms. Although relieved by food, pain may continue even after a meal. Loss of appetite, known as anorexia, as well as weight loss and vomiting are more common. Remissions may be infrequent or absent. Medical follow-up of gastric ulcers should continue for several years, because a small percentage of the erosions

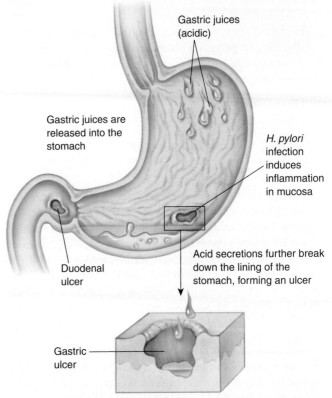

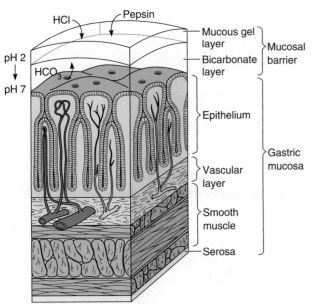

Figure 36.2 | Natural defenses against stomach acid

Figure 36.3 | Mechanism of peptic ulcer formation *Source: Pearson Education/PH College.*

become cancerous. The most severe ulcers may penetrate through the wall of the stomach and cause death. Whereas duodenal ulcers occur most frequently in the 30- to 50-year age group, gastric ulcers are more common over age 60.

Ulceration in the lower small intestine is known as Crohn's disease and erosions in the large intestine are called ulcerative colitis. These diseases, together categorized as inflammatory bowel disease, are discussed in Chapter 37 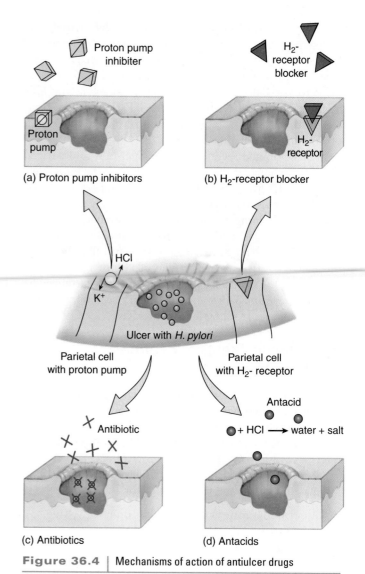.

36.4 Pathogenesis of Gastroesophageal Reflux Disease

Gastroesophageal reflux disease (GERD) is a common condition in which the acidic contents of the stomach move upward into the esophagus. This causes an intense burning (heartburn) and may lead to ulcers in the esophagus.

The cause of GERD is usually a weakening of the lower esophageal sphincter. The sphincter may no longer close tightly, allowing the contents of the stomach to move upward when the stomach contracts. GERD is associated with obesity, and losing weight may eliminate the symptoms. Many of the drugs prescribed for peptic ulcers are also used to treat GERD, with the goal being to reduce gastric acid secretion. Because drugs provide only symptomatic relief, surgery may become necessary to eliminate the cause of GERD.

36.5 Pharmacotherapy of Peptic Ulcer Disease

Before initiating pharmacotherapy, patients are usually advised to change lifestyle factors that contribute to PUD or GERD. For example, eliminating tobacco and alcohol use and reducing stress often cause an ulcer to go into remission.

For patients requiring pharmacotherapy, a wide variety of both prescription and OTC drugs are available. These drugs fall into four primary classes, plus one miscellaneous group.

- H_2-receptor antagonists
- Proton pump inhibitors
- Antacids
- Antibiotics
- Miscellaneous drugs

The goals of pharmacotherapy are to provide immediate relief from symptoms, promote healing of the ulcer, and prevent future recurrence of the disease. The choice of medication depends on the source of the disease (infectious versus inflammatory), the severity of symptoms, and the convenience of OTC versus prescription drugs. The mechanisms of action of the four major drug classes for PUD are shown in Figure 36.4.

H_2-Receptor Antagonists

The discovery of the H_2-receptor antagonists in the 1970s marked a major breakthrough in the treatment of PUD. Since then, they have become available OTC and are often drugs of choice in the treatment of peptic ulcer disease. These agents are shown in Table 36.1.

(a) Proton pump inhibitors

(b) H_2-receptor blocker

(c) Antibiotics

(d) Antacids

Figure 36.4 | Mechanisms of action of antiulcer drugs

NATURAL THERAPIES | **Ginger's Tonic Effects on the GI Tract**

The use of ginger (*Zingiber officinalis*) for medicinal purposes dates back to antiquity in India and China. The active ingredients of ginger, and those that create its spicy flavor and pungent odor, are located in its roots or rhizomes. It is sometimes standardized according to its active substances, gingerols and shogaols. It is sold in pharmacies as dried ginger root powder, at a dose of 250 to 1,000 mg and is readily available at most grocery stores for home cooking. Ginger is one of the best studied herbs, and it appears to be useful for a number of digestive-related conditions. Perhaps its widest use is for treating nausea, including that caused from motion sickness, pregnancy morning sickness, and postoperative procedures. It has been shown to stimulate appetite, promote gastric secretions, and increase peristalsis. Its effects appear to be from direct action on the GI tract, rather than on the CNS. Ginger has no toxicity when used at recommended doses. Overdoses may lead to CNS depression, inhibition of platelet aggregation, and cardiotonic effects.

Table 36.1	H₂-Receptor Antagonists
Drug	**Route and Adult Dose (max dose where indicated)**
cimetidine (Tagamet)	PO; 300–400 mg bid-qd or 800 mg at hs for active ulcers; 300 mg bid or 400 mg at hs for ulcer prophylaxis
famotidine (Pepcid, Mylanta AP)	PO; 20 mg bid or 40 mg at hs for active ulcers; 20 mg at hs for ulcer prophylaxis
nizatidine (Axid)	PO; 300 mg at hs for active ulcers; 150 mg at hs for ulcer prophylaxis
ⓟ ranitidine (Zantac)	PO; 100–150 mg bid or 300 mg at hs for active ulcer; 150 mg at hs for ulcer prophylaxis

36.6 Pharmacotherapy with H₂-Receptor Antagonists

Histamine has two types of receptors: H₁ and H₂. Activation of H₁-receptors produces the classic symptoms of allergy, whereas the H₂-receptors are responsible for increasing acid secretion in the stomach. Cimetidine (Tagamet), the first H₂-receptor antagonist, and other drugs in this class, are quite effective at suppressing the volume and acidity of stomach acid. These drugs are used to treat the symptoms of both PUD and GERD, and several agents in this class are available OTC for the treatment of heartburn. Side effects of the H₂-receptor blockers are minor and rarely cause discontinuation of therapy.

NURSING CONSIDERATIONS

The role of the nurse in H₂-receptor antagonist therapy involves careful monitoring of a patient's condition and providing education as it relates to the prescribed drug regimen. Because some H₂-receptor blockers are available without prescription, the nurse should assess the patient's use of OTC formulations to avoid duplication of doses. If using OTC formulations, patients should be advised to seek medical attention if symptoms persist or reoccur. Persistent pain or heartburn may be symptoms of more serious disease that requires medical treatment. Drugs in this class are usually well tolerated. Cimetidine is used less frequently than other H₂-receptor antagonists because of numerous drug-drug interactions (it inhibits hepatic drug-metabolizing enzymes) and because it must be taken up to four times a day. Safety during pregnancy and lactation for drugs in this class has not been established (pregnancy category B).

IV preparations of H₂-receptor antagonists are occasionally utilized. Because dysrhythmias and hypotension have occurred with IV cimetidine, ranitidine (Zantac) or famotidine (Pepcid) is utilized if the IV route is necessary.

CNS side effects such as dizziness, drowsiness, confusion, and headache are more likely to occur in elderly patients. The nurse should assess for kidney and liver function. These drugs are mainly excreted via the kidneys. Patients with diminished kidney function require smaller dosages and are more likely to experience adverse effects due to the accumulation of the drug in the blood. Although rare, these medications can cause hepatotoxicity. Long-term use of

H₂-receptor antagonists may lead to vitamin B₁₂ deficiency because they decrease absorption of the vitamin. Iron supplements may be needed, as this mineral is best absorbed in an acidic environment. The nurse should evaluate the CBC for possible anemia in patients with long-term use.

Patient education as it relates to H₂-receptor antagonists should include goals, reasons for obtaining baseline data such as vital signs, tests for cardiac and renal disorders, and possible side effects. See "Nursing Process Focus: Patients Receiving H₂-Receptor Antagonist Therapy" for specific teaching points.

Proton Pump Inhibitors

Proton pump inhibitors act by blocking the enzyme responsible for secreting hydrochloric acid in the stomach. They are widely used in the short-term therapy of peptic ulcer disease. These agents are shown in Table 36.2.

36.7 Pharmacotherapy with Proton Pump Inhibitors

Proton pump inhibitors are relatively new drugs that have become widely used for the treatment of peptic ulcer disease and GERD. Drugs in this class reduce acid secretion in the

Pr PROTOTYPE DRUG | RANITIDINE (Zantac)

ACTIONS AND USES

Ranitidine acts by blocking H_2-receptors in the stomach to decrease acid production. It has a higher potency than cimetidine that allows it to be administered once daily, usually at bedtime. Adequate healing of the ulcer takes approximately 4 to 8 weeks although those at high risk to PUD may continue on drug maintenance for prolonged periods to prevent reoccurrence. Gastric ulcers heal more slowly than duodenal ulcers, and thus require longer therapy. IV and IM forms are available for the treatment of stress-induced bleeding in acute situations. Ranitidine is pregnancy category B.

Administration Alert

■ May cause an increase in serum creatinine, AST, ALT alkaline phosphatase, and total bilirubin.

ADVERSE EFFECTS AND INTERACTIONS

Ranitidine does not cross the blood-brain barrier to any appreciable extent, so the confusion and CNS depression observed with cimetidine is not expected with ranitidine. Although rare, severe reductions in the number of red and white blood cells and platelets are possible, thus periodic blood counts may be performed. High doses may result in impotence or a loss of libido in men.

Although ranitidine has fewer drug-drug interactions than cimetidine, it interacts with several drugs. For example, ranitidine may reduce the absorption of cefpodoxime, ketoconazole, and itraconazole.

 See the companion website for a Nursing Process Focus specific to this drug.

Table 36.2	Proton Pump Inhibitors
Drug	**Route and Adult Dose (max dose where indicated)**
esomeprazole (Nexium)	PO; 20–40 mg qd
lansoprazole (Prevacid)	PO; 15–60 mg qd
Pr omeprazole (Prilosec)	PO; 20–60 mg qd-bid
pantoprazole (Protonix)	PO; 40 mg qd
rabeprazole (Aciphex)	PO; 20 mg qd

stomach by binding irreversibly to the enzyme H^+, K^+-ATPase. In the parietal cells of the stomach, this enzyme acts as a pump to release acid (also called H^+, or protons) onto the surface of the GI mucosa. The proton pump inhibitors reduce acid secretion to a greater extent than the H_2-receptor antagonists and have a longer duration of action. All agents in this class have similar efficacy and side effects. The side effects of proton pump inhibitors are generally infrequent and minor. The newer agents esomeprazole (Nexium) and pantoprazole (Protonix) offer the convenience of once-a-day dosing.

NURSING CONSIDERATIONS

The role of the nurse in proton pump inhibitor therapy involves careful monitoring of a patient's condition and providing education as it relates to prescribed drug regimen. Proton pump inhibitors are usually well tolerated for short-term use. With long-term use, liver function should be periodically monitored as well as serum gastrin, because oversecretion of gastrin occurs with constant acid suppression. Generally, proton pump inhibitors are not used during pregnancy and lactation; they range from pregnancy category B (rabeprazole)

to C (omeprazole and lansoprazole). The nurse should assess for drug-drug interactions. Proton pump inhibitors will affect the absorption of medications, vitamins, and minerals that need an acidic environment in the stomach. The nurse should obtain the patient's history of smoking, because smoking increases stomach acid production.

These drugs should be taken 30 minutes prior to eating, usually before breakfast. Proton pump inhibitors are unstable in an acidic environment and are enteric coated to be absorbed in the small intestine. These drugs may be administered at the same time as antacids. Proton pump inhibitors are usually administered in combination with clarithromycin (Biaxin) for the treatment of *H. pylori*.

The nurse should monitor for adverse effects such as diarrhea, headache, and dizziness. Proton pump inhibitors are a relatively new class of drug; therefore, the long-term effects have not been fully determined.

Patient education as it relates to proton pump inhibitors should include goals, reasons for obtaining baseline data such as vital signs, diagnostic procedures and laboratory tests, and possible side effects. Following are important points the nurse should include when teaching patients regarding proton pump inhibitors.

NURSING PROCESS FOCUS | PATIENTS RECEIVING H₂-RECEPTOR ANTAGONIST THERAPY

ASSESSMENT

Prior to administration:
- Obtain a complete health history including allergies, drug history, and possible drug interactions.
- Assess patient for signs of GI bleeding.
- Obtain vital signs.
- Assess level of consciousness.
- Obtain results of CBC, liver, and renal function tests.

POTENTIAL NURSING DIAGNOSES

- Risk for Falls, related to adverse effect of drug
- Deficient Knowledge, related to drug therapy
- Acute Pain, related to gastric irritation from ineffective drug therapy
- Imbalanced Nutrition: Less than Body Requirements, related to adverse effects of drug

PLANNING: PATIENT GOALS AND EXPECTED OUTCOMES

The patient will:
- Report episodes of drowsiness, dizziness
- Demonstrate an understanding of drug therapy
- Report reoccurrence of abdominal pain or discomfort during drug therapy
- Maintain body weight throughout course of treatment

IMPLEMENTATION

Interventions and (Rationales)	*Patient Education/Discharge Planning*
Monitor use of OTC drugs to avoid drug interactions especially with cimetidine therapy.	Instruct patient to consult with healthcare provider before taking other medications or herbal products.
Monitor level of abdominal pain or discomfort to assess effectiveness of drug therapy.	Advise patient that pain relief may not occur for several days after beginning therapy.
Monitor patient use of alcohol. (Alcohol can increase gastric irritation.)	Instruct patient to avoid alcohol use.
Discuss possible drug interactions. (Antacids can decrease the effectiveness of other drugs taken concurrently.)	Instruct patient to take H₂-receptor antagonists and other medications at least 1 hour before antacids.
Institute effective safety measures regarding falls. (Drugs may cause drowsiness or dizziness.)	Instruct patient to avoid driving or performing hazardous activities until drug effects are known.
Explain need for lifestyle changes. (Smoking and certain foods increase gastric acid secretion.)	Encourage patient to: ■ Stop smoking; provide information on smoke cessation programs ■ Avoid foods that cause stomach discomfort
Observe patient for signs of GI bleeding.	Instruct patient to immediately report episodes of blood in stool or vomitus or increase in abdominal discomfort.

EVALUATION OF OUTCOME CRITERIA

Evaluate the effectiveness of drug therapy by confirming that patient goals and expected outcomes have been met (see "Planning").

⊖⊙ See Table 36.1 for a list of drugs to which these nursing actions apply.

- Take medication before meals.
- Inform healthcare provider of significant diarrhea.
- Do not crush, break, or chew medication.
- Avoid smoking, alcohol use, and foods that cause gastric discomfort.
- Report GI bleeding, abdominal pain, and heartburn.

- Eat foods with beneficial bacteria, such as yogurt, or take acidophilus to replace "friendly" bacteria.
- Sleep with head elevated 30 degrees. A foam wedge or risers may be placed under the top of the bed frame to keep the head elevated.

Pr PROTOTYPE DRUG | OMEPRAZOLE (Prilosec)

ACTIONS AND USES

Omeprazole was the first proton pump inhibitor to be approved for peptic ulcer disease. It reduces acid secretion in the stomach by binding irreversibly to the enzyme H^+, K^+-ATPase. Although this agent can take 2 hours to reach therapeutic levels, its effects may last 72 hours. It is used for the short-term, 4- to 8-week therapy of peptic ulcers and GERD. Most patients are symptom free after 2 weeks of therapy. It is used for longer periods in patients who have chronic hypersecretion of gastric acid, a condition known as Zollinger-Ellison syndrome. It is the most effective drug for this syndrome. Omeprazole is only available in oral form.

Administration Alerts

- Administer before meals.
- Tablets should not be chewed, divided, or crushed.
- May be administered with antacids.
- Pregnancy category C.

ADVERSE EFFECTS AND INTERACTIONS

Adverse effects are generally minor and include headache, nausea, diarrhea, rash, and abdominal pain. The main concern with proton pump inhibitors is that long-term use has been associated with an increased risk of gastric cancer in laboratory animals. Because of this possibility, therapy is generally limited to 2 months.

Omeprazole interacts with several drugs. For example, concurrent use of diazepam, phenytoin, and CNS depressants will cause increased blood levels of these drugs. Concurrent use of warfarin may increase the likelihood of bleeding.

See the companion website for a Nursing Process Focus specific to this drug.

Table 36.3	Antacids
Drug	**Route and Adult Dose (max dose where indicated)**
aluminum hydroxide (Amphojel, others)	PO; 600 mg tid or qid
calcium carbonate (Titralac, Tums)	PO; 1–2 g bid-tid
calcium carbonate with magnesium hydroxide (Mylanta Gel-caps, Rolaids)	PO; 2–4 capsules or tablets PRN (max 12 tablets/day)
magnesium hydroxide (Milk of Magnesia)	PO; 2.4–4.8 g (30–60 ml)/d in 1 or more divided doses
magnesium hydroxide and aluminum hydroxide (Maalox)	PO; 2–4 tablets PRN (max 16 tablets/day)
magnesium hydroxide and aluminum hydroxide with simethicone (Mylanta, Maalox Plus, others)	PO; 10–20 ml PRN (max 120 ml/day) or 2–4 tablets prn (max 24 tablets/day)
magaldrate (Riopan)	PO; 480–1,080 mg (5–10 ml suspension or 1–2 tablets) qid (max 20 tablets or 100 ml/d)
sodium bicarbonate (Alka-Seltzer, baking soda) (see page 664 for the Prototype Drug box)	PO; 0.3–2.0 g qd-qid or 1/2 tsp of powder in glass of water

Antacids

Antacids are alkaline substances that have been used to neutralize stomach acid for hundreds of years. These agents, shown in Table 36.3, are readily available as OTC drugs.

36.8 Pharmacotherapy with Antacids

Prior to the development of H_2-receptor antagonists and proton pump inhibitors, antacids were the mainstay of peptic ulcer and GERD pharmacotherapy. Indeed, many patients still use these inexpensive and readily available OTC drugs. Antacids, however, are no longer recommended as the sole drug class for peptic ulcer disease.

Antacids are alkaline, inorganic compounds of aluminum, magnesium, sodium, or calcium. Combinations of aluminum hydroxide and magnesium hydroxide, the most common type, are bases, capable of rapidly neutralizing stomach acid. Chewable tablets and liquid formulations are available. Simethicone is sometimes added to antacid preparations because it reduces gas bubbles that cause bloating and discomfort. A few products combine antacids and H_2-receptor blockers into a single tablet; for example, Pepcid Complete contains calcium carbonate, magnesium hydroxide, and famotidine.

Unless taken in extremely large amounts, antacids are very safe. Antacids containing sodium, calcium, or magnesium can result in absorption of these minerals to the general circulation. This absorption is generally not a problem unless the patient is on a sodium-restricted diet or has other conditions such as diminished renal function that could result in accumulation of these minerals. In fact, some manufacturers advertise their antacid products as calcium supplements. Patients should follow the label instructions carefully and not take more than the recommended dosage.

NURSING CONSIDERATIONS

The role of the nurse in antacid therapy involves careful monitoring of a patient's condition and providing education as it relates to prescribed drug regimen. Antacids are for occasional use only and patients should seek medical attention if symptoms persist or reoccur. The nurse should obtain a medical history, including the use of OTC and prescription drugs. The nurse should assess the patient for signs of renal insufficiency; magnesium-containing antacids should be used with caution in these patients. Hypermagnesemia may occur because the kidneys are unable to excrete excess magnesium.

When used according to label directions, antacids have few side effects. Magnesium- and aluminum-based products may cause diarrhea, and those with calcium may cause constipation.

Patient education as it relates to antacids should include goals, reasons for obtaining baseline data such as vital signs and tests for cardiac and renal disorders, and possible side effects. Following are important points the nurse should include when teaching patients regarding antacids.

- Patients with renal failure should avoid magnesium-based antacids.
- Patients with heart failure or hypertension should be advised to avoid sodium-based antacids.

- Take antacids at least 2 hours before other oral medications. Antacids directly affect the acidity of the stomach and may interfere with drug absorption.
- Note number and consistency of stools, since antacids may alter bowel activity.
- Medication may make stools appear white.
- Shake liquid preparations thoroughly before dispensing.

Antibiotics for *H. Pylori*

The gram negative bacterium *Helicobacter pylori* is associated with 90% of all duodenal ulcers and 75% of all gastric ulcers. It is also strongly associated with gastric cancer. To more rapidly and completely eliminate peptic ulcers, several antibiotics are used to eradicate this bacterium.

36.9 Pharmacotherapy with Combination Antibiotic Therapy

H. pylori has adapted well as a human pathogen by devising ways to neutralize the high acidity surrounding it and by making chemicals called adhesins that allow it to stick tightly to the GI mucosa. *H. pylori* infections can remain active for life, if not treated appropriately. Elimination of this organism causes ulcers to heal more rapidly and to remain in remission longer. The following antibiotics are commonly used for this purpose.

- amoxicillin (Amoxil, others)
- clarithromycin (Biaxin)
- metronidazole (Flagyl)
- tetracycline (Achromycin, others)
- bismuth subsalicylate (Pepto-Bismol) or ranitidine bismuth citrate (Tritec)

Pr PROTOTYPE DRUG | ALUMINUM HYDROXIDE (Amphojel, others)

ACTIONS AND USES

Aluminum hydroxide is an inorganic agent used alone or in combination with other antacids such as magnesium hydroxide. Unlike calcium-based antacids that can be absorbed and cause systemic effects, aluminum compounds have minimal absorption. Their primary action is to neutralize stomach acid by raising the pH of the stomach contents. Unlike H$_2$-receptor antagonists and proton pump inhibitors, aluminum antacids do not reduce the volume of acid secretion. They are most effectively used in combination with other antiulcer agents for the symptomatic relief of heartburn due to PUD or GERD.

Administration Alerts

- Aluminum antacids should be administered at least 2 hours before or after other drugs because absorption could be affected.
- Pregnancy category C.

ADVERSE EFFECTS AND INTERACTIONS

When given in high doses, aluminum compounds may interfere with phosphate metabolism and cause constipation. They are often combined with magnesium compounds, which counteract the constipation. Like many other antacids, aluminum compounds should not be taken with other medications, as they may interfere with their absorption. Sodium polystyrene sulfonate may cause systemic alkalosis.

 See the companion website for a Nursing Process Focus specific to this drug.

Two or more antibiotics are given concurrently to increase the effectiveness of therapy and to lower the potential for bacterial resistance. The antibiotics are also combined with a proton pump inhibitor or an H_2-receptor antagonist. Bismuth compounds are sometimes added to the antibiotic regimen. Although technically not antibiotics, bismuth compounds inhibit bacterial growth and prevent *H. pylori* from adhering to the gastric mucosa. Antibiotic therapy generally continues for 7 to 14 days. Additional information on anti-infectives can be found in Chapters 21 and 22 ∞.

36.10 Miscellaneous Drugs for Peptic Ulcer Disease

Several additional drugs are beneficial in treating peptic ulcer disease. Sucralfate (Carafate) consists of sucrose (a sugar) plus aluminum hydroxide (an antacid). The drug produces a thick, gel-like substance that coats the ulcer, protecting it against further erosion and promoting healing. It does not affect the secretion of gastric acid. Little of the drug is absorbed from the GI tract. Other than constipation, side effects are minimal.

Misoprostol (Cytotec) is a prostaglandin-like substance that acts by inhibiting gastric acid secretion and stimulating the production of protective mucus. Its primary use is for the prevention of peptic ulcers in patients taking high doses of NSAIDs or glucocorticoids. Diarrhea and abdominal cramping are relatively common. Classified as a pregnancy category X drug, misoprostol is contraindicated in pregnant patients. In fact, misoprostol is sometimes used to terminate pregnancies, as discussed in Chapter 29 ∞.

Prior to the discovery of safer and more effective drugs, anticholinergics such as atropine were used to treat peptic ulcers. Pirenzepine (Gastozepine) is a cholinergic blocker (muscarinic) available in Canada that inhibits the autonomic receptors responsible for gastric acid secretion. Although the action of pirenzepine is somewhat selective to the stomach, other anticholinergic effects such as dry mouth and constipation are possible. It is rare to find anticholinergics used for treating peptic ulcer today.

CHAPTER REVIEW

Key Concepts

The numbered key concepts provide a succinct summary of the important points from the corresponding numbered section within the chapter. If any of these points are not clear, refer to the numbered section within the chapter for review. Expanded versions can be found on the companion website.

36.1 The digestive system is responsible for breaking down food, absorbing nutrients, and eliminating wastes. Transit time through the GI tract can affect drug action.

36.2 The stomach secretes enzymes and acid that accelerate the process of chemical digestion.

36.3 Peptic ulcer disease (PUD) is caused by an erosion of the mucosal layer of the stomach or duodenum. Gastric ulcers are more commonly associated with cancer and require longer follow-up.

36.4 Gastroesophageal reflux disease (GERD) is caused by acidic stomach contents entering the esophagus. GERD and PUD are treated with similar medications.

36.5 Peptic ulcer disease is best treated by a combination of lifestyle changes and pharmacotherapy.

36.6 H_2-receptor blockers slow acid secretion by the stomach and are often drugs of choice in treating PUD and GERD.

36.7 Proton pump inhibitors block the enzyme H^+, K^+-ATPase and are effective at reducing gastric acid secretion.

36.8 Antacids are effective at neutralizing stomach acid and are inexpensive OTC therapy for PUD and GERD.

36.9 Combinations of antibiotics are administered to eliminate *H. pylori*, the cause of many peptic ulcers.

36.10 Several miscellaneous drugs, including sucralfate, misoprostol, and pirenzepine are also beneficial in treating PUD.

Review Questions

1. Many common antacids are combinations of salts containing aluminum and magnesium. For which population of patients are such antacids contraindicated? What product(s) should be used instead?

2. Before starting drug therapy for PUD, the patient should attempt to make lifestyle modifications that are associated with this disorder. What is the nurse's role in assisting the patient to initiate such changes?

3. Explain the following statement: All H_2-receptor antagonists are antihistamines but not all antihistamines are H_2-receptor antagonists.

4. The use of amoxicillin (Amoxil) and clarithromycin (Biaxin) in treating PUD is to eliminate *H. pylori* from the GI tract. Why, even though the patient is feeling better midway through the treatment regimen, is it important to comply with the directions on the prescription bottle to take all of the medication?

Critical Thinking Questions

1. A patient with chronic hyperacidity of the stomach takes aluminum hydroxide (Amphojel) on a regular basis. The patient presents to the clinic with complaints of increasing weakness. What may the nurse's assessment find as the cause of this weakness?

2. Nurses who work at night are at higher risk for developing peptic ulcer disease. Why is this?

3. A patient who is on ranitidine (Zantac) for PUD smokes and drinks alcohol daily. Will the Zantac be effective for this patient? Why or why not?

 ## EXPLORE MediaLink

NCLEX review, case studies, and other interactive resources for this chapter can be found on the companion website at www.prenhall.com/adams. Click on "Chapter 36" to select the activities for this chapter. For animations, more NCLEX review questions, and an audio glossary, access the accompanying CD-ROM in this textbook.

CHAPTER 37

Drugs for Bowel Disorders, Nausea, and Vomiting

DRUGS AT A GLANCE

DRUGS FOR CONSTIPATION: LAXATIVES
Bulk forming
 psyllium mucilloid (Metamucil, others)
Stool softener/surfactant
Stimulant
Saline and osmotic
Miscellaneous agents

DRUGS FOR DIARRHEA: ANTIDIARRHEALS
Opioids
 diphenoxylate with atropine (Lomotil)
Miscellaneous agents

DRUGS FOR NAUSEA AND VOMITING
Anticholinergics
Antihistamines
Benzodiazepines
Cannabinoids
Glucocorticoids
Phenothiazine and phenothiazine-like
 prochlorperazine (Compazine)
Serotonin-receptor antagonists

DRUGS FOR SUPPRESSING APPETITE: ANOREXIANTS
 sibutramine (Meridia)

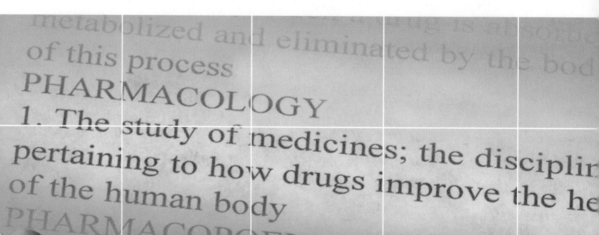

MediaLink   www.prenhall.com/adams

CD-ROM
Audio Glossary
NCLEX Review

Companion Website
NCLEX Review
Dosage Calculations
Case Study
Care Plans
Expanded Key Concepts

OBJECTIVES

After reading this chapter, the student should be able to:

1. Identify the major anatomical structures of the lower gastrointestinal tract.
2. Explain the pathogenesis of constipation and diarrhea.
3. Discuss conditions where the pharmacotherapy of bowel disorders is indicated.
4. Explain conditions where the pharmacotherapy of nausea and vomiting is indicated.
5. Describe the types of drugs used in the short-term management of obesity.
6. Describe the nurse's role in the pharmacologic management of bowel disorders, nausea, and vomiting.
7. For each of the drug classes listed in Drugs at a Glance, know representative drugs, explain the mechanism of drug action, describe primary actions, and identify important adverse effects.
8. Categorize drugs used in the treatment of bowel disorders, nausea, and vomiting based on their classification and mechanism of action.
9. Use the Nursing Process to care for patients who are receiving drug therapy for bowel disorders, nausea, and vomiting.

Bowel disorders, nausea, and vomiting are among the most common complaints for which patients seek medical consultation. These non-specific symptoms may be caused by any number of infectious, metabolic, inflammatory, neoplastic, or neuropsychologic disorders. In addition, nausea, vomiting, constipation, and diarrhea are the most common side effects of oral medications. Symptoms often resolve without the need for pharmacotherapy. When severe or prolonged, however, bowel disorders, nausea, and vomiting may lead to serious consequences unless drug therapy is initiated. This chapter will examine the pharmacotherapy of these common conditions associated with the gastrointestinal (GI) tract.

PHARMFACTS — Gastrointestinal Disorders

- Approximately 60 to 70 million Americans are affected by a digestive disease.
- At least 13% of all hospitalizations are related to digestive disorders.
- Approximately 140,000 new cases of colorectal cancer occur each year; it is the second leading cause of cancer deaths, killing more than 55,000 Americans.
- Irritable bowel syndrome affects 10% to 20% of adults.
- Americans spend over $33 billion annually on weight reduction products and services.
- The incidence of motion sickness peaks from ages 4 to 10, then begins to decline.
- About 25% of Americans (more than 1 million adults) who are using weight loss supplements are not overweight.

37.1 Normal Function of the Lower Digestive Tract

The lower portion of the GI tract consists of the small and large intestines, as shown in Figure 37.1. The first 10 inches of the small intestine, the duodenum, is the site where partially digested food from the stomach, known as chyme, mixes with bile from the gallbladder and digestive enzymes from the pancreas. It is sometimes considered part of the upper GI tract because of its close proximity to the stomach. The most common disorder of the duodenum, peptic ulcer, was discussed in Chapter 36 ⊙⊙.

The remainder of the small intestine consists of the jejunum and ileum. The jejunum is the site where most nutrient absorption occurs. The ileum empties its contents into the large intestine through the ileocecal valve. Peristalsis through

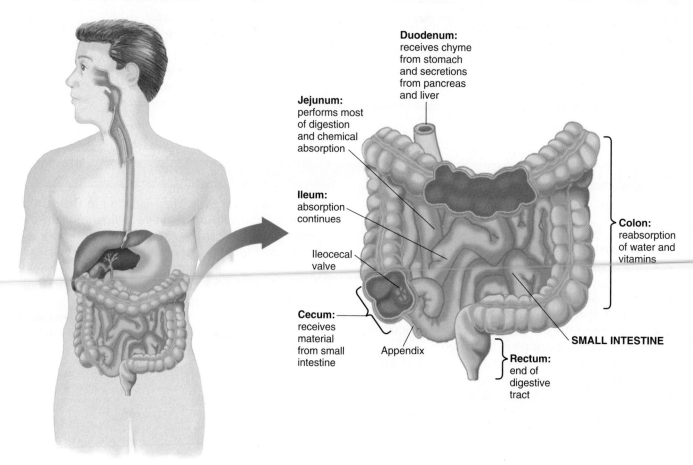

Figure 37.1 | The digestive system: functions of the small intestine and large intestine (colon) *Source: Pearson Education/PH College.*

the intestines is controlled by the autonomic nervous system. Activation of the parasympathetic division will increase peristalsis and speed materials through the intestine; the sympathetic division has the opposite effect. Travel time for chyme through the entire small intestine varies from 3 to 6 hours.

The large intestine, or colon, receives chyme from the ileum in a fluid state. The major function of the colon is to reabsorb water from chyme and to excrete the remaining material from the body. The colon harbors a substantial number of bacteria and fungi, the host flora, which serve a useful purpose by synthesizing B-complex vitamins and vitamin K. Disruption of the host flora in the colon can lead to diarrhea. With few exceptions, little reabsorption of nutrients occurs during the 12-to 24-hour journey through the colon.

CONSTIPATION

Constipation is identified by a decrease in the frequency and number of bowel movements. Stools may become dry, hard, and difficult to evacuate from the rectum.

37.2 Pathophysiology of Constipation

As waste material travels through the large intestine, water is reabsorbed. Reabsorption of the proper amount of water results in stools of a normal, soft-formed consistency. If the waste material remains in the colon for an extended period, however, too much water will be reabsorbed, leading to small, hard stools. Constipation may cause abdominal distention and discomfort, and flatulence.

The etiology of constipation may be related to a lack of exercise, insufficient food intake, especially insoluble dietary fiber, diminished fluid intake, or a medication regimen that includes drugs that reduce intestinal motility. Lifestyle modifications that incorporate positive dietary changes and physical activity should be considered before drugs are utilized. Foods that can cause constipation include alcoholic beverages, products with a high content of refined white flour, dairy products, and chocolate. The normal frequency of bowel movements varies widely among individuals, from two to three per day, to as few as one per week.

Occasional constipation is common and does not require drug therapy. Chronic, infrequent, and painful bowel movements, accompanied by severe straining, may justify initiation of treatment. In its most severe form, constipation can lead to a fecal impaction and complete obstruction of the bowel. Constipation occurs more frequently in older adults because fecal transit time through the colon slows with aging; this population also exercises less and has a higher frequency of chronic disorders that cause constipation.

Table 37.1	Laxatives and Cathartics
Drug	**Route and Adult Dose (max dose where indicated)**
Bulk Forming	
calcium polycarbophil (FiberCon, Fiberall, Mitrolan)	PO; 1 g qd prn
methylcellulose (Citrucel)	PO; 5–20 ml tid in 8–10 oz water
psyllium mucilloid (Metamucil, Naturacil, others)	PO; 1–2 tsp in 8 oz water qd prn
Saline and Osmotic	
magnesium hydroxide (Milk of Magnesia)	PO; 20–60 ml qd prn
polyethylene glycol (MiraLax)	PO; 17g in 8 oz of liquid qd for 2–4 days
sodium biphosphate (Fleet Phospho-Soda)	PO; 15–30 ml mixed in water qd prn
Stimulant	
bisacodyl (Dulcolax)	PO; 10–15 mg qd prn
castor oil (Emulsoil, Neoloid, Purge)	PO; 15–60 ml qd prn
phenolphthalein (Ex-Lax, Feen-a-Mint, Correctol)	PO; 60–240 mg qd prn
Stool Softener/Surfactant	
docusate (Surfak, Dialose, Colace, others)	PO; 50–500 mg qd
Miscellaneous Agent	
mineral oil	PO; 45 ml bid

Laxatives

Laxatives are drugs that promote bowel movements. Many are available OTC for the self-treatment of simple constipation. Laxatives are identified in Table 37.1.

37.3 Pharmacotherapy with Laxatives

Laxatives are drugs that promote evacuation of bowel or defecation. Cathartic is a related term that implies a stronger and more complete bowel emptying. A variety of prescription and OTC formulations are available, including tablets, liquids, and suppositories to treat existing constipation or to prevent this disorder.

Prophylactic laxative pharmacotherapy is appropriate postoperatively. Such treatment is indicated to preclude straining or bearing down during defecation—a situation that has the potential to precipitate increased intra-abdominal, intraocular, or blood pressure. Drugs, in conjunction with enemas, are often given to cleanse the bowel prior to diagnostic or surgical procedures of the colon or genitourinary tract. Cathartics are usually the drug of choice preceding diagnostic procedures of the colon, such as colonoscopy or barium enema.

When taken in prescribed amounts, laxatives have few side effects. These drugs are often classified into four primary groups and a miscellaneous category.

- Bulk-forming agents absorb water, thus adding size to the fecal mass. They are often taken prophylactically, to prevent constipation.

- Stool softeners or surfactants cause more water and fat to be absorbed into the stools. They are often used in patients who have undergone recent surgery.
- Stimulants irritate the bowel to increase peristalsis; may cause cramping in patients.
- Saline or osmotic laxatives are not absorbed in the intestine; they pull water into the fecal mass to create a more watery stool.
- Miscellaneous agents include mineral oil, which acts by lubricating the stool and the colon mucosa.

NURSING CONSIDERATIONS

The role of the nurse in laxative therapy involves careful monitoring of a patient's condition and providing education as it relates to the prescribed drug. Prior to pharmacotherapy with laxatives, the nurse must assess the abdomen for distention, bowel sounds, and bowel patterns. If there is absence of bowel sounds, peristalsis must be restored prior to laxative therapy. A patient with a sudden, unexplained change in bowel patterns should be evaluated, as it could indicate a serious condition such as colon cancer. The nurse should also assess for esophageal obstruction, intestinal obstruction, fecal impaction, and undiagnosed abdominal pain. Laxatives are contraindicated in all of these conditions due to the risk for causing bowel perforation. If diarrhea occurs, laxative use should be discontinued. There are many products to prevent and treat constipation. Because most are OTC medications there is a risk for misuse and overuse.

Bulk-forming laxatives are pregnancy category C, and should be used with caution during pregnancy and lactation. Because fiber absorbs water and expands providing "bulk," these agents must be taken with plenty of water. These laxatives will not be effective unless taken with one to two glasses of water. The nurse must assess the patient's ability to swallow as obstruction can occur if the product does not clear the esophagus or if a stricture exists. Bulk-forming products may take 24 to 48 hours to be effective and may be taken on a regular basis to prevent constipation.

Stool softeners are generally prescribed for patients who have experienced a sudden change in lifestyle that puts them at risk for constipation, such as a surgery, injury, or conditions such as MI where straining during defecation should be avoided. They are contraindicated during pregnancy and lactation (pregnancy category C). The nurse should assess for the development of diarrhea and cramping; if diarrhea develops, the medication should be withheld. Docusate is contraindicated in patients with abdominal pain accompanied by nausea and vomiting, fecal impaction, and in intestinal obstruction or perforation. Docusate sodium (Colace) should not be given to patients on sodium restriction. Docusate potassium (Dialose) should not be given to patients with renal impairment. Docusate increases systemic absorption of mineral oil, so these two medications should not be given concurrently. Docusate should not be taken with certain herbal products such as senna, cascara, rhubarb, or aloe, as it will increase their absorption and the risk of liver toxicity.

Stimulant laxatives act as irritants to the bowel and increase peristalsis. They are the quickest acting and most likely to cause diarrhea and cramping. Bowel rupture could occur if obstruction is present. Stimulant laxatives are not used during pregnancy and lactation (pregnancy category C). Because of their rapid and potent effects, the nurse must pay particular attention to responding to the patient's need to use a bedpan or quickly get to the bathroom. These products are also used as a "bowel prep" prior to bowel exams or surgeries, sometimes in combination with stimulant laxatives, osmotic laxatives, and enemas. As the patient will be NPO prior to the procedure, the nurse should assess for signs of dehydration and changes in vital signs. It may be necessary to initiate IV fluids. Herbal stimulant laxatives, such as cascara or senna, are common components of OTC weight-loss products and patients taking them may experience rebound, severe constipation if these medications are abruptly withdrawn.

Saline or osmotic laxatives pull water into the GI tract. Most are pregnancy category B. Dehydration may result when these medications are taken frequently or in excess if the patient has inadequate fluid intake. Osmotic laxatives are highly potent, work within hours, and are often a part of bowel prep.

Patient education as it relates to these medications should include goals and reasons for obtaining baseline data such as vital signs, abdominal assessment, and possible side effects. Following are other important points the nurse should include when teaching patients regarding laxatives.

- Follow label instructions carefully and do not take more than the recommended dose.
- If changes in bowel patterns persist or become more severe, seek medical attention.
- Take bulk-forming agents at a different time than other medications to ensure proper absorption.

See "Nursing Process Focus: Patients Receiving Laxative Therapy" for additional teaching points.

Pr Prototype Drug	**PSYLLIUM MUCILLOID (Metamucil, others)**

ACTIONS AND USES	**ADVERSE EFFECTS AND INTERACTIONS**
Psyllium is derived from a natural product, the seeds of the plantain plant. Like other bulk-forming laxatives, psyllium is an insoluble fiber that is indigestible and not absorbed from the GI tract. When taken with a sufficient quantity of water, psyllium swells and increases the size of the fecal mass. The larger the size of the fecal mass, the more the defecation reflex will be stimulated, thus promoting the passage of stool. Several doses of psyllium may be needed to produce a therapeutic effect. Frequent use of psyllium may effect a small reduction in blood cholesterol level.	Psyllium rarely produces side effects. It generally causes less cramping than the stimulant-type laxatives and results in a more natural bowel movement. If taken with insufficient water, it may cause obstructions in the esophagus or intestine. Psyllium should not be administered to patients with undiagnosed abdominal pain. Psyllium may decrease the absorption and effects of warfarin, digoxin, nitrofurantoin, antibiotics, and salicylates.
Administration Alerts	
■ Mix with 8 oz of water, fruit juice, or milk, and administer immediately.	
■ Follow each dose with an additional 8 oz of liquid.	
■ Observe elderly patients closely for possible aspiration.	
■ Pregnancy category C.	

 See the companion website for a Nursing Process Focus specific to this drug.

NURSING PROCESS FOCUS	PATIENTS RECEIVING LAXATIVE THERAPY

ASSESSMENT

Prior to administration:
- Obtain complete health history including allergies, drug history, and possible drug interactions.
- Assess bowel elimination pattern.
- Assess bowel sounds.

POTENTIAL NURSING DIAGNOSES

- Risk for Injury (intestinal obstruction), related to adverse effects from drug therapy
- Constipation

PLANNING: PATIENT GOALS AND EXPECTED OUTCOMES

The patient will:
- Report relief from constipation
- Demonstrate an understanding of the drug's action by accurately describing drug side effects and precautions
- Immediately report effects such as nausea, vomiting, diarrhea, abdominal pain, and lack of bowel movement

IMPLEMENTATION

Interventions and (Rationales)	*Patient Education/Discharge Planning*
■ Monitor frequency volume and consistency of bowel movements. (Changes in bowel habits can indicate a serious condition.)	Advise patient to: ■ Discontinue laxative use if diarrhea occurs ■ Notify healthcare provider if constipation continues ■ Take medication as prescribed ■ Increase fluids and dietary fiber, such as whole grains, fibrous fruits, and vegetables ■ Expect results from medication within 2 to 3 days after initial dose
■ Monitor patient's ability to swallow. (Bulk laxatives can swell and cause obstruction in the esophagus.)	■ Instruct patient to discontinue medication and notify healthcare provider if having difficulty swallowing.
■ Monitor patient's fluid intake. (Esophageal or intestinal obstruction may result if the patient does not take in adequate amounts of fluid with the medication.)	Instruct patient to: ■ Drink six 8-oz glasses of fluid per day ■ Mix medication in 8 full oz of liquid ■ Drink at least 8 oz of additional fluid

EVALUATION OF OUTCOME CRITERIA

Evaluate the effectiveness of drug therapy by confirming that patient goals and expected outcomes have been met (see "Planning").

See Table 37.1 for a list of drugs to which these nursing actions apply.

DIARRHEA

Diarrhea is an increase in the frequency and fluidity of bowel movements. Diarrhea is not a disease; it is a symptom of an underlying disorder.

37.4 Pathophysiology of Diarrhea

Occasionally, the large intestine does not reabsorb enough water from the fecal mass and stools become watery. Like constipation, occasional diarrhea is a common disorder that does not warrant drug therapy. When prolonged or severe, especially in children, diarrhea can result in significant loss of body fluids and pharmacotherapy is indicated. Prolonged diarrhea may lead to acid-base or electrolyte disorders (Chapter 44).

Diarrhea may be caused by certain medications, infections of the bowel, and substances such as lactose. Antibiotics often cause diarrhea by killing normal intestinal flora, thus giving rise to an overgrowth of opportunistic pathogenic organisms. It is vital to assess and treat the etiology of the diarrhea. Assessing the patient's recent travels, dietary habits, immune system competence, and recent drug history may provide information about the etiology of the diarrhea. Critically ill patients with a reduced immune response who are exposed to many antibiotics may have diarrhea related to pseudomembranous colitis, a condition that may lead to shock and death.

Ulceration in the distal portion of the small intestine, called **Crohn's disease**, and erosions in the large intestine, called **ulcerative colitis**, are common causes of diarrhea. Together these diseases, are categorized as inflammatory bowel disease, and are treated with anti-inflammatory medications (Chapter 30) ⊕. Particularly severe cases may require immunosuppressant drugs such as cyclosporine (Neoral, Sandimmune) or methotrexate (Folex, Mexate, others).

Irritable bowel syndrome (IBS), also known as spastic colon or mucous colitis, is a common disorder of the lower GI tract. Symptoms include abdominal pain, bloating, excessive gas, and colicky cramping. Bowel habits are frequently altered with diarrhea alternating with constipation, and there may be mucus in the stool. IBS is considered a functional bowel disorder, meaning that the normal operation of the digestive tract is impaired without the presence of detectable organic disease. It is not a precursor of more serious disease. Stress is often a precipitating factor along with dietary factors. Treatment is supportive with drug therapy targeted at symptomatic treatment. Tegaserod (Zelnorm) was recently approved for the short term pharmacotherapy of IBS in women presenting with constipation as the primary complaint. It acts by binding to 5-HT receptors in the GI tract, which stimulates the peristaltic reflex.

Antidiarrheals

For occasional mild cases of diarrhea, OTC products are effective at returning elimination patterns to normal. For chronic or severe cases, the opioids are the most efficacious of the antidiarrheal agents. The antidiarrheals are shown in Table 37.2.

37.5 Pharmacotherapy with Antidiarrheals

Pharmacotherapy related to diarrhea depends on the severity of the condition and identifiable etiologic factors. If the cause is an infectious disease, then an antibiotic or antiparasitic drug is indicated. Should the etiology be inflammatory in nature, anti-inflammatory drugs are warranted. When the cause appears to be due to a side effect of pharmacotherapy, the healthcare provider may discontinue the offending medication, lower the dose, or substitute an alternative drug.

The most effective drugs for the symptomatic treatment of diarrhea are the opioids which slow peristalsis in the colon, with only a slight risk of dependence. The most common opioid antidiarrheals are codeine and diphenoxylate with atropine (Lomotil). Diphenoxylate is a Schedule V agent that acts directly on the intestine to slow peristalsis, thereby allowing for more fluid and electrolyte absorption in the large intestine. The opioids cause CNS depression at high doses, and are generally reserved for more severe cases due to the potential for dependence.

OTC drugs for diarrhea act by a number of different mechanisms. Loperamide (Imodium) is an analog of meperidine, although it has no narcotic effects and is not classified as a controlled substance. Low dose loperamide is available OTC; higher doses are available by prescription. Other OTC treatments include bismuth subsalicylate (Pepto-Bismol), which acts to bind and absorb toxins. The psyllium and pectin (Kaopectate) preparations may also slow diarrhea, since they tend to absorb large amounts of fluid and form bulkier stools. Intestinal flora modifiers are supplements that help to correct the altered GI flora; a good source of healthy bacteria is yogurt with active cultures.

NURSING CONSIDERATIONS

The role of the nurse in antidiarrheal therapy involves careful monitoring of a patient's condition and providing education as it relates to the prescribed drug regimen. Antidiarrheal drugs should be given for symptomatic relief of diarrhea while the underlying etiology is treated. Because diarrhea can cause a loss of fluid and electrolytes, hydration status, serum potassium, magnesium, and bicarbonate should be assessed. The nurse should also assess for blood in the stool. The nurse needs to be especially observant of infants, children, and the elderly because diarrhea

Table 37.2	Antidiarrheals
Drug	**Route and Adult Dose (max dose where indicated)**
Opioids	
camphorated opium tincture (Paregoric)	PO; 5–10 ml q2h to qid prn
difenoxin with atropine (Motofen)	PO; 1–2 mg after each diarrhea episode (max 8 mg/d)
diphenoxylate with atropine (Lomotil)	PO; 1–2 tabs or 5–10 ml tid-qid
loperamide (Imodium)	PO; 4 mg as a single dose, then 2 mg after each diarrhea episode (max 16 mg/d)
Miscellaneous Agents	
bismuth salts (Pepto-Bismol)	PO; 2 tabs or 30 ml prn
furazolidone (Furoxone)	PO; 100 mg qid
kaolin-pectin (Kaopectate)	PO; 60–120 ml after each diarrhea episode

can quickly lead to dehydration and electrolyte imbalance. Because antidiarrheals are excreted in the liver and kidneys, hepatic and renal function should be assessed.

Antidiarrheals are not generally used during pregnancy and lactation. They should not be used in conditions where constipation should be avoided, such as pseudomembranous colitis or severe ulcerative colitis, because the drugs could worsen or mask these conditions. Toxic megacolon has occurred in patients with ulcerative colitis taking loperamide (Imodium). Because drowsiness may occur with opioids the nurse should assess the patient's ability to get out of bed safely. Antidiarrheals are contraindicated in patients with severe dehydration, electrolyte imbalance, liver and renal disorders, and glaucoma. Opioid antidiarrheals should be used with caution in patients with a history of drug abuse. Adverse reactions occur more frequently in children, especially those with Down syndrome.

Patient education as it relates to these drugs should include goals and reasons for obtaining baseline data such as vital signs, abdominal assessment, and possible side effects. Following are other important points the nurse should include when teaching patients regarding antidiarrheals.

■ Seek medical care for diarrhea that does not resolve within 2 days, if a fever develops, or dehydration occurs (infants, children, and the elderly are at greatest risk and may need medical attention sooner).
■ Discontinue medication once frequent or watery stools have stopped.
■ Seek medical care if the presence of blood is found in the stool.

See "Nursing Process Focus: Patients Receiving Antidiarrheal Therapy" for additional teaching points.

NAUSEA AND VOMITING

Nausea is an unpleasant, subjective sensation, usually in the midepigastrum, that is accompanied by weakness, diaphoresis, and hyperproduction of saliva. It is sometimes accompanied by dizziness. Intense nausea often leads to vomiting, or emesis, in which the stomach contents are forced upward into the esophagus and out of the mouth.

37.6 Pathophysiology of Nausea and Vomiting

Vomiting is a defense mechanism used by the body to rid itself of toxic substances. Vomiting is a reflex primarily controlled by a portion of the medulla of the brain, known as the vomiting center, which receives sensory signals from the digestive tract, the inner ear, and the cerebral cortex. Interestingly, the vomiting center is not protected by the blood-brain barrier, as is the vast majority of the brain. These neurons can directly sense the presence of toxic substances in the blood. Once the vomiting reflex is triggered, wavelike contractions of the stomach quickly propel its contents upward and out of the body.

SPECIAL CONSIDERATIONS

Cultural Remedies for Diarrhea

Because diarrhea is an age-old malady that affects all populations, different cultures have adopted tried-and-true symptomatic remedies for the condition. One preparation, used by people in many regions of the world, is cornstarch (a heaping teaspoonful) in a glass of tepid water. For centuries, mothers have boiled rice and given the diluted rice water to babies for diarrhea. The rationale behind these two therapies is that they work by absorbing excess water in the intestines, thus stopping the diarrhea. Although a rationale was not related in earlier times, people of many cultures found that eating grated apple that had turned brown alleviated symptoms. This apparently evolved into what today is known as the ABCs of diarrhea treatment: apples, bananas (just barely ripe), and carrots. The underlying principle is the pectin that is present in these foods oxidizes, producing the same ingredient found in many OTC diarrhea medicines.

Pr PROTOTYPE DRUG	**DIPHENOXYLATE WITH ATROPINE** (Lomotil)
ACTIONS AND USES	**ADVERSE EFFECTS AND INTERACTIONS**

ACTIONS AND USES

The primary antidiarrheal ingredient in Lomotil is diphenoxylate. Like other opioids, diphenoxylate slows peristalsis, allowing time for additional water reabsorption from the colon and more solid stools. It acts within 45 to 60 minutes. It is effective for moderate to severe diarrhea, but is not recommended for children. The atropine in Lomotil is not added for its anticholinergic effect, but to discourage patients from taking too much of the drug.

Administration Alert

■ Pregnancy category C.

ADVERSE EFFECTS AND INTERACTIONS

Unlike most opioids, diphenoxylate has no analgesic properties and has an extremely low potential for abuse. Some patients experience dizziness or drowsiness and care should be taken not to drive or operate machinery until the effects of the drug are known.

Diphenoxylate with atropine interacts with several other drugs. For example, other CNS depressants, including alcohol, will add to its CNS depressant effect. At higher doses, the anticholinergic effects of atropine may be observed, which include drowsiness, dry mouth, and tachycardia. When taken with MAO inhibitors, diphenoxylate may cause hypertensive crisis.

 See the companion website for a Nursing Process Focus specific to this drug.

NURSING PROCESS FOCUS	PATIENTS RECEIVING ANTIDIARRHEAL THERAPY

ASSESSMENT	POTENTIAL NURSING DIAGNOSES
Prior to administration: ■ Obtain complete health history including allergies, drug history, and possible drug interactions. ■ Assess sodium, chloride, and potassium levels. ■ Evaluate results of stool culture. ■ Assess for presence of dehydration. ■ Obtain vital signs and EKG.	■ Risk for Imbalanced Fluid Volume: Less than Body Requirements, related to fluid loss secondary to diarrhea ■ Risk for Injury (falls), related to drowsiness secondary to drug therapy

PLANNING: PATIENT GOALS AND EXPECTED OUTCOMES

The patient will:
■ Report relief of diarrhea
■ Demonstrate an understanding of the drug's action by accurately describing drug side effects and precautions
■ Immediately report effects such as persistent diarrhea, constipation, abdominal pain, blood in stool, confusion, dizziness, or fever

IMPLEMENTATION

Interventions and (Rationales)	Patient Education/Discharge Planning
■ Monitor frequency, volume, and consistency of stools. (This will determine the effectiveness of drug therapy.)	Advise patient to: ■ Record the frequency of stools ■ Note if any blood is present in stools ■ Report any abdominal pain or abdominal distention immediately
■ Minimize the risk of dehydration and electrolyte imbalance. (These may occur secondary to diarrhea.)	■ Instruct patient to increase fluid intake and drink electrolyte-enriched fluids.
■ Prevent accidental overdosage.	■ Advise patient who is using liquid preparations to use the dropper included to measure medication dosage. Do not use household measurements.
■ Monitor for dry mouth. (This is a side effect of medications.)	■ Advise patient to suck on ice, sour candy, or chew gum to relieve sensation of dry mouth.
■ Initiate safety measures to prevent falls. (These medications may cause drowsiness.)	Advise patient to: ■ Refrain from driving or performing hazardous activities until the effects of drug are known ■ Abstain from using alcohol or other CNS depressants
■ Monitor electrolyte levels.	Advise patient to: ■ Keep all laboratory appointments ■ Report weakness and muscle cramping

EVALUATION OF OUTCOME CRITERIA

Evaluate the effectiveness of drug therapy by confirming that patient goals and expected outcomes have been met (see "Planning").

See Table 37.2 for a list of drugs to which these nursing actions apply.

Nausea and vomiting are common symptoms associated with a wide variety of conditions such as GI infections, food poisoning, stress, nervousness, emotional imbalances, changes in body position (motion sickness), and extreme pain. Other conditions that promote nausea and vomiting are general anesthetic agents, migraine headache, trauma to the head or abdominal organs, inner ear disorders, and diabetes. Psychological factors play a significant role, as patients often become nauseated during periods of extreme stress or when confronted with unpleasant sights, smells, or sounds.

The nausea and vomiting experienced by many women during the first trimester of pregnancy is referred to as morning sickness. Should this become acute, with continual vomiting, this condition may lead to hyperemesis gravidarum, a situation in which the health and safety of the mother and developing baby can become severely compromised. Pharmacotherapy is only initiated after other antinausea measures have been found to be ineffective.

Many drugs, by their chemical nature, bring about nausea or vomiting as a side effect. The most extreme example of this occurs with the antineoplastic drugs, most of which cause intense nausea and vomiting.

A foremost problem secondary to nausea and vomiting is dehydration. When large amounts of fluids are vomited, water in the plasma moves from the blood to other body tissues, resulting in dehydration. Because the contents lost from the stomach are strongly acidic, vomiting may cause a change in the pH of the blood, resulting in metabolic alkalosis. With excessive loss, severe acid-base disturbances can lead to vascular collapse that results in death if medical intervention is not initiated. Dehydration is exceptionally dangerous for infants, small children, and the elderly, and is evidenced by dry mouth, sticky saliva, and reduced urine output that is dark yellow-orange to brown.

Nausea and vomiting may be prevented or alleviated with natural remedies or by the use of drugs from several different classes. The treatment goal for nausea or vomiting is removal of the cause, when feasible.

Antiemetics

Drugs from at least eight different classes are used to prevent nausea and vomiting. Many of these act by inhibiting dopamine or serotonin receptors in the brain. The antiemetics are shown in Table 37.3.

37.7 Pharmacotherapy with Antiemetics

A large number of antiemetics are available to treat nausea and vomiting, and selection of a particular agent depends on the experience of the healthcare provider and the cause of the nausea. For example, nausea due to motion sickness is effectively treated with the anticholinergics or antihistamines. Nausea and vomiting associated with antineoplastic agents is often treated with the phenothiazines, glucocorticoids, or serotonin-receptor blockers. Aprepitant (Emend) is the first of a new class of antiemetics, the neurokinin receptor antagonists, used to prevent nausea and vomiting following antineoplastic therapy. To prevent loss of the antiemetic medication due to vomiting, many of these agents are available through the IM, IV, and/or suppository routes.

Patients receiving antineoplastic drugs may receive three or more antiemetics to reduce the nausea and vomiting from chemotherapy. In fact, therapy with antineoplastic drugs is one of the most common reasons why antiemetic drugs are prescribed.

Motion sickness is a disorder affecting a portion of the inner ear known as the **vestibular apparatus** which is associated with significant nausea. The most common drug used for motion sickness is scopolamine (Transderm), which is usually administered as a transdermal patch. Antihistamines such as dimenhydrinate (Dramamine) and meclizine (Antivert) are also effective, but may cause significant drowsiness in some patients. Drugs used to treat motion sickness are most effective when taken 20 to 60 minutes before travel is expected.

On some occasions, it is desirable to *stimulate* the vomiting reflex with drugs called **emetics**. Indications for emetics include ingestion of poisons and overdoses of oral drugs. Ipecac syrup, given orally, or apomorphine, given SC, will induce vomiting in about 15 minutes.

NURSING CONSIDERATIONS

The role of the nurse in antiemetic therapy involves careful monitoring of a patient's condition and providing education as it relates to the prescribed drug regimen. The nurse should assess symptoms that precipitated the vomiting or that are occurring concurrently. If a patient becomes sedated and continues to vomit, a nasogastric tube insertion with suction may be indicated. Antiemetics are contraindicated in patients who are hypersensitive to the drugs, have bone marrow depression, are comatose, and experience vomiting of unknown etiology. These drugs are used with caution in patients with breast cancer. Patient safety is a concern, as drowsiness is a frequent side effect of antiemetics. Patients may be at risk for falls because of medication side effects and sensation of weakness from vomiting. Orthostatic hypotension is a side effect of some antiemetics.

Drugs used to stimulate emesis should only be used in emergency situations under the direction of a healthcare provider. They are used only when the patient is alert due to the risk of aspiration. When the patient is comatose, a gastric lavage tube is placed and attached to suction, to empty gastric contents.

Patient education as it relates to antiemetics should include goals and reasons for obtaining baseline data such as vital signs, abdominal assessment, and possible side effects. Following are important points the nurse should include when teaching patients regarding antiemetics.

- Use assistance to get out of bed until effects of medication are known.
- Avoid driving or performing hazardous tasks.
- If blood is vomited, or if the vomiting is associated with severe abdominal pain, notify the healthcare provider immediately.
- Do not use OTC antiemetics for prolonged periods; vomiting may be a symptom of a serious disorder that requires medical attention.
- Before inducing vomiting with an OTC emetic, check with the healthcare provider; some poisons and caustic chemicals should not be vomited.

Table 37.3	Selected Antiemetics	
Drug	**Route and Adult Dose (max dose where indicated)**	
Anticholinergic		
scopolamine (Hyoscine, Transderm-Scop)	Transdermal; 0.5 mg q 72 h	
Antihistamines		
cyclizine hydrochloride (Marezine)	PO; 50 mg q4-6h (max 200 mg/day)	
dimenhydrinate (Dramamine, others)	PO; 50–100 mg q4-6h (max 400 mg/day)	
diphenhydramine (Benadryl, others) (see 428 for the Prototype Drug box)	PO; 25–50 mg tid-qid (max 300 mg/day)	
hydroxyzine (Atarax, Vistaril)	PO; 25–100 mg tid or qid	
meclizine (Antivert, Bonine, others)	PO; 25–50 mg qd, take 1 h before travel	
Benzodiazepines		
diazepam (Valium) (see 164 for the Prototype Drug box)	IV/IM; 5–10 mg, repeat if needed at 10–15 min intervals up to 30 mg, then repeat if needed q2–4h	
lorazepam (Ativan) (see 150 for the Prototype Drug box)	IV; 1.0–1.5 mg prior to chemotherapy	
Cannabinoids		
dronabinol (Marinol)	PO; 5 mg/m^2 1–3 h before administration of chemotherapy, then q2–4h after chemotherapy for a total of 4–6 doses, dose may be increased by 2.5 mg/m^2 (max 15 mg/m^2)	
nabilone (Cesamet)	PO; 1–2 mg bid	
Glucocorticoids		
dexamethasone (Decadron)	PO; 0.25–4 mg bid-qid	
methylprednisolone (Medrol, Solu-Medrol, others)	PO; 4–48 mg/d in divided doses	
Neurokinin Receptor Antagonist		
aprepitant (Emend)	PO; 125 mg 1 h prior to chemotherapy	
Phenothiazine and Phenothiazine-like		
metoclopramide (Reglan, others)	PO; 2 mg/kg 1 h prior to chemotherapy	
perphenazine (Phenazine, Trilafon)	PO; 8–16 mg bid-qid	
prochlorperazine (Compazine, others)	PO; 5–10 mg tid or qid	
promethazine (Phenergan, others)	PO; 12.5–25 mg q4-qid	
thiethylperazine (Torecan)	PO; 10 mg qd-tid	
Serotonin Receptor Antagonists		
dolasetron (Anzemet)	PO; 100 mg 1 h prior to chemotherapy	
granisetron (Kytril)	IV; 10 μg/kg 30 minutes prior to chemotherapy	
ondansetron (Zofran)	PO; 4 mg tid prn	

WEIGHT LOSS

Hunger occurs when the hypothalamus recognizes the levels of certain chemicals (glucose) or hormones (insulin) in the blood. Hunger is a normal physiologic response that drives people to seek nourishment. Appetite is somewhat different than hunger. Appetite is a psychological response that drives food intake based on associations and memory. For example, people often eat, not because they are experiencing hunger, but because it is a particular time of day, or because they find the act of eating pleasurable or social.

Anorexiants

Despite the public's desire for effective drugs to induce weight loss, there are few such drugs on the market. The

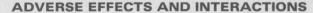

| **PROTOTYPE DRUG** | **PROCHLORPERAZINE** (Compazine) |

ACTIONS AND USES

Prochlorperazine is a phenothiazine, a class of drugs usually prescribed for psychoses, as discussed in Chapter 17 ⊘. The phenothiazines are the largest group of drugs prescribed for severe nausea and vomiting and prochlorperazine is the most frequently prescribed antiemetic in its class. Prochlorperazine acts by blocking dopamine receptors in the brain, which inhibits signals to the vomiting center in the medulla. It is frequently given by the rectal route, where absorption is rapid.

Administration Alerts

- Administer 2 hours before or after antacids and antidiarrheals.
- Pregnancy category C.

ADVERSE EFFECTS AND INTERACTIONS

Prochlorperazine produces dose-related anticholinergic side effects such as dry mouth, sedation, constipation, orthostatic hypotension, and tachycardia. When used for prolonged periods at higher doses, extrapyramidal symptoms resembling those of Parkinson's disease are a serious concern.

Prochlorperazine interacts with alcohol to increase CNS depression. Antacids and antidiarrheals inhibit absorption of prochlorperazine. When taken with phenobarbital, metabolism of prochlorperazine is increased.

🌐 *See the companion website for a Nursing Process Focus specific to this drug.*

| **NATURAL THERAPIES** | **Acidophilus for Diarrhea** |

Lactobacillus acidophilus is a probiotic bacterium normally found in the human alimentary canal and the vagina. It is considered to be protective flora, inhibiting the growth of potentially pathogenic species such as *E. coli*, *C. albicans*, *C. pylori*, and *G. vaginalis*. One mechanism used by *L. acidophilus* to limit the growth of other bacterial species is the generation of hydrogen peroxide, which is toxic to most cells.

The primary use of *L. acidophilus* is to restore the normal flora of the intestine following diarrhea, particularly from antibiotic therapy. This probiotic may also help to restore normal microflora in the vagina, although the evidence for this effect is not conclusive. *L. acidophilus* may be obtained by drinking acidophilus milk, or by eating yogurt or kefir containing live (or active) cultures. Those wishing to obtain *L. acidophilus* from yogurt should read the labels carefully, because not all products contain active cultures; frozen yogurt contains no active cultures. Supplements include capsules, tablets, and granules. Doses are not standardized, and tablet doses range from 50 to 500 mg.

approved agents are used for the treatment of obesity, although they produce only modest effects.

37.8 Pharmacotherapy with Anorexiants

Obesity may be defined as being more than 20% above the ideal body weight. Because of the prevalence of obesity in society and the difficulty most patients experience when following weight reduction plans for extended periods of time, drug manufacturers have long sought to develop safe drugs that induce weight loss. In the 1970s, amphetamine and dextroamphetamine (Dexedrine) were widely prescribed as anorexiants, to reduce appetite, however, these drugs, are addictive, and rarely prescribed for this purpose today. In the 1990s, the combination of fenfluramine and phentermine

(Fen-Phen) was widely prescribed, until fenfluramine was removed from the market for causing heart valve defects.

Attempts to produce drugs that promote weight loss by blocking lipid absorption resulted in orlistat (Xenical), which acts to block fat absorption in the GI tract. Unfortunately, orlistat may also decrease absorption of other substances, including fat-soluble vitamins and warfarin (Coumadin). To avoid having severe GI effects such as flatus with discharge, oily stool, abdominal pain, and discomfort, patients should restrict their fat intake. GI effects often diminish after 4 weeks of therapy. This drug produces only a very small increase in weight reduction compared to placebos.

Sibutramine (Meridia), a serotonin reuptake inhibitor, is the most widely prescribed appetite suppressant for the short-term control of obesity. Sibutramine is generally well tolerated with common side effects of dry mouth and headache. It may have significant interactions with other medications, which are usually related to the additive effect of serotonin reuptake inhibition. The patient should not take any OTC cold, cough, decongestant, or allergy medicine without notifying the healthcare provider, as these drugs may increase blood pressure. Anorexiants are prescribed for patients with a body mass index (BMI) of at least 30 or greater, or a BMI of 27 or greater, with other risk factors for disease such as hypertension, hyperlipidemia or diabetes.

NURSING CONSIDERATIONS

The role of the nurse in anorexiant therapy involves careful monitoring of a patient's condition and providing education as it relates to the prescribed drug regimen. With anorexiants, the nurse should focus on lifestyle changes that will have a greater effect on weight reduction in the long term. Drugs for weight loss have limited effectiveness and some have serious side effects.

Orlistat (Xenical) is contraindicated in pregnancy and lactation (pregnancy category B), malabsorption syndrome, cholestasis, and obesity due to organic causes. It is used with caution in patients with frequent diarrhea and those with known deficiencies of fat-soluble vitamins. The nurse should monitor blood glucose levels in patients with diabetes mellitus.

Amphetamine and other stimulant-type anorexiants can be dangerous due to cardiovascular side effects such as hypertension, tachycardia, and dysrhythmias and their potential for dependence. Use of these drugs must be closely monitored. These drugs should not be used during pregnancy or lactation.

Sibutramine (Meridia) should not be used during pregnancy or lactation (pregnancy category C). It is contraindicated in patients with cardiac conditions such as dysrhythmias, coronary artery disease, HF, and poorly controlled hypertension. It should not be administered concurrently with other serotonin reuptake inhibitors such as fluoxetine (Prozac). Sibutramine is used with caution in patients with a history of hypertension, seizures, and narrow angle glaucoma. Prior to and during administration, liver function tests, bilirubin levels, alkaline phosphatase levels, and lipid profiles should be obtained. The nurse should assess heart rate and blood pressure regularly and report sustained increases immediately.

Patient education as it relates to these drugs should include goals, reasons for obtaining baseline data such as vital signs, and possible side effects. Following are important points the nurse should include when teaching patients regarding anorexiants.

- Lifestyle modifications are necessary for sustained weight loss to occur; patient should be encouraged to seek support groups for long-term weight management.
- Maintain close medical follow-up with amphetamine medications.
- Do not take any OTC or herbal medications without healthcare provider approval.
- The nurse should advise patients taking orlistat (Xenical) of the following:
  - Take a multivitamin each day.
  - Dose may be omitted if there is no fat present in the meal or meal is skipped.
  - Excessive flatus and fecal leaking may occur when a high-fat meal is consumed.

 PROTOTYPE DRUG | **SIBUTRAMINE** (Meridia)

ACTIONS AND USES

Sibutramine (Meridia), a selective serotonin reuptake inhibitor (SSRI), is the most widely prescribed appetite suppressant for the short-term control of obesity. When combined with a reduced calorie diet, sibutramine may produce a gradual weight loss of at least 10% of initial body weight, over a period of a year. Sibutramine therapy is not recommended for longer than 1 year.

Administration Alerts

- Allow at least 2 weeks between discontinuing MAO inhibitors and starting Meridia.
- Pregnancy category C.

ADVERSE EFFECTS AND INTERACTIONS

Headache is the most common complaint reported during sibutramine therapy, although insomnia and dry mouth are also possible. It should be used with great care in patients with cardiac disorders, as it may cause tachycardia and raise blood pressure. It is a Schedule IV drug with low potential for dependence.

Sibutramine interacts with several other drugs. For example, decongestants, cough, and allergy medications may cause elevated blood pressure. Ketoconazole and erythromycin may inhibit the metabolism of sibutramine. Concurrent use with a MAOI or SSRI may cause serotonin syndrome.

 See the companion website for a Nursing Process Focus specific to this drug.

CHAPTER REVIEW

Key Concepts

The numbered key concepts provide a succinct summary of the important points from the corresponding numbered section within the chapter. If any of these points are not clear, refer to the numbered section within the chapter for review. Expanded versions can be found on the companion website.

37.1 The small intestine is the location for most nutrient and drug absorption. The large intestine is responsible for the reabsorption of water.

37.2 Constipation, the infrequent passage of hard, small stools, is a common disorder caused by slow motility of material through the large intestine.

37.3 Laxatives are drugs given to promote emptying of the large intestine by stimulating peristalsis, lubricating the fecal mass, or adding more bulk to the colon contents.

37.4 Diarrhea is an increase in the fluidity of feces that occurs when the colon fails to reabsorb enough water.

37.5 For simple diarrhea, OTC medications are effective. Opioids are the most effective drugs for controlling severe diarrhea.

37.6 Vomiting is a defense mechanism used by the body to rid itself of toxic substances. Nausea is an uncomfortable feeling that may precede vomiting.

37.7 Symptomatic treatment of nausea and vomiting includes drugs from many different classes, including phenothiazines, antihistamines, cannabinoids, corticosteroids, benzodiazepines, and serotonin receptor antagonists.

37.8 Anorexiants are drugs used for the short-term management of obesity, and these drugs produce only modest effects.

Review Questions

1. Bismuth compounds are used to treat several digestive disorders. What are they?

2. What type of teaching plan, including dietary modifications and pharmacologic products, might be developed to "wean" a person off chronic laxative use?

3. There are various classifications of drugs employed in the treatment of nausea and vomiting. Which class is considered to be of greatest benefit?

4. Anorexiants, used to treat obesity, are seldom effective for long-term weight loss. Why, then, are they prescribed?

Critical Thinking Questions

1. The patient has been taking diphenoxylate (Lomotil) for diarrhea for the past 3 days. The patient has had diarrhea five times today. What would be a nursing priority?

2. The healthcare provider has ordered morphine and prochlorperazine (Compazine) for a patient with postoperative pain. The patient insists that she is "needle phobic" and wants all the medication in one syringe. What is the nurse's response?

3. A patient comes to the clinic complaining of no bowel movement for 4 days (other than small amounts of liquid stool). The patient has been taking psyllium mucilloid (Metamucil) for his constipation and wants to know why this is not working. What is the nurse's response?

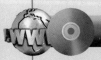 **EXPLORE MediaLink**

NCLEX review, case studies, and other interactive resources for this chapter can be found on the companion website at www.prenhall.com/adams. Click on "Chapter 37" to select the activities for this chapter. For animations, more NCLEX review questions, and an audio glossary, access the accompanying CD-ROM in this textbook.

DRUGS AT A GLANCE

VITAMINS
Lipid soluble
Pr *vitamin A*
Water soluble
Pr *folic acid (Folacin, Folvite)*

MINERALS
Macrominerals
Pr *magnesium sulfate*
Microminerals

NUTRITIONAL SUPPLEMENTS
Enteral nutrition
Parenteral nutrition

metabolized and eliminated by the bod
of this process
PHARMACOLOGY
1. The study of medicines; the discipli
pertaining to how drugs improve the he
of the human body
PHARMACOPEIA

MediaLink www.prenhall.com/adams

CD-ROM
Audio Glossary
NCLEX Review

Companion Website
NCLEX Review
Dosage Calculations
Case Study
Care Plans
Expanded Key Concepts

OBJECTIVES

After reading this chapter, the student should be able to:

1. Identify characteristics that differentiate vitamins from other nutrients.
2. Describe the functions of common vitamins and minerals.
3. Compare and contrast the properties of water-soluble and fat-soluble vitamins.
4. Identify diseases and conditions that may benefit from vitamin or mineral pharmacotherapy.
5. Describe the nurse's role in the pharmacologic management of nutritional disorders.
6. Compare and contrast the properties of macrominerals and trace minerals.
7. Identify differences among oligomeric, polymeric, modular, and specialized formulations for enteral nutrition.
8. Compare and contrast enteral and parenteral methods of providing nutrition.
9. Use the Nursing Process to care for patients who are receiving drug therapy for nutritional disorders.

The nutritional supplement business is a multibillion dollar industry. Although clever marketing often leads patients to believe that vitamin and dietary supplements are essential to maintain health, most people obtain all the necessary nutrients through a balanced diet. Once the body has obtained the amounts of vitamins, minerals, or nutrients it needs to carry on metabolism, the excess is simply excreted or stored. In certain conditions, however, dietary supplementation is necessary and will benefit the patient's health. This chapter focuses on these conditions and explores the role of vitamins, minerals, and nutritional supplements in pharmacology.

| PHARMFACTS | Vitamins, Minerals, and Nutritional Supplements |

- About 40% of Americans take vitamin supplements daily.
- There is no difference between the chemical structure of a natural vitamin and a synthetic vitamin, yet consumers pay much more for the natural type.
- Vitamin B_{12} is only present in animal products. Vegetarians may find adequate amounts in fortified cereals, nutritional supplements, or yeast.
- Administration of folic acid during pregnancy has been found to reduce birth defects in the nervous system of the baby.
- Patients who never go outside or never receive sun exposure may need vitamin D supplements.
- Vitamins technically cannot increase a patient's energy level. Energy can only be provided by adding calories in carbohydrates, proteins, and lipids.
- Heavy menstrual periods may result in considerable iron loss.

VITAMINS

Vitamins are essential substances needed in very small amounts to maintain homeostasis. Patients having a low or unbalanced dietary intake, those who are pregnant, or those experiencing a chronic disease may benefit from vitamin therapy.

38.1 Role of Vitamins in Maintaining Health

Vitamins are organic compounds required by the body in very small amounts for growth and for the maintenance of normal metabolic processes. Since the discovery of thiamine in 1911, over a dozen vitamins have been identified. Because scientists did not know the chemical structures of the vitamins when they were discovered, they assigned letters and numbers such as A, B_{12}, and C. These names are still widely used today.

An important characteristic of vitamins is that, with the exception of vitamin D, human cells cannot synthesize them. They, or their precursors known as provitamins, must be supplied in the diet. A second important characteristic is if the vitamin is not present in adequate amounts, then the body's metabolism will be disrupted and disease will result. Furthermore, the symptoms of the deficiency can be reversed by the administration of the missing vitamin.

Vitamins serve diverse and important roles. For example, the B complex vitamins are coenzymes essential to many metabolic pathways. Vitamin A is a precursor of retinal, a pigment needed for vision. Calcium metabolism is regulated by a hormone that is derived from vitamin D. Without vitamin K, abnormal prothrombin is produced and blood clotting is affected.

38.2 Classification of Vitamins

A simple way to classify vitamins is by their ability to mix with water. Those that dissolve easily in water are called water-soluble vitamins. Examples include vitamin C and the B vitamins. Those that dissolve in lipids are called fat or lipid-soluble and include vitamins A, D, E, and K.

The difference in solubility affects the way the vitamins are absorbed by the GI tract and stored in the body. The water-soluble vitamins are absorbed with water in the digestive tract and readily dissolve in blood and body fluids. When excess water-soluble vitamins are absorbed, they cannot be stored for later use and are simply excreted in the urine. Because they are not stored to any significant degree, they must be ingested daily, otherwise deficiencies will quickly develop.

Fat-soluble vitamins, on the other hand, cannot be absorbed in sufficient quantity in the small intestine unless they are ingested with other lipids. These vitamins can be stored in large quantities in the liver and adipose tissue. Should the patient not ingest sufficient amounts, fat-soluble vitamins are removed from storage depots in the body, as needed. Unfortunately, storage may lead to dangerously high levels of these vitamins, if they are taken in excessive amounts.

38.3 Recommended Dietary Allowances

Based on scientific research on humans and animals, the Food and Nutrition Board of the National Academy of Sciences has established levels for the dietary intake of vitamins and minerals called Recommended Dietary Allowances (RDAs). Canada publishes similar data called the Recommended Nutrient Intake (RNI). The RDA values represent the *minimum* amount of vitamin or mineral needed to prevent a deficiency in a healthy adult. The RDAs are revised periodically to reflect the latest scientific research. Current RDAs for vitamins are shown in Table 38.1.

The need for certain vitamins and minerals varies widely. Patients who are pregnant, have chronic disease, or exercise vigorously have different nutritional needs than the average adult. Recognizing and adjusting for these nutritional differences is essential to maintaining good health.

Vitamin, mineral, or herbal supplements should never substitute for a balanced diet. Sufficient intake of proteins, carbohydrates, and lipids is needed for proper health. Furthermore, although the label on a vitamin supplement may indicate that it contains 100% of the RDA for a particular vitamin, the body may absorb as little as 10% to 15% of the amount ingested. With the exception of vitamins A and D, it is not harmful for most patients to consume 2 to 3 times the recommended levels of vitamins.

38.4 Indications for Vitamin Pharmacotherapy

Most patients who eat a normal, balanced diet are able to obtain all the necessary nutrients they need, without vitamin supplementation. Indeed, megavitamin therapy is not only expensive, but also harmful to health if taken for prolonged periods. Hypervitaminosis, or toxic levels of vitamins, has been reported for vitamins A, C, D, E, B_6, niacin, and folic acid. In the United States, syndromes of vitamin excess may actually be more common than those of vitamin deficiency.

Vitamin deficiencies follow certain patterns. The following are general characteristics of vitamin deficiency disorders.

- Patients more commonly present with multiple vitamin deficiencies than with a single vitamin deficiency.
- Symptoms of deficiency are nonspecific, and often do not appear until the deficiency has been present for a prolonged period.
- Deficiencies in the United States are most often the result of poverty, fad diets, chronic alcohol or drug abuse, or prolonged parenteral feeding.

Certain patients and conditions require higher levels of vitamins. Infancy and childhood are times of potential deficiency due to the high growth demands placed on the body. In addition, requirements for all nutrients are increased during pregnancy and lactation. With normal aging, the absorption of food diminishes and the quantity of ingested food is often reduced, leading to a higher risk of vitamin deficiencies in elderly patients. Vitamin deficiencies in patients with chronic liver and kidney disease are well documented.

Certain drugs affect vitamin metabolism. Alcohol is known for its ability to inhibit the absorption of thiamine and folic acid. Alcohol abuse is the most common cause of thiamine deficiency in the United States. Folic acid levels may be reduced in patients taking phenothiazines, oral contraceptives, phenytoin (Dilantin), or barbiturates. Vitamin D deficiency can be caused by therapy with certain anticonvulsants. Inhibition of vitamin B_{12} absorption has been reported with a number of drugs including trifluoperazine (Stelazine), alcohol, and oral contraceptives. The nurse must be aware of these drug interactions and recommend vitamin therapy when appropriate.

Table 38.1	**Vitamins**			
Vitamin	**Function(s)**	**RDA**		**Common Cause(s) of Deficiency**
		Men	**Women**	
A	visual pigments, epithelial cells	1,000 mg RE*	800 mg RE	prolonged dietary deprivation, particularly where rice is the main food source; pancreatic disease; cirrhosis
B complex: biotin	coenzyme in metabolic	30 μg	30 μg	deficiencies are rare
cyanocobalamin B$_{12}$	coenzyme in nucleic acid metabolism	2 μg	2 μg	lack if intrinsic factor, inadequate intake of foods from animal origin
folate	coenzyme in amino acid and nucleic acid metabolism	200 μg	160–180 μg	pregnancy, alcoholism, cancer, oral contraceptive use
niacin B$_3$	coenzyme in metabolic reactions	15–20 mg	13–15 mg	prolonged dietary deprivation, particularly where Indian corn (maize) or millet is the main food source; chronic diarrhea; liver disease; alcoholism
pantothenic acid	coenzyme in metabolic reactions	5 mg	5 mg	deficiencies are rare
pyridoxine B$_6$	coenzyme in amino acid metabolism	2 mg	1.5–1.6 mg	alcoholism; oral contraceptive use; malabsorption diseases
riboflavin B$_2$	coenzyme in metabolic reactions	1.4–1.8 mg	1.2–1.3 mg	Inadequate consumption of milk or animal products; chronic diarrhea; liver disease; alcoholism
thiamine B$_1$	coenzyme in metabolic reactions	1.2–1.5 mg	1.0–1.1 mg	prolonged dietary deprivation, particularly where rice is the main food source; hyperthyroidism, pregnancy, liver disease; alcoholism
C	coenxyme and antioxidant	60 mg	60 mg	inadequate intake of fruits and vegetables; pregnancy, chronic inflammatory disease; burns; diarrhea; alcoholism
D	calcium and phosphate metabolism	5–10 mg	5–10 μg	low dietary intake; inadequate exposure to sunlight
E	antioxidant	10 TE**	8 mg TE	premature infants; malabsorption diseases
K	cofactor in blood clotting	65–80 μg	55–65 μg	newborns; liver disease; long-term parenteral nutrition; certain drugs such as cephalosporins and salicylates

* RE = retinoid equivalents

** TE = alpha-tocopherol equivalents

Lipid-Soluble Vitamins

The lipid- or fat-soluble vitamins are abundant in both plant and animal foods, and are relatively stable during cooking.

38.5 Pharmacotherapy with Lipid-Soluble Vitamins

Lipid-soluble vitamins are absorbed from the intestine with dietary lipids and are stored primarily in the liver. When consumed in high amounts, these vitamins can accumulate to toxic levels and produce hypervitaminosis. Because these are OTC agents, patients must be strongly advised to care-fully follow the instructions of the healthcare provider, or the label directions, for proper dosage. It is not unusual to find some OTC preparations that contain up 200% to 400% of the RDA. Medications containing lipid-soluble vitamins, and their doses, are given in Table 38.2.

Vitamin A, also known as retinol, is obtained from foods containing carotenes, precursors to vitamin A that are converted to retinol in the wall of the small intestine following absorption. The most abundant and biologically active carotene is beta carotene. During metabolism, each molecule of beta carotene yields two molecules of vitamin A. Good sources of dietary vitamin A include yellow and dark leafy vegetables, butter, eggs, whole milk, and liver.

Table 38.2	Lipid-Soluble Vitamins for Treating Nutritional Disorders
Drug	**Route and Adult Dose (max dose where indicated)**
vitamin A (Aquasol A)	PO; 500,000 IU/day for 3 d followed by 50,000 IU/d for 2 wk, then 10,000–20,000 IU d for 2 mo
	IM; 100,000 IU/d for 3 d followed by 50,000 IU/d for 2 wk
vitamin D: calcitriol (Calcijex, Rocaltrol)	PO; 0.25 µg/d, may be increased by 0.25 µg/day q4–8wk for dialysis patients or q2–4wk for hypoparathyroid patients if necessary
	IV; 0.5 µg three times/wk at the end of dialysis, may need up to 3 µg three times/wk
vitamin E: tocopherol (Aquasol E, Vita-Plus E, others)	PO/IM; 60–75 IU/d
vitamin K: phytonadione (AquaMEPHYTON)	PO/SC/IM; 2.5–10 mg (up to 25 mg), may be repeated after 6–8 hr if needed

Vitamin D is actually a group of chemicals sharing similar activity. Vitamin D_2, also known as **ergocalciferol**, is obtained from fortified milk, margarine, and other dairy products. Vitamin D_3 is formed in the skin by a chemical reaction requiring ultraviolet radiation. The pharmacology of the D vitamins, and a drug prototype for the active form of vitamin D, are detailed in Chapter 46 ⊙.

Vitamin E consists of about eight chemicals, called **tocopherols**, having similar activity. Alpha-tocopherol comprises 90% of the tocopherols, and is the only one of pharmacologic importance. Dosage is sometimes reported as milligrams of alpha-tocopherol equivalents (TE). Vitamin E is found in plant seed oils, whole grain cereals, eggs, and certain organ meats such as liver, pancreas, and heart. It is considered a primary antioxidant, preventing the formation of free radicals that damage cell membranes and cellular structures. Deficiency in adults has only been observed with severe malabsorption disorders; however, deficiency in premature neonates may lead to hemolytic anemia. Patients may self-administer vitamin E because it is thought to be useful in preventing heart disease and increasing sexual prowess. Unlike most other vitamins, therapeutic doses of vitamin E have not been clearly established although supplements available OTC suggest doses of 100 to 400 units per day. In addition to oral and IM preparations, a topical form is available to treat dry, cracked skin.

Vitamin K is also a mixture of several chemicals. Vitamin K_1 is found in plant sources, particularly green leafy vegetables, tomatoes, cauliflower, egg yolks, liver, and cheeses. Vitamin K_2 is synthesized by microbial flora in the colon. Deficiency states, caused by inadequate intake or by antibiotic destruction of normal intestinal flora, may result in delayed hemostasis. The body does not have large stores of vitamin K, and a deficiency may occur in only 1 to 2 weeks. Certain clotting factors (II, VII, IX, and X) are dependent upon vitamin K for their biosynthesis. Vitamin K is used as a treatment for patients with clotting disorders and is the antidote for warfarin (Coumadin) overdose. It is also given to infants at birth to promote blood clotting. Administration of vitamin K completely reverses deficiency symptoms.

SPECIAL CONSIDERATIONS

Vitamin Supplements and Patient Communication

In the current culture, many people take vitamin supplements. Product advertising promotes vitamin supplements as a means to maintain optimal health. If taken in recommended dosages, vitamin toxicity is not a concern in healthy people, however, some vitamin supplements should be taken with caution as they can interact with prescribed medications. Some products are fortified with vitamins or minerals. For example, certain manufacturers claim that their cereals and juices have 100% of the RDA for particular vitamins and minerals. People who take supplements may not consider these fortified foods as vitamin sources, and accidental overdosage can result.

Healthcare providers should adopt a nonjudgmental attitude that promotes trust and honest communication with the patient. In this way, the patient will be open about the use of vitamin and nutritional supplements. Acceptance and understanding are necessary to assist patients to take vitamins in a responsible way that does not compromise clinical drug treatment.

NURSING CONSIDERATIONS

The role of the nurse in drug therapy with fat-soluble vitamins involves careful monitoring of a patient's condition and providing education as it relates to the prescribed drug regimen. The nurse is responsible for assessing, counseling, and monitoring patients taking fat-soluble vitamins. Because these vitamins are available OTC, patients consider them relatively harmless. The nurse should teach patients that excessive vitamin intake can be harmful.

For all fat-soluble vitamins, the nurse should begin with assessment for deficiency. The symptoms of inadequate supply or storage of fat-soluble vitamins is dependent of the specific nutrient. For example, patients deficient in vitamin A frequently report problems with night vision, skin lesions, or mucous membrane dysfunction. A baseline visual acuity exam should be performed.

In severe vitamin D deficiency, patients experience skeletal abnormalities, such as rickets in children and osteomalcia in adults. The nurse should assess laboratory tests for serum levels of calcium, phosphorus, magnesium, alkaline phosphatase, and creatinine to determine electrolyte and mineral balance. An insufficient level of vitamin E has no obvious effects, but the vitamin is believed to protect cellular components from oxidation. Bleeding tendencies are characteristic of vitamin K deficiency. Patients should be assessed for impaired liver function, because fat-soluble vitamins are stored in the liver, and for malabsorption disorders that could prevent the absorption of the vitamins.

The nurse should also assess the patient's dietary intake. Patients should be instructed in foods that may supply the necessary fat-soluble vitamins essential for good health. When performing dietary counseling, it is critical that the nurse consider the socioeconomic status and culture of the patient when recommending foods that may be used to treat deficiency and to suggest foods that the patient can afford or will eat.

Fat-soluble vitamins stored in the liver can accumulate to toxic levels, causing accidental hypervitaminosis. Chronic overdose will affect many organs, including the liver. Excessive vitamin A intake taken during pregnancy can result in severe birth defects. Intravenous infusion of vitamin K is only used in emergency situations because it may cause bronchospasm, respiratory, and cardiac arrest. Large doses of vitamin E appear to be nontoxic; however, the nurse should monitor patients concurrently taking warfarin (Coumadin) for increased risk of bleeding.

Patient education as it relates to fat-soluble vitamins should include goals, reasons for obtaining baseline data such as lab tests for liver function and CBC, and possible side effects. Following are important points the nurse should include when teaching patients about fat-soluble vitamins:

- Take vitamins only as prescribed or as directed on the label. Do not double doses.
- Discontinue using the vitamin and notify your healthcare provider immediately if toxicity symptoms occur.
- Consult your healthcare provider before taking OTC drugs; they might contain additional fat-soluble vitamins and lead to toxicity.
- Include vitamin-rich foods in your diet, to decrease the need for vitamin supplements.

Water-Soluble Vitamins

The water-soluble vitamins consist of the B complex vitamins and vitamin C.

38.6 Pharmacotherapy with Water-Soluble Vitamins

The B complex group is composed of 12 different vitamins that are grouped together because they were originally derived from yeast and foods that counteracted the disease beriberi. They have very different chemical structures and serve different metabolic functions. The B vitamins are known by their chemical names as well as their vitamin number. For example, vitamin B_{12} is also called cyanocobalamin. Medications containing water-soluble vitamins, and their doses, are given in Table 38.3.

Pr PROTOTYPE DRUG | VITAMIN A (Aquasol A)

ACTIONS AND USES

Vitamin A is essential for general growth and development, particularly of the bones, teeth, and epithelial membranes. It is necessary for proper wound healing, essential for the biosynthesis of steroids, and is one of the pigments required for night vision. Vitamin A is indicated in deficiency states and during periods of increased need such as pregnancy, lactation, or debilitated states. Night blindness and slow wound healing can be effectively treated with as little as 30,000 IU of vitamin A given daily over a week. It is also prescribed for GI disorders, when absorption in the small intestine is diminished or absent. Topical forms are available for acne, psoriasis, and other skin disorders. Doses of vitamin A are sometimes measured in retinoid equivalents (RE). In severe deficiency states, up to 500,000 IU may be given per day for 3 days, gradually tapering off to 10,000 to 20,000 IU/day.

Administration Alerts

- Pregnancy category A at low doses
- Pregnancy category X at high doses.

ADVERSE EFFECTS AND INTERACTIONS

Adverse effects are not observed with low doses of vitamin A. Acute ingestion produces serious CNS toxicity, including headache, irritability, drowsiness, delirium, and possible coma. Long-term ingestion of high amounts causes drying and scaling of the skin, alopecia, fatigue, anorexia, vomiting, and leukopenia.

People taking vitamin A should avoid taking mineral oil and cholestyramine, as both may decrease the absorption of vitamin A.

NURSING PROCESS FOCUS | PATIENTS RECEIVING VITAMIN A (AQUASOL A)

ASSESSMENT

Prior to administration:
- Obtain complete health history including allergies, drug history, and possible drug interactions.
- Obtain complete physical examination.
- Assess for the presence/history of vitamin A deficiency such as inadequate dietary intake, malabsorption diseases, and impaired liver function.
- Obtain baseline vision acuity examination.
- Assess integrity of skin and mucous membranes.
- Obtain the following laboratory studies: serum vitamin A level, CBC, liver function profile, and serum protein/albumin levels

POTENTIAL NURSING DIAGNOSES

- Imbalanced Nutrition: Less than Body Requirements
- Disturbed Sensory Perception, related to vitamin A deficiency
- Risk for Impaired Skin Integrity
- Deficient Knowledge, related to drug therapy

PLANNING: PATIENT GOALS AND EXPECTED OUTCOMES

The patient will:
- Exhibit improvement in serum vitamin A level
- Demonstrate an understanding of the drug's action by accurately describing drug side effects and precautions
- Immediately report side effects such as increased nausea, vomiting, headache, loss of hair, lethargy, and malaise

IMPLEMENTATION

Interventions and (Rationales)	Patient Education/Discharge Planning
■ Monitor patient's diet to determine intake of vitamin A foods. (Deficiency state may be caused by poor dietary habits.)	Instruct patient to: ■ Maintain a dietary log for 48 hr ■ Eat foods rich in vitamin A such as egg yolks, butter, milk, liver, dark leafy vegetables, and orange fruits and vegetables
■ Periodically monitor visual acuity. (Vitamin A may cause miosis, papilledema, and nystagmus.)	■ Advise patient to report any changes in vision.
■ Monitor for symptoms of vitamin A toxicity. (Storage of excess vitamin A can lead to hypervitaminosis.)	Instruct patient to: ■ Watch for signs and symptoms of vitamin A overdose such as nausea, vomiting, anorexia, dry skin and lips, headache, and loss of hair ■ Immediately stop taking medication if signs of toxicity are noted
■ Monitor for signs of intracranial pressure. (Vitamin A may cause increased intracranial pressure if taken in large doses.)	Instruct patient to: ■ Follow dosage directions given by the healthcare provider or on the label ■ Immediately report any changes in neurologic status such as increased sleepiness, headaches, lethargy, and malaise
■ Assess for use of mineral oil. (Mineral oil inhibits the absorption of vitamin A.)	■ Advise patient to avoid laxatives that contain mineral oil.
■ Monitor for drug interactions with oral contraceptives. (Concurrent use of vitamin A and oral contraceptives can cause toxic levels of vitamin A.)	Instruct patient to: ■ Adhere to medication schedule and avoid double doses of the vitamin ■ Keep appointments for follow-up laboratory studies if taking oral contraceptives

EVALUATION OF OUTCOME CRITERIA

Evaluate the effectiveness of drug therapy by confirming that patient goals and expected outcomes have been met (see "Planning").

Table 38.3	Water-Soluble Vitamins for Treating Nutritional Disorders
Drug	**Route and Adult Dose (max dose where indicated)**
vitamin B_1: thiamine hydrochloride (Betalins, Biamine)	IV/IM; 50–100 mg tid
vitamin B_2: riboflavin	PO; 5–10 mg/d
vitamin B_3: niacin (Niac, Nicobid, Nicolar, others)	PO; 10–20 mg/d; IV/IM/SC; 25–100 mg two to five times/d
vitamin B_6: pyridoxine hydrochloride (Beesix, hexaBetalin, NesTrex)	PO/IM/IV; 2.5–10 mg/d times 3 wk, then may reduce to 2.5–5 mg/d
Pr vitamin B_9: folic acid (Folacin, Folvite)	PO/IM/SC/IV; ≤ 1 mg/d
vitamin B_{12}: cyanocobalamin (Betalin 12, Cobex, Cyanabin, others)	IM/Deep SC; 30 µg/d for 5–10 d, then 100–200 µg/mo
vitamin C: ascorbic acid (Ascorbicap, Cebid, Vita-C, others)	PO/IV/IM/SC; 150–500 mg/d in one to two doses

Vitamin B_1, or thiamine, is a precursor of an enzyme responsible for several steps in the oxidation of carbohydrates. It is abundant in both plant and animal products, especially whole grain foods, dried beans, and peanuts. Because of its abundance, thiamine deficiency in the United States is not common, except in alcoholics and in patients with chronic liver disease. Thiamine deficiency, or beriberi, is characterized by neurologic signs such as paresthesia, neuralgia, and progressive loss of feeling and reflexes. Chronic deficiency can result in heart failure. Severe deficiencies may require parenteral thiamine up to 100 mg/day. With pharmacotherapy, symptoms can be completely reversed in the early stages of the disease; however, permanent disability can result in patients with prolonged deficiency.

Vitamin B_2, or riboflavin, is a component of coenzymes that participate in a number of different oxidation-reduction reactions. Riboflavin is abundantly found in plant and meat products, including wheat germ, eggs, cheese, fish, nuts, and leafy vegetables. Like thiamine, deficiency of riboflavin is most commonly observed in alcoholics. Signs of deficiency include corneal vascularization and anemia, as well as skin abnormalities such as dermatitis and cheilosis. Most symptoms are resolved by administering 25 to 100 mg/day until improvement is noted.

Vitamin B_3, or niacin, is a key component of nicotinamide adenine dinucleotide (NAD) and nicotinamide adenine dinucleotide phosphate (NADP), two coenzymes that are essential for oxidative metabolism. Niacin is synthesized from the amino acid tryptophan and is widely distributed in both animal and plant foodstuffs, including beans, wheat germ, meats, nuts, and whole grain breads. Niacin deficiency, or pellagra, is most commonly seen in alcoholics, and in those areas of the world where corn is the primary food source. Early symptoms include fatigue, anorexia, and drying of the skin. Advanced symptoms include three classic signs: dermatitis, diarrhea, and dementia. Deficiency is treated with niacin at dosages ranging from 10 to 25 mg per day. When used to treat hyperlipidemia, niacin is given as nicotinic acid and doses are much higher—up to 3 g per day (Chapter 27) .

Vitamin B_6, or pyridoxine, consists of several closely related compounds, including pyridoxine itself, pyridoxal, and pyridoxamine. Vitamin B_6 is essential for the synthesis of heme, and is a primary coenzyme involved in the metabolism of amino acids. It is also needed for the synthesis of the neurotransmitter gamma-aminobutyric acid (GABA). Deficiency states can be the result of alcoholism, uremia, hypothyroidism, or heart failure. Certain drugs can cause vitamin B_6 deficiency, including isoniazid (INH), cycloserine (Seromycin), hydralazine (Apresoline), oral contraceptives, and pyrazinamide (PZA). Patients receiving these drugs may routinely receive B_6 supplementation. Deficiency symptoms include skin abnormalities, cheilosis, fatigue, and irritability. Symptoms reverse after administration of about 10 to 20 mg/day for several weeks.

Vitamin B_9, more commonly known as folate or folic acid, is metabolized to tetrahydrofolate, which is essential for normal DNA synthesis and for erythropoiesis. Folic acid is widely distributed in plant products, especially green leafy vegetables and citrus fruits. This vitamin is highlighted as a drug prototype in this chapter.

Vitamin B_{12}, or cyanocobalamin, is folate of a cobalt-containing vitamin that is a required coenzyme for a number of metabolic pathways. It also has important roles in cell replication, erythrocyte maturation, and myelin synthesis. Sources include lean meat, seafood, liver, and milk. Deficiency of vitamin B_{12} results in pernicious (megaloblastic) anemia. This vitamin is featured as a prototype drug in Chapter 28 .

Vitamin C, or ascorbic acid, is the most commonly purchased OTC vitamin. It is a potent antioxidant, and serves many functions including collagen synthesis, tissue healing, and maintenance of bone, teeth, and epithelial tissue. Many consumers purchase the vitamin for its ability to prevent the common cold, a function that has not been definitively proven. Deficiency of vitamin C, or scurvy, is caused by diets deficient in fruits and vegetables. Alcoholics, cigarette smokers, cancer patients, and those with renal failure are at highest risk to vitamin C deficiency. Symptoms include fatigue, bleeding gums and other hemorrhages, gingivitis, and poor wound healing. Symptoms can normally be reversed by the administration of 300 to 1,000 mg/day of vitamin C for several weeks.

Although there is a great deal of anecdotal evidence that vitamin C helps to fend off a cold, the claims are unsubstantiated; however, vitamin C may be useful as an immune stimulator and modulator in some circumstances. Several studies have shown that vitamin C can significantly reduce the duration and severity of colds in some people and reduce the incidence in others. It is thought that this is due, at least in part, to antihistamine activity of vitamin C. The best results were obtained with 2 g (or greater) daily doses. Preliminary evidence also suggests that vitamin C can be useful in improving respiratory infections.

NURSING CONSIDERATIONS

The role of the nurse in water-soluble vitamin therapy involves careful monitoring of a patient's condition and providing education as it relates to the prescribed drug regimen. Water-soluble vitamins are used for multiple reasons in healthcare. The nurse should determine the reason for the specific vitamin therapy being prescribed and assess for the presence or absence of the associated symptoms.

Thiamine is often administered to hospitalized patients who have severe liver disease. If thiamine deficiency is not corrected in these patients, irreversible brain damage may occur. There are no known adverse effects from oral administration of thiamine and parenteral administration rarely causes any type of adverse effect. Niacin may be administered in the treatment of niacin deficiency or as an adjunct in cholesterol-lowering therapy. Pyridoxine deficiency is also associated with poor nutritional status, chronic debilitating diseases, and alcohol abuse. Both niacin and pyridoxine may cause severe flushing. The nurse should inform the patient that this is an expected reaction and will not cause permanent harm. Most pa-

tients tolerate therapy with the B vitamins with few adverse effects.

Vitamin C, readily available as an OTC nutritional supplement, may cause diarrhea, nausea, vomiting, abdominal pain, and hyperuricemia in high doses. Patients with a history of kidney stones should be cautioned against using vitamin C, unless directed by a healthcare provider, because excessive intake may promote renal calculi formation. Patients taking vitamin C should be advised to increase fluid intake. Most patients are able to take vitamin C without experiencing serious side effects.

Patient education as it relates to water-soluble vitamins should include goals, reasons for obtaining baseline data such as lab tests for liver function and CBC, and possible side effects. Following are the important points the nurse should include when teaching patients about water-soluble vitamins.

- Niacin and pyridoxine may cause a feeling of warmth and flushing of skin, but this will diminish with continued therapy.
- Include vitamin-rich foods (whole grains, fresh vegetables, fresh fruits, lean meats, and dairy products) in the diet, to decrease the need for vitamin supplements.
- Water-soluble vitamins are not stored in the body and must be replenished daily.
- Take vitamins only as prescribed or as directed on the label. Do not double doses.

MINERALS

Minerals are inorganic substances needed in small amounts to maintain homeostasis. Minerals are classified as macrominerals or microminerals; the macrominerals must be ingested in larger amounts. A normal, balanced diet will provide the proper amounts of the required minerals in most patients. The primary minerals used in pharmacotherapy are shown in Table 38.4.

Pr PROTOTYPE DRUG | **FOLIC ACID** (Folacin, Folvite)

ACTIONS AND USES

Folic acid is administered to reverse symptoms of deficiency, which most commonly occurs in patients with inadequate intake, such as with chronic alcohol abuse. Because this vitamin is destroyed by high temperatures, people who overcook their food may experience folate deficiency. Pregnancy markedly increases the need for dietary folic acid; folic acid is given during pregnancy to promote normal fetal growth. Because insufficient vitamin B$_{12}$ creates a lack of activated folic acid, deficiency symptoms resemble those of vitamin B$_{12}$ deficiency. The megaloblastic anemia observed in folate-deficient patients, however, does not include the severe nervous system symptoms seen in patients with B$_{12}$ deficiency. Administration of 1 mg/day of oral folic acid often reverses the deficiency symptoms within 5 to 7 days. Folic acid is pregnancy category A.

ADVERSE EFFECTS AND INTERACTIONS

Side effects during folic acid therapy are uncommon. Patients may feel flushed following IV injections. Allergies to folic acid are possible.

Folic acid interacts with many drugs. For example, phenytoin, trimethoprim-sulfisoxazole, and other medications may interfere with the absorption of folic acid. Chloramphenicol may antagonize effects of folate therapy. Oral contraceptives, alcohol, barbiturates, methotrexate, and primidone may cause folate deficiency.

NURSING PROCESS FOCUS   **PATIENTS RECEIVING FOLIC ACID (FOLACIN, FOLVITE) Pr**

ASSESSMENT

Prior to administration:
- Obtain complete health history including allergies, drug history, and possible drug interactions.
- Obtain complete physical examination with special attention to symptoms related to anemic states such as pallor, fatigue, weakness, tachycardia, and shortness of breath.
- Obtain the following laboratory studies: folic acid levels, hemoglobin, hematocrit, and reticulocyte counts
- Obtain CBC to determine the type of anemia present. (Folic acid is not beneficial in normocytic anemia, refractory anemia, and aplastic anemia.)

POTENTIAL NURSING DIAGNOSES

- Imbalanced Nutrition: Less than Body Requirements
- Deficient Knowledge, related to drug therapy

PLANNING: PATIENT GOALS AND EXPECTED OUTCOMES

The patient will:
- Exhibit improvement in serum folic acid level
- Demonstrate an understanding of the drug's action by accurately describing drug side effects and precautions
- Immediately report side effects such as continued weakness and fatigue

IMPLEMENTATION

Interventions and (Rationales)	*Patient Education/Discharge Planning*
■ Monitor patient's dietary intake of folic acid-containing foods. (Deficiency state may be caused by poor dietary habits.)	Instruct patient to: ■ Eat foods high in folic acid such as vegetables, fruits, and organ meats ■ Consult with healthcare provider concerning amount of folic acid that should be in the diet
■ Encourage patient to conserve energy. (Anemia, caused by folic acid deficiency may lead to weakness and fatigue.)	Advise patient to: ■ Rest when tired and not to overexert ■ Plan activities to avoid fatigue
■ Encourage patient to take medication appropriately.	Instruct patient to: ■ Avoid use of alcohol because it increases folic acid requirements ■ Take only the amount of the drug prescribed

EVALUATION OF OUTCOME CRITERIA

Evaluate the effectiveness of drug therapy by confirming that patient goals and expected outcomes have been met (see "Planning").

38.7 Pharmacotherapy with Minerals

Minerals are essential substances that constitute about 4% of the body weight and serve many diverse functions. Some are present primarily as essential ions or electrolytes in body fluids; others are bound to organic molecules such as hemoglobin, phospholipids, or metabolic enzymes. Those minerals that function as critical electrolytes in the body, most notably sodium and potassium, are covered in more detail in Chapter 44 ⊙. Sodium chloride and potassium chloride are featured as drug prototypes in that chapter.

Because minerals are needed in very small amounts for human metabolism, a normal balanced diet will supply the necessary quantities for most patients. Like vitamins, excess amounts of minerals can lead to toxicity and patients should be advised not to exceed recommended doses. Mineral supplements, however, are indicated for certain disorders. Iron-deficiency anemia is the most common nutritional deficiency in the world, and is a common indication for iron supplements. Women at high risk of osteoporosis are advised to consume extra calcium, either in their diet or as a dietary supplement.

Table 38.4	Minerals for Treating Nutritional Disorders
Drug	**Route and Adult Dose (max dose where indicated)**
sodium bicarbonate (see page 664 for the Prototype Drug box) ⓒⓄ	PO; 0.3–2.0 g qd-qid or 1 tsp of powder in glass of water
potassium chloride (K-Dur, Micro-K, Klor-Con, others) (see page 662 for the Prototype Drug box) ⓒⓄ	PO; 10–100 mEq/h divided doses IV; 10–40 mEq/h diluted to at least 10–20 mEq/100 mL of solution (max 200–400 mEq/d)
Calcium Salts	
calcium carbonate (BioCal, Titralac, others)	PO; 1–2 g bid-tid
calcium chloride (Calciject, Calcitrans, Solucalcine)	IV; 0.5–1.0 g qd q3d
calcium citrate (Citracal)	PO; 1–2 g bid-tid
calcium gluceptate (Glu-calcium, Calcitrans)	IV; 1.1–4.4 g qd IM; 0.5–1.1 g qd
calcium phosphate tribasic (Posture)	PO; 1–2 g bid-tid
calcium gluconate (Kalcinate) (see page 683 for the Prototype Drug box) ⓒⓄ	PO; 1–2 g bid-qid
calcium lactate (Cal-Lac, Calcimax, others)	PO; 325 mg–1.3 g tid with meals
Iron Salts	
ferrous fumarate (Feco-T, Femiron, Feostat, others)	200 mg tid-qid
ferrous gluconate (Fergon, Simron)	325–600 mg qid, may be gradually increased to 650 mg qid as needed and tolerated
ferrous sulfate (Feosol, Fer-Iron, others) (see page 381 for the Prototype Drug box) ⓒⓄ	750–1,500 mg qd in one to three divided doses
iron dextran (Dexferrum, Imfed, Imferon)	IM/IV dose is individualized and determined from a table of correlations between patient's weight and hemoglobin per package insert; (max 100 mg (2 ml) of iron dextran within 24 hr)
iron sucrose injection (Venofer)	IV; 1 ml (20 mg) injected in dialysis line at rate of 1 ml/min up to 5 ml (100 mg) or infuse 100 mg in NS over 15 min one to three times/wk
Magnesium	
magnesium chloride (Chloromag, Slo-Mag)	PO; 270–400 mg qd
magnesium oxide (Mag-Ox, Maox, others)	PO; 400–1,200 mg/d in divided doses
ⓟ magnesium sulfate (Epsom Salt)	IV/IM; 0.5–3.0 g qd
Phosphorous	
monobasic potassium phosphate (K-Phos original)	PO; 1 g qid
monobasic potassium and sodium phosphates (K-Phos MF, K-Phos neutral)	PO; 250 mg qid (max 2 g phosphorous/d)
potassium phosphate (Neutra-Phos-K)	PO; 1.45 g qid IV; 10 mmol phosphorous/d
potassium and sodium phosphates (Neutra-Phos, Uro-KP neutral)	PO; 250 mg phosphorous qid
Zinc	
zinc acetate (Galzin)	PO; 50 mg tid
zinc gluconate	PO; 20–100 mg (20 mg lozenges may be taken to a max of six lozenges/d)
zinc sulfate (Orazinc, Zincate, others)	PO; 15–220 mg qd

Certain drugs affect normal mineral metabolism. Patients taking loop or thiazide diuretics can cause significant potassium loss. Corticosteroids and oral contraceptives are among several classes of drugs that can promote sodium retention. The uptake of iodine by the thyroid gland can be impaired by certain oral hypoglycemics and lithium carbonate (Eskalith). Oral contraceptives have been reported to lower the plasma levels of zinc and to increase those of copper. The nurse must be aware of these drug-related interactions and recommend changes to mineral intake when appropriate.

38.8 Pharmacotherapy with Macrominerals

Macrominerals (major minerals) are inorganic substances that must be obtained daily from dietary sources in amounts of 100 mg or higher. The macrominerals include calcium, chlorine, magnesium, phosphorous, potassium, sodium, and sulfur. As bone salts, calcium and phosphorous comprise approximately 75% of the total mineral content in the body. Recommended daily allowances have been established for each of the macrominerals except sulfur, as listed in Table 38.5.

Calcium is essential for nerve conduction, muscular contraction, and hemostasis. Much of the body's calcium is bound in the bony matrix of the skeleton. Hypocalcemia occurs when serum calcium falls below 4.5 mEq/L and may be caused by inadequate intake of calcium-containing foods, lack of vitamin D, chronic diarrhea, or decreased secretion of parathyroid hormone. Symptoms of hypocalcemia involve the nervous and muscular systems. The patient often becomes irritable and restless, and muscular twitches, cramps, spasms, and cardiac abnormalities are common. Long-term hypocalcemia may lead to fractures. Pharmacotherapy includes calcium compounds, which are available in many oral formulations including calcium carbonate, calcium citrate, calcium gluconate, or calcium lactate. In severe cases, IV preparations are administered. Calcium gluconate is featured as a prototype drug in Chapter 43 ∞.

Phosphorous is an essential mineral that is often bound to calcium in the form of calcium phosphate in bones. In addition to its role in bone formation, phosphorous is a component of ATP and nucleic acids. Phosphate (PO_4^{-2}) is an important buffer in the blood. Because of its close relationship to phosphate, phosphorous balance is normally considered the same as phosphate balance. Symptoms of hypophosphatemia include weakness, muscle tremor, anorexia, weak pulse, and bleeding abnormalities. When serum phosphorous falls below 1.5 mEq/L, phosphate therapy is usually administered. Sodium phosphate and potassium phosphate are available for phosphorous deficiencies.

Magnesium is the second most abundant intracellular cation. Like potassium, it is necessary for proper neuromuscular function. Magnesium serves a metabolic role in activating certain enzymes in the breakdown of carbohydrates and proteins. Hypomagnesemia is generally asymptomatic until serum magnesium falls below 1.0 mEq/L. Because it produces few symptoms in its early stages, it is sometimes described as the most common undiagnosed electrolyte abnormality. Patients may experience general weakness, dysrhythmias, hypertension, loss of deep tendon reflexes, and respiratory depression. These symptoms are sometimes mistaken for hypokalemia. Pharmacotherapy with magnesium sulfate can quickly reverse symptoms of hypomagnesemia. Magnesium sulfate is a CNS depressant and is sometimes given to either prevent or terminate seizures associated with eclampsia. Magnesium salts have additional applications as cathartics or antacids (magnesium citrate, magnesium hydroxide, and magnesium oxide) and as analgesics (magnesium salicylate).

Table 38.5	Macrominerals	
Mineral	**RDA**	**Function**
calcium	800–1,200 mg	forms bony matrix; regulates nerve conduction and muscle contraction
chloride	750 mg	major anion in body fluids; part of gastric acid secretion
magnesium	Men: 350–400 mg Women: 280–300 mg	cofactor for many enzymes; necessary for normal nerve conduction and muscle contraction
phosphorous	700 mg	forms bone matrix; part of ATP and nucleic acids
potassium	2.0 g	necessary for normal nerve conduction and muscle contraction; principal cation in intracellular fluid; essential for acid-base and electrolyte balance
sodium	500 mg	necessary for normal nerve conduction and muscle contraction; principal cation in extracellular fluid; essential for acid-base and electrolyte balance
sulfur	not established	component of proteins, B vitamins, and other critical molecules

NURSING CONSIDERATIONS

The role of the nurse in macromineral therapy involves careful monitoring of a patient's condition and providing education as it relates to the prescribed drug regimen. Macrominerals are used for multiple reasons in healthcare. The nurse should determine the reason for the specific macromineral therapy being prescribed and assess for the presence or absence of the associated symptoms.

Although minerals cause no harm in small amounts, larger doses can cause life-threatening adverse effects. Calcium is one of the most common minerals in use. To prevent and treat osteoporosis, it is recommended that adult women take 1,200 mg/day of calcium. Common side effects include mild GI distress and constipation. Prolonged therapy with calcium may increase the risk of hypercalcemia, especially in patients with decreased liver and renal function. Symptoms of hypercalcemia include nausea, vomiting, constipation, frequent urination, lethargy, and depression. Since calcium interacts with many drugs such as glucocorticoids, thiazide diuretics, and tetracyclines, the patient should inform the healthcare provider when using calcium supplements. The patient should also be advised to avoid zinc-rich foods such as legumes, nuts, sprouts, and soy that impair calcium absorption.

Phosphorus is a mineral sometimes used as a dietary supplement. Patients who are on a sodium- or potassium-restricted diet should not use phosphorus supplements. Most adverse effects of excess phosphate are mild and include GI distress, diarrhea, and dizziness. The patient should stop taking phosphorus at the first sign of seizure activity, as phosphorus can promote seizures. Antacids should be avoided because they may decrease serum phosphorus levels.

Magnesium sulfate is given to correct hypomagnesemia, evacuate the bowel in preparation for diagnostic examinations, and for seizures associated with eclampsia of pregnancy. The medication is given orally to replace magnesium and by the IM or IV routes to prevent or terminate eclampsia seizure. When given IV, it is important for the nurse to assess the neurologic status of the patient, because overdose can lead to reduced reflexes and muscle weakness. The nurse should monitor for LOC changes, deep tendon reflexes, thirst and confusion. Because of its effects on muscles and the heart, it is contraindicated in patients with myocardial damage, heart block, and recent cardiac arrest. It has a laxative effect when given orally, so it should not be given to patients with abdominal pain, nausea, vomiting, or intestinal obstruction. Magnesium sulfate should be used with caution in patients with impaired kidney function and those on cardiac glycosides.

Patient education as it relates to macromineral therapy should include goals, reasons for obtaining baseline data such as lab tests for liver function and CBC, and possible side effects. Following are the important points the nurse should include when teaching patients about minerals.

- Take minerals only as prescribed or as directed on the label. Overdose may lead to toxicity.
- Discontinue using the medication and notify the healthcare provider immediately if toxicity symptoms occur.
- Consult the healthcare provider before taking OTC drugs; they might contain additional minerals and lead to toxicity.
- Eat a well-balanced diet to eliminate or reduce the need for mineral supplements.

Pr **PROTOTYPE DRUG** | **MAGNESIUM SULFATE**

ACTIONS AND USES

Severe hypomagnesemia can be rapidly reversed by the administration of IM or IV magnesium sulfate. Hypomagnesemia has a number of causes, including loss of body fluids due to diarrhea, diuretics, or nasogastric suctioning; and prolonged parenteral feeding with magnesium-free solutions. After administration, magnesium sulfate is distributed throughout the body, and effects are observed within 30 minutes. Oral forms of magnesium sulfate are used as cathartics, when complete evacuation of the colon is desired. Its action as a CNS depressant has led to its occasional use as an anticonvulsant. Magnesium sulfate is pregnancy category A.

Administration Alerts

- Continuously monitor patient during IV infusion for early signs of decreased cardiac function.
- Monitor serum magnesium levels every 6 hours during parenteral infusion.
- When giving IV infusion, give required dose over 4 hours.

ADVERSE EFFECTS AND INTERACTIONS

IV infusions of magnesium sulfate require careful observation to avoid toxicity. Early signs of magnesium overdose include flushing of the skin, sedation, confusion, intense thirst, and muscle weakness. Extreme levels cause neuromuscular blockade with resultant respiratory paralysis and heart block and may cause circulatory collapse, complete heart block, and respiratory failure. Plasma magnesium levels should be monitored frequently. Patients receiving CNS depressants may experience increased sedation. Because of these potentially fatal adverse effects, the use of magnesium sulfate is restricted to severe magnesium deficiency. Mild to moderate hypomagnesemia is treated with oral forms of magnesium such as magnesium gluconate or magnesium hydroxide.

Administration of neuromuscular blocking agents with magnesium sulfate may increase respiratory depression and apnea.

NURSING PROCESS FOCUS	**PATIENTS RECEIVING MAGNESIUM SULFATE Pr**

ASSESSMENT

Prior to administration:
- Obtain complete health history including allergies, drug history, and possible drug interactions.
- Obtain complete physical examination with special attention to respiratory status and deep tendon reflexes.
- Assess for the presence/history of malnutrition, hypomagnesia, seizure activity, preeclampsia, and kidney disease.
- Obtain serum magnesium level and renal profile.

POTENTIAL NURSING DIAGNOSES

- Risk for Injury, related to disease conditions and adverse effects of drug
- Deficient Knowledge, related to drug therapy

PLANNING: PATIENT GOALS AND EXPECTED OUTCOMES

The patient will:
- Exhibit improvement in serum magnesium level
- Demonstrate an understanding of the drug's action by accurately describing drug side effects and precautions
- Immediately report side effects such as lowered pulse, dizziness, difficulty breathing, and weakness

IMPLEMENTATION

Interventions and (Rationales)	*Patient Education/Discharge Planning*
▪ Assess magnesium level to determine deficiency. (The therapeutic range is very narrow; toxic levels may develop quickly.)	▪ Instruct patient that magnesium sulfate should only be taken on the advice of a healthcare provider.
▪ Monitor vital signs frequently throughout intravenous infusion. (Magnesium sulfate depresses respirations, pulse rate, and rhythm.)	▪ Instruct patient to report any difficulty breathing, low pulse rate, or dizziness.
▪ Report urine output of <100 ml/hr to healthcare provider. (Patients who have impaired renal function will have decreased renal clearance, leading to toxicity.)	▪ Instruct patient to report any problems with urination or edema.
▪ Observe newborns for signs and symptoms of magnesium toxicity if the mother received magnesium sulfate during labor. (The neonate may have received some amount of magnesium that could cause skeletal muscle and cardiac muscle depression.)	▪ Advise laboring mothers who are receiving magnesium sulfate that the newborn will be monitored closely after birth.

EVALUATION OF OUTCOME CRITERIA

Evaluate the effectiveness of drug therapy by confirming that patient goals and expected outcomes have been met (see "Planning").

38.9 Pharmacotherapy with Microminerals

The nine microminerals, commonly called trace minerals, are required daily in amounts of 20 mg or less. The fact that they are needed in such small amounts does not diminish their role in human health; deficiencies in some of the trace minerals can result in profound illness. The functions of some of the trace minerals, such iron and iodine, are well established; the role of others are less completely understood. The RDA for each of the microminerals is shown in Table 38.6

Iron is an essential micromineral most commonly associated with hemoglobin. Excellent sources of dietary iron include meat, shellfish, nuts, and legumes. Excess iron in the body results in hemochromatosis, whereas lack of iron results in iron-deficiency anemia. The pharmacology of iron supplements is presented in Chapter 28, where ferrous sulfate is featured as a drug prototype ⬭ .

Iodine is a trace mineral needed to synthesize thyroid hormone. The most common source of dietary iodine is iodized salt. When dietary intake of iodine is low, hypothyroidism occurs and enlargement of the thyroid gland

Table 38.6	Microminerals	
Trace Mineral	**RDA**	**Function**
chromium	0.05–2.0 mg	potentiates insulin and is necessary for proper glucose metabolism
cobalt	0.1 μg	cofactor for vitamin B_{12} and several oxidative enzymes
copper	1.5–3.0 mg	cofactor for hemoglobin synthesis
fluorine	1.5–4.0 mg	influences tooth structure and possible effects on growth
iodine	150 μg	component of thyroid hormones
iron	Men: 10–12 mg Women: 10–15 mg	component of hemoglobin and some enzymes of oxidative phosphorylation
manganese	2–5 mg	cofactor in some enzymes of lipid, carbohydrate, and protein metabolism
molybdenum	75–250 mg	cofactor for certain enzymes
selenium	Men: 50–70 μg Women: 50–55 μg	antioxidant cofactor for certain enzymes
zinc	12–15 mg	cofactor of certain enzymes, including carbonic anhydrase; needed for proper protein structure, normal growth, and wound healing

(goiter) results. At high concentrations, iodine suppresses thyroid function. Lugol's solution, a mixture containing 5% elemental iodine and 10% potassium iodide, is given to hyperthyroid patients prior to thyroidectomy or during a thyrotoxic crisis. Sodium iodide acts by rapidly suppressing the secretion of thyroid hormone and is indicated for patients having an acute thyroid crisis. Radioactive iodine (I-131) is given to destroy overactive thyroid glands. Pharmacotherapeutic uses of iodine as a drug extend beyond the treatment of thyroid disease. Iodine is an effective topical antiseptic that can be found in creams, tinctures, and solutions. Iodine molecules such as iothalamate and diatrizoate are very dense and serve as diagnostic contrast agents in radiologic procedures of the urinary and cardiovascular systems. The role of potassium iodide in protecting the thyroid gland during acute radiation exposure is discussed in Chapter 3 ⊕.

Fluorine is a trace mineral found abundantly in nature, and is best known for its effects on bones and teeth. Research has validated that adding fluoride to the water supply in very small amounts (1 part per billion) can reduce the incidence of dental caries. This effect is more pronounced in children, as fluoride is incorporated into the enamel of growing teeth. Concentrated fluoride solutions can also be applied topically by dental professionals. Sodium fluoride and stannous fluoride are components of most toothpastes and oral rinses. Because high amounts of fluoride can be quite toxic, the use of fluoride-containing products should be closely monitored in children.

Zinc is a component of at least 100 enzymes, including alcohol dehydrogenase, carbonic anhydrase, and alkaline phosphatase. This trace mineral has a regulatory function in enzymes controlling nucleic acid synthesis and has been implicated to have roles in wound healing, male fertility, bone formation, and cell-mediated immunity. Zinc sulfate,

zinc acetate, and zinc gluconate are available to prevent and treat deficiency states. In addition, lozenges containing zinc are available OTC for treating sore throats and symptoms of the common cold.

NUTRITIONAL SUPPLEMENTS

The nurse will encounter a large number of patients who are undernourished. Major goals in resolving nutritional deficiencies are to identify the specific type of deficiency and supply the missing nutrients. Nutritional supplements may be needed for short-term therapy, or for the remainder of the patient's life.

38.10 Etiology of Undernutrition

When the patient is taking in or absorbing fewer nutrients than required for normal body growth and maintenance, undernutrition occurs. Successful pharmacotherapy relies upon the skills of the nurse in identifying the symptoms and causes of the patient's undernutrition.

Causes of undernutrition range from the simple to the complex, and include the following:

- Aging
- HIV-AIDS
- Alcoholism
- Burns
- Cancer
- Chronic inflammatory bowel disease
- Eating disorders
- Gastrointestinal disorders
- Chronic neurologic disease such as progressive dysphagia and multiple sclerosis
- Short-bowel syndrome

- Surgery
- Trauma

The most obvious cause for undernutrition is low dietary intake, although reasons for the inadequate intake must be assessed. Patients may have no resources to purchase food and may be suffering from starvation. Clinical depression leads many patients to shun food. Elderly patients may have poor-fitting dentures or difficulty chewing or swallowing after a stroke. In terminal disease, patients may be comatose or otherwise unable to take food orally. Although the etiologies differ, patients with insufficient intake will exhibit a similar pattern of general weakness, muscle wasting, and loss of subcutaneous fat.

When the undernutrition is caused by lack of one specific nutrient, vitamin, or mineral, the disorder is more difficult to diagnose. Patients may be on a fad diet lacking only protein, or just fat from their intake. Certain digestive disorders may lead to malabsorption of specific nutrients or vitamins. Patients may simply avoid certain foods such as green leafy vegetables, dairy products, or meat products, which can lead to specific nutritional deficiencies. Proper pharmcotherapy requires the expert knowledge and assessment skills of the nurse, so that the correct treatment can be administered.

38.11 Enteral Nutrition

A large number of nutritional supplements are available. A common method of classifying these agents is by their route of administration. Products that are administered via the gastrointestinal tract, either orally or through a feeding tube, are classified as enteral nutrition. Those that are administered by means of IV infusion are called parenteral nutrition.

When the patient's condition permits, enteral nutrition is best provided by oral consumption. Oral feeding allows natural digestive processes to occur, and requires less intense nursing care. It does, however, rely on patient compliance, since it is not feasible for the healthcare provider to observe the patient at every meal.

Tube feeding, or enteral tube alimentation, is necessary when the patient has difficulty swallowing or is otherwise unable to take meals orally. Various tube feeding routes are possible, including nasogastric, nasoduodenal, nasojejunal, gastrostomy, or jejunostomy. An advantage of tube feeding is that the nurse can precisely measure and record the amount of enteral nutrition the patient is receiving.

The particular enteral product is chosen to address the specific nutritional needs of the patient. Because of the wide diversity in their formulations, it is difficult to categorize enteral products, and several different methods are used. A simple method is to classify enteral products as oligomeric, polymeric, modular, or specialized formulations.

Oligomeric formulations are agents containing varying amounts of free amino acids and peptide combinations. Indications include partial bowel obstruction, irritable bowel syndrome, radiation enteritis, bowel fistulas, and short-bowel syndrome. Sample products include Vivonex T.E.N. and Peptamen Liquid.

Polymeric formulations are the most common enteral preparations. These products contain various mixtures of proteins, carbohydrates, and lipids. Indications include general undernutrition, although the patient must have a fully functioning GI tract. Sample products include Slenderized Compleat regular, Sustacal Powder, and Ensure-Plus.

Modular formulations contain a single nutrient, protein, lipid, or carbohydrate. Indications include a single nutrient deficiency, or they may be added to other formulations to provide more specific nutrient needs. Sample products include Casec, Polycose, Microlipid, and MCT Oil.

Specialized formulations are products that contain a specific nutrient combination for a particular condition. Indications include a specific disease state such as hepatic failure, renal failure, or a specific genetic enzyme deficiency. Sample products include Amin-Aid, Hepatic-Aid II, and Pulmocare.

Patients sometimes exhibit GI intolerance to enteral nutrition, usually expressed as vomiting, nausea, or diarrhea. Therapy is often started slowly, with small quantities so that side effects can be assessed. The nurse must be observant for drug interactions that occasionally occur when drugs are given along with enteral nutrition.

38.12 Total Parenteral Nutrition

When a patient's metabolic needs are unable to be met through enteral nutrition, total parenteral nutrition (TPN), or hyperalimentation, is indicated. For short-term therapy, peripheral vein TPN may be utilized. Because of the risk of phlebitis, however, long-term therapy often requires central vein TPN. Patients who have undergone major surgery or trauma and those who are severely undernourished are candidates for central vein TPN. Because the GI tract is not being utilized, patients with severe malabsorption disease may be treated successfully with TPN.

TPN is able to provide all of a patient's nutritional needs in a hypertonic solution containing amino acids, lipid emulsions, carbohydrate (as dextrose), electrolytes, vitamins, and minerals. The particular formulation may be specific to the disease state, such as renal failure or hepatic failure. TPN is administered through an infusion pump, so that nutrition can be precisely monitored. Patients in various settings such as acute care, long-term care, and home health care often benefit from TPN therapy. See "Nursing Process Focus: Patients Receiving Total Parenteral Nutrition" for more information.

MediaLink A.S.P.E.N.

NURSING PROCESS FOCUS | PATIENTS RECEIVING TOTAL PARENTERAL NUTRITION

ASSESSMENT

Prior to administration:
- Obtain complete health history including allergies, drug history, and possible drug interactions.
- Obtain complete physical examination.
- Assess for the presence/history of nutritional deficit such as inadequate oral intake, gastrointestinal disease, and increased metabolic need.
- Obtain the following laboratory studies: total protein/albumin levels, creatinine/BUN, CBC electrolytes, lipid profile, and serum iron levels

POTENTIAL NURSING DIAGNOSES

- Risk for Infection
- Imbalanced Nutrition: Less than Body Requirements
- Risk for Imbalanced Fluid Volume
- Deficient Knowledge, related to drug therapy

PLANNING: PATIENT GOALS AND EXPECTED OUTCOMES

The patient will:
- Exhibit improvement or stabilization of nutritional status
- Demonstrate an understanding of the drug's action by accurately describing drug side effects and precautions
- Immediately report side effects such as symptoms of hypoglycemia or hyperglycemia, fever, chills, cough, or malaise

IMPLEMENTATION

Interventions and (Rationales)	Patient Education/Discharge Planning
■ Monitor vital signs, observing for signs of infection such as elevated temperature. (Bacteria may grow in high glucose and high protein solutions.)	■ Instruct patient to report fever, chills, soreness or drainage of the infusion site, cough, and malaise.
■ Take extraordinary precautions to prevent infection. ■ Use strict aseptic technique with IV tubing, dressing changes, and TPN solution. ■ Refrigerate solution until 30 min before using. ■ Comply with healthcare facility protocol for tubing and filter changes.	■ Instruct patient that infusion site is high risk for infection development and the need for sterile dressings and aseptic technique with solutions and tubing.
■ Monitor blood glucose levels. Observe for signs of hyper- or hypoglycemia and administer insulin as directed. (Blood glucose levels may be affected if TPN is turned off, the rate reduced or if excess levels of insulin are added to the solution.)	Instruct patient to report symptoms of: ■ Hyperglycemia (excessive thirst, copious urination, and insatiable hunger) ■ Hypoglycemia (nervousness, irritability, and dizziness)
■ Monitor for signs of fluid overload. (TPN is a hypertonic solution and can create intravascular shifting of extracellular fluid.)	■ Instruct patient to report shortness of breath, heart palpitations, swelling, or decreased urine output.
■ Monitor renal status, including intake and output ratio, daily weight, and laboratory studies such as serum creatinine and BUN.	Instruct patient to: ■ Weigh self daily ■ Monitor intake and output ■ Report sudden increases in weight or decreased urinary output ■ Keep all appointments for follow-up care and laboratory testing
■ Maintain accurate infusion rate with infusion pump. ■ Make rate changes gradually and never discontinue TPN abruptly. ■ Increase or decrease flow rate by no more than 10% to prevent fluctuation in blood glucose levels.	Instruct patient: ■ About the importance of maintaining the prescribed rate of infusion ■ To never stop the TPN solution abruptly unless instructed by the healthcare provider

EVALUATION OF OUTCOME CRITERIA

Evaluate the effectiveness of drug therapy by confirming that patient goals and expected outcomes have been met (see "Planning").

CHAPTER REVIEW

Key Concepts

The numbered key concepts provide a succinct summary of the important points from the corresponding numbered section within the chapter. If any of these points are not clear, refer to the numbered section within the chapter for review. Expanded versions can be found on the companion website.

38.1 Vitamins are organic substances that are needed in small amounts to promote growth and maintain health. Deficiency of a vitamin will result in disease.

38.2 Vitamins are classified as lipid-soluble (A, D, E, and K) or water-soluble (C and B complex).

38.3 Failure to meet the Recommended Dietary Allowances (RDAs) for vitamins may result in deficiency disorders.

38.4 Vitamin therapy is indicated for conditions such as poor nutritional intake, pregnancy, and chronic disease states.

38.5 Deficiencies of vitamins A, D, E, or K are indications for pharmacotherapy with lipid-soluble vitamins.

38.6 Deficiencies of vitamins C, thiamine, niacin, riboflavin, folic acid, cyanocobalamin, or pyridoxine are indications for pharmacotherapy with water-soluble vitamins.

38.7 Minerals are inorganic substances needed in very small amounts to maintain normal body metabolism.

38.8 Pharmacotherapy with macrominerals includes agents containing calcium, magnesium, potassium, or phosphorous.

38.9 Pharmacotherapy with microminerals includes agents containing iron, iodine, fluorine, or zinc.

38.10 Undernutrition may be caused by low dietary intake, malabsorption disorders, fad diets, or wasting disorders such as cancer or AIDS.

38.11 Enteral nutrition, provided orally or through a feeding tube, is a means of meeting a patient's complete nutritional needs.

38.12 Total parenteral nutrition (TPN) is a means of supplying nutrition to patients via a peripheral vein (short term) or central vein (long term).

Review Questions

1. What are some patient conditions in which the RDA for a vitamin may not be sufficient?

2. What is the difference between a vitamin and a mineral?

3. Under what conditions might a patient be switched from enteral nutrition to TPN?

Critical Thinking Questions

1. A patient has been self-medicating with vitamin B$_3$ (niacin) for an elevated cholesterol level. The patient comes to the clinic with a severe case of redness and flushing and is concerned about an allergic reaction. What is the nurse's response?

2. A patient complains of a constant headache for the past several days. The only supplements the patient has been taking is megadoses of vitamins A, C, and E. What would be a priority for the nurse with this patient?

3. A patient presents to the healthcare provider with complaints of severe flank pain. This patient has a history of renal calculi. The only medication the patient takes is a multivitamin daily as well as vitamin C. What is the potential problem?

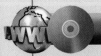 **EXPLORE MediaLink**

NCLEX review, case studies, and other interactive resources for this chapter can be found on the companion website at www.prenhall.com/adams. Click on "Chapter 38" to select the activities for this chapter. For animations, more NCLEX review questions, and an audio glossary, access the accompanying CD-ROM in this textbook.

The Endocrine and Genitourinary Systems

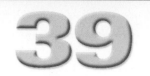
▪ DRUGS AT A GLANCE

HYPOTHALAMIC AND PITUITARY DRUGS
Hypothalamic agents
Anterior pituitary agents
Ⓟ *vasopressin injection (Pitressin)*

THYROID DRUGS
Thyroid agents
Ⓟ *levothyroxine (Synthroid)*
Antithyroid agents
Ⓟ *propylthiouracil (PTU)*

ADRENAL DRUGS
Glucocorticoids
Ⓟ *hydrocortisone (Aeroseb-HC, Alphaderm, others)*
Antiadrenal agents

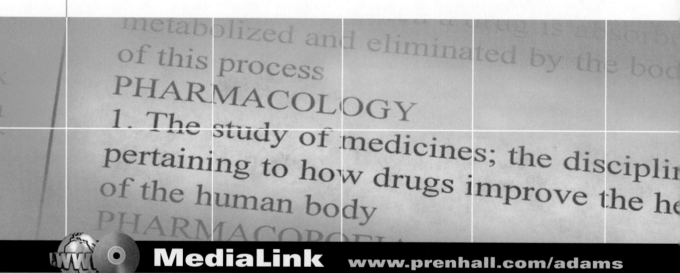

MediaLink www.prenhall.com/adams

CD-ROM
Audio Glossary
NCLEX Review

Companion Website
NCLEX Review
Dosage Calculations
Case Study
Care Plans
Expanded Key Concepts

OBJECTIVES

After reading this chapter, the student should be able to:

1. Describe the general structure and functions of the endocrine system.
2. Through the use of a specific example, explain the concept of negative feedback in the endocrine system.
3. Describe the clinical uses of the hypothalamic and pituitary hormones.
4. Explain the pharmacotherapy of diabetes insipidus.
5. Identify the signs and symptoms of hypothyroidism and hyperthyroidism.
6. Explain the pharmacotherapy of thyroid disorders.
7. Describe the signs and symptoms of Addison's disease and Cushing's syndrome.
8. Explain the pharmacotherapy of adrenal gland disorders.
9. Describe the nurse's role in the pharmacologic management of pituitary, thyroid, and adrenal disorders.
10. For each of the classes listed in Drugs at a Glance, identify representative drugs, explain the mechanism of drug action, primary actions, and important adverse effects.
11. Categorize drugs used in the treatment of endocrine disorders based on their classification and mechanism of action.
12. Use the Nursing Process to care for patients who are receiving drug therapy for pituitary, thyroid, and adrenal disorders.

Like the nervous system, the endocrine system is a major controller of homeostasis. Whereas a nerve exerts instantaneous control over a single muscle fiber or gland, a hormone from the endocrine system may affect all body cells and take as long as several days to produce an optimum response. Small amounts of hormones may produce profound effects on the body. Conversely, deficiencies of small quantities may produce equally as profound physiologic changes. This chapter examines common endocrine disorders and their pharmacotherapy. The reproductive hormones are covered in Chapters 40 and 41 ⌘.

39.1 The Endocrine System and Homeostasis

The endocrine system consists of various glands that secrete hormones, chemical messengers released in response to a change in the body's internal environment. The hormone attempts to return the body to homeostasis. For example, when the level of glucose in the blood rises above normal, the pancreas secretes insulin to return glucose levels to normal. The various endocrine glands and their hormones are illustrated in Figure 39.1.

After secretion, hormones enter the blood and are transported throughout the body. Some, such as insulin and thyroid hormone, have receptors on nearly every cell in the body. Others, such as parathyroid hormone (PTH) and oxytocin, have receptors on only a few specific types of cells.

In the endocrine system, it is common for one hormone to control the secretion of another hormone. In addition, it is common for the last hormone or action in the pathway to provide feedback to turn off the secretion of the first hormone. For example, as serum calcium falls, PTH is released; PTH causes an increase in serum calcium, which provides feedback to the parathyroid glands to shut off PTH secretion. This common feature of endocrine homeostasis is known as negative feedback.

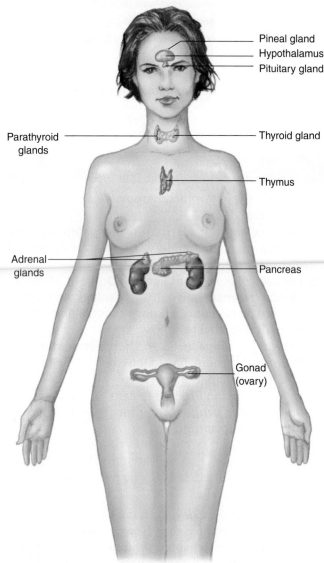

Pineal gland
Hypothalamus
Pituitary gland

Parathyroid glands

Thyroid gland

Thymus

Adrenal glands

Pancreas

Gonad (ovary)

Figure 39.1 | The endocrine system *Source: Pearson Education/PH College.*

39.2 The Hypothalamus and Pituitary Gland

Two endocrine structures in the brain deserve special recognition because they control many other endocrine glands. The hypothalamus secretes releasing hormones that travel via blood vessels a short distance to the anterior pituitary gland. These releasing hormones signal the pituitary which hormone is to be released. After secretion from the pituitary, the hormone travels to its target tissues to cause its effects. For example, the hypothalamus secretes thyrotropin-releasing hormone (TRH) that travels to the pituitary gland with the message to secrete thyroid-stimulating hormone (TSH). TSH then travels to its target organ, the thyroid gland, to stimulate the release of thyroid hormone. Although the pituitary is often called the master gland, the pituitary and hypothalamus are best visualized as an integrated unit.

The pituitary gland is comprised of two distinct regions. The anterior pituitary, or adenohypophysis, con-

sists of glandular tissue and secretes adrenocorticotropic hormone (ACTH), thyroid-stimulating hormone (TSH), growth hormone, prolactin, follicle-stimulating hormone (FSH), and leuteinizing hormone (LH). The posterior pituitary, or neurohypophysis, contains nervous tissue rather than glandular tissue. Neurons in the posterior pituitary store antidiuretic hormone (ADH) and oxytocin, which are released in response to nerve impulses from the hypothalamus. Hormones associated with the hypothalamus and pituitary gland are shown in Figure 39.2.

39.3 Indications for Hormone Pharmacotherapy

The goals of hormone pharmacotherapy vary widely. In many cases, the hormone is administered as replacement therapy for patients who are unable to secrete sufficient quantities of their own endogenous hormones. Examples of replacement therapy include the administration of thyroid hormone after the thyroid gland has been surgically removed, or supplying insulin to patients whose pancreas is not functioning. Replacement therapy usually supplies the physiologic, low level amounts of the hormone that would normally be present in the body. A summary of selected endocrine disorders and their drug therapy is shown in Table 39.1.

Some hormones are used in cancer chemotherapy. Examples include testosterone for breast cancer and estrogen for testicular cancer. The antineoplastic mechanism of action of these hormones is not known. When used as antineoplastics, the doses of the hormones far exceed those levels normally present in the body. Hormones are nearly always used in combination with other antineoplastic medications, as discussed in Chapter 35 ∞ .

Another goal of pharmacotherapy may be to produce an exaggerated response that is part of the normal action of the hormone, to achieve some therapeutic advantage. Supplying hydrocortisone to suppress inflammation is an example of taking advantage of the normal action of the glucocorticoids, but at higher amounts than would normally be present in the body. Supplying small amounts of estrogen or progesterone at specific times during the menstrual cycle can prevent ovulation and pregnancy. In this example, the patient is given natural hormones; however, they are taken at a time when levels in the body are normally low.

DISORDERS OF THE HYPOTHALAMUS AND PITUITARY GLAND

Because of its critical role in controlling other endocrine tissues, lack of adequate pituitary secretion can have multiple, profound effects on body function. Hypopituitarism can be caused by various tumors of the pituitary and associated brain regions, trauma, autoimmune disorders, or stroke. Pharmacotherapy involves administration of the missing hormone, perhaps for the life of the patient.

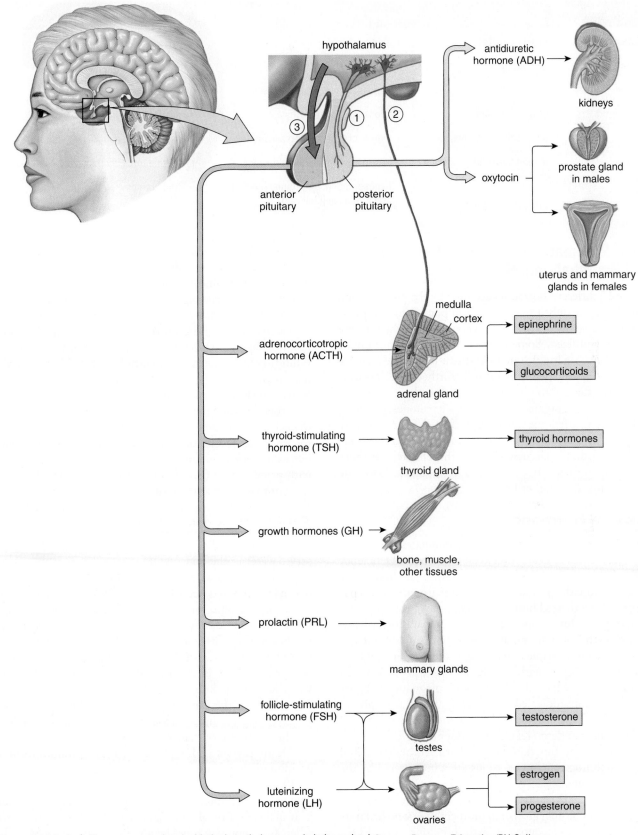

Figure 39.2 | Hormones associated with the hypothalamus and pituitary gland *Source: Pearson Education/PH College.*

Table 39.1	Selected Endocrine Disorders and Their Drug Treatment		
Gland	**Hormone(s)**	**Disorder**	**Drugs**
adrenal cortex	glucocorticoids	hypersecretion: Cushing's syndrome	antiadrenal agents
		hyposecretion: Addison's disease	glucocorticoids
pituitary	growth hormone	hyposecretion: dwarfism	somatrem and somatropin
	antidiuretic hormone	hyposecretion: diabetes insipidus	vasopressin, desmopressin, and lypressin
thyroid	thyroid hormone (T_3 and T_4)	hypersecretion: Grave's disease	propylthiouracil, methimazole, and I-131
		hyposecretion: myxedema (adults) and cretinism (children)	thyroid hormone

39.4 Pharmacotherapy with Pituitary and Hypothalamic Hormones

Of the 15 different hormones secreted by the pituitary and hypothalamus, only a few are used in pharmacotherapy, as listed in Table 39.2. There are several reasons why they are not widely utilized. Some of these hormones can only be obtained from natural sources and can be quite expensive when used in therapeutic quantities. Furthermore, it is usually more effective to give drugs that directly affect secretion at the target organs. Two pituitary hormones, prolactin and oxytocin, affect the female reproductive system and are discussed in Chapter 41 ⊝ . Corticotropin affects the adrenal gland, and is discussed later in this chapter. Of those remaining, growth hormone and antidiuretic hormone have the most clinical utility.

Growth Hormone

Growth hormone, or **somatotropin**, stimulates the growth and metabolism of nearly every cell in the body. Deficiency of this hormone in children results in dwarfism, however, it does not cause the profound mental impairment seen in patients lacking thyroid hormone. Somatrem (Protropin) and somatropin (Humatrope, others) are preparations of human growth hormone made by recombinant DNA techniques that are available as replacement therapy in children. If therapy is begun early in life, as much as 6 inches of growth may be achieved. Somatropin is pregnancy category C and is contraindicated in patients after the epiphyses have closed. This drug has many potential side effects and patients must undergo regular assessments of glucose tolerance and thyroid function during pharmacotherapy. All of the growth hormone preparations are administered by the parenteral route.

Prior to 2003, growth hormone therapy was not approved for promoting growth in short children who had normal levels of endogenous growth hormone. The FDA, however, has now approved growth hormone therapy to treat those who are healthy but unusually short. The height limit for treatment is defined as an expected adult height of less than 5 feet 3 inches for men and 4 feet 11 inches for women. It was found that growth hormone could add 1 to 3 inches in

height to children who took it for 4 to 6 years, and that the health risks for the children were not significant. The approval could significantly increase the number of children who receive growth hormone, although the annual cost of $30,000 to $40,000 a year may discourage many patients.

Octreotide (Sandostatin) is a synthetic growth hormone antagonist structurally related to growth hormone–inhibiting hormone (**somatostatin**). In addition to inhibiting growth hormone, octreotide promotes fluid and electrolyte reabsorption from the GI tract and prolongs intestinal transit time. It has limited applications in treating growth hormone excess in adults (acromegaly) and in treating the severe diarrhea sometimes associated with metastatic carcinoid tumors. Acromegaly may also be treated with pegvisomont (Somavert), a recently approved growth hormone receptor antagonist.

Antidiuretic Hormone

As its name implies, antidiuretic hormone (ADH) conserves water in the body. ADH is secreted from the posterior pituitary gland when the hypothalamus senses that plasma volume has decreased, or that the osmolality of the blood has become too high. ADH acts on the collecting ducts in the kidney to increase water reabsorption. **Diabetes insipidus** is a rare disease caused by a deficiency of ADH. Patients with this disorder have an intense thirst and produce very dilute urine due to the large volume of water lost by the kidneys. ADH is also called vasopressin, because it has the capability to raise blood pressure, when secreted in large amounts. Vasopressin is available as a drug for the treatment of diabetes insipidus.

Desmopressin (DDAVP) is the most common form of antidiuretic hormone in use. It has a duration of action of 8 to 20 hours, whereas vasopressin (Pitressin) and lypressin (Diapid) have durations of only 2 to 8 hours. Desmopressin is available as a nasal spray and is easily self-administered, whereas vasopressin must be administered IM or SC. The patient may also more easily increase or decrease the dosage depending on urine output. Desmopressin is also available in subcutaneous, intravenous, and oral forms. Desmopressin and lypressin do not have the intense vasoconstricting effects of vasopressin.

Table 39.2	Hypothalamic and Pituitary Agents
Drug	**Route and Adult Dose (max dose where indicated)**
Hypothalamic Agents	
gonadorelin acetate (Lutrepulse)	SC/IV; 100 mcg
gonadorelin hydrochloride (Factrel)	SC/IV; 100 mcg administered in women during the early phase of menstrual cycle (days 1 to 7) if it can be determined
nafarelin (Synarel)	Inhalation; two inhalations/d (200 μg/inhalation), one in each nostril beginning between days 2 and 4 of menstrual cycle (max 800 μg/d)
octreotide (Sandostatin)	SC; 100–600 μg/d in two to four divided doses; may switch to IM depot injection after 2 wk at 20 mg q4wk for 2 mo
protirelin (Thypinone)	IV; 500 μg bolus over a period of 15–30 sec
Anterior Pituitary Agents	
corticotropin (ACTH, Acthar)	IV; 10–25 U in 500 ml D5W infused over 8 hr
cosyntropin (Cortrosyn)	IM/IV; 0.25 mg injected over 2 min
menotropins (Pergonal, Humegon)	IM; 75–150 IU daily for the first 5 days of treatment; subsequent doses adjusted to individual response
somatrem (Protropin)	IM/SC (Child); Doses up to 0.1 mg/kg (0.2 U/kg) three times/wk with a minimum of 48 hr between doses
somatropin (Humatrope)	SC (Child); Humatrope 0.18 mg/kg/wk divided into equal doses on three alternate days
thyrotropin (thyroid-stimulating hormone, TSH)	IM/SC; 10 U daily for 1–3 d
Posterior Pituitary Agents	
desmopressin acetate (DDAVP, Stimate)	IV; 0.3μg/kg, repeated as needed; intranasal: 0.1 ml (10 μg) bid
lypressin (Diapid)	Intranasal; 1–2 sprays (2–4 pressor units) in each nostril qid
oxytocin (Pitocin) (see 621 for the Prototype Drug box)	IV; 1 mU/min, may increase by 1 mU/min q15min (max 20 mU/min)
vasopressin (Pitressin)	IM/SC; 5–10 U aqueous solution bid-qid (5–60 U/d) or 1.25–2.5 U in oil q2–3d

NURSING CONSIDERATIONS

The role of the nurse in antidiuretic hormone therapy involves careful monitoring of a patient's condition and providing education as it relates to the prescribed drug regimen. The therapeutic goal for patients receiving antidiuretic hormone therapy is focused on maintaining fluid and electrolyte status. For patients taking antidiuretic hormones, the nurse should assess for fluid and electrolyte imbalances and for urine specific gravity prior to administration. A low specific gravity indicates lack of urine concentration and suggests ADH deficiency. The nurse should periodically assess urine specific gravity during pharmacotherapy to determine if the therapeutic effect is being achieved. The nurse should also closely monitor the patient's vital signs, especially pulse and blood pressure, as antidiuretic hormone can affect plasma volume and is a potent vasoconstrictor.

Body weight, intake, and output must be monitored, because these drugs may cause excess water retention. The nurse should also monitor the neurologic status of the pa-tient. Symptoms of water intoxication may first present as headache accompanied by confusion and drowsiness. The use of vasopressin is contraindicated in patients with pre-existing heart disease. Furthermore, it should be used cautiously in elderly patients because of the possibility of undiagnosed heart disease.

Patient education as it relates to antidiuretic hormone should include goals, reasons for obtaining baseline data such as vital signs and tests for cardiac and renal disorders, and possible side effects. The patient should be instructed to check weight at least two times per week and report significant changes to the healthcare provider. See "Nursing Process Focus: Patients Receiving Antidiuretic Hormone Therapy" for additional points the nurse should include when teaching about this class of drug.

39.5 Normal Function of the Thyroid Gland

The thyroid gland secretes hormones that affect nearly every cell in the body. By stimulating the enzymes involved with glucose oxidation, thyroid gland hormones regulate

| **Pr PROTOTYPE DRUG** | **VASOPRESSIN INJECTION** (Pitressin) |

ACTIONS AND USES

Three ADH preparations are available for the treatment of diabetes insipidus: vasopressin (Pitressin), desmopressin (DDAVP, Stimate), and lypressin (Diapid). Vasopressin is a synthetic hormone that has a structure identical to that of human ADH. It acts on the renal collecting tubules to increase their permeability to water, thus enhancing water reabsorption. Although it acts within minutes, vasopressin has a short half-life that requires it to be administered three to four times per day. Vasopressin tannate is formulated in peanut oil to increase its duration of action. Vasopressin is usually given IM or IV, although an intranasal form is available for mild diabetes insipidus. Desmopressin has a longer duration of action than vasopressin, and results in fewer serious adverse effects. Desmopressin is occasionally used by the intranasal route for enuresis, or bed-wetting.

Administration Alerts

- Vasopressin tannate should never be administered IV because it is an oil.
- Vasopressin aqueous injection may be given by continuous IV infusion after it is diluted in normal saline or D5W.
- Pregnancy category X.

ADVERSE EFFECTS AND INTERACTIONS

Vasopressin has a strong vasoconstrictor action that is unrelated to its antidiuretic properties, thus hypertension is possible. The drug can precipitate angina episodes and myocardial infarction in patients with coronary artery disease. Excessive fluid retention can cause water intoxication: symptoms including headache, restlessness, drowsiness, and coma. Water intoxication can usually be avoided by teaching the patient to decrease water intake during vasopressin therapy.

Vasopressin injection interacts with several other drugs. For example, alcohol, epinephrine, heparin, lithium, and phenytoin may decrease the antidiuretic effects of vasopressin. Neostigmine may increase vasopressor actions. Carbamazepine and thiazide diuretics may increase antidiuretic activity.

 See the companion website for a Nursing Process Focus specific to this drug.

| **NATURAL THERAPIES** | **Treatments for Thyroid Disease** |

Thyroid disease is a serious condition that usually requires medical attention. As a preventative, one can consume substances that contain precursors to thyroid hormone. Since T_3 and T_4 both require iodine, dietary intake of this mineral must be sufficient. Iodized salt usually contains enough iodine for proper thyroid function, however, kelp or seafood, particularly shellfish, are additional, natural sources of iodine. T_3 and T_4 also contain the amino acid tyrosine, which is usually obtained from protein sources such as meat or eggs. Other rich sources of tyrosine include avocados, bananas, lima beans, and various seeds. Supplementation with L-tyrosine is usually not necessary.

A number of natural therapies have been used to treat overactive thyroid glands. Lemon balm (*Melissa officinalis*) is a beautiful perennial plant that has a slight lemon odor when the leaves are crushed. Although native to the Mediterranean region, it is widely cultivated in Europe, Asia, and North America. The traditional medicinal properties of the leaves as a sedative and antispasmodic have been reported for hundreds of years. It has been shown to block the antibodies responsible for destroying the thyroid gland in Grave's disease, although this effect has yet to be confirmed in clinical studies. Lemon balm is usually taken as a tea, several times daily, although capsules, extracts, and tinctures are available.

basal metabolic rate, the baseline speed by which cells perform their functions. By increasing cellular metabolism, thyroid hormone increases body temperature. The gland also helps to maintain blood pressure and regulate growth and development.

The thyroid gland has two basic types of cells that secrete different hormones. **Parafollicular cells** secrete calcitonin, a hormone that is involved with calcium homeostasis (Chapter 46) ⊙. **Follicular cells** in the gland secrete thyroid hormone, which is actually a combination of two different hormones: thyroxine (T_4) and triiodothyronine (T_3). Iodine is essential for the synthesis of these hormones, and is provided through the dietary intake of common iodized salt. The names of these hormones refer to the number of bound iodine atoms in each molecule, either three (T_3) or four (T_4).

Thyroxine is the major hormone secreted by the thyroid gland. At the target tissues, however, thyroxine is converted to T_3 through the enzymatic cleavage of one iodine atom. T_3 is thought to enter the target cells, where it binds to intracellular receptors within the nucleus.

Thyroid function is regulated through multiple levels of hormonal control. Falling thyroxine levels in the blood signal the hypothalamus to secrete thyroid-releasing hormone (TRH), or thyrotropin. TRH stimulates the pituitary gland

NURSING PROCESS FOCUS	**PATIENTS RECEIVING ANTIDIURETIC HORMONE THERAPY**

ASSESSMENT	**POTENTIAL NURSING DIAGNOSES**
Prior to administration: ■ Obtain complete health history including allergies, drug history, and possible drug interactions. ■ Obtain complete physical examination. ■ Assess for the presence/history of neurosurgery, pituitary tumors, head injury, and nocturia. ■ Obtain laboratory studies including urine specific gravity, urine/serum osmolarity, and serum electrolytes.	■ Risk for Imbalanced Fluid Volume, related to effect of drug therapy ■ Disturbed Sleep Pattern, related to frequent nocturia ■ Impaired Urinary Elimination, related to effects of drug therapy ■ Risk for Injury, related to side effects ■ Deficient Knowledge, related to drug therapy

PLANNING: PATIENT GOALS AND EXPECTED OUTCOMES

The patient will:
■ Exhibit normal fluid and electrolyte balance
■ Report uninterrupted sleep patterns
■ Identify and report side effects to healthcare provider
■ Demonstrate an understanding of the drug's action

IMPLEMENTATION

Interventions and (Rationales)	*Patient Education/Discharge Planning*
■ Monitor vital signs. (Changes may indicate alterations in body fluid status such as hyper- or hypovolemia.)	■ Instruct the patient to report irregular heartbeat, shortness of breath, dizziness, or headache.
■ Monitor cardiovascular status such as peripheral pulses, heart sounds, skin temperature and color, and EKG. (ADH has potent vasoconstriction properties and may cause hypertension and dyshythmias.)	■ Instruct the patient in the importance of follow-up care and to take medication exactly as prescribed.
■ Administer fluid replacement as directed. (IV infusions should be regulated to maintain body fluid balance.) ■ Encourage oral fluid intake to satisfy thirst only. (Excessive fluid intake may trigger a diabetes insipidus episode.)	Instruct patient to: ■ Monitor fluid balance and report vomiting, diarrhea, perfuse sweating, and frequent urination ■ Consume fluid to satisfy thirst and to report excessive unquenchable thirst
■ Monitor intake/output ratio and weigh patient daily. (ADH may result in fluid retention that can lead to water intoxication. Daily weight is an indicator of fluid retention.)	Instruct patient: ■ To weigh self daily and report excessive gains or losses ■ In titration techniques based on urinary output
■ Monitor for presence of nocturia or nocturnal enuresis. Determine the patient's ability to satisfy physiologic sleep needs. (Less frequent nighttime urination is an indication of the effectiveness of ADH therapy.)	Instruct patient to: ■ Keep a sleep log recording the number of times per night he or she is awakened to urinate ■ Avoid potentially hazardous activities due to possible drowsiness until therapeutic effect of drug is achieved ■ Have frequent rest periods or daytime naps if sleep deprivation is present until therapeutic effect is achieved
■ Monitor for symptoms of fluid volume overload such as headache, restlessness, shortness of breath, tachycardia, hypertension, and low urinary output. (These are signs of water intoxication.)	■ Instruct patient to report headaches, shortness of breath, palpitation, and low urine output.

continued

NURSING PROCESS FOCUS: *Patients Receiving Antidiuretic Hormone Therapy (continued)*

Interventions and (Rationales)	Patient Education/Discharge Planning
■ Monitor status of nasal mucous membranes if nasal preparations are prescribed. (Intranasal use can cause changes in the nasal mucosa, resulting in unpredictable drug absorption.)	Instruct patient: ■ To report worsening of condition since route of administration may need to be changed ■ To report drainage or irritation of the nasal mucosa if taking nasal preparation ■ In subcutaneous injection methods, as appropriate
■ Monitor laboratory studies, including urine and serum osmolarity, urine specific gravity, and serum electrolytes. (These assess fluid volume status.)	Instruct patient: ■ To measure urine specific gravity ■ In the importance of keeping all laboratory appointments

EVALUATION OF OUTCOME CRITERIA

Evaluate the effectiveness of drug therapy by confirming that patient goals and expected outcomes have been met (see "Planning").

See Table 39.2, under the heading "Posterior Pituitary Agents," for a list of drugs to which these nursing actions apply.

to secrete TSH, which then stimulates the thyroid gland to release thyroid hormone. Rising levels of thyroid hormone in the blood trigger a negative feedback response to shut off secretion of TRH and TSH. The negative feedback mechanism for the thyroid gland is shown in Figure 39.3.

Thyroid Agents

Thyroid disorders are common and drug therapy is often indicated. The correct dose of thyroid drug is highly individualized and requires careful, periodic adjustment. The medications used to treat thyroid disease are shown in Table 39.3.

39.6 Pharmacotherapy of Hypothyroidism

Hypothyroidism may result from either a poorly functioning thyroid gland or low secretion of TSH by the pituitary gland. The most common cause of hypothyroidism in the United States is chronic autoimmune thyroiditis, known as Hashimoto's disease. Early symptoms of hypothyroidism in adults, or myxedema, include fatigue, general weakness, muscle cramps, and dry skin. More severe symptoms include slurred speech, bradycardia, weight gain, decreased sense of taste and smell, and intolerance to cold environments. The etiology of myxedema may include autoimmune disease, surgical removal of the thyroid gland, or aggressive treatment with antithyroid drugs. At high doses, the antidysrhythmic drug amiodarone (Cordarone) can induce hypothyroidism in patients due to its high iodine content. Enlargement of the thyroid gland, or goiter, may be absent or present, depending on the cause of the disease. Hypothyroidism usually responds well to pharmacotherapy with natural or synthetic thyroid hormone.

NURSING CONSIDERATIONS

The role of the nurse in thyroid hormone therapy involves careful monitoring of a patient's condition and providing education as it relates to the prescribed drug regimen. The nurse should assess the patient for signs and symptoms of thyroid disease. The nurse should also assess and monitor the patient's vital signs as cardiovascular complications may occur as a result of drug therapy.

Levothyroxine (Synthroid) is a commonly used thyroid hormone replacement. The nurse should thoroughly assess cardiovascular function because this drug may cause cardiovascular collapse in patients with undiagnosed heart disease due to an increase in basal metabolic rate. This action may precipitate dysrhythmias in patients with undiagnosed heart disease, especially in elderly patients. The drug should also be used with caution with impaired renal function, because the increased metabolic rate increases the workload of the kidney. Patients with diabetes mellitus, diabetes insipidus, and Addison's disease experience a worsening of symptoms because of the initial increase in basal metabolism. The drug is contraindicated in patients with adrenal insufficiency.

Dessicated thyroid is made up of dried beef and pork thyroid glands. It is used less frequently than levothyroxine because it does not produce reliable results. Desiccated thyroid will cause the same cardiac complications as levothyroxine. Liothyronine sodium is a short-acting synthetic form of the natural thyroid hormone that can be administered IV to individuals with myxedema coma. The short duration of action allows for rapid dosage adjustments in critically ill patients. Thyroid hormones have their optimum effect when taken on an empty stomach. Patients should be taught the signs and symp-

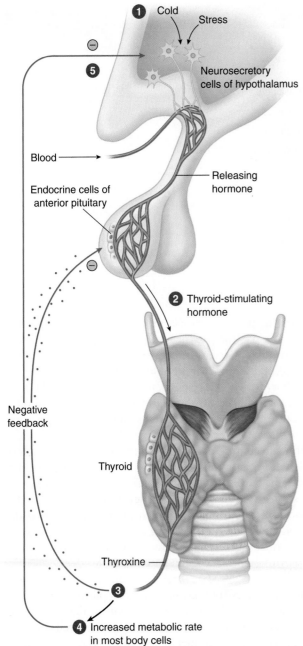

Figure 39.3 Feedback mechanisms of the thyroid gland: 1. stimulus; 2. release of TSH; 3. release of thyroid hormone; 4. increased BMR; 5. negative feedback

1 Cold
Stress

5

Neurosecretory cells of hypothalamus

Blood

Releasing hormone

Endocrine cells of anterior pituitary

2 Thyroid-stimulating hormone

Negative feedback

Thyroid

Thyroxine

3

4 Increased metabolic rate in most body cells

- Hypothyroidism is 10 times more common in women; hyperthyroidism is 5 to 10 times more common in women.
- The two most common thyroid diseases, Grave's disease and Hashimoto's thyroiditis, are autoimmune diseases and may have a genetic link.
- One of every 4,000 babies is born without a working thyroid gland.
- About 15,000 new cases of thyroid cancer are diagnosed each year.
- One of every five women over age 75 has Hashimoto's thyroiditis.
- Postpartum thyroiditis occurs in 5% to 9% of women after giving birth, and may recur in future pregnancies.
- Both hyperthyroidism and hypothyroidism can affect a woman's ability to become pregnant, and can cause miscarriages.

Antithyroid Agents

Medications are often used to treat the cause of hyperthyroidism or to relieve its distressing symptoms. The goal of antithyroid therapy is to lower the activity of the thyroid gland.

39.7 Pharmacotherapy of Hyperthyroidism

Hypersecretion of thyroid hormone results in symptoms that are the opposite of hypothyroidism: increased body metabolism, tachycardia, weight loss, elevated body temperature, and anxiety. The most common type of hyperthyroidism is called Grave's disease. Considered an autoimmune disease in which the body develops antibodies against its own thyroid gland, Grave's disease is about 8 times more common in men, and most often occurs between the ages of 30 and 40. Other causes of hyperthyroidism are adenomas of the thyroid, pituitary tumors, and pregnancy. If the cause of the hypersecretion is found to be a tumor, or if the disease cannot be controlled through pharmacotherapy, thyroidectomy is indicated.

Pharmacotherapy for hyperthyroidism is limited to three medications. Two of these, propylthiouracil (PTU) and methimazole (Tapazole), are called thioamides. These agents act by inhibiting the incorporation of iodine atoms into the chemical precursors to T_3 and T_4. Methimazole has a much longer half-life that offers the advantage of less frequent dosing, although side effects can be more severe. Although both thioamides are pregnancy category D agents, methimazole crosses the placenta more readily than propylthiouracil and is contraindicated in pregnant patients.

The third antithyroid drug, sodium iodide-131 (Iodotope) is a radioisotope used to destroy overactive thyroid glands by emitting ionizing radiation. Shortly after oral administration, I-131 accumulates in the thyroid gland,

---

toms of hyperthyroidism such as nervousness, weight loss, diarrhea, and intolerance to heat. The patient should notify the healthcare provider at the first sign of any of these symptoms.

Patient education as it relates to thyroid hormones should include goals, reasons for obtaining baseline data such as vital signs and tests for cardiac and renal disorders, and possible side effects. See "Nursing Process Focus: Patients Receiving Thyroid Hormone Replacement" for specific teaching points.

Table 39.3	Thyroid and Antithyroid Drugs
Drug	**Route and Adult Dose (max dose where indicated)**
Thyroid Agents	
levothyroxine (Levothroid, Synthroid, others)	PO; 100–400 µg/d
liothyronine (Cytomel, Triostat)	PO; 25–75 µg qd
liotrix (Euthroid, Thyrolar)	PO; 12.5–30 µg qd
thyroid (Thyrar, Thyroid USP)	PO; 60–100 mg qd
Antithyroid Agents	
methimazole (Tapazole)	PO; 5–15 mg tid
potassium iodide and iodine (Lugol's Solution, Thyro-Block)	PO; 0.1–1.0 ml tid
propylthiouracil (PTU)	PO; 100–150 mg tid
radioactive iodide (^{131}I, Iodotope)	PO; 0.8–150 mCi (curies are units of radioactivity)

SPECIAL CONSIDERATIONS

Shift Workers, Hypothyroidism and Drug Compliance

Many body processes such as temperature, blood pressure, levels of certain hormones, biochemical processes, and alertness fluctuate on a 24-hour schedule known as the circadian rhythm. Circadian processes are thought to be triggered by daylight. Normal circadian cycles may be interrupted in those people who work varied shifts. Likewise, medications that must be given at a specified time to enhance the potential effect can be a concern for shift workers.

Thyroid medication is best given at the same time each day; however, this can be a challenge to shift workers, especially if they rotate shifts. These drugs are best given after awakening in the morning as they can disturb sleep patterns. For a shift worker, the time of awakening may vary depending on the shift worked. It is essential that the patient be aware of this challenge and work with the healthcare provider to reach a medication schedule that allows optimization of the drug effects.

where it destroys follicular cells. The goal of pharmacotherapy with I-131 is to destroy just enough of the thyroid gland, so that levels of thyroid function return to normal. Full benefits may take several months. Although most patients require only a single dose, others may need additional treatments. Small diagnostic doses of I-131 are used in the nuclear medicine department to determine the degree of iodide uptake in the various parts of the thyroid gland. Nonradioactive sodium iodide is occasionally administered IV to manage an acute form of hyperthyroidism known as thyrotoxic crisis, or thyroid storm.

NURSING CONSIDERATIONS

The role of the nurse in antithyroid therapy involves careful monitoring of a patient's condition and providing edu-

cation as it relates to the prescribed regimen. The nurse should assess the patient for signs of hyperthyroidism. For all antithyroid drugs, the nurse should monitor the patient for complications that are associated with the drugs.

For patients receiving propylthiouracil (PTU), the nurse should monitor white blood cell count periodically because this drug may cause agranulocytosis. This condition puts the patient at greater risk for infection; therefore, efforts to control invasion of microbes should be strictly observed. Because the metabolism of this drug occurs in the liver, the nurse should assess for signs of jaundice and for elevations in liver transaminase levels. Concurrent medication use should be determined because many drug-drug interactions are possible with propylthiouracil. For example, anticoagulants may cause increased bleeding because propylthiouracil causes an antivitamin K effect.

Methimazole (Tapazole) is similar in structure to propylthiouracil but has a lower safety profile. Though rare, the nurse should monitor the patient for blood dyscrasias. The patient may develop agranulocytosis, as well as jaundice related to the hepatic metabolism of the drug. These adverse effects usually disappear when the drug is discontinued.

Radioactive iodine (I-131) is used to permanently decrease thyroid function. It is difficult to calculate the exact dose needed to achieve a euthyroid state; therefore, individuals who take this medication require periodic thyroid function tests. The nurse should instruct the patient in the signs and symptoms of hypothyroidism because many patients treated with I-131 will need thyroid hormone replacement therapy. Patients should not be in close contact with children or pregnant women for 1 week following administration of the drug, because the patient will be emitting small amounts of radiation. Physical distance should be increased for a few days to limit the possibility of exposing others to radiation. This drug is absolutely contraindicated in patients who are pregnant or lactating.

Patient education as it relates to antithyroid agents should include goals, reasons for obtaining baseline data

| **Pr** **PROTOTYPE DRUG** | **LEVOTHYROXINE** (Synthroid) |

ACTIONS AND USES

Levothyroxine is a synthetic form of thyroxine (T_4) used for replacement therapy in patients with low thyroid function. Actions are those of thyroid hormone, and include loss of weight, improved tolerance to environmental temperature, increased activity, and increased pulse rate. Doses are highly individualized. Therapy may take 3 weeks or longer before T_4 levels stabilize; Doses may require periodic adjustments for several months. Serum TSH levels are monitored to determine whether the patient is receiving sufficient levothyroxine—low TSH levels usually indicate that the dosage of T_4 needs to be increased. Levothyroxine is pregnancy category A.

Administration Alert

■ Administer medication at the same time every day, preferably in the morning to decrease incidence of drug-related insomnia.

ADVERSE EFFECTS AND INTERACTIONS

The difference between a therapeutic dose of levothyroxine and one that produces adverse effects is narrow. Care must be taken to avoid overtreatment with this drug. Adverse effects are those of hyperthyroidism and include palpitations, dysrhythmias, anxiety, insomnia, weight loss, and heat intolerance. Menstrual irregularities may occur in females, and long-term use of levothyroxine has been associated with osteoporosis in women.

Levothyroxine interacts with many other drugs; for example, cholestyramine and colestipol decrease absorption of levothyroxine. Concurrent administration of epinephrine and norepinephrine increases risk of cardiac insufficiency. Oral anticoagulants may potentiate hypoprothrombinemia.

Use with caution with herbal supplements, such as lemon balm, which may interfere with thyroid hormone action.

 See the companion website for a Nursing Process Focus specific to this drug.

such as vital signs and tests for cardiac and renal disorders, and possible side effects. See "Nursing Process Focus: Patients Receiving Antithyroid Therapy" for specific teaching points.

ADRENAL GLAND DISORDERS

Though small in size, the adrenal glands secrete hormones that affect every body tissue. Adrenal disorders range from excess hormone secretion to deficient hormone secretion. The specific pharmacotherapy depends on which portion of the adrenal gland is responsible for the abnormal secretion.

39.8 Normal Function of the Adrenal Gland

The adrenal glands secrete three essential classes of steroid hormones: the glucocorticoids, mineralocorticoids, and gonadocorticoids. Collectively, the glucocorticoids and mineralocorticoids are called corticosteroids or adrenocortical hormones.

The gonadotropins secreted by the adrenal cortex are mostly androgens, though small amounts of estrogens are also produced. The amounts of these adrenal sex hormones are normally far less than the levels secreted by the gonads. It is believed that they contribute to the onset of puberty. The adrenal glands also are the primary source of endogenous estrogen in postmenopausal women. Hypersecretion of gonadotropins, such as that caused from a tumor of the adrenal cortex, results in masculinization. The physiological effects of androgens are detailed in Chapter 42 .

Aldosterone accounts for over 95% of the mineralocorticoids secreted by the adrenals. The primary function of aldosterone is to promote sodium reabsorption and potassium excretion by the renal tubule, thus regulating plasma volume. When plasma volume falls, the kidney secretes renin, which results in the production of angiotensin II. Angiotensin II then causes aldosterone secretion, which promotes sodium and water retention. Certain adrenal tumors cause excessive secretion of aldosterone, a condition known as hyperaldosteronism, which is characterized by hypertension and hypokalemia.

Over 30 glucocorticoids are secreted from the adrenal cortex, including cortisol, corticosterone and cortisone. Cortisol, also called hydrocortisone, is secreted in the highest amount, and is the most important pharmacologically. Glucocorticoids affect the metabolism of nearly every cell, and prepare the body for long-term stress. The effects of glucocorticoids are diverse, and include the following:

■ Increase the level of blood glucose (hyperglycemic effect) by inhibiting insulin secretion and promoting gluconeogenesis, the synthesis of carbohydrates from lipid and protein sources

■ Increase the breakdown of proteins and lipids and their utilization as energy sources

■ Suppress the inflammatory and immune responses (Chapters 29 and 31)

■ Increase the sensitivity of vascular smooth muscle to norepinephrine and angiotensin II

■ Influence the CNS by affecting mood and maintaining normal brain excitability

| NURSING PROCESS FOCUS | PATIENTS RECEIVING THYROID HORMONE REPLACEMENT |

ASSESSMENT

Prior to administration:
- Obtain complete health history including allergies, drug history, and possible drug interactions.
- Obtain complete physical examination.
- Assess for the presence/history of symptoms of hypothyroidism.
- Obtain EKG and laboratory studies including T_4, T_3, and serum TSH levels.

POTENTIAL NURSING DIAGNOSES

- Activity Intolerance, related to disease process
- Fatigue, related to impaired metabolic status
- Deficient Knowledge, related to drug therapy
- Ineffective Health Maintenance, related to side effects of drug

PLANNING: PATIENT GOALS AND EXPECTED OUTCOMES

The patient will:
- Exhibit normal thyroid hormone levels
- Report a decrease in hypothyroid symptoms
- Experience no significant adverse effects from drug therapy
- Demonstrate an understanding of hypothyroidism and the need for life-long therapy

IMPLEMENTATION

Interventions and (Rationales)

- Monitor vital signs. (Changes in metabolic rate will be manifested as changes in blood pressure, pulse, and body temperature.)

- Monitor for decreasing symptoms related to hypothyroidism such as fatigue, constipation, cold intolerance, lethargy, depression, and menstrual irregularities. (Decreasing symptoms will determine that drug is achieving therapeutic affect.)

- Monitor for symptoms related to hyperthyroidism such as nervousness, insomnia, tachycardia, dysrhythmias, heat intolerance, chest pain, and diarrhea. (Symptoms of hyperthyroidism indicate the drug is at a toxic level.)

- Monitor T_3, T_4, and TSH levels. (This helps to determine the effectiveness of pharmacotherapy.)

- Monitor blood glucose levels especially in individuals with diabetes mellitus. (Thyroid hormone increase metabolic rate and glucose utilization may be altered.)

- Provide supportive nursing care to cope with symptoms of hypothyroidism such as constipation, cold intolerance, and fatigue until drug has achieved therapeutic effect.

- Monitor weight at least weekly. (Weight loss is expected due to increased metabolic rate. Weight changes help to determine the effectiveness of drug therapy.)

Patient Education/Discharge Planning

- Instruct patient to report dizziness, palpitations, and intolerance to temperature changes.

- Instruct patient about the signs of hypothyroidism and to report symptoms.

- Instruct patient about the signs of hyperthyroidism and to report symptoms.

- Instruct patient about the importance of ongoing monitoring of thyroid hormone levels and to keep all laboratory appointments.

- Instruct the diabetic patient to monitor blood glucose levels and adjust insulin doses as directed by the healthcare provider.

Instruct patient to:
- Increase fluid and fiber intake, and activity to reduce constipation
- Wear additional clothing and maintain a comfortable room environment for cold intolerance
- Plan activities and include rest periods to avoid fatigue

- Instruct patient to weigh weekly and to report significant changes.

continued

Pr PROTOTYPE DRUG | **PROPYLTHIOURACIL (PTU)**

ACTIONS AND USES

Propylthiouracil is administered to patients with hyperthyroidism. It acts by interfering with the synthesis of T_3 and T_4 in the thyroid gland. It also prevents the conversion of T_4 to T_3 in the target tissues. Its action may be delayed from several days to as long as 6 to 12 weeks. Effects include a return to normal thyroid function: weight gain, reduction in anxiety, less insomnia, and slower pulse rate. Due to its short half-life, PTU is usually administered several times a day.

Administration Alerts

■ Administer with meals to reduce GI distress.
■ Pregnancy category D.

ADVERSE EFFECTS AND INTERACTIONS

Overtreatment with propylthiouracil produces symptoms of hypothyroidism. Rash is the most common side effect. A small percentage of patients experience agranulocytosis, which is its most serious adverse effect. Periodic laboratory blood counts and TSH values are necessary to establish proper dosage.

Antithyroid medications interact with many other drugs. For example, propylthiouracil can reverse the efficacy of drugs such as aminophylline, anticoagulants, and cardiac glycosides.

 See the companion website for a Nursing Process Focus specific to this drug.

39.9 Control of Glucocorticoid Secretion

Control of glucocorticoid levels in the blood begins with corticotropin releasing factor (CRF), secreted by the hypothalamus. CRF travels to the pituitary where it causes the release of adrenocorticotropic hormone (ACTH). ACTH then travels through the blood and reaches the adrenal cortex, causing it to release glucocorticoids. When the level of cortisol in the blood rises, it provides negative feedback to the hypothalamus and pituitary to shut off further release of glucocorticoids. This negative feedback mechanism is shown in Figure 39.4.

ACTH is available as a medication in three different preparations: corticotropin injection (Acthar, ACTH), repository corticotropin (H. P. Acthar, ACTH-40, ACTH-80), and corticotropin zinc hydroxide (Cortrophin-Zinc). A fourth drug, cosyntropin (Cortrosyn) closely resembles ACTH. Although these preparations stimulate the adrenal gland to produce glucocorticoids, they are rarely used to correct corticosteroid deficiency. The ACTH agents cannot be given by the oral route and they produce numerous side effects. The primary use of these agents is to diagnose adrenal disorders. After administration of cosyntropin, plasma levels of cortisol are measured to determine if the adrenal gland responded to the ACTH stimulation.

Glucocorticoids

The glucocorticoids are used as replacement therapy for patients with adrenocortical insufficiency and to dampen inflammatory and immune responses. The glucocorticoids, shown in Table 39.4, are one of the most widely prescribed drug classes.

39.10 Pharmacotherapy with Glucocorticoids

Lack of adequate corticosteroid production, known as adrenocortical insufficiency, may be caused by hyposecretion of the adrenal cortex or by inadequate secretion of ACTH from the pituitary. Symptoms include hypoglycemia, fatigue, hypotension, increased skin pigmentation, and GI disturbances such as anorexia, vomiting, and diarrhea. Low

NURSING PROCESS FOCUS	PATIENTS RECEIVING ANTITHYROID THERAPY

ASSESSMENT

Prior to administration:
- Obtain complete health history including allergies, drug history, and possible drug interactions.
- Obtain complete physical examination.
- Assess for the presence/history of hyperthyroidism.
- Obtain laboratory studies including T_3/T_4 levels, TSH level, EKG, and CBC.

POTENTIAL NURSING DIAGNOSES

- Risk for Infection, related to drug-induced agranulocytosis
- Risk for Injury, related to side effects of drug therapy
- Ineffective Health Maintenance, related to adverse GI effects
- Deficient Knowledge, related to drug therapy

PLANNING: PATIENT GOALS AND EXPECTED OUTCOMES

The patient will:
- Exhibit a decrease in the symptoms of hyperthyroidism
- Exhibit normal thyroid hormone levels
- Exhibit no drug adverse effects such as agranulocytosis or gastrointestinal distress
- Demonstrate an understanding of the disease process and health maintenance strategies

IMPLEMENTATION

Interventions and (Rationales)	*Patient Education/Discharge Planning*
■ Monitor vital signs. (Changes in metabolic rate will be manifested as changes in blood pressure, pulse, and body temperature.)	Instruct patient: ■ To count pulse for a full minute and record pulse with every dose ■ In pulse rate parameters that require notification of the health-care provider (pulse rate more than . . . ; pulse rate greater than . . .) ■ To report dizziness, palpitations, and intolerance to temperature changes
■ Monitor thyroid function tests. (This is used to determine the effectiveness of the drug therapy.)	■ Instruct patient in the importance of follow-up care and to keep all laboratory appointments.
■ Monitor for signs of infection, including CBC, and WBC count. (Antithyroid drug may cause agranulocytosis.)	Instruct patient: ■ That antithyroid medication may affect the body's ability to defend against bacteria and viruses ■ To report sore throat, fever, chills, malaise, and weakness
■ Monitor weight at least weekly. (As a result of slower metabolism, weight gain is expected.)	■ Instruct patient to weigh weekly and to report significant changes.
■ Monitor for drowsiness. Ensure safe environment. (Antithyroid medications may cause drowsiness.)	■ Instruct patient that medication may cause drowsiness and to avoid hazardous activities until the effects of the drug are known.
■ Monitor for gastrointestinal distress. (Antithyroid medications may cause nausea/vomiting.)	■ Instruct patient to take antithyroid medication with food.
■ Monitor for a decrease in symptoms related to hyperthyroidism such as nervousness, insomnia, tachycardia, dysrythmias, heat intolerance, chest pain, and diarrhea. (This will determine if drug is at a therapeutic level.)	■ Instruct patient about the signs of hyperthyroidism and to report to the healthcare provider.
■ Monitor for symptoms related to hypothyroidism such as fatigue, constipation, cold intolerance, lethargy, depression, and menstrual irregularities. (These symptoms indicate drug is at a toxic level.)	■ Instruct patient about the signs of hypothyroidism and to report to the healthcare provider.

continued

NURSING PROCESS FOCUS: *Patients Receiving Antithyroid Therapy (continued)*

Interventions and (Rationales)	Patient Education/Discharge Planning
■ Monitor for activity intolerance. (Hyperthyroidism results in protein catabolism, overactivity, and increased metabolism leading to exhaustion.)	■ Instruct patient to schedule rest periods while performing activities of daily living until medication has achieved therapeutic effect.
■ Monitor dietary intake. Avoid foods with high iodine content such as soy, tofu, turnips, iodized salt, and some breads as directed. (Iodine increases the production of thyroid hormones, which is not desirable in these patients.)	■ Instruct patient about the use of iodized salt, shellfish, and OTC medications.
■ Monitor patient's response to drug therapy.	■ Instruct patient to keep log of responses to medication including pulse, weight, mood status, and energy level. Inform patient that stabilization of thyroid hormone levels may take several months.

EVALUATION OF OUTCOME CRITERIA

Evaluate the effectiveness of drug therapy by confirming that patient goals and expected outcomes have been met (see "Planning").

See Table 39.3, under the heading "Antithyroid Agents," for a list of drugs to which these nursing actions apply.

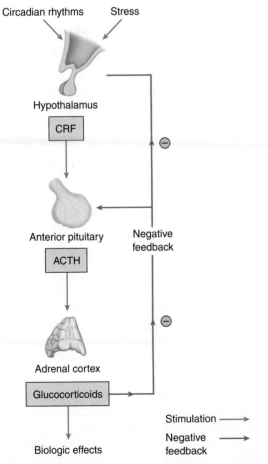

Figure 39.4 | Feedback control of the adrenal cortex

plasma cortisol, accompanied by high plasma ACTH levels, is diagnostic. Primary adrenocortical insufficiency, known as **Addison's disease**, is quite rare and includes a deficiency of both glucocorticoids and mineralocorticoids. Autoimmune destruction of both adrenal glands is the most common cause of Addison's disease.

Acute adrenocortical insufficiency may result when glucocorticoids are abruptly withdrawn from a patient who has been on long-term glucocorticoid therapy. When glucocorticoids are taken as medications for prolonged periods, they provide negative feedback to the pituitary to stop secreting ACTH. Without stimulation by ACTH, the adrenal cortex shrinks and stops secreting endogenous glucocorticoids, a condition known as adrenal atrophy. If the glucocorticoid medication is abruptly withdrawn, the shrunken adrenal glands will not be able to secrete sufficient glucocorticoids and symptoms of acute adrenocortical insufficiency will appear. Symptoms include nausea, vomiting, lethargy, confusion, and coma. Immediate administration of IV therapy with hydrocortisone is essential, as shock may quickly result if the symptoms remain untreated. Other possible causes of acute adrenocortical insufficiency include infection, trauma, and cancer.

For chronic corticosteroid insufficiency, replacement therapy is indicated. The goal of replacement therapy is to achieve the same physiologic level of hormones in the blood that would be present if the adrenal glands were functioning properly. Patients requiring replacement therapy usually need to take glucocorticoids their entire lifetime. Patients with adrenal insufficiency may also need a mineralocorticoid, such as fludrocortisone (Florinef).

Table 39.4	Selected Glucocorticoids
Drug	**Route and Adult Dose (max dose where indicated)**
Short Acting	
cortisone (Cortistan, Cortone)	PO; 20–300 mg qd
⊕hydrocortisone (Cortef, Hydrocortone, others)	PO; 2–80 mg tid-qid
Intermediate Acting	
methylprednisolone (Medrol)	PO; 2–60 mg qd-qid
prednisolone (Delta-Cortef, others)	PO; 5–60 mg qd-qid
prednisone (Deltasone, Meticorten, others) (see page 423 for the Prototype Drug box) ⊝⊚	PO; 5–60 mg qd-qid
triamcinolone (Aristocort, Kenacort, others)	PO; 4–48 mg qd-bid
Long Acting	
betamethasone (Celestone)	PO; 0.6–7.2 mg qd
dexamethasone (Decadron, Dexasone, others)	PO; 0.25–4.0 mg bid-qid

In addition to acute and chronic adrenal insufficiency, glucocorticoids are prescribed for a large number of other disorders. Their ability to quickly and effectively suppress the inflammatory and immune responses gives them tremendous therapeutic utility to treat a diverse set of conditions. Following are the indications for pharmacotherapy with glucocorticoids.

- Adrenal insufficiency
- Allergies, including seasonal rhinitis (Chapter 31) ⊝⊚
- Asthma (Chapter 29) ⊝⊚
- Chronic inflammatory bowel disease, including ulcerative colitis and Crohn's disease (Chapter 37) ⊝⊚
- Hepatic, neurologic, and renal disorders characterized by edema
- Neoplastic disease, including Hodgkin's disease, leukemias, and lymphomas (Chapter 35) ⊝⊚
- Posttransplant surgery (Chapter 30) ⊝⊚
- Rheumatic disorders, including rheumatoid arthritis, ankylosing spondylitis, and bursitis (Chapter 46) ⊝⊚
- Shock (Chapter 26) ⊝⊚
- Skin disorders, including contact dermatitis and rashes (Chapter 46) ⊝⊚

Cushing's syndrome occurs when high levels of glucocorticoids are present in the body over a prolonged period. Although hypersecretion of these hormones can occur due to pituitary or adrenal tumors, the most common cause of Cushing's syndrome is long-term therapy with high doses of glucocorticoid medications. Signs and symptoms include adrenal atrophy, osteoporosis, increased risk of infections, delayed wound healing, acne, peptic ulcers, and a redistribution of fat around the face (moon face), shoulders, and neck (buffalo hump). Mood and personality changes may occur, and the patient may become psychologically depend-

ent on the therapeutic effects of the drug. Some glucocorticoids, including hydrocortisone, also have mineralocorticoid activity and can cause retention of sodium and water. Because of their anti-inflammatory properties, glucocorticoids may mask signs of infection.

Glucocorticoids interact with many drugs. Because of their hyperglycemic effects, these agents may decrease the effectiveness of antidiabetic agents. Combining glucocorticoids with other ulcerogenic drugs such as aspirin and other NSAIDs markedly increases the risk of peptic ulcer disease. Administration with nonpotassium-sparing diuretics may lead to hypocalcemia and hypokalemia. The nurse must take special care when new drugs are added to the regimen of a patient taking glucocorticoids.

The following strategies are used to avoid serious adverse effects from glucocorticoids.

- Keep doses to the lowest possible amount that will achieve a therapeutic effect.
- Administer glucocorticoids every other day (alternate-day dosing) to limit adrenal atrophy.
- For acute conditions, give patients large amounts for a few days and then gradually decrease the drug dose until it is discontinued.
- Give the drugs locally by inhalation, intra-articular injections, or apply topically to the skin, eyes, or ears, when feasible, to diminish the possibility of systemic effects.

NURSING CONSIDERATIONS

The role of the nurse in glucocorticoid therapy involves careful monitoring of a patient's condition and providing education as it relates to the prescribed drug regimen. There are many glucocorticoid drugs available, including prednisone, methylprednisolone, dexamethasone, and the inhaled and topical glucocorticoid preparations. The nurse should assess the patient for signs and symptoms of infection as immunosuppression is a common effect of these drugs. The nurse should also monitor vital signs closely for temperature and blood pressure elevation. Pregnancy and lactation are contraindications for glucocorticoid therapy.

All patients receiving glucocorticoids at high doses for extended periods are at risk for Cushing's syndrome. Patients who take these medications are prone to many adverse effects. The nurse should use great care in starting an IV because of increased capillary fragility. Blood glucose should be monitored frequently because these drugs increase blood glucose. The nurse should observe the patient's emotional status because emotional lability often occurs. Patients should be protected from sources of infection because of the immunosuppressive effects of these drugs. Wound healing is decreased and the chance of peptic ulcer is increased.

Patient education as it relates to glucocorticoids should include goals, reasons for obtaining baseline data such as vital signs and tests for cardiac and renal disorders, and possible side effects. See "Nursing Process Focus: Patients Receiving Systemic Glucocorticoid Therapy" for specific teaching points.

39.11 Pharmacotherapy of Cushing's Syndrome

High levels of corticosteroids can cause Cushing's syndrome and numerous adverse effects when present for prolonged periods. When the cause of this hypersecretion is an adrenal tumor or perhaps an ectopic tumor secreting ACTH, drug therapy may be initiated to lower serum glucocorticoid levels. These antiadrenal agents inhibit the metabolic conversion of cholesterol to adrenal corticosteroids. They are not curative; their use is temporary until the tumor can be removed or otherwise treated with radiation or antineoplastics.

NURSING CONSIDERATIONS

The role of the nurse in antiadrenal therapy involves careful monitoring of a patient's condition and providing education as it relates to the prescribed drug regimen. The two drugs that are used to inhibit excessive corticosteroid synthesis are aminoglutethimide (Cytadren) and ketoconazole (Nizoral).

Aminoglutethimide is used to suppress adrenal function by blocking the initial step in the biochemical conversion of cholesterol to adrenal steroids. Synthesis of gonadotropins, mineralocorticoids, and glucocorticoids is affected and suppression of adrenal function usually occurs in 3 to 5 days. The

---

Pr PROTOTYPE DRUG | HYDROCORTISONE

ACTIONS AND USES

Structurally identical to the natural hormone cortisol, hydrocortisone is a synthetic corticosteroid that is the drug of choice for treating adrenocortical insufficiency. When used for replacement therapy, it is given at physiologic doses. Once proper dosing is achieved, its therapeutic effects should mimic those of endogenous corticosteroids. Hydrocortisone is also available for the treatment of inflammation, allergic disorders, and many other conditions. Intra-articular injections may be given to decrease severe inflammation in affected joints.

Hydrocortisone is available in six different formulations. Hydrocortisone base (Aeroseb-HC, Alphaderm, Cetacort, others) and hydrocortisone acetate (Anusol HC, Cortaid, Cortef Acetate) are available as oral preparations, creams, and ointments. Hydrocortisone cypionate (Cortef Fluid) is an oral suspension. Hydrocortisone sodium phosphate (Hydrocortone Phosphate) and hydrocortisone sodium succinate (A-Hydrocort, Solu-Cortef) are for parenteral use only. Hydrocortisone valerate (Westcort) is only for topical applications.

Administration Alerts

- Administer exactly as prescribed and at the same time every day.
- Administer oral formulations with food.
- Pregnancy category C.

ADVERSE EFFECTS AND INTERACTIONS

When used at physiologic doses for replacement therapy, adverse effects of hydrocortisone should not be evident. The patient and nurse must be vigilant, however, in observing for signs of Cushing's syndrome, which can develop with overtreatment. If taken for longer than 2 weeks, hydrocortisone should be discontinued gradually. Hydrocortisone possesses some mineralocorticoid activity, so sodium and fluid retention may be noted. A wide range of CNS effects have been reported, including insomnia, anxiety, headache, vertigo, confusion, and depression. Cardiovascular effects may include hypertension and tachycardia. Long-term therapy may result in peptic ulcer disease.

Hydrocortisone interacts with many drugs; for example, barbiturates, phenytoin, and rifampin may increase hepatic metabolism, thus decreasing hydrocortisone levels. Estrogens potentiate the effects of hydrocortisone. NSAIDs compound ulcerogenic effects. Cholestyramine and colestipol decrease hydrocortisone absorption. Diuretics and amphotericin B exacerbate hypokalemia. Anticholinesterase agents may produce severe weakness. Hydrocortisone may cause a decrease in immune response to vaccines and toxoids.

Use with caution with herbal supplements, such as aloe and buckthorn (a laxative), which may create a potassium deficiency with chronic use or abuse.

 See the companion website for a Nursing Process Focus specific to this drug.

NURSING PROCESS FOCUS | PATIENTS RECEIVING SYSTEMIC GLUCOCORTICOID THERAPY

ASSESSMENT

Prior to administration:
- Obtain complete health history including allergies, drug history, and possible drug interactions.
- Obtain complete physical examination, focusing on presenting symptoms.
- Determine the reason the medication is being administered.
- Obtain laboratory studies (long-term therapy) including serum sodium and potassium levels, hematocrit and hemoglobin levels, blood glucose level, and BUN.

POTENTIAL NURSING DIAGNOSES

- Risk for Infection, related to immunosuppression
- Risk for Injury, related to side effects of drug therapy
- Deficient Knowledge, related to drug therapy

PLANNING: PATIENT GOALS AND EXPECTED OUTCOMES

The patient will:
- Exhibit a decrease in the symptoms for which the drug is being given
- Exhibit no symptoms of infection
- Demonstrate an understanding of the drug's action, drug administration, and side effects

IMPLEMENTATION

Interventions and (Rationales)	*Patient Education/Discharge Planning*
■ Monitor vital signs. (Blood pressure may increase because of increased blood volume and potential vasoconstriction effect.)	■ Instruct patient to report dizziness, palpitations, or headaches.
■ Monitor for infection. Protect patient from potential infections. (Glucocorticoids increase susceptibility to infections by suppressing the immune response.)	Instruct patient to: ■ Avoid people with infection ■ Report fever, cough, sore throat, joint pain, increase weakness, and malaise ■ Consult with the healthcare provider before taking any immunizations
■ Monitor patient's compliance with drug regimen. (Sudden discontinuation of these agents can precipitate an adrenal crisis.)	Instruct patient: ■ To never suddenly stop taking the medication ■ In proper use of self-administering tapering dose pack ■ To take oral medications with food
■ Monitor for symptoms of Cushing's syndrome such as moon face, "buffalo hump" contour of shoulders, weight gain, muscle wasting, increased deposits of fat in the trunk. (Symptoms may indicate excessive use of glucocorticoids.)	Instruct patient: ■ To weigh self daily ■ That initial weight gain is expected; provide the patient with weight gain parameters that warrant reporting ■ That there are multiple side effects to therapy and that changes in health status should be reported
■ Monitor blood glucose levels. (Glucocorticoids cause an increase in gluconeogenesis and reduce glucose utilization.)	Instruct patient to: ■ Report symptoms of hyperglycemia such as excessive thirst, copious urination, and insatiable appetite ■ Adjust insulin dose based on blood glucose level as directed by the healthcare provider
■ Monitor skin and mucous membranes for lacerations, abrasions, or break in integrity. (Glucocorticoids impair wound healing.)	Instruct patient to: ■ Examine skin daily for cuts and scrapes and to cover any injuries with sterile bandage ■ Watch for symptoms of skin infection such as redness, swelling, and drainage ■ Notify the healthcare provider of any nonhealing wound or symptoms of infection

continued

NURSING PROCESS FOCUS: *Patients Receiving Systemic Glucocortoid Therapy (continued)*

Interventions and (Rationales)	Patient Education/Discharge Planning
■ Monitor gastrointestinal status for peptic ulcer development. (Glucocorticoids decrease gastric mucous production and predispose patient to peptic ulcers.)	■ Instruct patient to report GI side effects such as heartburn, abdominal pain, or tarry stools.
■ Monitor serum electrolytes. (Glucocorticoids cause hypernatremia and hypokalemia.)	Instruct patient to: ■ Consume a diet high in protein, calcium, and potassium but low in fat and concentrated simple carbohydrates ■ Keep all laboratory appointments
■ Monitor changes in musculoskeletal system. (Glucocorticoids decrease bone density and strength and cause muscle atrophy and weakness.)	Instruct patient: ■ To participate in exercise or physical activity, to help maintain bone and muscle strength ■ The drug may cause weakness in bones and muscles, avoid strenuous activity that may cause injury
■ Monitor emotional stability. (Glucocorticoids may produce mood and behavior changes such as depression or feeling of invulnerability.)	■ Instruct patient that mood changes may be expected and to report mental status changes to the healthcare provider.

EVALUATION OF OUTCOME CRITERIA

Evaluate the effectiveness of drug therapy by confirming that patient goals and expected outcomes have been met (see "Planning").

See Table 39.4 for a list of drugs to which these nursing actions apply.

effectiveness of aminoglutethimide declines over time; thus, therapy is usually limited to 3 months. Aminoglutethimide also blocks the conversion of androgens to estrogens in peripheral tissues. Because of this antiestrogen effect, an unlabeled use of this drug is to treat forms of breast cancer that have a positive estrogen receptor test. When the patient is receiving this drug, the nurse should assess and monitor CBC results because hematologic abnormalities may occur such as leukopenia and thrombocytopenia. The nurse should also assess and monitor the patient's stress level because increased stress may precipitate adrenal insufficiency. The nurse should monitor the patient's blood pressure, both lying and standing, because the drug may cause orthostatic hypotension from decreased aldosterone production. Patients should be cautioned while ambulating, because dizziness may occur that could result in falls. Aminoglutethimide is pregnancy category D and is thus contraindicated during pregnancy.

Ketoconazole (Nizoral) is classified as an antifungal but it also inhibits the synthesis of adrenal steroid hormones. To be effective as a steroid hormone inhibitor, it must be given in doses much higher than used in the treatment of fungal infections. At these high doses it may cause hepatic dysfunction related to the metabolism of the drug in the liver. The nurse should assess hepatic function prior to be-

ginning therapy. The nurse should monitor the patient for jaundice, bleeding, pale stools, or dark urine. Ketoconazole is contraindicated for patients with liver disorders, or history of alcohol abuse. Nausea and vomiting are common side effects. If nausea is a problem, the medication may be taken with food. This medication should be administered with water or fruit juice because it is better absorbed in an acidic environment.

Patient education as it relates to antiadrenal drugs should include goals, reasons for obtaining baseline data such as vital signs and tests for cardiac and renal disorders, and possible side effects. Following are important points the nurse should include when teaching patients regarding antiadrenal drugs.

- Report signs of jaundice, abnormal bleeding, or changes in the color of stools or urine.
- Take temperature regularly and report elevations.
- Change positions slowly to avoid dizziness and effects of orthostatic hypotension.
- Take medication with fruit juice.
- Limit or avoid alcohol consumption while taking these drugs.
- Notify healthcare provider if pregnancy occurs or is suspected.

CHAPTER REVIEW

Key Concepts

The numbered key concepts provide a succinct summary of the important points from the corresponding numbered section within the chapter. If any of these points are not clear, refer to the numbered section within the chapter for review. Expanded versions can be found on the companion website.

39.1 The endocrine system maintains homeostasis by using hormones as chemical messengers that are secreted in response to changes in the internal environment.

39.2 The hypothalamus secretes releasing hormones, which direct the anterior pituitary gland as to which hormones should be released.

39.3 Hormones are used as replacement therapy, as antineoplastics, and for their natural therapeutic effects such as their suppression of body defenses.

39.4 Only a few pituitary and hypothalamic hormones, including growth hormone and ACTH, have clinical applications as drugs.

39.5 The thyroid gland secretes thyroxine and triiodothyronine, which control the basal metabolic rate and affect every cell in the body.

39.6 Hypothyroidism may be treated by administering thyroid hormone.

39.7 Hyperthyroidism is treated by administering agents that decrease the activity of the thyroid gland or that kill overactive thyroid cells.

39.8 The adrenal cortex secretes glucocorticoids, gonadotropins, and mineralocorticoids. The glucocorticoids mobilize the body for long-term stress and influence carbohydrate, lipid, and protein metabolism in most cells.

39.9 Glucocorticoid release is controlled by ACTH from the pituitary.

39.10 Adrenocortical insufficiency may be acute or chronic. Glucocorticoids are prescribed for adrenocortical insufficiency and a wide variety of other conditions.

39.11 Antiadrenal drugs may be used to treat Cushing's syndrome by inhibiting corticosteroid synthesis. Their use is usually limited to 3 months of therapy.

Review Questions

1. Why are hypothalamic and pituitary hormones not widely used in pharmacotherapeutics?

2. If thyroid hormone is secreted by the thyroid gland, how can a deficiency in this hormone be caused by disease in the hypothalamus or pituitary?

3. Why does administration of glucocorticoids for extended periods result in adrenal atrophy, and what strategies can be used to lessen the risk of adrenal atrophy?

Critical Thinking Questions

1. A 5-year-old girl requires treatment for diabetes insipidus acquired following a case of meningitis. The child has suffered serious complications including blindness and mental retardation. Her diabetes insipidus is being treated with intranasal desmopressin and the child's mother has been asked to help evaluate the drug's effectiveness using urine volumes and urine specific gravity. Discuss the changes that would indicate that the drug is effective.

2. A 17-year-old boy with a history of severe asthma is admitted to the intensive care unit. He is comatose, appears much younger than his listed age, and has a short stature. The nurse notes that the asthma has been managed with prednisone for 15 days, until 3 days ago. The patient's father is extremely anxious and says that he was unable to refill his son's prescription for medicine until he got his "paycheck." What is the nurse's role in this situation?

3. A 9-year-old boy has been diagnosed with growth hormone deficiency. His parents have decided to proceed with a prescribed regimen of somatropin (Humatrope). Outline the basic information the parent's need to know regarding this regimen, side effects, and evaluation of effectiveness.

EXPLORE MediaLink

NCLEX review, case studies, and other interactive resources for this chapter can be found on the companion website at www.prenhall.com/adams. Click on "Chapter 39" to select the activities for this chapter. For animations, more NCLEX review questions, and an audio glossary, access the accompanying CD-ROM in this textbook.

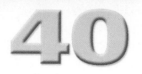

CHAPTER 40

Drugs for Pancreatic Disorders

DRUGS AT A GLANCE

INSULINS
Pr *regular insulin (Humulin R, Novolin R, Pork Regular Iletin II, Regular Purified Pork Insulin)*

ORAL HYPOGLYCEMICS
Pr *glipizide (Glucotrol, Glucotrol XL)*

PANCREATIC ENZYME REPLACEMENT
Pr *pancrelipase (Lipancreatin, Pancrease, Zymase)*

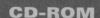 **MediaLink** www.prenhall.com/adams

CD-ROM

Animation:
   Mechanism in Action: Glipizide (Glucotrol)
Audio Glossary
NCLEX Review

Companion Website

NCLEX Review
Dosage Calculations
Case Study
Care Plans
Expanded Key Concepts

OBJECTIVES

After reading this chapter, the student should be able to:

1. Describe the endocrine and exocrine functions of the pancreas.
2. Compare and contrast type 1 and type 2 diabetes mellitus.
3. Compare and contrast types of insulin.
4. Describe the signs and symptoms of insulin overdose and underdose.
5. Describe the nurse's role in the pharmacologic management of pancreatic disorders.
6. For each of the drug classes listed in Drugs at a Glance, identify representative drug examples, explain the mechanism of drug action, primary actions, and important adverse effects.
7. Explain the pharmacotherapy of pancreatitis.
8. Use the Nursing Process to care for patients receiving drug therapy for pancreatic disorders.

The pancreas serves unique and vital functions by supplying essential digestive enzymes while also secreting the hormones responsible for glucose homeostasis. From a pharmacologic perspective, the most important disorder associated with the pancreas is diabetes mellitus. Millions of people have diabetes, a disease caused by genetic and environmental factors which impairs the cellular utilization of glucose. Because glucose is essential to every cell in the body, the effects of diabetes are widespread. Diabetes merits special consideration in pharmacology because the nurse will encounter many patients with this disorder. This chapter examines diabetes mellitus and acute and chronic pancreatitis.

40.1 Normal Functions of the Pancreas

Located behind the stomach and between the duodenum and spleen, the pancreas is an essential organ to both the digestive and endocrine systems. It is responsible for the secretion of several enzymes into the duodenum that assist in the chemical digestion of nutrients. This is its exocrine function. Clusters of cells in the pancreas, called islets of Langerhans, are responsible for its endocrine function: the secretion of glucagon and insulin. Alpha cells secrete glucagon and beta cells secrete insulin (Figure 40.1). As with other endocrine organs, the pancreas secretes these hormones directly into blood capillaries, where they are available for transport to body tissues. Insulin and glucagon play key roles in keeping glucose levels within a normal range within the blood.

Insulin secretion is regulated by a number of chemical, hormonal, and neural factors. One important regulator is the level of glucose in the blood. After a meal when blood glucose levels rise, the islets of Langerhans are stimulated to secrete insulin which causes glucose to leave the blood and enter cells. High insulin levels and falling blood glucose levels provide negative feedback to the pancreas to stop secreting insulin.

Insulin affects carbohydrate, lipid, and protein metabolism in most cells of the body. One of its most important actions is to assist in glucose transport; without insulin, glucose cannot enter cells. A cell may be literally swimming in glucose, but it cannot enter and be used as an energy source by the cell without insulin present. Insulin is said to have a hypoglycemic effect, because its presence causes glucose to leave the blood and serum glucose to fall. The brain is an important exception, not requiring insulin for glucose transport.

Islet cells in the pancreas also secrete glucagon. Glucagon is best thought of as an antagonist to insulin, because its actions are opposite to those of insulin. When levels of glucose are low, glucagon is secreted. Its primary function is to maintain adequate levels of glucose in the blood between meals. Glucagon has a hyperglycemic effect, because its presence causes blood glucose to rise. Figure 40.2

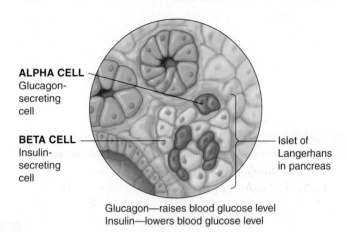

ALPHA CELL
Glucagon-
secreting
cell

BETA CELL
Insulin-
secreting
cell

Islet of
Langerhans
in pancreas

Glucagon—raises blood glucose level
Insulin—lowers blood glucose level

Figure 40.1 | Glucagon- and insulin-secreting cells in the islets of Langerhans *Source: Pearson Education/PH College.*

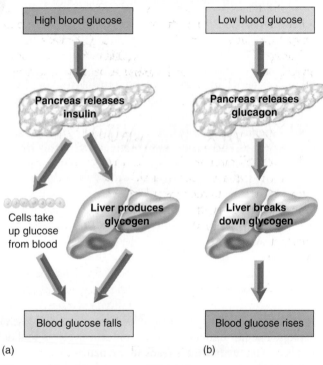

High blood glucose

Low blood glucose

Pancreas releases
insulin

Pancreas releases
glucagon

Cells take
up glucose
from blood

Liver produces
glycogen

Liver breaks
down glycogen

Blood glucose falls

Blood glucose rises

(a)

(b)

Figure 40.2 | Insulin, glucagon, and blood glucose

illustrates the relationships among blood glucose, insulin, and glucagon.

Blood glucose levels are usually kept within a normal range by insulin and glucagon, however, other hormones and drugs can affect glucose metabolism. Hyperglycemic hormones include epinephrine, thyroid hormones, growth hormone, and corticosteroids. Common drugs that can raise blood glucose levels include phenytoin, NSAIDs, and diuretics. Drugs with a hypoglycemic effect include alcohol, lithium, ACE inhibitors, and beta-adrenergic blockers. The nurse must ensure that blood glucose levels are periodically monitored in patients receiving medications that exhibit hypoglycemia or hypoglycemic effects.

DIABETES MELLITUS

Worldwide, approximately 135 million people are thought to have diabetes mellitus (DM); by 2025, this number is expected to increase to 300 million (Hjelm, 2003). The etiology of DM includes a combination of genetic and environmental factors. The recent increase in the frequency of the disease is probably the result of trends toward more sedentary and stressful lifestyles, increasing consumption of highly caloric foods with resultant obesity, and increased longevity.

Diabetes mellitus is a group of metabolic diseases in which there is deficient insulin secretion or decreased sensitivity of insulin receptors on target cells resulting in hyperglycemia. Diabetes mellitus includes type 1, type 2, gestational diabetes, and other specific types such as those found in Cushing's syndrome or that are chemically induced. Discussion in this chapter is limited to type 1 and type 2 DM.

40.2 Etiology and Characteristics of Type 1 Diabetes Mellitus

Type 1 diabetes mellitus is one of the most common diseases of childhood. Type 1 diabetes was previously called - *juvenile-onset diabetes*, because it is often diagnosed between the ages of 11 and 13. Because the symptoms of Type 1 diabetes can occur for the first time in adulthood, this is not the most accurate name for this disorder. This type of diabetes is also referred to as insulin-dependent diabetes mellitus.

Type 1 DM results from a lack of insulin secretion by the pancreas. The cause of this deficient secretion is thought to be an interaction of genetic, immunologic, and environmental factors, with beta cells being destroyed by antibodies. (Beta cells within the islets of Langerhans secrete insulin.) Another subType 1s said to be idiopathic as no evidence of autoimmune disease is identifiable. Children and siblings of those with the disease have a higher risk of acquiring the disorder.

The signs and symptoms of type 1 DM are consistent from patient to patient, with the most diagnostic sign being sustained hyperglycemia. Following are the typical signs and symptoms of type 1 DM.

- Hyperglycemia—fasting blood glucose greater than 126 mg/dl on at least two separate occasions
- Polyuria—excessive urination
- Polyphagia—increase in hunger
- Polydipsia—increased thirst
- Glucosuria—high levels of glucose in the urine
- Weight loss
- Fatigue

Untreated DM produces long-term damage to arteries which leads to heart disease, stroke, kidney disease, and blindness. Lack of adequate circulation to the feet often causes gangrene of the toes, which may require amputation.

- Of the 16 million Americans who have diabetes, 5 million probably are unaware that they have the disease.
- Each day, over 2,000 people are diagnosed with diabetes.
- Diabetes causes almost 200,000 deaths each year; it is the sixth leading cause of death.
- Diabetes is the leading cause of blindness in adults; each year 12,000 to 24,000 people lose their sight because of diabetes.
- Diabetes is responsible for 50% of nontraumatic lower limb amputations; 56,000 amputations are performed each year on diabetics.
- Costs for diabetes treatment exceed $100 billion annually—$1 in every $7 of healthcare expenditures.
- Diabetes is the leading cause of end-stage renal disease, accounting for about 40% of new cases.

Nerve degeneration is common and produces symptoms ranging from tingling in the fingers or toes to complete loss of sensation of a limb. Because glucose is unable to enter cells, lipids are utilized as an energy source and ketoacids are produced as waste products. These ketoacids can give the patient's breath an acetone-like, fruity odor. More importantly, high levels of ketoacids lower the pH of the blood, causing diabetic ketoacidosis (DKA), and may progress to coma and possible death if untreated.

Insulin

Insulin was first made available as a medication in 1922. Prior to that time, type 1 diabetics were unable to adequately maintain normal blood glucose, experienced many complications, and usually died at a young age. Increased insulin availability and improvements in insulin products, personal blood glucose monitoring devices, and the insulin pump have made it possible for patients to maintain more exact control of their blood glucose levels.

40.3 Pharmacotherapy with Insulin

Therapy of type 1 DM requires treatment with insulin in conjunction with proper meal planning and exercise. Food must be eaten regularly, every 4 to 5 hours, as skipping meals can have profound effects on blood glucose. Regular, moderate exercise increases the cellular responsiveness to insulin, lowering the amount of insulin needed to maintain normal blood glucose levels. During heavy prolonged exercise, such as in competitive sports, individuals may become hypoglycemic and need to consume food or drink to raise their blood sugar to normal levels. Those regularly engaging in strenuous activities should eat food or consume a sports drink prior to commencing the activity as a preventative measure.

The treatment goal with insulin therapy is to maintain blood glucose levels within strict, normal limits. Several types of insulin are available, differing in their onset and duration of action. Until the 1980s, the source of all insulin was beef or pork pancreas. Almost all insulin today, however, is human insulin obtained through recombinant DNA technology. While some patients may still use pork or beef insulin, human insulin is more effective, causes fewer allergies, and has a lower incidence of resistance.

The route of administration for insulin is subcutaneous, although research is being conducted to discover more convenient routes such as an insulin nasal spray. Doses of insulin are highly individualized for each patient; some patients may need two or more injections daily. Two different compatible types of insulin are sometimes mixed, using a standard method, to obtain the desired therapeutic effects. Regular insulin, which is clear, is always drawn up in the syringe first, followed by the cloudy insulin. Some patients have an insulin pump. This pump is usually abdominally anchored and is programmed to give small doses of insulin subcutaneous into the abdomen at predetermined intervals with larger boluses possible at mealtime by setting the dose manually. Common insulin preparations are given in Table 40.1.

The hormone glucagon is administered as a replacement therapy for some diabetic patients when they are in a hypoglycemic state and have impaired glucagon secretion. Glucagon (1 mg) can be given IV, IM, or SC to reverse hypoglycemic symptoms in 20 minutes or less, depending on the route.

NURSING CONSIDERATIONS

The role of the nurse in insulin therapy involves careful monitoring of a patient's condition and providing education as it relates to the prescribed drug regimen. The nurse must be familiar with the onset, peak, and duration of action of the insulin(s) prescribed, as well as any other important aspects of the specific insulin, and convey this information to the patient.

The nurse should assess the patient for signs and symptoms of hypoglycemia as well as the adequacy of glucose monitoring. The most likely time for hypoglycemia is when insulin reaches its peak effect, during exercise, or during acute illness. The nurse should obtain food for the patient and determine that the patient is ready to eat, before administering insulin. The nurse should assess the patient's level of understanding of the symptoms of insulin reaction, hypoglycemia, and diabetic ketoacidosis. The nurse will need to do sufficient teaching to ensure that patients can recognize key symptoms and that they know what action to take in response to them. Contraindications to insulin include sensitivity to an ingredient in the formulation, and hypoglycemia that would be worsened by administration of insulin. Use with caution in patients with pregnancy, severe stress, and infection. Patients with these conditions usually have increased insulin requirements and must be monitored more carefully.

Two of the most frequently prescribed types of insulin are NPH and regular insulin. Intermediate or NPH (isophane) insulin is used to provide a longer-acting source of insulin as compared to regular insulin and other types of short-acting insulin. The onset of action for NPH insulin is between 1 and 4 hours and peak effect occurs in 8 to 12

Table 40.1	Insulin Preparations
Drug	**Route and Adult Dose (max dose where indicated)**
Insulin Analogs	
insulin aspart (NovoLog)	SC; 0.25–0.7 U/kg/d given 5–10 min before each meal
insulin glargine (Lantus) *long*	For type 1 diabetes: SC; if not taking insulin, 10 U at hs qd; if taking NPH or ultralente insulin qd, give same dose at hs; if taking NPH insulin bid, give 80% of total daily dose at hs
	For type 2 diabetes: if already taking oral hypoglycemic drugs, start with 10 U SC at hs qd and adjust according to patient's needs
insulin lispro (Humalog) *rapid*	SC; 5–10 U given 0–15 min ac
Insulin Mixtures	
NPH 70% Regular 30% (Humulin 70/30, Novolin 70/30)	IM/SC; Individualized doses
NPH 50% Regular 50%	IM/SC; Individualized doses
Short-acting Insulin	
insulin injection (Regular Iletin II, Humulin R, Novolin R)	SC; 5–10 U given 15–30 min ac and hs
Intermediate-acting Insulin	
isophane insulin suspension (NPH, NPH Iletin II, Humulin N, Novolin N)	IM/SC; Individualized doses
insulin zinc suspension (Lente Iletin II, Lente L, Humulin L, Novolin L)	IM/SC; Individualized doses
Long-acting Insulin	
extended insulin zinc suspension (Humulin U, Ultralente)	IM/SC; Individualized doses

SPECIAL CONSIDERATIONS

Psychosocial and Cultural Impacts on the Young Diabetic

For the child or adolescent who is diabetic, there are psychosocial and cultural considerations in terms of compliance with medication and dietary regimens. Even if diagnosed early in life (with learned behaviors regarding the disease parameters), the elementary school years can be difficult for some children. Social events such as birthday parties, field trips, and after-school snacktime where sweet treats are the norm serve as a physical and psychological temptation. During adolescence, when the teen wants to fit in with a peer group, the diabetic regimen can become more difficult. It is during this time that failure to take insulin or to follow dietary guidelines becomes an issue that may impact present and future health in a negative manner. Some teens may have insulin pumps and can more easily take extra insulin to cover foods not usually on their diet. The ability to do this helps teens feel less different from peers, but carried to excess this practice can also lead to problems. The nurse plays a vital role in patient-family education and referrals to community agencies that may assist in helping the young person keep blood sugar in control while preserving self-esteem.

hours. Its duration is 18 to 24 hours. NPH insulin is normally given 30 minutes before the first meal of the day, but in some instances a second, smaller dose is prescribed before the evening meal or at bedtime. Many patients are prescribed insulin that is premixed, such as 70% NPH with 30% regular or rapid acting. If the patient is prescribed a premixed insulin solution, it is important that proper instruction is given, especially if the patient will be using additional regular or rapid-acting insulin in a sliding scale manner.

Under some circumstances regular insulin may be given IV, but other types of insulin, including NPH, are to be given only as SC injections. Intermediate insulin cannot be given IV.

Rapid-acting insulin lispro (Humalog) is being used more frequently. The onset of action is 10 to 15 minutes, which is much faster than the onset of 30 to 60 minutes associated with regular insulin. The peak effect of rapid-acting insulin lispro occurs in 30 to 60 minutes and its duration of action is 5 hours or less. It is often used with insulin infusion pumps.

Insulin glargine (Lantus) is a newer agent that is a recombinant human insulin analog. It must not be mixed in the syringe with any other insulin and must be administered SC. Insulin glargine appears to have a constant long duration hypoglycemic effect with no defined peak effect. It is prescribed once daily, at bedtime.

Long-acting insulin is prescribed for some patients. Protamine zinc (PZI) (Iletin II) has an onset of 4 to 8 hours, a peak effect at 14 to 24 hours, with duration of 36 hours. Extended insulin zinc suspension (Ultralente) has an onset of 4 to 6 hours, a peak of 10 to 30 hours, and duration of 36 hours. A mixed insulin, Novolin Mix (70% N and 30% R) has an onset of 4 to 8 hours, a peak effect of 16 to 18 hours, and duration greater than 36 hours.

When administering insulin, the nurse must ensure that the units on the syringe match the units on the insulin vial. For example, when U100 insulin is ordered, the vial must be U100 and the syringe must also be calibrated for U100. Although U100 and U50 are the most often used strengths of insulin, U500 is available for patients who have developed insulin resistance and need a much higher dose to manage blood glucose. When giving U500 insulin, a syringe calibrated for U500 is necessary.

The adverse effects of insulin therapy are mostly related to hypoglycemia, hyperinsulinemia, or hyperglycemia. Other adverse effects of which the nurse should be aware include localized allergic reactions at the injection site, generalized urticaria (swollen raised areas that itch and usually disappear in 24 hours), and swollen lymph glands. Some patients will experience Somogyi phenomenon, a rapid decrease in blood glucose, usually during the night, which stimulates the release of hormones that elevate blood glucose (epinephrine, cortisol, glucagon) resulting in elevated morning blood glucose. Additional insulin above the patient's normal dose may produce a rapid rebound hypoglycemia. Patients experiencing Somogyi phenomenon require education about the condition and will need to work with a healthcare provider to find the optimum insulin regimen.

Symptoms of insulin reaction or hypoglycemia occur when a patient with type 1 DM has more insulin in the blood than is needed for the amount of circulating blood glucose. This may occur when the insulin level peaks, during exercise, when the patient receives too much insulin due to a medication error, or if the patient skips a meal. Some of the symptoms of hypoglycemia are the same as those of diabetic ketoacidosis. Those that differ and help to make the determination that a patient is hypoglycemic include pale, cool, and moist skin, with blood glucose less than 50 mg/dl and a sudden onset of symptoms. Left untreated, severe hypoglycemia may cause death.

Symptoms of diabetic ketoacidosis that differ from those of hypoglycemia include flushed dry warm skin, fruity breath, blurred vision, Kussmaul's respirations, and a blood glucose greater than 300 mg/dl. Diabetic ketoacidosis usually develops over several days. Left untreated, the patient with diabetic ketoacidosis can eventually enter a coma and die.

Following are important points the nurse should include when teaching patients regarding insulin therapy.

- Closely monitor blood glucose, as directed by healthcare provider.
- Carry a source of simple sugar in case of hypoglycemic reactions.
- When in doubt if symptoms indicate hypoglycemia or hyperglycemia, treat for hypoglycemia. Hypoglycemia progresses rapidly while hyperglycemia is slow in progression.
- Rotate insulin sites to prevent lipodystrophy.
- Do not inject insulin into areas that are raised, swollen, dimpled, or itching.
- Keep insulin vials that are currently in use at room temperature, as it is less irritating to the skin.
- When not needed, refrigerate insulin to keep it stable.
- Strictly follow the prescribed diet unless otherwise instructed.
- Wear a medic alert bracelet to alert emergency personnel of DM. Notify caregivers, coworkers, and others who may be able to render assistance.
- Monitor blood glucose before each meal and before insulin administration to prevent hypoglycemic reactions.
- Use only an insulin syringe, calibrated the same as the strength of the insulin, to administer insulin.
- Use only the type of insulin prescribed by the healthcare provider.

40.4 Etiology and Characteristics of Type 2 Diabetes Mellitus

There are a number of differences between type 2 and type 1 DM. Type 2 diabetes mellitus usually begins in middle-age adults and has been referred to as age-onset diabetes or maturity onset diabetes. These are inaccurate descriptions of this disorder, however, because increasing numbers of children are being diagnosed with type 2 DM. Children who develop type 2 diabetes are most often overweight and sedentary. Hispanic children are in a high-risk group for type 2 diabetes, perhaps because many Hispanic diets are high in carbohydrates and fats. Approximately 90% of all diabetics are type 2.

Unlike type 1 DM, type 2 patients are capable of secreting insulin, although in relatively deficient amounts. The fundamental problem in type 2 DM, however, is that insulin receptors in the target tissues have become insensitive or resistant to the hormone. Thus, the small amount of insulin secreted does not bind to its receptors as efficiently, and less effect is achieved.

Another important difference is that proper diet and exercise can sometimes increase the sensitivity of insulin receptors to the point that drug therapy is unnecessary for type 2 DM. Many patients with type 2 DM are obese and will need a medically supervised plan to reduce weight gradually and exercise safely. This is an important lifestyle change for such patients; they will need to maintain these changes for a lifetime. Patients with poorly managed type 2 DM often suffer from the same complications as patients with type 1 diabetes (e.g., retinopathy, neuropathy, and nephropathy).

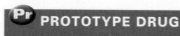 **PROTOTYPE DRUG** | **REGULAR INSULIN** (Humulin R, Novolin R, Pork Regular Iletin II, Regular Purified Pork Insulin)

ACTIONS AND USES

Regular insulin is prepared from pork pancreas or as human insulin through recombinant DNA technology. It is classified as short-acting insulin, with an onset of 30 to 60 minutes, a peak effect at 2 to 3 hours, and a duration of 5 to 7 hours. Its primary action is to promote the entry of glucose into cells. For the emergency treatment of acute ketoacidosis, it may be given SC or IV. Regular insulin is also available as Humulin 70/30 (a mixture of 30% regular insulin and 70% isophane insulin) or as Humulin 50/50 (a mixture of 50% of both regular and isophane insulin). Regular insulin is pregnancy category B.

Administration Alerts

- Hypoglycemic reactions may occur quickly if regular insulin is not supported by sufficient food or is given when patient is hypoglycemic.
- Regular insulin is the only type of insulin that may be used for IV injection.
- Injection sites must be rotated. When the patient is hospitalized, use sites not normally used while the patient is at home.
- Administer approximately 30 minutes before meals so insulin will be absorbed and available when the patient begins to eat.

ADVERSE EFFECTS AND INTERACTIONS

The most serious adverse effect from insulin therapy is hypoglycemia. Hypoglycemia may result from taking too much insulin, not properly timing the insulin injection with food intake, or skipping a meal. Dietary carbohydrates must have reached the blood when insulin is injected, otherwise the drug will remove too much glucose and signs of hypoglycemia—tachycardia, confusion, sweating, and drowsiness—will ensue. If severe hypoglycemia is not quickly treated with glucose, convulsions, coma, and death may follow.

Regular insulin interacts with many drugs. For example, the following substances may potentiate hypoglycemic effects: alcohol, salicylates, MAO inhibitors, anabolic steroids, and guanethidine. The following substances may antagonize hypoglycemic effects: corticosteroids, thryoid hormones, and epinephrine. Serum glucose levels may be increased with furosemide or thiazide diuretics. Symptoms of hypoglycemic reaction may be masked with beta-adrenergic blockers.

Use with caution with herbal supplements, such as garlic and ginseng, which may potentiate the hypoglycemic effects of insulin.

 See the companion website for a Nursing Process Focus specific to this drug.

Oral Hypoglycemics

Type 2 diabetes is usually controlled with oral hypoglycemic agents, which are prescribed after diet and exercise have failed to reduce blood glucose to normal levels. In severe, unresponsive cases, insulin may also be necessary for type 2 diabetics or it may be required temporarily during times of stress such as illness or loss.

40.5 Pharmacotherapy with Oral Hypoglycemics

All oral hypoglycemics have the common action of lowering blood glucose levels when taken on a regular basis. Many have the potential to cause hypoglycemia; thus, periodic laboratory tests are conducted to monitor blood glucose levels. Oral hypoglycemics are not effective for type 1 DM. The oral hypoglycemics are shown in Table 40.2.

Classification of oral hypoglycemic drugs is based on their chemical structures and mechanisms of action. The five classes of oral hypoglycemic medications used for type 2 diabetes are sulfonylureas, biguanides, thiazolidinediones, alpha-glucosidase inhibitors, and meglitinides. Therapy is usually initiated with a single agent. If therapeutic goals are not achieved, two agents are administered concurrently. Failure to achieve normal blood glucose levels with two oral hypoglycemics usually indicates a need for insulin.

The sulfonylureas were the first oral hypoglycemics available, and are divided into first and second generation categories. Although drugs from both generations have equal efficacy, the second generation drugs have fewer drug-drug interactions. A first generation sulfonylurea, tolbutamide (Orinase) has the shortest duration of action and is quickly converted to inactive metabolites; therefore, it is sometimes prescribed for patients who have kidney dysfunction, when other more potent antidiabetic drugs are contraindicated. The sulfonylureas act by stimulating the release of insulin from islet cells and by increasing the sensitivity of insulin receptors on target cells. The most common adverse effect of sulfonylureas is hypoglycemia, which is usually caused by taking too much medication or not eating enough food. Persistent hypoglycemia from these agents may be prolonged and require administration of dextrose to return glucose to normal levels. Other side effects include hypersensitivity reactions, GI distress, hepatotoxicity, and hematologic disorders. When alcohol is taken with these agents, some patients report an Antabuse-like reaction and experience flushing, palpitations, and nausea.

The biguanides such as metformin (Glucophage) act by decreasing the hepatic production of glucose (gluconeogenesis) and reducing insulin resistance. They do not promote insulin release from the pancreas. Most side effects are minor and related to GI effects such as anorexia, nausea, and diarrhea. Unlike the sulfonylureas, biguanides alone do not

NURSING PROCESS FOCUS | PATIENTS RECEIVING INSULIN THERAPY

ASSESSMENT

Prior to administration:
- Obtain complete health history including allergies, drug history, and possible drug interactions.
- Assess vital signs. If the patient has a fever or elevated pulse, assess further to determine the cause, as infection can alter the amount of insulin required.
- Assess blood glucose level.
- Assess appetite and presence of symptoms that indicate the patient may not be able to consume or retain the next meal.
- Assess subcutaneous areas for potential insulin injection sites.
- Assess knowledge of insulin and ability to self-administer insulin.

POTENTIAL NURSING DIAGNOSES

- Risk for Injury (hypoglycemia), related to adverse effects of drug therapy
- Deficient Knowledge, related to need for self-injection
- Risk for Imbalanced Nutrition, related to adverse effects of drug therapy
- Risk for Infection, related to blood glucose elevations and impaired circulation

PLANNING: PATIENT GOALS AND EXPECTED OUTCOMES

The patient will:
- Immediately report irritability, dizziness, diaphoresis, hunger, behavior changes, and changes in LOC
- Demonstrate ability to self-administer insulin
- Demonstrate an understanding of lifestyle modifications necessary for successful maintenance of drug therapy

IMPLEMENTATION

Interventions and (Rationales)	*Patient Education/Discharge Planning*
■ Increase frequency of blood glucose monitoring if the patient is experiencing fever, nausea, vomiting, or diarrhea. (Illness usually requires adjustments in insulin doses.)	■ Instruct patient to increase blood glucose monitoring when experiencing fever, nausea, vomiting, or diarrhea.
■ Check urine for ketones if blood glucose is over 300. (Ketones will spill into the urine at this glucose level and provide an early sign of diabetic ketoacidosis.)	Teach patient: ■ How to check urine for ketones ■ That ketoacidosis normally develops slowly but is a serious problem that needs to be corrected
■ Monitor weight on a routine basis. (Changes in weight will alter insulin needs.)	■ Instruct patient to weigh self on a routine basis at the same time each day, and to report significant changes (e.g., plus or minus 10 lb).
■ Monitor vital signs. (Increased pulse and blood pressure are early signs of hypoglycemia. Patients with diabetes may have circulatory problems and/or impaired kidney function that can increase blood pressure.)	■ Teach patient how to take blood pressure, and pulse and to report significant changes.
■ Monitor potassium level. (Insulin causes potassium to move into the cell and may cause hypokalemia.)	■ Instruct patient to report the first sign of heart irregularity.
■ Check blood glucose and feed patient some form of simple sugar at the first sign of hypoglycemia. (Using a simple sugar will raise blood sugar immediately.)	Advise patient: ■ That exercise may increase insulin needs ■ To check blood glucose before and after exercise and to keep a simple sugar on their person while exercising ■ Before strenuous exercise, to eat some form of simple sugar or complex carbohydrate as a prophylaxis against hypoglycemia

EVALUATION OF OUTCOME CRITERIA

Evaluate the effectiveness of drug therapy by confirming that patient goals and expected outcomes have been met (see "Planning").

🔗 See Table 40.1 for a list of drugs to which these nursing actions apply.

Table 40.2	Oral Hypoglycemics
Drug	**Route and Adult Dose (max dose where indicated)**
Alpha-glucosidase Inhibitors	
acarbose (Precose)	PO; 25–100 mg tid (max 300 mg/d)
miglitol (Glyset)	PO; 25–100 mg tid (max 300 mg/d)
Biguanide	
metformin HCl (Glucophage)	PO; 500 mg qd-tid (max 3 g/d)
Meglitinides	
nateglinide (Starlix)	PO; 60–120 mg tid
repaglinide (Prandin)	PO; 0.5–4.0 mg bid-qid
Sulfonylureas, First Generation	
acetohexamide (Dimelor, Dymelor)	PO; 250 mg qd (max 1,500 mg/d)
chlorpropamide (Diabinese, Novopropamide)	PO; 100–250 mg qd (max 750 mg/d)
tolazamide (Tolamide, Tolinase)	PO; 100–500 mg qd-bid (max 1 g/d)
tolbutamide (Orinase)	PO; 250–1,500 mg qd-bid (max 3 g/d)
Sulfonylureas, Second Generation	
glimepiride (Amaryl)	PO; 1–4 mg qd (max 8 mg/d)
glipizide (Glucotrol)	PO; 2.5–20 mg qd-bid (max 40 mg/d)
glyburide (DiaBeta, Micronase, Glynase)	PO; 1.25–10 mg qd-bid (max 20 mg/d)
Thiazolidinediones	
pioglitazone (Actos)	PO; 15–30 mg qd (max 45 mg/d)
rosiglitazone (Avandia)	PO; 2–4 mg qd-bid (max 8 mg/d)
Combination Drugs	
glipizide/metformin (Metaglip)	PO; 2.5/250 mg qd (max 10 mg glipizide and 2,000 mg metformin/d)
glyburide/metformin (Glucovance)	PO; 1.25 mg/250 mg qd-bid (max 20 mg glyburide and 2,000 mg metformin/d)
rosiglitazone/metformin (Avandamet)	PO; Variable dose (max 8 mg rosiglitazone and 1,000 mg metformin/d)

cause hypoglycemia or weight gain. Although rare, drugs in this class have been reported to cause lactic acidosis in patients with impaired liver function due to accumulation of medication in the liver.

The alpha-glucosidase inhibitors such as acarbose (Precose) act by blocking the enzyme in the small intestine responsible for breaking down complex carbohydrates into monosaccharides. Because carbohydrates must be in the monosaccharide form to be absorbed, digestion of glucose is delayed. These agents are usually well tolerated and have minimal side effects. The most common side effects are GI in nature, such as abdominal cramping, diarrhea, and flatulence. Liver function should be monitored, as a small incidence of liver impairment has been reported. Although alpha-glucosidase inhibitors, do not produce hypoglycemia when used alone, hypoglycemia may occur when these agents are combined with insulin or a sulfonylurea. Concurrent use of garlic and ginseng may increase the hypoglycemic action of alpha-glucosidase inhibitors.

The thiazolidinediones, or glitazones, reduce blood glucose by decreasing insulin resistance and inhibiting hepatic gluconeogenesis. The most common adverse effects are fluid retention, headache, and weight gain. Hypoglycemia does not occur. Liver function should be monitored because thiazolidinediones may be hepatotoxic; troglitazone (Rezulin) was withdrawn from the market because of drug-related deaths due to hepatic failure.

The meglitinides are the newest class of oral hypoglycemics that act by stimulating the release of insulin from islet cells. They have equal efficacy to the sulfonylureas, and are well tolerated. Repaglinide (Prandin) is well tolerated, although hypoglycemia is a potentially serious adverse effect.

Since the various oral hypoglycemics work in different ways to lower blood sugar and have different properties, combinations of antidiabetic agents have been developed to maximize the therapeutic effects and minimize adverse effects. One popular combination drug is glyburide/metformin

NATURAL THERAPIES — Stevia for Hyperglycemia

Stevia (*Stevia rebaudiana*) is an herb indigenous to Paraguay that may be helpful to diabetics. The FDA has not approved its first use, as a sweetener. The powdered extract is readily available as a food supplement, however, and can be used in place of sugar. Its sweetening power is 300 times that of sugar, but it does not appear to have a negative effect on blood glucose or insulin secretion. In animal experiments, Stevia significantly elevated the glucose clearance, an effect that may be beneficial to diabetics. The nurse should strongly encourage all diabetic patients to discuss this supplement and other herbal products with the healthcare provider before taking them.

(Glucovance), which comes in various strengths such as 1.25/250, 2.5/500, and 5/500.

NURSING CONSIDERATIONS

The role of the nurse in oral hypoglycemic therapy involves careful assessment and monitoring of a patient's condition and providing education as it relates to the prescribed drug regimen. The assessment of the patient with type 2 diabetes includes a physical examination, health history, psychosocial history, and lifestyle history. A thorough assessment is needed because diabetes can affect multiple body systems. Psychosocial factors and lifestyle, as well as knowledge base regarding diabetes, can affect the patient's ability to keep his or her blood glucose within the normal range. Lifestyle factors and health history help to determine the type of drug prescribed.

Most patients need information about the benefits of keeping blood glucose levels within a normal range. Blood glucose should be monitored daily; urinary ketones should be monitored if blood glucose is over 300. The nurse should also monitor intake and output and review lab studies for liver function abnormalities. The nurse should monitor the patient for signs and symptoms of illness or infection, as illness can affect the patient's medication need. These drugs should be used cautiously in those with impaired renal and hepatic function, and those who are malnourished, because these conditions interfere with absorption and metabolism of the oral hypoglycemics. Caution should be taken in patients with pituitary or adrenal disorders due to hormones from these sources affecting blood glucose levels. Oral hypoglycemics are contraindicated in hypersensitivity, ketoacidosis, or diabetic coma. They are also contraindicated in patients who are pregnant or lactating as safety has not been established and these drugs may be secreted in breast milk.

The American Diabetes Association and the American Association of Clinical Endocrinologists recommend that type 2 diabetics maintain a preprandial blood glucose level below 110 mg/dl. In healthy persons, the beta cells secrete insulin in response to small increases in blood glucose, which is referred to as an acute insulin response. This response is diminished at 115 mg/dl, and the higher the glucose level the less likely it is that the beta cells will respond by secreting insulin. Because type 2 diabetics need to secrete some insulin, keeping the blood glucose level below 110 before meals optimizes secretion of insulin.

Oral hypoglycemics should be administered as directed by the healthcare provider. Some oral antidiabetic drugs are given 30 minutes before breakfast so that the drug will have reached the plasma when the patient begins to eat. Others such as acarbose (Precose) and miglitol (Glyset) are given with each meal.

Type 2 diabetics need to recognize the symptoms of **hyperosmolar nonketotic coma (HNKC)**, which is a life-threatening emergency. Like diabetic ketoacidosis in the type 1 diabetic, HNKC develops slowly and is caused by insufficient circulating insulin. It is seen most often in older adults. The skin appears flushed, dry, and warm like in diabetic ketoacidosis. Unlike diabetic ketoacidosis, HNKC does not affect breathing. Blood glucose levels may rise over 600 mg/dl and reach 1,000 to 2,000 mg/dl. HNKC has a higher mortality rate than DKA.

Patient education as it relates to oral hypoglycemic drugs should include goals for pharmacotherapy, importance of diet and exercise, reasons for obtaining baseline data such as vital signs and cardiac and renal function tests, and recognizing symptoms of hypoglycemia. Following are other important points the nurse should include when teaching patients regarding these drugs.

- Always carry a source of simple sugar in case of hypoglycemic reactions.
- Wear a medic alert bracelet to alert emergency personnel of the diabetes. Notify caregivers, coworkers, and others who may be able to render assistance.
- Avoid the use of alcohol to avoid an Antabuse-like reaction.
- Maintain specified diet and exercise regimen while on antidiabetic drugs as these activities will help to keep blood glucose within a normal range.
- Swallow tablets whole and do not crush sustained-release tablets.
- Take medication 30 minutes before breakfast, or as directed by the healthcare provider.

EXOCRINE DISORDERS OF THE PANCREAS

The pancreas is responsible for the secretion of essential digestive enzymes. Because lack of secretion will result in malabsorption disorders, replacement therapy is sometimes warranted.

40.6 Pancreatic Enzymes

Lobules of acinar cells comprise the exocrine portion of the pancreas, which secretes over 1 L of pancreatic juice daily. The enzymatic portion of pancreatic juice contains the proenzymes procarboxypeptidase, chymotrypsinogen, and trypsinogen. Although these enzymes are present in the pancreas and associated

Pr PROTOTYPE DRUG | GLIPIZIDE (Glucotrol, Glucotrol XL)

ACTIONS AND USES

Glipizide is a second generation sulfonylurea offering advantages of higher potency, once-a-day dosing, fewer side effects, and fewer drug-drug interactions than some of the first generation drugs in this class. Glipizide stimulates the pancreas to secrete more insulin and also increases the sensitivity of insulin receptors at target tissues. Some degree of pancreatic function is required for glipizide to lower blood glucose. Maximum effects are achieved if the drug is taken 30 minutes prior to the first meal of the day.

Administration Alerts

- Sustained-release tablets must be swallowed whole and not crushed or chewed.
- Sulfonylureas including glipizide should not be given after the last meal of the day.
- Administer medication as directed by the healthcare provider.
- Pregnancy category C.

ADVERSE EFFECTS AND INTERACTIONS

Hypoglycemia is less frequent with glipizide than with first generation sulfonylureas. Elderly patients are prone to hypoglycemia because many have decreased renal and hepatic function, which can cause an increase in the amount of medication circulating in the blood. For this reason, elderly patients are often prescribed a reduced dosage.

Patients should stay out of direct sunlight, as rashes and photosensitivity are possible. Some patients experience mild, GI-related effects such as nausea, vomiting, or loss of appetite. Glipizide and other sulfonylureas have the potential to interact with a number of drugs; thus, the patient should always consult with a healthcare provider before adding a new medication or herbal supplement. Ingestion of alcohol will result in distressing symptoms that include headache, flushing, nausea, and abdominal cramping.

Glipizide interacts with several drugs. For example, there is a cross-sensitivity with sulfonamides and thiazide diuretics. Oral anticoagulants, chloramphenicol, clofibrate, and MAO inhibitors may potentiate the hypoglycemic actions of glipizide.

Use with caution with herbal supplements, such as ginseng and garlic, which may increase hypoglycemic effects.

 See the companion website for a Nursing Process Focus specific to this drug.

---

ducts, they are in an inactive state. Once reaching the small intestine, they are converted to their active forms: carboxypeptidase, chymotrypsin, and trypsin. This delay in activation prevents digestion of pancreatic tissue by these enzymes. Three other pancreatic enzymes—lipase, amylase, and nuclease—are secreted in their active form but require the presence of bile for optimum activity. Pancreatic juice also contains significant amounts of bicarbonate ion, which helps to neutralize the highly acidic chyme from the stomach.

Secretions from the acinar cells flow into the main pancreatic duct. This duct joins with the common bile duct; the pancreatic juice and bile mix before emptying into the duodenum. The hepatopancreatic sphincter (sphincter of Oddi) controls the emptying of bile into the duodenum.

40.7 Pharmacotherapy of Pancreatitis

Pancreatitis results when amylase and lipase remain in the pancreas, rather than being released into the duodenum. The enzymes escape from the acinar cells into the surrounding tissue, causing inflammation in the pancreas, or pancreatitis. Pancreatitis can be either acute or chronic.

Acute pancreatis usually occurs in middle-age adults and is often associated with gallstones in women and alcoholism in men. The patient usually recovers from the illness and regains normal function of the pancreas. Some patients with acute pancreatitis have reoccurring attacks and progress to chronic pancreatitis.

Symptoms of acute pancreatitis present suddenly, often after eating a fatty meal or consuming excessive amounts of alcohol. The most common symptom is a continuous severe pain in the epigastric area often radiating to the back. Other signs and symptoms of acute pancreatitis include nausea and vomiting, abdominal rigidity and distention, decreased bowel sounds, fever, increased pulse rate, hypotension, and cool, clammy skin. Within 24 hours, the skin may appear slightly jaundiced. Lab reports may reveal elevated serum amylase and lipase as well as hypocalcemia.

Many patients with acute pancreatitis require only bedrest and withholding food and fluids by mouth for a few days for the symptoms to subside. For patients with acute pain, meperidine (Demerol) brings effective relief. Several other medications are used in the treatment of acute pancreatitis depending on assessment findings and the experience of the prescribing clinician. Some healthcare providers use antibiotics to prevent infection whereas others believe this may contribute to drug-resistant organisms or may increase morbidity. To reduce or neutralize gastric secretions, H_2 blockers such as cimetidine (Tagamet) or proton pump inhibitors such as omeprazole (Prilosec) may be prescribed. To decrease the amount of pancreatic enzymes secreted, carbonic anhydrase inhibitors such as acetazolamide (Diamox) or antispasmodics such as dicyclomine (Bentyl) may be prescribed. In particularly severe cases, IV fluids and total parenteral nutrition may be necessary.

About 70% to 80% of all cases of chronic pancreatitis are associated with alcoholism. Alcohol is thought to

NURSING PROCESS FOCUS	PATIENTS RECEIVING ORAL HYPOGLYCEMIC THERAPY

ASSESSMENT DATA	POTENTIAL NURSING DIAGNOSES
Prior to administration: ■ Obtain complete health history including allergies, drug history, and possible drug interactions. ■ Assess for pain location and level. ■ Assess knowledge of drug. ■ Assess ability to conduct blood glucose testing.	■ Risk for Injury (hypoglycemia), related to adverse effects of drug therapy ■ Pain (abdominal), related to adverse effects of drug ■ Deficient Knowledge, related to drug therapy ■ Deficient Knowledge, related to blood glucose testing

PLANNING: PATIENT GOALS AND EXPECTED OUTCOMES

The patient will:
■ Describe signs and symptoms that should be reported immediately, including nausea, diarrhea, jaundice, rash, headache, anorexia, abdominal pain, tachycardia, seizures, and confusion
■ Demonstrate an ability to accurately self-monitor blood glucose; maintain blood glucose within a normal range

IMPLEMENTATION

Interventions and (Rationales)	Patient Education/Discharge Planning
■ Monitor blood glucose at least daily and monitor urinary ketones if blood glucose is over 300. (Ketones will spill into the urine at high blood glucose levels and provide an early sign of diabetic ketoacidosis.)	■ Teach patient how to monitor blood glucose and test urine for ketones, especially when ill.
■ Monitor for signs of lactic acidosis if patient is receiving a biguanide. (Mitochondrial oxidation of lactic acid is inhibited and lactic acidosis may result.)	■ Instruct patient to report signs of lactic acidosis such as hyperventilation, muscle pain, fatigue, increased sleeping.
■ Review lab tests for any abnormalities in liver function. (These drugs are metabolized in the liver and may cause elevations in AST and LDH. Metformin decreases absorption of vitamin B_{12} and folic acid, which may result in deficiencies of these substances.)	■ Instruct patient to report the first sign of yellow skin, pale stools, or dark urine.
■ Obtain accurate history of alcohol use, especially if patient is receiving a sulfonylurea or biguanide. (These drugs may cause a Antabuse-like reaction.)	■ Advise patient to abstain from alcohol and to avoid liquid OTC medications, which may contain alcohol.
■ Monitor for signs and symptoms of illness or infection. (Illness may increase blood glucose levels.)	■ Instruct patient to report the first signs of fatigue, muscle weakness, and nausea. ■ Discuss importance of adequate rest and healthy routines.
■ Monitor blood glucose frequently especially at the beginning of therapy and in elderly patients. ■ Monitor patients carefully who also take a beta-blocker, because early signs of hypoglycemia may not be apparent.	Teach patient: ■ Signs and symptoms of hypoglycemia, such as hunger, irritability, sweating ■ At first sign of hypoglycemia, to check blood glucose and eat a simple sugar; if symptoms do not improve, call 911 ■ To monitor blood glucose before breakfast and supper ■ Not to skip meals and to follow a diet specified by the healthcare provider
■ Monitor weight, weighing at the same time of day each time. (Changes in weight will impact the amount of drug needed to control blood glucose.)	■ Instruct patient to weigh each week, at the same time of day, and report any significant loss or gain.
■ Monitor vital signs. (Increased pulse and blood pressure are early signs of hypoglycemia.)	■ Teach patient how to take accurate blood pressure, temperature, and pulse.

continued

NURSING PROCESS FOCUS: *Patients Receiving Oral Hypoglycemic Therapy (continued)*

Interventions and (Rationales)	*Patient Education/Discharge Planning*
■ Monitor skin for rashes and itching. (These are signs of an allergic reaction to the drug.)	■ Advise patient of the importance of immediately reporting skin rashes and itching that is unaccounted for by dry skin.
■ Monitor activity level. (Dose may require adjustment with change in physical activity.)	■ Advise patient to increase activity level which will help lower blood glucose. ■ Advise patient to closely monitor blood glucose when involved in vigorous physical activity.

EVALUATION OF OUTCOME CRITERIA

Evaluate the effectiveness of drug therapy by confirming that patient goals and expected outcomes have been met (see "Planning").

See Table 40.2 for a list of drugs to which these nursing actions apply.

SPECIAL CONSIDERATIONS

Psychosocial and Community Impacts of Alcohol-Related Pancreatitis

Patients with acute pancreatitis are most often middle-age and those with chronic pancreatitis are most often in their 50s or 60s. Patients whose pancreatitis is associated with gallstones may receive a different type and amount of support from significant others, the community, and even from nurses as compared with those who have pancreatitis associated with alcoholism. Nurses will need to examine their feelings and attitudes related to alcoholism in general and to patients with pancreatitis-associated alcoholism in particular, and will need to adopt attitudes to help the patient attain treatment goals.

Patients who abuse alcohol often need referral to community agencies to manage their addiction and/or remain in recovery. Family members may also need referral to community agencies for help in dealing with altered family processes due to the patient's drinking and any role they may have played in enabling the patient to abuse alcohol.

promote the formation of insoluble proteins that occlude the pancreatic duct. Pancreatic juice is prevented from flowing into the duodenum and remains in the pancreas to damage cells and cause inflammation. Other causes include spasms of the hepatopancreatic sphincter that cause it to remain closed, and strictures or stones in the duct system. Symptoms include chronic epigastric or left upper quadrant pain, anorexia, nausea, vomiting, and weight loss. Steatorrhea, the passing of bulky, foul-smelling fatty stools, occurs late in the course of the disease. Chronic pancreatitis eventually leads to pancreatic insufficiency that may necessitate insulin therapy as well as replacement of pancreatic enzymes.

Drugs prescribed for the treatment of acute pancreatitis may also be prescribed in cases of chronic pancreatitis. In addition, the patient with chronic pancreatitis may require insulin and is likely to need antiemetics and a pancreatic enzyme supplement such as pancrelipase (Cotazym, Pancrease, others) or pancreatin (Creon, Pankreon, other) to digest fats, proteins, and complex carbohydrates.

NURSING CONSIDERATIONS

The role of the nurse in pancreatic enzyme replacement therapy involves careful monitoring of a patient's condition and providing education as it relates to the prescribed drug regimen. Assessment of the patient with acute or chronic pancreatitis should include a complete assessment, physical examination, health history, psychosocial history, and lifestyle history. The nurse should obtain information about alcohol and other drugs, tobacco use, and dietary habits. Spicy foods, gas-forming foods, cola drinks, coffee, and tea stimulate gastric and pancreatic secretions and the nurse should assess the patient for intake of these foods.

The nurse should assess for and monitor the presence, amount, and type of pain as well as breathing patterns which may be rapid and shallow due to pain. The nurse should assess the symmetry of the chest wall and the movement of the chest and diaphragm as the patient with pancreatitis is at risk for atelectasis and can develop pleural effusion as a result of ineffective breathing patterns. The nurse should monitor blood gases as hypoventilation can result in hypercapnia. The patient may have other abnormal findings such as elevated serum and urinary amylase, and elevated serum bilirubin. The nurse should also monitor the patient's nutritional status, presence of signs of infection, and hydration status which may be impaired due to nausea and vomiting. Contraindications include a history of allergy to pork protein or enzymes because the drug has a porcine

PROTOTYPE DRUG | PANCRELIPASE (Cotazym, Pancrease, others)

ACTIONS AND USES

Pancrelipase contains lipase, protease, and amylase of porcine origin. This agent facilitates the breakdown and conversion of lipids into glycerol and fatty acids, starches into dextrin and sugars, and proteins into peptides. Given orally, it acts locally in the GI tract, is not absorbed, and is excreted in the feces. It is used as replacement therapy for patients with insufficient pancreatic exocrine secretions. Pancrelipase is available in powder, tablet, and delayed-release capsule formulations.

On an equal weight basis, pancrelipase is more potent than pancretin with 12 times the lipolytic activity. It also contains at least 4 times as much trypsin and amylase.

Administration Alerts

- Do not crush or open enteric-coated tablets.
- Give the drug before or with meals, or as directed by the health-care provider.
- Pregnancy category C.

ADVERSE EFFECTS AND INTERACTIONS

Side effects of pancrelipase are uncommon, since the enzymes are not absorbed. The most common side effects are GI symptoms of nausea, vomiting, and/or diarrhea; and can cause metabolic symptom of hyperuricosuria.

Pancrelipase interacts with iron, which may result in decreased absorption of iron.

 See the companion website for a Nursing Process Focus specific to this drug.

(pork) origin. Safety in pregnancy and lactation has not been established.

Patient education as it relates to pancreatic enzymes should include goals, reasons for obtaining baseline data such as vital signs and tests for cardiac and renal disorders, and possible side effects. The nurse should assess the patient's knowledge base regarding pancreatitis and any medication prescribed to treat it. The patient should be advised to report pain and seek relief before it becomes too intense; severe pain as well as restlessness and anxiety can increase pancreatic enzyme secretions. The nurse should teach the patient that sitting up, leaning forward, or curling in a fetal position will often decrease pain. The nurse should explain the importance of bedrest and a calm environment in decreasing metabolic rate, pain, and pancreatic secretions.

Following are other important points the nurse should include when teaching patients regarding pancreatic enzyme replacement.

- Eliminate all alcohol intake, as alcohol can initiate acute attacks of pancreatitis.
- Avoid smoking.
- Avoid spicy foods, gas-forming foods, cola drinks, coffee, and tea.
- Take pancreatic enzymes with meals or snacks.
- Weigh self and report significant changes to the health-care provider.
- Observe stools for color, frequency, and consistency and report abnormalities.
- Restrict fat intake and eat smaller and more frequent meals.
- Report episodes of nausea and vomiting.

CHAPTER REVIEW

Key Concepts

The numbered key concepts provide a succinct summary of the important points from the corresponding numbered section within the chapter. If any of these points are not clear, refer to the numbered section within the chapter for review. Expanded versions can be found on the companion website.

40.1 The pancreas is both an endocrine and an exocrine gland. Insulin is released when blood glucose increases and glucagon when blood glucose decreases.

40.2 Type 1 diabetes mellitus (DM) is caused by a lack of insulin secretion and is characterized by serious, chronic conditions affecting the cardiovascular and nervous systems.

40.3 Type 1 DM is treated by dietary restrictions, exercise, and insulin injections. The many types of insulin preparations vary as to their onset of action, time to peak effect, and duration.

40.4 Type 2 DM is caused by a lack of sensitivity of insulin receptors at the target cells and a deficiency in insulin secretion. If untreated, the same chronic conditions result as in type 1 DM.

40.5 Type 2 DM is controlled through lifestyle changes and oral hypoglycemic drugs.

40.6 The pancreas secretes several enzymes essential to digestion, which are secreted in an inactive form until they leave the pancreas.

40.7 Pancreatitis results when pancreatic enzymes are trapped in the pancreas and not released into the duodenum. Pharmacotherapy includes replacement enzymes and supportive drugs for pain, gastric acid reduction, or infections.

Review Questions

1. What are the major differences between types 1 and 2 DM?

2. Why are oral hypoglycemic drugs ineffective at treating type 1 DM?

3. What nursing action(s) helps to prevent lipodystrophies in diabetic patients?

4. What are common indications for receiving pancreatic enzyme replacement therapy?

Critical Thinking Questions

1. A 28-year-old woman who is pregnant with her first child is diagnosed with gestational DM. She is concerned about the fact that she might have to take "shots." She tells the nurse at the public health clinic that she doesn't think she can self-administer an injection and asks if there is a pill that will control her blood sugar. She has heard her grandfather talk about his pills to control his "sugar." What should the nurse explain to this patient?

2. A 4-year-old boy has been diagnosed with cystic fibrosis. The child's parents reported a history of frequent bulky and greasy stools, abdominal pain, and many episodes of recurrent bronchitis. The child is prescribed pancrelipase (Pancrease) 4,000 U orally with each meal as part of his treatment program. A lower dose is given prior to snacks. Relate this drug therapy to this child's pathophysiology.

3. When reviewing a patient's insulin administration record, the nurse notes that the patient is routinely rotating injection sites from arm to leg to abdomen. The nurse also notes that the patient continues to have fluctuation in his blood glucose levels despite receiving the same amount of insulin. What does the nurse need to explain to this patient about site rotation?

EXPLORE MediaLink

NCLEX review, case studies, and other interactive resources for this chapter can be found on the companion website at www.prenhall.com/adams. Click on "Chapter 40" to select the activities for this chapter. For animations, more NCLEX review questions, and an audio glossary, access the accompanying CD-ROM in this textbook.

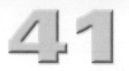
■ DRUGS AT A GLANCE

ORAL CONTRACEPTIVES

Estrogen-progestin combinations

Pr *Monophasic*
   (ethinyl estradiol with norethindrone)
   (Ortho-Novum 1/35)

   Biphasic
   Triphasic

Progestin-only agents

DRUGS FOR EMERGENCY CONTRACEPTION AND PHARMACOLOGIC ABORTION

HORMONE REPLACEMENT THERAPY

Estrogens and estrogen/progestin combinations

Pr *conjugated estrogens (Premarin) and
   conjugated estrogens with
   medroxyprogesterone (Prempro)*

DRUGS FOR DYSFUNCTIONAL UTERINE BLEEDING

Progestins

Pr *medroxyprogesterone (Provera)*

UTERINE STIMULANTS AND RELAXANTS

Oxytocics (stimulants)

Pr *oxytocin (Pitocin, Syntocinon)*

Ergot alkaloids

Prostaglandins

Tocolytics (relaxants)

   Beta₂-adrenergic agonists
   Other tocolytics

DRUGS FOR FEMALE INFERTILITY AND ENDOMETRIOSIS

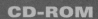

MediaLink www.prenhall.com/adams

CD-ROM

Animation:

   Mechanism in Action: Ethinyl estradiol
   (Ortho-Novum)

Audio Glossary

NCLEX Review

Companion Website

NCLEX Review

Dosage Calculations

Case Study

Care Plans

Expanded Key Concepts

OBJECTIVES

After reading this chapter, the student should be able to:

1. Describe the roles of the hypothalamus, pituitary, and ovaries in maintaining female reproductive function.
2. Explain the mechanisms by which estrogens and progestins prevent conception.
3. Explain how drugs may be used to provide emergency contraception and to terminate early pregnancy.
4. Describe the role of drug therapy in the treatment of menopausal and postmenopausal symptoms.
5. Identify the role of the female sex hormones in the treatment of cancer.
6. Discuss the uses of progestins in the therapy of dysfunctional uterine bleeding.
7. Compare and contrast the use of uterine stimulants and relaxants in the treatment of antepartum and postpartum patients.

8. Explain how drug therapy may be used to treat female infertility.
9. Describe the nurse's role in the pharmacologic management of disorders and conditions of the female reproductive system.
10. For each of the classes shown in Drugs at a Glance, identify representative drugs, explain the mechanism of drug action, primary actions, and important adverse effects.
11. Categorize drugs used in the treatment of female reproductive disorders and conditions based on their classification and mechanism of action.
12. Use the Nursing Process to care for patients who are receiving drug therapy for disorders and conditions of the female reproductive system.

Hormones from the pituitary gland and gonads provide for the growth and maintenance of the female reproductive organs. Endogenous hormones can be supplemented with natural or synthetic hormones to achieve a variety of therapeutic goals, ranging from replacement therapy, to prevention of pregnancy, to milk production. This chapter examines drugs used to treat disorders and conditions associated with the female reproductive system.

41.1 Hypothalamic and Pituitary Regulation of Female Reproductive Function

Regulation of the female reproductive system is achieved by hormones from the hypothalamus, pituitary gland, and ovary. The hypothalamus secretes gonadotropin-releasing hormone (GnRH), which travels a short distance to the pituitary to stimulate the secretion of follicle-stimulating hormone (FSH) and luteinizing hormone (LH). Both of these pituitary hormones act upon the ovary and cause immature ovarian follicles to begin developing. The rising and falling levels of pituitary hormones create two interrelated cycles that occur on a periodic, monthly basis, the ovarian and uterine cycles. The hormonal changes that occur during the ovarian and uterine cycles are illustrated in Figure 41.1.

Under the influence of FSH and LH, several ovarian follicles begin the maturation process each month during a woman's reproductive years. On approximately day 14 of the ovarian cycle, a surge of LH secretion causes one follicle to expel its oocyte, a process called ovulation. The ruptured follicle, minus its oocyte, remains in the ovary and is transformed into the hormone-secreting corpus luteum. The oocyte, on the other hand, begins its journey through the uterine tube and eventually reaches the

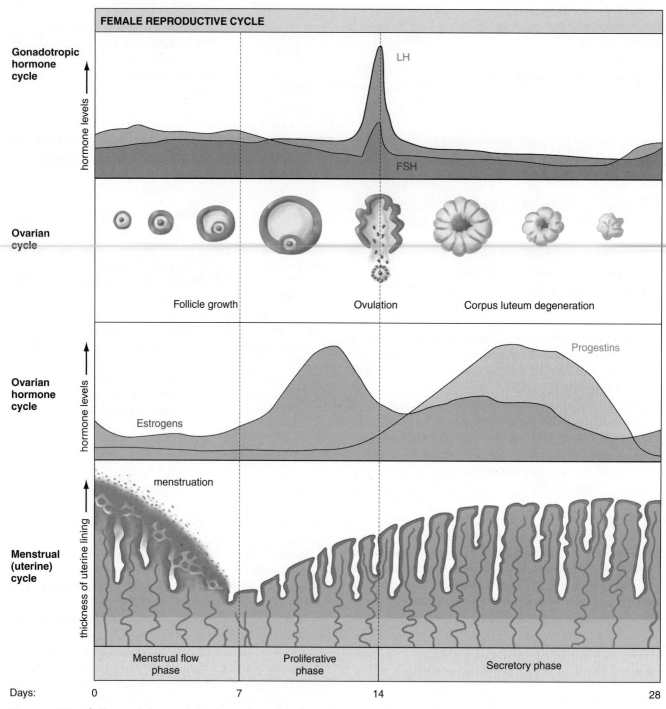

Figure 41.1 | Hormonal changes during the ovarian and uterine cycles *Source: Pearson Education/PH College.*

uterus. If conception does not occur, the outer lining of the uterus degenerates, and is shed to the outside during menstruation.

41.2 Ovarian Control of Female Reproductive Function

As ovarian follicles mature they secrete the female sex hormones **estrogen** and **progesterone**. Estrogen is actually a generic term for three different hormones: estradiol, es-

trone, and estriol. Estrogen is responsible for the maturation of the female reproductive organs and for the appearance of the secondary sex characteristics. In addition, estrogen has numerous metabolic effects on nonreproductive tissues, including the brain, kidneys, blood vessels, and skin. For example, estrogen helps to maintain low blood cholesterol levels and facilitates calcium uptake by bones to help maintain proper bone density (Chapter 46)⊕. When women enter menopause at about age 50 to 55, the ovaries stop secreting estrogen.

PHARMFACTS	Female Reproductive Conditions

- There is a wide range of ages when women reach menopause: 8 of 100 women will stop menstruating before age 40, and 5 of 100 women will continue beyond age 60.
- About half the cases of dysfunctional uterine bleeding are diagnosed in women over 45 years of age; however, 20% of cases occur under the age of 20.
- The primary reason why a woman may become pregnant while on oral contraceptives is skipping a dose.
- A nonsmoking woman aged 25 to 29 has a 2 in 100,000 chance of dying from complications due to oral contraceptives. The risk of a woman in this age group dying in an automobile accident is 74 in 100,000.
- Oral contraceptives have more benefits than simply contraception. It is estimated that each year they prevent the following:
  51,000 cases of pelvic inflammatory disease
  9,900 hospitalizations for ectopic pregnancy
  27,000 cases of iron deficiency anemia
  20,000 hospitalizations for certain types of nonmalignant breast disease

In the last half of the ovarian cycle, the corpus luteum secretes a class of hormones called progestins, the most abundant of which is progesterone. In combination with estrogen, progesterone promotes breast development and regulates the monthly changes of the uterine cycle. Under the influence of estrogen and progesterone, the uterine endometrium becomes vascular and thickens in preparation for receiving a fertilized egg. High progesterone and estrogen levels in the final third of the uterine cycle provide negative feedback to shut off GnRH, FSH, and LH secretion. This negative feedback loop is illustrated in Figure 41.2. Without stimulation from FSH and LH, estrogen and progesterone levels fall sharply, the endometrium is shed, and menstrual bleeding begins.

CONTRACEPTION

ORAL CONTRACEPTIVES

Oral contraceptives are drugs used to prevent pregnancy. Most oral contraceptives are a combination of estrogens and progestins. In small doses, they prevent fertilization by inhibiting ovulation. Selected oral contraceptives are shown in Table 41.1.

41.3 Estrogens and Progestins as Oral Contraceptives

The most widespread pharmacologic use of the female sex hormones is to prevent pregnancy. When used appropriately, they are nearly 100% effective. Most oral contraceptives contain a combination of estrogen and progestin; a few preparations contain only progestin. The most common estrogen used for contraception is ethinyl estradiol, and the most common progestin is norethindrone.

A large number of oral contraceptive preparations are available, differing in dose and by type of estrogen and progestin. Selection of a specific formulation is individualized to each patient, and determined by which drug gives the best contraceptive protection with the fewest side effects. Daily doses of estrogen in oral contraceptives have declined from 150 μg, 40 years ago, to about 35 μg in modern formulations. This reduction has resulted in a decrease in estrogen-related adverse effects.

Typically, drug administration of an oral contraceptive begins on day 5 of the ovarian cycle, and continues for 21 days. During the other 7 days of the month, the patient takes a placebo. While the placebo serves no pharmacologic purpose, it does encourage the patient to take the pills on a daily basis. Some of these placebos contain iron, which replaces iron lost from menstrual bleeding. If a daily dose is missed, two pills taken the following day usually provide adequate contraception. If more than one day is missed, the patient should observe other contraceptive precautions, such as using condoms, until the oral contraceptive doses can be resumed at the beginning of the next monthly cycle. Figure 41.3 shows a typical monthly oral contraceptive packet with the 28 pills.

The estrogen-progestin oral contraceptives act by providing negative feedback to the pituitary to shut down the secretion of LH and FSH. Without the influence of these pituitary hormones, the ovarian follicle cannot mature and ovulation is prevented. The estrogen-progestin agents also reduce the likelihood of implantation by making the uterine endometrium less favorable to receive an embryo. In addition to their contraceptive function, these agents are sometimes prescribed to promote timely and regular monthly cycles, and to reduce the incidence of dysmenorrhea.

The three types of estrogen-progestin formulations are monophasic, biphasic, and triphasic. The most common is the monophasic, which delivers a constant amount of estrogen and progestin throughout the menstrual cycle. In biphasic agents, the amount of estrogen in each pill remains constant, but the amount of progestin is increased toward the end of the menstrual cycle to better nourish the uterine lining. In triphasic formulations, the amounts of both estrogen and progestin vary in three distinct phases during the 28-day cycle.

The progestin-only oral contraceptives, sometimes called minipills, prevent pregnancy primarily by producing a thick, viscous mucus at the entrance to the uterus that discourages penetration by sperm. They also tend to inhibit implantation of a fertilized egg. Minipills are less effective than estrogen-progestin combinations, having a failure rate of 1% to 4%. Their use also results in a higher incidence of menstrual irregularities such as amenorrhea, prolonged bleeding, or breakthrough spotting. They are generally

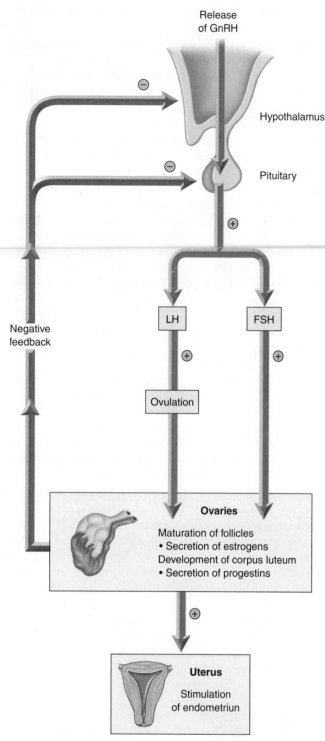

Release
of GnRH

Hypothalamus

Pituitary

Negative
feedback

LH

FSH

Ovulation

Ovaries

Maturation of follicles
• Secretion of estrogens
Development of corpus luteum
• Secretion of progestins

Uterus

Stimulation
of endometriun

Figure 41.2 | Negative feedback control of the female reproductive hormones

reserved for patients who are at high risk to side effects from estrogen.

Several long-term formulations of oral contraceptives are available. A deep IM injection of medroxyprogesterone acetate (Depo-Provera) provides 3 months of con-

traceptive protection. The Norplant system consists of six small, plastic tubes filled with levonorgestrel implanted subcutaneously under the inner aspect of the upper arm that provides contraception for up to 5 years. Ortho-Evra is a new transdermal patch containing ethinyl estradiol and norelgestromin that is worn on the skin. The patch is changed every 7 days for the first 3 weeks, followed by no patch during week 4. NovaRing is a 2-inch-diameter ring containing estrogen and progestin that is inserted into the vagina to provide 3 weeks of contraceptive protection. The ring is removed during week 4, and a new ring is inserted during the first week of the next menstrual cycle. Merena consists of a polyethylene cylinder, placed in the uterus, that releases levonorgestrel. This drug acts locally to prevent conception over 5 years. The efficacy of these long-term formulations is similar to that of oral contraceptives. They offer a major advantage for women who are likely to forget their daily pill, or who prefer a greater ease of use.

The nurse must be alert for drugs that interact with estrogen or progesterone. A number of anticonvulsants and antibiotics can reduce the effectiveness of oral contraceptives, thus increasing a woman's risk of pregnancy. Because oral contraceptives can reduce the effectiveness of warfarin (Coumadin), insulin, and certain oral hypoglycemic agents, dosage adjustment may be necessary.

The risk of cancer following long-term oral contraceptive use has been extensively studied. Because some studies have shown a small increase in breast cancer incidence, oral contraceptives are contraindicated in patients with known or suspected breast cancer. The incidences of endometrial cancer and ovarian cancer, however, are significantly reduced after long-term oral contraceptive administration. It is likely that the relationship between the long-term use of these drugs and cancer will continue to be a controversial and frequently researched topic.

NURSING CONSIDERATIONS

The role of the nurse in oral contraceptive therapy involves careful monitoring of a patient's condition and providing education as it relates to the prescribed drug regimen. Oral contraception is the most effective form of birth control and there are many products available to prevent pregnancy. Oral contraception is contraindicated for women with a history of stroke, MI, coronary artery disease, thromboembolic disorders, or estrogen-dependent tumors due to increases in estrogen levels and risk of thrombus formation. Pregnancy should be ruled out before initiating oral contraceptive therapy. The nurse should obtain a complete health history including personal or familial history of breast cancer, liver tumors, and hemorrhagic disorders, because these conditions contraindicate the use of oral contraceptives. Risks and ad-

Table 41.1	Selected Oral Contraceptives		
Trade Name	**Type**	**Estrogen**	**Progestin**
Alesse	monophasic	ethinyl estradiol; 20 µg	levonorgestrel; 0.1 mg
Desogen	monophasic	ethinyl estradiol; 30 µg	desogestrel; 0.15 mg
Loestrin 1.5/30 Fe	monophasic	ethinyl estradiol; 30 µg	norethindrone; 1.5 mg
Lo/Ovral	monophasic	ethinyl estradiol; 30 µg	norgestrel; 0.3 mg
Ortho-Cyclen	monophasic	ethinyl estradiol; 35 µg	norgestimate; 0.25 mg
Yasmin	monophasic	ethinyl estradiol; 30 µg	drospirenone; 3 mg
Ortho-Novum 10/11	biphasic	ethinyl estradiol; 35 µg	norethindrone; 0.5 mg (phase 1)
		ethinyl estradiol; 35 µg	norethindrone; 1.0 mg (phase 2)
Ortho-Novum 7/7/7	triphasic	ethinyl estradiol; 35 µg	norethindrone; 0.5 mg (phase 1)
		ethinyl estradiol; 35 µg	norethindrone; 0.75 mg (phase 2)
		ethinyl estradiol; 35 µg	norethindrone; 1.0 mg (phase 3)
Ortho Tri-Cyclen	triphasic	ethinyl estradiol; 35 µg	norgestimate; 0.5 mg (phase 1)
		ethinyl estradiol; 35 µg	norgestimate; 0.75 mg (phase 2)
		ethinyl estradiol; 35 µg	norgestimate; 1.0 mg (phase 3)
Tri-Levlen	triphasic	ethinyl estradiol; 35 µg	levonorgestrel; 0.05 mg (phase 1)
		ethinyl estradiol; 40 µg	levonorgestrel; 0.075 mg (phase 2)
		ethinyl estradiol; 30 µg	levonorgestrel; 0.125 mg (phase 3)
Triphasil	triphasic	ethinyl estradiol; 30 µg	norgestrel; 0.05 mg (phase 1)
		ethinyl estradiol; 40 µg	norgestrel; 0.075 mg (phase 2)
		ethinyl estradiol; 30 µg	norgestrel; 1.25 mg (phase 3)
Micronor	progestin only	none	norethindrone; 0.35 mg
Nor-Q.D.	progestin only	none	norethindrone; 0.35 mg
Ovrette	progestin only	none	norgestrel; 0.075 mg

verse effects are greater for women who smoke and are older than 35 years of age. Oral contraceptives should be used with caution in patients with hypertension, cardiac or renal disease, liver dysfunction, diabetes, gallbladder disease, and a history of depression.

The nurse should monitor for side effects of oral contraceptives. Blood pressure should be monitored as these medications can cause mild to moderate hypertension. The nurse should frequently assess vital signs and monitor for symptoms of thrombophlebitis, such as pain, redness, and tenderness of the calves. Oral contraceptives can mimic certain symptoms of pregnancy including breast tenderness, nausea, bloating, and chloasma. The nurse should reassure the patient that these side effects do not indicate pregnancy. Oral contraceptives may increase the risk of certain types of breast cancer, so the nurse should be sure that patients know how to perform breast self-exams and are aware of the routine scheduling of mammograms appropriate for their age bracket.

Patient education as it relates to oral contraceptives should include goals, reasons for assessing cardiovascular status, and possible side effects. See "Nursing Process Focus: Patients Receiving Oral Contraceptives" for specific teaching points.

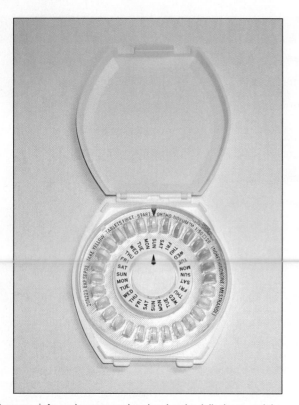

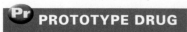

Figure 41.3 | An oral contraceptive showing the daily doses and the different formulation taken in the last 7 days of the 28-day cycle

EMERGENCY CONTRACEPTION AND PHARMACOLOGIC ABORTION

Emergency contraception is the prevention of implantation following unprotected intercourse. Pharmacologic abortion is the removal of an embryo by the use of drugs, after implantation has occurred. The treatment goal is to provide effective, immediate prevention or termination of pregnancy. Agents used for these purposes are shown in Table 41.2.

41.4 Drugs for Emergency Contraception and Termination of Early Pregnancy

Statistics suggest that over half the pregnancies in the United States are unplanned. Some of these occur due to the inconsistent use or failure of contraceptive devices; even oral contraceptives have a failure rate of 0.3% to 1%. Emergency contraception following unprotected intercourse offers a means of protecting against unwanted pregnancies. The goal is to prevent implantation of a fertilized ovum.

Emergency contraception can be accomplished pharmacologically by a number of methods. Taking 0.75 mg of levonorgestrel in two doses, 12 hours apart, has been shown to prevent conception. A combination of ethinyl estradiol and levonorgestrel (Preven) is also effective, though nausea

---

MediaLink | **Mechanism in Action Ortho-Novum**

| **Pr** PROTOTYPE DRUG | **ETHINYL ESTRADIOL WITH NORETHINDRONE** (Ortho-Novum 1/35) |

ACTIONS AND USES

Ortho-Novum is typical of the monophasic oral contraceptives, containing fixed amounts of estrogen (0.035 mg) and progesterone (1 mg) for 21 days, followed by placebo tablets for 7 days. It is nearly 100% effective at preventing conception. Ortho-Novum is also available in biphasic and triphasic preparations. All preparations prevent ovulation by negative feedback control targeted at the hypothalamic-pituitary axis. When the right combination of estrogens and progestins is present in the bloodstream, the release of FSH and LH is inhibited, thus preventing ovulation. Noncontraceptive benefits of Ortho-Novum include improvement in menstrual cycle regularity and decreased incidence of dysmenorrhea.

Administration Alerts

- Tablets must be taken exactly as directed.
- If dose is missed, take as soon as remembered, or take two tablets the next day.
- Pregnancy category X.

ADVERSE EFFECTS AND INTERACTIONS

Common side effects include edema, unexplained loss of vision, diplopia, intolerance to contact lenses, gall bladder disease, nausea, abdominal cramps, changes in urinary function, dysmenorrhea, breast fullness, fatigue, skin rash, acne, headache, weight gain, midcycle breakthrough bleeding, vaginal candidiasis, photosensitivity, and changes in urinary patterns. Cardiovascular side effects may include hypertension and thromboembolic disorders.

Ethinyl estradiol interacts with many drugs. For example, rifampin, some antibiotics, barbiturates, anticonvulsants, and antifungals decrease efficacy of oral contraceptives, so increased risk of breakthrough bleeding and increased risk of pregnancy may occur. Ortho-Novum may also decrease the effects of oral anticoagulants.

Use with caution with herbal supplements. For example, breakthrough bleeding has been reported with concurrent use of St. John's wort.

 See the companion website for a Nursing Process Focus specific to this drug.

NURSING PROCESS FOCUS	PATIENTS RECEIVING ORAL CONTRACEPTIVE THERAPY

ASSESSMENT

Prior to administration:
- Obtain health history to include cigarette smoking.
- Obtain drug history to determine possible drug interactions and allergies.
- Assess cardiovascular status including hypertension, history of MI, CVA, and thromboembolic disease.
- Determine if patient is pregnant or lactating.

POTENTIAL NURSING DIAGNOSES

- Deficient Knowledge, related to drug therapy
- Nausea, related to side effects of drug
- Noncompliance, related to medication regimen

PLANNING: PATIENT GOALS AND EXPECTED OUTCOMES

The patient will:
- Report effective birth control
- Demonstrate an understanding of the drug's action by accurately describing drug side effects and precautions
- Take medication exactly as ordered to prevent pregnancy
- Immediately report effects such as symptoms of thrombophlebitis, difficulty breathing, visual disturbances, and severe headache

IMPLEMENTATION

Interventions and (Rationales)	*Patient Education/Discharge Planning*
■ Monitor for the development of breast or other estrogen-dependent tumors. (Estrogen may cause tumor growth or proliferation.)	■ Instruct patient to immediately report if first degree relative is diagnosed with any estrogen-dependent tumor.
■ Monitor for thrombophlebitis or other thromboembolic disease. (Estrogen predisposes to thromboembolic disorders by increasing levels of clotting factors.)	■ Instruct patient to immediately report pain in calves, limited movement in legs, dyspnea, sudden severe chest pain, headache, seizures, anxiety, or fear.
■ Monitor for cardiac disorders and hypertension. (These drugs increase blood levels of angiotensin and aldosterone, which increase blood pressure.)	Instruct patient to: ■ Report immediately signs of possible cardiac problems such as chest pain, dyspnea, edema, tachycardia or bradycardia, and palpitations ■ Monitor blood pressure regularly ■ Report symptoms of hypertension such as headache, flushing, fatigue, dizziness, palpitations, tachycardia, nosebleeds
■ Encourage patient not to smoke. (Smoking increases risk of thromboembolic disease.)	Instruct patient to: ■ Be aware that the combination of oral contraceptives and smoking greatly increases risk of cardiovascular disease, especially MI ■ Be aware that the risk increases with age (>35) and with number of cigarettes smoked (15 or more/day)
■ Monitor blood and urine glucose levels. (These drugs increase serum glucose levels.)	■ Instruct patient to monitor urine and blood glucose regularly and contact healthcare provider if hyperglycemia or hypoglycemia occur.
■ Monitor patient's knowledge level of proper administration. (Incorrect use may lead to pregnancy.)	Instruct patient to: ■ Discontinue medication and notify healthcare provider if significant bleeding occurs at midcycle ■ Take missed dose as soon as remembered or take two tablets the next day. If three consecutive tablets are missed, begin a new compact of tablets, starting 7 days after last tablet was taken ■ Contact healthcare provider if two consecutive periods are missed, as pregnancy may have occurred

continued

NURSING PROCESS FOCUS: *Patients Receiving Oral Contraceptive Therapy (continued)*

Interventions and (Rationales)	Patient Education/Discharge Planning
■ Encourage compliance with follow-up treatment. (Follow-up is necessary to avoid serious adverse effects.)	Instruct patient to: ■ Schedule annual PAP smears ■ Perform self-breast exams monthly and obtain routine mammograms as recommended by the healthcare provider

EVALUATION OF OUTCOME CRITERIA

Evaluate the effectiveness of drug therapy by confirming that patient goals and expected outcomes have been met (see "Planning").

See Table 41.1 for a list of drugs to which these nursing actions apply.

Table 41.2	Agents for Emergency Contraception and Pharmacologic Abortion
Drug	**Route and Adult Dose (max dose where indicated)**
Agents for Emergency Contraception	
ethinyl estradiol (Estinyl, Feminore)	PO; 5 mg/d for 5 consecutive days beginning within 72h of intercourse
ethinyl estradiol and levonorgestrel (Preven)	PO; 1 tablet (0.25 mg levonorgestrel and 0.05 mg ethinyl estradiol) taken as soon as possible but within 72 h of unprotected intercourse, followed by two pills 12 h later
Levonorgestrel	PO; 2 tablets within 72h of unprotected intercourse, 2 tablets 12h later
Agents for Pharmacologic Abortion	
carboprost tromethamine (Hemabate)	IM; initial: 250 μg (1 mL) repeated at 1 1/2–3 1/2h intervals if indicated by uterine response. Dosage may be increased to 500 μg (2 mL) if uterine contractility is inadequate after several doses of 250 μg (1 mL), not to exceed total dose of 12 mg or continuous administration for more than 2 d
dinoprostone (Cervidil, Prepidil, Prostin E$_2$)	Intravaginal; insert suppository high in vagina, repeat q2–5h until abortion occurs or membranes rupture (max: total dose 240 mg)
methotrexate with misoprostol	IM; methotrexate (50 mg/m^2) followed 5 days later by Intravaginal 800 μg of misoprostol
mifepristone (Mifeprix) with misoprostol	PO; day one: 600 mg of Mifepristone; day three (if abortion has not occurred): 400 μg of misoprostol

and vomiting are common and an antiemetic drug may be indicated to reduce these unpleasant side effects. Most estrogen-progestin oral contraceptive agents are also effective for emergency contraception, if given at sufficient doses and with correct timing. Administration of ethinyl estradiol alone for 5 days is effective, though it causes nausea and vomiting in many patients. All of these agents should be administered as soon as possible after unprotected intercourse; if taken more than 72 hours later, they become less effective. When used accordingly, these drugs act by preventing ovulation; they do not cause abortion.

Once the ovum has been fertilized, several pharmacologic choices are available to terminate the pregnancy. A single dose of mifepristone (Mifiprex, RU486) followed 36 to 48 hours later by a single dose of misoprostol (Cytotec) is a frequently used regimen. Mifepristone is a synthetic steroid that blocks progesterone receptors in the uterus. If given within 3 days of intercourse, mifepristone alone is almost 100% effective at preventing pregnancy. Given up to 9 weeks after conception, mifepristone aborts the implanted embryo. Misoprostol is a prostaglandin that causes uterine contractions, thus increasing the effectiveness of the pharmacologic abortion.

Although mifepristone-misoprostol should never be substituted for effective means of contraception such as abstinence or oral contraceptives, these medications do offer women a safer alternative to surgical abortion. The primary adverse effect is cramping that occurs soon after taking misoprostol. The most serious adverse effect is prolonged bleeding, which may continue for 1 to 2 weeks after dosing.

A few other agents may be used to promote pharmacologic abortion. Methotrexate, an antineoplastic agent, combined with intravaginal misoprostol, usually induces abortion within 24 hours. The prostaglandins carboprost and dinoprostone induce strong uterine contractions that can expel an implanted embryo up to the second trimester.

MENOPAUSE

Menopause is characterized by a progressive decrease in estrogen secretion by the ovaries resulting in the permanent cessation of menses. Menopause is neither a disease nor a disorder, but is a natural consequence of aging that is often accompanied by number of unpleasant symptoms.

41.5 Hormone Replacement Therapy

Over the past 20 years, healthcare providers have commonly prescribed hormone replacement therapy (HRT) to treat unpleasant symptoms of menopause and to prevent the long-term consequences of estrogen loss listed in Table 41.3. In 2001, over 66 million prescriptions for Premarin and Prempro were filled, and sales of the two drugs exceeded $2 billion.

Two recent studies have raised questions regarding the safety of HRT for menopause. Data from this research suggest that patients taking HRT may have an increased risk of coronary artery disease, stroke, and venous thromboembolism. The potential adverse effects documented in these studies were significant enough to suggest that the potential benefits of long-term HRT may not outweigh the risks for many women. Although there is consensus that HRT does offer relief from the immediate, distressing menopausal symptoms, it is now recommended that women *not* undergo HRT to prevent coronary heart disease. In addition, although HRT appears to prevent osteoporotic bone fractures, women are now encouraged to discuss alternatives with their healthcare provider, as discussed in Chapter 46 ⊘. Undoubtedly, research will continue to provide valuable information on the long-term effects of HRT. Until then, the choice of HRT to treat menopausal symptoms remains a highly individualized one, between the patient and her healthcare provider.

In addition to their use in treating menopausal symptoms, estrogens are used for female hypogonadism, primary ovarian failure, and as replacement therapy following surgical removal of the ovaries, usually combined with a progestin. The purpose of the progestin is to counteract some of the adverse effects of estrogen on the uterus. When used alone, estrogen increases the risk of uterine cancer. Estrogen without progestin is only considered appropriate for patients who have had a hysterectomy.

High doses of estrogens are sometimes used to treat prostate and breast cancer. Prostate cancer is usually dependent on androgens for growth; administration of estrogens will suppress androgen secretion. As an antineoplastic

Table 41.3	Potential Consequences of Estrogen Loss Related to Menopause
Stage	**Symptoms/Conditions**
Early Menopause	
	mood disturbances, depression, irritability
	insomnia
	hot flashes
	irregular menstrual cycles
	headaches
Midmenopause	
	vaginal atrophy, increased infections, painful intercourse
	skin atrophy
	stress urinary incontinence
	sexual disinterest
Postmenopause	
	cardiovascular disease
	osteoporosis
	Alzheimer's-like dementia
	colon cancer

hormone, estrogen is rarely used alone. It is one of many agents used in combination for the chemotherapy of cancer, as discussed in Chapter 35 ⊚ .

NURSING CONSIDERATIONS

For the use of estrogen-containing products as oral contraceptives, refer to "Nursing Process Focus: Patients Receiving Oral Contraceptives".

The role of the nurse in HRT involves careful monitoring of a patient's condition and providing education as it relates to the prescribed drug regimen. Conjugated estrogens are contraindicated for use in breast cancer (except in patients being treated for metastatic disease), and any estrogen-dependent cancer in the patient's history. These conditions put the patient at a higher risk for developing cancer. Conjugated estrogen is contraindicated in pregnancy or for use in women who intend to become pregnant in the immediate future, because it can cause fetal harm. It is also contraindicated for patients with a history of thromboembolic disease.

Cautious use of estrogen therapy must be exercised in a patient whose first degree relative has a history of breast or genital cancer. Estrogen monotherapy places the woman at higher risk for cancer of the female reproductive organs.

Caution must also be used in patients with CAD, hypertension, cerebrovascular disease, fibrocystic breast disease, breast nodules, or abnormal mammograms.

When treating symptoms of menopause, estrogens are prescribed for the shortest time possible and at the lowest possible dose to decrease the risk of serious adverse reactions. These hormones should be taken exactly as ordered. When used for cancer, the male patient may develop secondary female characteristics, such as higher voice, sparse body hair, and increased breast size. Impotence may occur.

The nurse should monitor for side effects of HRT. Due to the risk of thromboembolism, the nurse should monitor the patient closely for signs and symptoms of thrombus or embolus, such as pain in calves, limited movement in legs, dyspnea, sudden severe chest pain, or anxiety. Estrogens can also cause depression, decreased libido, headache, fatigue, and weight gain. Because current controversy surrounds the long-term use of these drugs as HRT, it is imperative for women to be aware of current research and discuss treatment alternatives with their healthcare provider before beginning pharmacotherapy.

Patient education as it relates to HRT should include goals, reasons for assessing cardiovascular status, and possible side effects. See "Nursing Process Focus: Patients Receiving Hormone Replacement Therapy" for specific teaching points.

Pr PROTOTYPE DRUG | **CONJUGATED ESTROGENS** (Premarin) and **CONJUGATED ESTROGENS WITH MEDROXYPROGESTERONE** (Prempro)

ACTIONS AND USES

Premarin contains a mixture of different estrogens. It exerts several positive metabolic effects, including an increase in bone density and a reduction in LDL cholesterol. It may also lower the risk of coronary artery disease and colon cancer in some patients. When used as postmenopausal replacement therapy, estrogen is typically combined with a progestin, as in Prempro. Conjugated estrogens may be administered by the IM or IV route for abnormal uterine bleeding due to hormonal imbalance.

Administration Alerts

- Use a calibrated dosage applicator for administration of vaginal cream.
- For IM or IV administration of conjugated estrogens, reconstitute by first removing approximately 5 ml of air from the dry-powder vial, then slowly inject the diluent to the vial, aiming it at the side of the vial. Gently agitate to dissolve; do not shake.
- Administer IV push slowly, at a rate of 5 mg/min.
- Both are pregnancy category X.

ADVERSE EFFECTS AND INTERACTIONS

Adverse effects of Prempro or Premarin include nausea, fluid retention, edema, breast tenderness, abdominal cramps and bloating, acute pancreatitis, appetite changes, skin eruptions, mental depression, decreased libido, headache, fatigue, nervousness, and weight gain. Effects are dose dependent. Estrogens, when used alone, have been associated with a higher risk of uterine cancer. Although adding a progestin may exert a protective effect by lowering the risk of uterine cancer, recent studies suggest the progestin may increase the risk of breast cancer following long-term use. The risks of adverse effects increase in patients over age 35.

Drug interactions include a decreased effect of tamoxifen, enhanced corticosteroid effects, decreased effects of anticoagulants, especially warfarin. The effects of estrogen may be decreased if taken with barbiturates or rifampin and there is a possible increased effect of tricyclic antidepressants if taken with estrogens.

Use with caution with herbal supplements. For example, red clover and black cohosh may interfere with estrogen therapy. Effects of estrogen may be enhanced if combined with ginseng.

 See the companion website for a Nursing Process Focus specific to this drug.

NURSING PROCESS FOCUS   PATIENTS RECEIVING HORMONE REPLACEMENT THERAPY

ASSESSMENT	POTENTIAL NURSING DIAGNOSES
Prior to administration: ■ Obtain complete health history including personal or familial history of breast cancer, gall bladder disease, diabetes mellitus, liver or kidney disease. ■ Obtain drug history to determine possible drug interactions and allergies. ■ Assess cardiovascular status including hypertension, history of MI, CVA, and thromboembolic disease. ■ Determine if patient is pregnant or lactating.	■ Excess Fluid Volume, related to edema secondary to side effect of drug ■ Ineffective Tissue Perfusion, related to development of thrombophlebitis, pulmonary or cerebral embolism

PLANNING: PATIENT GOALS AND EXPECTED OUTCOMES

The patient will:
■ Report relief from symptoms of menopause
■ Demonstrate an understanding of the drug's action by accurately describing drug side effects and precautions
■ Immediately report such effects as symptoms of thrombophlebitis, difficulty breathing, visual disturbances, severe headache, and seizure activity

IMPLEMENTATION

Interventions and (Rationales)	*Patient Education/Discharge Planning*
■ Monitor for thromboembolic disease. (Estrogen increases risk for thromboembolism.)	■ Instruct patient to report shortness of breath, feeling of heaviness, chest pain, severe headache, warmth, or swelling in affected part, usually the legs or pelvis.
■ Monitor for abnormal uterine bleeding. (If undiagnosed tumor is present, these drugs can increase its size and cause uterine bleeding.)	■ Instruct patient to report excessive uterine bleeding or that which occurs between menstruations.
■ Monitor breast health. (Estrogens promote the growth of certain breast cancers.)	■ Instruct patient to have regular breast exams, perform monthly BSE and obtain routine mammograms, as recommended by healthcare provider.
■ Monitor for vision changes. (These drugs may worsen myopia or astigmatism and cause intolerance of contact lenses.)	Instruct patient to: ■ Obtain regular eye exams during HRT ■ Report changes in vision ■ Report any difficulty in wearing contact lenses
■ Encourage patient not to smoke. (Smoking increases risk of cardiovascular disease.)	■ Instruct patient to avoid smoking and participate in smoking cessation programs, if necessary.
■ Encourage patient to avoid caffeine. (Estrogens and caffeine may lead to increased CNS stimulation.)	Instruct patient to: ■ Restrict caffeine consumption ■ Recognize common foods that contain caffeine: coffee, tea, carbonated beverages, chocolate, certain OTC medications ■ Report unusual nervousness, anxiety, and insomnia
■ Monitor glucose levels. (Estrogens may increase blood glucose levels.)	Instruct patient to: ■ Monitor blood and urine glucose frequently, if diabetic ■ Report any consistent changes in blood glucose
■ Monitor for seizure activity. (Estrogen-induced fluid retention may increase risk of seizures.)	■ Instruct patient to be alert for possibility of seizures, even at night, and report any seizure-type symptoms

continued

NURSING PROCESS FOCUS: *Patients Receiving Hormone Replacement Therapy (continued)*

Interventions and (Rationales)	*Patient Education/Discharge Planning*
■ Monitor patient's understanding and proper self-administration. (Improper administration may increase incidence of adverse effects.)	Instruct patient to: ■ Administer proper dose, form, and frequency of medication ■ Take with food to decrease GI irritation ■ Take daily dose at HS to decrease occurrence of side effects ■ Document menstruation and any problems that occur

EVALUATION OF OUTCOME CRITERIA

Evaluate the effectiveness of drug therapy by confirming that patient goals and expected outcomes have been met (see "Planning").

See Table 41.4, under the heading "Estrogens," for a list of drugs to which these nursing actions apply.

SPECIAL CONSIDERATIONS

Estrogen Use and Psychosocial Issues

Because undesirable side effects may occur with estrogen use, the nurse should communicate these prior to implementation of drug therapy. The nurse can explore the patient's reaction to these potential risks. An assessment of the patient's emotional support system should also be made before initiating drug therapy. Hirsutism, loss of hair, or a deepening of the voice can occur in the female patient. The male patient may develop secondary female characteristics such as a higher voice, lack of body hair, and increased breast size. Impotence may also develop and is typically viewed as a concern by most men.

Patients should be taught that these adverse effects are reversible and may subside with adjustment of dosage or discontinuation of estrogen therapy. This knowledge may allow both male and female patients to remain compliant when adverse effects occur. During therapy, patients may need emotional support to assist in dealing with these body image issues. The nurse can encourage this support, discuss these issues with family members, and refer patients for counseling. For the female patient, the nurse can refer to an aesthetician for hair removal or wig fitting. The male patient and his sexual partner may need a referral to deal with issues surrounding impotence and its effect on their relationship.

UTERINE ABNORMALITIES

Dysfunctional uterine bleeding is a condition in which hemorrhage occurs on a noncyclic basis or in abnormal amounts. It is the health problem most frequently reported by women and a common reason for hysterectomy. Progestins are the drugs of choice for treating uterine abnormalities.

41.6 Pharmacotherapy with Progestins

Secreted by the corpus luteum, the function of endogenous progesterone is to prepare the uterus for implantation of the embryo and pregnancy. If implantation does not occur, levels of progesterone fall dramatically and menses begins. If pregnancy occurs, the ovary will continue to secrete progesterone to maintain a healthy endometrium until the placenta develops sufficiently to begin producing the hormone. Whereas the function of estrogen is to cause proliferation of the endometrium, progesterone limits and stabilizes endometrial growth.

Dysfunctional uterine bleeding can have a number of causes, including early abortion, pelvic neoplasms, thyroid disorders, pregnancy, and infection. Types of dysfunctional uterine bleeding include the following conditions.

- Amenorrhea—absence of menstruation
- Oligomenorrhea—infrequent menstruation
- Menorrhagia—prolonged or excessive menstruation
- Breakthrough bleeding—hemorrhage between menstrual periods
- Postmenopausal bleeding—hemorrhage following menopause

Dysfunctional uterine bleeding is often caused by a hormonal imbalance between estrogen and progesterone. Although estrogen increases the thickness of the endometrium, bleeding occurs sporadically unless balanced by an adequate amount of progesterone secretion. Administration of a progestin in a pattern starting 5 days after the onset of menses and continuing for the next 20 days can sometimes help to reestablish a normal, monthly cyclic pattern. Oral contraceptives may also be prescribed for this disorder.

In cases of heavy bleeding, high doses of conjugated estrogens may be administered for 3 weeks prior to adding medroxyprogesterone for the last 10 days of therapy. Treatment with nonsteroidal anti-inflammatory drugs (NSAIDs) sometimes helps to reduce bleeding and ease painful menstrual flow. If aggressive hormonal therapy fails to stop the heavy bleeding, dilation and curettage (D&C) may be necessary.

Progestins are occasionally prescribed for the treatment of metastatic endometrial carcinoma. In these cases, they

Table 41.4	Selected Estrogens and Progestins
Drug	**Route and Adult Dose (max dose where indicated)**
Estrogens	
estradiol (Estraderm, Estrace)	PO; 1–2 mg qd
estradiol cypionate (dep-Gynogen, Depogen)	IM; 1–5 mg q3–4 wks
estradiol valerate (Delestrogen, Duragen-10, Valergen)	IM; 10–20 mg q4 wks
estrogen, conjugated (Premarin)	PO; 0.3–1.25 mg qd for 21 days each month
estropipate (Ogen)	PO; 0.75–6 mg qd for 21 days each month
ethinyl estradiol (Estinyl, Feminone)	PO; 0.02–0.05 mg qd for 21 days each month
Progestins	
medroxyprogesterone (Provera, Cycrin)	PO; 5–10 mg qd on days 1–12 of menstrual cycle
norethindrone acetate (Norlutate)	PO; 5 mg qd for 2 weeks; increase by 2.5 mg/d q2 weeks (max 15 mg/d)
norethindrone (Micronor, Nor-Q.D.)	PO; 0.35 mg qd beginning on day 1 of menstrual cycle
progesterone micronized (Prometrium)	PO; 400 mg at hs for 10 days
Estrogen-Progestin Combinations	
conjugated estrogens, equine/medroxyprogesterone acetate (Prempro)	PO; 0.625 mg/d continuously or in 25 day cycles
estradiol/norgestimate (Ortho-Prefest)	PO; 1 tablet of 1 mg estradiol for 3 days, followed by 1 tablet of 1 mg estradiol combined with 0.09 mg norgestimate for 3 days. Regimen is repeated continuously without interruption
ethinyl estradiol/norethindrone acetate (Femhrt)	PO; 5 μg (1 tablet) qd

are used for palliation, usually in combination with other antineoplastics. Selected progestins and their dosages are shown in Table 41.4.

NURSING CONSIDERATIONS

The role of the nurse in progestin therapy involves careful monitoring of a patient's condition and providing education as it relates to the prescribed drug regimen. Before administering progesterone, the nurse should obtain baseline data including blood pressure, weight, and pulse. Laboratory tests including CBC, liver function, serum glucose, and an electrolyte profile should be obtained. Progestin is contraindicated for use in patients with a personal or close family history of breast or genital malignancies, thromboembolic disorders, impaired liver function, and undiagnosed vaginal bleeding. It is also contraindicated in pregnancy or lactation. Patients with allergies to peanuts should avoid the use of Prometrium, because the oral capsules contain peanut oil. Progestin must be used with caution in women with a history of depression, anemia, diabetes, asthma, seizure disorders, cardiac or kidney disorders, migraine headaches, previous ectopic pregnancies,

history of sexually transmitted infections, unresolved abnormal Pap smears, or previous pelvic surgeries.

The nurse should monitor for side effects of these hormones. Susceptible patients may experience acute intermittent porphyria as a reaction to progesterone, thus the nurse should assess for severe, colicky abdominal pain, vomiting, distention, diarrhea, and constipation. Common side effects of progesterone include breakthrough bleeding, nausea, abdominal cramps, dizziness, edema, and weight gain. The nurse should also monitor for amenorrhea; sudden, severe headache; and signs of pulmonary embolism such as sudden severe chest pain and dyspnea; and report such symptoms to the healthcare provider immediately. Because progesterone can cause photosensitivity and phototoxicity, the nurse should monitor for pruritus, sensitivity to light, acne, rash, and alopecia. Phototoxic reactions cause serious sunburn within 5 to 18 hours after sun exposure.

Patient education as it relates to progestins should include goals, reasons for assessing cardiovascular status, and possible side effects. See "Nursing Process Focus: Patients Receiving Progestin Therapy" for specific teaching points.

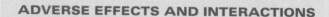

Pr PROTOTYPE DRUG | MEDROXYPROGESTERONE ACETATE (Provera)

ACTIONS AND USES

Medroxyprogesterone is a synthetic progestin with a prolonged duration of action. Like its natural counterpart, the primary target tissue for medroxyprogesterone is the endometrium of the uterus. It inhibits the effect of estrogen on the uterus, thus restoring normal hormonal balance. Applications include dysfunctional uterine bleeding and secondary amenorrhea. Medroxyprogesterone may also be given IM for the palliation of metastatic uterine or renal carcinoma.

Administration Alerts

- Give PO with meals to avoid gastric distress.
- Observe IM sites for abscess: presence of lump and discoloration of tissue.
- Pregnancy category X.

ADVERSE EFFECTS AND INTERACTIONS

The most common side effects are breakthrough bleeding and breast tenderness. Weight gain, depression, hypertension, nausea, vomiting, and dysmenorrheal and vaginal candidiasis may also occur. The most serious side effects relate to increased risk for thromboembolic disease.

Serum levels of medroxyprogesterone are decreased by aminoglutethimide, barbiturates, primidone, rifampin, rifabutin, and topiramate.

Use with caution with herbal supplements. For example, St. John's wort may cause intermenstrual bleeding and loss of efficacy.

See the companion website for a Nursing Process Focus specific to this drug.

NATURAL THERAPIES | Chaste Berry for PMS and Menopause

The chaste tree (*Vitex Agnus-castus*) is a shrub common to river banks in the southern Mediterranean region. The dried berries have been used for thousands of years, with recorded references dating to Hippocrates.

Chaste berries contain a number of active substances, some of which are antiadrenogenic and exert effects similar to progesterone. Extracts have a physiological effect on premenstrual syndrome, as well as the unpleasant symptoms of menopause. Women who take the herbal remedy report that PMS symptoms such as bloating, breast fullness, headache, irritability, mood swings, and anger reduce by 50%. There is better regulation of the menstrual cycle, and less bleeding. When used during menopause, it may help to reverse vaginal changes and diminished libido. It is also reported to increase milk production in lactating women. Adverse effects are minor and include GI upset, rash, and headaches.

LABOR AND BREASTFEEDING

OXYTOCICS AND TOCOLYTICS

Oxytocics are agents that stimulate uterine contractions to promote the induction of labor. Tocolytics, are used to inhibit uterine contractions during premature labor. These agents are shown in Table 41.5.

41.7 Pharmacologic Management of Uterine Contractions

The most widely used oxytocic is the natural hormone oxytocin, which is secreted by the posterior portion of the pituitary gland. The target organs for oxytocin are the uterus and the breast. It is secreted in increasingly larger amounts as the growing fetus distends the uterus. As blood levels of oxytocin rise, the uterus is stimulated to contract, thus promoting labor and the delivery of the baby and the placenta. As pregnancy progresses, the number of oxytocin receptors in the uterus increases, making it more sensitive to the effects of the hormone. Parenteral oxytocin (Pitocin) may be given to initiate labor. Doses in an IV infusion are increased gradually, every 15 to 60 minutes, until a normal labor pattern is established. After delivery, an IV infusion of oxytocin may be given to control postpartum uterine bleeding by temporarily impeding blood flow to this organ.

In postpartum patients, oxytocin is released in response to suckling, whereby it causes milk to be ejected (let down) from the mammary glands. Oxytocin does not increase the volume of milk production. This function is provided by the pituitary hormone prolactin, which increases the synthesis of milk. The actions of oxytocin during breastfeeding are illustrated in Figure 41.4. When given for milk letdown, oxytocin (Pitocin) is given intranasally several minutes before breastfeeding or pumping is anticipated.

Several prostaglandins are also used as uterine stimulants. Unlike most hormones that travel through the blood to affect distant tissues, prostaglandins are local hormones that act directly at the site where they are secreted. Although the body makes dozens of different prostaglandins, only a few have clinical utility. Dinoprostone (Cervidil), prostaglandin E_2, is used to initiate labor, to prepare the cervix for labor, or to expel a fetus that has died. Mifepristone (Mifiprex, RU486), a synthetic analog of prostaglandin E_1, is used for emergency contraception and for pharmacologic abortion, as described earlier in this chapter. Carboprost (Hemabate), 15-methyl-prostaglandin F_2 alpha, can induce pharmacologic abortion and may be indicated for controlling postpartum bleeding.

NURSING PROCESS FOCUS	PATIENTS RECEIVING PROGESTIN THERAPY

ASSESSMENT

Prior to administration:
- Obtain complete health history including personal or familial history of breast, endometrial or renal cancer, liver or kidney disease, dysfunctional uterine bleeding, endometrial hyperplasia.
- Obtain drug history to determine possible drug interactions and allergies.
- Assess cardiovascular status including history of thromboembolic disease.

POTENTIAL NURSING DIAGNOSES

- Deficient Knowledge, related to drug therapy
- Nausea, related to side effect of drug
- Noncompliance, related to drug regiman

PLANNING: PATIENT GOALS AND EXPECTED OUTCOMES

The patient will:
- Report relief from dysfunctional uterine bleeding or amenorrhea
- Demonstrate an understanding of the drug's action by accurately describing drug side effects and precautions
- Immediately report effects such as signs of embolism; sudden, severe headache; edema; vision changes; and phototoxicity

IMPLEMENTATION

Interventions and (Rationales)	Patient Education/Discharge Planning
■ Monitor lab tests including liver function, blood glucose, sodium, and chloride levels. (Progestins can affect electrolyte balance and liver function.)	■ Instruct patient to obtain periodic lab tests and monitor glucose levels closely if diabetic.
■ Monitor for vision changes. (Progestins may cause retinal emboli or cerebrovascular thrombosis.)	■ Instruct patient to report unexplained partial or complete loss of vision, ptosis, or diplopia.
■ Monitor for fluid imbalance. (Progestins cause fluid retention and weight gain.)	■ Instruct patient to monitor for edema or weight gain by weighing self weekly and recording; especially patients who have asthma, seizure disorders, cardiac or kidney impairment, or migraines.
■ Monitor for integumentary effects of medication. (Progestins have multiple effects on the skin and associated structures.)	Instruct patient to: ■ Report itching, photosensitivity, acne, rash, and hair overgrowth or hair loss ■ Avoid exposure to UV light and prolonged periods of time in the sun ■ Use sunscreen (>SPF 12) when outdoors ■ Recognize that these changes are temporary and will improve upon discontinuation of this medication

EVALUATION OF OUTCOME CRITERIA

Evaluate the effectiveness of drug therapy by confirming that patient goals and expected outcomes have been met (see "Planning").

See Table 41.4, under the heading "Progestins," for a list of drugs to which these nursing actions apply.

Tocolytics are uterine relaxants prescribed to *inhibit* the uterine contractions experienced during premature labor. Suppressing labor allows additional time for the fetus to develop and may permit the pregnancy to reach normal term. Premature birth is a leading cause of infant death. Typically, the mother is given a monitor with a sensor that records uterine contractions and this information is used to determine the doses and timing of tocolytic medications.

Two beta$_2$-adrenergic agonists are used as uterine relaxants. Ritodrine (Yutopar) may be given by the oral or IV route to suppress labor contractions. It is more effective when administered before labor intensifies, and its use normally

Table 41.5	Uterine Stimulants and Relaxants
Drug	**Route and Adult Dose (max dose where indicated)**
STIMULANTS (OXYTOCICS)	
oxytocin (Pitocin, Syntocinon)	IV (antepartum); 1 mU/min starting dose to a maximum of 20 mU/min
Ergot Alkaloids	
ergonovine maleate (Ergotrate Maleate)	PO; 1 tablet (0.2 mg) tid-qid after childbirth for a maximum of 1 week
methylergonovine maleate (Methergine)	PO; 0.2–0.4 mg bid-qid
Prostaglandins	
carboprost tromethamine (Hemabate)	IM; initial; 250 μg (1 mL) repeated at 1 1/2–3 1/2 h intervals if indicated by uterine response
dinoprostone (Cervidil, Prepidil, Prostin E$_2$)	Intravaginal; 10 mg
misoprostol (Cytotec)	PO; 400 μg as a single dose
RELAXANTS (TOCOLYTICS)	
Beta$_2$-Adrenergic Agonists	
ritodrine hydrochloride (Yutopar)	IV; 50–100 μg/min starting dose, increased by 50 μg/min q10 min
terbutaline sulfate (Brethine)	IV; 10 μg/min (max 80 μg/min)
Other Tocolytics	
magnesium sulfate (see p. 558)	IV; 1–4 g in 5% dextrose by slow infusion
nifedipine (Procardia) (see p. 270)	PO; 10 mg as a single dose

results in only a 1- to 2-day prolongation of pregnancy. Terbutaline is another beta$_2$-agonist that may be used for uterine relaxation, though it is not approved for this purpose in the United States. The benefits of tocolytics must be carefully weighed against their potential adverse effects, which include tachycardia in both the mother and the fetus.

NURSING CONSIDERATIONS

The role of the nurse in uterine stimulant therapy involves careful monitoring of both the mother and child's condition and providing education as it relates to the administered drug. The healthcare provider must evaluate the patient for fetal presentation, especially for the presence of cephalopelvic disproportion.

To safely administer oxytocin, the fetus must be viable and vaginal delivery must be possible. If invasive cervical cancer, active herpes genitalis, or cord prolapse exists, oxytocin is contraindicated. Oxytocin is also contraindicated in patients with a history of previous uterine or cervical surgery including cesarean section. This drug is not used if the patient is a grand multipara, older than 35 years of age, or has a history of uterine sepsis or traumatic birth. Previous sensitivity or allergic reaction to an ergot derivative contraindicates the use of oxytocin. Dinoprostone use is con-

traindicated in patients with active cardiac, pulmonary, renal, or hepatic disease. These medications must be used cautiously with vasoconstrictive drugs.

The nurse should monitor for side effects of these hormone-based medications. Because oxytocin increases the frequency and force of uterine contractions, the patient in labor must be assessed frequently for elevations in blood pressure, heart rate, and fetal heart rate. The infusion must be discontinued if fetal distress is detected to prevent fetal anoxia. The nurse should administer oxygen and have the mother change position to improve fetal oxygenation. Hypertensive crisis may occur if local or regional anesthesia is used in combination with oxytocin.

Uterine hyperstimulation is characterized by contractions that are less than 2 minutes apart, with greater force than 50 mm Hg, or last longer than 90 seconds. Oxytocin should be discontinued immediately if hyperstimulation occurs. The nurse should monitor fluid balance because prolonged IV infusion of oxytocin may cause water intoxication. Symptoms of water intoxication must be assessed and reported immediately and include drowsiness, listlessness, headache, confusion, anuria, and weight gain. Side effects of oxytocin include anxiety, maternal dyspnea, hypotension or hypertension, nausea, vomiting, neonatal jaundice, and maternal or fetal dysrhythmias.

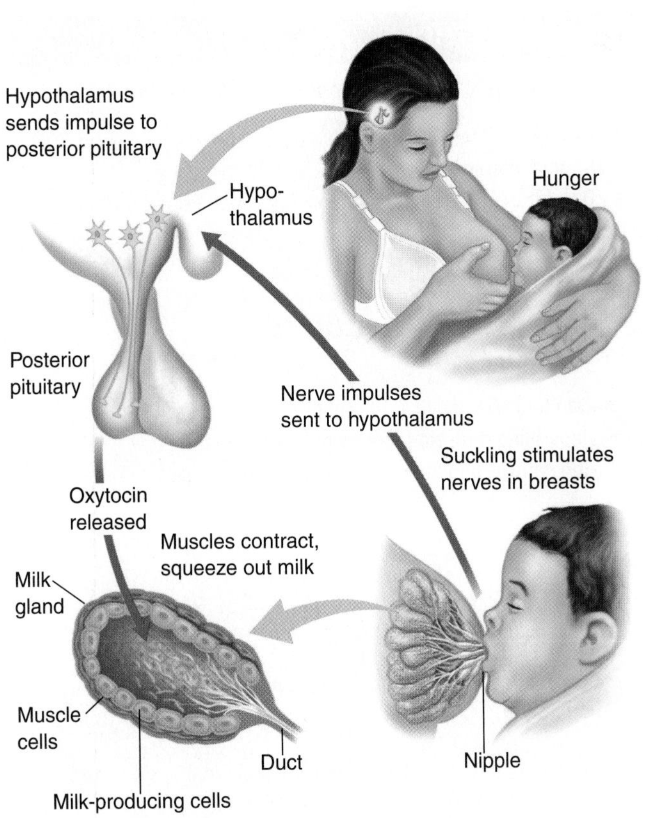

Hypothalamus sends impulse to posterior pituitary

Hypo- thalamus

Hunger

Posterior pituitary

Nerve impulses sent to hypothalamus

Oxytocin released

Suckling stimulates nerves in breasts

Muscles contract, squeeze out milk

Milk gland

Muscle cells

Duct

Nipple

Milk-producing cells

Figure 41.4 | Oxytocin and breastfeeding

See "Nursing Process Focus: Patients Receiving Oxytocin" for specific teaching points regarding this prototype drug.

FEMALE INFERTILITY

Infertility is defined as the inability to become pregnant after at least 1 year of frequent, unprotected intercourse. Infertility is a common disorder, with as many as 25% of couples experiencing difficulty in conceiving children at some point during their reproductive lifetimes. It is estimated that females contribute to approximately 60% of the infertility disorders. Agents used to treat infertility are shown in Table 41.6.

41.8 Pharmacotherapy of Female Fertility

Causes of female infertility are varied, and include lack of ovulation, pelvic infection, and physical obstruction of the uterine tubes. Extensive testing is often necessary to determine the exact cause of the infertility. For women whose infertility has been determined to have an endocrine etiology, pharmacotherapy may be of value. Endocrine disruption of reproductive function can occur at the level of the hypothalamus, pituitary, or ovary, and pharmacotherapy is targeted to the specific cause of the dysfunction.

Lack of regular ovulation is a cause of infertility that can be successfully treated with drug therapy. Clomiphene

---

Pr PROTOTYPE DRUG | **OXYTOCIN (Pitocin, Syntocinon)**

ACTIONS AND USES

Oxytocin is a natural hormone secreted by the posterior pituitary that is a drug of choice for inducing labor. Oxytocin is given by several different routes depending on its intended action. Given by IV infusion antepartum, oxytocin induces labor by increasing the frequency and force of contractions of uterine smooth muscle. It is timed to the final stage of pregnancy, after the cervix is dilated, membranes have ruptured, and presentation of the fetus has occurred. Oxytocin may also be administered postpartum to reduce hemorrhage after expulsion of the placenta, and to aid in returning normal muscular tone to the uterus. A second route of administration is intranasally to promote the ejection of milk from the mammary glands. Milk letdown occurs within minutes after applying spray or drops to the nostril during breastfeeding.

Administration Alerts

- Dilute 10 U oxytocin in 1,000 cc IV fluid prior to administration. For postpartum administration, may add up to 40 U in 1,000 cc IV fluid.
- Incidence of allergic reactions is higher when given IM or by IV injection, rather than IV infusion
- Pregnancy category X.

ADVERSE EFFECTS AND INTERACTIONS

When given IV, vital signs of the fetus and mother are monitored continuously to avoid complications in the fetus, such as dysrhythmias or intracranial hemorrhage. Serious complications in the mother may include uterine rupture, seizures, or coma. Risk of uterine rupture increases in women who have delivered five or more children. Though experience has shown the use of oxytocin to be quite safe, labor should only be induced by this drug when there are demonstrated risks to the mother or fetus in continuing the pregnancy.

Oxytocin interacts with several drugs. For example, vasoconstrictors used concurrently with oxytocin cause severe hypertension.

Use with caution with herbal supplements. For example, ephedra or ma-huang used with oxytocin may lead to hypertension.

NURSING PROCESS FOCUS	PATIENTS RECEIVING OXYTOCIN

ASSESSMENT

Prior to administration:

- Obtain complete health history including past and present gynecologic and obstetric history.
- Obtain drug history to determine possible drug interactions and allergies.

POTENTIAL NURSING DIAGNOSES

- Excess Fluid Volume, related to water intoxication due to ADH effects of drug
- Risk for Injury to Fetus, related to strong uterine contractions

PLANNING: PATIENT GOALS AND EXPECTED OUTCOMES

The patient will:

- Report increase in force and frequency of uterine contractions and/or letdown of milk for breastfeeding
- Demonstrate an understanding of the drug's action by accurately describing drug side effects and precautions
- Immediately report effects such as listlessness, headache, confusion, anuria, hypotension, nausea, vomiting, and weight gain

IMPLEMENTATION

Interventions and (Rationales)	Patient Education/Discharge Planning
■ Monitor fetal heart rate. (Increase in force and frequency of uterine contractions may cause fetal distress.)	■ Instruct patient about the purpose and importance of fetal monitoring.
■ Monitor maternal status including blood pressure, pulse, and frequency, duration, and intensity of contractions.	■ Instruct patient about the importance of monitoring maternal status.
■ Monitor fluid balance. (Prolonged IV infusion may cause water intoxication.)	■ Instruct patient to report drowsiness, listlessness, headache, confusion, anuria, weight gain.
■ Monitor for postpartum/postabortion hemorrhage. (Oxytocin can be used to control postpartum bleeding.)	Instruct patient: ■ About the importance of being monitored frequently after delivery or after abortion ■ To report severe vaginal bleeding or increase in lochia
■ Monitor lactation status. (Oxytocin causes milk ejection within minutes after administration.)	Instruct patient: ■ That oxytocin does not increase milk production ■ To monitor for decreased breast pain, redness, hardness, if taking oxytocin to decrease breast engorgement

EVALUATION OF OUTCOME CRITERIA

Evaluate the effectiveness of drug therapy by confirming that patient goals and expected outcomes have been met (see "Planning").

(Clomid, Serophene) is a drug of choice for female infertility that acts as an antiestrogen. Clomiphene stimulates the release of LH, resulting in the maturation of more ovarian follicles than would normally occur. The rise in LH level is sufficient to induce ovulation in about 90% of treated patients. The pregnancy rate of patients taking clomiphene is high, and twins occur in about 5% of treated patients. Therapy is usually begun with a low dose of 50 mg for 5 days, following menses. If ovulation does not occur, the dose is increased to 100 mg for 5 days, then to 150 mg. If ovulation still is not induced, human chorionic gonadotropin (HCG)

is added to the regimen. Made by the placenta during pregnancy, HCG is similar to LH and can mimic the LH surge that normally causes ovulation. The use of clomiphene assumes that the pituitary gland is able to respond by secreting LH, and that the ovaries are responsive to LH. If either of these assumptions is false, other treatment options should be considered.

If the endocrine disruption is at the pituitary level, therapy with human menopausal gonadotropin (HMG) or gonadotropin-releasing hormone (GnRH) may be indicated. These therapies are generally indicated only after

Table 41.6	Agents for Female Infertility
Drug	**Mechanism**
bromocriptine mesylate (Parlodel)	Reduction of high prolactin levels
clomiphene (Clomid, Serophene)	Promote follicle maturation and ovulation
danazol (Danocrine)	Control of endometriosis
Human FSH (purified from the urine of postmenopausal women)	Promote follicle maturation and ovulation
urofollitropin (Fertinex, Metrodin)	
Recombinant FSH	Promote follicle maturation and ovulation
follitropin alfa (Gonal-F)	
follitropin beta (Follistim)	
GnRH and GnRH Analogs	Promote follicle maturation and ovulation or control of endometriosis
cetrorelix acetate (cetrotide)	
leuprolide acetate (Lupron, Lupron Depot)	
nafarelin acetate (Synarel)	
ganirelix acetate (Antagon)	
gonadorelin acetate (Lutrepulse)	
goserelin acetate (Zoladex)	
human chorionic gonadotropin-HCG (A.P.L., Chorex, Choron 10, Profasi HP, Pregnyl)	Promote follicle maturation and ovulation
human menopausal gonadotropin-menotropins (Pergonal, Humegon, Repronex)	Promote follicle maturation and ovulation

clomiphene has failed to induce ovulation. HMG is a combination of FSH and LH extracted from the urine of postmenopausal women, who secrete large amounts of these hormones. Also called menotropins (Pergonal, Humegon), HMG acts on the ovaries to increase follicle maturation, and results in a 25% incidence of multiple pregnancies. Successful therapy with HMG assumes that the ovaries are responsive to LH and FSH. Newer formulations use recombinant DNA technology to synthesize gonadotropins containing nearly pure FSH, rather than extracting the FSH-LH mixture from urine.

Given IV, gonadorelin (Factrel) is a synthetic analog of GnRH that is prescribed for patients unresponsive to clomiphene (Clomid, Serophene). GnRH analogs take over the function of the hypothalamus, and attempt to restart normal hormonal rhythms. Other medications used to stimulate ovulation are bromocriptine (Parlodel) and human chorionic gonadotropin (HCG).

Endometriosis, a common cause of infertility, is characterized by the presence of endometrial tissue in nonuterine locations such as the pelvis and ovaries. Being responsive to hormonal stimuli, this abnormal tissue can cause pain, dysfunctional bleeding, and dysmenorrhea. Leuprolide (Lupron) is a GnRH agonist that produces an initial release of LH and FSH, followed by suppression due to the negative feedback effect on the pituitary. Many women experience relief from the symptoms of endometriosis after 3 to 6 months of leuprolide therapy, and the benefits may extend well beyond the treatment period. Leuprolide is also indicated for the palliative therapy of prostate cancer. As an alternative choice, danazol (Danocrine) is an anabolic steroid that suppresses FSH production, which in turn shuts down both ectopic and normal endometrial activity. While leuprolide is only given by the parenteral route, danazol is given orally.

CHAPTER REVIEW

Key Concepts

The numbered key concepts provide a succinct summary of the important points from the corresponding numbered section within the chapter. If any of the points are not clear, refer to the numbered section within the chapter for review. Expanded versions can be found on the companion website.

41.1 Female reproductive function is controlled by GnRH from the hypothalamus, and FSH and LH from the pituitary.

41.2 Estrogens are secreted by ovarian follicles and are responsible for the secondary sex characteristics of the female. Progestins are secreted by the corpus luteum and prepare the endometrium for implantation.

41.3 Low doses of estrogens and progestins prevent conception by blocking ovulation.

41.4 Drugs may be administered within 72 hours after unprotected sex to prevent implantation of the fertilized egg. Other agents may be given to stimulate uterine contractions to expel the implanted embryo.

41.5 Estrogen-progestin combinations are used for hormone replacement therapy during and after menopause; however, their long-term use may have serious adverse effects.

41.6 Progestins are prescribed for dysfunctional uterine bleeding. High doses of progestins are also used as antineoplastics.

41.7 Oxytocics are drugs that stimulate uterine contractions and induce labor. Tocolytics slow uterine contractions to delay labor.

41.8 Medications may be administered to stimulate ovulation, to increase female fertility.

Review Questions

1. Why is a progestin usually prescribed along with estrogen in oral contraceptives, and when treating postmenopausal symptoms?

2. What is the difference between the effects of prolactin and oxytocin on the breast?

3. Explain why lack of sufficient pituitary secretion can cause female infertility. Describe several pharmacologic approaches to treating infertility due to pituitary hyposecretion.

Critical Thinking Questions

1. A 28-year-old female has a 3-year history of pelvic pain, dyspareunia, and infertility. She has been diagnosed with endometriosis and is prescribed leuprolide (Lupron) once a month per intramuscular injection. Discuss the mechanism of action of leuprolide in managing the patient's endometriosis.

2. A labor and delivery nurse places one-fourth tablet (crushed) of misoprostol (Cytotec) on the cervix of a patient who is being induced because she is 2 weeks past her due date. After several hours, the patient begins to have contractions and the nurse notes late decelerations on the monitor. The nurse flushes the drug out of the patient's vagina with saline per hospital protocol. Is it possible that the misoprostol stimulated these uterine contractions? Why or why not?

3. A nurse is assessing a 32-year-old postpartum patient and notes 2+ pitting edema of the ankles and pretibial area. The patient denied having "swelling" prior to delivery. The nurse reviews the patient's chart and notes that she was induced with oxytocin (Pitocin) over a 23-hour period. Is there any relationship between this drug regimen and the patient's current presentation? What additional assessments should be made?

EXPLORE MediaLink

NCLEX review, case studies, and other interactive resources for this chapter can be found on the companion website at www.prenhall.com/adams. Click on "Chapter 41" to select the activities for this chapter. For animations, more NCLEX review questions, and an audio glossary, access the accompanying CD-ROM in this textbook.

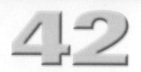

CHAPTER 42

Drugs for Disorders and Conditions of the Male Reproductive System

■ DRUGS AT A GLANCE

AGENTS FOR MALE HYPOGONADISM

Androgens

Pr *testosterone base (Andro)*

AGENTS FOR MALE INFERTILITY

AGENTS FOR ERECTILE DYSFUNCTION

Phosphodiesterase-5 inhibitors

Pr *sildenafil (Viagra)*

AGENTS FOR BENIGN PROSTATIC HYPERPLASIA

Alpha₁-adrenergic blockers

5-alpha reductase inhibitors

Pr *finasteride (Proscar)*

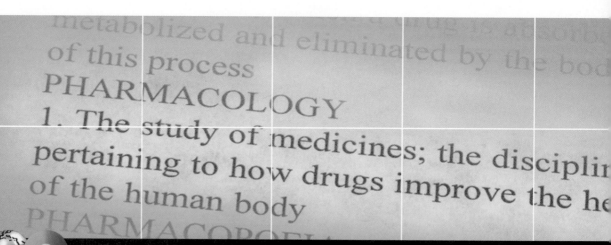

OBJECTIVES

After reading this chapter, the student should be able to:

1. Describe the roles of the hypothalamus, pituitary, and testes in maintaining male reproductive function.
2. Explain the role of androgens in the treatment of male hypogonadism.
3. Describe the misuse and dangers associated with the use of anabolic steroids to enhance athletic performance.
4. Discuss the use of androgens as antineoplastic agents.
5. Explain the limited role of drugs in the therapy of male infertility.
6. Describe the role of drug therapy in the treatment of erectile dysfunction.
7. Describe the nurse's role in the pharmacologic management of disorders and conditions of the male reproductive system.
8. Identify the static and functional components of benign prostatic hyperplasia (BPH), and how they lead to patient symptoms.
9. For each of the drugs/classes listed in Drugs at a Glance, identify representative drugs, explain the mechanism of drug action, primary actions, and important adverse effects.
10. Categorize drugs used in the treatment of male reproductive disorders and conditions based on their classification and mechanism of action.
11. Use the Nursing Process to care for patients who are receiving drug therapy for disorders and conditions of the male reproductive system.

Like the female, male reproductive function is regulated by a small number of hormones from the hypothalamus, pituitary, and gonads. Because hormonal secretion in the male is regular throughout the adult lifespan, pharmacologic treat- ment of reproductive disorders in the male is less complex, and more limited, than in the female. This chapter examines drugs used to treat disorders and conditions of the male reproductive system.

PHARMFACTS — Male Reproductive Conditions and Disorders

- Erectile dysfunction affects 10 to 15 million Americans— about 1 in 4 men over age 65.
- BPH affects 50% of men over age 60, and 90% of men over age 80.
- BPH is the most common benign neoplasm affecting middle-age and elderly men.
- Approximately 30% of men are subfertile and at least 2% of men are totally infertile.
- Smoking over 20 cigarettes a day has shown to reduce both the sperm count and sperm motility.

42.1 Hypothalamic and Pituitary Regulation of Male Reproductive Function

The same pituitary hormones that control reproductive function in the female (Chapter 41) also affect the male. Although the name follicle-stimulating hormone (FSH) applies to its target in the female ovary, this same hormone regulates sperm production in the male. In males, leuteinizing hormone (LH), sometimes called interstitial cell-stimulating hormone (ICSH), regulates the production of testosterone.

Although secreted in small amounts by the adrenal glands in females, androgens are considered male sex hormones.

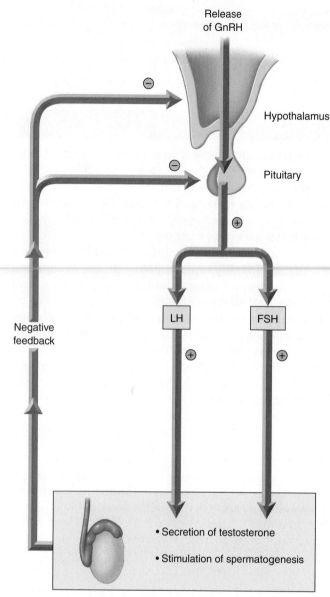

The testes secrete testosterone, the primary androgen responsible for maturation of the male sex organs and the secondary sex characteristics of the male. Unlike the cyclic secretion of estrogen and progesterone in the female, the secretion of testosterone is relatively constant in the adult male. Should the level of testosterone in the blood rise above normal, negative feedback is provided to the pituitary to shut off the secretion of LH and FSH. The relationship between the hypothalamus, pituitary, and the male reproductive hormones is illustrated in Figure 42.1.

Like estrogen, testosterone has metabolic effects in tissues outside the reproductive system. Of particular note is its ability to build muscle mass, which contributes to differences in muscle strength and body composition between males and females.

MALE HYPOGONADISM

ANDROGENS

Androgens include testosterone and related hormones that control many aspects of male reproductive function. Therapeutically they are used to treat hypogonadism and certain cancers. These agents are shown in Table 42.1.

42.2 Pharmacotherapy with Androgens

Lack of sufficient testosterone secretion by the testes can result in male **hypogonadism**. Insufficient testosterone secretion may be caused by disorders of the pituitary or the testes. Deficiency in FSH and LH secretion by the pituitary will result in a lack of stimulus to the testes to produce androgens. Lack of FSH and LH secretion may have a number of causes, including Cushing's syndrome, thyroid disorders, estrogen-secreting tumors, and therapy with GnRH agonists such as leuprolide (Lupron). Hypogonadism may be congenital, or acquired later in life.

Hypogonadism may also occur in patients with normal pituitary function, if the testes are diseased or otherwise un-

Figure 42.1 | Hormonal control of the male reproductive hormones

Table 42.1	Selected Androgens
Drug	**Route and Adult Dose (max dose where indicated)**
danazol (Danocrine)	PO; 200–400 mg bid for 3–6 months
fluoxymesterone (Halotestin)	PO; 2.5–20 mg qd for replacement therapy
methyltestosterone (Android, Testred)	PO; 10–50 mg qd
nandrolone phenpropionate (Durabolin, Hybolin)	IM; 50–100 mg q wk
testolactone (Teslac)	PO; 250 mg qid
testosterone (Andro 100, Histerone, Testoderm)	PO; 10–25 mg q 2–3 days
testosterone cypionate (Depotest, Andro-Cyp, Depo-Testosterone)	IM; 50–400 mg q2–4 wk
testosterone enanthate (Andro L.A., Delatest, Delatestryl)	IM; 50–400 mg q2–4 wk

responsive to FSH-LH. Examples of conditions that may cause testicular failure include mumps, testicular trauma or inflammation, and certain autoimmune disorders.

Symptoms of male hypogonadism include a diminished appearance of the secondary sex characteristics of the male: sparse axillary, facial, and pubic hair; increase in subcutaneous fat; and small testicular size. In adult males, lack of testosterone can lead to erectile dysfunction, low sperm counts, and decreased libido, or interest in intercourse. Nonspecific complaints may include fatigue, depression, and reduced muscle mass. In young males, lack of sufficient testosterone secretion may lead to delayed puberty.

Pharmacotherapy for male hypogonadism includes replacement therapy with testosterone or other androgens. Androgen therapy promotes normal gonadal development and often restores normal reproductive function. Secondary male sex characteristics reappear, a condition called masculinization or virilization.

Testosterone is available in a number of different formulations. Testosterone cypionate (Depotest, others) and testosterone enanthate (Andro LA) are slowly absorbed after IM injections, which are given every 2 to 4 weeks. Testosterone pellets (Testopel) are implanted SC, and last 3 to 6 months. Several skin patch products are available, which release testosterone over a 24-hour period. Testoderm patches are applied to the scrotal area, whereas Testoderm TTS and Androderm patches are applied to the arm, back, or upper buttocks. Two gel systems are available as Testim and Androgel which are applied to the shoulders, upper arm, or abdomen. The alcohol-based gels dry quickly and the testosterone is absorbed into the skin and released slowly to the blood. A new formulation is a buccal tablet (Striant) that adheres to the gum surface to release the drug over a 12 hour period.

Androgens have important physiological effects outside the reproductive system. Testosterone promotes the synthesis of erythropoietin, which explains why males usually have a slightly higher hematocrit than females. Testosterone has a profound anabolic effect on skeletal muscle, which is the rationale for giving this drug to debilitated patients who have muscle wasting disease.

Anabolic steroids are testosterone-like compounds with hormonal activity that are taken inappropriately by athletes who hope to build muscle mass and strength, thereby obtaining a competitive edge. When taken in large doses for prolonged periods, anabolic steroids can produce significant adverse effects, some of which may persist for months after discontinuation of the drugs. These agents tend to raise cholesterol levels and may cause low sperm counts and impotence in men. In female athletes, menstrual irregularities are likely, with an obvious increase in masculine appearance. Permanent liver damage may result. Behavioral changes include aggression and psychological dependence. The use of anabolic steroids to improve athletic performance is illegal and strongly discouraged by healthcare providers and athletic associations. Most androgens are classified as Schedule III drugs due to their abuse potential.

High doses of androgens are occasionally used as a palliative measure to treat certain types of breast cancer, in combination with other antineoplastics. Because most prostate carcinomas are testosterone dependent, androgens should not be prescribed for older males unless the possibility of prostate cancer has been ruled out. Patients with prostate carcinoma are sometimes given a GnRH agonist such as leuprolide (Lupron) to reduce circulating testosterone levels.

NURSING CONSIDERATIONS

The role of the nurse in androgen therapy involves careful monitoring of a patient's condition and providing education as it relates to the prescribed drug regimen. The nurse should conduct a physical assessment for evidence of decreased hormone production, such as decreased or absent body hair, small testes, impaired sexual functioning, or delayed signs of puberty. The nurse should also assess the patient's emotional status as depression and mood swings may be symptoms of decreased hormone secretion. The nurse should monitor lab results, especially liver enzymes, if the patient has a history of anabolic steroid use. Contraindications to androgen therapy include prostatic or male breast cancer, renal disease, cardiac and liver dysfunction, hypercalcemia, BPH, and hypertension. Androgens must be used cautiously in prepubertal males, older adults, and in acute intermittent porphyria.

The nurse should monitor for side effects of male patients taking androgens. See "Nursing Process Focus: Patients Receiving Androgen Therapy". Some adverse reactions found to occur in females as a result of androgen use include deepening of the voice, increased acne or oily

PROTOTYPE DRUG | **TESTOSTERONE BASE** (Andro, others)

ACTIONS AND USES

The primary therapeutic use of testosterone is for the treatment of hypogonadism in males by promoting virilization, including enlargement of the sexual organs, growth of facial hair, and a deepening of the voice. In adult males, testosterone administration will increase libido and restore masculine characteristics that may be deficient. Testosterone base acts by stimulating RNA synthesis and protein metabolism. High doses may suppress spermatogenesis.

Administration Alerts

- Place patch on hair-free, dry skin of the abdomen, back, thigh, upper arm or as directed.
- Alternate patch site q24h, rotating sites every 7 days.
- Give IM injection into gluteal muscles.
- Pregnancy category X.

ADVERSE EFFECTS AND INTERACTIONS

An obvious side effect of testosterone therapy is virilization, which is usually only of concern when the drug is taken by female patients. Increased libido may also occur. Salt and water are often retained, causing edema, and a diuretic may be indicated. Liver damage is rare, although a potentially serious adverse effect with some of the orally administered androgens. Acne and skin irritation is common during therapy.

Testosterone base interacts with several drugs. For example, when taken concurrently with oral anticoagulants, testosterone base may potentiate hypoprothrombinemia. Insulin requirements may decrease, and the risk of hepatotoxicity may increase when used with echinacea.

Use with caution with herbal supplements.

See the companion website for a Nursing Process Focus specific to this drug.

---

skin, increased hair growth, enlarged clitoris, and irregular menses.

Patient education as it relates to androgen therapy should include goals, reasons for obtaining baseline data such as vital signs and tests for cardiac and renal disorders. See "Nursing Process Focus: Patients Receiving Androgen Therapy" for specific teaching points.

MALE INFERTILITY

It is estimated that 30% to 40% of couples' infertility is caused by difficulties with the male reproductive system. Male infertility may have psychological etiology, which must be ruled out before pharmacotherapy is considered.

42.3 Pharmacotherapy of Male Infertility

Like female infertility, male infertility may have a number of complex causes. Oligospermia, the presence of less than 20 million sperm/ml of ejaculate is considered abnormal. Azoospermia, the complete absence of sperm in an ejaculate, may indicate an obstruction of the vas deferens or ejaculatory duct which can be corrected surgically. Infections such as mumps, chronic tuberculosis, and sexually transmitted diseases can contribute to infertility. The possibility of erectile dysfunction must be considered, and treated as discussed in Section 42.4. Infertility may occur with or without signs of hypogonadism.

The goal of endocrine pharmacotherapy of male infertility is to increase sperm production. Therapy often begins with IM injections of human chorionic gonadotropin (HCG), three times per week over 1 year. Although secreted by the placenta, the effects of HCG in the male are identical to those of LH: increasing testosterone secretion

and stimulating spermatogenesis. Sperm counts are conducted periodically to assess therapeutic progress. If HCG is unsuccessful, therapy with menotropins (Pergonal) may be attempted. Menotropin consists of a mixture of purified FSH and LH. For infertile patients exhibiting signs of hypogonadism, testosterone therapy also may be indicated.

Other pharmacologic approaches to treating male infertility have been attempted. Antiestrogens such as tamoxifen (Nolvadex) and clomiphene (Clomid) have been used to block the negative feedback of estrogen (from the adrenal glands) to the pituitary and hypothalamus, thus increasing the levels of FSH and LH. Testolactone (Teslac), an aromatase inhibitor, has been administered to block the metabolic conversion of testosterone to estrogen. Various nutritional supplements, such as using zinc to improve sperm production, L-arginine to improve sperm motility, and vitamins C and E as antioxidants to reduce reactive intermediates, have been tested. Unfortunately these and other attempts have not been conclusively shown to have any positive effect on male infertility.

Drug therapy of male infertility is not as successful as pharmacotherapy in the female, because only about 5% of infertile males have an endocrine etiology for their disorder. Many years of therapy may be required. Because of the expense and the large number of injections needed, other means of conception may be explored, such as in vitro fertilization or intrauterine insemination.

ERECTILE DYSFUNCTION

Erectile dysfunction, or impotence, is a common disorder in men. The defining characteristic of this condition is the consistent inability to either obtain an erection or to sustain an erection long enough to achieve successful intercourse.

 MediaLink Resources for Male Infertility

NURSING PROCESS FOCUS   PATIENTS RECEIVING ANDROGEN THERAPY

ASSESSMENT

Prior to administration:
- Obtain complete health history including male breast or prostatic cancer; BPH; cardiac, kidney, or liver disease; diabetes; and hypercalcemia.
- Obtain lab results including renal function tests, BUN, creatinine, and PSA.
- Obtain drug history to determine possible drug interactions and allergies.

POTENTIAL NURSING DIAGNOSES

- Disturbed Body Image, related to effects of decreased or increased hormone function
- Sexual Dysfunction, related to effects of drug therapy or decreased hormone function
- Disturbed Sleep Pattern, related to effects of drug therapy
- Deficient Knowledge, related to disease process and drug therapy

PLANNING: PATIENT GOALS AND EXPECTED OUTCOMES

The patient will:
- Demonstrate improvement of the underlying condition for which testosterone was ordered
- Demonstrate an understanding of the drug's action by accurately describing drug side effects and precautions, and importance of follow-up care

IMPLEMENTATION

Interventions and (Rationales)	*Patient Education/Discharge Planning*
• Monitor serum cholesterol levels. (Elevated cholesterol levels secondary to testosterone administration may increase patient's risk of cardiovascular disease.)	Instruct patient to: • Have cholesterol levels measured periodically during therapy • Modify factors that may lower risk of hypercholesterolemia: decrease fat in diet, increase exercise, decrease consumption of red meat
• Monitor calcium levels. (Testosterone can cause hypercalcemia.)	Instruct patient to: • Have calcium levels checked during therapy • Recognize and report symptoms of increased serum calcium, including deep bone and flank pain, anorexia, nausea/vomiting, thirst, constipation, lethargy, and psychoses
• Monitor bone growth in children and adolescents. (Premature epiphyseal closing may occur, leading to growth retardation.)	• Instruct pediatric caregiver to have bone age determinations on the child every 6 months.
• Monitor input, output, and patient weight. (Testosterone can cause retention of salt and water, leading to edema.)	• Instruct patient to check weight twice weekly and report increases, particularly if accompanied by dependent edema.
• Monitor blood glucose, especially in diabetics. (Testosterone therapy may change glucose tolerance.)	Instruct patient to: • Monitor blood glucose daily and report significant changes to healthcare provider • Recognize that adjustments may need to be made in hypoglycemic medications and diet
• Monitor proper self-administration.	Instruct patient to: • Mark calendar so medication can be taken/given at appropriate intervals • Apply transdermal patch to dry, clean scrotal skin that has been dry shaved and not to use chemical depilatories • Notify female partner of transdermal patch; there is a chance of absorbing testosterone, resulting in mild virilization • Avoid showering or swimming for at least 1 hour after gel application

EVALUATION OF OUTCOME CRITERIA

Evaluate the effectiveness of drug therapy by confirming that patient goals and expected outcomes have been met (see "Planning").

See Table 42.1 for a list of drugs to which these nursing actions apply.

42.4 Pharmacotherapy of Erectile Dysfunction

The incidence of erectile dysfunction increases with advancing age, although it may occur in a male adult of any age. Certain diseases, most notably atherosclerosis, diabetes, stroke, and hypertension, are associated with a higher incidence of the condition. Psychogenic causes may include depression, fatigue, guilt, or fear of sexual failure. In some men, a number of common drugs cause impotence as a side effect, including thiazide diuretics, phenothiazines, serotonin reuptake inhibitors, tricyclic antidepressants, propranolol (Inderal), and diazepam (Valium). Loss of libido may be due to low testosterone secretion.

Penile erection has both neuromuscular and vascular components. Autonomic nerves dilate arterioles leading to the major erectile tissues of the penis, called the **corpora cavernosa**. The corpora have vascular spaces that fill with blood to cause rigidity. The vasoconstriction of veins draining blood from the corpora allows the penis to remain rigid long enough for successful penetration. After ejaculation, the veins dilate, blood leaves the corpora, and the penis quickly loses its rigidity. Organic causes of erectile dysfunction may include damage to the nerves or blood vessels involved in the erection reflex.

The marketing of sildenafil (Viagra), an inhibitor of the enzyme phosphodiesterase-5, has revolutionized the medical therapy of erectile dysfunction. When sildenafil was approved as the first pharmacologic treatment for erectile dysfunction in 1998, it set a record for pharmaceutical sales for any new drug in U.S. history. Prior to the discovery of sildenafil, rigid or inflatable penile prostheses were implanted into the corpora. As an alternative to prostheses, drugs such as alprostadil (Caverject) or the combination of papaverine plus phentolamine were injected directly into the corpora cavernosa just prior to intercourse. Injections caused pain in many patients and reduced the spontaneity associated with pleasurable intercourse. These alternative therapies are rare today, though they may be used for patients in whom sildenafil is contraindicated.

The nurse should be aware that sildenafil does not cause an erection; it merely enhances the erection caused by physical contact or other sexual stimuli. In addition, sildenafil is not as effective in promoting erections in men who do not have erectile dysfunction. Despite considerable research interest, no effects of sildenafil have been shown on female sexual function, and this drug is not approved for use by women.

Recently, a second phosphodiesterase-5 inhibitor, vardenafil (Levitra), was approved by the FDA. Vardenafil acts by the same mechanism as sildenafil but has a faster onset and slightly longer duration of action. The two drugs exhibit similar types of side effects. Tadalafil (Cialis) is a third phosphodiesterase-5 inhibitor that is in widespread use in Europe and has entered the final stages of FDA approval. Tadalafil acts within 30 minutes and is reported to have a prolonged duration lasting from 24 to 36 hours.

NURSING CONSIDERATIONS

The role of the nurse in pharmacotherapy with erectile dysfunction agents involves careful monitoring of a patient's condition and providing education as it relates to the prescribed drug regimen. The nurse should obtain a complete physical examination including history of impaired sexual function, cardiovascular disease, and presence of emotional disturbances. The nurse should obtain and monitor results of lab tests related to liver function. Sildenafil and vardenafil are contraindicated with the use of organic nitrates and nitroglycerin, because they potentiate effect of nitrates, leading to severe hypotension. Nitrates are also found in recreational drugs, including amyl nitrate or nitrite, commonly called "poppers." Coadministration of vardenafil and alpha-adrenergic blockers can also lead to profound hypotension. These agents are contraindicated in patients with severe cardiovascular disease and in the presence of anatomic deformities of the penis.

Cautious use should be observed in the patient with hepatic dysfunction because these drugs are metabolized in the liver, and drug accumulation may lead to toxicity. Patients with cirrhosis or severe decreased liver function should start with lower doses. Leukemia, sickle cell anemia, multiple myeloma, ulcer, and retinitis pigmentosa patients should also use sildenafil cautiously.

The nurse should monitor for side effects including vision changes such as blurred vision, being unable to differentiate between green and blue, objects having a blue tinge to them, and photophobia. The nurse should also observe safety precautions until known if sensory-perceptual alterations will occur, so falls and other accidents can be avoided. The patient should be monitored for presence of headache, dizziness, flushing, rash, nasal congestion, diarrhea, dyspepsia, UTI, chest pain, or indigestion.

Patient education as it relates to erectile dysfunction agents should include the goals, reasons for obtaining baseline data such as vital signs and tests for cardiac and renal disorders, and possible side effects. For patients receiving sildenafil or vardenafil, following are the important teaching points.

- Do not take more than one dose in a 24-hour period.
- Have vital signs, including blood pressure, checked routinely.
- Take sildenafil 1 hour prior to sexual activity and vardenafil 25 to 40 minutes prior to sexual activity.
- If taking nitrates or alpha blockers, do not use erectile dysfunction agents.
- Do not share medication.
- Do not take more than the recommended dose, as this increases the risk of side effects.

BENIGN PROSTATIC HYPERPLASIA

Benign prostatic hyperplasia (BPH) is an enlargement of the prostate gland that occurs in most men of advanced age.

Pr PROTOTYPE DRUG | SILDENAFIL (Viagra)

ACTIONS AND USES

Sildenafil acts by relaxing smooth muscle in the corpus cavernosum, thus allowing increased blood flow into the penis. The increased blood flow results in a firmer and longer lasting erection in about 70% of men taking the drug. The onset of action is relatively rapid, less than 1 hour, and its effects last 2 to 4 hours. Sildenafil blocks the enzyme phosphodiesterase-5.

Administration Alerts

■ Avoid administration of sildenafil with meals, especially high-fat meals, because absorption is decreased.

■ Avoid grapefruit juice when administering sildenafil.

ADVERSE EFFECTS AND INTERACTIONS

The most serious adverse effect, hypotension, occurs in patients concurrently taking organic nitrates for angina. Common side effects include headache, dizziness, flushing, rash, nasal congestion, diarrhea, dyspepsia, UTI, chest pain, or indigestion. Priapism, a sustained erection lasting longer than 6 hours has been reported with sildenafil use and may lead to permanent damage to penile tissues.

Sildenafil interacts with many drugs. Cimetidine, erythromycin, and ketoconazole will increase serum levels of sildenafil and necessitate lower drug doses. Protease inhibitors (ritonavir, amprenavir, others) will cause increased sildenafil levels, which may lead to toxicity. Rifampin may decrease sildenafil levels, leading to decreased effectiveness.

 See the companion website for a Nursing Process Focus specific to this drug.

It is a nonmalignant disorder that progressively decreases the outflow of urine by obstructing the urethra, causing difficult urination. BPH is not considered to be a precursor to prostate carcinoma.

BPH is characterized by increased urinary frequency (usually with small amounts of urine), increased urgency to urinate, postvoid leakage, excessive nighttime urination, decreased force of the urine stream, and a sensation that the bladder did not empty completely. The urinary outlet obstruction can lead to serious complications such as urinary infections or uremia. In severe cases, a surgical procedure called transurethral resection is needed to restore the patency of the urethra. BPH is illustrated in Figure 42.2.

ANTIPROSTATIC AGENTS

Only a few drugs are available for the pharmacotherapy of BPH. Early in the course of the disease, drug therapy may be of benefit. These agents are shown in Table 42.2.

42.5 Pharmacotherapy of Benign Prostatic Hyperplasia

Although most of the symptoms of BPH are caused by static pressure of the enlarged prostate on the urethra, approximately 40% of the pressure has a functional component caused by increased smooth muscle tone in the region. Alpha$_1$-adrenergic receptors are located in smooth muscle cells in the neck of the urinary bladder, and in the prostate gland. The role of these receptors in normal physiology is not completely understood. When activated, however, the alpha$_1$-adrenergic receptors provide resistance to urine outflow from the bladder and inhibit the micturition reflex.

Only a few drugs are available to treat benign enlargement of the prostate. Although the drugs have limited efficacy, they have some value in treating mild disease, as an alternative to

NATURAL THERAPIES | Saw Palmetto

Saw palmetto *(Serona repens)* is a bushy palm that grows in the coastal regions of the southern United States. The portion having medicinal properties is the berries of the plant. Like finasteride, saw palmetto is thought to help stop a cascade of prostate-damaging enzymes that may create BPH. It also occupies binding sites on the prostate that are typically occupied by dihydrotestosterone (DHT), an enzyme that may trigger BPH. It may reduce prostate swelling and inflammation by blocking estradiol, a type of estrogen that can cause prostate cells to multiply. Several clinical studies have suggested that saw palmetto is as effective as finasteride at treating mild to moderate BPH and produces fewer side effects.

Saw palmetto contains a variety of sterols and free fatty acids that are thought to be responsible for its beneficial actions, although the sterol beta-sitosterol has recently been proposed as the major active ingredient. Doses range from 160–320 mg/day of standardized extract or 2–3 mg/day of dried berries.

surgery. Because pharmacotherapy alleviates the symptoms but does not cure the disease, these medications must be taken the remainder of the patient's life, or until surgery is indicated. The most common drug for BPH is finasteride (Proscar), a 5-alpha-reductase inhibitor featured as the prototype.

Although primarily used for hypertension, several alpha$_1$-adrenergic blockers have been approved for BPH. The selective alpha$_1$-blockers relax smooth muscle in the prostate gland, bladder neck, and urethra, thus easing the urinary obstruction. Doxazosin (Cardura) and terazosin (Hytrin) are of particular value to patients who have both hypertension and BPH; these two disorders occur concurrently in about 25% of men over age 60. A third alpha$_1$-blocker, tamsulosin (Flomax), has no effect on blood pressure and its only indication is BPH. Drugs in this class improve urine flow and reduce other bothersome symptoms of BPH within 1 to 2 weeks

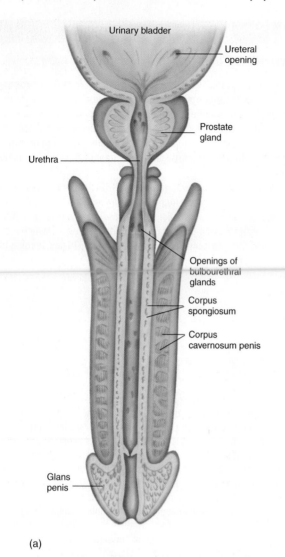

(a)

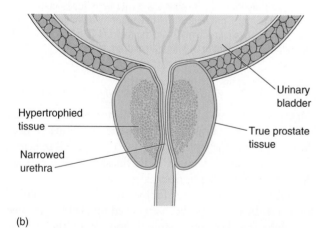

(b)

Figure 42.2 | Benign prostatic hyperplasia: (a) normal prostate with penis; (b) benign prostatic hyperplasia *Source: Pearson Education/PH College.*

after administration. Primary adverse effects include headache, fatigue, and dizziness. Doxazosin and terazosin are not associated with an increased risk of sexual dysfunction, but ejaculatory dysfunction has been reported with tamsulosin. Reflex tachycardia due to stimulation of baroreceptors is common with alpha-blockers. Additional information on the alpha-blockers presented in Chapter 21 ∞ .

NURSING CONSIDERATIONS

The role of the nurse in drug therapy with antiprostatic agents involves careful monitoring of a patient's condition and providing education as it relates to the prescribed drug regimen. The nurse should obtain a complete physical examination including history of cardiovascular disease and sexual dysfunction. The nurse should also assess changes in urinary elimination including urinary retention, nocturia, dribbling, difficulty starting urinary stream, frequency, and urgency. If the patient is prescribed alpha-blockers for treatment of prostatic hypertrophy, the patient's vital signs should be assessed, especially blood pressure and heart rate. The patient may experience hypotension with the first few doses and orthostatic hypotension may persist throughout treatment. The first dose phenomenon, especially syncope, can occur. The nurse should monitor the patient for evidence of orthostatic hypotension, dizziness, and GI disturbances. The elderly are especially prone to the hypotensive and hypothermic effects related to vasodilation caused by these drugs. Alpha-blockers should be used cautiously in patients with asthma or heart failure because they cause bradycardia and bronchoconstriction.

Exercise caution in patients with decreased hepatic function, because the drugs are metabolized in the liver. Patients with obstructive uropathy should use finasteride cautiously. The nurse should monitor the emotional status of patients taking alpha-blockers, as depression is a common side effect. The nurse should inform the patient that it may take 6 to 12 months of treatment before the drug relieves symptoms of BPH. Improvement will last only as long as the medication is continued.

The nurse should monitor for side effects of the antiprostatic agent. Side effects include impotence, decreased volume of ejaculate, or decreased libido. The nurse should inform the patient to report these occurrences to the healthcare provider.

Patient education related to antiprostatic agents should include goals, reasons for obtaining baseline data such as vital signs and tests for cardiac and renal disorders, and possible side effects.

For patients receiving an alpha-blocker, following are the important teaching points.

■ Report increased difficulty with urinary voiding.
■ Report significant side effects.
■ Take medication at bedtime, and take the first dose immediately before getting into bed.
■ Always arise slowly, avoiding sudden posture changes.

See "Patients Receiving Finasteride (Proscar)" for specific points the nurse should include when teaching patients regarding this drug.

Table 42.2	Agents for Benign Prostatic Hyperplasia
Drug	**Route and Adult Dose (max dose where indicated)**
Alpha Adrenergic Blockers	
doxazosin (Cardura) (see page 278 for the Protoype Drug box) ⊖	PO; 1–8 mg qd
prazosin (Minipress)	PO; 1 mg qid or bid
tamsulosin (Flomax)	PO; 0.4 mg qd 30 min after a meal 0.8 mg qd (max/)
terazosin (Hytrin)	PO; start with 1 mg hs, then 1–5 mg/d (max 20 mg/d)
5-Alpha Reductase Inhibitor	
finasteride (Proscar)	PO; 5 mg qd

Pr PROTOTYPE DRUG | FINASTERIDE (Proscar)

ACTIONS AND USES

Finasteride acts by inhibiting 5-alpha-reductase, the enzyme responsible for converting testosterone to one of its metabolites, 5-alpha-dihydrotestosterone. This metabolite causes proliferation of prostate cells and promotes enlargement of the gland. Because it inhibits the metabolism of testosterone, finasteride is sometimes called an antiandrogen. Finasteride promotes shrinkage of enlarged prostates and subsequently helps to restore urinary function. It is most effective in patients with larger prostates. This drug is also marketed as Propecia, which is prescribed to promote hair regrowth in patients with male-pattern baldness. Doses of finasteride are 5 times higher when prescribed for BPH than when prescribed for baldness.

Administration Alerts

- Tablets may be crushed for oral administration.
- The pregnant nurse should avoid handling crushed medication as it may be absorbed through the skin and cause harm to a male fetus.

ADVERSE EFFECTS AND INTERACTIONS

Finasteride causes various types of sexual dysfunction in up to 16% of patients, including impotence, diminished libido, and ejaculatory dysfunction.

No clinically significant drug interactions have been established.

Use with caution with herbal supplements. For example, saw palmetto may potentiate the effects of finasteride.

NURSING PROCESS FOCUS | PATIENTS RECEIVING FINASTERIDE (Proscar)

ASSESSMENT

Prior to administration:
- Obtain complete health history including liver disease and altered urinary functioning.
- Obtain drug history to determine possible drug interactions and allergies.
- Determine if patient has a female partner who is pregnant or who is planning to become pregnant.

POTENTIAL NURSING DIAGNOSES

- Noncompliance, related to side effects of drug
- Deficient Knowledge, related to drug therapy
- Sexual Dysfunction, related to adverse reaction to drug therapy

PLANNING: PATIENT GOALS AND EXPECTED OUTCOMES

The patient will:
- Experience a decreased size of enlarged prostate gland
- Demonstrate an understanding of the drug's action by accurately describing drug side effects and precautions, and importance of follow-up care

IMPLEMENTATION

Interventions and (Rationales)	*Patient Education/Discharge Planning*
■ Monitor urinary function. (Finasteride may interfere with PSA test results.)	Instruct patient to: ■ Schedule a digital rectal exam and PSA test periodically during therapy ■ Recognize and report symptoms of BPH: urinary retention, hesitancy, difficulty starting stream, decreased diameter of stream, nocturia, dribbling, frequency ■ Avoid all fluids in evenings, especially caffeine-containing fluids and alcohol, to avoid nocturia ■ Drink adequate fluids early in day, to decrease chances of kidney stones and UTI
■ Monitor female partner for pregnancy. (Finasteride is teratogenic to the male fetus.)	Instruct patient and/or female partner to: ■ Avoid semen of man using finasteride ■ Avoid touching crushed tablets of finasteride, to prevent transdermal absorption, and the transfer of medication through placenta to fetus ■ Use a reliable barrier contraceptive during therapy
■ Monitor patient's commitment to the medication regimen. (Maximum therapeutic effects may take several months.)	Instruct patient and/or female partner to: ■ Continue medication even if no decrease in symptoms for 6 to 12 months, or no increase in hair growth for 3 months ■ Recognize that lifelong therapy may be necessary to control symptoms of BPH
■ Monitor for adverse reactions.	■ Instruct patient and/or female partner to report impotence, decreased volume of ejaculate, or decreased libido.

EVALUATION OF OUTCOME CRITERIA

Evaluate the effectiveness of drug therapy by confirming that patient goals and expected outcomes have been met (see "Planning").

CHAPTER REVIEW

Key Concepts

The numbered key concepts provide a succinct summary of the important points from the corresponding numbered section within the chapter. If any of these points are not clear, refer to the numbered section within the chapter for review. Expanded versions can be found on the companion website.

42.1 FSH and LH from the pituitary regulate the secretion of testosterone, the primary hormone contributing to the growth, health, and maintenance of the male reproductive system.

42.2 Androgens are used to treat hypogonadism in males, and breast cancer in females. Anabolic steroids are frequently abused by athletes, and can result in serious adverse effects with long-term use.

42.3 Male infertility is difficult to treat pharmacologically; medications include HCG, menotropins, testolactone, and antiestrogens.

42.4 Erectile dysfunction is a common disorder that may be successfully treated with sildenafil (Viagra), an inhibitor of the enzyme phosphodiesterase-5.

42.5 In its early stages, benign prostatic hyperplasia may be treated successfully with drug therapy, including finasteride (Proscar) and alpha$_1$-adrenergic blockers.

Review Questions

1. Why is sildenafil used to treat erectile dysfunction rather than testosterone?

2. Why is the treatment of male infertility less successful than the treatment of female infertility?

3. Why is treatment with alpha$_1$-adrenergic blockers more successful at alleviating symptoms of BPH than 5-alpha-reductase inhibitors, in men with only slightly enlarged prostates?

Critical Thinking Questions

1. A 78-year-old widower has come to see his healthcare provider. The nurse practitioner interviews the patient about his past medical history and current health concerns. The patient states that he is planning to marry "a very nice lady," but is concerned about his sexual performance. He asks about a prescription for sildenafil (Viagra). What additional historical data does the nurse need to collect given this patient's age?

2. A 16-year-old male goes out for the football team. He is immediately impressed with the size of several junior and senior lineman. One older student offers to "hook him up"

with a source for androstenedione (Andro). From a developmental perspective, explain why this young man may be susceptible to anabolic steroid abuse. Can anabolic steroid abuse impact his stature?

3. A 68-year-old man has been diagnosed with benign prostatic hyperplasia (BPH). As the nurse prepares to educate him about his prescription for finasteride (Proscar), he says that he has been hearing about the benefits of saw palmetto, an herbal preparation. Discuss the mechanism of action of finasteride and compare it to that of saw palmetto.

EXPLORE MediaLink

NCLEX review, case studies, and other interactive resources for this chapter can be found on the companion website at www.prenhall.com/adams. Click on "Chapter 42" to select the activities for this chapter. For animations, more NCLEX review questions, and an audio glossary, access the accompanying CD-ROM in this textbook.

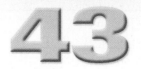
■ DRUGS AT A GLANCE

LOOP (HIGH-CEILING) DIURETICS

THIAZIDE AND THIAZIDELIKE DIURETICS
Pₜ *chlorothiazide (Diuril)*

POTASSIUM-SPARING DIURETICS
Pₜ *spironolactone (Aldactone)*

MISCELLANEOUS AGENTS
Carbonic anhydrase inhibitors
Osmotic diuretics

metabolized and eliminated by the bod
of this process
PHARMACOLOGY
1. The study of medicines; the disciplin
pertaining to how drugs improve the he
of the human body

MediaLink   www.prenhall.com/adams

CD-ROM
Animation:
    Basic Function of the Kidney
Audio Glossary
NCLEX Review

Companion Website
NCLEX Review
Dosage Calculations
Case Study
Care Plans
Expanded Key Concepts

OBJECTIVES

After reading this chapter, the student should be able to:

1. Explain the role of the urinary system in maintaining fluid, electrolyte, acid, and base balance.
2. Explain the processes that occur as filtrate travels through the nephron.
3. Describe the adjustments in pharmacotherapy that must be considered in patients with renal failure.
4. Identify indications for diuretics.
5. Identify the general side effects expected during pharmacotherapy with diuretics.
6. Compare and contrast the loop, thiazide, and potassium-sparing diuretics.

7. Describe the nurse's role in the pharmacologic management of renal disorders, and in diuretic therapy.
8. For each of the classes shown in Drugs at a Glance, identify representative drugs, explain the mechanism of drug action, primary actions, and important adverse effects.
9. Categorize drugs used in the treatment of urinary system disorders based on their classification and mechanism of action.
10. Use the Nursing Process to care for patients who are receiving drug therapy for renal disorders, and diuretic therapy.

The kidneys serve an amazing role in maintaining proper homeostasis. By filtering a volume equivalent to all the body's extracellular fluid every 100 minutes, the kidneys are able to make immediate adjustments to fluid volume, electrolyte composition, and acid-base balance. The purpose of this chapter is to examine agents that influence kidney function by increasing urine output. Chapter 44 will cover agents that more specifically affect fluid, electrolyte, and acid-base imbalances⬤ .

PHARMFACTS Renal Disorders

- Over 12,000 kidney transplants are performed annually.
- Over 47,000 people are on a waiting list for kidney transplants.
- One of every 750 people is born with a single kidney. A single kidney is larger and more vulnerable to injury from heavy contact sports.
- Urinary tract infection (UTI) is more common in women: 20% to 30% of females experience recurrent infections.
- About 260,000 Americans suffer from chronic kidney failure and 50,000 die annually from causes related to the disease.
- Type 2 diabetes is the leading cause of chronic kidney failure, accounting for 30% to 40% of all new cases each year.
- Hypertension is the second leading cause of chronic kidney failure, accounting for about 25% of all new cases each year.

43.1 Functions of the Kidneys

When most people think of the kidneys, they think of excretion. Although this is certainly true, the kidneys have (MediaLink Basic Function of the Kidney Animation) many other homeostatic functions. The kidneys are the primary organs for regulating fluid balance, electrolyte composition, and acid-base balance of body fluids. They also secrete the enzyme renin, which helps to regulate blood pressure (Chapter 21) and erythropoietin, a hormone that stimulates red blood cell production (Chapter 28)⬤ . In addition, the kidneys are responsible for the production of calcitriol, the active form of vitamin D, which helps maintain bone homeostasis (Chapter 46)⬤ . It is not surprising that the overall health of the patient is strongly dependent on proper functioning of the kidneys.

The urinary system consists of two kidneys, two ureters, one urinary bladder, and a urethra. Each kidney contains over 1 million **nephrons**, the functional units of the kidney. As blood enters a nephron, it is filtered through a semipermeable membrane known as **Bowman's capsule**. Water and other small molecules readily pass through Bowman's capsule and enter the first section of the nephron, the **proximal tubule**. Once in the nephron, the fluid is called **filtrate**. After leaving the proximal tubule, the filtrate travels through the **loop of Henle** and, subsequently, the **distal tubule**. Nephrons empty their filtrate into common collecting ducts, and then into larger and larger collecting portions inside the kidney. Fluid leaving the collecting ducts and entering subsequent portions of the kidney is called urine. Parts of the nephron are illustrated in Figure 43.1.

water entering the filtrate each day, 45.5 gal are reabsorbed, leaving only 1.5 L to be excreted in the urine. Glucose, amino acids, and essential ions such as sodium, chloride, calcium, and bicarbonate are also reabsorbed.

Certain ions and molecules too large to pass through Bowman's capsule may still enter the urine by crossing from the blood to the filtrate using a process known as **secretion**. Potassium, phosphate, hydrogen, and ammonium ions and many organic acids enter the filtrate through this mechanism.

Reabsorption and secretion are critical to the pharmacokinetics of many drugs. Some drugs are reabsorbed, whereas others are secreted into the filtrate. For example, approximately 90% of a dose of penicillin G enters the urine through secretion. The processes of reabsorption and secretion are shown in Figure 43.1.

43.2 Renal Reabsorption and Secretion

When filtrate passes through Bowman's capsule, its composition is the same as plasma minus large proteins, such as albumin, that are too large to pass through the filter. As it travels through the nephron, the composition of filtrate changes dramatically. Some substances in the filtrate pass across the walls of the nephron to reenter the blood, a process known as **reabsorption**. Water is the most important molecule reabsorbed in the tubule. For every 47 gal of

RENAL FAILURE

Renal failure is the decrease in kidney function resulting in an inability to maintain electrolyte and fluid balance and excrete nitrogenous waste products. Renal failure may be acute or chronic, and may result from disorders of other body systems or be intrinsic to the kidney itself. The primary treatment goal is to maintain blood flow through the kidney and adequate urine output.

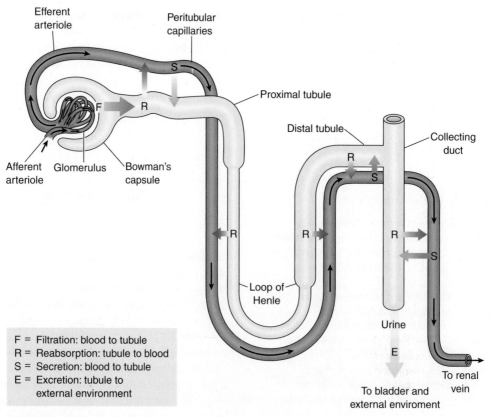

F = Filtration: blood to tubule
R = Reabsorption: tubule to blood
S = Secretion: blood to tubule
E = Excretion: tubule to external environment

Figure 43.1 | The nephron

43.3 Pharmacotherapy of Renal Failure

Before pharmacotherapy may be considered in a patient with renal failure, an accurate diagnosis of the kidney impairment is necessary. The basic diagnostic test is a urinalysis, which examines urine for the presence of blood cells, proteins, pH, specific gravity, ketones, glucose, and microorganisms. Although it is easy to perform, the urinalysis is nonspecific and does not identify the etiology of the kidney disease. Many diseases can cause abnormal urinalysis values. To provide a more definitive diagnosis, diagnostic imaging such as computed tomography, sonography, or magnetic resonance imaging may be necessary. Renal biopsy may be performed to obtain a more specific diagnosis.

Renal failure is classified as acute or chronic. Acute renal failure requires immediate treatment because retention of nitrogenous waste products in the body such as urea and creatinine, known as azotemia, can result in death if untreated. The most common cause of acute renal failure is renal hypoperfusion: lack of sufficient blood flowing through the kidneys. Hypoperfusion can lead to permanent damage to kidney cells. To correct this type of renal failure, the cause of the hypoperfusion must be quickly identified and corrected. Potential causes include heart failure, dysrhythmias, hemorrhage, and dehydration.

Chronic renal failure occurs over a period of months or years. Over half of the cases of chronic renal failure occur in patients with long-standing hypertension or diabetes mellitus. Due to its long development and nonspecific symptoms, chronic renal failure may go undiagnosed for many years, until the impairment becomes irreversible. In end-stage renal disease, dialysis and kidney transplantation become treatment alternatives.

Pharmacotherapy of renal failure attempts to cure the cause of the dysfunction. Diuretics are given to increase urine output and cardiovascular drugs are commonly administered to treat underlying hypertension or heart failure. Dietary management is often necessary to prevent worsening of renal impairment. Depending on the stage of the disease, dietary management may include protein restriction and reduction of sodium, potassium, phosphorous, and magnesium. A summary of the pharmacologic agents used to treat kidney failure is given in Table 43.1.

The nurse serves a key role in recognizing and responding to renal failure. Once a diagnosis is established, all nephrotoxic medications should be either discontinued or used with extreme caution. Common nephrotoxic drugs include NSAIDs, aminoglycoside antibiotics, amphotericin B, many antineoplastic agents and ACE inhibitors in volume-depleted patients. Because the kidneys excrete most drugs, medications will require a significant dosage reduction in patients with moderate to severe renal failure. The importance of this cannot be overemphasized: administering the "average" dose to a patient in severe renal failure can have mortal consequences.

DIURETICS

Diuretics are drugs that adjust the volume and/or composition of body fluids. They are of particular value in the treatment of renal failure, hypertension, and removing edema fluid in patients with heart failure.

43.4 Mechanism of Action of Diuretics

A diuretic is a drug that increases urine output. Mobilizing excess fluid in the body for the purpose of excretion is particularly desirable in the following conditions.

- Hypertension
- Heart failure
- Kidney failure
- Liver failure or cirrhosis
- Pulmonary edema

Table 43.1	Pharmacologic Management of Renal Failure	
Complication	**Pathogenesis**	**Treatment**
Anemia	Hypoperfusion of kidneys results in less erythropoietin synthesis	erythropoietin (epoetin alfa, Procrit, Epogen)
Hyperkalemia	Kidneys are unable to adequately excrete potassium	Dietary restriction of potassium; polystyrene sulfate (Kayexalate) with sorbitol
Hyperphosphatemia	Kidneys are unable to adequately excrete phosphate	Dietary restriction of phosphate; Phosphate binders such as calcium carbonate (Os-Cal 500, others), calcium acetate (PhosLo) or sevelamer HCl (Renagel)
Hypervolemia	Hypoperfusion of kidneys leads to water retention	Dietary restriction of sodium Loop diuretics in acute conditions, thiazide diuretics in mild conditions
Hypocalcemia	Hyperphosphatemia leads to loss of calcium	Usually corrected by reversing the hyperphosphatemia but additional calcium supplements may be necessary
Metabolic acidosis	Kidneys are unable to adequately excrete metabolic acids	sodium bicarbonate or sodium citrate

Most diuretics act by blocking sodium (Na^+) reabsorption in the nephron, thus sending more Na^+ to the urine. Chloride ion (Cl^-) follows sodium. Because water molecules also tend to travel with sodium ions, blocking the reabsorption of Na^+ will increase the volume of urination, or diuresis. Some drugs, such as furosemide (Lasix), act by preventing the reabsorption of sodium in the loop of Henle. Because of the abundance of sodium in the filtrate within the loop of Henle, furosemide is capable of producing large increases in urine output. Other drugs, such as the thiazides, act on the distal tubule. Because most Na^+ has already been reabsorbed from the filtrate by the time it reaches the distal tubule, the thiazides produce less diuresis than furosemide. The sites in the nephron at which the various diuretics act are shown in Figure 43.2.

It is common practice to combine two or more drugs in the pharmacotherapy of hypertension and fluid retention disorders. The primary rationales for combination therapy are that the incidence of side effects is decreased and the pharmacologic effect may be enhanced. For patient convenience, some of these drugs are combined in single tablet formulations. Examples of single tablet diuretic combinations include the following:

- Aldactazide: hydrochlorothiazide and spironolactone
- Apresazide: hydrochlorothiazide and hydralazine
- Dyazide: hydrochlorothiazide and triamterene
- Maxzide: hydrochlorothiazide and triamterene

43.5 Pharmacotherapy with Loop Diuretics

The most effective diuretics are called loop or high-ceiling diuretics. Drugs in this class act by blocking the reabsorption of sodium and chloride in the loop of Henle. When given IV, they have the ability to cause large amounts of fluid to be excreted by the kidney in a very short time. Loop diuretics are used to reduce the edema associated with heart failure, hepatic cirrhosis, or chronic renal failure. Furosemide and torsemide are also approved for hypertension. The loop diuretics are shown in Table 43.2.

Furosemide is the most commonly prescribed loop diuretic. A drug profile for furosemide was given in Chapter 22 ☞ . Unlike the thiazide diuretics, furosemide is able to increase urine output even when blood flow to the kidneys is diminished, which makes it of particular value in patients with renal failure. Torsemide has a longer half-life than furosemide, which offers the advantage of once-a-day dosing. Bumetanide (Bumex) is 40 times more potent than furosemide, but has a shorter duration of action.

The rapid excretion of large amounts of water has the potential to produce serious adverse effects such as dehydration and electrolyte imbalances. Signs of dehydration include thirst, dry mouth, weight loss, and headache. Hypotension, dizziness, and fainting can result from the fluid loss. Excess potassium loss may result in dysrhythmias;

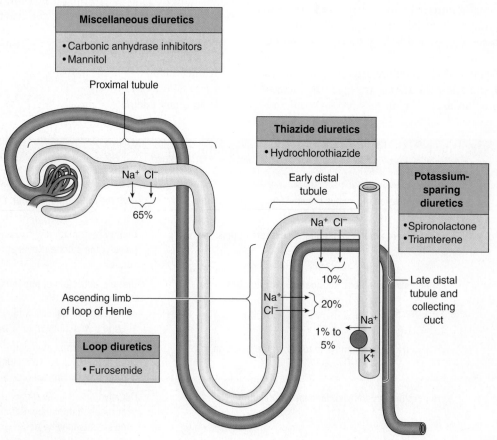

Figure 43.2 | Sites of action of the diuretics

Table 43.2	Loop Diuretics
Drug	**Route and Adult Dose (max dose where indicated)**
bumetanide (Bumex)	PO; 0.5–2 mg qd, may repeat at 4–5 h intervals if needed (max 10 mg/d) IV/IM: 0.5–1 mg over 1–2 min, repeated q2–3h prn (max 10 mg/d)
ethacrynic acid (Edecrin)	PO; 50–100 mg 1–2 qd-bid, may increase by 25–50 mg prn up to 400 mg/d IV; 0.5–1 mg/kg or 50 mg up to 100 mg, may repeat if necessary
furosemide (Lasix) (see page 293 for the Prototype Drug box)	PO; 20–80 mg in 1 or more divided doses (max 600 mg/d) IV/IM; 20–40 mg in 1 or more divided doses up to 600 mg/d
torsemide (Demadex)	PO/IV; 10–20 mg qd (max 200 mg/d)

potassium supplements may be indicated to prevent hypokalemia. Potassium loss is of particular concern to patients who are also taking digoxin (Lanoxin). Although rare, ototoxicity is possible and other ototoxic drugs such as the aminoglycoside antibiotics should be avoided during loop diuretic therapy. Because of the potential for serious side effects, the loop diuretics are normally reserved for patients with moderate to severe fluid retention, or when other diuretics have failed to achieve therapeutic goals.

NURSING CONSIDERATIONS

The role of the nurse in loop diuretic therapy involves careful monitoring of a patient's condition and providing education as it relates to the prescribed drug regimen. Prior to initiation of therapy, the nurse should obtain baseline values for weight, blood pressure (sitting and supine), pulse, respiration, and electrolytes. Any sites of edema and its extent should be recorded. The nurse should measure abdominal girth for patients with fluid in the abdomen (ascites). Loop diuretics should be used with caution in patients with cardiovascular disease, renal impairment, diabetes mellitus, or a history of gout. They should also be used with caution in patients who are pregnant, or concurrently taking digoxin, lithium, ototoxic drugs, NSAIDs, or other antihypertensives.

Blood pressure and pulse rate should be monitored regularly. Should a substantial drop in blood pressure occur, the medication should be withheld and the pressure reported to the physician. Intake and output should be monitored, including weighing the patient daily and evaluating for decreased edema. Potassium levels should be monitored closely, as loop diuretics cause potassium depletion. The nurse should closely observe elderly patients for weakness, hypotension, and confusion. The nurse should monitor lab results for electrolyte imbalance, elevated BUN, hyperglycemia, and anemia, which can be side effects of diuretics. The nurse should monitor vital signs and intake and output carefully to establish effectiveness of the medication. Rapid and excessive diuresis can result in dehydration, hypovolemia, and circulatory collapse.

Patient education as it relates to loop diuretics should include goals, reasons for obtaining baseline data such as vital signs and tests for renal disorders, and possible side effects. Following are important points the nurse should include when teaching patients regarding loop diuretics.

SPECIAL CONSIDERATIONS

Diuretic Therapy in Elderly Patients

Diuretic therapy is commonly used to treat elderly patients with chronic diseases such as heart failure. The target goal for diuretic therapy is removal of excess fluid, to reduce the cardiac workload. This can be a problem for the elderly for several reasons. Diuretics can cause frequent urination, which can be inconvenient and increase the likelihood of incontinence in an elderly person. With the threat of this embarrassment, the older adult may opt for less participation in activities, resulting in social isolation. Depression may result. In addition to these risks, diuretics can cause electrolyte imbalances, making the elderly person susceptible to faintness, dizziness, and falls. Again, fear of these adverse effects can promote isolation. Nurses must assess for these concerns and work with the patient on alternatives to help the elderly take diuretic therapy and maintain the quality of their lives.

- Weigh self daily, preferably in the morning before eating.
- Maintain a weight record.
- Monitor blood pressure and report substantial pressure drops.
- Make position changes slowly, because diuretics in combination with other drugs can cause dizziness.
- Report any hearing loss.
- Monitor blood glucose diligently (for diabetic patients).
- Report tenderness or swelling in joints which may indicate gout.

43.6 Pharmacotherapy with Thiazide Diuretics

The thiazides comprise the largest, most commonly prescribed class of diuretics. These drugs act on the distal tubule to block Na^+ reabsorption and increase potassium and water excretion. Their primary use is for the treatment of mild to moderate hypertension, however, they are also indicated for edema due to mild to moderate heart failure, liver failure, and renal failure. They are less efficacious than the loop diuretics and are not effective in patients with severe renal failure. The thiazide diuretics are shown in Table 43.3.

All the thiazide diuretics have equivalent efficacy and safety profiles. They differ, however, in their potency and duration of action. Four drugs, chlorthalidone (Hygroton), indapamide (Lozol), metolazone (Mykrox, Zaroxolyn), and quinethazone (Hydromox) are not true thiazides, though they are included with this drug class because they have similar actions and side effects.

Other than lack of ototoxicity, the side effects of the thiazides are identical to those of the loop diuretics, though their frequency is less. The nurse should assess for signs and symptoms of dehydration and excessive loss of sodium, potassium, or chloride ions. Concurrent therapy with digoxin requires careful monitoring to avoid excessive potassium loss. Diabetic patients should be made aware that thiazide diuretics sometimes raise blood glucose levels.

NURSING CONSIDERATIONS

The role of the nurse in thiazide diuretic therapy involves careful monitoring of a patient's condition and providing education as it relates to the prescribed drug regimen. Prior to administering diuretics, the nurse should assess for hypotension and withhold the medication if low blood pressure is present. The nurse should assess for hypersensitivity to thiazides or sulfonamides, anuria, and hypokalemia because thiazides are contraindicated in patients with these conditions. They should be used with caution in patients who are allergic to sulfa, are diabetic, or have impaired renal or hepatic function. Baseline lab tests such as CBC, electrolytes, BUN, creatinine, uric acid, and blood glucose should be obtained. All diuretics, including thiazide diuretics, reduce circulating blood volume that may cause orthostatic hypotension and changes in serum electrolyte levels. The nurse should examine the skin and mucous membranes for turgor and moisture, because diuretics are notorious for causing dehydration. The nurse should monitor vital signs, especially blood pressure, when caring for patients taking thiazides. The Nursing Process Focus in Chapter 21 provides a quick guide to the care of all individuals receiving diuretic therapy ⊙.

Because the effectiveness of diuretic therapy is measured in weight loss and fluid output, the patient should be weighed at the same time of day, wearing the same type of clothing. A weight gain of more than 2 lb should be reported, as it may indicate fluid retention. The nurse must carefully monitor intake and output to determine hydration status and effectiveness of the medication. Conditions such as diarrhea, vomiting, or profuse sweating will increase fluid loss and put the patient at greater risk for dehydration.

Like loop diuretics, the thiazides cause potassium depletion, thus patients should be monitored for signs of hypokalemia. Dietary intake of high sodium foods may negate the effects of thiazide diuretic in reducing blood pressure or relieving excessive fluid volume.

Table 43.3	Thiazide and Thiazidelike Diuretics
Drug	**Route and Adult Dose (max dose where indicated)**
Short Acting	
℞chlorothiazide (Diuril)	PO; 250 mg–1 g/d in 1–2 divided doses. IV; 250 mg–1 g/d in 1–2 divided doses
hydrochlorothiazide (HydroDIURIL, HCTZ) (see page 267 for the Prototype Drug box) ⊙	PO; 25–200 mg/d in 1–3 divided doses
Intermediate Acting	
bendroflumethiazide (Naturetin)	PO; 2.5–20 mg/d in 1–2 divided doses
benzthiazide (Aquatag, Exna, Hydrex)	PO; 25–200 mg/d or qod
hydroflumethiazide (Diucardin, Saluron)	PO; 25 mg–200 mg/d in 1–2 divided doses
metolazone (Zaroxolyn, Mykrox)	PO; 5–20 mg qd
quinethazone (Hydromox)	PO; 50–100 mg qd
Long Acting	
chlorthalidone (Hygroton)	PO; 50–100 mg qd
indapamide (Lozol)	PO; 2.5–5 mg qd
methyclothiazide (Aquatensen, Enduron)	PO; 2.5–10 mg qd
polythiazide (Renese)	PO; 1–4 mg qd
trichlormethiazide (Metahydrin, Naqua, Niazide, Diurese)	PO; 1–4 mg qd–bid

Some thiazide diuretics may cause hyperglycemia and glycosuria in diabetic patients. Blood glucose levels should be monitored closely and dosage adjustments of hypoglycemic drugs may be indicated. Also, some patients with gout may experience hyperuricemia secondary to thiazide's interference with uric acid excretion. The nurse should monitor uric acid levels and assess for symptoms of gout such as pain, swelling, and redness in the joints.

Patient education as it relates to thiazides should include goals, reasons for obtaining baseline data such as vital signs and lab work, and possible side effects. Following are important points the nurse should include when teaching patients regarding thiazides.

■ Monitor blood pressure on a regular basis; withhold medication and report a blood pressure below specific written parameters.
■ Weigh every 2 to 3 days and report changes of more than 2 lb.
■ Consume foods that are high in potassium content such as oranges, peaches, bananas, dried apricots, potatoes, tomatoes, and broccoli.
■ Avoid food high in sodium content, such as canned foods, "fast" foods, and frozen dinners.
■ Protect skin from exposure to direct sunlight because these medications can cause photosensitivity.
■ Take thiazide diuretics in the morning when possible, to prevent the need to get up through the night to urinate.
■ Keep a symptom log during the initial phase of therapy to assist the healthcare provider in tailoring dosages as needed.

■ Use additional health promotional activities, in addition to diuretics, to help reduce blood pressure, such as smoking cessation, exercise, weight control, stress management, and moderate consumption of alcohol, if any.

See "Nursing Process Focus: Patients Receiving Diuretic Therapy" for the complete nursing process applied to caring for patients receiving diuretic therapy.

43.7 Pharmacotherapy with Potassium-Sparing Diuretics

Hypokalemia is one of the most serious adverse effects of the thiazide and loop diuretics. The therapeutic advantage of the potassium-sparing diuretics is that a mild diuresis can be obtained without affecting blood potassium levels. The potassium-sparing diuretics are shown in Table 43.4.

Normally, sodium and potassium are exchanged in the distal tubule; Na^+ is reabsorbed back into the body and K^+ is secreted into the tubule. Potassium-sparing diuretics block this exchange, causing sodium to stay in the tubule and ultimately leave through the urine. When sodium is blocked, the body retains more K^+. Because most of the sodium has already been removed before the filtrate reaches the distal tubule, potassium-sparing diuretics produce only a mild diuresis. Their primary use is in combination with thiazide or loop diuretics, to minimize potassium loss.

Unlike the loop and thiazide diuretics, patients taking potassium-sparing diuretics should not take potassium

---

Pr PROTOTYPE DRUG	CHLOROTHIAZIDE (Diuril)

ACTIONS AND USES

The most common indication for chlorothiazide is mild to moderate hypertension. It may be combined with other antihypertensives in the multidrug therapy of severe hypertension. It is also prescribed to treat fluid retention due to heart failure, liver disease, and corticosteroid or estrogen therapy. When given orally, it may take as long as 4 weeks to obtain the optimum therapeutic effect. When given IV, results are seen in 15 to 30 min.

Administration Alerts

■ Give oral doses in the morning to avoid interrupted sleep due to nocturia.
■ Give IV at a rate of 0.5 g over 5 min when administering intermittently.
■ When administering IV, take special care to avoid extravasation as this drug is highly irritating to tissues.
■ Pregnancy category C.

ADVERSE EFFECTS AND INTERACTIONS

Excess loss of water and electrolytes can occur during chlorothiazide pharmacotherapy. Symptoms include thirst, weakness, lethargy, muscle cramping, hypotension, and tachycardia. Due to the potentially serious consequences of hypokalemia, patients concurrently taking digoxin should be carefully monitored. The intake of potassium-rich foods should be increased, and potassium supplements may be indicated.

Chlorothiazide interacts with several drugs. For example, when administered with amphotericin B or corticosteroids, hypokalemic effects are increased. Antidiabetic medications such as sulfonylureas and insulin may be less effective when taken with chlorothiazide. Cholestyramine and colestipol decrease absorption of chlorothiazide. Concurrent adminisitration with digoxin may cause digitoxin toxicity due to increased potassium and magnesium loss. Alcohol potentiates the hypotensive action of some thiazide diuretics and caffeine may increase diuresis.

Use with caution with herbal supplements, such as licorice, which, in large amounts, will create an additive effect of hypokalemia. Aloe may increase potassium loss.

 See the companion website for a Nursing Process Focus specific to this drug.

Table 43.4	Potassium-sparing Diuretics
Drug	**Route and Adult Dose (max dose where indicated)**
amiloride hydrochloride (Midamor)	PO; 5 mg qd (max 20 mg/d)
spironolactone (Aldactone)	PO; 25–400 mg qd-bid
triamterene (Dyrenium)	PO; 100 mg bid (max 300 mg/d)

supplements or be advised to add potassium-rich foods to their diet. Intake of excess potassium when taking these medications may lead to hyperkalemia.

NURSING CONSIDERATIONS

The role of the nurse in potassium-sparing diuretic therapy involves careful monitoring of a patient's condition and providing education as it relates to the prescribed drug regimen. The nurse must constantly monitor the patient for signs of hyperkalemia, such as irritability, anxiety, abdominal cramping, and irregularities in pulse, because these diuretics prevent potassium from being excreted. The nurse should also assess for anuria, acute renal insufficiency, and impaired kidney function because potassium-sparing diuretics are contraindicated in these conditions. They should be used with caution in patients who have a BUN of 40 mg/dl or greater, and in patients with liver disease. As with thiazide diuretics, the nurse should monitor blood pressure before administering these drugs, as they cause a reduction in circulating blood volume and decreased blood pressure. Electrolyte levels, especially potassium and sodium, and renal function tests, should be obtained before initiating therapy and frequently during early therapy. The nurse should also assess for signs of hypersensitivity reaction, such as fever, sore throat, malaise, joint pain, ecchymoses, profound fatigue, shortness of breath, and pallor.

Some potassium-sparing diuretics cause dizziness when first prescribed, so the nurse must be careful to ensure patient safety when changing position and ambulating. The patient should be instructed to continue taking the medication even though he or she may be feeling well.

Patients taking potassium-sparing diuretics may experience decreased libido. Additional hormonal side effects that may occur with these diuretics include hirsutism in females, gynecomastia, impotence in males, irregular menses, amenorrhea, and postmenopausal bleeding. The nurse should report these side effects to the healthcare provider immediately, and provide emotional support.

Follow-up care is critical with patients taking potassium-sparing diuretics. The patient should have weekly blood pressure monitoring and EKG tests as directed by the healthcare provider, especially if therapy is prolonged.

Patient education as it relates to potassium-sparing diuretics should include goals, reasons for obtaining baseline data such as vital signs and lab tests for electrolytes, and

possible side effects. Following are important points the nurse should include when teaching patients regarding potassium-sparing diuretics.

- Report signs of hyperkalemia immediately, including irritability, anxiety, abdominal cramping, and irregular heart beat.
- Avoid using salt substitutes that are potassium based.
- Avoid eating excess amounts of foods high in potassium such as oranges, peaches, potatoes, tomatoes, broccoli, bananas, and dried apricots.
- Avoid performing tasks that require mental alertness until effects of medication are known.
- Do not abruptly discontinue taking the diuretic unless recommended by the healthcare provider.
- Take medication exactly as ordered and keep all appointments for follow-up care.
- Keep a symptom log during the initial phase of therapy to assist the healthcare provider in tailoring dosages as needed.
- Use additional health promotional activities to help reduce blood pressure, such as smoking cessation, exercise, weigh control, stress management, and moderate consumption of alcohol, if any.

See "Nursing Process Focus: Patients Receiving Diuretic Therapy" for the complete nursing process applied to caring for patients receiving diuretic therapy.

43.8 Miscellaneous Diuretics for Specific Indications

A few diuretics, shown in Table 43.5, cannot be classified as loop, thiazide, or potassium-sparing agents. These diuretics have limited and specific indications. Three of these drugs inhibit carbonic anhydrase, an enzyme that affects acid-base balance by its ability to form carbonic acid from water and carbon dioxide. For example, acetazolamide (Diamox) is a carbonic anhydrase inhibitor used to decrease intraocular fluid pressure in patients with open angle glaucoma (Chapter 48) 🔗. Unrelated to its diuretic effect, acetazolamide also has applications as an anticonvulsant and in treating motion sickness.

The osmotic diuretics also have very specific applications. For example, mannitol is used to maintain urine flow in patients with acute renal failure or during prolonged surgery. Since this agent is not reabsorbed in the tubule, it is

Pr PROTOTYPE DRUG | SPIRONOLACTONE (Aldactone)

ACTIONS AND USES

Spironolactone acts by blocking sodium reabsorption in the distal tubule. It accomplishes this by inhibiting aldosterone, the hormone secreted by the adrenal cortex that is responsible for increasing the renal reabsorption of sodium in exchange for potassium, thus causing water retention. When blocked by spironolactone, sodium and water excretion is increased and the body retains more potassium. The other two potassium-sparing diuretics do not exert an antialdosterone effect, but instead act by directly inhibiting the sodium-potassium exchange mechanism in the renal tubule.

Administration Alerts

■ Give with food to increase absorption of drug.
■ Do not give potassium supplements.
■ Pregnancy category D.

ADVERSE EFFECTS AND INTERACTIONS

Spironolactone does such an efficient job of retaining potassium that hyperkalemia may develop. The probability of hyperkalemia is increased if the patient takes potassium supplements or is concurrently taking ACE inhibitors. Signs and symptoms of hyperkalemia include muscle weakness, ventricular tachycardia, or fibrillation. When serum potassium levels are monitored carefully and maintained within normal values, side effects from spironolactone are uncommon.

Spironolactone interacts with several drugs. For example, when combined with ammonium chloride, acidosis may occur. Aspirin and other salicylates may decrease the diuretic effect of the medication. Concurrent use of spironolactone and digoxin may decrease the effects of digoxin. When taken with potassium supplements, ACE inhibitors, and ARBS, hyperkalemia may result.

 See the companion website for a Nursing Process Focus specific to this drug.

Table 43.5	Miscellaneous Diuretics
Drug	**Route and Adult Dose (max dose where indicated)**
Carbonic Anhydrase Inhibitors	
acetazolamide (Diamox)	PO; 250–375 mg qd
dichlorphenamide (Daranide, Oratrol)	PO; 25–50 mg qd-tid
methazolamide (Neptazane)	PO; 50–100 mg bid-tid
Osmotic Type	
mannitol (Osmitrol)	IV; 100 g infused over 2–6h
urea (Ureaphil)	IV; 1.0–1.5 g/kg over 1–2.5h

able to maintain the flow of filtrate even in cases with severe renal hypoperfusion. Mannitol can also be used to lower intraocular pressure in certain types of glaucoma. It is a highly potent diuretic that is only given by the IV route. Unlike other diuretics that draw excess fluid away from tissue spaces, mannitol can worsen edema and thus must be used with caution in patients with preexisting heart failure or pulmonary edema.

NATURAL THERAPIES | Cranberry for Urinary Tract Infections

Since the mid-1800s, cranberry has been used for the prevention of urinary tract infections. Cranberry causes an increase in the urine acidity, which discourages the growth of pathogenic microorganisms. A component in cranberries stops bacteria from adhering to bladder walls. Well-controlled studies have yet to clearly demonstrate that cranberry juice can lower the pH enough to actually kill organisms; however, anecdotal evidence remains strong in support of the treatment. The only reported adverse effect from cranberry is increased diarrhea when large quantities are ingested. If a juice form is used, unsweetened juices are preferred over sweetened. Dehydrated extracts of cranberries and blueberries are also available in capsule or tablet form.

 MediaLink | The Florida Health Site

| NURSING PROCESS FOCUS | PATIENTS RECEIVING DIURETIC THERAPY |

ASSESSMENT

Prior to administration:
- Obtain complete health history (mental and physical), including data on recent surgeries or trauma.
- Obtain vital signs; assess in context of patient's baseline values.
- Obtain patient's medication history, including nicotine and alcohol consumption to determine possible drug allergies and/or interactions.
- Obtain blood and urine specimens for laboratory analysis.

POTENTIAL NURSING DIAGNOSES

- Excess Fluid Volume, related to excessive diuresis secondary to diuretic use
- Risk for Deficient Fluid Volume
- Impaired Urinary Elimination, related to diuretic use

PLANNING: PATIENT GOALS AND EXPECTED OUTCOMES

The patient will:
- Exhibit normal fluid balance and maintain electrolyte levels within normal limits during drug therapy
- Demonstrate an understanding of the drug's action by accurately describing drug side effects and precautions
- Immediately report effects such as symptoms of hyperkalemia or hypokalemia and hypersensitivity

IMPLEMENTATION

Interventions and (Rationales)	*Patient Education/Discharge Planning*
■ Monitor laboratory values. (Diuretics can cause electrolyte imbalances.)	■ Instruct patient to inform laboratory personnel of diuretic therapy when providing blood or urine samples.
■ Monitor vital signs, especially blood pressure. (Diuretics reduce blood volume, resulting in lowered blood pressure.)	Instruct patient to: ■ Monitor blood pressure as specified by the healthcare provider and ensure proper use of home equipment ■ Withhold medication for severe hypotensive readings as specified by the healthcare provider (e.g., "hold for levels below 88/50")
■ Observe for changes in level of consciousness, dizziness, fatigue, and postural hypotension. (Reduction in blood volume due to diuretic therapy may produce changes in LOC or syncope.)	Instruct patient to: ■ Immediately report any change in consciousness, especially feeling faint ■ Avoid abrupt changes in posture; rise slowly from prolonged periods of sitting/lying down ■ Obtain blood pressure readings in sitting, standing, and supine positions
■ Monitor for fluid overload by measuring intake, output, and daily weights. (Intake, output, and daily body weight are indications of the effectiveness of duretic therapy.)	Instruct patient to: ■ Immediately report any severe shortness of breath, frothy sputum, profound fatigue and edema in extremities, potential signs of heart failure, or pulmonary edema ■ Accurately measure intake, output, and body weight and report weight gain of 2 lb or more within 2 days or decrease in output ■ Avoid excessive heat which contributes to fluid loss through perspiration ■ Consume adequate amounts of *plain water*
■ Monitor potassium intake. (Potassium is vital to maintaining proper electrolyte balance and can become depleted with thiazide or loop diuretics.)	For patients receiving loop or thiazide diuretics, encourage foods high in potassium. For patients receiving potassium-sparing diuretics: ■ Instruct patient to avoid foods high in potassium ■ Consult with healthcare provider before using vitamin/mineral supplements or electrolyte-fortified sports drinks

continued

NURSING PROCESS FOCUS: *Patients Receiving Diuretic Therapy (continued)*

Interventions and (Rationales)	Patient Education/Discharge Planning
■ Observe for signs of hypersensitivity reaction.	Instruct patient or caregiver to report: ■ Difficulty breathing, throat tightness, hives or rash, or bleeding ■ Flulike symptoms: shortness of breath, fever, sore throat, malaise, joint pain, profound fatigue
■ Monitor hearing and vision. (Loop diuretics are ototoxic. Thiazide diuretics increase serum digitalis levels; elevated levels produce visual changes.)	■ Instruct patient to report any changes in hearing or vision such as ringing or buzzing in the ears, becoming "hard of hearing" or experiencing dimness of sight, seeing halos, or having "yellow vision".
■ Monitor reactivity to light exposure. (Some diuretics cause photosensitivity.)	Instruct patient to: ■ Limit exposure to the sun ■ Wear dark glasses and light-colored loose-fitting clothes when outdoors

EVALUATION OF OUTCOME CRITERIA

Evaluate the effectiveness of drug therapy by confirming that patient goals and expected outcomes have been met (see "Planning").

See Tables 43.1 through 43.4 for lists of drugs to which these nursing actions apply.

CHAPTER REVIEW

Key Concepts

The numbered key concepts provide a succinct summary of the important points from the corresponding numbered section within the chapter. If any of these points are not clear, refer to the numbered section within the chapter for review. Expanded versions can be found on the companion website.

43.1 The kidneys regulate fluid volume, electrolytes, and acid-base balance.

43.2 As filtrate travels through the nephron, its composition changes dramatically as a result of the processes of reabsorption and secretion.

43.3 The dosage levels for most medications must be adjusted in patients with renal failure. Diuretics may be used to maintain urine output, while the cause of the hypoperfusion is treated.

43.4 Diuretics are drugs that increase urine output, usually by blocking sodium reabsorption.

43.5 The most efficacious diuretics are the loop or high-ceiling agents that block the reabsorption of sodium in the loop of Henle.

43.6 The thiazides act by blocking sodium reabsorption in the distal tubule of the nephron, and are the most widely prescribed class of diuretics.

43.7 Though less efficacious than the loop diuretics, potassium-sparing diuretics are used in combination with other agents, and help to prevent hypokalemia.

43.8 Several less commonly prescribed classes such as the osmotic diuretics and the carbonic anhydrase inhibitors have specific indications in reducing intraocular fluid pressure (acetazolamide) or reversing severe renal hypoperfusion (mannitol).

Review Questions

1. How does the composition of filtrate differ from that of blood?

2. Why are drugs that block sodium reabsorption at the loop of Henle more efficacious than those that act on the distal tubule?

3. Explain why hypokalemia is a common side effect of the hydrochlorothiazide, yet hyperkalemia is more common with spironolactone. What advice should the patient be given to avoid potassium imbalances?

Critical Thinking Questions

1. A 43-year-old male is diagnosed with hypertension following an annual physical examination. The patient is thin and states that he engages in fairly regular exercise but describes his job as highly stressful. He also has a positive family history of hypertension and stroke. The healthcare provider initiates therapy with losartan (Cozaar). After 2 months, the patient has noted no appreciable difference in blood pressure values. The healthcare provider switches the patient to Hyzaar, which proves to be very effective. Why is the new therapy more effective?

2. A 78-year-old female is admitted to the intensive care unit with a diagnosis of heart failure. The nurse administers furosemide (Lasix) 40 mg IV push. What assessments should the nurse make to determine the effectiveness of this therapy?

3. A 17-year-old male is admitted to the ICU following a car-train collision. The patient sustained a depressed skull fracture and is on a ventilator. Two days after surgery, there are obvious signs of increasing intracranial pressure. The nurse administers a 32 g 15% solution of mannitol (Osmitrol) per IV over 30 minutes. The patient's mother asks the nurse to explain why her son needs this drug. What explanation should the nurse offer?

EXPLORE MediaLink

NCLEX review, case studies, and other interactive resources for this chapter can be found on the companion website at www.prenhall.com/adams. Click on "Chapter 43" to select the activities for this chapter. For animations, more NCLEX review questions, and an audio glossary, access the accompanying CD-ROM in this textbook.

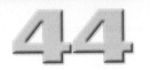

CHAPTER 44

Drugs for Fluid, Electrolyte, and Acid-Base Disorders

◼ DRUGS AT A GLANCE

FLUID REPLACEMENT AGENTS
Colloids
Pr *dextran 40 (Gentran 40, Hyskon, 10% LMD, Rheomacrodex)*
Crystalloids

ELECTROLYTES
Pr *sodium chloride*
Pr *potassium chloride*

ACID-BASE AGENTS
Pr *sodium bicarbonate*
Pr *ammonium chloride*

metabolized and eliminated by the body.
of this process
PHARMACOLOGY
1. The study of medicines; the discipline
pertaining to how drugs improve the heal
of the human body
PHARMACOPEIA

MediaLink www.prenhall.com/adams

CD-ROM
Animations:
    Fluid Balance
    Acids
Audio Glossary
NCLEX Review

Companion Website
NCLEX Review
Dosage Calculations
Case Study
Care Plans
Expanded Key Concepts

KEY TERMS

acidosis *page 663*
alkalosis *page 664*
anion *page 656*
buffer *page 662*
cation *page 656*
colloids *page 654*
crystalloids *page 654*

electrolytes *page 656*
extracellular fluid (ECF) compartment
page 652
hyperkalemia *page 660*
hypernatremia *page 658*
hypokalemia *page 660*
hyponatremia *page 658*

intracellular fluid (ICF) compartment
page 652
osmolality *page 653*
osmosis *page 653*
pH *page 661*
tonicity *page 653*

OBJECTIVES

After reading this chapter, the student should be able to:

1. Describe conditions in which therapy with IV fluids may be indicated.
2. Explain how changes in the osmolality or tonicity of a fluid can cause water to move to a different compartment.
3. Compare and contrast colloids and crystalloids used in IV therapy.
4. Explain the importance of electrolyte balance in the body.
5. Identify causes of sodium imbalance and the medications used to treat these conditions.
6. Identify causes of potassium imbalance and the medications used to treat these conditions.

7. Discuss common causes of alkalosis and acidosis and the medications used to treat these disorders.
8. Describe the nurse's role in the pharmacologic management of fluid, electrolyte, and acid-base disorders.
9. For each of the classes listed in Drugs at a Glance, identify representative drugs, explain the mechanism of drug action, primary actions, and important adverse effects.
10. Categorize drugs used in the treatment of fluid, electrolyte, and acid-base disorders based on their classification and mechanism of action.
11. Use the Nursing Process to care for patients who are receiving drug therapy for fluid, electrolyte, and acid-base disorders.

The maintenance of normal fluid volume, electrolyte composition, and acid-base balance is essential to life. Conditions such as hemorrhage and dehydration must be quickly treated, otherwise fluids and electrolytes will be rapidly depleted.

Disorders of acid-base balance may be acute, as in diabetic ketoacidosis, or they may proceed more slowly, over a period of months. Fortunately, safe and effective drugs are available to quickly reverse most symptoms of fluid volume, electrolyte, or acid-base imbalance.

FLUID BALANCE

Body fluids travel between compartments, which are separated by semipermeable membranes. Control of water balance in the various compartments is essential to homeostasis. Fluid imbalances are frequent indications for pharmacotherapy.

44.1 Body Fluid Compartments

The bulk of body fluid consists of water, which serves as the universal solvent in which most of the body's nutrients, electrolytes, and minerals are dissolved. Water alone is responsible for about 60% of the total body weight.

In a simple model, water in the body can be located in one of two places, or compartments. The intracellular fluid (ICF) compartment, which contains water that is *inside* cells, accounts for about two-thirds of the total body water. The remaining one-third of body fluid resides *outside* cells in the extracellular fluid (ECF) compartment. The ECF compartment is further divided into two parts: fluid in the *plasma* and fluid in the *interstitial spaces* between cells. The relationship between these fluid compartments is illustrated in Figure 44.1.

A continuous exchange and mixing of fluids occurs between the various compartments, which are separated by membranes. The plasma membranes of the cells separate the ICF from the ECF. The capillary membranes separate

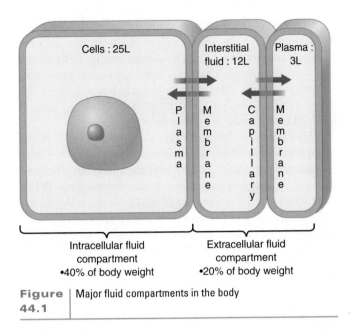

Figure 44.1 | Major fluid compartments in the body

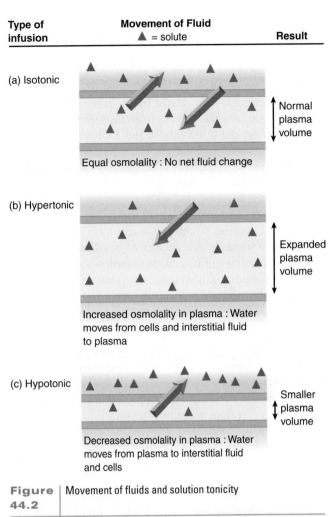

Figure 44.2 | Movement of fluids and solution tonicity

plasma from the interstitial fluid. Although water travels freely among the compartments, the movement of large molecules and those with electrical charges are governed by processes of diffusion and active transport. Movement of ions and drugs across membranes is a primary concern of pharmacokinetics (Chapter 5)⊕ .

44.2 Osmolality, Tonicity, and the Movement of Body Fluids

Osmolality and tonicity are two related terms central to understanding fluid balance in the body. Large changes in the osmolality or tonicity of a body fluid can cause significant shifts in water balance between compartments. The nurse will often administer IV fluids to compensate for these changes.

The **osmolality** of a fluid is determined by the number of dissolved particles, or solutes, in 1 kg (1 L) of water. In most body fluids, three solutes determine the osmolality: sodium, glucose, and urea. Sodium is the greatest contributor to osmolality due to its abundance in most body fluids. The normal osmolality of body fluids ranges from 275 to 295 milliosmols per kilogram (mOsm/kg).

The term **tonicity** is sometimes used interchangeably with osmolality although, they are somewhat different. Whereas osmolality is a laboratory value that can be precisely measured, tonicity is a general term used to describe the *relative* concentration of IV fluids. Tonicity is the ability of a solution to cause a change in water movement across a membrane due to osmotic forces. The tonicity of the plasma is used as the reference point when administering IV solutions: Normal plasma is considered isotonic. Solutions that are isotonic have the same concentration of solutes (same osmolality) as the blood. Hypertonic solutions have a greater concentration of solutes than plasma, whereas hypotonic solutions have a lesser concentration of solutes than plasma.

Through **osmosis**, water moves from areas of low solute concentration (low osmolality), to areas of high solute concentration (high osmolality). If a hypertonic (hyperosmolar) IV solution is administered, the plasma gains more solutes than the interstitial fluid. Water will move, by osmosis, from the interstitial fluid to the plasma. Water will move the opposite direction, from plasma to interstitial fluid, if a hypotonic solution is administered. Isotonic solutions will produce no net fluid shift. These movements are illustrated in Figure 44.2.

44.3 Regulation of Fluid Intake and Output

The average adult has a water intake of approximately 2500 ml/day, most of which comes from food and beverages. Water output is achieved through the kidneys, lungs, skin, feces, and sweat. To maintain water balance, water intake must equal water output. Gains or losses of water can be estimated by changes in total body weight.

The most important physiologic regulator of fluid intake is the thirst mechanism. The sensation of thirst occurs when osmoreceptors in the hypothalamus sense a hypertonic ECF. As saliva secretion diminishes and the mouth dries, the individual is driven to ingest liquid. As the ingested water is absorbed, the osmolality of the ECF falls and the thirst center in the hypothalamus is no longer stimulated.

The kidneys are the primary regulators of fluid output. Through the renin-angiotensin mechanism (Chapter 21), the hormone aldosterone is secreted by the adrenal cortex ⊂⊃. Aldosterone causes the kidneys to retain sodium and water, thus increasing the osmolality of the ECF. A second hormone, antidiuretic hormone (ADH), is released during periods of high plasma osmolality. ADH acts directly on the distal tubules of the kidney to increase water reabsorption.

Failure to properly balance intake with output can result in fluid volume disorders that are indications for pharmacologic intervention. Fluid deficit disorders can cause dehydration or shock, which are treated by administering oral or intravenous fluids. Fluid excess disorders are treated with diuretics (Chapter 43) ⊂⊃. When treating fluid volume disorders, the ultimate goal is to diagnose and correct the *cause* of the disorder, while administering supporting fluids and medications to stabilize the patient.

FLUID REPLACEMENT AGENTS

Loss of fluids from the body can result in dehydration and shock. Fluid replacement solutions are used to maintain blood volume and support blood pressure.

44.4 Intravenous Therapy with Crystalloids and Colloids

When fluid output exceeds fluid intake, volume deficits may result. Shock, dehydration, or electrolyte loss may occur; large deficits are fatal, unless treated. The following are some common reasons for fluid loss.

- Loss of GI fluids due to vomiting, diarrhea, chronic laxative use, or GI suctioning
- Excessive sweating during hot weather, athletic activity, or prolonged fever
- Severe burns
- Trauma resulting in significant blood loss
- Excessive renal fluid loss due to diuretic therapy or uncontrolled diabetic ketoacidosis

The immediate goal in treating a volume deficit disorder is to replace the missing fluid. In nonacute circumstances, this may be achieved by administering fluids via the oral route or through a nasogastric tube. In acute situations, intravenous fluid therapy is indicated. Regardless of the route, careful attention must be paid to restoring normal levels of electrolytes, as well as fluid volume.

Intravenous replacement fluids are of two basic types: colloids and crystalloids. Colloids are proteins or other large molecules that remain in the blood for a long time because they are too large to cross the capillary membranes. While circulating, they draw water molecules from the cells and tissues into the plasma through their ability to increase plasma osmolality and osmotic pressure. These agents are sometimes called plasma volume expanders. They are particularly important in treating hypovolemic shock due to burns, hemorrhage, or surgery. Several of these products contain dextran, a synthetic polysaccharide. Dextran infusions can double the plasma volume within a few minutes, though its effects last only about 12 hours. Plasma protein fraction contains 83% albumin and 17% plasma globulins. Plasma protein fraction and albumin are also indicated in patients with hypoproteinemia. Selected colloid solutions are given in Table 44.1.

Crystalloids are IV solutions that contain electrolytes and other agents that are used to replace lost fluids, and to promote urine output. Unlike colloids, crystalloid solutions are capable of quickly diffusing across membranes, leaving the plasma and entering the interstitial fluid and ICF. Isotonic, hypotonic, and hypertonic solutions are available. Some crystalloids contain dextrose, a form of glucose, commonly in concentrations of 2.5%, 5%, or 10%. Dextrose is added to provide nutritional value: 1 L of 5% dextrose supplies 170 calories. In addition, water is formed during the metabolism of dextrose, adding to the rehydration of the patient.

Infusion of crystalloids will increase total fluid volume in the body, but the compartment which is most expanded depends on the solute (sodium) concentration. Infusion of hypertonic crystalloids will draw water from the cells and tissues and expand plasma volume. Hypotonic crystalloids will cause water to move out of the plasma to the tissues and cells; thus, these solutions are not considered efficient plasma volume expanders. Selected crystalloid solutions are given in Table 44.2.

Table 44.1	Selected Colloid IV Solutions (Plasma Volume Expanders)
Drug	**Tonicity**
5% albumin	isotonic
dextran 40 in normal saline	isotonic
dextran 40 in D5W	isotonic
dextran 70 in normal saline	isotonic
hetastarch 6% in normal saline	isotonic
plasma protein fraction	isotonic

Table 44.2	Selected Crystalloid IV Solutions
Drug	**Tonicity**
normal saline (0.9% NaCl)	isotonic
hypertonic saline (3% NaCl)	hypertonic
hypotonic saline (0.45% NaCl)	hypotonic
lactated Ringer's	isotonic
plasma-lyte 148	isotonic
plasma-lyte 56	hypotonic
Dextrose Solutions	
5% dextrose in water (D5W)	isotonic*
5% dextrose in normal saline	hypertonic
5% dextrose in 0.2% saline	isotonic
5% dextrose in lactated Ringer's	hypertonic
5% dextrose in plasma-lyte 56	hypertonic

* Because dextrose is metabolized quickly, the solution is sometimes considered hypotonic.

NURSING CONSIDERATIONS

The role of the nurse in fluid replacement therapy involves careful monitoring of a patient's condition and providing education as it relates to the prescribed drug regimen. Prior to administration of colloids, or plasma volume expanders, the nurse should obtain a complete health history, drug history, and a physical examination. Lab tests, including CBC, serum electrolytes, BUN, and creatinine, should be obtained. The nurse should also evaluate the patient's fluid balance before initiating therapy. Administration of colloid solutions to dehydrated patients can lead to renal failure.

Colloidal solutions are contraindicated in patients with renal failure, hypervolemic conditions, severe HF, thrombocytopenia, and those with clotting abnormalities. They should be used with caution in patients with active hemorrhage, severe dehydration, chronic liver disease, or impaired renal function. The nurse should carefully monitor vital signs and observe the patient for the first 30 minutes of the infusion for hypersensitivity reactions. The nurse should stop the infusion at the first sign of hypersensitivity.

Some colloidal solutions decrease platelet adhesion and lead to decreased coagulation. Plasma expanders will lower hematocrit and hemoglobin levels because of increased intravascular volume. The nurse should report a hematocrit below 30% to the physician immediately.

The primary nursing responsibility when caring for the patient receiving plasma volume expanders is monitoring fluid volume status. The patient should be closely monitored for both fluid volume deficit and fluid volume excess. Vital signs and hemodynamic monitoring should be as-sessed frequently during the infusion, until the patient's condition stabilizes. The patient's neurologic status and urinary output should also be closely assessed, as these two systems are critically dependent on proper fluid balance. The infusion of the solutions can create a multitude of problems for the critically ill patient.

These medications are most often used to treat shock, so the patient may not be alert. However, caregivers may need emotional support from the nurse, including updates about the patient's condition and psychosocial support.

Patient education as it relates to colloidal solutions should include goals, reasons for obtaining baseline data such as vital signs and lab tests, and possible side effects. Following are important points the nurse should include when teaching patients and families about colloidal solutions.

- Immediately report any signs of bleeding such as easy bruising, blood in the urine, or dark, tarry stools.
- Immediately report flushing, shortness of breath, or itching, which could indicate hypersensitivity to the medication.
- Immediately report shortness of breath, cough, chest congestion, or heart palpitations, which could indicate circulatory overload.

ELECTROLYTES

Electrolytes are small, charged molecules essential to homeostasis. Too little or too much of an electrolyte may result in serious disease and must be quickly corrected. Table 44.3 lists inorganic substances and their electrolytes that are important to human physiology.

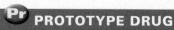

PROTOTYPE DRUG | **DEXTRAN 40** (Gentran 40, Hyskon, 10% LMD, Rheomacrodex)

ACTIONS AND USES

Dextran 40 is a polysaccharide that is too large to pass through capillary walls. It is identical to dextran 70, except dextran 40 has a lower molecular weight. Dextran 40 acts by raising the osmotic pressure of the blood, thereby causing fluid to move from the tissues to the vascular spaces. Given as an IV infusion, it has the capability of expanding plasma volume within minutes after administration. Cardiovascular responses include increased blood pressure, increased cardiac output, and improved venous return to the heart. Dextran 40 is excreted rapidly by the kidneys. Indications include fluid replacement for patients experiencing hypovolemic shock due to hemorrhage, surgery, or severe burns. When given for acute shock it is infused as rapidly as possible until blood volume is restored.

Dextran 40 also reduces platelet adhesiveness, and improves blood flow through its ability to reduce blood viscosity. These properties have led to its use in preventing deep vein thromboses and pulmonary emboli.

Administration Alerts

- Emergency administration may be given 1.2 to 2.4 g/min.
- Nonemergency administration should be infused no faster than 240 mg/min.
- Once opened, discard unused portion because dextran contains no preservatives.
- Pregnancy category C.

ADVERSE EFFECTS

Vital signs should be monitored continuously to avoid hypertension caused by the plasma volume expansion. Signs of fluid overload such as tachycardia, peripheral edema, distended neck veins, dyspnea, or cough should be reported immediately. Because of its extensive renal excretion, dextran 40 is contraindicated in patients with renal failure. Due to its ability to quickly draw water from tissues, it is also contraindicated in patients with severe dehydration. A small percentage of patients are allergic to dextran 40, with urticaria being the most common sign.

There are no clinically significant interactions.

 See the companion website for a Nursing Process Focus specific to this drug.

44.5 Normal Functions of Electrolytes

Chapter 26 discusses the role of minerals in health and wellness ⊂⊃. In certain body fluids, some of these minerals become ions and possess a charge. Small, inorganic molecules possessing a positive or negative charge are called **electrolytes**. Positively charged electrolytes are called **cations**; those with a negative charge are **anions**.

Inorganic compounds are held together by ionic bonds. When placed in aqueous solution, these bonds break and the compound undergoes dissociation or ionization. The resulting ions have charges and are able to conduct electricity, hence the name *electrolyte*. Electrolyte levels are measured in units of milliequivalents per liter (mEq/L).

Electrolytes are essential to many body functions, including nerve conduction, membrane permeability, muscle contraction, water balance, and bone growth and remodeling. Levels of electrolytes in body fluids must be maintained within narrow ranges. As electrolytes are lost due to normal excretory functions, they must be compensated by adequate intake, otherwise electrolyte imbalances can result. The major body electrolyte imbalance states are shown in Table 44.4. Calcium, phosphorous, and magnesium im-

balances are discussed in Chapter 38; the role of calcium in bone homeostasis is presented in Chapter 43 ⊂⊃.

44.6 Pharmacotherapy of Sodium Imbalances

Sodium is the major electrolyte in extracellular fluid. Due to its central roles in neuromuscular function, acid-base balance, and overall fluid distribution, sodium imbalances can have serious consequences. Although definite sodium monitors or sensors have yet to be discovered in the body, the regulation of sodium balance is well understood.

Sodium balance and water balance are intimately connected. As sodium levels increase in a body fluid, solute particles accumulate, and the osmolality increases. Water will move toward this area of relatively high osmolality. In simplest terms, water travels toward or with sodium. The physiologic consequences of this relationship cannot be overstated: As water content of the plasma increases, so does blood volume and blood pressure. Thus, sodium movement provides an important link between water retention, blood volume, and blood pressure.

NURSING PROCESS FOCUS | PATIENTS RECEIVING FLUID REPLACEMENT THERAPY

ASSESSMENT

Prior to administration:
- Obtain complete health history including allergies, drug history, and possible drug interactions.
- Obtain complete physical examination.
- Assess for the presence of fluid volume deficit.
- Obtain the following laboratory studies: CBC, serum electrolytes, renal function (BUN and serum creatinine).

POTENTIAL NURSING DIAGNOSES

- Deficient Fluid Volume
- Risk for Decreased Cardiac Output
- Risk for Injury, related to side effects of drug therapy

PLANNING: PATIENT GOALS AND EXPECTED OUTCOMES

The patient will:
- Exhibit signs of normal fluid volume such as stable blood pressure and adequate urinary output
- Demonstrate an understanding of the drug's action by accurately describing drug side effects and precautions
- Immediately report effects such as itching, shortness of breath, flushing, cough, and heart palpitations

IMPLEMENTATION

Interventions and (Rationales)

- Monitor hemodynamic status every 15 to 60 min, including blood pressure, urinary output, and invasive pressure monitoring devices. (Plasma volume expanders cause rapid movement of water into the circulatory system.)

- Monitor for hypersensitivity reactions such as urticaria, pruritus, dyspnea, flushing, and anaphylaxis.

- Monitor for signs of circulatory overload such as dyspnea, cyanosis, cough, crackles, wheezes, and neck vein distention. (Medication may cause fluid overload quickly.)

- Monitor for changes in CBC results. (Plasma volume expanders can inhibit coagulation and lower hematocrit and hemoglobin levels. Report reduction of hematocrit below 30%.)

Patient Education/Discharge Planning

Instruct patient about:
- Reason that vital signs and other assessments are being monitored frequently
- Expected outcomes of plasma volume expansion therapy

- Instruct patient to report itching, shortness of breath, or flushing as symptoms occur.

- Instruct patient to report shortness of breath, cough, or heart palpitation as soon as such symptoms occur.

- Instruct patient of the need for frequent laboratory studies.

EVALUATION OF OUTCOME CRITERIA

Evaluate the effectiveness of drug therapy by confirming that patient goals and expected outcomes have been met (see "Planning").

See Table 44.1 for a list of drugs to which these nursing actions apply.

Table 44.3	Electrolytes Important to Human Physiology		
Compound	**Formula**	**Cation**	**Anion**
calcium chloride	$CaCl_2$	Ca^{+2}	$2Cl^-$
disodium phosphate	Na_2HPO_4	$2Na^+$	HPO_4^{-2}
potassium chloride	KCl	K^+	Cl^-
sodium bicarbonate	$NaHCO_3$	Na^+	HCO_3^-
sodium chloride	$NaCl$	Na^+	Cl^-
sodium sulfate	Na_2SO_4	$2Na^+$	SO_4^{-2}

Table 44.4	Electrolyte Imbalances		
Ion	**Condition**	**Abnormal Serum Value (mEq/L)**	**Supportive Treatment***
calcium	hypercalcemia	>11	hypotonic fluid or calcitonin
	hypocalcemia	<4	calcium supplements or vitamin D
chloride	hyperchloremia	>112	hypotonic fluid
	hypochloremia	<95	hypertonic salt solution
magnesium	hypermagnesemia	>4	hypotonic fluid
	hypomagnesemia	<0.8	magnesium supplements
phosphate	hyperphosphatemia	>6	dietary restriction
	hypophosphatemia	<1	phosphate supplements
potassium	hyperkalemia	>5	hypotonic fluid, buffers, or dietary restriction
	hypokalemia	<3.5	potassium supplements
sodium	hypernatremia	>145	hypotonic fluid or dietary restriction
	hyponatremia	<135	hypertonic salt solution or sodium supplement

*For all electrolyte imbalances, the primary therapeutic goal is to identify and correct the *cause* of the imbalance.

In healthy individuals, sodium intake is equal to sodium output, which is under the regulation of the kidneys. High levels of aldosterone secreted by the adrenal cortex promote sodium and water retention by the kidneys. Inhibition of aldosterone promotes sodium and water excretion. When a patient ingests high amounts of sodium, aldosterone secretion decreases and more sodium enters the urine. This relationship is illustrated in Figure 44.3.

Sodium excess, or **hypernatremia**, is a serum sodium level of greater than 145 mEq/L. The most common cause of hypernatremia is kidney disease, resulting in decreased sodium excretion. Hypernatremia may also be caused by excessive intake of sodium, either through dietary consumption or by overtreatment with IV fluids containing sodium chloride or sodium bicarbonate. Another cause of hypernatremia is high net water losses, such as that occurring from inadequate water intake, watery diarrhea, fever, or burns. In addition, high doses of glucocorticoids or estrogens promote sodium retention.

A high serum sodium level increases the osmolality of the plasma and draws fluid from interstitial spaces and cells, thus causing cellular dehydration. Manifestations of hypernatremia include thirst, fatigue, weakness, muscle twitching, convulsions, weight gain, and dyspnea. For minor hypernatremia, a low-salt diet may be effective in returning serum sodium to normal levels. In patients with acute hypernatremia, however, treatment goals are to rapidly return the osmolality of the plasma to normal, and to excrete the excess sodium. If the patient is hypovolemic, the administration of hypotonic fluids such as 5% D5W or 0.45% NaCl will increase plasma volume, while at the same time reducing plasma osmolality. For the patient who is hypervolemic, diuretics may be used to remove sodium from the body.

Sodium deficiency, or **hyponatremia**, is a serum sodium level of less than 135 mEq/L. Hyponatremia may occur through excessive dilution of the plasma, or by increased sodium loss due to disorders of the skin, GI tract, or kidneys. Excessive ADH secretion, or administration of hypotonic IV solutions, can increase plasma volume and lead to hyponatremia. Significant loss of sodium by the skin may occur in burn patients, and in those with excessive sweating or prolonged fever. Gastrointestinal losses occur from vomiting, diarrhea, or GI suctioning and renal sodium loss may occur with diuretic use and in certain advanced kidney disorders. Early symptoms of hyponatremia include nausea, vomiting, anorexia, and abdominal cramping. Later signs include altered neurologic function such as confusion, lethargy, convulsions, and muscle twitching or tremors. Tachycardia, hypotension, and dry skin and mucous membranes may also occur. Hyponatremia is usually treated with solutions of sodium chloride.

NURSING CONSIDERATIONS

The role of the nurse in sodium replacement therapy involves careful monitoring of a patient's condition and providing education as it relates to the prescribed drug regimen. Because sodium and body water are so closely related, the nurse's primary role when caring for patients with sodium imbalances is monitoring fluid balance. Hyponatremia is seldom caused from inadequate dietary intake;

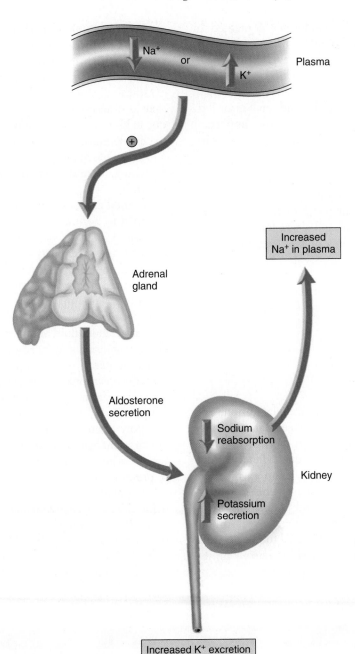

Figure 44.3 | Renal regulation of sodium and potassium balance

however, in rare instances, this may occur with individuals following sodium-restricted diets or receiving diuretic therapy. In most cases, infusion of 0.45% or 0.9% sodium solutions are used to restore extracellular fluid balance.

Prior to and during administration of sodium solutions, the nurse should assess sodium and electrolyte balance. When assessing for hyponatremia, the nurse should observe for signs of nausea, vomiting, muscle cramps, tachycardia, dry mucous membranes, and headache. The nurse must also be alert for signs indicating hypernatremia such as weakness, restlessness, irritability, seizures, coma, hypertension, tachycardia, fluid accumulation, pulmonary edema, and respiratory arrest.

Serum sodium levels, urine specific gravity, and serum and urine osmolarity should be monitored closely when administering hypertonic solutions. The patient should be taught to report any symptoms that may relate to fluid overload during infusion of hypertonic saline solutions. The symptoms of this condition include shortness or breath, palpitation, headache, and restlessness.

Side effects of sodium chloride when given as an electrolyte replacement are rare. Some patients have self-induced hypernatremia by taking salt tablets, believing they will replace sodium lost due to sweating. Those who sweat profusely due to working outdoors or exercising can avoid heat-related problems if they consume adequate amounts of water or balanced electrolyte solutions contained in sports drinks. The patient should only consume salt tablets when instructed by the healthcare provider.

Patient education as it relates to sodium replacement should include goals, reasons for obtaining baseline data such as vital signs and tests for cardiac and renal disorders, and possible side effects. Following are the important points the nurse should include when teaching patients regarding sodium replacements.

- Avoid taking sodium chloride (salt) tablets to replace sodium lost through perspiration.
- Drink adequate amounts of water or balanced sports drinks to replenish lost fluids and electrolytes.
- Immediately report symptoms of low sodium such as nausea, vomiting, muscle cramps, rapid heart rate, and headache.
- Immediately report symptoms of high sodium such as weakness, restlessness, irritability, seizures, hypertension, and fluid retention.

44.7 Pharmacotherapy of Potassium Imbalances

Potassium is the most abundant intracellular cation, and serves important roles in regulating intracellular osmolality and in maintaining acid-base balance. Potassium levels must be carefully balanced between adequate dietary intake and renal excretion. Like sodium, potassium excretion is influenced by the effect of aldosterone on the kidney. In fact, the renal excretion of sodium and potassium ions is closely linked—for every sodium ion that is reabsorbed, one potassium ion is secreted into the renal tubules. Serum potassium levels must be maintained within narrow limits; excess or deficiency states can be serious or fatal.

Hyperkalemia is a serum potassium level greater than 5 mEq/L, which may be caused by high consumption of potassium-rich foods or dietary supplements, particularly when patients are taking potassium-sparing diuretics such as spironolactone (Chapter 43)⊙. Excess potassium may also accumulate when renal excretion is diminished due to kidney pathology. The most serious consequences of hyperkalemia are related to cardiac function; dysrhythmias and heart block are possible. Other symptoms are muscle twitching, fatigue, paresthesias, dyspnea, cramping, and diarrhea.

In mild cases of hyperkalemia, potassium levels may be returned to normal by restricting major dietary sources of potassium such as bananas, dried fruits, peanut butter, broccoli, and green leafy vegetables. If the patient is taking a potassium-sparing diuretic, the dose must be lowered or an alternate drug may be considered. In severe cases, serum potassium levels may be temporarily lowered by administering glucose and insulin, which cause potassium to leave the extracellular fluid and enter cells. Calcium gluconate or calcium chloride may be administered on an emergency basis to counteract potential potassium toxicity on the heart. Sodium bicarbonate is sometimes infused to correct any acidosis that may be concurrent with the hyperkalemia. Elimination of excess potassium may be enhanced by giving polystyrene sulfonate orally or rectally. This agent, which exchanges sodium ion for potassium ion in the intestine, is given concurrently with a laxative such as sorbitol to promote rapid evacuation of the potassium.

Hypokalemia occurs when serum potassium level falls below 3.5 mEq/L. Hypokalemia is a relatively common adverse effect resulting from high doses of loop diuretics such as furosemide (Lasix). In addition, strenuous muscular activity and severe vomiting or diarrhea can result in significant potassium loss. Because the body does not have large

---

Pr PROTOTYPE DRUG	SODIUM CHLORIDE (NaCl)

ACTIONS AND USES

Sodium chloride is administered during periods of hyponatremia when serum levels fall below 130 mEq/L. Sodium chloride is available in several concentrations to treat different levels of hyponatremia. Normal saline consists of 0.9% NaCl, and is used to treat mild hyponatremia. When serum sodium falls below 115 mEq/L, a 3% NaCl solution may be infused. Other concentrations include 0.45% and 0.22%, and both hypotonic and isotonic solutions are available. The decision on which NaCl concentration to administer is driven by the severity of the sodium deficiency. Infusions of high concentrations of NaCl are contraindicated in patients with congestive heart failure or with impaired renal function.

Administration Alert

- Pregnancy category C.

ADVERSE EFFECTS

Patients receiving NaCl infusions must be monitored frequently to avoid symptoms of hypernatremia. Symptoms of excessive sodium include lethargy, confusion, muscle tremor or rigidity, hypotension, and restlessness. Because some of these symptoms are also common to hyponatremia, the healthcare provider must rely on periodic lab assessments to be certain sodium values lie within the normal range. When infusing 3% NaCl solutions, the nurse should continuously check for signs of pulmonary edema.

There are no clinically significant drug interactions.

 See the companion website for a Nursing Process Focus specific to this drug.

Laxatives and Fluid-Electrolyte Balance

With aging, peristalsis slows, food intake diminishes, and physical activity declines; and these factors can change bowel movement regularity. Many older adults believe they must have a bowel movement every day, and take daily laxatives. Chronic use of laxatives may result in fluid depletion and hyperkalemia. Stimulant laxatives, in particular, are the most frequently prescribed class of laxatives and these agents alter electrolyte transport in the intestinal mucosa. The elderly are especially susceptible to fluid and electrolyte depletion with chronic laxative use. The nurse should teach the patient to drink plenty of fluids when taking a laxative, and that overuse of laxatives can result in adverse side effects and that they should be used only as directed. The nurse should recommend that older patients increase exercise (as tolerated) and add insoluble fiber to the diet to maintain elimination regularity.

stores of potassium, adequate daily intake is necessary. Neurons and muscle fibers are most sensitive to potassium loss, and muscle weakness, lethargy, anorexia, dysrhythmias, and cardiac arrest are possible consequences. Mild hypokalemia is treated by increasing the dietary intake of potassium-rich foods, whereas more severe deficiencies require higher doses of oral or parenteral potassium supplements.

NURSING CONSIDERATIONS

The role of the nurse in potassium replacement therapy involves careful monitoring of a patient's condition and providing education as it relates to the prescribed drug regimen. Potassium imbalances are probably the most common electrolyte disturbance that patients experience. Quick recognition of potassium imbalance will prevent life-threatening complications such as dysrhythmias, heart blocks, and cardiac arrest.

Potassium supplements are contraindicated in conditions that predispose the patient to hyperkalemia, such as severe renal impairment and use of potassium-sparing diuretics. Potassium supplements are also contraindicated in acute dehydration, heat cramps, and patients with digitalis intoxication with AV node disturbance. They should be used with caution in patients with kidney disease, cardiac disease, and systemic acidosis.

Oral potassium administration is used for the prevention and treatment of mild deficiency. Oral forms, especially tablets and capsules which can produce high local concentrations of potassium, are irritating to the GI tract and may cause peptic ulcers. This is less likely with the use of tablets and capsules that contain microencapsulated particles. To minimize GI irritation, the nurse should instruct the patient to administer oral forms with meals. Prior to oral or IV administration of potassium chloride, serum potassium level should be measured. The nurse should check for the most recent potassium level before administering any form

of potassium. Too much potassium can be just as dangerous for the patient as too little potassium. In either case, the consequences can be fatal.

Intravenous potassium administration is used for patients with severe deficiency or those who cannot tolerate oral forms. The nurse should monitor serum potassium levels throughout treatment to reduce the risk of hyperkalemia. The nurse should assess renal function prior to and during treatment and, if renal failure develops, the infusion should be stopped immediately. The nurse should monitor for EKG changes, which can be an early indication of developing hyperkalemia. Patients who experience potassium imbalances must be taught to avoid the underlying problems, comply with medication regimen, and use dietary interventions to correct and maintain normal electrolyte balance.

Patient education as it relates to potassium replacement should include goals, reasons for obtaining baseline data such as vital signs and tests for cardiac and renal disorders, and possible side effects. Following are important points the nurse should include when teaching patients regarding potassium replacements.

- Report symptoms of hypokalemia such as weakness, fatigue, lethargy, or anorexia.
- Report symptoms of hyperkalemia such as nausea, abdominal cramping, oliguria, weakness, changes in heart rate, and numbness or tingling of arms or legs.
- Report decreased urinary output, since this can lead to hyperkalemia.
- Keep all lab appointments to assess serum potassium level.
- If taking a potassium supplement, avoid potassium-rich foods and salt substitutes that are potassium based.
- Take potassium supplements with food to decrease GI distress.

ACID-BASE BALANCE

Unless quickly corrected, acidosis and alkalosis can have serious and even fatal consequences. Acidic and basic agents may be given to rapidly correct pH imbalances in body fluids.

44.8 Buffers and the Maintenance of Body pH

The degree of acidity or alkalinity of a solution is measured by its **pH**. A pH of 7.0 is defined as neutral, above 7.0 as basic or alkaline, and below 7.0 as acidic. To maintain homeostasis, the pH of plasma and most body fluids must be kept within the narrow range of 7.35 to 7.45. Nearly all proteins and enzymes in the body function optimally within this narrow range of pH values. A few enzymes, most notably those in the digestive tract, require pH values outside the 7.35 to 7.45 range to function properly. The correction of acid-base imbalance is illustrated in Figure 44.4.

The body generates significant amounts of acid during normal metabolic processes. Without sophisticated means

PROTOTYPE DRUG | POTASSIUM CHLORIDE (KCI)

ACTIONS AND USES

Potassium chloride is the drug of choice for treating or preventing hypokalemia. It is also used to treat mild forms of alkalosis. Oral formulations include tablets, powders, and liquids, usually heavily flavored due to the unpleasant taste of the drug. Because the drug can cause peptic ulcers, the supplement should be diluted with plenty of water. When given IV, potassium preparations must be administered slowly, since bolus injections can overload the heart and cause cardiac arrest. Because pharmacotherapy with loop or thiazide diuretics is the most common cause of potassium loss, patients taking these diuretics are usually instructed to take oral potassium supplements to prevent hypokalemia. Potassium chloride is pregnancy category A.

Administration Alerts

- Always give oral medication while patient is upright to avoid esophagitis.
- Tablets should not be crushed or chewed.
- Dilute liquid forms before giving through a nasogastric tube.
- Never administer IV push or in concentrated amounts, and do not exceed 10 mEq/hr in IV rate.
- Be extremely careful to avoid extravasation and infiltration.

See the companion website for a Nursing Process Focus specific to this drug.

ADVERSE EFFECTS AND INTERACTIONS

Nausea and vomiting are common, because potassium chloride irritates the GI mucosa. The drug may be taken with meals or antacids to lessen gastric distress. The most serious side effects of potassium chloride are related to the possible accumulation of excess potassium. Hyperkalemia may occur if the patient takes potassium supplements concurrently with potassium-sparing diuretics. Kidney function should be assessed periodically. Since the kidneys perform over 90% of the body's potassium excretion, reduced renal function can rapidly lead to hyperkalemia, particularly in patients taking potassium supplements.

Potassium supplements interact with potassium-sparing diuretics and ACE inhibitors to increase the risk for hyperkalemia.

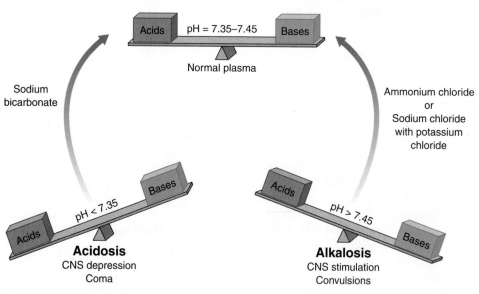

Figure 44.4 | Acid-base imbalances

of neutralizing these metabolic acids, the overall pH of body fluids would quickly fall below the normal range. Buffers are chemicals that help maintain normal body pH by neutralizing strong acids and bases. The two primary buffers the body uses to keep pH within normal limits are bicarbonate ions and phosphate ions.

The body uses two mechanisms to remove acid. The CO_2 produced during body metabolism is efficiently removed by the lungs during exhalation. The kidneys remove excess acid in the form of hydrogen ion (H^+) by excreting it in the urine. If retained in the body, CO_2 and/or H^+ would lower body pH. Thus, the lung and the kidney collaborate in the removal of acids to maintain normal acid-base balance.

44.9 Pharmacotherapy of Acidosis

Acidosis occurs when the pH of the plasma falls below 7.35, which is confirmed by measuring arterial pH, partial pressure of carbon dioxide (PCO_2), and plasma bicarbonate levels. Diagnosis must differentiate between respiratory etiology and metabolic (renal) etiology. Occasionally, the cause has mixed respiratory and metabolic components. The most profound symptoms of acidosis affect the central nervous system, and include lethargy, confusion, and CNS depression leading to coma. A deep, rapid respiration rate indicates an attempt by the lungs to rid the body of excess acid. Common causes of acidosis are shown in Table 44.5.

NURSING CONSIDERATIONS

The role of the nurse in drug therapy of acidosis involves careful monitoring of a patient's condition and providing education as it relates to the prescribed drug regimen. The focus of nursing care is directed toward correction and maintenance of acid-base status. The nurse should assess the arterial blood gas analysis, which reports pH, carbon dioxide levels (PCO_2), bicarbonate levels (HCO_3^-), and oxygenation status (PO_2 and O_2 saturation). The nurse should also assess the patient for symptoms associated with acidosis such as sleepiness, coma, disorientation, dizziness, headache, seizures, and hypoventilation. The nurse will further assess the patient for causative factors that could produce acidosis such as diabetes mellitus, shock, diarrhea, and vomiting. Acidosis is frequently corrected when the underlying disease condition is successfully managed.

The patient receiving sodium bicarbonate is prone to alkalosis, especially if an excessive amount has been administered. The nurse should monitor the patient for symptoms of alkalosis such as irritability, confusion, cyanosis, slow respirations, irregular pulse, and muscle twitching. These symptoms would warrant withholding the medication and notifying the healthcare provider.

There are several contraindications and precautions related to the administration of sodium bicarbonate. Patients who have lost chloride due to vomiting or continuous GI suctioning, and patients receiving diuretic therapy that may cause hypochloremia, should not be given sodium bicarbonate. Patients who have hypocalcemia should not receive sodium bicarbonate because it may produce alkalosis. Due to the sodium content of this drug, it should be used judiciously in patients with cardiac disease and renal impairment.

Sodium bicarbonate may also be used to alkalinize the urine. This process is useful in the treatment of overdoses of certain acidic medications such as aspirin and phenobarbital. When IV sodium bicarbonate is given, it causes the urine to become more alkaline. Less acid is reabsorbed in the renal tubules, so more acid and acidic medicine is excreted. This process is known as ion trapping. The nurse should closely monitor the patient's acid-base status and report symptoms of imbalance to the healthcare provider. The nurse should provide care directed toward supporting critical body functions such as cardiovascular, respiratory, and neurologic status that may be impaired secondary to the drug overdose.

Sodium bicarbonate (baking soda) is used as a home remedy to neutralize gastric acid, relieving heartburn, or sour stomach. Although occasional use is acceptable, the nurse should be aware that patients may misinterpret cardiac symptoms as heartburn and may overuse sodium bicarbonate, leading to systemic alkalosis.

Table 44.5	Causes of Alkalosis and Acidosis	
ACIDOSIS	**ALKALOSIS**
Respiratory Origins of Acidosis	**Respiratory Origin of Alkalosis**
• hypoventilation or shallow breathing	• hyperventilation due to asthma, anxiety, or high altitude
• airway constriction	
• damage to respiratory center in medulla	
Metabolic Origins of Acidosis	**Metabolic Origins of Alkalosis**
• severe diarrhea	• constipation for prolonged periods
• kidney failure	• ingestion of excess sodium bicarbonate
• diabetes mellitus	• diuretics that cause potassium depletion
• excess alcohol ingestion	• severe vomiting
• starvation	

Patient education as it relates to sodium bicarbonate should include goals, reasons for obtaining baseline data such as vital signs and electrolyte levels, and possible side effects. Following are important points the nurse should include when teaching patients regarding sodium bicarbonate.

- Contact a healthcare provider immediately if gastric discomfort continues, or is accompanied by chest pain, dyspnea, or diaphoresis.
- Use alternative OTC antacids to prevent the problem of excess sodium or bicarbonate being absorbed into systemic circulation.
- Do not use any antacid, including sodium bicarbonate, for greater than 2 weeks without consulting the healthcare provider.

44.10 Pharmacotherapy of Alkalosis

At plasma pH values above 7.45, alkalosis develops. Like acidosis, alkalosis may have both respiratory and metabolic causes, as shown in Table 44.5. Also like acidosis, the central nervous system is greatly affected. Symptoms of CNS stimulation occur including nervousness, hyperactive reflexes, and convulsions. Slow, shallow breathing indicates that the body is attempting to retain acid and lower internal pH. In mild cases, alkalosis may be corrected by administering sodium chloride combined with potassium chloride. This combination increases the renal excretion of bicarbonate ion, which indirectly increases the acidity of the blood. More severe alkalosis may be treated with infusions of ammonium chloride.

NATURAL THERAPIES | Sea Vegetables for Acidosis

Sea vegetables, or seaweeds, are a form of marine algae that grow in the upper levels of the ocean, where sunlight can penetrate. Examples of these edible seaweeds include kelp, arame, and nori, which are used a great deal in Asian cooking. Sea vegetables are found in coastal locations throughout the world. Kelp, or Laminaria, is found in the cold waters of the North Atlantic and Pacific oceans.

Sea vegetables contain a multitude of vitamins, as well as protein. Their most notable nutritional aspect, however, is their mineral content. Plants from the sea contain more minerals than most other food sources, including calcium, magnesium, phosphorous, iron, potassium, and all essential trace elements. Because they are so rich in minerals, seaweeds act as alkalizers for the blood, helping to rid the body of acid conditions (acidosis). Laminaria is a particularly rich source of iron.

NURSING CONSIDERATIONS

The role of the nurse in drug therapy with ammonium chloride involves careful monitoring of a patient's condition and providing education as it relates to the prescribed drug regimen. The major treatment for both metabolic alkalosis and respiratory alkalosis is to first attempt to correct the underlying disease condition creating the imbalance. The administration of ammonium chloride is only used in clinical practice when the alkalosis is so severe that the pH must be restored quickly to prevent life-threatening consequences. This drug is contraindicated in the presence of liver disease, since its acidifying action depends on proper liver functioning to convert ammonium ions to urea.

During the intravenous infusion of ammonium chloride, the nurse must continually assess for metabolic acidosis and ammonium toxicity. Symptoms of toxic levels of ammonium include pallor, sweating, irregular breathing, retching,

---

Pr PROTOTYPE DRUG | SODIUM BICARBONATE

ACTIONS AND USES

Sodium bicarbonate is the drug of choice for correcting acidosis. After dissociation, the bicarbonate ion acts by directly raising the pH of body fluids. Sodium bicarbonate may be given orally, if acidosis is mild, or IV in cases of acute disease. Although sodium bicarbonate neutralizes gastric acid, it is rarely used to treat peptic ulcers due to its tendency to cause uncomfortable gastric distension. After absorption, sodium bicarbonate makes the urine more basic, which aids in the renal excretion of acidic drugs such as barbiturates and salicylates.

Administration Alerts

- Do not add oral preparation to calcium-containing solutions.
- Pregnancy category C.

ADVERSE EFFECTS AND INTERACTIONS

Most of the side effects of sodium bicarbonate therapy are the result of metabolic alkalosis caused by too much bicarbonate ion. Symptoms may include confusion, irritability, slow respiration rate, and vomiting. Simply discontinuing the sodium bicarbonate infusion often reverses these symptoms; however, potassium chloride or ammonium chloride may be administered to reverse the alkalosis. During sodium bicarbonate infusions, serum electrolytes should be carefully monitored, as sodium levels may give rise to hypernatremia and fluid retention. In addition, high levels of bicarbonate ion passing through the kidney tubules increase potassium secretion, and hypokalemia is possible.

Sodium bicarbonate interacts with several drugs. For example, it may decrease absorption of ketoconazole, and may decrease elimination of dextroamphetamine, ephedrine, pseudoephedrine, and quinidine. Sodium bicarbonate may increase elimination of lithium, salicylates, and tetracyclines.

 See the companion website for a Nursing Process Focus specific to this drug.

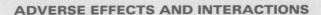

Pr PROTOTYPE DRUG | AMMONIUM CHLORIDE

ACTIONS AND USES

Severe alkalosis may be reversed by the administration of acidic agents such as ammonium chloride. During the hepatic conversion of ammonium chloride to urea, Cl^- and H^+ are formed, and the pH of body fluids decreases. Ammonium chloride acidifies the urine, which is beneficial in treating certain urinary tract infections. Historically, it has been used as a diuretic, though safer and more efficacious agents have made its use for this indication obsolete. By acidifying the urine, ammonium chloride promotes the excretion of alkaline drugs such as amphetamines. When given for acidosis, the IM or IV route is preferred.

Administration Alerts

- IV solution should be infused slowly (no more than 5 ml/min) to prevent ammonia toxicity.
- Pregnancy category B.

ADVERSE EFFECTS AND INTERACTIONS

Ammonium chloride is generally infused slowly, to minimize the potential for producing acidosis. The nurse should observe for signs of CNS depression characteristic of acidosis. Ammonium chloride may interact with several drugs; for example, it may cause crystalluria when taken with aminosalicylic acid. Ammonium chloride increases excretion of amphetamines, flecainide, mexiletine, methadone, ephedrine, and pseudoephedrine, and decreases urinary excretion of sulfonylureas and salicylates.

See the companion website for a Nursing Process Focus specific to this drug.

---

bradycardia, twitching, and convulsions. If the patient exhibits any of these symptoms, the nurse should immediately stop the infusion and contact the healthcare provider.

The nurse must also closely monitor the patient's renal status during the administration of ammonium chloride, because the excretion of this drug depends on normal kidney function. The nurse should monitor intake and output ratios, body weight, electrolyte status, and renal function studies for any sign of renal impairment.

When ammonium chloride is administered IV, the nurse should closely monitor the intravenous infusion site, because this drug is extremely irritating to veins and may cause severe inflammation. The drug must be infused slowly, no more than 5 ml/min, to prevent ammonia toxicity.

Like sodium bicarbonate, ammonium chloride is used as an ionic trapping agent in the treatment of drug overdoses. Ammonium chloride acidifies urine, which increases the excretion of alkaline substances such as amphetamines, phencyclidine (PCP/angel dust), or other basic substances. Overdoses of alkaline substances can greatly compromise the cardiovascular, respiratory, and neurologic status and the nursing role for this type of patient will be directed to-

ward monitoring the patient's acid-base status and supporting critical body functions.

Patient education as it relates to ammonium chloride should include goals, reasons for obtaining baseline data such as vital signs and renal status, and possible side effects. Following are the important points the nurse should include when teaching patients and families regarding ammonium chloride.

- Report pain at IV site.
- If medication is taken orally, report anorexia, nausea, vomiting, and thirst.
- If medication is given parenterally, report rash, headache, bradycardia, drowsiness, confusion, depression, and excitement alternating with coma.
- Take ammonium chloride tablets for no longer than 6 days.
- Report severe GI upset, fever, chills, and changes in urine or stool color.
- Take medication after meals or use enteric-coated tablets to decrease GI upset; swallow tablets whole.

MediaLink Understanding Acid-Base Balance

CHAPTER REVIEW

Key Concepts

The numbered key concepts provide a succinct summary of the important points from the corresponding numbered section within the chapter. If any of these points are not clear, refer to the numbered section within the chapter for review. Expanded versions can be found on the companion website.

44.1 There is a continuous exchange of fluids across membranes separating the intracellular and extracellular fluid compartments. Large molecules and those that are ionized are less able to cross membranes.

44.2 Changes in the osmolality of body fluids can cause water to move to different compartments.

44.3 Water balance is achieved through complex mechanisms that regulate fluid intake and output. The greatest contributor to osmolality is sodium, although glucose and urea also contribute.

44.4 Intravenous fluid therapy using crystalloids and colloids is used to replace lost fluids. Colloids such as dextran have the ability to rapidly expand plasma volume.

44.5 Electrolytes are charged substances that are essential to nerve conduction, membrane permeability, water balance, and other critical body functions.

44.6 Sodium is essential to maintain osmolality, water balance, and acid-base balance. Hypernatremia may be corrected with hypotonic IV fluids or diuretics and hyponatremia is corrected with infusions of sodium chloride.

44.7 Potassium is essential for proper nervous and muscle function, as well as maintaining acid-base balance. Hyperkalemia may be treated with glucose and insulin, or by administration of polystyrene sulfonate.

44.8 The body uses buffers to maintain overall pH within narrow limits.

44.9 Pharmacotherapy of acidosis, a plasma pH below 7.35, includes the administration of sodium bicarbonate.

44.10 Pharmacotherapy of alkalosis, a plasma pH above 7.45, includes the administration of ammonium chloride, or sodium chloride with potassium chloride.

Review Questions

1. How does a colloid IV fluid differ from a crystalloid?

2. Do the terms *osmolality* and *tonicity* have the same meaning? Explain by using examples how each term is properly used.

3. Compare and contrast the typical symptoms of hypernatremia and hyponatremia. How are they treated pharmacologically?

4. Compare and contrast the typical symptoms of hyperkalemia and hypokalemia. How are they treated pharmacologically?

5. Compare and contrast the typical symptoms of acidosis and alkalosis. How are they treated pharmacologically?

Critical Thinking Questions

1. A 72-year-old male with a history of heart failure presents to the emergency room complaining of weakness and "palpitations." The patient has been managed on furosemide (Lasix) and Lanoxin at home. His current EKG reveals atrial fibrillation, and serum electrolytes reveal a potassium of 2.5 mEq/L. The physician orders an IV solution of 1,000 cc Ringer's lactate with 40 mEq KCl to infuse over 8 hr. What are the issues the nurse must consider to safely administer this drug?

2. An 18-year-old woman is admitted to the labor and delivery unit for observation with a blood pressure of 186/108. She has 3–4+ pitting edema of the lower extremities and states that her hands and face are "swollen." The CBC reveals an elevated hemoglobin and hematocrit. The certified nurse midwife diagnoses the patient with pregnancy-induced hypertension and orders an IV of D5LR. In addition, she requests that the nurse "push oral fluids." The nurse considers whether the midwife's order should be questioned. Discuss the appropriateness of this order.

EXPLORE MediaLink

NCLEX review, case studies, and other interactive resources for this chapter can be found on the companion website at www.prenhall.com/adams. Click on "Chapter 44" to select the activities for this chapter. For animations, more NCLEX review questions, and an audio glossary, access the accompanying CD-ROM in this textbook.

The Integumentary System, Musculoskeletal System, and Eyes/Ears

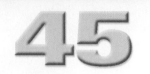
◾ DRUGS AT A GLANCE

CENTRALLY ACTING MUSCLE RELAXANTS
Pr *cyclobenzaprine (Cycoflex, Flexeril)*

DIRECT-ACTING ANTISPASMOTICS
Pr *dantrolene sodium (Dantrium)*

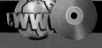

MediaLink   www.prenhall.com/adams

CD-ROM
Animation:
   Mechanism in Action: Cyclobenzaprine
   (Cycoflex)
Audio Glossary
NCLEX Review

Companion Website
NCLEX Review
Dosage Calculations
Case Study
Care Plans
Expanded Key Concepts

OBJECTIVES

After reading this chapter, the student should be able to:

1. Identify the different body systems contributing to muscle movement.
2. Discuss nonpharmacologic therapies used to treat muscle spasms and spasticity.
3. Explain the goals of pharmacotherapy with skeletal muscle relaxants.
4. Describe the nurse's role in the pharmacologic management of muscle spasms.
5. Compare and contrast the roles of the following drug categories in treating muscle spasms and spasticity: centrally acting skeletal muscle relaxants and direct-acting antispasmotics.
6. For each of the drug classes listed in Drugs at a Glance, know representative drugs, explain their mechanism of action, primary actions, and important adverse effects.
7. Use the Nursing Process to care for patients who are receiving drug therapy for muscle spasms.

Disorders associated with movement are some of the most difficult conditions to treat because their underlying mechanisms may span at least four important systems in the body: the nervous, muscular, endocrine, and skeletal systems. Proper body movement depends not only on intact neural pathways, but also on proper functioning of muscles, which in turn depends on on the levels of minerals such as sodium, potassium, and calcium in the bloodstream. This chapter focuses on the pharmacotherapy of muscular disorders associated with muscle spasms and spasticity. Many of the drugs used to treat muscle spasms are distinct from those used for spasticity.

MediaLink NIAMSD

MUSCLE SPASMS

Muscle spasms are involuntary contractions of a muscle or group of muscles. The muscles become tightened, develop a fixed pattern of resistance, and result in a diminished level of functioning.

45.1 Causes of Muscle Spasms

Muscle spasms are a common condition usually associated with excessive usage and local injury to the skeletal muscle. Other causes of muscle spasms include overmedication with antipsychotic drugs (Chapter 17)⊕, epilepsy, hypocalcemia, pain, and debilitating neurologic disorders. Patients with muscle spasms may experience inflammation, edema and pain at the affected muscle, loss of coordination, and reduced mobility. When a muscle goes into spasm, it freezes in

PHARMFACTS   Muscle Spasms

- Over 12 million people worldwide have muscle spasms.
- Muscle spasms severe enough for drug therapy are often found in patients who have had other debilitating disorders such as stroke, injury, neurodegenerative diseases, and cerebral palsy.
- Cerebral palsy is usually associated with events that occur before or during birth, but may be acquired during the first few months or years of life as the result of head trauma or infection.
- Dystonia affects about 250,000 people in the United States; it is the third most common movement disorder, following essential tremor and Parkinson's disease.
- Researchers have recognized multiple forms of inheritable dystonia and identified at least 10 genes or chromosomal locations responsible for the various manifestations.

a contracted state. A single, prologed contraction is a **tonic spasm**, whereas multiple, rapidly repeated contractions are **clonic spasms**. Treatment of muscle spasms involves both nonpharmacologic and pharmacologic therapies.

45.2 Pharmacologic and Nonpharmacologic Treatment of Muscle Spasms

When treating a patient with complaints of muscle spasms, a careful history and physical exam should be done to determine the etiology. After a determination has been made, nonpharmacologic therapies are normally used in conjunction with medications. Nonpharmacologic measures may include immobilization of the affected muscle, application of heat or cold, hydrotherapy, ultrasound, supervised exercises, massage, and manipulation.

Pharmacotherapy for muscle spasm may include combinations of analgesics, anti-inflammatory agents and centrally acting skeletal muscle relaxants. Most skeletal muscle relaxants relieve symptoms of muscular stiffness and rigidity resulting from muscular injury. They help to improve mobility in cases when patients have restricted movements. The therapeutic goals are to minimize pain and discomfort, increase range of motion, and improve the patient's ability to function independently.

CENTRALLY ACTING SKELETAL MUSCLE RELAXANTS

45.3 Treating Muscle Spasms at the Level of the Central Nervous System

Many antispasmodic drugs treat muscle spasms at the level of the central nervous system (CNS). Although the exact mechanisms of centrally acting muscle relaxant drugs are not fully known, it is believed that they generate their effect within the brain and/or spinal cord by inhibiting upper motor neuron activity, causing sedation, or altering simple reflexes.

Skeletal muscle relaxants are used to treat local spasms resulting from muscular injury and may be prescribed alone or in combination with other medications to reduce pain and increase range of motion. Commonly used centrally acting medications include baclofen (Lioresal), cyclobenzaprine (Cycoflex, Flexeril), tizanidine (Zanaflex), and benzodiazepines such as diazepam (Valium), clonazepam (Klonopin), and lorazepam (Ativan), as summarized in Table 45.1. All of the centrally acting agents have the potential to cause sedation.

Baclofen (Lioresal), structurally similar to the inhibitory neurotransmitter gamma amino butyric acid (GABA), produces its effect by a mechanism that is not fully known. It inhibits neuronal activity within the brain and possibly the spinal cord, although there is some question as to whether the spinal effects of baclofen are associated with GABA. It may be used to reduce muscle spasms in patients with multiple sclerosis, cerebral palsy, or spinal cord injury. Common side effects of baclofen are drowsiness, dizziness, weakness, and fatigue. Baclofen is often a drug of first choice due to its wide safety margin.

Tizanidine (Zanaflex) is a centrally acting alpha$_2$-adrenergic agonist inhibiting motor neurons mainly at the spinal cord level. Patients receiving high doses report drowsiness; thus, it also affects some neural activity in the brain. Though uncommon, one adverse effect of tizanidine is hallucinations. The most frequent side effects are dry mouth, fatigue, dizziness, and sleepiness. Tizanidine is as efficacious as baclofen and is considered by some to be a drug of first choice.

As discussed in Chapter 14, benzodiazepines inhibit both sensory and motor neuron activity by enhancing the effects of

Table 45.1	Centrally Acting Skeletal Muscle Relaxants
Drug	**Route and Adult Dose (max dose where indicated)**
baclofen (Lioresal)	PO; 5 mg tid (max 80 mg/d)
cyclobenzaprine hydrochloride (Cycoflex, Flexeril)	PO; 10–20 mg bid-qid (max 60 mg/d)
carisoprodol (Soma)	PO; 350 mg tid
chlorphenesin (Maolate)	PO; 800 mg tid until effective; reduce to 400 mg qid or less
chlorzoxazone (Paraflex, Parafon Forte)	PO; 250–500 mg tid-qid (max 3 g/d)
clonazepam (Klonopin)	PO; 0.5 mg tid (max 20 mg/d)
diazepam (Valium) (see page 164 for the Prototype Drug Box) ⬤⬤	PO; 4–10 mg bid-qid; IM/IV; 2–10 mg, repeat if needed in 3–4 h; IV pump; administer emulsion at 5 mg/min
lorazepam (Ativan) (see page 150 for the Prototype Drug Box) ⬤⬤	PO; 1–2 mg bid-tid (max 10 mg/d)
metaxalone (Skelaxin)	PO; 800 mg tid-qid (max of 10 d)
methocarbamol (Robaxin)	PO; 1.5 g qid for 2–3 d, then reduce to 1 g qid
orphenadrine citrate (Banflex, Flexon, Myolin, Norflex)	PO; 100 mg bid
tizanidine (Zanaflex)	PO; 4–8 mg tid-qid (max 36 mg/d)

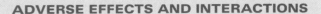

Pr **PROTOTYPE DRUG** | **CYCLOBENZAPRINE** (Cycoflex, Flexeril)

ACTIONS AND USES

Cyclobenzaprine relieves muscle spasms of local origin without interfering with general muscle function. This drug acts by depressing motor activity primarily in the brainstem, but with limited effects occurring also in the spinal cord. It increases circulating levels of norepinephrine, blocking presynaptic uptake. Its mechanism of action is similar to tricyclic antidepressants (Chapter 16)⊙ . It causes muscle relaxation in cases of acute muscle spasticity, but it is not effective in cases of cerebral palsy or diseases of the brain and spinal cord. This medication is meant to provide therapy for only 2 to 3 weeks.

Administration Alerts

- Pregnancy category B.
- The drug is not recommended for pediatric use.
- Maximum effects may take 1 to 2 weeks.

 See the companion website for a Nursing Process Focus specific to this drug.

ADVERSE EFFECTS AND INTERACTIONS

Adverse reactions to cyclobenzaprine include drowsiness, blurred vision, dizziness, dry mouth, rash, and tachycardia. It should be used with caution in patients with MI, dysrhythmias, or severe cardiovascular disease. One reaction, although rare, is swelling of the tongue. Alcohol, phenothiazines, and other CNS depressants may cause additive sedation. Cyclobenzaprine should not be used within 2 weeks of a MAO inhibitor since hyperpyretic crisis and convulsions may occur.

NATURAL THERAPIES | **Cayenne for Muscular Tension**

Cayenne (*Capsicum annum*), also known as chili pepper, paprika, or red pepper, has been used as a remedy for muscle tension. Applied in a cream base, it is commonly used to relieve muscle spasms in the shoulder and areas of the arm. Capsaicin, the active ingredient in cayenne, diminishes the chemical messengers that travel through the sensory nerves, therefore decreasing the sensation of pain. Its effect accumulates over time so creams containing capsaicin need to be applied regularly to be effective. Although no known medical condition exists that would prevent the use of cayenne, it should never be applied over broken skin. External use of full-strength cayenne should be limited to no more than 2 days because it may cause skin inflammation, blisters, and ulcers. It also needs to be kept away from eyes and mucous membranes to avoid burns. Hands must be washed thoroughly after usage. Commercial, OTC creams containing capsaicin are available and are discussed in Chapter 46⊙ .

GABA⊙ . Common adverse side effects include drowsiness and ataxia (loss of coordination). Benzodiazepines are usually prescribed for muscle relaxation when baclofen and tizanidine fail to produce adequate relief.

SPASTICITY

Spasticity is a condition in which certain muscle groups remain in a continuous state of contraction, usually as a result of damage to the CNS. The contracted muscles become stiff with increased muscle tone. Other signs and symptoms may include mild to severe pain, exaggerated deep tendon reflexes, muscle spasms, scissoring (involuntary crossing of the legs), and fixed joints.

45.4 Causes and Treatment of Spasticity

Spasticity usually results from damage to the motor area of the cerebral cortex which controls muscle movement. Etiologies most commonly associated with this condition include neurologic disorders such as cerebral palsy, severe head injury, spinal cord injury or lesions, and stroke. **Dystonia**, a chronic neurologic disorder, is characterized by involuntary muscle contraction that forces body parts into abnormal, occasionally painful movements or postures. It affects the muscle tone of the arms, legs, trunk, neck, eyelids, face, or vocal cords. Spasticity can be distressing and greatly impact an individual's quality of life whether the condition is short or long term. In addition to causing pain, impaired physical mobility influences the ability to perform activities of daily living (ADLs) and diminishes the patient's sense of independence.

Effective treatment for spasticity includes both physical therapy and medications. Medications alone are not adequate in reducing the complications of spasticity. Regular and consistent physical therapy exercises have been shown to decrease the severity of symptoms. Types of treatment includes muscle stretching to help prevent contractures, muscle group strengthening exercises, and repetitive motion exercises for improvement of accuracy. In extreme cases, surgery for tendon release or to sever the nerve-muscle pathway has occasionally been used. Drugs effective in the treatment of spasticity include several classifications of antispasmodics that act in the CNS, or at neuromuscular junctions.

DIRECT-ACTING ANTISPASMODICS

45.5 Treating Muscle Spasms Directly at the Muscle Tissue

Drugs effective in the treatment of spasticity include two centrally acting drugs, baclofen (Lioresal) and diazepam

(Valium), and dantrolene (Dantrium), a direct-acting drug. The direct-acting drugs produce an antispasmodic effect at the level of the neuromuscular junction, as shown in Figure 45.1.

Dantrolene relieves spasticity by interfering with the release of calcium ions in skeletal muscle. Other direct-acting drugs include botulinum toxin type A (Botox, Dysport) and botulinum toxin type B (Myobloc), used to offer significant relief of symptoms to people with dystonia; and quinine sulfate (Quinamm, Quiphile), which is used to treat leg cramps. Direct-acting drugs are summarized in Table 45.2.

Botulinum toxin is an unusual drug because, in higher quantities, it acts as a poison. *Clostridium botulinum* is the bacteria responsible for food poisoning or botulism. At lower doses, however, this drug is safe and effective as a muscle relaxant for patients with dystonia. It produces its effect by blocking the release of acetylcholine from cholinergic nerve terminals (Chapter 13) .

Because of the extreme weakness associated with botulinum, therapies may be needed to improve muscle strength. To circumvent major problems with mobility or posture, botulinum toxin is often applied to small muscle groups. Sometimes this drug is administered with centrally acting oral medications to increase functional use of a range of muscle groups.

Drawbacks to botulinum therapy are its delayed and limited effects. The treatment is mostly effective within 6 weeks and lasts for only 3 to 6 months. Another drawback is pain; botulinum is injected directly into the muscle. Pain associated with injections is usually blocked by a local anesthetic.

NURSING CONSIDERATIONS

The role of the nurse in antispasmodic therapy involves careful monitoring of a patient's condition and providing education as it relates to the prescribed drug regimen. The nurse should assess compliance with drug use, side effects,

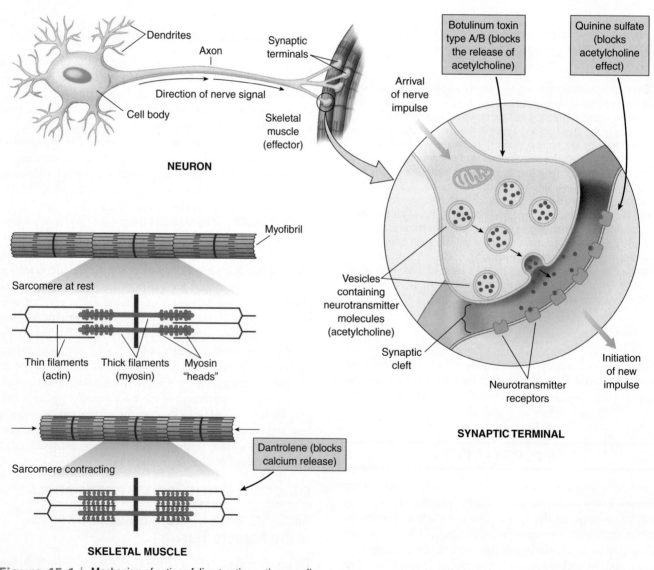

Figure 45.1 | Mechanism of action of direct-acting antispasmodics

Table 45.2	Direct-Acting Antispasmodic Drugs
Drug	**Route and Adult Dose (max dose where indicated)**
botulinum toxin type A (Botox, Dysport)	25 U injected directly into target muscle (max 30 day dose should not exceed 200 U)
botulinum toxin type B (Myobloc)	2,500–5,000 U/dose injected directly into target muscle; doses should be divided among muscle groups
dantrolene sodium (Dantrium)	PO; 25 mg qd; increase to 25 mg bid-qid; may increase every 4–7 d up to 100 mg bid-tid
quinine sulfate (Quinamm, Quiphile)	PO; 260–300 mg at hs

SPECIAL CONSIDERATIONS

The New Fountain of Youth?

Seen as the new fountain of youth, botulinum toxin type A (Botox Cosmetic) injections were approved by the FDA for the temporary improvement in the appearance of moderate to severe frown lines (vertical lines between the brows) in adult patients aged 65 years or less. It works to relax frown muscles by blocking nerve impulses that trigger wrinkle-causing muscle contractions, creating a smooth appearance between the brows. Administered in a few tiny injections of purified protein, this minimally invasive treatment is simple and quick, and delivers dramatic results with minimal discomfort. Results can be seen as early as 24 to 48 hours and the effect lasts up to 4 months. Injections should not be repeated more than once every 3 months. Side effects include headache, nausea, flulike symptoms, temporary eyelid drooping, mild pain, erythema at the injection site, and muscle weakness. According to the American Society for Aesthetic Plastic Surgery (ASAPS), Botox injections are the fastest growing cosmetic procedure in the industry. In 2001, more than 1.6 million people received injections, an increase of 46% over the previous year. Plastic surgery events known as Botox parties—also seminars, evenings, and socials—are seen to be a key element of Botox marketing in much of the United States.

and expected outcomes. Centrally acting drugs such as cyclobenzaprine and chlorzoxazone should be avoided in patients with liver disease. All centrally acting drugs cause CNS depression as evidenced by drowsiness and dizziness; therefore, patients should be advised to avoid hazardous activities such as driving until the effects of the drug are known. Patients should also be advised to avoid alcohol, benzodiazepines, opioids, and antihistamines as they can intensify the CNS depressant effects of the drugs. The nurse should warn patients against abrupt discontinuation of treatment because this may result in seizures.

Although dantrolene is a direct-acting muscle relaxant, it has similar effects and precautions as centrally acting drugs and is contraindicated in patients with liver disease, compromised pulmonary function, or cardiac dysfunction. The nurse should also be aware that a patient with spasticity may not be able to self-medicate and caregiver assistance may be required.

Patient education as it relates to central and direct-acting antispasmodics should include goals, reasons for obtaining baseline data such as health history and blood work, and side effects and interactions. See "Nursing Process Focus: Patients Receiving Drugs for Muscle Spasms or Spasticity" for specific points the nurse should include when teaching patients regarding this class of drugs.

Pr PROTOTYPE DRUG | DANTROLENE SODIUM (Dantrium)

ACTIONS AND USES

Dantrolene is often used for spasticity, especially for spasms of the head and neck. It directly relaxes muscle spasms by interfering with the release of calcium ions from storage areas inside skeletal muscle cells. It does not affect cardiac or smooth muscle. Dantrolene is especially useful for muscle spasms when they occur after spinal cord injury or stroke and in cases of cerebral palsy, multiple sclerosis, and occasionally for the treatment of muscle pain after heavy exercise. It is also used for the treatment of malignant hyperthermia.

Administration Alerts

■ Use oral suspension within several days, as it does not contain a preservative.
■ IV solution has a high pH and therefore is extremely irritating to tissue.
■ Pregnancy category C.

ADVERSE EFFECTS AND INTERACTIONS

Adverse effects include muscle weakness, drowsiness, dry mouth, dizziness, nausea, diarrhea, tachycardia, erratic blood pressure, photosensitivity, and urinary retention.

Dantrolene interacts with many other drugs. For example, it should not be taken with OTC cough preparations and antihistamines, alcohol, or other CNS depressants. Verapamil and other calcium channel blockers taken with dantrolene increase the risk of ventricular fibrillation and cardiovascular collapse. Patients with impaired cardiac or pulmonary function or hepatic disease should not take this drug.

 See the companion website for a Nursing Process Focus specific to this drug.

NURSING PROCESS FOCUS | **PATIENTS RECEIVING DRUGS FOR MUSCLE SPASMS OR SPASTICITY**

ASSESSMENT

Prior to administration:
- Obtain complete health history including allergies, drug history, and possible drug interactions.
- Obtain complete physical examination.
- Establish baseline level of consciousness and vital signs.

POTENTIAL NURSING DIAGNOSES

- Pain (acute/chronic), related to muscle spasms
- Impaired Physical Mobility, related to acute/chronic pain
- Risk for Injury, related to drug side effects
- Deficient Knowledge, related to drug therapy

PLANNING: PATIENT GOALS AND EXPECTED OUTCOMES

The patient will:
- Report a decrease in pain, increase in range of motion, and reduction of muscle spasm
- Exhibit no adverse effects from the therapeutic regimen
- Demonstrate an understanding of the therapeutic regimen

IMPLEMENTATION

Interventions and (Rationales)	*Patient Education/Discharge Planning*
■ Monitor LOC and vital signs. (Some skeletal muscle relaxants alter the patient's LOC. Others within this class may alter blood pressure and heart rate.)	Instruct patient to: ■ Avoid driving and other activities requiring mental alertness until effects of the medication are known ■ Report any significant change in sensorium, such as slurred speech, confusion, hallucinations, or extreme lethargy ■ Report palpitations, chest pain, dyspnea, unusual fatigue, weakness, and visual disturbances ■ Avoid using other CNS depressants such as alcohol that will intensify sedation
■ Monitor pain. ■ Determine location, duration, and precipitating factors of the patient's pain. (Drugs should diminish patients pain.)	Instruct patient: ■ To report the development of new sites of muscle pain ■ In relaxation techniques, deep breathing, and meditation methods to facilitate relaxation and reduce pain
■ Monitor for withdrawal reactions. (Abrupt withdrawal of baclofen may cause visual hallucinations, paranoid ideation, and seizures.)	■ Advise patient to not abruptly discontinue treatment.
■ Monitor muscle tone, range of motion, and degree of muscle spasm. (This will determine effectiveness of drug therapy.)	■ Instruct patient to perform gentle range of motion, only to the point of mild physical discomfort, throughout the day.
■ Provide additional pain relief measures such as positional support, gentle massage, and moist heat or ice packs. (Drugs alone may not be sufficient in providing pain relief.)	■ Instruct patient in complimentary pain interventions such as positioning, gentle massage, and the application of heat or cold to the painful area.
■ Monitor for side effects such as drowsiness, dry mouth, dizziness, nausea, vomiting, faintness, headache, nervousness, diplopia, and urinary retention (cyclobenzaprine).	Instruct the patient to: ■ Report side effects ■ Take medication with food to decrease GI upset ■ Report signs of urinary retention such as a feeling of urinary bladder fullness, distended abdomen, and discomfort
■ Monitor for side effects such as muscle weakness, dry mouth, dizziness, nausea, diarrhea, tachycardia, erratic blood pressure, photosensitivity, and urinary retention. (These adverse effects occur with certain drugs in this class.)	Instruct patient: ■ That frequent mouth rinses, sips of water, and sugarless candy or gum may help with dry mouth ■ That medication may cause a decrease in muscle strength and dosage may need to be reduced ■ To use sunscreen and protective clothing when outdoors

continued

NURSING PROCESS FOCUS: Patients Receiving Drugs for Muscle Spasms or Spasticity (continued)

EVALUATION OF OUTCOME CRITERIA

Evaluate the effectiveness of drug therapy by confirming that patient goals and expected outcomes have been met (see "Planning").

See Tables 45.1 and 45.2 for lists of drugs to which these nursing actions apply.

CHAPTER REVIEW

Key Concepts

The numbered key concepts provide a succinct summary of the important points from the corresponding numbered section within the chapter. If any of these points are not clear, refer to the numbered section within the chapter for review. Expanded versions can be found on the companion website.

45.1 Muscle spasms, involuntary contractions of a muscle or group of muscles, most commonly occur because of localized trauma to the skeletal muscle.

45.2 Muscle spasms can be treated through nonpharmacologic and pharmacologic therapies.

45.3 Many muscle relaxants treat muscle spasms at the level of the CNS, generating their effect within the brain and/or spinal cord, usually by inhibiting upper motor neuron activity, sedation, or alteration of simple reflexes.

45.4 Spasticity, a condition in which selected muscles are continuously contracted, results from damage to the CNS. Effective treatment for spasticity includes both physical therapy and medications.

45.5 Some antispasmodic drugs used for spasticity act directly on muscle tissue, relieving spasticity by interfering with the release of calcium ions.

Review Questions

1. Compare the cause of localized muscle spasms and spasticity. What is the main goal of antispasmodic therapy for each condition?

2. Compare the two general ways that antispasmodic drugs relieve muscle spasms and symptoms of spasticity.

Critical Thinking Questions

1. A 46-year-old male quadriplegic has been experiencing severe spasticity in the lower extremities, making it difficult for him to maintain position in his electric wheelchair. Prior to the episodes of spasticity, the patient was able to maintain a sitting posture. The risks and benefits of therapy with dantrolene (Dantrium) have been explained to him and he has decided that the benefits outweigh the risks. What assessments should the nurse make to determine whether the treatment is beneficial?

2. A 52-year-old breast cancer survivor is taking tamoxifen (Nolvadex) and has experienced leg and foot cramps "almost nightly." She states that these cramps have markedly decreased the quality of her sleep and that she is ready to "just stop taking" the tamoxifen, to end the leg cramps. The nurse is aware that tamoxifen is considered important in the chemoprevention of breast cancer. What variety of treatment modalities can be offered this patient to promote her comfort and decrease the chance that she will stop therapy?

3. A 32-year-old cotton farmer injured his lower back while unloading a truck at a farm cooperative. His healthcare provider started him on cyclobenzaprine (Flexeril) 10 mg tid for 7 days and referred him to outpatient physical therapy. After 4 days, the patient reports back to the office nurse that he is constipated and having trouble emptying his bladder. Discuss the cause of these side effects.

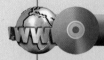

EXPLORE MediaLink

NCLEX review, case studies, and other interactive resources for this chapter can be found on the companion website at www.prenhall.com/adams. Click on "Chapter 45" to select the activities for this chapter. For animations, more NCLEX review questions, and an audio glossary, access the accompanying CD-ROM in this textbook.

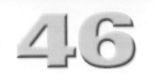
DRUGS AT A GLANCE

CALCIUM SUPPLEMENTS AND VITAMIN D THERAPY

- calcium gluconate (Kalcinate)
- calcitriol (Calcijex, Rocaltrol)

BONE RESORPTION INHIBITORS

Hormonal agents

- raloxifene (Evista)

Bisphosphonates

- etidronate disodium (Didronel)

DISEASE-MODIFYING DRUGS OF IMPORTANCE FOR RHEUMATOID ARTHRITIS

- hydroxychloroquine sulfate (Plaquenil Sulfate)

URIC ACID INHIBITORS

- colchicine

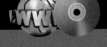

MediaLink www.prenhall.com/adams

CD-ROM

Animation:

   Mechanism in Action: Calcitriol (Calcijex)

Audio Glossary

NCLEX Review

Companion Website

NCLEX Review

Dosage Calculations

Case Study

Care Plans

Expanded Key Concepts

OBJECTIVES

After reading this chapter, the student should be able to:

1. Identify important symptoms or disorders associated with an imbalance of calcium, vitamin D, parathyroid hormone, and calcitonin.

2. Discuss drug treatments for hypocalemia, osteomalacia, and rickets.

3. Describe the nurse's role in the pharmacologic management of disorders caused by calcium and vitamin D deficiency.

4. Identify important disorders characterized by weak, fragile bones and abnormal joints.

5. Explain nonpharmacologic therapies used to treat bone and joint disorders.

6. Describe the nurse's role in the pharmacologic management of disorders related to bones and joints.

7. For each of the drug classes listed in Drugs at a Glance, know representative drugs, explain their mechanisms of action, primary actions, and/or important adverse effects.

8. Use the Nursing Process to care for patients receiving drug therapy for bone and joint disorders.

The skeletal system and joints are at the core of body movement and must be free of any defect that could affect stability of the other systems. Disorders associated with bones and joints may affect a patient's ability to fulfill daily activities and lead to immobility.

This chapter focuses on the pharmacotherapy of important skeletal disorders such as osteomalacia, osteoporosis, arthritis, and gout. Drugs used to treat important bone and joint disorders are mentioned in view of the major mobility problems that would occur without medical intervention. The importance of calcium balance and the action of vitamin D are stressed as they relate to the proper structure and function of bones.

46.1 Normal Calcium Physiology and Vitamin D

One of the most important minerals in the body responsible for bone formation is calcium. Levels of calcium in the blood are controlled by two endocrine glands: the parathyroid glands, which secrete parathyroid hormone (PTH), and the thyroid gland, which secretes calcitonin, as shown in Figure 46.1.

PTH stimulates bone cells called osteoclasts. These cells accelerate the process of **bone resorption**, demineralization that breaks down bone into its mineral components. Once bone is broken down or resorbed, calcium becomes available to be transported and used elsewhere in the body. The opposite of this process is **bone deposition**, which is

bone building. This process, which removes calcium from the blood, is stimulated by the hormone calcitonin.

PTH and calcitonin control calcium homeostasis in the body by influencing three major targets: the bones, kidneys, and gastrointestinal (GI) tract. The GI tract is mainly influenced by parathyroid hormone and involves vitamin D. Vitamin D and calcium metabolism are intimately related: Calcium disorders are often associated with vitamin D disorders.

Vitamin D is unique among vitamins in that the body is able to synthesize it from precursor molecules. In the skin, the inactive form of vitamin D, called **cholecalciferol**, is synthesized from cholesterol. Exposure of the skin to sunlight or ultraviolet light increases the level of cholecalciferol in the blood. Cholecalciferol can also be obtained

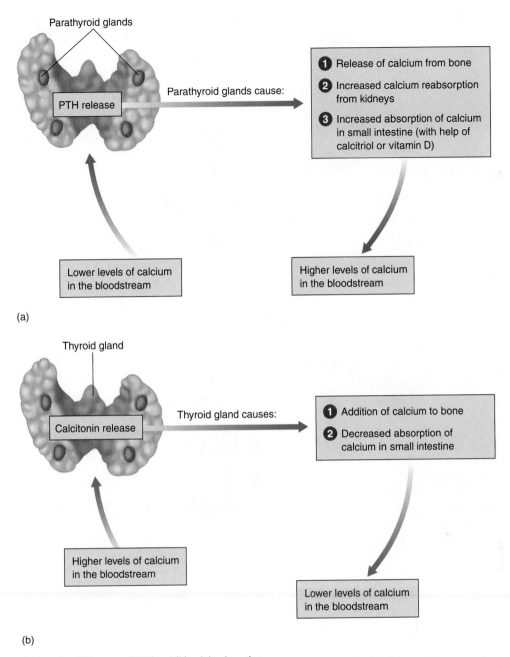

Parathyroid glands

PTH release

Parathyroid glands cause:

1 Release of calcium from bone
2 Increased calcium reabsorption from kidneys
3 Increased absorption of calcium in small intestine (with help of calcitriol or vitamin D)

Lower levels of calcium in the bloodstream

Higher levels of calcium in the bloodstream

(a)

Thyroid gland

Calcitonin release

Thyroid gland causes:

1 Addition of calcium to bone
2 Decreased absorption of calcium in small intestine

Higher levels of calcium in the bloodstream

Lower levels of calcium in the bloodstream

(b)

Figure 46.1 | (a) Parathyroid hormone (PTH) and (b) calcitonin action

from dietary products such as milk or other foods fortified with vitamin D. Figure 46.2 illustrates the metabolism of vitamin D.

Following its absorption or formation, cholecalciferol is converted to an intermediate vitamin form called **calcifediol**. Enzymes in the kidneys metabolize calcifediol to **calcitriol**, the active form of vitamin D. Parathyroid hormone stimulates the formation of calcitriol at the level of the kidneys. Patients with extensive kidney disease are unable to adequately synthesize calcitriol.

The primary function of calcitriol is to increase calcium absorption from the GI tract. Dietary calcium is absorbed better in the presence of active vitamin D and

parathyroid hormone, resulting in higher levels of calcium in the blood.

The importance of proper calcium balance in the body cannot be overstated. Calcium ion influences the excitability of all neurons. When calcium concentrations are too high (hypercalcemia), sodium permeability decreases across cell membranes. This is a dangerous state because nerve conduction depends on the proper influx of sodium into cells. When calcium levels in the bloodstream are too low (hypocalcemia), cell membranes become hyperexcitable. If this situation becomes severe, convulsions or muscle spasms may result. Calcium is also important for the normal functioning of other body processes such as blood coagulation and muscle contraction.

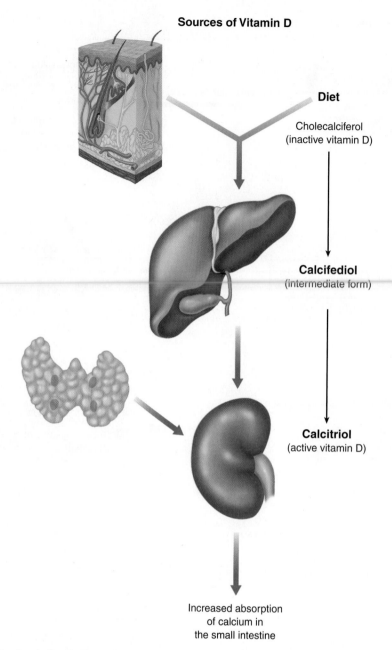

Sources of Vitamin D

Diet

Cholecalciferol
(inactive vitamin D)

Calcifediol
(intermediate form)

Calcitriol
(active vitamin D)

Increased absorption
of calcium in
the small intestine

Figure 46.2 | Pathway for vitamin D activation and action

CALCIUM-RELATED DISORDERS

Diseases and conditions of calcium and vitamin D metabolism include hypocalcemia, osteomalacia, osteoporosis, and Paget's disease. Therapies for calcium disorders include calcium supplements, vitamin D supplements, bisphosphonates, and several miscellaneous agents.

46.2 Pharmacotherapy of Hypocalcemia

Hypocalcemia is not a disease, but a sign of underlying pathology; therefore, diagnosis of the cause of hypocalcemia is essential. One common etiology is hyposecretion of PTH, as occurs when the thyroid and parathyroid glands are surgically removed. Digestive-related malabsorption

disorders and vitamin D deficiencies also result in hypocalcemia. When taking a medical history, the nurse should assess for lack of adequate intake of calcium-containing foods.

Symptoms of hypocalcemia are those of nerve and muscle excitability. Muscle twitching, tremor, or cramping may be evident. Numbness and tingling of the extremities may occur and convulsions are possible. Confusion and abnormal behavior may be observed. Severe hypocalcemia requires IV administration of calcium salts, whereas less severe hypocalcemia can often be reversed with oral supplements.

The two major forms of calcium are complexed and elemental. Most calcium supplements are in the form of complexed calcium. These products are often compared on the basis of their ability to release elemental calcium into the bloodstream. The greater the ability of complexed calcium to release elemental calcium, the more potent is the supplement. Elemental calcium may be obtained from dietary sources such as dark green vegetables, canned salmon, and fortified products including tofu, orange juice, and milk.

NURSING CONSIDERATIONS

The role of the nurse in calcium supplement therapy involves careful monitoring of a patient's condition and providing education as it relates to the prescribed drug regimen. The nurse should carefully evaluate and monitor patients taking calcium supplements. Before treatment begins, the nurse should obtain a thorough health history, including medications taken and a complete physical to include CBC and electrolyte profile, vital signs, and an ECG to establish baseline data. Lab tests and vital signs should be repeated throughout the treatment to determine effectiveness of the medication. Patients with known hypercalcemia, digitalis toxicity, dysrhythmias, or renal calculi should not take calcium gluconate. Calcium supplements should be used cautiously with patients who have severe renal or respiratory disease, pregnant or lactating women, and children.

Patient education as it relates to calcium supplements should include goals, reasons for obtaining baseline data, and possible side effects. Following are important points the nurse should include when teaching patients and caregivers about these supplements.

- Report signs or symptoms of hypercalcemia: drowsiness, lethargy, weakness, headache, anorexia, nausea and vomiting, increased urination, and thirst.
- Report signs or symptoms of hypocalcemia: seizures, muscle spasms, facial twitching, or paresthesias.
- Report side effects of medication such as nausea, vomiting, constipation, and difficulty urinating.
- Take safety precautions to prevent falling or fractures.

- Participate in active and passive ROM exercises, as tolerated.
- Consume calcium-rich foods, including milk and dairy products, dark green vegetables, soy beans, and canned fish with bones such as salmon.
- Avoid excessive intake of zinc-rich foods such as nuts, legumes, seeds, sprouts, and tofu, as zinc decreases calcium absorption.
- Avoid taking antacids that contain calcium or consuming calcium-fortified juices or foods without first notifying the healthcare provider.

46.3 Pharmacotherapy of Osteomalacia

Osteomalacia, referred to as rickets in children, is a disorder characterized by softening of bones without alteration of basic bone structure. The cause of osteomalacia and rickets is a lack of vitamin D and calcium in the diet, usually as a result of kidney failure or malabsorption of calcium from the GI tract. Signs and symptoms include hypocalcemia, muscle weakness, muscle spasms, and diffuse bone pain, especially in the hip area. Patients may also experience pain in the arms, legs, and spinal column. Classic signs of rickets in children include bowlegs and a pigeon breast. Children may also develop a slight fever and become restless at night.

Tests performed to verify osteomalacia include bone biopsy, bone radiographs, computerized tomography (CT) scan of the vertebral column, and determination of serum calcium, phosphate, and vitamin D levels. Many of these tests are routine for bone disorders and are performed as needed to determine the extent of bone health.

In extreme cases, surgical correction of disfigured limbs may be required. Drug therapy for children and adults consists of calcium supplements and vitamin D. A summary of drugs used for these conditions is provided in Table 46.1.

Pr PROTOTYPE DRUG	CALCIUM GLUCONATE (Kalcinate)
ACTIONS AND USES	**ADVERSE EFFECTS AND INTERACTIONS**
Calcium gluconate and other calcium compounds are used to correct hypocalcemia, and for osteoporosis and Paget's disease. The objective of calcium therapy is to return serum levels of calcium to normal. People at high risk for developing these conditions include postmenopausal women, those with little physical activity over a prolonged period, and patients taking certain medications such as corticosteroids, immunosuppressive drugs, and some antiseizure medications. Calcium gluconate is available in tablets or as a 10% solution for IV injection. Calcium gluconate is pregnancy category B.	The most common adverse effect of calcium gluconate is hypercalcemia, brought on by taking too much of this supplement. Symptoms include drowsiness, lethargy, weakness, headache, anorexia, nausea and vomiting, increased urination, and thirst. IV administration of calcium may cause hypotension, bradycardia, dysrhythmia, and cardiac arrest. Concurrent use of cardiac glycosides increases the risk of dysrhythmia. Magnesium may compete for GI absorption. Calcium decreases the absorption of tetracyclines.
Administration Alerts	
■ Give oral calcium supplements with meals or within 1 hr following meals. ■ If IV, administer slowly to avoid cardiac abnormalities.	

 See the companion website for a Nursing Process Focus specific to this drug.

MediaLink ⊕ National Institute of Arthritis, Musculoskeletal and Skin Diseases

NURSING PROCESS FOCUS   PATIENTS RECEIVING CALCIUM SUPPLEMENTS

ASSESSMENT

Prior to administration:
- Obtain complete health history including allergies, drug history, and possible drug interactions.
- Obtain baseline ECG.
- Obtain baseline vital signs, especially apical pulse for rate and rhythm, and blood pressure.
- Obtain lab work to include CBC and electrolytes, especially calcium.

POTENTIAL NURSING DIAGNOSES

- Risk for Injury, related to loss of bone mass and side effects of drug
- Deficient Knowledge, related to drug therapy

PLANNING: PATIENT GOALS AND EXPECTED OUTCOMES

The patient will:
- Have normal serum calcium levels (8.5–11.5 mg/dl)
- Demonstrate an understanding of the drug's action by accurately describing drug side effects and precautions, and measures to take to decrease any side effects
- Immediately report side effects and adverse reactions

IMPLEMENTATION

Interventions and (Rationales)	Patient Education/Discharge Planning
■ Monitor electrolytes throughout therapy. (Calcium and phosphorus levels tend to vary inversely. Low magnesium levels tend to coexist with low calcium levels.)	■ Teach patient of importance of routine lab studies, so deviations from normal can be corrected immediately.
■ Monitor for signs and symptoms of hypercalcemia. (Overtreatment may lead to excessive serum calcium levels.)	■ Instruct patient to report signs or symptoms of hypercalcemia: drowsiness, lethargy, weakness, headache, anorexia, nausea and vomiting, increased urination, and thirst.
■ Initiate seizure precautions for patients at risk for hypocalcemia. (Low calcium levels may cause seizures.)	■ Teach patient to be aware of signs of hypocalcemia, such as seizures, muscle spasms, facial twitching, and paresthesias.
■ Monitor for musculoskeletal difficulties. (Calcium gluconate is used to treat osteoporosis, rickets, osteomalacia.)	Instruct patient to: ■ Take special precautions to prevent fractures ■ Report episodes of sudden pain, joints out of alignment, inability of patient to assume normal positioning
■ Monitor intake and output. Use cautiously in patient with renal insufficiency. (Calcium is excreted by the kidneys.)	■ Instruct patient to report any difficulty in urination and measure I&O.
■ Monitor cardiac functioning. (Possible side effects may include short QT wave, heart block, hypotension, dysrhythmia, or cardiac arrest with IV administration.)	■ Inform patient to recognize and report palpitations or shortness of breath to healthcare provider.
■ Monitor injection site during intravenous administration for infiltration. (Extravasation may lead to necrosis.)	■ Instruct patient to report any pain at IV site.
■ Monitor diet. (Consuming calcium-rich foods may increase effect of drug. Consuming foods rich in zinc may decrease calcium absorption.)	■ Advise patient to: consume calcium-rich foods and avoid zinc-rich foods

EVALUATION OF OUTCOME CRITERIA

Evaluate the effectiveness of drug therapy by confirming that patient goals and expected outcomes have been met (see "Planning").

Table 46.1	Calcium Supplements and Vitamin D Therapy
Drug	**Route and Adult Dose**
Calcium Supplements (All Doses are in Terms of Elemental Calcium.)	
calcium acetate (Phos-Ex, PhosLo)	PO; 1–2 g bid-tid
calcium carbonate (BioCal, Calcite-500, others)	PO; 1–2 g bid-tid
calcium chloride	IV; 0.5–1 g qd q3d
calcium citrate (Citracal)	PO; 1–2 g bid-tid
calcium gluceptate	IV; 1.1–4.4 g qd
	IM; 0.5–1.1 g qd
Pr calcium gluconate (Kalcinate)	PO; 1–2 g bid-qid
calcium lactate	PO; 325 mg–1.3 g tid with meals
calcium phosphate tribasic (Posture)	PO; 1–2 g bid-tid
Vitamin D Supplements	
calcifediol (Calderol)	PO; 50–100 µg qd or qod
Pr calcitriol (Calcijex, Rocaltrol)	PO; 0.25 µg qd
ergocalciferol (Deltalin, Calciferol)	PO/IM; 25–125 µg qd for 6–12 wk

Inactive, intermediate, and active forms of vitamin D are also available as medications. The amount of vitamin D a patient needs will often vary depending on how much he or she is exposed to sunlight. After age 70, the average recommended intake of vitamin D increases from 400 to 600 IU/day. Because vitamin D is needed to absorb calcium from the GI tract, many supplements combine vitamin D and calcium into a single tablet.

NURSING CONSIDERATIONS

The role of the nurse in vitamin D therapy involves careful monitoring of a patient's condition and providing education as it relates to the prescribed drug regimen. The nurse should carefully evaluate and monitor patients taking this lipid-soluble vitamin because accumulation can lead to toxicity. Before a patient begins treatment, the nurse should obtain a thorough health history. Patients with known impaired liver function should be closely monitored during vitamin D therapy. Before treatment begins, the nurse should obtain a history of medications taken and a complete physical examination to establish baseline data. Liver function tests may be done to establish baseline data for patients on long-term therapy.

Periodic physicals should be done to determine the effectiveness of the drug. Patients should be monitored for side effects such as hypercalcemia, headache, weakness, dry mouth, thirst, increased urination, and muscle or bone pain. Periodic electrolyte levels should be obtained, as vitamin D therapy may lead to abnormal serum levels of calcium, magnesium, and phosphate.

Patient education as it relates to vitamin D supplements should include goals, reasons for obtaining baseline data, and possible side effects. Following are important points the nurse should include when teaching patients and caregivers about vitamin D.

- Consume dietary sources of vitamin D such as fortified milk.
- Take exactly as directed, because vitamin D can build to toxic levels if taken in excess quantities. Signs of overdose include fatigue, weakness, nausea, vomiting, and impairment of kidney function.
- Exposure to sunlight, 20 minutes a day, has been shown to supply enough vitamin D to prevent disease such as rickets.
- Avoid alcohol and other hepatotoxic drugs.
- Report use of any medication and avoid taking supplements containing lipid-soluble vitamins unless advised to do so by a healthcare provider.

46.4 Pharmacotherapy of Osteoporosis

Osteoporosis is the most common metabolic bone disease, responsible for as many as 1.5 million fractures annually. This disorder is usually asymptomatic, until the bones become brittle enough to fracture or for a vertebrae to collapse. In some cases, a lack of dietary calcium and vitamin D contribute to bone deterioration. In other cases, osteoporosis is due to disrupted bone homeostasis. Simply stated, bone resorption outpaces bone deposition and patients develop weak bones. Following are risk factors for osteoporosis.

- Postmenopause
- High alcohol or caffeine consumption
- Anorexia nervosa
- Tobacco use
- Physical inactivity

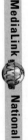

MediaLink National Osteoporosis Foundation

PROTOTYPE DRUG   **CALCITRIOL** (Calcijex, Rocaltrol)

ACTIONS AND USES

Calcitriol is the active form of vitamin D, available in both oral and IV formulations. It promotes the intestinal absorption of calcium and elevates serum levels of calcium. This medication is used in cases when patients have impaired kidney function or have hypoparathyroidism. Calcitriol reduces bone resorption and is useful in treating rickets. The effectiveness of calcitriol depends on the patient receiving an adequate amount of calcium; therefore, it is usually prescribed in combination with calcium supplements.

Administration Alerts

- Protect capsules from light and heat.
- Pregnancy category C.

ADVERSE EFFECTS AND INTERACTIONS

Common side effects include hypercalcemia, headache, weakness, dry mouth, thirst, increased urination, and muscle or bone pain. Thiazide diuretics may enhance effects of vitamin D, causing hypercalcemia. Too much vitamin D may cause dysrhythmia in patients receiving cardiac glycosides. Magnesium supplements should not be given concurrently due to increased risk of hypermagnesemia.

 See the companion website for a Nursing Process Focus specific to this drug.

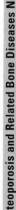

PHARMFACTS   **Osteoporosis**

- Osteoporosis is the most prevalent bone disorder in America.
- On a yearly basis, 28 million patients are either diagnosed with osteoporosis or are considered to be at extreme risk for this disorder.
- Women are 4 times more likely to develop osteoporosis than men. Many women with osteoporosis are of postmenopausal age.
- After the age of 50, one of every two women and one of every eight men are likely to develop a fracture related to osteoporosis.

- Testosterone deficiency, particularly in elderly men
- Lack of adequate vitamin D or calcium in the diet
- Drugs such as corticosteroids, some anticonvulsants, and immunosuppressants that lower calcium levels in the bloodstream

The most common risk factor associated with the development of osteoporosis is the onset of menopause. When women reach menopause, estrogen secretion declines and bones become weak and fragile. One theory to explain this occurence is that normal levels of estrogen may limit the life span of osteoclasts, the bones cells that resorb bone. When estrogen levels become low, osteoclast activity is no longer controlled, and bone demineralization is accelerated, resulting in loss of bone density. In women with osteoporosis, fractures often occur in the hips, wrists, forearms, or spine. The metabolism of calcium in osteoporosis is illustrated in Figure 46.3.

Many drug therapies are available for osteoporosis. These include calcium and vitamin D therapy, estrogen replacement therapy, estrogen receptor modulators, statins, slow-release sodium fluoride, biphosphonates, and calcitonin. Many of these drug classes are also used for other bone disorders or conditions unrelated to the skeletal system. Selected drugs for osteoporosis are listed in Table 46.2.

Hormone Replacement Therapy

Until recently, hormone replacement therapy (HRT) with estrogen was one of the most common treatments for osteoporosis in postmenopausal women. Because of increased risks of uterine cancer, thromboembolic disease, breast cancer, and other chronic disorders, the use of HRT in treating osteoporosis is no longer recommended. Additional information on HRT and the effects of estrogen may be found in Chapter 41 🔗 .

Calcitonin

Calcitonin, a natural product obtained from salmon, is approved for the treatment of osteoporosis in women who are more than 5 years postmenopause. It is available by nasal spray or SC injection. Calcitonin increases bone density and reduces the risk of vertebral fractures. Side effects are generally minor; the nasal formulation may irritate the nasal mucosa and allergies are possible. Parenteral forms may produce nausea and vomiting. In addition to treating osteoporosis, calcitonin is indicated for Paget's disease and hypercalcemia.

Selective Estrogen Receptor Modulators

Selective estrogen receptor modulators (SERMs) comprise a relatively new class of drugs used in the prevention and treatment of osteoporosis that bind to estrogen receptors. SERMS may be estrogen agonists or antagonists, depending on the specific drug and the tissue involved. For example, raloxifene (Evista) blocks estrogen receptors in the uterus and breast; thus, it has no estrogen-like proliferative effects on these tissues that might promote cancer. Raloxifene does, however, decrease bone resorption, thus increasing bone density, making fractures less likely. Like estrogen, it has a cholesterol-lowering effect.

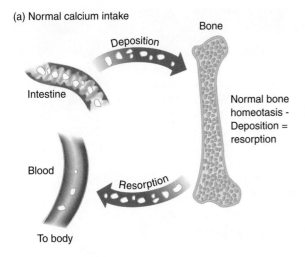

(a) Normal calcium intake

Bone

Deposition

Intestine

Normal bone homeotasis - Deposition = resorption

Blood

Resorption

To body

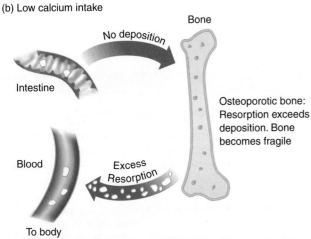

(b) Low calcium intake

Bone

No deposition

Intestine

Osteoporotic bone: Resorption exceeds deposition. Bone becomes fragile

Blood

Excess Resorption

To body

Figure 46.3 | Calcium metabolism in osteoporosis

NURSING CONSIDERATIONS

The role of the nurse in drug therapy with hormones and estrogen modulators (SERMs) involves careful monitoring of a patient's condition and providing education as it relates to the prescribed drug regimen. The nurse should carefully evaluate and monitor patients taking this class of medications, and obtain a thorough health history. The nurse should also obtain a history of medications taken and a complete physical including liver function studies and a bone scan to determine the progression of the disease, and to establish baseline data. Annual checkups and periodic bone density scans should be repeated throughout therapy to determine the effectiveness of the drug. Raloxifene is a pregnancy category X drug, and is thus contraindicated in pregnant patients.

Patients with a known history of thromboembolism, who are pregnant or lactating, taking hormone replacement, or are premenopausal should not take these drugs. SERMs should be used carefully when taking the following drugs: clofibrate, diazepam, diazoxide, ibuprofen, indomethacin, and naproxen.

Patient education as it relates to SERMs should include goals, reasons for obtaining baseline data, and possible side effects. Following are important points the nurse should include when teaching patients and caregivers about SERMs.

- Report side effects that may indicate thromboembolic disease, especially sudden chest pain, dyspnea, pain in calves, and swelling in the legs.
- Consume supplements of calcium and vitamin D, as directed by the healthcare provider.
- Participate in active weight-bearing exercises such as stair climbing or lifting weights.
- Avoid prolonged periods of immobility.
- Take special safety precautions to prevent falling or fractures.
- Discuss the possibility of using a "hip protector" to prevent hip fractures due to accidental falls.

Bisphosphonates

The most common drug class for osteoporosis is the **bisphosphonates**. These drugs are structural analogs of pyrophosphate, a natural inhibitor of bone resorption. Bisphosphonates inhibit bone resorption by suppressing osteoclast activity thus increasing bone density and reducing the incidence of fractures. Examples include etidronate (Didronel), alendronate (Fosamax), tiludronate (Skelid), and pamidronate (Aredia), which is available as an injectable drug. Adverse effects include GI problems such as nausea, vomiting, abdominal pain, and esophageal irritation. Because these drugs are poorly absorbed, they should be taken on an empty stomach, as tolerated by the patient.

Table 46.2	Bone Resorption Inhibitor Drugs
Drug	**Route and Adult Dose**
Hormonal agents	
calcitonin—human (Cibacalcin); calcitonin—salmon (Calciman, Miacalcin)	Paget's disease: SC; human, 0.5 mg qd SC/IM: salmon, 100 IU qd; Hypercalcemia: SC/IM: salmon, 4 IU/kg bid
Pr raloxifene hydrochloride (Evista)	PO; 60 mg qd
Bisphosphonates	
alendronate sodium (Fosamax)	osteoporosis treatment: PO; 10 mg qd; osteoporosis prevention: PO; 5 mg qd; Paget's disease: PO; 40 mg qd for 6 mo
Pr etidronate disodium (Didronel)	PO; 5–10 mg/kg qd for 6 mo or 11–20 mg/kg qd for 3 mo
pamidronate disodium (Aredia)	IV; 15–90 mg in 1000 ml NS or D5W over 4–24 h
risedronate sodium (Actonel)	PO; 30 mg qd at least 30 min before the first drink or meal of the day for 2 mo
tiludronate disodium (Skelid)	PO; 400 mg qd taken with 6–8 oz of water 2 h before or after food for 3 mo

Pr PROTOTYPE DRUG | RALOXIFENE (Evista)

ACTIONS AND USES

Raloxifene is a selective estrogen receptor modulator (SERM). It decreases bone resorption and increases bone mass and density by acting through the estrogen receptor. Raloxifene is primarily used for the prevention of osteoporosis in postmenopausal women. This drug also reduces serum total cholesterol and LDL (low-density lipoprotein) without lowering HDL (high-density lipoprotein) or triglycerides.

Administration Alerts

- Take drug exactly as prescribed.
- May be taken with or without food.
- Pregnancy category X.

ADVERSE EFFECTS AND INTERACTIONS

Common side effects are hot flashes, migraine headache, flulike symptoms, endometrial disorder, breast pain, and vaginal bleeding. Patients should not take cholesterol-lowering drugs or estrogen replacement therapy concurrently with this medication.

Warfarin use may lead to decreased prothrombin time. Decreased raloxifene absorption will result from concurrent use of ampicillin or cholestyramine. Use of raloxifene with other highly protein-bound drugs (ibuprofen, indomethacin, diazepam, etc.) may interfere with binding sites.

See the companion website for a Nursing Process Focus specific to this drug.

Recent studies suggest that once-weekly dosing may give the same bone density benefits as daily dosing, due to the extended duration of drug action of the bisphosphonates.

NURSING CONSIDERATIONS

The role of the nurse in bisphosphonate drug therapy involves careful monitoring of a patient's condition and providing education as it relates to the prescribed drug regimen. The nurse should carefully evaluate and monitor patients taking this class of medication and obtain a thorough health history. The nurse should obtain a drug history and a complete physical to include CBC, pH, chemistry panel and renal function studies, vital signs (especially heart rate for rate and rhythm), and bone density testing to establish baseline data. These tests should be repeated throughout the treatment to determine the progress of pharmacotherapy.

Patients with known hypersensitivity, children, and those with colitis and severe renal disease should not take these drugs. Bisphosphonates should be used carefully with patients who are pregnant or lactating and those with mild renal disease. Preexisting vitamin D deficiency or hypocalcemia should be corrected before beginning bisphosphate therapy. Therapeutic effects may not be evident for several months.

Patient education as it relates to bisphosphonates should include goals, reasons for obtaining baseline data, and possible side effects. Following are important points the nurse should include when teaching patients and caregivers about bisphosphonates:

- Recognize signs of hypocalcemia, such as seizures, muscle spasms, facial twitching, and paresthesias.
- Report any difficulty in urination, a decrease in urinary

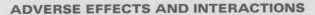

Pr **PROTOTYPE DRUG**	**ETIDRONATE** (Didronel)

ACTIONS AND USES	**ADVERSE EFFECTS AND INTERACTIONS**
Bisphosphonates are a common treatment for post-menopausal osteoporosis. Etidronate is available in oral and IV forms and has the capability of strengthening bones with continued use by slowing bone resorption. Effects begin 1 to 3 months after therapy starts and may continue for months after therapy is stopped. This drug lowers serum alkaline phosphatase, the enzyme associated with bone turnover, without major adverse effects. Etidronate is also used for Paget's disease and to treat hypercalcemia due to malignancy.	Common side effects of etidronate are diarrhea, nausea, vomiting, esophageal irritation, and a metallic or altered taste perception. Pathologic fractures may occur if the drug is taken longer than 3 months.
Administration Alerts	Calcium supplements may decrease absorption of etidronate; therefore, concomitant use of these drugs should be avoided. Food-drug interactions are common. Milk and other dairy products, and medications such as calcium, iron, antacids, other mineral supplements, must be reviewed before beginning bisphosphonate therapy because they have the potential to decrease the effectiveness of bisphosphonates.
■ Take drug on an empty stomach 2 hours before a meal.	
■ Pregnancy category B (PO); C (parenteral).	

See the companion website for a Nursing Process Focus specific to this drug.

function, or other side effects such as nausea, vomiting, diarrhea, or bone pain.

■ Take medication on an empty stomach and wait at least 30 minutes before eating.

■ Consume calcium-rich foods, including milk and milk products, dark green vegetables, canned fish with bones such as salmon, and soy beans.

■ Take special safety precautions to prevent falling or fractures.

■ Report any episodes of sudden onset of pain, warmth or inflammation over bony areas, or restricted activity.

■ Participate in active and passive ROM exercises as possible.

■ Properly store medication; keep away from children.

46.5 Pharmacotherapy of Paget's Disease

Paget's disease, or osteitis deformans, is a chronic, progressive condition characterized by enlarged and abnormal bones. With this disorder, the processes of bone resorption and bone formation occur at a high rate. Excessive bone turnover causes the new bone to be weak and brittle; deformity and fractures may result. The patient may be asymptomatic, or have only vague, nonspecific complaints for many years. Symptoms include pain of the hips and femurs, joint inflammation, headaches, facial pain, and hearing loss if bones around the ear cavity are affected. Nerves along the spinal column may be pinched due to compression between the vertebrae.

Paget's disease is sometimes confused with osteoporosis because some of the symptoms are similar. In fact, medical treatments for osteoporosis are similar to those for Paget's disease. The cause of Paget's disease, however, is quite different. The enzyme alkaline phosphatase is elevated in the blood because of the extensive bone turnover, and the disease is usually confirmed by early detection of this enzyme in the blood. Calcium is also liberated because of its close association with phosphate. If diagnosed early enough, symptoms can be treated successfully. If the diagnosis is made late in the progress of the disease, permanent skeletal abnormalities may develop, and other disorders may appear, including arthritis, kidney stones, and heart disease.

Bisphosphonates are drugs of choice for the pharmacotherapy of Paget's disease. Therapy is usually cyclic, with bisphosphonates administered until serum alkaline phosphatase levels return to normal, followed by several months without the drugs. When serum alkaline phosphatase becomes elevated, therapy is begun again. The pharmacologic goals are to slow the rate of bone reabsorption and encourage the deposition of strong bone. Calcitonin nasal spray is used as an option for patients who cannot tolerate bisphosphonates. Surgery may be indicated in cases of severe bone deformity, degenerative arthritis, or fracture. Patients with Paget's disease should maintain adequate dietary sources of calcium and vitamin D on a daily basis, and adequate exposure to sunlight is important.

JOINT DISORDERS

Joint conditions such as osteoarthritis, rheumatoid arthritis, and gout are frequent indications for pharmacotherapy. Osteoarthritis (OA) is a degenerative, age-onset disease characterized by wearing away of cartilage at articular joint surfaces. Rheumatoid arthritis (RA) is a systemic autoimmune disorder characterized by disfigurement and inflammation of multiple joints that occurs at an earlier age than osteoarthritis. Gout is a metabolic disorder that is a form of acute arthritis characterized by joint pain caused by the accumulation of uric acid in the bloodstream or joint cavities. Because joint pain is common to all three disorders, analgesics and anti-inflammatory drugs are important components of pharmacotherapy. A few additional drugs are specific to the particular joint pathology.

MediaLink The Paget Foundation

NURSING PROCESS FOCUS — PATIENTS RECEIVING BISPHOSPHONATES

ASSESSMENT

Prior to administration:
- Obtain complete health history including allergies, drug history and possible drug interactions.
- Assess for presence/history of pathologic fractures, hypocalcemia, and hypercalcemia.
- Assess nutritional status.
- Obtain lab work to include CBC, pH, electrolytes and renal function studies (BUN, creatinine, uric acid), serum calcium and phosphorous.

POTENTIAL NURSING DIAGNOSES

- Deficient Knowledge, related to drug therapy
- Risk for Imbalanced Fluid Volume, related to adverse reaction to drug
- Nausea, related to side effects of drug
- Pain, acute, bone, related to adverse drug reaction
- Ineffective Therapeutic Regimen Management, related to the fact that therapeutic response may take 1–3 months

PLANNING: PATIENT GOALS AND EXPECTED OUTCOMES

Patient will:
- Demonstrate decreased progression of osteoporosis or Paget's disease
- Demonstrate decreased risk for pathologic fractures
- Remain free of side effects or adverse reactions
- Demonstrate understanding of dietary needs/modifications
- Maintain adequate fluid volume

IMPLEMENTATION

Interventions and (Rationales)	Patient Education/Discharge Planning
■ Monitor for pathologic fractures and bone pain. (Drug may cause defective mineralization of newly formed bone.)	■ Instruct patient to report any sudden bone or joint pain, inability to correctly position self, swelling over bone or joint.
■ Monitor for GI side effects. (There may be problems with absorption if patient has persistent nausea or diarrhea.)	■ Advise patient that new onset nausea or diarrhea may be symptom of adverse reaction, and to report immediately.
■ Monitor calcium lab values: Serum calcium levels should be 9–10mg/dl. (Through inhibition of bone resorption, drug causes blood levels of calcium to fall.)	Advise patient to: ■ Have lab studies performed prior to beginning bisphosphonate therapy and periodically during therapy ■ Report symptoms of hypocalcemia (muscle spasms, facial grimacing, convulsions, irritability, depression, psychoses) ■ Report symptoms of hypercalcemia (increased bone pain, anorexia, nausea/vomiting, constipation, thirst, lethargy, fatigue, confusion, depression)
■ Monitor kidney function, especially creatinine level. (Etidronate cannot be used in patients whose creatinine is >5.) ■ Monitor BUN, vitamin D, urinalysis, and serum phosphate and magnesium levels.	■ Instruct patient to report any urinary changes, such as decreased urine production, increased urination.
■ Monitor dietary habits. (Diet must have adequate amounts of vitamin D, calcium, and phosphate.)	■ Advise patient to include good food sources of vitamin D, calcium, and phosphate, including dairy products and green leafy vegetables.
■ Monitor compliance with recommended regimen. (Patient may discontinue drug due to apparent lack of response.)	Advise patient: ■ That therapy should continue for 6 months maximum, but full therapeutic response may take 1–3 months ■ That effects continue several months after drug is discontinued ■ To avoid vitamins, mineral supplements, antacids and high-calcium products within 2 hours of taking bisphosphonates

EVALUATION OF OUTCOME CRITERIA

Evaluate the effectiveness of drug therapy by confirming that patient goals and expected outcomes have been met (see "Planning").

☞ *See Table 46.2, under "Bisphosphonates", for a list of drugs to which these nursing actions apply.*

46.6 Pharmacotherapy of Arthritis

Arthritis is a general term meaning inflammation of a joint. There are several types of arthritis, each having somewhat different characteristics based on the etiology. Osteoarthritis is the most common type and produces symptoms that include localized pain and stiffness, joint and bone enlargement, and limitations in movement. It is not accompanied by the degree of inflammation associated with other forms of arthritis. The etiology of osteoarthritis is thought to be due to excessive wear and tear of weight-bearing joints; the knee, spine, and hip are particularly affected. Many consider this disorder to be a normal part of the aging process. A patient with osteoarthritis is shown in Figure 46.4.

The goals of pharmacotherapy for osteoarthritis include reduction of pain and inflammation. Due to their safety and efficacy, the COX-2 inhibitors are the preferred therapy for osteoarthritis. Topical medications (capsaicin cream and balms), NSAIDs (including aspirin), acetaminophen, and tramadol (Ultram) are also of value for treatment of pain associated with osteoarthritis. In acute cases, intra-articular glucocorticoids may be used on a temporary basis.

A new type of drug therapy for patients with moderate osteoarthritis who do not respond adequately to analgesics is now available. Sodium hyaluronate (Hyalgan) is a preparation of a chemical normally found in high amounts within synovial fluid. Administered by injection directly into the knee joint, this drug replaces or supplements the body's natural hyaluronic acid that deteriorated due to the inflammation of osteoarthritis. Treatment consists of three to five injections, one injection per week. By coating the articulating cartilage surface, Hyalgan helps to provide a barrier thus preventing friction and further inflammation of the joint. Information given to the patient prior to administration should include side effects such as pain and/or

swelling at the injection site and the avoidance of any strenuous activities for approximately 48 hours after injection.

Rheumatoid arthritis (RA) is the second most common form of arthritis, and has an autoimmune etiology. In RA, **autoantibodies** called rheumatoid factors activate complement and draw leukocytes into the area, where they attack normal cells. This results in persistent injury and the formation of inflammatory fluid within the joints. Joint capsules, tendons, ligaments, and skeletal muscles may also be affected. Unlike OA, which causes local pain in affected joints, patients with RA may develop systemic manifestations that include infections, pulmonary disease, pericarditis, abnormal numbers of blood cells, and symptoms of metabolic dysfunction such as fatigue, anorexia, and weakness. A patient with RA is shown in Figure 46.5.

Pharmacotherapy for RA includes the same classes of analgesics and anti-inflammatory drugs used for osteoarthritis. Additional drugs are sometimes used to control the severe inflammation and the immune aspects of the disease. Additional therapies include the following:

- Glucocorticoids
- Disease-modifying drugs: hydroxychloroquine (Plaquenil), gold salts, sulfasalazine (Azulfidine), D-penicillamine (Cuprimine)
- Immunosuppressants: methotrexate (Rheumatrex), leflunomide (Arava), azathioprine (Imuran), cyclosporine (Neoral), cyclophosphamide (Cytoxan)
- Tumor necrosis factor blockers: etanercept (Enbrel), infliximab (Remicade)

These additional therapies are taken as a second course of treatment after pain and anti-inflammatory medications. Several months may be required before maximum therapeutic effects are achieved. Because many of these drugs can be toxic, patients should be closely monitored. Adverse effects vary depending on the type of drug. These agents are shown in Table 46.3.

Nonpharmacologic therapies for the pain of arthritis are common. The use of nonimpact and passive ROM exercises to maintain flexibility along with rest is encouraged. Splinting may help keep joints positioned correctly

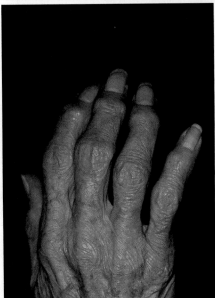

Figure 46.4 | Patient with osteoarthritis

| PHARMFACTS | Arthritis |

- Between 20 and 40 million patients in the United States are affected by osteoarthritis.
- After age 40, more than 90% of the population has symptoms of osteoarthritis in major weight-bearing joints. After 70 years of age, almost all patients have symptoms of osteoarthritis.
- Of the world's population, 1% has rheumatoid arthritis, which most often affects patients between 30 and 50 years of age. Women are 3 to 5 times more likely to develop rheumatoid arthritis than men.
- Between 1% and 3% of the U.S. population is affected by gout. Most of the patients are men between the ages of 30 and 60. Most women are affected after menopause.

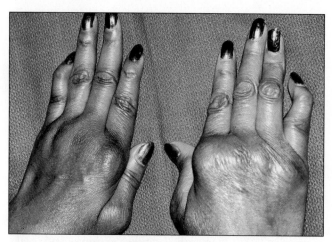

Figure 46.5 | Patient with rheumatoid arthritis *Source: Courtesy of Dr. Jason L. Smith.*

NATURAL THERAPIES — Glucosamine and Chondroitin for Osteoarthritis

Glucosamine sulfate is a natural substance that is an important building block of cartilage. With aging, glucosamine is lost with the natural thinning of cartilage. As cartilage wears down, joints lose their normal cushioning ability, resulting in the pain and inflammation of osteoarthritis. Glucosamine sulfate is available as an OTC dietary supplement. Some studies have shown it to be more effective than a placebo in reducing mild arthritis and joint pain. It is purported to promote cartilage repair in the joints. Although reliable long-term studies are not available, glucosamine is marketed as a safe and inexpensive alternative to prescription anti-inflammatory drugs.

Chondroitin sulfate is another dietary supplement purported to promote cartilage repair. It is a natural substance that forms part of the matrix between cartilage cells. Chondroitin is usually combined with glucosamine in specific arthritis formulas.

and relieve pain. Other therapies commonly used to relieve pain and discomfort include thermal therapies, meditation, visualization, distraction techniques, and massage therapy. Knowledge of proper body mechanics and posturing may offer some benefit. Physical and occupational therapists are usually active in helping patients minimize pain through these approaches. Surgical techniques such as joint replacement and reconstructive surgery may become necessary when other methods are ineffective.

46.7 Pharmacotherapy of Gout

Gout is due to an accumulation of uric acid crystals that occurs from increased metabolism of DNA or RNA, or from the reduced excretion of uric acid by the kidneys. Uric acid is the final breakdown product of DNA and RNA metabolism. One metabolic step that is important to the pharmacotherapy of this disease is the conversion of hypoxanthine to uric acid by the enzyme xanthine oxidase. An elevated blood level of uric acid is called hyperuricemia.

Gout may be classified as primary or secondary. Primary gout, caused by genetic errors in uric acid metabolism, is most commonly observed in Pacific Islanders. Secondary gout is caused by diseases or drugs that increase the metabolic turnover of nucleic acids, or that interfere with uric acid excretion. Examples of drugs that may cause gout include thiazide diuretics, aspirin, cyclosporine, and alcohol, when ingested on a chronic basis. Conditions that can cause secondary gout include diabetic ketoacidosis, kidney failure, and diseases associated with a rapid cell turnover such as leukemia, hemolytic anemia, and polycythemia.

Acute gouty arthritis occurs when needle-shaped uric acid crystals accumulate in joints, resulting in red, swollen, and inflamed tissue. Attacks have a sudden onset, often occur at night, and may be triggered by diet, injury, or other stresses. Gouty arthritis most often occurs in the big toes, heels, ankles, wrists, fingers, knees, and elbows. Of the patients with gout, 90% are men.

The goals of gout pharmacotherapy are twofold: termination of acute attacks and prevention of future attacks. NSAIDs are the drugs of choice for treating the pain and inflammation of acute attacks. Indomethacin (Indocin) is a

Table 46.3	Disease-Modifying Drugs for Rheumatoid Arthritis
Drug	**Route and Adult Dose (max dose where indicated)**
auranofin (Ridaurd)	PO; 3–6 mg qd-bid; may increase up to 3 mg tid after 6 mo
aurothioglucose (Gold thioglucose, Solganal)	IM; 10 mg wk 1; 25 mg wk 2; then 50 mg/wk to a cumulative dose of 1 g;
azathioprine (Imuran)	PO; 0.5–1.0 mg/kg/d (max 2.5 mg/kg/d)
gold sodium thiomalate (Myochrysine)	IM; 10 mg wk 1; 25 mg wk 2, then 25–50 mg/wk to a cumulative dose of 1 g
hydroxychloroquine sulfate (Plaquenil Sulfate)	PO; 400–600 mg qd
leflunomide (Arava)	PO; Loading dose 100 mg/d for 3 d; maintenance dose 10–20 mg qd
methotrexate (Mexate, Folex) (see p. 508 for the Prototype Drug box)	PO; 2.5–5 mg q12 h for three doses each week
penicillamine (Cubrimine, Depen)	PO; 125–250 mg qd (max 1–1.5 g/day)
sulfasalazine (Azulfidine)	PO; 250–500 mg qd (max 8 g/day)

Pr **PROTOTYPE DRUG** | **HYDROXYCHLOROQUINE SULFATE** (Plaquenil)

ACTIONS AND USES

Hydroxychloroquine is prescribed for rheumatoid arthritis and lupus erythematosus in patients who have not responded well to other anti-inflammatory drugs. This agent relieves the severe inflammation characteristic of these disorders. For full effectiveness, hydroxychloroquine is most often prescribed with salicylates and glucocorticoids. This drug is also used for prophylaxis and treatment of malaria (Chapter 33) ⊖⊃ .

Administration Alerts

■ Take at the same time every day.

■ Administer with milk to decrease GI upset.

■ Store drug in safe place, as it is very toxic to children.

■ Pregnancy category C.

ADVERSE EFFECTS AND INTERACTIONS

Adverse symptoms include blurred vision, GI disturbances, loss of hair, headache, and mood and mental changes. Hydroxychloroquine has possible ocular effects that include blurred vision, photophobia, diminished ability to read, and blacked out areas in the visual field.

Antacids with aluminum and magnesium may prevent absorption. This drug interferes with the patient's response to rabies vaccine. Hydroxychloroquine may increase the risk of liver toxicity when administered with hepatotoxic drugs; alcohol use should be eliminated during therapy. It also may lead to increased digoxin levels.

 See the companion website for a Nursing Process Focus specific to this drug.

Table 46.4	Uric Acid-Inhibiting Drugs for Gout and Gouty Arthritis
Drug	**Route and Adult Dose (max dose where indicated)**
allopurinol (Lopurin, Zyloprim)	PO (primary); 100 mg qd; may increase by 100 mg/wk (max 800 mg/day); PO (secondary); 200–800 mg qd for 2–3 d or longer
colchicine	PO; 0.5–1.2 mg followed by 0.5–0.6 mg q 1–2 h until pain relief (max 4 mg/attack)
probenecid (Benemid, Probalan)	PO; 250 mg bid for 1 wk; then 500 mg bid (max 3 g/d)
sulfinpyrazone (Anturan)	PO; 100–200 mg bid for 1 wk; then increase to 200–400 mg bid

NSAID that has been widely used for acute gout, although the newer COX-2 inhibitors are also prescribed.

The uric acid inhibitors such as colchicine probenecid (Benemid), sulfinpyrazone (Anturane), and allopurinol (Lopurin) are also used for acute gout. Uric acid inhibitors block the accumulation of uric acid within the blood or uric acid crystals within the joints. When uric acid accumulation is blocked, symptoms associated with gout diminish. About 80% of the patients using uric acid inhibitors experience GI complaints such as abdominal cramping, nausea, vomiting, and/or diarrhea. These agents are summarized in Table 46.4. Glucocorticoids are useful for the short-term therapy of acute gout, particularly when the symptoms are in a single joint and the medication is delivered intraarticularly.

Prophylaxis of gout includes dietary management, avoidance of drugs that worsen gout, and treatment with antigout medications. Patients should avoid high purine foods such as meat, legumes, alcoholic beverages, mushrooms, and oatmeal, because nucleic acids will be formed when they are metabolized. Prophylaxis therapy includes drugs that lower serum uric acid. Probenecid and sulfinpyrazone are uricosuric drugs that increase the excretion of uric acid by blocking its reabsorption in the kidney. Allopurinol blocks xanthine oxidase, thus inhibiting the formation of

uric acid. Prophylactic therapy is used for patients who suffer frequent and acute gout attacks. Drugs for gout are shown in Table 46.4.

NURSING CONSIDERATIONS

The role of the nurse in drug therapy with antigout agents involves careful monitoring of a patient's condition and providing education as it relates to the prescribed drug regimen. The nurse should carefully evaluate and monitor patients taking this class of drugs and obtain a thorough health history. The nurse should obtain a drug history and a complete physical examination to include lab studies, which include CBC, platelets, liver and renal function studies, uric acid levels, and urinalysis. Vital signs should also be taken to establish baseline data. These tests should be repeated throughout the treatment to assess the effectiveness of the drug.

Patients with known hypersensitivity, pregnancy, or severe GI, renal, hepatic, or cardiac disease should not take antigout agents. These drugs should be used carefully in children and cautiously with patients who have blood dyscrasias or mild liver disease.

Patient education as it relates to antigout drugs should include goals, reasons for obtaining baseline data, and

PROTOTYPE DRUG | COLCHICINE

ACTIONS AND USES

Colchicine inhibits inflammation and reduces pain associated with gouty arthritis. It may be taken prophylactically for acute gout or in combination with other uric acid-inhibiting agents. Colchicine works by inhibiting the synthesis of microtubules, subcellular structures responsible for helping white blood cells infiltrate an area.

Administration Alerts

- Take on an empty stomach, when symptoms first appear.
- Pregnancy category C. Parenteral doses must not be given to pregnant women.

ADVERSE EFFECTS AND INTERACTIONS

Side effects such as nausea, vomiting, diarrhea, and GI upset are more likely to occur at the beginning of therapy. These side effects are related to disruption of microtubules responsible for cell proliferation. Colchicine may also directly interfere with the absorption of vitamin B_{12}.

Colchicine interacts with many drugs. For example, NSAIDs may increase GI symptoms and cyclosporine may increase bone marrow suppression. Erythromycin may increase colchicine levels. Phenylbutazone may increase the risk for blood dyscrasias. Loop diuretics may decrease colchicine effects. Alcohol or products that contain alcohol may cause skin rashes and enhance liver damage.

NURSING PROCESS FOCUS | PATIENTS RECEIVING COLCHICINE Pr

ASSESSMENT

Prior to administration:
- Obtain complete health history including allergies, drug history, and possible drug interactions.
- Obtain baseline vital signs.
- Obtain lab work to include CBC, platelets, uric acid levels, renal and liver function tests, and urinalysis.

POTENTIAL NURSING DIAGNOSES

- Activity Intolerance, related to joint pain
- Disturbed Body Image, related to joint swelling
- Deficient Knowledge, related to effects and side effects of drug therapy

PLANNING: PATIENT GOALS AND EXPECTED OUTCOMES

The patient will:
- Report a decrease in pain and an increase in function in affected joints
- Demonstrate an understanding of the drug's action by accurately describing drug side effects and precautions, and measures to take to decrease any side effects
- Immediately report side effects and adverse reactions

IMPLEMENTATION

Interventions and (Rationales)	Patient Education/Discharge Planning
Monitor lab results throughout therapy. (Agranulocytosis and thrombocytopenia may occur.) Perform Coombs test for hemolytic anemia.	Teach patient importance of routine lab studies, so deviations from normal can be corrected immediately.
Monitor for signs of toxicity.	Instruct patient to report weakness, abdominal pain, nausea, and/or diarrhea.
Monitor for signs of renal impairment such as oliguria. Record intake and output.	Instruct patient to report a decrease in urinary output and to increase fluid intake to 3–4 L/day.
Ensure that medication is administered correctly.	Inform patient to take medication on an empty stomach. Medication should be taken at first sign of gout attack.
Monitor for pain and mobility. (This is used to assess effectiveness of medication.)	Teach patient to report an increase or decrease in discomfort and swelling.

EVALUATION OF OUTCOME CRITERIA

Evaluate the effectiveness of drug therapy by confirming that patient goals and expected outcomes have been met (see "Planning").

possible side effects. Following are important points the nurse should include when teaching patients and caregivers about antigout agents.

- Take the medication exactly as ordered.
- Report side effects such as rash, headache, anorexia, lower back pain, pain on urination, hematuria, and decrease in urinary output to the healthcare provider.
- Increase fluid intake to 3 to 4 L/day.
- Decrease or eliminate alcohol consumption; alcohol increases uric acid levels.

- Limit foods that will cause the urine to be more alkaline, to decrease chance of stone formation, such as milk, fruits, carbonated drinks, most vegetables, molasses, and baking soda.
- Avoid taking aspirin and large doses of vitamin C; they enhance stone formation.
- Use effective birth control during drug therapy and notify the healthcare provider of any suspicion of pregnancy.

CHAPTER REVIEW

Key Concepts

The numbered key concepts provide a succinct summary of the important points from the corresponding numbered section within the chapter. If any of these points are not clear, refer to the numbered section within the chapter for review. Expanded versions can be found on the companion website.

46.1 Adequate levels of calcium in the body are necessary to properly transmit nerve impulses, to prevent muscle spasms, and to provide stability and movement. Adequate levels of vitamin D, parathyroid hormone, and calcitonin are also necessary for these functions.

46.2 Hypocalcemia is a serious condition that requires immediate therapy with calcium supplements, often concurrently with vitamin D.

46.3 Pharmacotherapy of osteomalacia, softening of bones, includes calcium and vitamin D supplements.

46.4 Pharmacotherapy of osteoporosis includes bisphosphonates, estrogen modulator drugs, and calcitonin.

46.5 Pharmacotherapy of patients with Paget's disease includes bisphosphonates and calcitonin.

46.6 For osteoarthritis, the main drug therapy is pain medication that includes aspirin, acetaminophen, NSAIDs, COX-2 inhibitors, or stronger analgesics. Drug therapy for rheumatoid arthritis includes NSAIDs, COX-2 inhibitors, glucocorticoids, immunosuppressants, and disease-modifying drugs.

46.7 Gout is characterized by a buildup of uric acid in either the blood or the joint cavities. Drug therapy centers around agents that inhibit uric acid buildup or enhance its excretion.

Review Questions

1. Give examples where unusually low or high levels of blood calcium affect normal body functioning.

2. What are the major drug therapies used for osteoporosis?

3. Identify the two major types of arthritis. What are the differences between the pharmacotherapy of these disorders?

4. What are the differences in pharmacotherapy between gouty arthritis and other arthritic disorders?

Critical Thinking Questions

1. A young woman calls the triage nurse in her healthcare provider's office with questions concerning her mother's medication. The mother, age 76, has been taking alendronate (Fosamax) after a bone density study revealed a decrease in bone mass. The daughter is worried that her mother may not be taking the drug correctly. She asks for

information to make sure that her mother is taking the drug correctly to minimize any chance for side effects. What information should the triage nurse incorporate in a teaching plan regarding the oral administration of alendronate?

2. A community health nurse has decided to discuss the benefits of oral calcium supplements with an 82-year-old female patient. The patient had a stroke 6 years ago and requires help with most ADLs. She rarely leaves home since her husband died 18 months ago and has lost 25 pounds because she "just can't get interested" in her meals. She refuses to drink milk. What considerations must the nurse make before recommending calcium supplementation?

3. A 36-year-old man comes to the emergency department complaining of severe pain in the first joint of his right big toe. The triage nurse inspects the toe and notes that the joint is red, swollen, and exquisitely tender. Recognizing this as a typical presentation for acute gouty arthritis, what historical data should the nurse obtain relevant to this disease process?

EXPLORE MediaLink

NCLEX review, case studies, and other interactive resources for this chapter can be found on the companion website at www.prenhall.com/adams. Click on "Chapter 46" to select the activities for this chapter. For animations, more NCLEX review questions, and an audio glossary, access the accompanying CD-ROM in this textbook.

CHAPTER 47

Drugs for Skin Disorders

DRUGS AT A GLANCE

ANTI-INFECTIVES
Antibacterials, antifungals, and antivirals

ANTIPARASITICS
Scabicides
Pr lindane (Kwell)
Pediculicides

DRUGS FOR SUNBURN AND OTHER MINOR BURNS
Local anesthetics
Pr benzocaine (Solarcaine, others)

DRUGS FOR ACNE AND ROSACEA
Benzoyl peroxide
Retinoids
Pr isotretinoin/13-cis-retinoic acid (Accutane)
Antibiotics
Other agents

DRUGS FOR DERMATITIS
Topical glucocorticoids

DRUGS FOR PSORIASIS
Topical glucocorticoids
Topical immunomodulators
Systemic agents

metabolized and eliminated by the body.
of this process

PHARMACOLOGY

1. The study of medicines; the discipline
pertaining to how drugs improve the heal
of the human body

PHARMACOPEIA

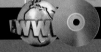 **MediaLink** www.prenhall.com/adams

CD-ROM
Audio Glossary
NCLEX Review

Companion Website
NCLEX Review
Dosage Calculations
Case Study
Care Plans
Expanded Key Concepts

OBJECTIVES

After reading this chapter, the student should be able to:

1. Identify the skin layers and associated structures.
2. Explain the process by which superficial skin cells are replaced.
3. Identify important drug therapies for bacterial, fungal, or viral infections; mite and lice infestations; sunburn; acne vulgaris; rosacea; dermatitis; and psoriasis.
4. Describe the nurse's role in the pharmacologic management of skin disorders.
5. For each of the classes listed in Drugs at a Glance, know representative drugs, explain the mechanism of drug action, primary actions, and important adverse effects.
6. Use the Nursing Process to care for patients who are receiving drug therapy for skin disorders.

The integumentary system consists of the skin, hair, nails, sweat glands, and oil glands. The largest and most visible of all organs, the skin normally provides an effective barrier between the outside environment and the body's internal organs. At times, however, external conditions become too extreme or conditions within the body change, resulting in unhealthy skin. When this occurs, pharmacotherapy may be utilized to improve the skin's condition. The purpose of this chapter is to examine the broad scope of skin disorders and the drugs used for skin pharmacotherapy.

47.1 Structure and Function of the Skin

To understand the actions of drugs used for skin disorders, it is necessary to have a thorough understanding of skin structure. The skin is composed of three primary layers: the epidermis, dermis, and subcutaneous layer. The epidermis is the visible, outermost layer that comprises only about 5% of the skin depth. The middle layer is the dermis or cutis, which comprises about 95% of the entire skin thickness. The subcutaneous layer lies beneath the dermis. Some textbooks consider the subcutaneous layer as being separate from the skin, and not one of its layers.

Each layer of skin is distinct in form and function and provides the basis for how drugs are injected or topically applied (Chapter 4) ∞. The epidermis has either four or five sublayers depending on its thickness. The five layers from the innermost to outermost are stratum basale (also referred to as the stratum germinativum), stratum spinosum, stratum granulosum, stratum lucidum, and the strongest layer, stratum corneum. The stratum corneum is referred to as the horny layer because of the abundance of the protein keratin, also found in the hair, hooves, and horns of many mammals. Keratin forms a barrier to repel bacteria and foreign matter, and most substances cannot

penetrate it. The largest amount of keratin is found in those areas subject to mechanical stress, for example, the soles of the feet and the palms of the hands.

The deepest sublayer of the epidermis, stratum basale, supplies the epidermis with new cells after older superficial cells have been damaged or lost through normal wear. Over their lifetime, these newly created cells migrate from the stratum basale to the outermost layers of the skin. As these cells are pushed to the surface they are flattened and covered with a water-insoluble material, forming a protective seal. The average time it takes for a cell to move from the stratum basale to the body surface is about 3 weeks. Specialized cells within the deeper layers of the epidermis, called melanocytes, secrete the dark pigment melanin, which offers a degree of protection from the sun's ultraviolet rays. The number and type of melanocytes determine the pigment of the skin. The more melanin, the darker the skin color. In areas where the melanocytes are destroyed, there are milk-white areas of depigmented skin referred to as **vitiligo**.

The second primary layer of skin, the dermis, consists of dense, irregular connective tissue. The dermis provides a foundation for the epidermis and accessory structures such as hair and nails. Most receptor nerve endings, oil glands, sweat glands, and blood vessels are found within the dermis.

Beneath the dermis is the subcutaneous layer, or hypodermis, that consists mainly of adipose tissue which cushions, insulates, and provides a source of energy for the body. The amount of subcutaneous tissue varies in an individual, and is determined by nutritional status and heredity.

47.2 Causes of Skin Disorders

Of the many types of skin disorders, some have vague, generalized signs and symptoms and others have specific and easily identifiable causes. Pruritus, or itching, is a general condition associated with dry, scaly skin, or it may be a symptom of mite or lice infestation. Inflammation, a characteristic of burns and other traumatic disorders, occurs when damage to the skin is extensive. Local erythema or redness accompanies inflammation and many other skin disorders. Additional symptoms including bleeding, bruises, and infections may result from trauma to deeper tissues.

Although difficult to classify, skin disorders may be grouped into three general categories: infectious, inflammatory, or neoplastic. Bacterial, fungal, viral, and parasitic infections of the skin are relatively common, and are frequent targets for anti-infective pharmacotherapy. Inflammatory disorders encompass a broad range of pathology that includes acne, burns, eczema, dermatitis, and psoriasis. Pharmacotherapy of inflammatory skin disorders includes many of the agents discussed in Chapter 31 ⊜ , such as glucocorticoids. Neoplastic disease includes malignant melanoma and basal cell carcinoma which are treated with the therapies described in Chapter 35 ⊜ . A summary of these disorders is given in Table 47.1.

Not all skin disorders are localized to the skin. A number of systemic conditions associated with other organ systems can cause changes in the color and integrity of the skin. During patient assessment, the nurse must observe for skin abnormalities, including color, sizes, types, and character of any lesions. Skin turgor and moisture are examined,

as this may indicate possible dehydration. If skin conditions are noted, a complete history and physical assessment is needed to identify potential systemic causes such as liver or renal impairment, primary or metastatic tumors, recent injury, and poor nutritional status. The relationship between the integumentary system and other body systems is depicted in Figure 47.1. Common symptoms associated with a range of conditions are shown in Table 47.2.

Although there are many skin disorders, some warrant only localized or short-term pharmacotherapy. Examples include lice infestation, sunburn with minor irritation, and acne. Eczema, dermatitis, and psoriasis are more serious disorders requiring extensive and sometimes prolonged therapy.

SKIN INFECTIONS

The skin has a normal population of microorganisms or flora that includes a diverse collection of viruses, fungi, and bacteria. The intact skin provides an effective barrier against infection from these organisms. The skin is very dry, and keratin is a poor energy source for microbes. Although perspiration often provides a wet environment, its high salt content discourages microbial growth. Furthermore, the outer layer is continually being sloughed off, and the microorganisms go with it.

47.3 Pharmacotherapy of Bacterial, Fungal, and Viral Skin Infections

Bacterial skin diseases can occur when the skin is punctured or cut, or when the outer layer is abraded through trauma or removed through severe burns. Some bacteria also infect hair follicles. The two most common bacterial infections of the skin are caused by *Staphylococcus* and *Streptococcus*, which are normal skin inhabitants. *S. aureus* is responsible for furuncles, carbuncles, and abscesses of the skin. Both *S. aureus* and *S. pyogenes* can cause impetigo, a skin disorder commonly occurring in school-age children.

Table 47.1	Classification of Skin Disorders
Type	**Examples**
infectious	Bacterial infections such as boils, impetigo, infected hair follicles; fungal infections such as ringworm, athlete's foot, jock itch, nail infection; parasitic infections such as mosquito bites, ticks, mites, lice; viral infections such as cold sores, fever blisters (herpes simplex), chickenpox, warts, shingles (herpes zoster), measles (rubeola), and German measles (rubella).
inflammatory	Injury and exposure to the sun such as sunburn and other environmental stresses; disorders marked by a combination of overactive glands, increased hormone production, and/or infection such as acne, blackheads, whiteheads, rosacea; disorders marked by itching, cracking, and discomfort such as eczema (atopic dermatitis), other forms of dermatitis (contact dermatitis, seborrheic dermatitis, stasis dermatitis), and psoriasis.
neoplastic	There are several types of skin cancers: squamous cell carcinoma, basal cell carcinoma, and malignant melanoma. Malignant melanoma is the most dangerous. Benign neoplasms include keratosis and keratoacanthoma.

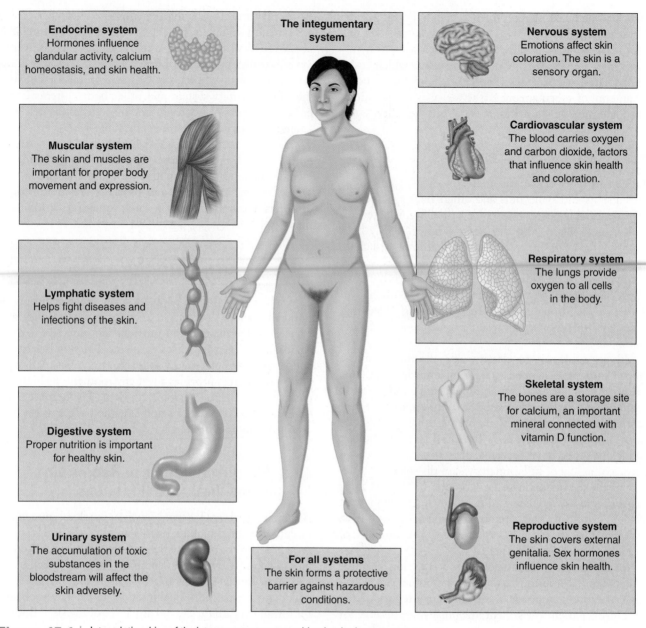

Figure 47.1 | Interrelationships of the integumentary system with other body systems

Although many skin bacterial infections are self-limiting, others may be serious enough to require pharmacotherapy. When possible, pharmacotherapy utilizes topical agents applied directly to the infection site. Topical agents offer the advantage of causing fewer side effects and many are available OTC for self-treatment. If the infection is deep within the skin, affects large regions of the body, or has the potential to become systemic, then oral or parenteral therapy is indicated. Chapter 32 provides a complete discussion of antibiotic therapy ⊕ . Some of the more common topical antibiotics include the following:

- Bacitracin ointment (Baciguent)
- Chloramphenicol cream (Chloromycetin)
- Erythromycin ointment (EryDerm, others)
- Gentamicin cream and ointment (Garamycin)
- Neomycin cream and ointment (Myciguent)
- Tetracycline (Topicycline)

Fungal infections of the skin or nails commonly occur in dark areas covered by clothing such as tinea pedis (athlete's foot) and tinea cruris (jock itch). Tinea capitis (ringworm of the scalp) and tinea unguium (nails) are also common. These pathogens generally are responsive to therapy with topical antifungal agents. More serious fungal infections of the skin and mucous membranes, such as *Candida albicans* infections that occur in immunocompromised patients, require systemic antifungals (Chapter 33) ⊕ .

Some viral infections of the skin are considered diseases of childhood. These include varicella (chickenpox), rubeola (measles), and rubella (German measles). Usually self-limiting and nonspecific, treatment of these infections is

Table 47.2	Signs and Symptoms Associated with Changing Health, Age, or Weakened Immune System
Sign	**Description**
discoloration of the skin	Discoloration is often a sign of an underlying medical disorder (for example, anemia, cyanoisis, fever, jaundice, and Addison's disease); some medications have photosensitive properties, making the skin sensitive to the sun and causing erythema.
delicate skin, wrinkles, and hair loss	Many degenerative changes occur in the skin; some are found in elderly patients; others are genetically related (fragile epidermis, wrinkles, reduced activity of oil and sweat glands, male pattern baldness, poor blood circulation); hair loss may also be linked to medical procedures, for example, radiation and chemotherapy.
seborrhea/oily skin and bumps	This condition as usually associated with younger patients; examples include cradle cap in infants and an oily face, chest, arms, and back in teenagers and young adults; pustules, cysts, papules, and nodules represent lesions connected with oily skin.
scales, patches, and itchy areas	Some symptoms may be related to a combination of genetics, stress, and immunity; other symptoms are due to a fast turnover of skin cells; some symptoms develop for unknown reasons.
warts, skin marks, and moles	Some skin marks are congenital; others are acquired or may be linked to environmental factors.
tumors	Tumors may be genetic or may occur because of exposure to harmful agents or conditions.

PHARMFACTS Skin Disorders

- An estimated 3 million people with new cases of lice infestation are treated each year in the United States.
- Nearly 17 million people in the United States have acne, making it the most common skin disease.
- More than 15 million people in the United States have symptoms of dermatitis.
- Of infants and young children, 10% experience symptoms of dermatitis; roughly 60% of these infants continue to have symptoms into adulthood.
- Psoriasis affects between 1% and 2% of the U.S. population. This disorder occurs in all age groups—adults mainly—affecting about the same number of men as women.

directed at controlling the extent of skin lesions. Viral infections of the skin in adults include herpes zoster (shingles) and herpes simplex (cold sores and genital lesions). Pharmacotherapy of severe viral skin lesions may include antiviral therapy with acyclovir (Zovirax), as discussed in Chapter 34 ⊙⊙ .

SKIN PARASITES

Common skin parasites include mites and lice. Scabies is an eruption of the skin caused by the female mite, *Sarcoptes scabiei*, which burrows into the skin to lay eggs, which hatch after about 5 days. Scabies mites are barely visible without magnification and are smaller than lice. Scabies lesions most commonly occur between the fingers, on the extremities, axillary and gluteal folds, around the trunk, and in the pubic area, as shown in Figure 47.2. The major symptom is intense itching; vigorous scratching may lead to secondary

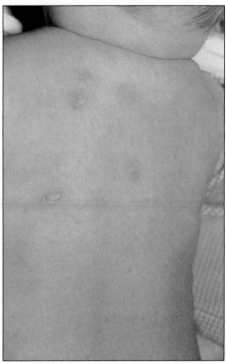

Figure 47.2 Scabies *Source: Courtesy of Dr. Jason L. Smith.*

infections. Scabies is readily spread through contact with upholstery and shared bed and bath linens.

Lice, scientific name *Pediculus*, are small parasites ranging from 1 to 4 mm in length and are readily spread by infected clothing or close personal contact. They require human blood for survival and will die within 24 hours without the blood of a human host. Lice (singular = louse)

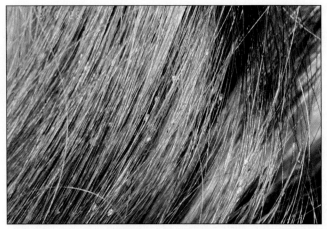

Figure 47.3 | Pediculus capitis *Source: Courtesy of Dr. Jason L. Smith.*

often infest the pubic area or the scalp and lay eggs, referred to as **nits**, which attach to body hairs. Head lice are referred to as *Pediculus capitis* (Figure 47.3), body lice as *Pediculus corpus*, and pubic lice as *Phthirus pubis*. The pubic louse is referred to as a crab louse, because it looks like a tiny crab when viewed under the microscope. Individuals with pubic lice will sometimes say that they have "crabs." Pubic lice may produce sky blue macules on inner thighs or lower abdomen. The bite of the louse and the release of saliva into the wound lead to intense itching followed by vigorous scratching. Secondary infections can result from scratching.

47.4 Pharmacotherapy with Scabicides and Pediculicides

Scabicides are drugs that kill mites and **pediculicides** are drugs that kill lice. Some drugs are effective against both types of parasites. The choice of drug may depend on where the infestation is located, as well as other factors such as age, pregnancy, or breastfeeding.

The traditional drug of choice for both mites and lice is lindane (Kwell, Scabene). Lindane is absorbed directly into lice, mites, and their eggs, producing seizures and death of the parasites. Lindane is available in cream, lotion, and shampoo. Other agents include permethrin (Nix, Elimite), a combination scabicide/pediculicide; crotamiton (Eurax), a scabicide; and malathion (Ovide), a pediculicide. All scabicides and pediculicides must be used strictly as directed, because their excessive use can cause serious systemic effects and/or skin irritation. Drugs for the treatment of lice or mites must not be applied to the mouth, open skin lesions, or eyes, as this will cause severe irritation.

To ensure the effectiveness of pharmacotherapy, patients should inspect hair shafts after treatment, checking for nits by combing with a fine-toothed comb after the hair is dry. This must be conducted daily for at least 1 week after treatment. Some strains of lice and mites have become resistant to common medications, adding to the impor-

tance of checking the patient several times during the postapplication period to be sure all the parasites have been killed. Because nits may be present in bedding, carpets, combs, brushes, seams of clothing, and upholstery, all material coming in close contact with the patient must be washed in hot water or treated with medication.

NURSING CONSIDERATIONS

The role of the nurse in scabicide and pediculicide therapy involves careful monitoring of a patient's condition and providing education as it relates to the prescribed regimen. Before applying a scabicide or pediculicide, the nurse should assess the patient's skin and hair, examining for signs of lice, nits, or scabies to verify the need for the medication. Lice may not be obvious on the body but may be found in seams of clothing that contact the axilla, neckline, groin, or beltline. The nurse should assess the skin for abrasions, cuts, rashes, and areas of inflammation, to determine areas that might be prone to irritation to the medication or increase its absorption rate.

The nurse should obtain a complete history including when the condition began; what treatment, if any, has already been tried including OTC and home remedies; any patient allergies; and if anyone in the family has a similar infestation. The nurse should assess the patient for history of epilepsy as these drugs can lower the seizure threshold in some patients.

The nurse should also assess females of childbearing age to determine if the patient is pregnant or nursing. Scabicides and pediculicides are used with caution in these patients and precautions should be taken to protect the nursing infant. Lindane (Kwell) is contraindicated in premature infants and should not be applied to children younger than 2 years of age due to increased risk of CNS toxicity. In children ages 2 to 10, lindane is used with caution and sometimes only after other agents such as permethrin (Nix) and crotamiton (Eurax) have failed to achieve therapeutic goals. The nurse should keep in mind that children and the elderly may need reduced dosages. Instructions for applying these drugs must be carefully followed. If overapplied, wrongly applied, or accidentally ingested, the patient may experience headaches; nausea or vomiting; irritation of the nose, ears, or throat; dizziness; tremors; restlessness; or convulsions.

The nurse should wear gloves when applying lindane. Lesions should be cleansed with antibacterial soap and tepid water three times a day to promote healing and reduce chances of secondary infection. The skin should be dried before applying medication.

Patient education as it relates to scabicides and pediculicides should include goals and reasons for obtaining baseline data such as vital signs and tests for cardiac and renal disorders. Following are important points the nurse should include when teaching patients regarding scabicides/ pediculicides.

- Keep medication out of the reach of children as it is highly toxic if swallowed or inhaled.
- If breastfeeding, use another source of milk for a minimum of 4 days after using lindane or similar drugs.
- Keep room temperature in the range of 68° to 72°F with low room humidity to reduce itching and drying of skin.

- Prevent reinfestation from household animals, including frequent bathing of pets and making sure their bedding is washed in hot water or sprayed with a pediculicide or scabicide.
- If the child is in daycare, notify caregivers of treatment so that other infected children may be identified.

See "Nursing Process Focus: Patients Receiving Lindane (Kwell)" for specific points the nurse should include when teaching patients regarding this drug.

SUNBURN AND MINOR BURNS

Burns are a unique type of stress that may affect all layers of the skin. Minor, first degree burns affect only the outer layers of the epidermis, are characterized by redness, and are analogous to sunburn. Sunburn results from overexposure to ultraviolet light, and is associated with light skin complexions, prolonged exposure to the sun during the more hazardous hours of the day (10 A.M. until 3 P.M.), and lack of protective clothing when outdoors. Nonpharmacologic approaches to sunburn prevention include the appropriate use of sunscreens and sufficient clothing. Chronic sun exposure can result in serious conditions, including eye injury, cataracts, and skin cancer.

47.5 Pharmacotherapy of Sunburn and Minor Skin Irritation

The best treatment for sunburn is prevention. Patients must be reminded of the acute and chronic hazards of exposure to direct sunlight. Liberal application of a lotion or oil having a very high SPF (sun protection factor) to areas of skin directly exposed to sunlight is strongly recommended.

Pr PROTOTYPE DRUG | **LINDANE** (Kwell)

ACTIONS AND USES

Lindane is marketed as a cream or lotion for mites, and as a shampoo for head lice. Lindane cream or lotion takes longer to produce its effect; therefore, it is usually left on the body for about 8 to 12 hours before rinsing. Lindane shampoo is usually applied and left on for at least 5 minutes before rinsing. Patients should be aware that penetration of the skin with mites causes itching, which lasts up to 2 or 3 weeks even after the parasites have been killed. Lindane kills mites and lice by overstimulating their nervous system.

Treatment may be reapplied in 24 hours when there is evidence of live lice or in 7 days for continued evidence that live mites are present.

Administration Alerts

- Do not use for premature infants and children less than 2 years of age.
- Do not use on areas of skin that have abrasions, rash, or inflammation.
- Pregnancy category C.

ADVERSE EFFECTS AND INTERACTIONS

CNS adverse effects include restlessness, dizziness, tremors, or convulsions (usually after misuse or accidental ingestion), and local irritation. If inhaled, lindane may cause headaches, nausea, vomiting, or irritation of the ears, nose, or throat.

No clinically significant interactions have been established.

NURSING PROCESS FOCUS | PATIENTS RECEIVING LINDANE (KWELL)

ASSESSMENT

Prior to administration:
- Obtain complete health history including allergies, drug history, and possible drug interactions.
- Assess vital signs.
- Assess skin for presence of lice and/or mite infestation, skin lesions, raw or inflamed skin, and open cuts.
- Obtain history of seizure disorders.
- Obtain patient's age.
- Assess pregnancy and lactation status.
- Obtain social history of close contacts, including household members and sexual partners.

POTENTIAL NURSING DIAGNOSES

- Deficient Knowledge, related to no previous contact with lice or mites or treatment
- Treatment Regimen Noncompliance, related to knowledge deficit, embarrassment
- Risk for Impaired Skin Integrity, related to lesions and itching

PLANNING: PATIENT GOALS AND EXPECTED OUTCOMES

- Patient and significant others will be free of lice or mites and experience no reinfestation.
- Patient will express an understanding of how lice and mites are spread, proper administration of lindane, necessary household hygiene, and the need to notify household members, sexual partners, other close contacts such as classmates of infestation.
- Skin will be intact and free of secondary infection and/or irritation.

IMPLEMENTATION

Interventions and (Rationales)	Patient Teaching/Discharge Planning
■ Monitor for presence of lice or mites. (This determines the effectiveness of drug therapy.)	Instruct patient and caregiver to: ■ Examine for nits on hair shafts; lice on skin or clothes; inner thigh areas; seams of clothes that come in contact with axilla, neckline, or beltline ■ Examine for mites between the fingers, on the extremities, axillary and gluteal folds, around the trunk, and in the pubic area
■ Apply lindane properly. (Proper application is critical to elimination of infestation.)	Instruct patient and caregiver: ■ To wear gloves during application, especially if applying lindane to more than one person, or if pregnant ■ That all skin lotions, creams, and oil-based hair products should be removed completely by scrubbing the whole body well with soap and water, and drying the skin prior to application ■ To apply lindane to clean and dry affected body area as directed, using no more than 2 oz per application ■ That eyelashes can be treated with the application of petroleum jelly twice a day for 8 days followed by combing to remove nits ■ To use fine-tooth comb to comb affected hair following lindane application to the hair and scalp to treat all household members and sexual contacts simultaneously ■ To recheck affected hair or skin daily for 1 week after treatment
■ Inform patient and caregivers about proper care of clothing and equipment. (Contaminated articles can cause reinfestation.)	Instruct patient and caregiver to: ■ Wash all bedding and clothing in hot water, and to dry-clean all nonwashable items which came in close contact with patient ■ Clean combs and brushes with lindane shampoo and rinse thoroughly

EVALUATION OF OUTCOME CRITERIA

Evaluate the effectiveness of drug therapy by confirming that patient goals and expected outcomes have been met (see "Planning").

The symptoms of sunburn include erythema, intense pain, nausea, vomiting, chills, and headache. These symptoms usually resolve within a matter of hours or days, depending on the severity of the exposure. Once sunburn has occurred, medications can only alleviate the symptoms; they do not speed recovery time.

Treatment for sunburn consists of addressing symptoms with soothing lotions, rest, prevention of dehydration, and topical anesthetic agents, if needed. Treatment is usually done on an outpatient basis. Topical anesthetics include benzocaine (Solarcaine), dibucaine (Nupercainal), and tetracaine HCl (Pontocaine). These medications may also provide minor relief from insect bites and pruritus. In more severe cases, oral analgesics such as aspirin or ibuprofen may be indicated.

NURSING CONSIDERATIONS

The role of the nurse in drug therapy for sunburn and minor skin irritation involves careful monitoring of a patient's condition and providing education as it relates to the prescribed drug regimen. The nurse should assess the location and extent of injury when patients present with severe sunburn. Benzocaine (Solarcaine) is contraindicated if serious burns are present. The nurse should also assess for secondary infection, as topical anesthetics are contraindicated if infection is present in area of sunburn. The assessment should include sunburn and tanning history, the amount of time the patient usually spends in the sun, how easily the patient tends to burn, and what sun protection the patient uses including the SPF rating of sunscreen products. If an anesthetic is indicated, the nurse should obtain an allergy history to such medications. Topical benzocaine may cause a hypersensitivity reaction. For patients using the medica-

tion for the first time, a trial application on a small area of skin should be conducted to check for allergy. If no adverse reaction has occurred after 30 to 60 minutes, the medication may be applied to the entire area of sunburn.

Patient education as it relates to topical regional anesthetics should include goals, reasons for obtaining baseline data such as vital signs, cardiac and renal disorders, and possible side effects. It is important that nurses educate patients about the safe use of topical regional anesthetic agents, appropriate treatment of sunburn, and prevention of overexposure to the sun. Following are important points the nurse should include when teaching patients about topical regional anesthetics.

- If severe pain persists, notify the healthcare provider.
- Avoid applying medication to broken skin or in presence of local infection.
- Prevent sunburn by decreasing exposure to sunlight or by increasing the SPF number of the sun protection product.
- Drink plenty of water to avoid dehydration.
- Refrigerate topical lotions so that they provide greater cooling when applied to the affected areas.

ACNE AND ROSACEA

Acne vulgaris is a common condition affecting 80% of adolescents. Although acne occurs most often in teenagers, it is not unusual to find patients with acne over 30 years of age, a condition referred to as mature acne or acne tardive. Acne vulgaris is more common in males but tends to persist longer in females.

The etiology of acne vulgaris is unknown, although factors associated with this condition include seborrhea, the overproduction of sebum by oil glands, and abnormal

---

Pr PROTOTYPE DRUG | BENZOCAINE (Solarcaine, Others)

ACTIONS AND USES	ADVERSE EFFECTS AND INTERACTIONS
Benzocaine is an ester type local anesthetic that provides temporary relief for pain and discomfort in cases of sunburn, pruritus, minor wounds, and insect bites. Its pharmacologic action is caused by local anesthesia of skin receptor nerve endings. Preparations are also available to treat specific areas such as the ear, mouth, throat, rectal, and genital areas.	Benzocaine has a low toxicity; however, some individuals are sensitive, and allergic reactions and anaphylaxis are possible. There are some reports of methemoglobinemia in infants. Benzocaine may interfere with the activity of some antibacterial sulfonamides.

Administration Alerts

- Benzocaine should not be used for treatment of patients with open lesions, traumatized mucosal areas, or a history of sensitivity to local anesthetics.
- Patients should use preparations only in areas of the body for which the medication is intended.
- Pregnancy category C.

 See the companion website for a Nursing Process Focus specific to this drug.

formation of keratin that blocks oil glands. The bacterium *Propionibacterium acnes* grows within oil gland openings and changes sebum to an acidic and irritating substance. As a result, small inflamed bumps appear on the surface of the skin. Other factors associated with acne include androgens, which play a role in controlling the activity of sebaceous glands, and below normal production of linoleic acid in sebum.

Acne lesions include open and closed comedones. Blackheads, or open comedones, occur when sebum has plugged the oil gland, causing it to become black because of the presence of melanin granules. Whiteheads, or closed comedones, develop just beneath the surface of the skin and appear white rather than black.

Rosacea is another skin disorder with lesions affecting mainly the face. Unlike acne, which most commonly affects teenagers, rosacea is a progressive disorder with an onset between 30 and 50 years of age. Rosacea is characterized by small papules or inflammatory bumps without pus that swell, thicken, and become painful, as shown in Figure 47.4. The face takes on a reddened or flushed appearance, particularly around the nose and cheek area. With time, the redness becomes more permanent and lesions resembling acne appear. The soft tissues of the nose may thicken, giving the nose a reddened, bullous, irregular swelling called rhinophyma.

Rosacea is exacerbated by factors such as sunlight, stress, increased temperature, and agents that dilate facial blood vessels including alcohol, spicy foods, skin care products, and warm beverages. It affects more women than men, although men more often develop rhinophyma.

47.6 Pharmacotherapy of Acne and Acne-Related Disorders

Medications used for acne and related disorders are available OTC and by prescription. Because of their increased toxicity, prescription agents are reserved for severe, persistent cases. These drugs are shown in Table 47.3.

Benzoyl peroxide (Benzalin, Fostex, others) is the most common topical OTC medication for acne. Benzoyl perox-

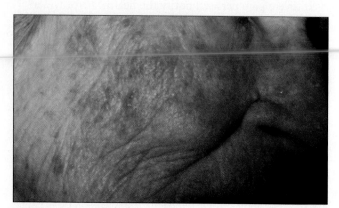

Figure 47.4 Rosacea *Source: Courtesy of Dr. Jason L. Smith.*

Table 47.3	Drugs for Acne and Acne-Related Disorders
Drug	**Remarks**
OTC Agent	
benzoyl peroxide (Benzacin, Benzamyclin, others)	Sometimes combined with tetracycline, erythromycin or clindamycin in severe cases, to fight bacterial infection.
Prescription Agents (Topical)	
adapalene (Differin)	Retinoid-like compound used to treat acne formation.
azelaic acid (Azelex, Finacea, others)	For mild to moderate inflammatory acne.
sulfacetamide sodium (Cetamide, Klaron, others)	For sensitive skin; sometimes combined with sulfur to promote peeling, as in the condition rosacea; also used for conjunctivitis.
tretinoin (Retin-A, others)	To prevent clogging of pore follicles; also used for the treatment of acute promyelocytic leukemia and wrinkles.
Prescription Agents (Oral)	
ethinyl estradiol (Estinyl)	Oral contraceptives are sometimes used for acne; combination drugs may be helpful, for example, ethinyl estradiol plus norgestimate (Ortho Tri-Cyclen-28)
doxycycline (Doryx, Vibramycin)	Antibiotic; refer to Chapter 32 ⊙.
isotretinoin/13-cis-retinoic acid (Accutane)	For acne with cysts or acne formed in small, rounded masses; pregnancy category X.
tetracycline hydrochloride (Achromycin, Panmycin, Sumycin) (see page 449 for the Prototype Drug box) ⊙	Antibiotic; refer to Chapter 32 ⊙.

ide has a keratolytic effect, which helps to dry out and shed the outer layer of epidermis. Other effects include possible sebum-suppressing action and antimicrobial activity that lasts up to 48 hours following application. This medication may be dispensed as a topical lotion, cream, or gel and is available in various percent concentrations. Other keratolytic agents used for severe acne include resorcinol, salicylic acid, and sulfur.

Retinoids are newer agents, usually by prescription only, that are effective against severe acne. Tretinoin (Retin-A) is a vitamin A derivative with an irritant action that decreases comedone formation and increases extrusion of comedones from the skin. Another use of tretinoin is for wrinkle removal. Other retinoids include isotretinoin (Accutane), an oral medication which is a vitamin A metabolite that aids in reducing the size of sebaceous glands, thereby decreasing oil production and the occurrence of clogged pores. Isotretinoin is not recommended during pregnancy because of possible harmful effects to the fetus. A common reaction to retinoids is sensitivity to sunlight. Additional retinoid-like agents and related compounds used to treat acne include the following prescription medications: adapalene (Differin), azelaic acid (Azelex), and sulfacetamide (Cetamide, Klaron, others).

Antibiotics are sometimes used in combination with acne medications to lessen the severe redness and inflammation associated with the disorder. Doxycycline (Vibramycin, others) and tetracycline (Achromycin) have been the traditional antibiotics used in acne therapy.

Ethinyl estradiol (Ortho Tri-Cyclen-28) is an estrogen commonly found in oral contraceptives that is also used to help clear the skin of acne. For the actions and contraindications of this and related hormones, see Chapter 41 .

Pharmacotherapy for rosacea includes a number of drugs given for acne vulgaris, including isotretinoin (Accutane), topical azelaic acid 20% cream (Finacea, Finevin), sulfacetamide preparations, and systemic antibiotics. In addition, patients with rosacea may be prescribed metronidazole 0.75% to 1% topical preparation (MetroGel, MetroCream), an antibacterial, and antiprotozoal preparation. Crotamiton (Eurax) 10% cream or lotion may also be prescribed if hair follicle mites are present. In addition to medications, some patients have vascular or carbon dioxide laser surgery for rhinophyma.

NURSING CONSIDERATIONS

The role of the nurse in drug therapy for acne-related disorders includes careful monitoring of a patient's condition and providing education as it relates to the prescribed drug regimen. The nurse working with teenagers with acne first needs to establish rapport, as many patients may be embarrassed or have an altered body image or self-esteem disturbance because of the acne. Establishing rapport early will help the nurse when obtaining the health history and physical assessment. The nurse should record when the acne began, what treatments have been tried, and with what success. Most acne sufferers will have attempted many OTC therapies before seeing a healthcare provider for a prescription drug, and may

continue to use these preparations in addition to new prescriptions. Because some medications prescribed for acne are not recommended for the pregnant patient, the nurse should ask women of childbearing age of their pregnancy status.

The nurse should wear gloves when examining the skin. As with all dermatologic conditions, the nurse should have the patient undress so he or she can observe as much of the skin surface as is possible. The acne on exposed areas such as the face may present somewhat differently than acne on the back or elsewhere. In some instances, patients are not aware of the extent of their skin disorder.

Isotretinoin (Accutane) is contraindicated with a history of severe depression and suicidal ideation, and patients should sign a consent regarding understanding of suicide risks prior to treatment. Concurrent use of isotretinoin and carbamazepine will decrease blood levels of carbamazepine, which may lead to increased seizure activity. Concurrent use of isotretinoin and hypoglycemic agents may lead to loss of glycemic control as well as increased risk for cardiovascular disease, secondary to elevated triglyceride levels.

A patch test should be done before the acne drug is used for the first time. When applying ointment, lotion, or cream to the skin, cleanse and completely dry the skin and apply the medication to a small area to test for sensitivity. A very small amount of a topical medication about the size of a pea is enough to cover the face adequately. Topical medication should not be applied to the eyes, mouth, or mucous membranes.

Because isotretinoin (Accutane) may cause severe birth defects or spontaneous abortions, female patients must have a negative pregnancy test result within 2 weeks of beginning treatment. Tetracycline or minocycline use may increase risk of pseudo-tumor cerebri, manifested by headache, papilledema, or decreased vision.

Patient education as it relates to drugs used to treat acne should include goals and reasons for obtaining baseline data such as vital signs and tests for cardiac and renal disorders. Patient teaching and understanding is vital to the proper use of acne drugs. Following are the important points the nurse should include when teaching patients about drugs used for the treatment of acne.

- Inform the healthcare provider of all OTC medications taken for acne.
- Take acne medications correctly and for the prescribed length of time.
- Avoid foods that seem to make acne worse. Keep a food log to determine which foods tend to worsen the condition.
- Avoid products that will irritate the skin such as cologne, perfumes, and other alcohol-based products.
- If severe skin irritation or inflammation develops during therapy, discontinue use and call the healthcare provider.

DERMATITIS

Dermatitis is an inflammatory skin disorder characterized by local redness, pain, and pruritus. Intense scratching may

| PROTOTYPE DRUG | ISOTRETINOIN/13-CIS-RETINOIC ACID (Accutane) |

ACTIONS AND USES

The principal action of isotretinoin is regulation of skin growth and turnover. As cells from the stratum germinativum grow toward the skin's surface, skin cells are lost from the stratum pore openings, and their replacement is slowed. Isotretinoin also decreases oil production by reducing the size and number of oil glands. Symptoms take 4 to 8 weeks to improve and maximum therapeutic benefit may take 5 to 6 months. This drug is most often used in cases of cystic acne or severe keratinization disorders.

Administration Alerts

- Do not use in patients with a history of severe depression and suicidal ideation.
- Pregnancy category X.
- Take with meals to minimize GI distress.

ADVERSE EFFECTS AND INTERACTIONS

Isotretinoin is a toxic metabolite of retinol or vitamin A. Common adverse effects are conjunctivitis, dry mouth, inflammation of the lip, dry nose, increased serum concentrations of triglycerides (by 50% to 70%), bone and joint pain, and photosensitivity. Liver function, serum glucose, and serum triglyceride tests should be performed when taking isotretinoin.

Isotretinoin interacts with vitamin A supplements, which increase toxicity. In addition, tetracycline or minocycline use may increase risk of pseudo-tumor cerebri. Concurrent use of hypoglycemic agents may lead to loss of glycemic control as well as increased risk for cardiovascular disease, secondary to elevated triglyceride levels. Concurrent use with carbamazepine will decrease blood levels of carbamazepine, which may lead to increased seizure activity.

| NATURAL THERAPIES | Burdock Root for Acne and Eczema |

Burdock root, *Arctium lappa*, comes from a thick, flowering plant sometimes found on the roadsides of Britain and North America. It contains several active substances such as bitter glycosides and flavonoids, and it has a range of potential actions in the body: anti-infective, diuretic, mild laxative, and skin detoxifier. It is sometimes described as an attacker of skin disorders from within because it fights bacterial infections, reduces inflammation, and treats some stages of eczema, particularly the dry and scaling phases. Some claim that it is also effective against boils and sores.

Burdock root is considered safe, having few side effects or drug interactions. It contains 50% inulin, a fiber widely distributed in vegetables and fruits, and is consumed as a regular part of the daily diet in many Asian countries. In many cases, burdock root is combined with other natural products for a better range of effectiveness. Such products include sarsaparilla (*Smilax officinalis*), yellow dock (*Rumex crispus*), licorice root (*Glycyrrhiza glabra*), echinacea (*Echinacea purpurea*), and dandelion (*Taraxacum officinale*).

lead to excoriation, scratches that break the skin surface and fill with blood or serous fluid to form crusty scales. Dermatitis may be acute or chronic.

Atopic dermatitis, or eczema, is a chronic, inflammatory skin disorder with a genetic predisposition. Patients presenting with eczema will often have a family history of asthma and hay fever as well as allergies to a variety of irritants such as cosmetics, lotions, soaps, pollens, food, and dust. About 75% of patients with atopic dermatitis will have had an initial onset before 1 year of age. In those babies predisposed to eczema, breastfeeding seems to offer protection, as it is rare for a breastfed child to develop eczema before the introduction of other foods. In infants and small children, lesions usually begin on the face and scalp, then progress to other parts of the body. A frequent and prominent symptom in infants is the appearance of red cheeks.

Contact dermatitis can be caused by a hypersensitivity response resulting from exposure to specific natural or synthetic allergens, such as plants, chemicals, latex, drugs, metals, or foreign proteins. Accompanying the allergic reaction may be various degrees of cracking, bleeding, or small blisters.

Seborrheic dermatitis is sometimes seen in newborns and in teenagers after puberty, and is characterized by yellowish, oily and crusted patches of skin that appear in areas of the face, scalp, chest, back, or pubic area. Bacterial infection or dandruff may accompany these symptoms.

Stasis dermatitis, a condition found primarily in the lower extremities, results from poor venous circulation. Redness and scaling may be observed in areas where venous circulation is impaired or where deep venous blood clots have formed.

47.7 Pharmacotherapy of Dermatitis

Pharmacotherapy of dermatitis is symptomatic and involves lotions and ointments to control itching and skin flaking. Antihistamines may be used to control inflammation, and analgesics or topical anesthetics may be prescribed for pain relief.

Topical glucocorticoids are the most effective treatment for dermatitis. As shown in Table 47.4, there are many formulations of glucocorticoids available in different potencies. Creams, lotions, solutions, gels, and pads are specially formulated to penetrate deep into the skin layers for relief of local inflammation, burning, and itching. Long-term glucocorticoid use, however, may lead to irritation, redness, and thinning of the skin membranes. If absorption occurs, topical glucocorticoids may produce undesirable systemic effects including adrenal insufficiency, mood changes, serum imbalances, and bone defects, as discussed in Chapter 39 .

NURSING PROCESS FOCUS | PATIENTS RECEIVING ISOTRETINOIN (ACCUTANE)

ASSESSMENT

Prior to administration:
- Obtain complete health history including allergies, drug history, and possible drug interactions.
- Obtain pregnancy and lactation status.
- Assess for history of psychiatric disorders.
- Assess vital signs to obtain baseline information.

POTENTIAL NURSING DIAGNOSES

- Disturbed Body Image, related to presence of acne and possible worsening of symptoms after treatment begins
- Decisional Conflict, related to desire for pregnancy, and necessity of preventing pregnancy during therapy with isotretinoin
- Noncompliance, related to length of treatment time, failure to use effective contraception
- Impaired Skin Integrity, related to inflammation, redness, scaling, secondary to treatment

PLANNING: PATIENT GOALS AND EXPECTED OUTCOMES

The patient will:
- Experience decreased acne, without side effects or adverse reactions
- Demonstrate acceptance of body image
- Demonstrate an understanding of the drug's action by accurately describing drug side effects and precautions

IMPLEMENTATION

Interventions and (Rationales)	Patient Education/Discharge Planning
■ Monitor lab studies during treatment, including blood glucose.	■ Instruct patient on importance of lab studies prior to therapy and periodically during therapy and doing home blood glucose monitoring if diabetic.
■ Discuss potential adverse reactions to drug therapy. (Understanding of drug effects is important for compliance.)	Instruct patient: ■ To use two forms of reliable birth control for 1 month before beginning treatment, during treatment, and for 1 month following completion of treatment ■ Not to donate blood during treatment and for a minimum of 4 weeks after completion of treatment; isotretinoin in donated blood could cause fetal damage if given to a pregnant woman ■ To talk with pediatrician about alternative methods of feeding if breastfeeding ■ To avoid use of vitamin A products
■ Monitor for cardiovascular problems. (Use isotretinoin with caution in patients with heart block, especially if patient is also taking a beta-blocker.)	■ Discuss with patient importance of complete disclosure regarding medical history and medications.
■ Monitor emotional health. (Patient may become depressed secondary to acne itself, length of treatment, possibility of worsening symptoms at beginning of treatment, changed body image, or drug itself.)	Instruct patient ■ To report signs of depression immediately and discontinue isotretinoin ■ Regarding signs and symptoms of depression ■ To report any feelings of suicide ideation
■ Monitor CBC, blood lipid levels, glucose levels, liver function tests, eye exam, GI status, urinalysis.	■ Teach patient importance of a complete workup prior to starting isotretinoin therapy and periodically during course of treatment.
■ Monitor for vision changes. (Corneal opacities and/or cataracts may develop as result of isotretinoin use. Dryness of eyes during treatment is common. Night vision may be diminished during treatment.)	Instruct patient: ■ To report any decreased vision and discontinue use of isotretinoin ■ To avoid driving at night if possible ■ That use of artificial tears may relieve dry eyes ■ That use of contact lenses may need to be discontinued during therapy

continued

NURSING PROCESS FOCUS: *Patients Receiving Isotretinoin (Accutane) (continued)*

Interventions and (Rationales)	Patient Education/Discharge Planning
■ Monitor alcohol use. (Alcohol use with isotretinoin leads to increased triglyceride levels.)	Advise patient to: ■ Eliminate or greatly reduce alcohol use, including alcohol-containing preparations such as mouthwashes or OTC medications ■ Read labels for alcohol content
■ Monitor skin problems. (This will determine the effectiveness of drug therapy.)	Advise patient: ■ That acne may worsen during beginning of treatment ■ To monitor skin for improvement in 4 to 8 weeks; if no improvement is noted, patient should contact primary healthcare provider
■ Monitor for side effects.	■ Instruct patient to be aware of and to report headache (especially if accompanied by nausea and vomiting), fatigue, depression, lethargy, severe diarrhea, rectal bleeding, abdominal pain, dry mouth, hematuria, proteinuria, liver dysfunction (jaundice, pruritus, dark urine).

EVALUATION OF OUTCOME CRITERIA

Evaluate the effectiveness of drug therapy by confirming that patient goals and expected outcomes have been met (see "Planning").

PSORIASIS

Psoriasis is a chronic, noninfectious, inflammatory disorder characterized by red raised patches of skin covered with flaky, thick, silver scales called plaques, as shown in Figure 47.5. These plaques shed the scales, which are sometimes grayish. The reason for the appearance of plaques is an extremely fast skin turnover rate, with skin cells reaching the surface in 4 to 7 days instead of the usual 14 days. Plaques are ultimately shed from the surface, while the underlying skin becomes inflamed and irritated.

The various forms of psoriasis are described in Table 47.5. Lesion size varies and the shape tends to be round. Lesions are usually discovered on the scalp, elbows, knees, and extensor surfaces of the arms and legs, sacrum, and occasionally around the nails. The etiology of psoriasis is unknown, but about 50% of the cases involve a family history of the disorder. One theory of causation is that psoriasis is an autoimmune condition. In psoriasis, certain overactive immune cells release cytokines that cause the increased production of skin cells.

47.8 Pharmacotherapy of Psoriasis

A number of prescription and OTC drugs are available for the treatment of psoriasis, including both topical and systemic agents, as shown in Table 47.6. A primary treatment is topical glucocorticoids, such as betamethasone (Diprosone) ointment, lotion, or cream and hydrocortisone acetate (Cortaid, Caldecort, others) cream or ointment. Topical glucocorticoids reduce the inflammation associated with fast skin turnover.

Another class of preparations is the topical immunomodulators (TIMS), which are agents that suppress the immune system. One example is tacrolimus (Protopic) ointment. Other agents applied topically are retinoid-like compounds such as calcipotriene (Dovonex), a synthetic vitamin D ointment, cream, or scalp solution; and tazarotene (Tazorac), a vitamin A derivative gel or cream. These drugs provide the same benefits as topical glucocorticoids, but exhibit a lower incidence of adverse effects. Calcipotriene may produce hypercalcemia if applied over large areas of the body or used in higher doses than recommended. This drug is usually not used on an extended basis.

The most often prescribed systemic drug for severe psoriasis is methotrexate. Methotrexate (Folex) is used in the treatment of a variety of disorders, including carcinomas and rheumatoid arthritis, in addition to being used for the treatment of psoriasis. Methotrexate is discussed as a prototype drug in Chapter 35 ☞. Other systemic drugs for psoriasis include acitretin (Soriatane) and etretinate (Tegison). These drugs are taken orally to inhibit excessive skin cell growth.

Other drugs used for different disorders, but which provide relief of severe psoriatic symptoms, are hydroxyurea (Hydrea) and cyclosporine (Sandimmune, Neoral). Hydroxyurea is a sickle cell anemia drug. Cyclosporine is an

Table 47.4	**Topical Glucocorticoids for Dermatitis and Related Symptoms**
Generic Name	**Trade Names**
Highest Level of Potency	
betamethasone	Benisone, Diprosone, Valisone
clobetasol	Dermovate, Temovate
diflorasone	Florone, Maxiflor, Psorcon
Middle Level of Potency	
amcinonide	Cyclocort
desoximetasone	Topicort, Topicort LP
fluocinonide	Lidex, Lidex-E, others
halcinonide	Halog
mometasone	Elocon
triamcinolone	Aristocort, Kenalog, others
Lower Level of Potency	
clocortolone	Cloderm
fluocinolone	Fluolar, Synalar, others
flurandrenolide	Cordran, Cordran SP
fluticasone	Flonase
hydrocortisone	Hytone, Locoid, Westcort, others
Lowest Level of Potency	
aclometasone	Aclovate
desonide	DesOwen, Tridesilon
dexamethasone	Decaderm, Decadron, others

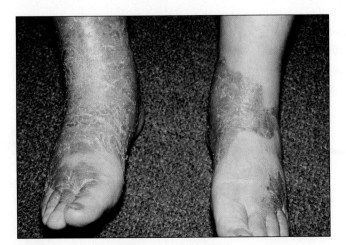

Figure 47.5 | Psoriasis *Source: Courtesy of Dr. Jason L. Smith.*

immunosuppressive agent that was presented as a prototype in Chapter 30⚭ . In addition, etanercept (Enbrel) and infliximab (Remicade), which are approved for other autoimmune conditions, have been found to improve symptoms of psoriasis. Etanercept and infliximab are tumor necrosis factor (TNF) blockers.

Other skin therapy techniques may be used with or without additional psoriasis medications. These include various forms of tar treatment (coal tar) and anthralin, which are applied to the skin's surface. Tar and anthralin inhibit DNA synthesis and arrest abnormal cell growth.

Phototherapy with UVB (ultraviolet B) and UVA (ultraviolet A) are used in cases of severe psoriasis. UVB therapy is less hazardous than UVA therapy. UVB has a wavelength similar to sunlight and it reduces widespread lesions that normally resist topical treatments. With close supervision, this type of phototherapy can be administered at home. Keratolytic pastes are often applied between treatments. The second type of phototherapy is

Table 47.5	Types of Psoriasis		
Form of Psoriasis	**Description of Form**	**Most Common Location of Lesions**	**Comments**
Guttate (droplike) or eruptive psoriasis	Lesions smaller than those of psoriasis vulgaris	Upper trunk and extremities	More common in early-onset psoriasis; can appear and resolve spontaneously a few weeks following a streptococcal respiratory infection
Psoriasis annularis	Ring-shaped lesions with clear centers		Rare
Psoriatic arthritis	Resembles rheumatoid arthritis	Fingers and toes at distal interphalangeal joints; can affect skin and nails	About 20% of patients with psoriasis also have arthritis
Psoriasis vulgaris	Lesions are papules that form into erythematous plaques with thick, silver or grey plaques, which bleed when removed; plaques in dark-skinned individuals often appear purple	Skin over scalp, elbows, and knees; lesions possible anywhere on the body	Most common form; requires long-term specialized management
Psoriatic erythrodema or exfoliative psoriasis	Generalized scaling; erythema without lesions	All body surfaces	
Pustular psoriasis	Eruption of pustules. Presence of fever	Trunk and extremities; can appear on palms, soles, and nail beds	

Table 47.6	Drugs for Psoriasis and Related Disorders
Drug	**Route and Adult Dose (max dose where indicated)**
Topical Medications	
calcipotriene (Dovonex)	Topically to lesions qd-bid
tazarotene (Tazorac)	Acne; apply thin film to clean dry area qd Plaque psoriasis; apply thin film qd in the evening
Systemic Medications	
acitretin (Soriatane)	PO; 10–50 mg qd with the main meal
cyclosporine (Sandimmune, Neoral)	PO; 1.25 mg/kg bid (max 4 mg/kg/d)
etretinate (Tegison)	PO; 0.75–1 mg/kg qd (max 1.5 mg/kg/d)
hydroxyurea (Hydrea)	PO; 80 mg/kg q3d or 20–30 mg/kg qd
methotrexate (Mexate, Folex) (see page 508 for the Prototype Drug box)	PO; 2.5–5 mg bid for three doses each week (max 25–30 mg/wk)

referred to as PUVA therapy because psoralens are often administered in conjunction with phototherapy. Psoralens are oral or topical agents that, when exposed to UV light, produce a photosensitive reaction. This reaction reduces the number of lesions, but unpleasant side effects such as headache, nausea, and skin sensitivity still occur, limiting the effectiveness of this therapy. Immunosuppressant drugs such as cyclosporine are not used in conjunction with PUVA therapy because they increase the risk of skin cancer.

CHAPTER REVIEW

Key Concepts

The numbered key concepts provide a succinct summary of the important points from the corresponding numbered section within the chapter. If any of these points are not clear, refer to the numbered section within the chapter for review. Expanded versions can be found on the companion website.

47.1 Three layers of skin, epidermis, dermis, and subcutaneous layer, provide effective barrier defenses for the body.

47.2 Skin disorders that may benefit from pharmacotherapy are acne, sunburns, infections, dermatitis, and psoriasis.

47.3 When the skin integrity is compromised, bacteria, viruses, and fungi can gain entrance and cause infections. Anti-infective therapy may be indicated.

47.4 Scabicides and pediculicides are used to treat parasitic mite and lice infestations, respectively.

47.5 The pharmacotherapy of sunburn includes the symptomatic relief of pain using soothing lotions, topical anesthetics, and analgesics.

47.6 The pharmacotherapy of acne includes treatment with benzoyl peroxide, retinoids, and antibiotics. Therapies for rosacea include retinoids and metronidazole.

47.7 The most effective treatment for dermatitis is topical glucocorticoids.

47.8 Both topical and systemic drugs, including glucocorticoids, immunomodulators, and methotrexate, are used to treat psoriasis.

Review Questions

1. Name examples of drugs used to treat mite and lice infestations. What precautions should be taken when using these drugs?

2. What is the major purpose of drugs used to treat acne and related skin conditions? Give examples of both topical and systemic drugs.

3. In most cases, which drug category is used to treat symptoms of dermatitis and psoriasis? What other drug therapies and techniques are used to provide a measure of relief for these symptoms?

Critical Thinking Questions

1. A senior nursing student is participating in well-baby screenings at a public health clinic. While examining a 4-month-old infant, the student notes an extensive, confluent diaper rash. The baby's mother is upset and asks the student nurse about the use of OTC corticosteroid ointment and wonders how she should apply the cream. How should the student nurse respond?

2. A 14-year-old girl has been placed on oral doxycycline (Doxy-Caps) for acne vulgaris because she has not responded to topical antibiotic therapy. After 3 weeks of therapy, the patient returns to the dermatologist's office complaining about episodes of nausea and epigastric pain. The nurse learns that the patient is "so busy with school activities" that she often

forgets a morning dose and "doubles up" on the drug before bedtime. Devise a teaching plan relevant to drug therapy that takes into consideration the major side effects of this drug and the cognitive abilities of this patient.

3. A 37-year-old woman is referred to a dermatologist for increasing redness and painful "acne" lesions. The patient is frustrated with her attempts to camouflage her "teenage face" with makeup. She relates to the nurse that she had acne as a teen but had no further problem until the last 11 months. After consultation, the dermatologist suggests a 3-month trial of isotretinoin (Accutane). What are the specific reproductive considerations for this patient? What information should this patient be provided in relation to reproductive concerns?

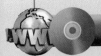

EXPLORE MediaLink

NCLEX review, case studies, and other interactive resources for this chapter can be found on the companion website at www.prenhall.com/adams. Click on "Chapter 47" to select the activities for this chapter. For animations, more NCLEX review questions, and an audio glossary, access the accompanying CD-ROM in this textbook.

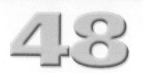

■ DRUGS AT A GLANCE

DRUGS FOR GLAUCOMA
Cholinergic agonists
Nonselective sympathomimetics
Prostaglandins
℗ *latanoprost (Xalatan)*
Beta-adrenergic blockers
℗ *timolol (Timoptic, Timoptic XE)*
Alpha₂-adrenergic agonists
Carbonic anhydrase inhibitors
Osmotic diuretics

**DRUGS FOR OPHTHALMIC EXAMINATIONS
AND MINOR EYE CONDITIONS**
Anticholinergics
Sympathomimetics
Lubricants

DRUGS FOR EAR CONDITIONS
Antibiotics
Cerumen softeners

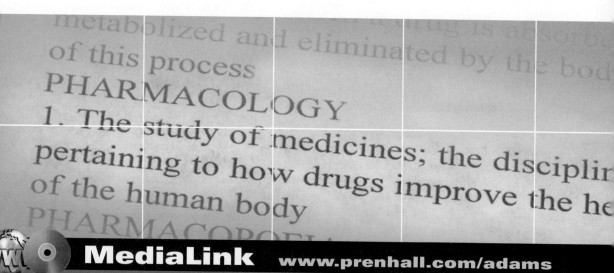

MediaLink www.prenhall.com/adams

CD-ROM
Animation:
  Mechanism in Action: Pilocarpine
  (Adsorbocarpine)
Audio Glossary
NCLEX Review

Companion Website
NCLEX Review
Dosage Calculations
Case Study
Care Plans
Expanded Key Concepts

OBJECTIVES

After reading this chapter, the student should be able to:

1. Describe eye anatomy relevant to glaucoma development.
2. Identify the major risk factors associated with glaucoma.
3. Compare and contrast the two principle types of glaucoma and explain their reasons for development.
4. Explain the two major mechanisms by which drugs reduce intraocular pressure.
5. Describe the nurse's role in the pharmacologic management of eye and ear disorders.
6. Identify examples of drugs for treating glaucoma and explain their basic actions and adverse effects.
7. Identify examples of drugs that dilate or constrict pupils, relax ciliary muscles, constrict ocular blood vessels, or moisten eye membranes.
8. Identify examples of drugs for treating ear conditions.
9. Use the Nursing Process to care for patients who are receiving drug therapy for eye and ear disorders.

The eye is vulnerable to a variety of conditions, many of which can be prevented, controlled, or reversed with proper treatment. A simple scratch can cause the patient almost unbearable discomfort as well as concern about the effect the damage may have on vision. Other eye disorders may be more bearable, but extremely dangerous—including glaucoma, a leading cause of blindness. The first part of this chapter covers various drugs used for the treatment of glaucoma. Drugs used routinely by ophthalmic healthcare providers are also discussed. The remaining part of the chapter presents drugs used for treatment of ear disorders, including infections, inflammation, and the buildup of ear wax.

48.1 Anatomy of the Eye

A firm knowledge of basic eye anatomy, shown in Figures 48.1 and 48.2, is required to understand eye disorders and their pharmacotherapy. A fluid called **aqueous humor** is found in the anterior cavity of the eye. The anterior cavity has two divisions, the anterior chamber, which extends from the cornea to the iris, and the posterior chamber, which lies between the iris and the lens. The aqueous humor originates in the posterior chamber from a muscular structure called the ciliary body.

Aqueous humor helps to retain the shape of the eye and circulates to bring nutrients to the area and remove wastes. From its origin in the ciliary body, aqueous humor flows through the pupil and into the anterior chamber. Within the anterior chamber and around the periphery is a network of spongy connective tissue, or trabecular meshwork, which contains an opening called the canal of Schlemm. The aqueous humor drains into the canal of Schlemm and out of the anterior chamber into the venous system, thus completing its circulation. Under normal circumstances, the rate of aqueous humor production is equal to its outflow; thus, the intraocular pressure (IOP) is maintained within a normal range.

GLAUCOMA

When the IOP rises above 20 mm Hg, the patient has **glaucoma**. Glaucoma often exists as a primary condition without an identifiable cause and is most frequently found in persons over age 60. In some cases, this disorder is due to genetic factors; it can be congenital in infants and children. Glaucoma can also be secondary to eye trauma, infection, inflammation, hemorrhage, tumor, or cataracts. Some medications may contribute to the development of glaucoma, including long-term use of topical glucocorticoids, some antihypertensives, antihistamines, and antidepressants. The major risk factors associated with glaucoma include high blood pressure, migraine headaches, refractive disorders

MediaLink | Glaucoma Research Foundation

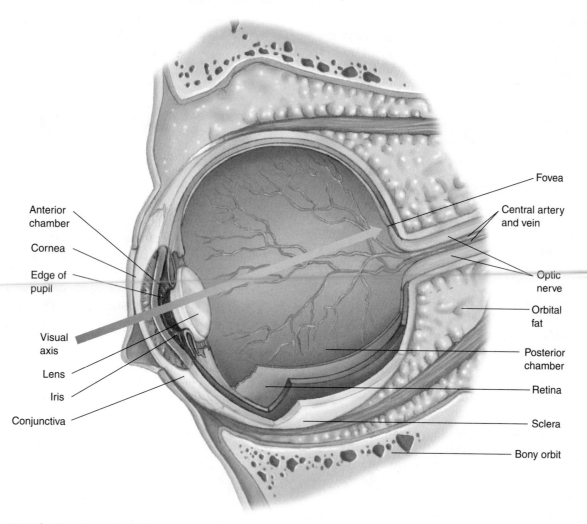

Figure 48.1 | Internal structures of the eye *Source: Pearson Education/PH College.*

such as nearsightedness or farsightedness, and normal aging. Glaucoma is the leading cause of preventable blindness.

48.2 Types of Glaucoma

Tonometry is an ophthalmic technique that tests for glaucoma by measuring intraocular pressure. Other routine refractory and visual field tests may uncover signs of glaucoma. One problem with diagnosis is that patients with glaucoma typically do not experience symptoms and therefore do not schedule regular eye exams. In some cases, glaucoma occurs so gradually that patients do not notice a problem until late in the disease process.

As shown in Figure 48.2, the two principal types of glaucoma are closed-angle glaucoma and open-angle glaucoma. Both disorders result from the same problem: a buildup of aqueous humor in the anterior cavity. This buildup is caused either by excessive production of aqueous humor or by a blockage to its outflow. In either case, IOP increases, leading to progressive damage to the optic nerve. As degeneration of the optic nerve is occurring, the patient will first notice a loss of visual field, and then a loss of cen-

tral visual acuity, and lastly total blindness. Major differences between closed-angle glaucoma and open-angle glaucoma include how quickly the IOP develops and whether there is narrowing of the anterior chamber angle between the iris and cornea.

Closed-angle glaucoma, also called acute glaucoma or narrow-angle glaucoma, is uncommon. The incidence is higher in older adults and in persons of Asian descent.

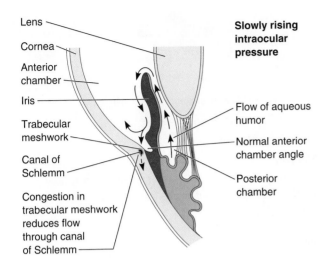

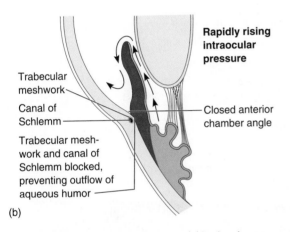

Figure 48.2 Forms of primary adult glaucoma: (a) in chronic open-angle glaucoma, the anterior chamber angle remains open, but drainage of aqueous humor through the canal of Schlemm is impaired; (b) in acute angle-closure glaucoma, the angle of the iris and anterior chamber narrows, obstructing the outflow of aqueous humor

This acute type of glaucoma is usually unilateral and caused by stress, impact injury, or medications. Pressure inside the anterior chamber increases suddenly, with the iris being pushed over the area where the aqueous humor normally drains. The displacement of the iris is due in part to the pupils having dilated or the lens accommodated, causing the narrowed angle to close. Signs and symptoms, caused by acute obstruction of the outflow of aqueous humor from the eye, include intense headaches, difficulty concentrating, bloodshot eyes, blurred vision, and a bulging iris. Closed-angle glaucoma constitutes an emergency situation.

Open-angle glaucoma, or chronic simple glaucoma, is the most common type accounting for 90% of the cases. It is usually bilateral; and intraocular pressure develops slowly, over a period of years. It is called "open-angle" because the iris does not cover the trabecular meshwork. Patients may be asymptomatic.

48.3 General Treatment of Glaucoma

All of the approaches to glaucoma therapy are directed to the goal of increasing the circulation of aqueous humor that has been reduced (in the case of chronic open-angle glaucoma) or prevented (in the case of closed-angle glaucoma). In cases of acute closed-angle glaucoma, surgery such as gonioplasty, laser iridotomy, and peripheral iridectomy may be performed to return the iris back to its original position. In gonioplasty, an argon laser makes laser burns at the periphery of the iris. When the burn scars heal, tension is created that draws the iris away from the cornea, thus widening the angle. Iridectomy involves the laser creation of a number of small perforations in the iris, which allow the aqueous humor to drain in the normal pathway. Iridectomy involves removal of a small section of the iris to increase the flow of aqueous humor. Although surgery is often performed in acute closed-angle glaucoma, the majority of cases of open-angle glaucoma are treated with medication.

48.4 Pharmacotherapy of Glaucoma

Pharmacotherapy for glaucoma works by one of two mechanisms: increasing the outflow of aqueous humor at the canal of Schlemm or decreasing the formation of aqueous humor at the ciliary body. Many agents for glaucoma act by affecting the autonomic nervous system (see Chapter 13) . Agents for glaucoma, as shown in Table 48.1, include the following classes.

- Cholinergic agonists
- Nonselective sympathomimetics
- Prostaglandins
- Beta-adrenergic blockers
- Alpha$_2$-adrenergic agonists
- Carbonic anhydrase inhibitors
- Osmotic diuretics

Cholinergic Agonists

Drugs that activate cholinergic receptors in the eye produce **miosis**, constriction of the pupil, and contraction of the ciliary muscle. These agents are sometimes called **miotics**. These actions change the trabecular meshwork to allow greater outflow of aqueous humor and a lowering of the IOP. Agents such as carbachol (Isopto Carbachol, Miostat) and pilocarpine (Adsorbocarpine, Isopto Carpine) act *directly* on cholinergic receptors. Demecarium (Humorsol), echothiophate (Phospholine Iodide), isoflurophate (Floropryl), and physostigmine act *indirectly* by blocking acetylcholinesterase (AchE), the enzyme responsible for breaking down the neurotransmitter acetylcholine. The indirect-acting AchE inhibitors produce essentially the same effects as direct-acting drugs, except they have a longer duration of action. Because of greater toxicity and longer action, these drugs are normally used only in patients with open-angle glaucoma who do not respond to other agents. The antidote for serious drug toxicity from cholinergic agonists is pralidoxime chloride (Z-PAM). The cholinergic agonists are applied topically to the eye.

MediaLink Mechanism in Action Pilocarpine

Table 48.1	Selected Drugs for Glaucoma
Drug	**Route and Adult Dose**
Cholinergic Agonists	
carbachol (Isopto Carbachol, Miostat)	1–2 drops 0.75–3% solution in lower conjunctival sac q4h–tid
demecarium bromide (Humorsol)	1–2 drops 0.125–0.25% solution twice per week
echothiophate iodide (Phosphaline Iodide)	1 drop 0.03–0.25% solution qd-bid
physostigmine sulfate (Eserine sulfate)	1 drop 0.25–0.5% solution qd-qid
ⓟ pilocarpine hydrochloride (Adsorbocarpine, Isopto Carpine, and others)	acute glaucoma: 1 drop 1–2% solution every 5–10 minutes for 3–6 doses; chronic glaucoma: 1 drop 0.5–4% solution every 4–12 hours
Sympathomimetics	
dipivefrin HCl (Propine)	1 drop 0.1% solution bid
epinephryl borate (Epinal, Eppy/N)	1–2 drops 0.25–2% solution qd-bid
Prostaglandins	
bimatoprost (Lumigan)	1 drop 0.03% solution qd in the evening
latanoprost (Xalatan)	1 drop (0.005%) solution qd in the evening
travaprost (Travatan)	1 drop 0.004% solution qd in the evening
unoprostone isopropyl (Rescula)	1 drop 0.15% solution bid
Beta-Adrenergic Blockers	
betaxolol (Betaoptic)	1 drop 0.5% solution bid
carteolol (Ocupress)	1 drop 1% solution bid
levobunolol (Betagan)	1–2 drops 0.25–0.5% solution qd-bid
metipranolol (OptiPranolol)	1 drop 0.3% solution bid
timolol (Timoptic, Timoptic XE)	1–2 drops of 0.25–0.5% solution qd-bid; gel (salve): apply qd
Alpha$_2$-Adrenergic Agonists	
apraclonidine (Iopidine)	1 drop 0.5% solution bid
brimonidine tartrate (Alphagan)	1 drop 0.2% solution tid
Carbonic Anhydrase Inhibitors	
ⓟ acetazolamide (Diamox)	PO; 250 mg qd-qid
brinzolamide (Azopt)	1 drop 1% solution tid
dichlorphenamide (Daranide, Oratrol)	PO; 100–200 mg followed by 100 mg bid
methazolamide (Neptazane)	PO; 50–100 mg bid or tid
Osmotic Diuretics	
glycerin anhydrous (Ophthalgan)	PO; 1–1.8 g/kg 1–1.5 h before ocular surgery; may repeat q5h
isosorbide (Ismotic)	PO; 1–3 g/kg bid–qid
mannitol (Osmitrol)	IV; 1.5–2 mg/kg as a 15–25% solution over 30–60 minutes

Nonselective Sympathomimetics

Sympathomimetics activate the sympathetic nervous system. Dipivefrin (Propine) and epinephryl borate (Epinal, others) are nonselective sympathomimetics administered topically for open-angle glaucoma. Epinephrine produces mydriasis (pupil dilation) and increases the outflow of aqueous humor, resulting in a lower IOP. Dipivefrin is con- verted to epinephrine in the eye. Should epinephrine reach the systemic circulation, it increases blood pressure and heart rate.

Prostaglandins

Latanoprost (Xalatan) is a prostaglandin analog available as a 0.005% eye drop solution, which decreases aqueous hu-

Pr **PROTOTYPE DRUG** | **LATANOPROST** (Xalatan)

ACTIONS AND USES	**ADVERSE EFFECTS AND INTERACTIONS**
Latanoprost is a prostaglandin analog believed to reduce intraocular pressure (IOP) by increasing the outflow of aqueous humor. The recommended dose is one drop in the affected eye(s) in the evening. It is metabolized to its active form in the cornea, reaching its peak effect in about 12 hours. It is used to treat open-angle glaucoma and elevated IOP. *Administration Alerts* ■ Remove contact lens before instilling eye drops. Do not reinsert contact for 15 minutes. ■ Avoid touching the eye or eyelashes with any part of eyedropper to avoid contamination of one area to another. ■ Wait 5 minutes before/after instillation of a different eye prescription to administer eye drop(s). ■ Pregnancy category C.	Adverse effects include ocular symptoms such as conjunctival edema, tearing, dryness, burning, pain, irritation, itching, sensation of foreign body in eye, photophobia, and/or visual disturbances. The eyelashes on the treated eye only may grow, thicken, and/or darken. Changes may occur in pigmentation of the iris of the treated eye and in the periocular skin. The most common systemic side effect is a flulike upper respiratory infection. Rash, asthenia, or headache may occur. Latanoprost interacts with thimerosal: If mixed with eye drops containing thimerosal, precipitation may occur.

 See the companion website for a Nursing Process Focus specific to this drug.

mor formation and increases outflow in open-angle glaucoma. Latanoprost (Xalatan) is presented in this chapter as a prototype drug. Other prostaglandins used in the treatment of glaucoma include bimatoprost (Lumigan), travaprost (Travatan), and unoprostone isopropyl (Rescula). The main side effect of these medications is heightened pigmentation, usually a brown color of the iris in patients with lighter colored eyes. These drugs cause cycloplegia, local irritation, and stinging of the eyes. Because of these effects, prostaglandins are normally administered just before the patient goes to bed.

Beta-Adrenergic Blockers

Beta-adrenergic blockers are drugs of choice for open-angle glaucoma. These include betaxolol (Betoptic), carteolol (Ocupress), levobunolol (Betagan), metipranolol (OptiPranolol), and timolol (Timoptic, Timoptic XE). These drugs act by decreasing the production of aqueous humor, thus reducing IOP. They generally produce fewer ocular adverse effects than cholinergic agonists or sympathomimetics. The topical administration of beta-blockers for glaucoma treatment does not result in significant systemic absorption. Should absorption occur, however, systemic side effects may include bronchoconstriction, bradycardia, and hypotension.

Alpha₂-Adrenergic Agonists

Alpha₂-adrenergic agonists are prescribed less frequently than the other antiglaucoma medications. These drugs include apraclonidine (Iopidine), which is used for short-term therapy, and brimonidine (Alphagan P), which is approved for long-term therapy. These drugs produce minimal cardiovascular and pulmonary side effects. The most

significant side effects are headache, drowsiness, dry mucosal membranes, blurred vision, and irritated eyelids.

Carbonic Anhydrase Inhibitors

Carbonic anhydrase inhibitors may be administered topically or systemically to reduce IOP in cases of open-angle glaucoma. They act by decreasing the production of aqueous humor. Usually these medications are used as a second choice if beta-blockers have not produced therapeutic results. Examples include acetazolamide (Diamox), brinzolamide (Azopt), dichlorphenamide (Daranide, Oratrol), dorzolamide (Trusopt), and methazolamide (Neptazane). Patients must be cautioned when taking these medications because they contain sulfur and may cause an allergic reaction. Because these drugs are diuretics and can reduce IOP quickly, serum electrolytes should be monitored during treatment.

Osmotic Diuretics

Osmotic diuretics are occasionally used in cases of eye surgery or acute closed-angle glaucoma. Examples include glycerin anhydrous (Ophthalgan), isosorbide (Ismotic), and mannitol (Osmitrol). Because they have an ability to quickly reduce plasma volume (Chapter 27), they are effective in reducing the formation of aqueous humor🔗. Side effects include headache, tremors, dizziness, dry mouth, fluid and electrolyte imbalances, and thrombophlebitis or venous clot formation near the site of IV administration.

NURSING CONSIDERATIONS

The role of the nurse in drug therapy for glaucoma involves careful monitoring of a patient's condition and providing education as it relates to the prescribed drug regimen. The initial assessment of a patient with glaucoma includes a general health history to determine past and current medical problems and medication regimen. The nurse should determine if the patient has a history of second or third degree heart block, bradycardia, heart failure, or COPD. Antiglaucoma agents that affect the autonomic nervous system may be contraindicated for patients with these conditions, because of possible drug absorption into the systemic circulation.

Several preparations used in glaucoma have a potential risk of cardiorespiratory side effects that will occur if the medication is systemically absorbed. Prior to starting drug therapy, a baseline blood pressure and pulse should be established. When a beta-blocker is used, the patient should be taught how to check pulse and blood pressure before medication administration. The nurse should review the parameters of the pulse and blood pressure with the patient and family members and establish guidelines when the healthcare provider should be notified. Because the safety of ophthalmic preparations as beta-blockers during pregnancy or lactation has not been established, the nurse should obtain information concerning the possibility of pregnancy or breastfeeding.

A key factor in preventing further ocular pathology is patient compliance with the medication regimen. The nurse should determine any factors that could decrease compliance such as insufficient financial resources, lack of knowledge, lack of dexterity or skill in inserting eye drops, or remembering the dosing schedule. Fear and anxiety about potential blindness and disability may also be evident in the patient diagnosed with glaucoma. It is crucial that the nurse allow the patient to verbalize feelings and provide emotional support to the patient and family. An explanation of the how the disease can be controlled may facilitate compliance as well as alleviate the patient's anxiety.

Patient education as it relates to drugs to treat glaucoma should include goals, reasons for obtaining baseline data such as vital signs and tests for cardiac and respiratory disorders, possible side effects, and safe administration of eye medications.

Frequently the person with glaucoma is elderly so a caregiver will administer the eye drops or gels. The nurse should review the proper method for administering eye medications given in Chapter 4 ⊕ . Following are the important points the nurse should include when teaching patients and caregivers regarding ophthalmic solutions used in glaucoma therapy.

- The patient is at risk for falls and accidents secondary to decreased vision. Assess for environmental hazards and simple methods to ensure safety.
- Visual difficulty is often worse immediately following instillation of eye drops as vision may be blurred. Remain still until the blurring diminishes.
- Report side effects including eye irritation, conjunctival edema, burning, stinging, redness, blurred vision, pain, irritation, itching, sensation of foreign body in the eye, photophobia, or visual disturbances.

- Remove contact lenses before instilling drops and wait at least 15 minutes before reinserting them to allow the medication sufficient contact with the eye.
- Report any reactions to the medication as well as any possibility of pregnancy.

See "Nursing Process Focus: Patients Receiving Ophthalmic Solutions for Glaucoma" for additional patient teaching points.

48.5 Pharmacotherapy for Eye Exams and Minor Eye Conditions

Some drugs are specifically designed to enhance eye examinations during ophthalmic procedures. **Cycloplegic drugs** paralyze the ciliary muscles and prevent the lens from moving during assessment. **Mydriatic drugs** dilate the pupils to allow better observation of retinal structures. These agents include anticholinergics, such as atropine (Isopto Atropine) and tropicamide (Mydriacyl), and sympathomimetics such as phenylephrine (Mydfrin). Cycloplegics cause severe blurred vision and a loss of near vision. Mydriatics cause intense photophobia and pain in response to bright light.

Anticholinergic mydriatics can worsen glaucoma by impairing aqueous humor outflow and thereby increasing IOP. In addition, anticholinergics have the potential for producing central side effects such as confusion, unsteadiness, or drowsiness. Examples of cycloplegic, mydriatic, and lubricant drugs are listed in Table 48.2.

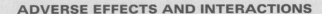

| **Pr** **PROTOTYPE DRUG** | **TIMOLOL** (Timoptic, Timoptic XE) |

ACTIONS AND USES

Timolol is a nonselective beta-adrenergic blocker available as a 0.25% or 0.5% ophthalmic solution. Timolol reduces elevated intraocular pressure (IOP) in chronic open-angle glaucoma by reducing the formation of aqueous humor. The usual dose is one drop in the affected eye(s) twice a day. Timoptic XE allows for once-a-day dosing. Treatment may require 2 to 4 weeks for maximum therapeutic effect. It is also available in tablets, which are prescribed to treat mild hypertension.

Administration Alerts

- Proper administration lessens the danger of the drug being absorbed systemically, which can mask symptoms of hypoglycemia.
- Pregnancy category C.

ADVERSE EFFECTS AND INTERACTIONS

The most common side effects are local burning and stinging upon instillation. In most patients there is no significant systemic absorption to cause adverse effects as long as timolol is applied correctly. If significant systemic absorption occurs, however, drug interactions could occur. Anticholinergics, nitrates, reserpine, methyldopa, and/or verapamil use could lead to increased hypotension and bradycardia. Indomethacin and thyroid hormone use could lead to decreased antihypertensive effects of timolol. Epinephrine use could lead to hypertension followed by severe bradycardia. Theophylline use could lead to decreased bronchodilation.

 See the companion website for a Nursing Process Focus specific to this drug.

| **NATURAL THERAPIES** | **Bilberry for Eye Health** |

Bilberry (*Vaccinium myrtillus*), a plant whose leaves and fruit are used medicinally, is found in central and northern Europe, Asia, and North America. It has been shown in clinical studies to increase conjunctival capillary resistance in patients with diabetic retinopathy, thereby providing protection against hemorrhage of the retina. One compound in bilberry, anthocyanosides, has a collagen stabilizing effect. Increased synthesis of connective tissue (including collagen) is one of the contributing factors that may lead to blindness caused by diabetic retinopathy. It has also been used to reduce eye inflammation and improve night vision. Billberry may be taken as a tea to treat nonspecific diarrhea and topically to treat inflammation of the mucous membranes of the mouth and throat.

Drugs for minor irritation and dryness come from a broad range of classes including antimicrobials, local anesthetics, glucocorticoids, and nonsteroidal anti-inflammatory drugs (NSAIDs). In each case, a range of drug preparations may be employed including drops, salves, optical inserts, and injectable formulations. Some agents only provide lubrication to the eye's surface, whereas others are designed to penetrate and affect a specific area of the eye.

EAR CONDITIONS

The ear has two major sensory functions: hearing and maintenance of equilibrium and balance. As shown in Figure 48.3, three structural areas, the outer ear, middle ear, and inner ear, carry out these functions.

Otitis, inflammation of the ear, most often occurs in the outer and middle ear compartments. External otitis, commonly called swimmer's ear, is inflammation of the outer ear that is most often associated with water exposure. Otitis media, inflammation of the middle ear, is most often associated with upper respiratory infections, allergies, or auditory tube irritation. Of all ear infections, the most difficult ones to treat are inner ear infections. Mastoiditis, or inflammation of the mastoid sinus, can be a serious problem because if left untreated it can result in hearing loss.

OTIC PREPARATIONS

48.6 Pharmacotherapy with Otic Preparations

The basic treatment for ear infection is topical antibiotics in the form of ear drops. Chloramphenicol (Chloromycetin, Pentamycetin) is the most commonly used topical otic antibiotic. Systemic antibiotics may be needed in cases when outer ear infections are extensive or in patients with middle or inner ear infections.

In cases of otitis media, drugs for pain, edema, and itching may also be necessary. Glucocorticoids are often combined with antibiotics or other drugs when inflammation is present. Examples of these drugs are listed in Table 48.3.

Mastoiditis is frequently the result of chronic or reoccuring bacterial otitis media. The infection moves into the bone and surrounding structures of the middle ear. Antibiotics are usually given for a trial period. If the antibiotics are not effective and symptoms persist, surgery such as mastoidectomy or meatoplasty may be indicated.

Cerumen (ear wax) softeners are also used for proper ear health. When cerumen accumulates, it narrows the ear canal, and may interfere with hearing. This is especially true for older patients and may be part of the changes associated with aging. Healthcare providers working with the elderly should be trained to take appropriate measures

MediaLink National Library of Medicine

NURSING PROCESS FOCUS   PATIENTS RECEIVING OPHTHALMIC SOLUTIONS FOR GLAUCOMA

ASSESSMENT

Prior to drug administration:
- Obtain complete health history including allergies, drug history, and possible drug interactions.
- Obtain complete physical examination focusing on visual acuity and visual field assessments.
- Assess for the presence/history of ocular pain.

POTENTIAL NURSING DIAGNOSES

- Risk for Injury, related to visual acuity deficits
- Self-care Deficit, related to impaired vision
- Pain, related to disease process

PLANNING: PATIENT GOALS AND EXPECTED OUTCOMES

The patient will:
- Exhibit no progression of visual impairment
- Demonstrate an understanding of the disease process
- Safely function within own environment without injury
- Report absence of pain

IMPLEMENTATION

Interventions and (Rationales)	Patient Education/Discharge Planning
Monitor visual acuity, blurred vision, papillary reactions, extraocular movements, and ocular pain.	Instruct patient to report changes in vision and headache.
Monitor the patient for specific contraindications for prescribed drug. (There are many physiologic conditions in which ophthalmic solutions may be contraindicated.)	Instruct patient to inform healthcare provider of all health-related problems and prescribed medications.
Remove contact lenses before administration of ophthalmic solutions.	Instruct patient to remove contact lenses prior to administering eye drops and wait 15 minutes before reinsertion.
Administer ophthalmic solutions using proper technique.	Instruct patient in the proper administration of eye drops. ■ Wash hands prior to eye drop administration. ■ Avoid touching the tip of the container to the eye which may contaminate the solution. ■ Administer the eye drop in the conjunctival sac. ■ Apply pressure over the lacrimal sac for 1 minute. ■ Wait 5 minutes before administering other ophthalmic solutions. ■ Schedule glaucoma medications around daily routines such as waking, mealtimes, and bedtime to lessen the chance of missed doses.
Monitor for ocular reaction to the drug such as conjunctivitis and lid reactions.	Instruct patient to report itching, drainage, ocular pain, or other ocular abnormalities.
Assess intraocular pressure readings. (These are used to determine effectiveness of drug therapy.)	Instruct patient that intraocular pressure readings will be done prior to beginning treatment and periodically during treatment.
Monitor color of iris and periorbital tissue of treated eye.	Instruct patient that: ■ More brown color may appear in the iris and in the periorbital tissue of treated eye only ■ Any pigmentation changes develop over months to years
Monitor for systemic absorption of ophthalmic preparations. (Ophthalmic drugs for glaucoma can cause serious cardiovascular and respiratory complications if the drug is systemically absorbed.)	Instruct patient to immediately report palpitations, chest pain, shortness of breath, and irregularities in pulse.

continued

NURSING PROCESS FOCUS: **Patients Receiving Ophthalmic Solutions for Glaucoma (continued)**

Interventions and (Rationales)	*Patient Education/Discharge Planning*
■ Monitor and adjust environmental lighting to aid in patient's comfort. (People who have glaucoma are sensitive to excessive light, especially extreme sunlight.)	Instruct patient to: ■ Adjust environmental lighting as needed to enhance vision or reduce ocular pain ■ Wear darkened glasses as needed
■ Encourage compliance with treatment regimen.	Instruct patient: ■ To adhere to medication schedule for eye drop administration ■ About the importance of regular follow-up care with ophthalmologist

EVALUATION OF OUTCOME CRITERIA

Evaluate the effectiveness of drug therapy by confirming that patient goals and expected outcomes have been met (see "Planning").

See Table 48.1 for a list of drugs to which these nursing actions apply.

Table 48.2	**Drugs for Mydriasis, Cycloplegia, and Lubrication of the Eye**
Drug	**Route and Adult Dose**
Mydriatics: Sympathomimetics	
hydroxyamphetamine (Paredrine)	1 drop 1% solution before eye exam
phenylephrine HCl (Mydfrin, Neo-Synephrine)	1 drop 2.5% or 10% solution before eye exam
Cycloplegics: Anticholinergics	
atropine sulfate (Isopto Atropine, others)	1 drop 0.5% solution qd
cyclopentolate (Cyclogyl, Pentalair)	1 drop 0.5–2% solution 40–50 min before eye exam
homatropine (Isopto Homatropine, others)	1–2 drops 2% or 5% solution before eye exam
scopolamine hydrobromide (Isopto Hyoscine)	1–2 drops 0.25% solution 1h before eye exam
tropicamide (Mydriacyl, Tropicacyl)	1–2 drops 0.5–1% solution before eye exam
Lubricants	
lanolin alcohol (Lacri-lube)	Apply a thin film to the inside of the eyelid
methylcellulose (Methulose, Visculose, others)	1–2 drops prn
naphazoline HCl (Albalon Allerest, ClearEyes, others)	1–3 drops 0.1% solution every 3–4 hours prn
oxymetazoline HCl (OcuClear, Visine LR)	1–2 drops 0.025% solution qid
polyvinyl alcohol (Liquifilm, others)	1–2 drops prn
tetrahydrozoline HCl (Collyrium, Murine Plus, Visine, others)	1–2 drops 0.05% solution bid-tid

when removing impacted cerumen. This procedure usually involves instillation of an ear wax softener and then a gentle lavage of the wax-impacted ear with tepid water using an aesepto-type syringe to gently insert the water. An instrument called an ear loop may be used to help remove ear wax, but should be used only by healthcare providers who are skilled in using it. Nurses should advise patients not to perform ear wax removal, especially in children, due to the potential for damage to the eardrum.

NURSING CONSIDERATIONS

The role of the nurse in drug therapy with otic preparations involves careful monitoring of a patient's condition and providing education as it relates to the prescribed drug regimen. Before any of the otic preparations are administered, the nurse should assess the patient's baseline hearing/auditory status. The nurse should assess the patient's symptoms and any current medical conditions. Because the structure of the inner ear

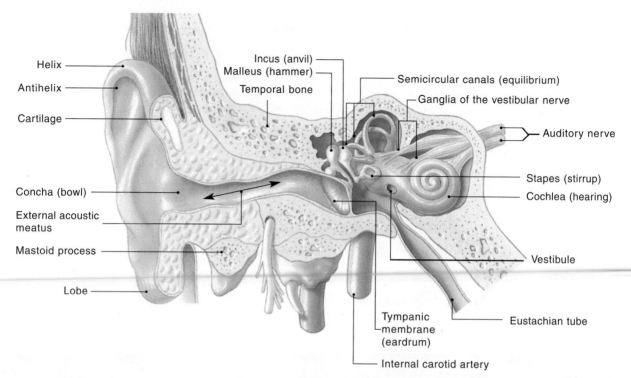

Figure 48.3 | Structures of the external ear, middle ear, and inner ear *Source: Pearson Education/PH College.*

Table 48.3	Otic Preparations
Drug	**Route and Adult Dose**
acetic acid and hydrocortisone (Vosol HC)	3 to 5 drops q 4h-qid for 24 hours, then 5 drops tid-qid
aluminum sulfate and calcium acetate (Domeboro)	2 drops 2% solution tid-qid
benzocaine and antipyrine (Auralgan)	Fill ear canal with solution tid for 2 or 3 days
carbamide peroxide (Debrox)	1–5 drops 6.5% solution bid for 4 days
ciprofloxacin hydrochloride and hydrocortisone (Cipro)	3 drops of the suspension instilled into ear bid for 7 days
polymixin B, neomycin and hydrocortisone (Cortisporin)	4 drops in ear tid-qid
triethanolamine polypeptide oleate 10% condensate (Cerumenex)	Fill ear canal with solution; wait 10–20 minutes

changes according to the patient's age, the nurse should have a thorough understanding of the anatomy of the ear.

The nurse should obtain information regarding hypersensitivity to hydrocortisone, neomycin sulfate, or polymyxin B. The use of these medications is contraindicated in the presence of perforated eardrum. Chloramphenicol ear drops are contraindicated in hypersensitivity and eardrum perforation. Side effects include burning, redness, rash, swelling, and other signs of topical irritation.

When instilling otic preparations, the ear should be thoroughly cleansed and the cerumen removed through irrigation. Eardrops should be warmed to body temperature before instillation (but not higher than body temperature). The nurse should administer wax emulsifiers according to manufacturer's guidelines or healthcare provider's orders.

Patient education as it relates to otic preparations should include goals, reasons for obtaining baseline data such as hearing/auditory tests, and possible side effects. Following are important points the nurse should include when teaching patients regarding otic preparations.

- Lay down while instilling chloramphenicol drops, as dizziness may occur. Also, do not touch dropper to the ear.
- Administer ear drops at body temperature by running warm water over the bottle.
- With adults and children older than 3 years, the pinna should be held up and back during instillation. With children younger than 3 years of age, the pinna should be gently pulled down and back during instillation.
- Massage the area around the ear gently after instillation to promote thorough administration to the ear canal.
- Lie on the opposite side of the affected ear for 5 minutes after instillation.

CHAPTER REVIEW

Key Concepts

The numbered key concepts provide a succinct summary of the important points from the corresponding numbered section within the chapter. If any of these points are not clear, refer to the numbered section within the chapter for review. Expanded versions can be found on the companion website.

48.1 Knowledge of basic eye anatomy is fundamental for an understanding of eye disorders and pharmacotherapy.

48.2 Glaucoma develops because the flow of aqueous humor in the anterior eye cavity becomes disrupted, leading to increasing intraocular pressure (IOP). Two principle types of glaucoma are closed-angle glaucoma and open-angle glaucoma.

48.3 General therapy of glaucoma may require laser surgery to correct the underlying pathology.

48.4 Drugs used for glaucoma decrease IOP by increasing the outflow of aqueous humor or by decreasing the formation of aqueous humor.

48.5 Mydriatic or pupil-dilating drugs and cycloplegic or ciliary muscle relaxing drugs are routinely used for eye examinations.

48.6 Otic preparations treat infections, inflammation, and ear wax buildup.

Review Questions

1. Which components of the eye are specifically affected by glaucoma?

2. Describe two major approaches for controlling intraocular pressure in glaucoma patients. What major drug classes are used in each case?

3. List examples of commonly used drugs for minor eye irritation and injury. What are the major actions of cycloplegic and mydriatic drugs?

4. Identify areas of the ear where microbial infections are most likely. What kind of otic preparations treat infections, inflammation, and ear wax buildup?

Critical Thinking Questions

1. A 3-year-old girl is playing nurse with her dolls. She picks up her mother's flexible metal necklace and places the tips of the necklace in her ears for her "stethoscope." A few hours later, she cries to her mother that her "ears hurt." The child's mother takes her to see the advanced practice nurse (APN) at an after-hours clinic. An examination reveals abrasions in the outer ear canal and some dried blood. The APN prescribes corticosporin otic drops. What does the healthcare provider need to teach the mother about instillation of this medication?

2. A 64-year-old man has been diagnosed with primary open-angle glaucoma. He has COPD following a 40-year history of smoking. Is he a candidate for treatment with timolol maleate (Timoptic)? Why or why not? Is there a preferred agent?

3. To determine her ability to administer glaucoma medications, the nurse asks the 82-year-old patient to instill her own medications prior to discharge. The nurse notes that the patient is happy to cooperate and watches as the patient quickly drops her head back, opens her eyes, and drops the medication directly onto her cornea. The patient blinks several times, smiles at the nurse, and says, "There, it is no problem at all!" What correction should the nurse make in the patient's technique?

EXPLORE MediaLink

NCLEX review, case studies, and other interactive resources for this chapter can be found on the companion website at www.prenhall.com/adams. Click on "Chapter 48" to select the activities for this chapter. For animations, more NCLEX review questions, and an audio glossary, access the accompanying CD-ROM in this textbook.

Glossary

A delta fibers nerves that transmit sensations of sharp pain

Absence seizure seizure with a loss or reduction of normal activity, including staring and transient loss of responsiveness

Absorption the process of moving a drug across body membranes

Acetylcholine primary neurotransmitter of the parasympathetic nervous system; also present at somatic neuromuscular junctions and at sympathetic preganglionic nerves

Acetylcholinesterase (AchE) enzyme that degrades acetylcholine within the synaptic cleft, enhancing effects of the neurotransmitter

Acidosis condition of having too much acid in the blood; plasma pH below 7.35

Acne vulgaris condition characterized by small inflamed bumps that appear on the surface of the skin

Acquired immunodeficiency syndrome (AIDS) infection caused by the human immunodeficiency virus (HIV)

Acquired resistance when a microbe is no longer affected by a drug following anti-infective pharmacotherapy

Action potential electrical changes in the membrane of a muscle or nerve cell due to changes in membrane permeability

Activated partial thromboplastin time (aPTT) blood test used to determine how long it takes clots to form, to regulate heparin dosage

Active immunity resistance resulting from a previous exposure to an antigen

Acute gouty arthritis condition where uric acid crystals accumulate in the joints of the big toes, ankles, wrists, fingers, knees, or elbows, resulting in red, swollen, or inflamed tissue

Acute radiation syndrome life-threatening symptoms resulting from acute exposure to ionizing radiation, including nausea, vomiting, severe leukopenia, thrombocytopenia, anemia, and alopecia

Addiction the continued use of a substance despite its negative health and social consequences

Addison's disease hyposecretion of glucocorticoids and aldosterone by the adrenal cortex

Adenohypophysis anterior portion of the pituitary gland

Adolescence person from 13 to 16 years of age

Adrenergic relating to nerves that release norepinephrine or epinephrine

Adrenergic antagonist drug that blocks the actions of the sympathetic nervous system

Adrenocorticotropic hormone (ACTH) hormone secreted by the anterior pituitary that stimulates the release of glucocorticoids by the adrenal cortex

Aerobic pertaining to an oxygen environment

Aerosol suspension of minute liquid droplets or fine solid particles suspended in a gas

Affinity chemical attraction that impels certain molecules to unite with others to form complexes

Afterload pressure that must be overcome for the ventricles to eject blood from the heart

Agonist drug that is capable of binding with receptors to induce a cellular response

Akathisia inability to remain still; constantly moving

Aldosterone hormone secreted by the adrenal cortex that increases sodium reabsorption in the distal tubule of the kidney

Alimentary canal hollow tube in the digestive system that starts in the mouth and includes the esophagus, stomach, small intestine, and large intestine

Alkalosis condition of having too many basic substances in the blood; plasma pH above 7.45

Alkylation process by which certain chemicals attach to DNA and change its structure and function

Allergic reaction acquired, hyperresponse of body defenses to a foreign substance (allergen)

Allergic rhinitis syndrome of sneezing, itchy throat, watery eyes, and nasal congestion resulting from exposure to antigens; also known as hay fever

Alopecia hair loss

Alpha-receptor type of subreceptor found in the sympathetic nervous system

Alzheimer's disease most common dementia characterized by loss of memory, delusions, hallucinations, confusion, and loss of judgment

Amenorrhea lack of normal menstrual periods

Amide type of chemical linkage found in some local anesthetics involving carbon, nitrogen, and oxygen (-NH-CO-)

Amyloid plaques abnormal protein fragments related to neuronal damage; a sign of Alzheimer's disease observed during autopsy

Anabolic steroids compounds resembling testosterone with hormonal activity commonly abused by athletes

Anaerobic pertaining to an environment without oxygen

Analgesic drug used to reduce or eliminate pain

Anaphylactic shock type of shock caused by an acute allergic reaction

Anaphylaxis acute allergic response to an antigen that results in severe hypotension and may lead to life-threatening shock if untreated

Anastomoses natural communication networks among the coronary arteries

Androgens steroid sex hormones that promote the appearance of masculine characteristics

Anemia lack of adequate numbers of red blood cells or deceased oxygen-carrying capacity of the blood

Angina pectoris acute chest pain upon physical or emotional exertion due to inadequate oxygen supply to the myocardium

Angiotensin II chemical released in response to falling blood pressure that causes vasoconstriction and release of aldosterone

Angiotensin-converting enzyme (ACE) enzyme responsible for converting angiotensin I to angiotensin II

Anions negatively charged ions

Anorexia loss of appetite

Anorexiant drug used to suppress appetite

Antacid drug that neutralizes stomach acid

Antagonism type of drug interaction where one drug inhibits the effectiveness of another

Antagonist drug that blocks the response of another drug

Antepartum prior to the onset of labor

Anthrax microorganism that can cause severe disease and high mortality in humans

Antibiotic substance produced by a microorganism that inhibits or kills other microorganisms

Antibody protein produced by the body in response to an antigen; used interchangeably with the term immunoglobulin

Anticholinergic drug that blocks the actions of the parasympathetic nervous system

Anticoagulant agent that inhibits the formation of blood clots

Antidiuretic hormone (ADH) hormone produced by the hypothalamus and secreted by the posterior pituitary that stimulates the kidneys to conserve water

Antiemetic drug that prevents vomiting

Antifibrinolytic drug used to prevent and treat excessive bleeding from surgical sites

Antigen foreign organism or substance that induces the formation of antibodies by the immune system

Anti-infective general term for any medication that is effective against pathogens

Antipyretic drug that lowers body temperature

Antiretroviral drug that is effective against retroviruses

Antithrombin III protein that prevents abnormal clotting by inhibiting thrombin

Antitussive drug used to suppress cough

Anxiety state of apprehension and autonomic nervous system activation resulting from exposure to a nonspecific or unknown cause

Anxiolytics drugs that relieve anxiety

Apoprotein protein component of a lipoprotein

Apothecary system of measurement older system of measurement using drams; rarely used

Aqueous humor fluid that fills the anterior and posterior chambers of the eye

Aromatase inhibitor hormone inhibitor that blocks the enzyme aromatase, which normally converts adrenal androgen to estradiol

ASAP order as soon as possible order that should be available for administration to the patient within 30 minutes of the written order

Assessment appraisal of a patient's condition that involves gathering and interpreting data

Asthma chronic inflammatory disease of the lungs characterized by airway obstruction

Astringent effect drops or sprays used to shrink swollen mucous membranes, or to loosen secretions and facilitate drainage

Atherosclerosis condition characterized by a buildup of fatty plaque and loss of elasticity of the walls of the arteries

Atonic seizure very-short-lasting seizure during which the patient may stumble and fall for no apparent reason

Atrioventricular (AV) node cardiac tissue that receives electrical impulses from the SA node and conveys them to the ventricles

Atrioventricular bundle cardiac tissue that receives electrical impulses from the AV node and sends them to the bundle branches; also known as the bundle of His

Attention-deficit disorder (ADD) inability to focus attention on a task for a sufficient length of time

Attention-deficit hyperactivity disorder (ADHD) disorder typically diagnosed in childhood and adolescence characterized by hyperactivity as well as attention, organization, and behavior control issues

Aura sensory cue such as bright lights, smells, or tastes that precede a migraine

Autoantibodies proteins called rheumatoid factors released by B lymphocytes that tear down the body's own tissue

Automaticity ability of certain myocardial cells to spontaneously generate an action potential

Autonomic nervous system portion of the peripheral nervous system that gives involuntary control over smooth muscle, cardiac muscle, and glands

Autonomy ability to make decisions unaided by others

Azole term for the major class of drugs used to treat mycoses

Azoospermia complete absence of sperm in an ejaculate

Azotemia accumulation of nitrogenous waste products in the kidneys that can result in death if untreated

Bacilli bacteria that are oblong in shape; also called rods

Bacteriocidal substance that kills bacteria

Bacteriostatic substance that inhibits the growth of bacteria

Balanced anesthesia use of multiple medications to rapidly induce unconsciousness, cause muscle relaxation, and maintain deep anesthesia

Baroreceptors nerves located in the walls of the atria, aortic arch, vena cava, and carotid sinus that sense changes in blood pressure

Basal metabolic rate resting rate of metabolism in the body

Baseline data patient information that is gathered before pharmacotherapy is implemented

B cell lymphocyte responsible for humoral immunity

Beneficence ethical principle of doing good

Benign not life threatening or fatal

Benign prostatic hypertrophy/hyperplasia (BPH) nonmalignant enlargement of the prostate gland

Benzodiazepines major class of drugs used to treat anxiety disorders

Beriberi deficiency of thiamine

Beta-lactam ring chemical structure found in most penicillins and some cephalosporins

Beta-lactamase (penicillinase) enzyme present in certain bacteria that is able to inactivate many penicillins and some cephalosporins

Beta-receptor type of subreceptor found in the sympathetic nervous system

Bile acid resin drug that bind bile acids, thus lowering cholesterol

Bioavailability ability of a drug to reach the bloodstream and its target tissues

Biologic response modifiers substances that are able to enhance or stimulate the immune system

Biologics substances that produce biologic responses within the body; they are synthesized by cells of the human body, animal cells, or microorganisms

Bioterrorism intentional use of infectious biologic agents, chemical substances, or radiation to cause widespread harm or illness

Bipolar disorder (manic depression) syndrome characterized by extreme and opposite moods, such as euphoria and depression

Bisphosphonates class of drugs that block bone resorption by inhibiting osteoclast activity

Blood-brain barrier anatomical structure that prevents certain substances from gaining access to the brain

Bone deposition opposite of bone resorption; the process of depositing mineral components into bone

Bone resorption process of bone demineralization or the breaking down of bone into mineral components

Botanical plant extract used to treat or prevent illness

Bowman's capsule portion of the nephron that filters blood and receives the filtrate from the glomerulus

Bradykinesia difficulty initiating movement and controlling fine muscle movements

Bradykinin chemical released by cells during inflammation that produces pain and side effects similar to those of histamine

Breakthrough bleeding hemorrhage at abnormal times during the menstrual cycle

Broad-spectrum antibiotic anti-infective that is effective against many different gram positive and gram negative organisms

Bronchospasm rapid constriction of the airways

Buccal route tablet or capsule that is placed in the oral cavity between the gum and the cheek

Buffer chemical that helps maintain normal body pH by neutralizing strong acids or bases

Bundle branches electrical conduction pathway in the heart leading from the AV bundle and through the wall between the ventricles

C fibers nerves that transmit dull, poorly localized pain

Calcifediol substance formed in the first step of vitamin D formation

Calcineurin intracellular messenger molecule to which immunosuppressants bind

Calcitonin hormone secreted by the thyroid gland that increases the deposition of calcium in bone

Calcitriol substance that is transformed in the kidneys during the second step of the conversion of vitamin D to its active form

Calcium channel blocker drug that blocks the flow of calcium ions into myocardial cells

Calcium ion channel pathway in a plasma membrane through which calcium ions enter and leave

Camptothecin class of antineoplastics that inhibits the enzyme topoisomerase

Cancer/carcinoma malignant disease characterized by rapidly growing, invasive cells that spread to other regions of the body and eventually kill the host

Capsid protein coat that surrounds a virus

Carbonic anhydrase enzyme that forms carbonic acid by combining carbon dioxide and water

Cardiac output amount of blood pumped by a ventricle in 1 minute

Cardiogenic shock type of shock caused when the heart is diseased such that it cannot maintain circulation to the tissues

Cardioversion/defibrillation conversion of fibrillation to a normal heart rhythm

Carotene class of yellow-red pigments that are precursors to vitamin A

Catecholamines class of agents secreted in response to stress that includes epinephrine, norepinephrine and dopamine

Cathartic substance that causes complete evacuation of the bowel

Cations positively charged ions

CD4 receptor protein that accepts HIV and allows entry of the virus into the T4 lymphocyte

Central nervous system (CNS) division of the nervous system consisting of the brain and spinal cord

Cerebrovascular accident/stroke/brain attack acute condition of a blood clot or bleeding in a vessel in the brain

Chemical name strict chemical nomenclature used for naming drugs established by the International Union of Pure and Applied Chemistry (IUPAC)

Chemoreceptors nerves located in the aortic arch and carotid sinus that sense changes in oxygen content, pH, or carbon dioxide levels in the blood

Chemotherapy drug treatment of cancer

Chief cells cells located in the mucosa of the stomach that secrete pepsinogen, an inactive form of the enzyme pepsin that chemically breaks down proteins

Cholecalciferol vitamin D_3 formed in the skin by exposure to ultraviolet light

Cholinergic relating to nerves that release acetylcholine

Chronic bronchitis recurrent disease of the lungs characterized by excess mucus production, inflammation, and coughing

Chronic obstructive pulmonary disease (COPD) generic term used to describe several pulmonary conditions characterized by cough, mucus production, and impaired gas exchange

Chronotropic effect change in the heart rate

Chyme semifluid, partly digested food that is passed from the stomach to the duodenum

Clinical investigation second stage of drug testing that involves clinical phase trials

Clinical phase trials testing of a new drug in selected patients

Clonic spasm multiple, rapidly repeated muscular contractions

Closed-angle glaucoma acute glaucoma that is caused by decreased outflow of aqueous humor from the anterior chamber

Clotting factors substances contributing to the process of blood hemostasis

Coagulation process of blood clotting

Coagulation cascade complex series of steps by which blood flow stops

Cocci bacteria that are spherical in shape

Colloids type of IV fluid consisting of large organic molecules that are unable to cross membranes

Colony-stimulating factors hormones that regulate the growth and maturation of specific WBC populations

Combination drug drug product with more than one active generic ingredient

Comedome type of acne that develops just beneath the surface of the skin (whiteheads) or as a result of a plugged oil gland (blackhead)

Complement a series of proteins involved in the nonspecific defense of the body that promote antigen destruction

Complementary and alternative medicine (CAM) treatments that consider the health of the whole person and promote disease prevention

Complementary and alternative therapies treatments considered outside the realm of conventional Western medicine

Compliance taking a medication in the manner prescribed by the healthcare provider, or, in the case of OTC drugs, following the instructions on the label

Conjugates side chains that, during metabolism, make drugs more water soluble and more easily excreted by the kidney

Constipation infrequent passage of abnormally hard and dry stools

Contractility the strength by which the myocardial fibers contract

Controlled substance in the United States, a drug whose use is restricted by the Comprehensive Drug Abuse Prevention and Control Act; in Canada, a drug subject to guidelines outlined in Part III, Schedule G of the Canadian Food and Drugs Act

Convulsions uncontrolled muscle contractions or spasms that occur in the face, torso, arms, or legs

Coronary arterial bypass graft (CABG) surgical procedure performed to restore blood flow to the myocardium by using a section of the saphenous vein or internal mammary artery to go around the obstructed coronary artery

Coronary arteries vessels that bring oxygen and nutrients to the myocardium

Corpus cavernosum tissue in the penis that fills with blood during an erection

Corpus luteum ruptured follicle that remains in the ovary after ovulation and secretes progestins

Corpus striatum area of the brain responsible for unconscious muscle movement; a point of contact for neurons projecting from the substantia nigra

Crohn's disease chronic inflammatory bowel disease affecting the ileum and sometimes the colon

Cross-tolerance when tolerance to one drug makes the patient tolerant to another drug

Crystalloids type of IV fluid resembling blood plasma minus proteins that is capable of crossing membranes

Culture set of beliefs, values, religious rituals, and customs shared by a group of people

Culture and sensitivity test laboratory exam used to identify bacteria and to determine which antibiotic is most effective

Cushing's syndrome condition of having too much corticosteroids in the blood, caused by excessive secretion by the adrenal glands or by overdosage with corticosteroid medication

Cyclooxygenase (COX–1 and COX–2) key enzyme in the prostaglandin metabolic pathway that is blocked by aspirin and other NSAIDs

Cycloplegic drugs drugs that relax or temporarily paralyze ciliary muscles and cause blurred vision

Cytokine chemical produced by white blood cells, such as interleukins, leukotrienes, interferon, and tumor necrosis factor, that guide the immune response

Cytotoxic T cell lymphocyte responsible for cell-mediated immunity that kills target cells directly or by secreting cytokines

Defecation evacuation of the colon; bowel movement

Delusions false ideas and beliefs not founded in reality

Dementia degenerative disorder characterized by progressive memory loss, confusion, and the inability to think or communicate effectively

Dependence strong physiologic or psychologic need for a substance

Depolarization reversal of charge of the plasma membrane charge such that the inside is made less negative

Depression disorder characterized by depressed mood, lack of energy, sleep disturbances, abnormal eating patterns, and feelings of despair, guilt, and misery

Dermatitis inflammatory condition of the skin characterized by itching and scaling

Dermatophytic superficial fungal infection

Designer drugs substances produced in a laboratory and intended to mimic the effects of other psychoactive controlled substances

Diabetes insipidus excessive urination due to lack of secretion of antidiuretic hormone

Diabetes mellitus, type 1 metabolic disease characterized by hyperglycemia caused by a lack of secretion of insulin by the pancreas

Diabetes mellitus, type 2 chronic metabolic disease caused by insufficient secretion of insulin by the pancreas, and a lack of sensitivity of insulin receptors

Diabetic ketoacidosis a type of metabolic acidosis due to an excess of ketone bodies, most often occuring when diabetes mellitus is uncontrolled

Diarrhea abnormal frequency and liquidity of bowel movements

Diastolic pressure blood pressure during the relaxation phase of heart activity

Dietary fiber ingested substance that is neither digested nor absorbed that contributes to the fecal mass

Dietary supplement nondrug substance regulated by the DSHEA

Dietary Supplement Health and Education Act of 1994 (DSHEA) primary law in the United States regulating herb and dietary supplements

Digestion the process by which the body breaks down ingested food into small molecules that can be absorbed

Distal tubule portion of the nephron that collects filtrate from the loop of Henle

Distribution the process of transporting drugs through the body

Diuretic substance that increases urine output

Dopamine type D2 receptor receptors for dopamine in the basal nuclei of the brain that are associated with schizophrenia and antipsychotic drugs

Dromotropic effect change in the conduction speed across the myocardium

Drug general term for any substance capable of producing biological responses in the body

Drug-protein complex drug that has bound reversibly to plasma proteins, particularly albumin, that makes the drug unavailable for distribution to body tissues

Dry powder inhaler (DPI) device used to convert a solid drug to a fine powder for the purpose of inhalation

Dysentery severe diarrhea that may include bleeding

Dysfunctional uterine bleeding hemorrhage that occurs at abnormal times or in excessive quantity during the menstrual cycle

Dyslipidemia abnormal (excess or deficient) levels of lipoproteins in the blood

Dysrhythmia abnormality in cardiac rhythm

Dystonia severe muscle spasms, particularly of the back, neck, tongue, and face; characterized by abnormal tension starting in one area of the body and progressing to other areas

Ectopic foci, pacemakers cardiac tissue outside the normal cardiac conduction pathway that generates action potentials

Eczema also called atopic dermatitis, a skin disorder with unexplained symptoms of inflammation, itching, and scaling

Efficacy the ability of a drug to produce a desired response

Electrocardiogram (ECG) device that records the electrical activity of the heart

Electroconvulsive therapy (ECT) used to treat serious and life-threatening mood disorders in patients who are unresponsive to pharmacotherapy

Electroencephalogram (EEG) diagnostic test that records brainwaves through electrodes attached to the scalp

Electrolytes charged substances in the blood such as sodium, potassium, calcium, chloride, and phosphate

Embolus blood clot carried in the bloodstream

Emesis vomiting

Emetic drug used to induce vomiting

Emphysema terminal lung disease characterized by permanent dilation of the alveoli

Endogenous opioids chemicals produced naturally within the body that decrease or eliminate pain; they closely resemble the actions of morphine

Endometriosis presence of endometrial tissue in nonuterine locations such as the pelvis and ovaries; a common cause of infertility

Endothelium the inner lining of a blood vessel

Enteral nutrition nutrients supplied orally or by feeding tube

Enteral route drugs given orally, and those administered through nasogastric or gastrostomy tubes

Enteric coated tablets that have a hard, waxy coating designed to dissolve in the alkaline environment of the small intestine

Enterohepatic recirculation recycling of drugs and other substances by the circulation of bile through the intestine and liver

Enzyme induction process in which a drug changes the function of the hepatic microsomal enzymes and increases metabolic activity in the liver

Epilepsy disorder of the CNS characterized by seizures and/or convulsions

Ergocalciferol activated form of vitamin D

Ergosterol lipid substance in fungal cell membranes

Erythema redness associated with skin irritation

Erythrocytic stage phase in malaria during which infected red blood cells rupture, releasing merozoites and causing fever and chills

Erythropoietin hormone secreted by the kidney that regulates the process of red blood cell formation, or erythropoiesis

Ester type of chemical linkage found in some local anesthetics involving carbon and oxygen (-CO-O-)

Estrogen class of steroid sex hormones secreted by the ovary

Ethical dilemma when two moral principles appear to be in conflict

Ethics branch of philosophy that deals with distinguishing between right and wrong, and the moral consequences of human actions

Ethnic people having a common history and similar genetic heritage

Evaluation, systematic objective assessment of the effectiveness and impact of interventions

Excoriation scratches that break the skin surface and fill with blood or serous fluid to form crusty scales

Excretion the process of removing substances from the body

Expectorant drug used to increase bronchial secretions

External otitis commonly called swimmer's ear, an inflammation of the outer ear

Extracellular fluid (ECF) compartment body fluid lying outside of cells, which includes plasma and interstitial fluid

Extrapyramidal side effects symptoms of acute dystonia, akathisia, Parkinsonism, and tardive dyskinesia often caused by antipsychotic drugs

Febrile seizure tonic-clonic motor activity lasting 1 to 2 minutes with rapid return of consciousness that occurs in conjunction with elevated body temperature

Ferritin one of two protein complexes that maintains iron stores inside cells (hemosiderin is the other)

Fetal-placental barrier special anatomical structure that inhibits many chemicals and drugs from entering the fetus

Fibrillation type of dysrhythmia in which the chambers beat in a highly disorganized manner

Fibrin an insoluble protein formed from fibrinogen by the action of thrombin in the blood clotting process

Fibrinogen blood protein that is converted to fibrin by the action of thrombin in the blood coagulation process

Fibrinolysis removal of a blood clot

Fidelity the obligation to be faithful to agreements and fulfill promises

Fight-or-flight response characteristic set of signs and symptoms produced when the sympathetic nervous system is activated

Filtrate fluid in the nephron that is filtered at Bowman's capsule

First-pass effect mechanism whereby drugs are absorbed across the intestinal wall and enter into the hepatic portal circulation

Five rights of drug administration principles that offer simple and practical guidance for nurses to use during drug preparation, delivery, and administration

Folic acid/folate B vitamin that is a coenzyme in protein and nucleic acid metabolism

Follicle-stimulating hormone (FSH) hormone secreted by the anterior pituitary gland that regulates sperm or egg production

Follicular cells cells in the thyroid gland that secrete thyroid hormone

Food and Drug Administration (FDA) U.S. agency responsible for the evaluation and approval of new drugs

Formulary lists of drugs and drug recipes commonly used by pharmacists

Frank-Starling law the greater the degree of stretch on the myocardial fibers, the greater will be the force by which they contract

Frequency response curve graphical representation that illustrates interpatient variability in responses to drugs

Fungi kingdom of organisms that includes mushrooms, yeasts, and molds

Gamma-aminobutyric acid (GABA) neurotransmitter in the CNS

Ganglion collection of neuron cell bodies located outside the CNS

Gastroesophageal reflux disease (GERD) the regurgitation of stomach contents into the esophagus

General anesthesia medical procedure that produces unconsciousness and loss of sensation throughout the entire body

Generalized anxiety disorder (GAD) difficult to control, excessive anxiety that lasts 6 months or more, focuses on a variety of life events, and interferes with normal day-to-day functions

Generalized seizures seizures that travel throughout the entire brain

Generic name nonproprietary name of a drug assigned by the government

Genetic polymorphism changes in enzyme structure and function due to mutation of the encoding gene

Glucocorticoid class of hormones secreted by the adrenal cortex that help the body respond to stress

Glycoprotein IIb/IIIa enzyme that binds fibrinogen and von Willebrand's factor to begin platelet aggregation and blood coagulation

Goal any object or objective that the patient or nurse seeks to attain or achieve

Gonadotropin-releasing hormone a hormone secreted by the hypothalamus that stimulates the secretion of follicle-stimulating hormone (FSH) and luteinizing hormone (LH)

Gout metabolic disorder characterized by the accumulation of uric acid in the bloodstream or joint cavities

Graded dose response relationship between and measurement of the patient's response obtained at different doses of a drug

Gram-negative bacteria that do not retain a purple stain because they have an outer envelope

Gram-positive bacteria that stain purple because they have no outer envelope

Grave's disease syndrome caused by hypersecretion of thyroid hormone

Growth fraction the ratio of the number of replicating cells to resting cells in a tumor

H$^+$, K$^+$-ATPase enzyme responsible for pumping acid onto the mucosal surface of the stomach

H$_1$-receptor sites located on smooth muscle cells in the bronchial tree and blood vessels that are stimulated by histamine to produce bronchodilation and vasodilation

H$_2$-receptor sites located on cells of the digestive system that are stimulated by histamine to produce gastric acid

H$_2$-receptor antagonist drug that inhibits the effects of histamine at its receptors in the GI tract

Hallucination seeing, hearing, or feeling something that is not real

Heart failure (HF) disease in which the heart muscle cannot contract with sufficient force to meet the body's metabolic needs

Helicobacter pylori bacterium associated with a large percentage of peptic ulcer disease

Helminth type of flat, round, or segmented worm

Helper T cell lymphocyte that coordinates both the humoral and cell-mediated immune responses and that is the target of the human immunodeficiency virus

Hematopoiesis process of erythrocyte production which begins with primitive stem cells that reside in bone marrow

Hemophilia hereditary lack of a specific blood clotting factor

Hemorrhagic stroke type of stroke caused by bleeding from a blood vessel in the brain

Hemosiderin one of two protein complexes that maintains iron stores inside cells (ferritin is the other)

Hemostasis the slowing or stopping of blood flow

Hepatic microsomal enzyme system as it relates to pharmacotherapy, liver enzymes that inactivate drugs and accelerate their excretion; sometimes called the P-450 system

Hepatitis viral infection of the liver

Herb plant with a soft stem that is used for healing or as a seasoning

High-density lipoprotein (HDL) lipid-carrying particle in the blood that contains high amounts of protein and lower amounts of cholesterol; considered to be "good" cholesterol

Highly active antiretroviral therapy (HAART) drug therapy for HIV infection which includes high doses of multiple medications that are given concurrently

Hippocampus region of the brain responsible for learning and memory; a part of the limbic system

Histamine chemical released by mast cells in response to an antigen that causes dilation of blood vessels, bronchoconstriction, tissue swelling, and itching

HIV-AIDS acronym for human immunodeficiency virus-acquired immune deficiency syndrome; characterized by profound immunosuppression that leads to opportunistic infections and malignancies not commonly found in patients with functioning immune defenses

HMG-CoA reductase primary enzyme in the biochemical pathway for the synthesis of cholesterol

Holistic viewing a person as an integrated biological, psychosocial, cultural, communicating whole, existing and functioning within the communal environment

Hormone chemicals secreted by endocrine glands that act as chemical messengers to affect homeostasis

Hormone replacement therapy (HRT) drug therapy, consisting of estrogen and progestin combinations; used to treat symptoms associated with menopause

Host flora normal microorganisms found in or on a patient

Household system of measurement older system of measurement using teaspoons, tablespoons, and cups

Humoral immunity branch of the immune system that produces antibodies

Hydrolysis breakdown of a substance into simpler compounds by the addition or taking up of water

Hypercholesterolemia high levels of cholesterol in the blood

Hyperemia increase in blood supply to a part or tissue space causing swelling, redness, and pain

Hyperglycemia high glucose level in the blood

Hyperkalemia high potassium level in the blood

Hyperlipidemia excess amount of lipids in the blood

Hypernatremia high sodium level in the blood

Hyperosmolar nonketotic coma life-threatening metabolic condition that occurs in people with type 2 diabetes

Hypertension high blood pressure

Hypervitaminosis excess intake of vitamins

Hypnotic drug that causes sleep

Hypoglycemia low glucose level in the blood

Hypogonadism below normal secretion of the steroid sex hormones

Hypokalemia low potassium level in the blood

Hyponatremia low sodium level in the blood

Hypovolemic shock type of shock caused by loss of fluids such as occurs during hemorrhage, extensive burns, or severe vomiting or diarrhea

Idiosyncratic response unpredictable and unexplained drug reaction

Ileum third portion of the small intestine extending from the jejunum to the ileocecal valve

Illusions distorted perceptions of actual sensory stimuli

Immune response specific reaction of the body to foreign agents involving B and/or T lymphocytes

Immunosuppressant any drug, chemical, or physical agent that lowers the immune defense mechanisms of the body

Impotence inability to obtain or sustain an erection; also called erectile dysfunction

Infant child under the age of 1 year

Infertility inability to become pregnant after at least 1 year of frequent, unprotected intercourse

Inflammation nonspecific body defense that occurs in response to an injury or antigen

Influenza common viral infection; often called flu

Inotropic agent drug or chemical that changes the force of contraction of the heart

Inotropic effect change in the strength or contractility of the heart

Insomnia the inability to fall asleep or stay asleep

Interferon type of cytokine secreted by T cells in response to antigens to protect uninfected cells

Interleukin class of cytokines synthesized by lymphocytes, monocytes, macrophages, and certain other cells, that enhance the capabilities of the immune system

Intervention action that produces an effect or that is intended to alter the course of a disease or condition

Intracellular fluid (ICF) compartment body fluid that is inside cells; accounts for about two-thirds of the total body water

Intracellular parasite infectious microbe that lives inside host cells

Intradermal (ID) medication administered into the dermis layer of the skin

Intramuscular (IM) delivery of medication into specific muscles

Intravenous (IV) medications and fluids administered directly into the bloodstream

Intrinsic factor chemical substance secreted by the parietal cells in the stomach that is essential for the absorption of vitamin B_{12}

Ionizing radiation radiation that is highly penetrating and can cause serious biologic effects

Irritable bowel syndrome inflammatory disease of the small or large intestine, characterized by intense abdominal cramping and diarrhea

Islets of Langerhans cell clusters in the pancreas responsible for the secretion of insulin and glucagon

Jejunum middle portion of small intestine between the duodenum and the ileum

Justice ethical principle that persons who have similar circumstances should be treated alike

Kaposi's sarcoma vascular cancer that first appears on the skin and then invades internal organs; frequently occurs in AIDS patients

Kappa receptor type of opioid receptor

Keratolytic action that promotes shedding of old skin

Ketoacids acidic waste products of lipid metabolism that lower the pH of the blood

Latent phase period of HIV infection during which there are no symptoms

Laxative drug that promotes defecation

Lecithin phospholipid that is an important component of cell membranes

Leukemia cancer of the blood characterized by overproduction of white blood cells

Leukotrienes chemical mediators of inflammation stored and released by mast cells; effects are similar to those of histamine

Leutinizing hormone (LH) secreted by the pituitary gland, triggers ovulation in the female and stimulates sperm production in the male

Libido interest in sexual activity

Limbic system area in the brain responsible for emotion, learning, memory, motivation, and mood

Lipodystrophy atrophy increase or decrease of subcutaneous fat at an insulin injection site, resulting in an indenture or a raised area

Lipoprotein substance carrying lipids in the bloodstream that is composed of proteins bound to fat

Liposome small sacs of lipids designed to carry drugs inside them

Loading dose comparatively large dose given at the beginning of treatment to rapidly obtain the therapeutic effect of a drug

Local anesthesia loss of sensation to a limited part of the body without loss of consciousness

Loop of Henle portion of the nephron between the proximal and distal tubules

Low-density lipoprotein (LDL) lipid-carrying particle that contains relatively low amounts of protein and high amounts of cholesterol; considered to be "bad" cholesterol

Low-molecular-weight heparins (LMWH) drugs closely resembling heperan that inhibit blood clotting

Lymphoma cancer of lymphatic tissue

Macromineral (major mineral) inorganic compound needed by the body in amounts of 100 mg or more daily

Maintenance dose dose that keeps the plasma drug concentration continuously in the therapeutic range

Malaria tropical disease characterized by severe fever and chills caused by the protozoan *Plasmodium*

Malignant life threatening or fatal

Mania condition characterized by an expressive, impulsive, excitable, and overreactive nature

Mast cell connective tissue cell located in tissue spaces that releases histamine following injury

Mastoiditis inflammation of the mastoid sinus

Mechanism of action how a drug exerts its effects

Median effective dose (ED$_{50}$) dose required to produce a specific therapeutic response in 50% of a group of patients

Median lethal dose (LD$_{50}$) often determined in preclinical trials, the dose of drug that will be lethal in 50% of a group of animals

Median toxicity dose (TD$_{50}$) dose that will produce a given toxicity in 50% of a group of patients

Medication drug after it has been administered

Medication administration record (MAR) documentation of all pharmacotherapies received by the patient

Medication error any preventable event that may cause or lead to inappropriate medication use or patient harm while the medication is in the control of the healthcare provider, patient, or consumer

Menopause period of time when females stop secreting estrogen and menstrual cycles cease

Menorrhagia prolonged or excessive menstruation

Metabolism total of all biochemical reactions in the body

Metastasis travel of cancer cells from their original site to a distant tissue

Metered dose inhaler (MDI) device used to deliver a precise amount of drug to the respiratory system

Methadone maintenance treatment of opioid dependence by using methadone

Methylxanthine chemical derivative of caffeine

Metric system of measurement most common system of drug measurement that uses grams and liters

Micromineral (trace mineral) inorganic compound needed by the body in amounts of 20 mg or less daily

Middle-age adulthood person from 40 to 65 years of age

Migraine severe headache preceded by auras that may include nausea and vomiting

Minimum effective concentration the amount of drug required to produce a therapeutic effect

Miosis constriction of the pupil

Miotics drugs that cause pupil constriction

Monoamine oxidase (MAO) enzyme that destroys norepinephrine in the nerve terminal

Monoamine oxidase inhibitors (MAO inhibitors) drugs inhibiting monoamine oxidase, an enzyme that terminates the actions of neurotransmitters such as dopamine, norepinephrine, epinephrine, and serotonin

Mood disorder change in behavior such as clinical depression, emotional swings, or manic depression

Mood stabilizer drug that levels mood that is used to treat bipolar disorder and mania

Mu receptor type of opioid receptor

Mucolytic drug used to loosen thick mucus

Mucosa layer inner lining of the alimentary canal that provides a surface area for the various acids, bases, and enzymes to break down food

Muscarinic type of cholinergic receptor found in smooth muscle, cardiac muscle, and glands

Muscle spasms involuntary contractions of a muscle or group of muscles that become tightened, develop a fixed pattern of resistance, and result in a diminished level of functioning

Mutation permanent, inheritable change to DNA

Myasthenia gravis motor disorder caused by a destruction of nicotinic receptors on skeletal muscles and characterized by profound muscular fatigue

Mycoses diseases caused by fungi

Mydriatic drugs agents that cause pupil dilation

Myocardial infarction blood clot blocking a portion of a coronary artery that causes necrosis of cardiac muscle

Myocardial ischemia lack of blood supply to the myocardium due to a constriction or obstruction of a blood vessel

Myoclonic seizure seizures characterized by brief, sudden contractions of a group of muscles

Myxedema condition caused by insufficient secretion of thyroid hormone

Narcotic natural or synthetic drug related to morphine; may be used as a broader legal term referring to hallucinogens, CNS stimulants, marijuana, and other illegal drugs

Narrow-spectrum antibiotic anti-infective that is effective against only one or a small number of organisms

Nausea uncomfortable wave-like sensation that precedes vomiting

NDA review third stage of new drug evaluation by the FDA

Nebulizer device used to convert liquid drugs into a fine mist for the purpose of inhalation

Negative feedback in homeostasis, when the first hormone in a pathway is shut off by the last hormone or product in the pathway

Negative symptoms in schizophrenia, symptoms that subtract from normal behavior including a lack of interest, motivation, responsiveness, or pleasure in daily activities

Neoplasm an abnormal swelling or mass, same as tumor

Nephron structural and functional unit of the kidney

Nerve agents chemicals used in warfare or by bioterrorists that can affect the central nervous system and cause death

Neurofibrillary tangles bundles of nerve fibers found in the brain of patients with Alzheimer's disease on autopsy

Neurogenic shock type of shock resulting from brain or spinal cord injury

Neurohypophysis posterior portion of the pituitary gland

Neurolept analgesia type of general anesthesia that combines fentanyl with droperidol to produce a state in which patients are conscious, though insensitive to pain and unconnected with surroundings

Neuroleptic malignant syndrome potentially fatal condition caused by certain antipsychotic medications characterized by an extremely high body temperature, drowsiness, changing blood pressure, irregular heartbeat, and muscle rigidity

Neuromuscular blocker drug used to cause total muscle relaxation

Neuropathic pain caused by injury to nerves and typically described as burning, shooting, or numb pain

Nicotinic type of cholinergic receptor found in ganglia of both the sympathetic and parasympathetic nervous systems

Nit egg of the louse parasite

Nitrogen mustards alkylating agents used to treat a variety of tumors

Nociceptors receptors connected with nerves that receive and transmit pain signals to the spinal cord and brain

Nonmaleficence ethical obligation to not harm the patient

Nonspecific body defenses defenses such as inflammation that protect the body from invasion by general hazards

Nonspecific cellular responses drug action that is independent of cellular receptors, and not associated with other mechanisms, such as changing the permeability of cellular membranes, depressing membrane excitability, or altering the activity of cellular pumps

Norepinephrine (NE) primary neurotransmitter in the sympathetic nervous system

Nosocomial infections infection acquired in a healthcare setting such as a hospital, physician's office, or nursing home

Nurse Practice Act legislation designed to protect the public by defining the legal scope of practice

Nursing diagnosis clinical-based judgment about the patient and his or her response to health and illness

Nursing process a five-part systematic decision-making method that includes assessment, nursing diagnosis, planning, implementation, and evaluation

Objective data information gathered through physical assessment, laboratory tests, and other diagnostic sources

Obsessive-compulsive disorder recurrent, intrusive thoughts or repetitive behaviors that interfere with normal activities or relationships

Older adulthood person over age 65

Oligomenorrhea infrequent menstruation

Oligospermia presence of less than 20 million sperm in an ejaculate

Oncogenes genes responsible for the conversion of normal cells into cancer cells

Open-angle glaucoma chronic, simple glaucoma caused by hindered outflow of aqueous humor from the anterior chamber

Opiate substance closely related to morphine extracted from the poppy plant

Opioid substance obtained from the unripe seeds of the poppy plant; natural or synthetic morphinelike substance

Orthostatic hypotension fall in blood pressure that occurs when changing position from recumbent to upright

Osmolality number of dissolved particles or solutes, in 1 kg (1 L) of water

Osmosis process by which water moves from areas of low solute concentration (low osmolality) to areas of high solute concentration (high osmolality)

Osteoarthritis disorder characterized by degeneration of joints, particularly the fingers, spine, hips, and knees

Osteomalacia rickets in children; caused by vitamin D deficiency characterized by softening of the bones without alteration of basic bone structure

Osteoporosis condition in which bones lose mass and become brittle and susceptible to fracture

Otitis media inflammation of the middle ear

Ototoxicity having an adverse effect on the organs of hearing

Outcome objective measures of goals

Ovulation release of an egg by the ovary

Oxytocin hormone secreted by the posterior pituitary gland that stimulates uterine contractions and milk ejection

Paget's disease disorder of bone formation and resorption characterized by weak, enlarged, and deformed bones

Palliation form of cancer chemotherapy intended to alleviate symptoms rather than cure the disease

Pancreatitis inflammaton of the pancreas which may be acute or chronic

Panic disorder anxiety disorder characterized by intense feelings of immediate apprehension, fearfulness, terror, or impending doom, accompanied by increased autonomic nervous system activity

Parafollicular cells cells in the thyroid gland that secrete calcitonin

Paranoia having an extreme suspicion and delusion that one is being followed, and that others are trying to inflict harm

Parasympathetic nervous system portion of the autonomic nervous system that is active during periods of rest and which results in the rest or relaxation response

Parasympathomimetics drugs that mimic the actions of the parasympathetic nervous system

Parenteral route dispensing of medications via a needle into the skin layers

Parietal cells cells in the stomach mucosa that secrete hydrochloric acid

Parkinson's disease degenerative disorder of the nervous system caused by a deficiency of the brain neurotransmitter dopamine that results in disturbances of muscle movement

Parkinsonism having tremor, muscle rigidity, stooped posture, and a shuffling gait

Partial (focal) seizures seizures that start on one side of the brain and travel a short distance before stopping

Partial agonist medication that produces a weaker, or less efficacious, response than an agonist

Passive immunity immune defense that lasts 2 to 3 weeks; obtained by administering antibodies

Pathogen organism that is capable of causing disease

Pathogenicity ability of an organism to cause disease in humans

Pediculicides medications that kill lice

Pegylation process that attaches polyethylene glycol (PEG) to an interferon to extend its pharmacologic activity

Pellagra deficiency of niacin

Peptic ulcer erosion of the mucosa in the alimentary canal, most commonly in the stomach and duodenum

Percutaneous transluminal coronary angioplasty (PTCA) procedure by which a balloon-shaped catheter is used to compress fatty plaque against an arterial wall for the purpose of restoring normal blood flow

Perfusion blood flow through a tissue or organ

Peripheral edema swelling in the limbs, particularly the feet and ankles, due to an accumulation of interstitial fluid

Peripheral nervous system division of the nervous system containing all nervous tissue outside the CNS, including the autonomic nervous system

Peripheral resistance the amount of friction encountered by blood as it travels through the vessels

Peristalsis involuntary wavelike contraction of smooth muscle lining the alimentary canal

Pernicious (megaloblastic) anemia type of anemia usually caused by lack of secretion of intrinsic factor

pH a measure of the acidity or alkalinity of a solution

Pharmacodynamics the study of how the body responds to drugs

Pharmacogenetics the area of pharmacology that examines the role of genetics in drug response

Pharmacokinetics the study of how drugs are handled by the body

Pharmacologic classification method for organizing drugs on the basis of their mechanism of action

Pharmacology the study of medicines; the discipline pertaining to how drugs improve or maintain health

Pharmacopoeia medical reference indicating standards of drug purity, strength, and directions for synthesis

Pharmacotherapy treatment or prevention of disease by means of drugs

Phobias fearful feelings attached to situations or objects such as snakes, spiders, crowds, or heights

Phosphodiesterase enzyme in muscle cells that cleaves phosphodiester bonds; its inhibition increases myocardial contractility

Phospholipid type of lipid that contains two fatty acids, a phosphate group, and a chemical backbone of glycerol

Photosensitivity condition that occurs when the skin is highly sensitive to sunlight

Physical dependence condition of experiencing unpleasant withdrawal symptoms when a substance is discontinued

Planning links strategies, or interventions to established goals and outcomes

Plaque fatty material that builds up in the lining of blood vessels and may lead to hypertension, stroke, myocardial infarction, or angina

Plasma cell cell derived from B lymphocytes that produces antibodies

Plasma half-life ($t_{1/2}$) the length of time required for a drug to decrease its concentration in the plasma by one-half after administration

Plasmid small piece of circular DNA found in some bacteria that is able to transfer resistance from one bacterium to another

Plasmin enzyme formed from plasminogen that dissolves blood clots

Plasminogen protein that prevents fibrin clot formation; precuror of plasmin

Polarized condition in which the inside of a cell is more negatively charged than the outside of the cell

Polyene antifungal class containing amphotericin B and nystatin

Polypharmacy the taking of multiple drugs concurrently

Positive symptoms in schizophrenia, symptoms that add on to normal behavior including hallucinations, delusions, and a disorganized thought or speech pattern

Postmarketing surveillance evaluation of a new drug after it has been approved and used in large numbers of patients

Postpartum occurring after childbirth

Postsynaptic neuron in a synapse, the nerve that has receptors for the neurotransmitter

Posttraumatic stress disorder type of anxiety that develops in response to reexperiencing a previous life event that was psychologically traumatic

Potassium ion channel pathway in a plasma membrane through which potassium ions enter and leave

Potency the strength of a drug at a specified concentration or dose

Preclinical investigation procedure implemented after a drug has been licensed for public use, designed to provide information on use and on occurrence of side effects

Preload degree of stretch of the cardiac muscle fibers just before they contract

Prenatal preceding birth

Preschool child child from 3 to 5 years of age

Presynaptic neuron nerve that releases the neurotransmitter into the synaptic cleft when stimulated by an action potential

PRN order (Latin: *pro re nata*) medication is administered as required by the patient's condition

Prodrug drug that becomes more active after it is metabolized

Progesterone hormone secreted by the corpus luteum and placenta responsible for building up the uterine lining in the second half of the menstrual cycle and during pregnancy

Prolactin hormone secreted by the anterior pituitary gland that stimulates milk production in the mammary glands

Prostaglandins class of local hormones that promotes local inflammation and pain when released by cells in the body

Protease viral enzyme that is responsible for the final assembly of the HIV virions

Prothrombin blood protein that is converted to thrombin in blood coagulation

Prothrombin activator enzyme in the coagulation cascade that converts prothrombin to thrombin; also called prothrombinase

Prothrombin time blood test used to determine the time needed for plasma to clot for the regulation of warfarin dosage

Proton pump inhibitors drugs that inhibit the enzyme H^+, K^+-ATPase

Prototype drug well-understood model drug to which other drugs in a pharmacologic class may be compared

Protozoan single-celled animal

Provitamins inactive chemicals that are converted to vitamins in the body

Proximal tubule portion of the nephron that collects filtrate from Bowman's capsule

Pruritus itching associated with dry, scaly skin

Psoralen drug used along with phototherapy for the treatment of psoriasis and other severe skin disorders

Psychedelics substances that alter perception and reality

Psychological dependence intense craving for a drug that drives people to continue drug abuse withdrawn

Psychology science that deals with normal and abnormal mental processes and their impact on behavior

Purine building block of DNA and RNA, either adenine or guanine

Purkinje fibers electrical conduction pathway leading from the bundle branches to all portions of the ventricles

Pyrimidine building block of DNA and RNA, either thymine or cytosine in DNA and cytosine and uracil in RNA

Rapid eye movement (REM) sleep stage of sleep characterized by quick, scanning movements of the eyes

Reabsorption movement of filtered substances from the kidney tubule back into the blood

Rebound congestion condition of hypersecretion of mucus following use of intranasal sympathomimetics

Rebound insomnia increased sleeplessness that occurs when long-term antianxiety or hypnotic medication is discontinued

Receptor the structural component of a cell to which a drug binds in a dose-related manner, to produce a response

Recommended Dietary Allowance (RDA) amount of vitamin or mineral needed each day to avoid a deficiency in a healthy adult

Red-man syndrome rash on the upper body caused by certain anti-infectives

Reflex tachycardia temporary increase in heart rate that occurs when blood pressure falls

Refractory period time during which the myocardial cells rest and are not able to contract

Releasing hormone hormone secreted by the hypothalamus that affects secretions in the pituitary gland

Renin-angiotensin system series of enzymatic steps by which the body raises blood pressure

Respiration exchange of oxygen and carbon dioxide in the lungs; also the process of deriving energy from metabolic reactions

Rest-and-digest response signs and symptoms produced when the parasympathetic nervous system is activated

Reticular activating system (RAS) responsible for sleeping and wakefulness and performs an alerting function for the cerebral cortex; includes the reticular formation, hypothalamus and part of the thalamus

Reticular formation portion of the brain affecting awareness and wakefulness

Retinoid compound resembling Vitamin A used in the treatment of severe acne and psoriasis

Reverse cholesterol transport the process by which cholesterol is transported away from body tissues to the liver

Reverse transcriptase viral enzyme that converts RNA to DNA

Reye's syndrome potentially fatal complication of infection associated with aspirin use in children

Rheumatoid arthritis systemic autoimmune disorder characterized by inflammation of multiple joints

Rhinophyma reddened, bullous, irregular swelling of the nose

Rosacea chronic skin disorder characterized by clusters of papules on the face

Routine order orders not written as STAT, ASAP, NOW, or PRN

Salicylism poisoning due to aspirin and aspirinlike drugs

Sarcoma cancer of connective tissue such as bone, muscle, or cartilage

Scabicides drugs that kill scabies mites

Scabies skin disorder caused by the female mite burrowing into the skin and laying eggs

Scheduled drug in the United States, a term describing a drug placed into one of five categories based on its potential for misuse or abuse

Schizoaffective disorder psychosis with symptoms of both schizophrenia and mood disorders

Schizophrenia psychosis characterized by abnormal thoughts and thought processes, withdrawal from other people and the outside environment, and apparent preoccupation with one's own mental state

School-age child child from 6 to 12 years of age

Scurvy deficiency of vitamin C

Seborrhea skin condition characterized by overactivity of oil glands

Second messenger cascade of biochemical events that initiates a drug's action by either stimulating or inhibiting a normal activity of the cell

Secretion in the kidney, movement of substances from the blood into the tubule after filtration has occurred

Sedative substance that depresses the CNS to cause drowsiness or sleep

Sedative-hypnotic drug with the ability to produce a calming effect at lower doses while having the ability to induce sleep at higher doses

Seizure symptom of epilepsy characterized by abnormal neuronal discharges within the brain

Selective estrogen receptor modulator (SERM) drug that produces an action similar to estrogen in body tissues; used for the treatment of osteoporosis in postmenopausal women

Selective serotonin reuptake inhibitor (SSRI) drug that selectively inhibits the reuptake of serotonin into nerve terminals; used mostly for depression

Septic shock type of shock caused by severe infection in the bloodstream

Serotonin syndrome set of signs and symptoms associated with overmedication with antidepressants that includes altered mental status, fever, sweating and lack of muscular coordination

Shock condition in which there is inadequate blood flow to meet the body's metabolic needs

Single order medication that is to be given only once, and at a specific time, such as a preoperative order

Sinoatrial (SA) node pacemaker of the heart located in the wall of the right atrium that controls the basic heart rate

Sinus rhythm number of beats per minute normally generated by the SA node

Situational anxiety anxiety experienced by people faced with a stressful environment

Sleep debt lack of sleep

Sociology study of human behavior within the context of groups and societies

Sodium ion channel pathway in a plasma membrane through which sodium ions enter and leave

Somastatin synonym for growth hormone inhibiting factor from the hypothalamus

Somatic nervous system nerve division that provides voluntary control over skeletal muscle

Somatotropin another name for growth hormone

Somogyi phenomenon rapid decrease in blood glucose which stimulates the release of hormones (epinephrine, cortisol, glucagon) resulting in an elevated morning blood glucose

Spasticity inability of opposing muscle groups to move in a coordinated manner

Spirilla bacteria that have a spiral shape

Spirituality the capacity to love, to convey compassion and empathy, to give and forgive, to enjoy life, and to find peace of mind and fulfillment in living

Stable angina type of angina that occurs in a predictable pattern, usually relieved by rest

Standards of care the skills and learning commonly possessed by members of a profession

Standing order order written in advance of a situation, which is to be carried out under specific circumstances

STAT order any medication that is needed immediately, and is to be given only once

Status epilepticus condition characterized by repeated seizures or one prolonged seizure attack that continues for at least 30 minutes

Steatorrhea stool containing high content of fat as occurs in some malabsorption syndromes

Stem cell cell that resides in the bone marrow, and is capable of maturing into any type of blood cell

Steroid type of lipid which consists of four rings that comprise certain hormones and drugs

Sterol nucleus ring structure common to all steroids

Strategic National Stockpile (SNS) program designed to ensure the immediate deployment of essential medical materials to a community in the event of a large-scale chemical or biologic attack

Stroke volume amount of blood pumped out by a ventricle in a single beat

Subcutaneous (SC or SQ) medication delivered beneath the skin

Subjective data information gathered regarding what a patient states or perceives

Sublingual route medication that is placed under the tongue, and allowed to dissolve slowly

Substance abuse self-administration of a drug that does not conform to the medical or social norms within the patient's given culture or society

Substance P neurotransmitter within the spinal cord involved in the neural transmission of pain

Substantia nigra location in the brain where dopamine is synthesized that is responsible for regulation of unconscious muscle movement

Superficial mycoses fungal diseases of the hair, skin, nails, and mucous membranes

Superinfection new infection caused by an organism different from the one causing the initial infection; usually a side effect of antiinfective therapy

Surgical anesthesia stage 3 of anesthesia, where most major surgery occurs

Sustained release tablets or capsules designed to dissolve slowly over an extended time

Sympathetic nervous system portion of the autonomic system that is active during periods of stress and results in the fight-or-flight response

Sympathomimetic drug that stimulates or mimics the sympathetic nervous system

Synapse junction between two neurons consisting of a presynaptic nerve, a synaptic cleft, and a postsynaptic nerve

Synaptic transmission the process by which a neurotransmitter reaches receptors to regenerate the action potential

Systemic mycoses fungal diseases affecting internal organs

Systolic pressure blood pressure during the contraction phase of heart activity

Tardive dyskinesia unusual tongue and face movements such as lip-smacking and wormlike motions of the tongue that occur during pharmacotherapy with certain antipsychotics

Taxoids antineoplastic drugs obtained from the Pacific Yew tree

T cell type of lymphocyte that is essential for the cell-mediated immune response

Tension headache common type of head pain caused by stress and relieved by nonnarcotic analgesics

Teratogen drug or other agent that causes developmental birth defects

Tetrahydrocannabinol (THC) the active chemical in marijuana

Therapeutic classification method for organizing drugs on the basis of their clinical usefulness

Therapeutic index the ratio of a drug's LD_{50} to its ED_{50}

Therapeutic range the dosage range or serum concentration that achieves the desired drug effects

Therapeutics the branch of medicine concerned with the treatment of disease and suffering

Three checks of drug administration in conjunction with the five rights, these ascertain patient safety and drug effectiveness

Thrombin enzyme that causes clotting by forming thrombin

Thrombocytopenia reduction in the number of circulating platelets

Thromboembolic disorder condition in which the patient develops blood clots

Thrombolytics drugs used to dissolve existing blood clots

Thrombopoietin hormone produced by the kidneys that controls megakaryocyte activity

Thrombotic stroke type of stroke caused by a blood clot blocking an artery in the brain

Thrombus blood clot obstructing a vessel

Thyrotoxic crisis acute form of hyperthyroidism that is a medical emergency; also called thyroid storm

Tissue plasminogen activator (tPA) natural enzyme and a drug that dissolves blood clots

Titer measurement of the amount of a substance in the blood

Tocolytic drug used to inhibit uterine contractions

Tocopherol generic name for vitamin E

Toddlerhood child from 1 to 3 years of age

Tolerance process of adapting to a drug over a period of time, and subsequently requiring higher doses to achieve the same effect

Tonic spasm single, prolonged muscular contraction

Tonic-clonic seizure seizure characterized by intense jerking motions and loss of consciousness

Tonicity the ability of a solution to cause a change in water movement across a membrane due to osmotic forces

Tonometry technique for measuring intraocular tension and pressure

Topoisomerase enzyme that assists in the repair of DNA damage

Total parenteral nutrition (TPN) nutrition provided through a peripheral or central vein

Toxic concentration level of drug that will result in serious adverse effects

Toxin chemical produced by a microorganism that is able to cause injury to its host

Toxoid substance that has been chemically modified to remove its harmful nature but is still able to elicit an immune response in the body

Trade name proprietary name of a drug assigned by the manufacturer; also called the brand name or product name

Transferrin protein complex that transports iron to the sites in the body where it is needed

Transplant rejection when the immune system recognizes a transplanted tissue as being foreign and attacks it

Tricyclic antidepressant (TCA) class of drugs used in the pharmacotherapy of depression

Triglyceride type of lipid that contains three fatty acids and a chemical backbone of glycerol

Tubercles cavitylike lesions in the lung characteristic of infection by *Mycobacterium tuberculosis*

Tumor abnormal swelling or mass

Tyramine form of the amino acid tyrosine that is found in foods such as cheese, beer, wine and yeast products

Ulcerative colitis inflammatory bowel disease of the colon

Undernutrition lack of adequate nutrition to meet the metabolic demands of the body

Unstable angina severe angina that occurs frequently, and which is not relieved by rest

Urinalysis diagnostic test that examines urine for the presence of blood cells, proteins, pH, specific gravity, ketones, glucose, and microorganisms

Vaccination immunization receiving a vaccine or toxoid to prevent disease

Vaccine biologic material that confers protection against infection; preparation of microorganism particles that is injected into a patient to stimulate the immune system, with the intention of preventing disease

Variant angina chest pain that is caused by acute spasm of the coronary arteries rather than by physical or emotional exertion

Vasomotor center area of the medulla that controls baseline blood pressure

Vendor Managed Inventory (VMI) supplies and pharmaceuticals that are shipped after a chemical or biological threat has been identified

Ventilation process by which air is moved into and out of the lungs

Veracity the ethical obligation to tell the truth

Very low–density lipoprotein (VLDL) lipid-carrying particle that is converted to LDL in the liver

Vestibular apparatus portion of the inner ear responsible for the sense of position

Vinca alkaloids chemicals obtained from the periwinkle plant that have antineoplastic activity

Virion particle of a virus capable of causing an infection

Virulence the severity of disease that a pathogen is able to cause

Virulization appearance of masculine secondary sex characteristics

Virus nonliving particle containing nucleic acid that is able to cause disease

Vitamins organic compounds required by the body in small amounts

Vitiligo milk-white areas of depigmented skin

Vomiting center area in the medulla that controls the vomiting reflex

Von Willebrand's disease decrease in quantity or quality of von Willebrand factor (vWF), which acts as a carrier of factor VIII and has a role in platelet aggregation

Withdrawal physical signs of discomfort associated with the discontinuation of an abused substance

Withdrawal syndrome symptoms that result when a patient discontinues taking a substance upon which he or she was dependent

Yeast type of fungus that is unicellular and divides by budding

Young adulthood person from 18 to 40 years of age

Zollinger-Ellison syndrome disorder of having excess acid secretion in the stomach resulting in peptic ulcer disease

Appendix A

Canadian Drugs and Their U.S. Equivalents

U.S. Drug Name	Canadian Drug Name
acebutolol hydrochloride (Sectral)	Monitan
acetaminophen (Tylenol)	Abenal, Atasol, Campain, others
acetazolamide (Diamox)	Acetazolam, Apo-Acetazolamide
acetohexamide (Dymelor)	Dimelor
albuterol (Proventil, Salbutamol)	Gen-Salbutamol, Novosalmol
allopurinol (Lopurin, Zyloprim)	Alloprin A, Apo-allopurinol-A
altretamine, hexamethylmelamine (Hexalen)	Hexastat
aminophylline (Truphylline)	Paladron, Corophyllin
amitriptyline hydrochloride (Elavil)	Apo-Amitripyline, Levate, Novotriptyn
amoxicillin (Amoxil, Trimox, Wymox)	Apo-Amoxi
ampicillin (Polycillin, Omnipen)	Novo-Ampicillin, Penbritin
asparaginase (Elspar)	Kidrolase A
aspirin (ASA, others)	Novasen, Astrin, Entrophen, others
atenolol (Tenormin)	Apo-Atenolol
atropine sulfate (Isopto Atropine, others)	Atropair
bacampicillin hydrochloride (Spectrobid)	Penglobe
benztropine mesylate (Cogentin)	Apo-Benzotropine, Bensylate, PMS Benzotropine
betamethasone (Celestone, Betacort, others)	Betnelan, Betaderm, others
bretylium tosylate (Bretylol)	Bretylate
brompheniramine maleate (Codimal-A, Dimetapp)	Dimetane
calcium carbonate (BioCal, Calcite-500, others)	Apo-Cal, Calsan, Caltrate
carbamazepine (Tegretol)	Apo-Carbamazine, Mazepine
carbenicillin indanyl (Geocillin, Geopen)	Geopen Oral
cephalexin (Keflex)	Ceporex, Novolexin
cetirizine (Zyrtec)	Reactine
chloral hydrate (Noctec)	Novochlorhydrate
chloramphenicol (Chlorofair, Chloromycetin, Chloroptic, Fenicol)	Novochlorocap, Pentamycetin
chlordiazepoxide hydrochloride (Librium)	Medilium, Novopoxide, Solium
chlorthalidone (Hygroton)	Novothalidone, Uridon
chlorpropamide (Chloronase, Diabinese, Glucamide)	Apo-Chlorpropamide, Novopropamide
chlorpheniramine maleate (Chlor-Trimeton, others)	Chlor-Tripolon, Novopheniram
chlorpromazine hydrochloride (Thorazine)	Largactil, Novochlorpromazine
cimetidine (Tagamet)	Apo-Cimetidine, Novocimetine, Peptol

U.S. Drug Name	Canadian Drug Name
cisplatin (Platinol)	Abiplatin
clindamycin hydrochloride (Cleocin)	Dalacin C
clonazepam (Klonopin)	Rivotril
clonidine hydrochloride (Catapres)	Dixaril
clorazepate dipotassium (Tranxene)	Novoclopate
clotrimazole (Gyne-Lotrimin, Mycelex, Femizole)	Canesten, Clotrimaderm, Myclo-Gyne
cloxacillin (Tegopen)	Apo-Cloxi, Novocloxin
codeine	Paveral
colchicine	Novocolchicine
colestipol (Colestid)	Cholestabyl
cyclizine hydrochloride (Marezine)	Marzine
cyclophosphamide (Cytoxan, Neosar)	Procytox
cyproheptadine hydrochloride (Periactin)	Vimicon
danazol (Danocrine)	Cyclomen
dexamethasone (Decadron, Dexasone, Hexadrol, Maxidex)	Deronil, Oradexon
dextroamphetamine sulfate (Dexedrine)	Oxydess II
diazepam (Valium)	Apo-Diazepam, Diazemuls, E-Pam
diethylstilbestrol (DES, Stilbestrol)	Honval
diltiazem (Cardizem, Dilacor, Tiamate, Tiazac)	Apo-Dilitaz
dimenhydrinate (Dramamine)	Apo-Dimenhydrinate, Gravol
diphenhydramine hydrochloride (Benadryl, others)	Allerdryl
dipyridamole (Persantine)	Apo-Dipyridamole
disopyramide phosphate (Norpace, Napamide)	Rythmodan
docusate (Surfak, Dialose, Colace)	Regulax
dopamine hydrochloride (Dopastat, Intropin)	Revimine
doxepin hydrochloride (Sinequan)	Triadapin
doxycycline hyclate (Doryx, Doxy, Monodox, Vibramycin)	Apo-Doxy, Doxycin
econazole nitrate (Spectazole)	Ecostatin
epinephrine (Adrenalin, Bronkaid, Primatene)	SusPhrine
ergocalciferol (Deltalin, Calciferol)	Ostoforte, Radiostol
ergotamine tartrate (Ergostat)	Gynergen
erythromycin (E-mycin, Erythrocin)	Novorythro, Erythromid, Apo-Erythro-S
estradiol valerate (Delestrogen, Duragen-10, Valergen)	Femogex
flucytosine (Ancobon)	Ancotil
fluoxymesterone (Halotestin)	Ora Testryl

U.S. Drug Name	Canadian Drug Name
flurazepam (Dalmane)	Apo-Flurazepam, Novoflupam
furosemide (Lasix)	Furomide
gentamicin sulfate (Garamycin, G-mycin, Jenamicin)	Cydomycin
glyburide (DiaBeta, Micronase, Glynase)	Euglucon
griseofulvin (Fulvicin)	Grisovin-FP
haloperidol (Haldol)	Peridol
heparin sodium (Hep-lock)	Calcilean, Hepalean
hydralazine hydrochloride (Apresoline)	Novo-Hylazin
hydrochlorothiazide (HydroDIURIL, HCTZ)	Apo-Hydro, Urozide
hydrocodone bitartrate (Hycodan)	Robidone
hydrocortisone (Cetacort, Cortaid, Solu-Cortef)	Rectocort, Cortiment
hydroxyzine (Atarax, Vistaril)	Apo-Hydroxyzine
ibuprofen (Advil, Motrin, others)	Amersol
imipramine hydrochloride (Tofranil)	Impril, Novopramine
indapamide (Lozol)	Lozide
isoniazid (INH, Laniazid, Nydrazid, Teebaconin)	Isotamine, PMS Isoniazid
isosorbide dinitrate (Isordil, Sorbitrate, Dilatrate-SR)	Coronex, Novosorbide
ketoprofen (Actron, Orudis, Oruvail)	Rhodis
lidocaine hydrochloride (Xylocaine)	Xylocard
lithium carbonate (Eskalith)	Carbolith, Duralith, Lithizine
lorazepam (Ativan)	Apo-Lorazepam
loxapine succinate (Loxitane)	Loxapac
meclizine (Antivert, Bonine)	Bonamine
methyldopa (Aldomet)	Apo-Methyldopa
methyltestosterone (Android, Testred)	Metandren
metoclopramide (Reglan)	Emex, Maxeran
metoprolol tartrate (Toprol, Lopressor)	Betaloc, Norometoprol, Apo-Metoprolol
morphine sulfate (Astramorph PF, Duramorph, others)	Epimorph, Statex
naproxen (Naprosyn, Anaprox)	Apo-Naproxen, Naxen, Novonaprox
nifedipine (Procardia, Adalat)	Apo-Nifed, Novo-Nifedin
nitrofurantoin (Furadantin, Furalan, Furanite, Macrobid, Macrodantin)	Apo-Nitrofurantoin, Nephronex, Novofuran
norethindrone acetate	Aygestin, Norlutate
nystatin (Mycostatin, Nilstat, Nystex)	Nadostine, Nyaderm
omeprazole (Prilosec)	Losec
oxazepam (Serax)	Ox-Pam, Zapex
oxymetazoline hydrochloride (Afrin 12 Hour, Neo-Synephrine 12 Hour, others)	Nafrine

U.S. Drug Name	Canadian Drug Name
penicillin G sodium/potassium (Pentids)	Megacillin
penicillin V (Pen-Vee K, Veetids, Betapen-VK)	Apo-Pen-VK, Nadopen-V
pentamidine isoethionate (Pentam 300, Nebupent)	Pentacarinat
pentobarbital sodium (Nembutal)	Novopentobarb
phenylephrine hydrochloride (Mydfrin, Neo-Synephrine)	AK-Dilate Dionephrine
pilocarpine hydrochloride (Adsorbocarpine, Isopto Carpine, others)	Pilocarpine, Miocarpine
prednisolone (Delta-Cortef, Key-Pred, Prelone, others)	Diopred, Inflamase, Pediapred
prednisone (Deltasone, Meticorten)	Apo-Prednisone, Winpred
primidone (Mysoline)	Apo-Primidone
probenecid (Benemid, Probalan)	Benuryl
procarbazine hydrochloride (Matulane)	Natulan
prochlorperazine (Compazine)	Prorazin, Stemetil
procyclidine hydrochloride (Kemadrin)	Procyclid
promethazine (Pentazine, Phenazine, Phenergan, others)	Histantil
propoxyphene hydrochloride (Darvon) Propoxyphene Napsylate (Darvon-N)	Novopropoxyn
propranolol hydrochloride (Inderal)	Apo-Propranolol, Detensol, Novopranol
propylthiouracil (PTU)	Propyl-Thyracil
protriptyline hydrochloride (Vivactil)	Triptil
psyllium hydrophilic mucilloid (Metamucil, Naturcil)	Karasil
pyrazinamide (PZA)	Tebrazid
quinidine sulfate (Quinidex)	Apo-Quinidine, Novoquinidin
quinine sulfate (Quinamm)	Novoquinine
ranitidine (Zantac)	Apo-Ranitidine
rifampin (Rifadin, Rimactane)	Rofact
scopolamine (Hyoscine, Transderm-Scop)	Transderm-V
secobarbital (Seconal)	Novosecobarb
spironolactone (Aldactone)	Novospiroton
sulfasalazine (Azulfidine)	PMS Sulfasalazine, others
sulfinpyrazone (Anturan)	Antazone, Anturane, others
tamoxifen citrate (Nolvadex)	Nolvadex-D, Tamofen
testosterone (Andro 100, Histerone, Testoderm)	Malogen
testosterone enanthate (Testone LA, Delatest, Delatestryl)	Malogex
tetracycline hydrochloride (Achromycin, Panmycin, Sumycin)	Novotetra

U.S. Drug Name	Canadian Drug Name
theophylline (Theo-Dur)	Pulmopylline, Somophyllin-12
thioguanine (TG)	Lanvis
thioridazine hydrochloride (Mellaril)	Novoridazine
tolbutamide (Orinase)	Mobenol, Novobutamide
trifluoperazine hydrochloride (Stelazine)	Novoflurazine, Solazine, Terfluzine
trihexyphenidyl hydrochloride (Artane)	Aparkane, Apo-Trihex, Novohexidyl

U.S. Drug Name	Canadian Drug Name
tripelennamine hydrochloride (PBZ-SR, Pelamine)	Pyribenzamine
Tums	Apo-Cal
valproic acid (Depakene)	Epival
verapamil hydrochloride (Calan, Isoptin, Verelan)	Novo-Veramil, Nu-Verap
vinblastine sulfate (Velban)	Velbe
warfarin sodium (Coumadin)	Warfilone

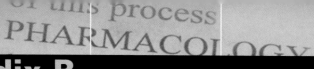

Top 200 Drugs Ranked by Number of Prescriptions

Rank	Market Name	Generic Name	Rank	Market Name	Generic Name
1.	Hydrocodone w/APAP	hydrocodone w/APAP	47.	Augmentin	amoxicillin/clavulanate
2.	Lipitor	atorvastatin	48.	Nexium	esomeprazole
3.	Atenolol	atenolol	49.	Accupril	quinapril
4.	Synthroid	levothyroxine	50.	Lisinopril	lisinopril
5.	Premarin	conjugated estrogens	51.	Effexor XR	venlafaxine
6.	Zithromax	azithromycin	52.	Singulair	montelukast
7.	Furosemide	furosemide	53.	Zestril	lisinopril
8.	Amoxicillin	amoxicillin	54.	Potassium Chloride	potassium chloride
9.	Norvasc	amlodipine	55.	Clonazepam	clonazepam
10.	Hydrochlorothiazide	hydrochlorothiazide	56.	Naproxen	naproxen
11.	Alprazolam	alprazolam	57.	Warfarin	warfarin
12.	Albuterol Aerosol	albuterol	58.	Trazodone	trazodone
13.	Zoloft	sertraline	59.	Cipro	ciprofloxacin
14.	Paxil	paroxetine	60.	Flonase	fluticasone
15.	Zocor	simvastatin	61.	Cyclobenzaprine	cyclobenzaprine
16.	Prevacid	lansoprazole	62.	Verapamil HCl	verapamil
17.	Ibuprofen	ibuprofen	63.	Enalapril	enalapril
18.	Triamterene/HCTZ	triamterene/HCTZ	64.	Albuterol Sulfate	albuterol
19.	Toprol XL	metoprolol	65.	Isosorbide Mononitrate	isosorbide mononitrate S.A.
20.	Cephalexin	cephalexin	66.	Levaquin	levofloxacin
21.	Celebrex	celecoxib	67.	Diazepam	diazepam
22.	Zyrtec	cetirizine	68.	Glucotrol XL	glipizide
23.	Levoxyl	levothyroxine	69.	Coumadin	warfarin
24.	Allegra	fexofenadine	70.	Plavix	clopidogrel
25.	Ortho Tri-Cyclen	norgestimate/ethinyl estradiol	71.	Diflucan	fluconazole
			72.	Advair Diskus	salmeterol/fluticasone
26.	Celexa	citalopram	73.	Protonix	pantoprazole
27.	Prednisone	prednisone	74.	Lotrel	amlodipine/benazepril
28.	Prilosec	omeprazole	75.	Amoxil	amoxicillin
29.	Vioxx	rofecoxib	76.	Diovan	valsartan
30.	Claritin	loratadine	77.	Glyburide	glyburide
31.	Fluoxetine	fluoxetine	78.	Carisoprodol	carisoprodol
32.	Acetaminophen/Codeine	acetaminophen/codeine	79.	Altace	ramipril
33.	Ambien	zolpidem	80.	Allopurinol	allopurinol
34.	Metoprolol Tartrate	metoprolol	81.	Estradiol	estradiol
35.	Lorazepam	lorazepam	82.	Avandia	rosiglitazone maleate
36.	Fosamax	alendronate	83.	Actos	pioglitazone
37.	Propoxyphene N/APAP	propoxyphene N/APAP	84.	Lotensin	benazepril
38.	Metformin	metformin	85.	Clarinex	desloratadine
39.	Ranitidine HCl	ranitidine	86.	Medroxyprogesterone	medroxyprogesterone
40.	Amitriptyline	amitriptyline	87.	Oxycodone/APAP	oxycodone/APAP
41.	Viagra	sildenafil citrate	88.	Doxycycline Hyclate	doxycycline
42.	Prempro	conj. estrogens/ medroxyprogesterone	89.	Lanoxin	digoxin
			90.	Cozaar	losartan
43.	Trimox	amoxicillin	91.	Nasonex	mometasone
44.	Neurontin	gabapentin	92.	Diltiazem HCl	diltiazem
45.	Wellbutrin SR	bupropion HCL	93.	Clonidine	clonidine
46.	Pravachol	pravastatin			

Rank	Market Name	Generic Name	Rank	Market Name	Generic Name
94.	Prinivil	lisinopril	144.	Remeron	mirtazapine
95.	Digitek	digoxin	145.	Famotidine	famotidine
96.	Methylprednisolone	methylprednisolone	146.	Metronidazole	metronidazole
97.	Evista	raloxifene	147.	Bextra	valdecoxib
98.	Folic Acid	folic acid	148.	Avapro	irbesartan
99.	Glucophage XR	metformin	149.	Glipizide	glipizide
100.	Penicillin VK	penicillin VK	150.	Buspirone	buspirone
101.	Flovent	fluticasone propionate	151.	Nystatin	nystatin
102.	Risperdal	risperidone	152.	Skelaxin	metaxalone
103.	Cotrim	TMZ-SMZ	153.	Serevent	salmeterol
104.	Promethazine	promethazine	154.	Dilantin	phenytoin
105.	Diovan HCT	valsartan / HCTZ	155.	Promethazine/Codeine	promethazine / codeine
106.	Aciphex	rabeprazole	156.	Necon	ethinyl estradiol / norethindrone
107.	Zyprexa	olanzapine			
108.	Allegra-D	fexofenadine / pseudoephedrine	157.	Captopril	captopril
109.	Levothroid	levothyroxine	158.	Clindamycin	clindamycin
110.	Doxazosin	doxazosin	159.	Aspirin	aspirin
111.	Xalatan	latanoprost	160.	Seroquel	quetiapine
112.	Gemfibrozil	gemfibrozil	161.	Acyclovir	acyclovir
113.	Flomax	tamsulosin	162.	Macrobid	nitrofurantoin
114.	Temazepam	temazepam	163.	Claritin D 12HR	loratadine/ pseudoephedrine
115.	Ultram	tramadol			
116.	Hyzaar	losartan/HCTZ	164.	Amoxicillin/Clavulanate	amoxicillin/clavulanate
117.	OxyContin	oxycodone	165.	Adderall XR	amphetamine mixed salts
118.	Humulin N	human insulin NPH	166.	Biaxin XL	clarithromycin
119.	Depakote	divalproex (Valproic acid)	167.	Trivora-28	levonorgestrel / ethinyl estradiol
120.	Concerta	methylphenidate XR			
121.	Klor-Con	potassium chloride	168.	Ortho-Cyclen	norgestimate/ ethinyl estradiol
122.	Glucovance	glyburide / metformin			
123.	Imitrex Oral	sumatriptan	169.	Cefzil	cefprozil
124.	Terazosin	terazosin	170.	Humulin 70/30	human insulin 70/30
125.	Claritin D 24HR	loratadine/pseudoephedrine	171.	Detrol LA	tolterodine
126.	Cartia XT	diltiazem	172.	Coreg	carvedilol
127.	Amaryl	glimepiride	173.	Tiazac	diltiazem
128.	Spironolactone	spironolactone	174.	Biaxin	clarithromycin
129.	Tricor	fenofibrate	175.	Tramadol	tramadol
130.	Ortho-Novum	norethindrone/ ethinyl estradiol	176.	Nasacort AQ	triamcinolone acetonide
			177.	Humalog	insulin lispro
131.	Hydroxyzine HCl	hydroxyzine	178.	Ultracet	tramadol/acetaminophen
132.	Monopril	fosinopril	179.	Endocet	oxycodone/APAP
133.	Combivent	ipratropium / albuterol	180.	Bactroban	mupirocin
134.	Meclizine	meclizine	181.	Veetids	penicillin VK
135.	Triamcinolone Acetonide	triamcinolone	182.	Trimethoprim/ Sulfamethoxazole	TMZ-SMZ
136.	Klor-Con M20	potassium chloride			
137.	Metoclopramide	metoclopramide	183.	Timolol Maleate	timolol maleate
138.	Minocycline	minocycline	184.	Rhinocort Aqua	budesonide
139.	Bisoprolol/HCTZ	bisoprolol/HCTZ	185.	Claritin Reditabs	loratadine
140.	Propranolol	propranolol	186.	Nortriptyline	nortriptyline
141.	Glucophage	metformin	187.	Aviane	levonorgestrel/ ethinyl estradiol
142.	Propacet	propoxyphene N/APAP			
143.	Valtrex	valacyclovir	188.	Actonel	risedronate
			189.	Topamax	topiramate

Rank	Market Name	Generic Name	Rank	Market Name	Generic Name
190.	Microgestin Fe	norethindrone/ ethinyl estradiol	195.	Tetracycline	tetracycline
191.	Tamoxifen	tamoxifen	196.	Apri	desogestrel/ ethinyl estradiol
192.	Mircette	desogestrel/ ethinyl estradiol	197.	Zestoretic	lisinopril/HCTZ
193.	Nifedipine	nifedipine	198.	Diclofenac	diclofenac
194.	Ditropan XL	oxybutynin	199.	Augmentin ES-600	amoxicillin/clavulanate
			200.	Carbidopa/Levodopa	carbidopa/levodopa

Source: Data from PharmaTrends 2002, *NDCHealth, Inc. www.rxlist.com/top 200.htm*

BIBLIOGRAPHY AND REFERENCES

General References

Audesirk, T., Audesirk, G., & Beyers, B. E. (2002) *Biology: Life on earth* (6th ed.). Upper Saddle River, NJ: Prentice Hall.

Beers, M. H., & Berkow, R. (Eds.). (2001). *Merck manual: Diagnosis and therapy* (17th ed.). Whitehouse Station, NJ: Merck & Co., Inc.

Holland, N., & Adams, M. (2003). *Core concepts in pharmacology.* Upper Saddle River, NJ: Prentice Hall.

Krogh, D. (2002). *Biology: A guide to the natural world* (2nd ed.). Upper Saddle River, NJ: Prentice Hall.

LeMone, P., & Burke, K. M. (2004). *Medical-surgical nursing: Critical thinking in client care* (3rd ed.). Upper Saddle River, NJ: Prentice Hall.

Martini, F. H. (2004). *Fundamentals of human anatomy and physiology* (6th ed.). San Francisco: Benjamin Cummings.

Medical Economics Staff (Ed.). (2000). *Physician's desk reference for herbal medicines* (2nd ed.). Montvale, NJ: Medical Economics.

————. (2001). *Physician's desk reference for nutritional supplements* (24th ed.). Montvale, NJ: Medical Economics.

————. (2004). *Physician's desk reference* (58th ed.). Montvale, NJ: Medical Economics.

Mulvihill, M. L., Zelman, P., Holdaway, P., Tompary, E., & Turchany, J. (2001). *Human diseases: A systemic approach* (5th ed.). Upper Saddle River, NJ: Prentice Hall.

Rice, J. (1999). *Medical terminology with human anatomy* (4th ed.). Upper Saddle River, NJ: Prentice Hall.

Silverthorn, D. U. (2001). *Human physiology: An integrated approach* (2nd ed.). Upper Saddle River, NJ: Prentice Hall.

Wilson, B. A., Shannon, M. T., & Strang, C. L. (2004). *Nurse's drug guide 2004.* Upper Saddle River, NJ: Prentice Hall.

Chapter 1

Carrico, J. M. (2000). Human Genome Project and pharmacogenomics: Implications for pharmacy. *J Am Pharm Assoc 40*(1), 115–116.

Newton, G. D., Pray, W. S., & Popovich, N. G. (2001). New OTC drugs and devices 2000: A selective review. *J Am Pharm Assoc 41*(2), 273–282.

Nies, A. S. (2001). Principles of therapeutics. In J. G. Hardman, L. E. Limbird, & A. G. Goodman, (Eds.), *The pharmacological basis of therapeutics* (pp. 45–66). New York: McGraw-Hill.

Olsen, D. P. (2000). The patient's responsibility for optimum healthcare. *Dis Manage Health Outcomes 7*(2), 57–65.

Chapter 2

Bond, C. A., Raehl, C. L., & Franke, T. (2001). Medication errors in United States hospitals. *Pharmacotherapy 21*(9), 1023–1036.

Brass, E. P. (2001). Drug therapy: Changing the status of drugs from prescription to over-the-counter availability. *N Engl J Med 345*, 810–816.

Brown, S. D., & Landry, F. J. (2001). Recognizing, reporting, and reducing adverse drug reactions. *South Med J 94*(4), 370–373.

Gaither, C. A., Kirking, D. M., Ascione, F. J., & Welage, L. S. (2001). Consumers' views on generic medications. *J Am Pharm Assoc 41*(5), 729–736.

Kacew, S. (1999). Effects of over-the-counter drugs on the unborn child: What is known and how should this influence prescribing? *Paedriatr Drugs 1*(2), 75–80.

Phillips, K. A., Veenstra, D. L., Oren, E., Lee, J. K., & Sardee, W. (2001). Potential role of pharmacogenomics in reducing adverse drug reactions: A systematic review. *JAMA 286*, 2270–2279.

Chapter 3

Barbera, J., Macintyre, A., Gostin, L., Inglesby, T., O'Toole, T., Diatele, C., Tonat, K., & Layton, M. (2001). Large-scale quarantine following biological terrorism in the United States: Scientific examination, logistic and legal limits, and possible consequences. *JAMA 286*(21), 2711–2717.

Bartlett, J. G., Sifton, D. W., & Kelly, G. L. (Eds.). (2002). *PDR guide to biological and chemical warfare response.* Montvale, NJ: Medical Economics.

Blendon, R. J., Des Roches, C. M., Benson, J. M., Herrmann, M. J., Taylor-Clark, K., & Weldon, K. J. (2003). The public and the smallpox threat. *N Engl J Med 348*(5), 426–432.

Bozeman, W. P., Dilbero, D., & Schauben, J. L. (2002). Biologic and chemical weapons of mass destruction. *Emerg Med Clin North Am 20*(4), xii, 975–993.

Cangemi, C. W. (2002). Occupational response to terrorism. *AAOHN J 50*(4), 190–196.

Chyba, C. F. (2001). Biological security in a changed world. *Science 293*(5539), 2349.

Crupi, R. S., Asnis, D. S., Lee, C. C., Santucci, T., Marino, M. J., & Flanz, B. J. (2003). Meeting the challenge of bioterrorism: Lessons learned from West Nile virus and anthrax. *Am J Emerg Med 21*(1), 77–79.

Donnellan, C. (2002). New law funds nursing's role in bioterrorism response. The ANA establishes the National Nurses Response Team. *Am J Nurs 102*(8), 23.

Fidler, D. P. (2001). The malevolent use of microbes and the rule of law: Legal challenges presented by bioterrorism. *Clinical Infectious Diseases 33*(5), 686–689.

Henderson, D. A., Inglesby, T. V., & O'Toole, T. (2002). *Bioterrorism: Guidelines for medical and public health management.* Chicago, IL: American Medical Association.

Hughes, J. M. (2001). Emerging infectious diseases: A CDC perspective. *Emerging Infectious Diseases 7*(3 Suppl), 494–496.

Khan, A. S., Swerdlow, D. L., & Juranek, D. D. (2001). Precautions against biological and chemical terrorism directed at food and water supplies. *Public Health Reports 116*(1), 3–14.

Kimmel, S. R., Mahoney, M. C., & Zimmerman, R. K. (2003). Vaccines and bioterrorism: Smallpox and anthrax. *J Fam Pract 52*(1 Suppl), S56–S61.

McLaughlin, S. (2001). Thinking about the unthinkable. Where to start planning for terrorism incidents. *Health Facilities Management 14*(7), 26–30, 32.

Morse, A. (2002). Bioterrorism preparedness for local health departments. *J Community Health Nurs 19*(4), 203–211.

Mortimer, P. P. (2003). Can postexposure vaccination against smallpox succeed? *Clin Infect Dis 36*(5), 622–629.

O'Connell, K. P., Menuey, B. C., & Foster, D. (2002). Issues in preparedness for biologic terrorism: A perspective for critical care nursing. *AACN Clin Issues 13*(3), 452–469.

O'Toole, T. (2001). Emerging illness and bioterrorism: Implications for public health. *Journal of Urban Health 78*(2), 396–402.

Rose, M. A., & Larrimore, K. L. (2002). Knowledge and awareness concerning chemical and biological terrorism: Continuing education implications. *J Contin Educ Nurs 33*(6), 253–258.

Salazar, M. K., & Kelman, B. (2002). Planning for biological disasters. Occupational health nurses as "first responders." *AAOHN J 50*(4), 174–181.

Spencer, R. C., & Lightfoot, N. F. (2001). Preparedness and response to bioterrorism. *Journal of Infection 43*(2), 104–110.

Stephenson, J. (2003). Smallpox vaccine program launched amid concerns raised by expert panel, unions. *JAMA 289*(6), 685–686.

Stillsmoking, K. (2002). Bioterrorism—are you ready for the silent killer? *AORN J 76*(3), 434, 437–442, 444–446.

Tasota, F. J., Henker, R. A., & Hoffman, L. A. (2002). Anthrax as a biological weapon: An old disease that poses a new threat. *Crit Care Nurse 22*(5), 21–32, 34.

Chapter 4

Armitage, G., & Knapman, H. (2003). Adverse events in drug administration: A literature review. *J Nurs Manag 11*(2), 130–140.

Bankston, J., Deshotels, J. M., Daughtry, L., & Metules, T. J. (Eds). (2001). Same trigger, less deadly. *SJS 64*(10), 39–41.

Berman, A. J., Kozier, B., & Snyder, S. (2002). *Kozier and Erb's techniques in clinical nursing* (5th ed.). Upper Saddle River, NJ: Prentice Hall.

Billups, S. J., Malone, D. C., & Carter, B. L. (2000). The relationship between drug therapy noncompliance and patient characteristics, health-related quality of life, and health care costs. *Pharmacotherapy 20*(8), 941–949.

Blais, K. K., Hayes, J., Kozier, B., & Erb, G. (2002). *Professional nursing practice: Concepts and perspectives* (4th ed.). Upper Saddle River, NJ: Prentice Hall.

Deedwania, P. C. (2002). The changing face of hypertension: Is systolic blood pressure the final answer? *Arch Int Med 162*(5), 506–508.

Koo, M. M., Krass, I., & Aslani, P. (2003). Factors influencing consumer use of written drug information. *Ann Pharmacother 37*(2), 259–267.

Kozma, C. M. (2002). Why aren't we doing more to enhance medication compliance? *Manag Care Interface 15*(1), 59–60.

Lesaffre, E., & de Klerk, E. (2000). Estimating the power of compliance-improving methods. *Control Clin Trials 21*(6), 540–551.

Madlon, K., Diane, J., & Mosch, F. S. (2000). Liquid medication dosing errors. *J of Family Practice 49*(1), 741–744.

Olsen, J. L., Giangrasso, A. P., & Shrimpton, D. M. (2004). *Medical dosage calculations* (8th ed.). Upper Saddle River, NJ: Prentice Hall.

Seal. R. (2000). How to promote drug compliance in the elderly. *Community Nurse 6*(1), 41–42.

Smith, D. I. (2001). Taking control of your medicines. Newsletter 1(1). Consumer Health Information Corporation, www.consumer-health.com

Smith, S., Duell, D., & Martin, B. (2000). *Clinical nursing skills: Basic to advanced skills* (5th ed.). Upper Saddle River, NJ: Prentice Hall Health.

Urquhart, J. (2000). Erratic patient compliance with prescribed drug regimens: Target for drug delivery systems. *Clin Pharmacol Ther 67*(4), 331–334.

Wooten, J. (2001). Toxic epidermal necrolysis. *Nursing 2001 64*(10), 35–38.

Chapter 5

Bateman, D. N. (2001). Introduction to pharmacokinetics and pharmacodynamics. *J of Toxicol: Clin Toxicol 39*(3), 207.

Bhattaram, V. B., Graefe, U., Kohlert, C., Veit, M., & Derendorf, H. (2002). Pharmacokinetics and bioavailability of herbal medicinal products. *Phytomedicine 9*, 1–33.

Doucet, J., Jego, D., Noel, D., Geffroy, C. E., Capet, C., Coquard, A., Couffin, E., Fauchais, A. L., Chassagne, P., Mouton-Schleifer, D., & Bercoff, E. (2002). Preventable and nonpreventable risk factors for adverse drug events related to hospital admission in the elderly. *Clin Drug Invest 22*(6), 385–392.

Hardman, J. G., Limbird, I. E., & Goodman, A. G. (Eds.). *The pharmacological basis of therapeutics* (10th ed.). New York: McGraw-Hill.

Kanneh, K. (2002). Paediatric pharmacological principles: An update part 2. Pharmacokinetics: Absorption and distribution. *Paediatric Nursing 14*(9), 39–44.

Kanneh, K. (2002). Paediatric pharmacological principles: An update part 3. Pharmacokinetics: Metabolism and excretion. *Paediatric Nursing 14*(10), 39–43.

Levy, R. H., Thummel, K. E., Trager, W. F., Hansten, P. D., & Eichelbaum, M. (Eds.). (2000). *Metabolic drug interactions.* Philadelphia: Lippincott, Williams & Wilkins.

Rollins, D. E. (2000). Clinical pharmacokinetics. In A. R. Gennaro (Ed.), *Remington: The science and practice of pharmacy* (chapter 59, pp. 1145–1155). Philadelphia: Lippincott, Williams & Wilkins.

Scott, G. N., & Elmer, G. W. (2002). Update on natural product-drug interactions. *Am J Health-Syst Pharm 59*(4), 339–347.

Suggs, D. M. (2000). Pharmacokinetics in children: History, considerations, and applications. *J Am Acad Nurse Pract 12*(6), 236–240.

White, R. J., & Park, G. (2001). Safe drug prescribing in the critically ill. In G. Park & M. Shelly (Eds.), *Pharmacology of the critically ill* (chapter 2). London: BMI Books.

Wilkinson, G. R. (2001). Pharmacokinetics: The dynamics of drug absorption, distribution and elimination. In J. G. Hardman, L. E. Limbard & A. G. Goodman (Eds.), *The pharmacological basis of therapeutics* (10th ed.). New York: McGraw-Hill.

Chapter 6

Berg, M. J. (2002, August 31–September 5). *Does sex matter?* 62nd International Pharmaceutical Federation. Congress, Nice, France. Title also appears in *Medscape Pharmacists 3*(2).

Bottles, K. (2001). A revolution in genetics: Changing medicine, changing lives. *Physician Exec 27*, 58–63.

du Souich, P. (2001). In human therapy, is the drug-drug interaction or the adverse drug reaction the issue? *Can J Clin Pharmacol 8*, 153–161.

Ginsburg, G. S., & McCarthy, J. J. (2001). Personalized medicine: Revolutionizing drug discovery and patient care. *Trends Biotechnol 19*, 491–496.

Hughes, R. (2001). *A manual of pharmacodynamics.* New Delhi, India: B. Jain Publishers.

Kramer, T. (2003). Side effects and therapeutic effects. *Medscape General Medicine 5*(1).

Kuo, G. M. (2003). Pharmacodynamic basis of herbal medicine. *Ann Pharmacother 37*(2), 308.

Ma, M. K., Woo, M. A., & McLeod, H. L. (2002). Genetic basis of drug metabolism. *Am J Healthsys Pharm 59*(21), 2061–2069.

Nies, A. S. (2001). Principles of therapeutics. In J. G. Hardman, L. E. Limbird, and A. G. Goodman (Eds.), *The pharmacological basis of therapeutics* (pp. 45–66). New York: McGraw-Hill.

Nightingale, C. H., Murakawa, T., & Ambrose, P. G. (Eds.). (2002). *Antimicrobial pharmacodynamics in theory and clinical practice.* New York: Marcel Dekker.

Relling, M. V., & Dervieux, T. (2001). Pharmacogenetics and cancer therapy. *Nat Rev Cancer 1*, 99–108.

Roses, A. D. (2001). Pharmacogenetics. *Hum Mol Genet 10*, 2261–2267.

Ross, E. M., & Kenakin, T. P. (2001). Pharamcodynamics: Mechanisms of drug action and the relationship between drug concentration and effect. In J. G. Hardman, L. E. Limbird, & A. G. Goodman, (Eds.), *The pharmacological basis of therapeutics* (pp. 31–44). New York: McGraw-Hill.

Ross, J. S., & Ginsburg, G. S. (2003). The integration of molecular diagnostics with therapeutics. *Am J Clin Pathol 119*(1), 26–36.

Steimer, W., & Potter, J. M. (2001). Pharmacogenetic screening and therapeutic drugs. *Clin Chim Acta 315*, 137–155.

Wortman, M. (2001). Medicine gets personal. *Technology Review* (January/February), 72–78.

Chapter 7

American Academy of Pediatrics, Committee on Drugs. (2001). The transfer of drugs and other chemicals into human breast milk. *Pediatrics 3*, 776–782.

Auerbach, K. G. (2000). Breastfeeding and maternal medication use. *J of Ob, Gyn, and Neo Nur 28*(5), 554–563.

Beers, M. H., & Berkow, R. (Eds.). (2000). *The Merck manual of geriatrics* (3rd ed.). Whitehouse Station, NJ: Merck & Company, Inc.

Bressler, R., & Katz, M. (2003). *Geriatric pharmacology* (2nd ed.). New York: McGraw-Hill Professional.

Briggs, G. G. (2002). Drug effects on the fetus and breast-fed infant. *Clin Ob and Gyn 45* (1), 6–21, 170–171.

Crome, P., & Ford, G. (Eds.). (2000). *Drugs and the older population.* London: Imperial College Press.

Dellasega, C., Klinefelter, J. M., & Halas, C. J. (2000). Psychoactive medications and the elderly patient. *Clin Rev 10*(6), 53–74.

Kearney, M. H. (1997). Drug treatment for women: Traditional models and new directions. *J of Ob, Gyn, and Neo Nurs 26*(4), 459–468.

Heinrich, J. (2001). Pediatric drug research: Substantial increase in studies of drugs for children but some challenges remain. Testimony before the Committee on Health, Education, Labor and Pensions, U.S. Senate, Washington, DC.

Leipzig, R. M. (Ed.). (2003). *Drug prescribing for older adults: An evidence-based approach.* Philadelphia: American College of Physicians.

Loughran, S. (1996). Nursing pharmacology. Medication use in the elderly: A population at risk. *MEDSURG Nursing 5*(2), 121–124.

Nice, F. J., Snyder, J. L., & Kotansky, B. C. (2000). Breastfeeding and over-the-counter medications. *J of Hum Lact 16*(4), 319–331.

O'Mahony, D., & Martin, U. (1999). *Practical therapeutics for the older patient.* Indianapolis: John Wiley & Sons, Inc.

Rosenbaum, M., & Irwin, K. (1998). Pregnancy, drugs, and harm reduction. In *Drug addiction research and the health of women* (pp. 309–318). Rockville, MD: United States Department of Health and Human Services. National Institutes of Health.

Spencer, J. P., Gonzalez, L. S., III, & Barnhart, D. J. (2001). Medications in the breast-feeding mother. *Amer Fam Phys 64*, 19–126.

Turkoski, B. B. (1999). Pharmacology. Meeting the challenge of medication reactions in the elderly. *Ortho Nursing 18*(5), 85–95.

Chapter 8

Bakker, D. A., Blais, D., Reed, E., Vaillancourt, C., Gervais, S., & Beaulieu, P. (1999). Descriptive study to compare patient recall of information: Nurse-taught versus video supplement. *Can Oncol Nurs J 9*(3), 115–120.

Carpenito, L. J. (2000). *Nursing diagnosis: Application to nursing practice* (8th ed.). Philadelphia: J. B. Lippincott.

Gardner, P. (2003). *Nursing process in action.* New York: Thompson Delmar Learning.

Hogan, M. A., Bowles, D., & White, J. E. (2003). *Nursing fundamentals: Reviews & rationales.* Upper Saddle River, NJ: Prentice Hall.

Jahraus, D., Sokolosky, S., Thurston, N., & Guo, D. (2002). Evaluation of an education program for patients with breast cancer receiving radiation therapy. *Cancer Nurs 24*(4), 266–275.

Jarvis, C. (2000). *Physical examination and health assessment* (3rd ed.). Philadelphia: Mosby.

Kozier, B., Erb, G., Berman, A. J., & Burke, K. (2000). *Fundamentals of nursing: Concepts, process, and practice* (6th ed.). Upper Saddle River, NJ: Prentice Hall.

McFarland, G. K., & McFarland, E. A. (1997). *Nursing diagnosis & intervention: Planning for patient care* (3rd ed.). St. Louis: Mosby.

North American Nursing Diagnosis Association. (2003). *Nursing diagnoses: Definitions and classification 2003–2004.* Philadelphia: Author.

Smith, S. F., Duell, D. J., & Martin, B. C. (2000). *Clinical nursing skills* (5th ed.). Upper Saddle River, NJ: Prentice Hall.

Chapter 9

Bates, D. W., Clapp, M., Federico, F., Goldmann, D., Kaushal, R., Landrigan, C., & McKenna, K. J. (2001). Medication errors and adverse drug events in pediatric inpatients. *JAMA 285*(16), 2114–2120.

Burns, J. P., Mitchell, C., Griffith, J. L., & Truog, R. D. (2001). End-of-life care in the pediatric intensive care: Attitudes and practices of pediatric critical care physicians and nurses. *Crit Care Med 29*(3), 658–664.

Cohen, M. R. (2000). Preventing medication errors related to prescribing. In M. R. Cohen (Ed.), *Medication errors. Causes, preventions and risk management.* Sudbury, MA: Jones and Bartlett Publishers.

Federal Drug Administration. (2001, October 1). Med error reports to FDA show a mixed bag. Drug Topics, www.drugtopics.com

Guido, G. W. (2001). *Legal and ethical issues in nursing* (3rd ed.). Upper Saddle River, NJ: Prentice Hall.

Kozier, B., Erb, G., Berman, A. J., & Burke, K. (2000). *Fundamentals of nursing* (8th ed.). Upper Saddle River, NJ: Prentice Hall.

Lazarou, J., Pomeranz, B. H., & Corey, P. N. (1998). Incidence of adverse drug reactions in hospitalized patients. A meta-analysis of prospective studies. *JAMA 279*(15), 1200–1205.

Mitchell, A. (2001). Challenges in pediatric pharmacotherapy: Minimizing medication errors. *Medscape Pharm 2*(1), 1–8.

Murphy, R. N. (1997). Legal and practical impact of clinical practice guidelines on nursing and medical practice. *Nurse Pract 22*(3), 138, 147–148.

National Coordinating Council for Medication Error Reporting and Prevention. Taxonomy of medication errors (1998), and

Recommendations to correct error-prone aspects of prescription writing (1996). www.nccmerp.org (accessed 2003, February 4).

Phillips, J., Beam, S., Brinker, A., Holquist, C., Honig, P., Lee, L. Y., & Pamer, C. (2001). Retrospective analysis of mortalities associated with medication errors. *Am J Health-Syst. Pharm 58,* 1835–1841.

Waldo, B. H. (1999). Preventing adverse drug reactions through administration. *Nurs Econ 17,* 276–279.

Chapter 10

Andrus, M. R., & Roth, M. T. (2002). Health literacy: A review. *Pharmacotherapy 22*(3), 282–302.

Bushy, A. (1999). Social and cultural factors affecting health care and nursing practice. In J. Lancaster, *Nursing issues in leading and managing change* (pp. 267–292). St. Louis: Mosby.

Chen, J. (2002, October 20–23). *The role of ethnicity in medication use.* Presented at the American College of Clinical Pharmacy 2002 Annual Meeting, Albuquerque, NM.

Chin, J. L. (2000). Viewpoint: Culturally Competent Health Care. *Public Health Reports 115*(1), 25–33.

Crow, K., & Matheson, L. (2000). Informed consent and truth-telling: Cultural directions for healthcare providers. *J Nurs Administr 30*(3), 148–152.

Davidhizar, R. (2002). Strategies for providing culturally appropriate pharmaceutical care to the Hispanic patient. *Hosp Pharm 37*(5), 505–510.

Gallagher, R. M. (2002). *The pain-depression conundrum: Bridging the body and mind.* Medscape clinical update based on session presented at the 21st Annual Scientific Meeting of the American Pain Society. Medscape Clinical Update at http://www.medscape.com/viewprogram/2030

Humma, L. M., & Terra, S. G. (2002). Pharmacogenetics and cardiovascular disease: Impact on drug response and applications to disease management. *Am J Health-Syst Pharm 59*(13), 1241–1252.

Kudzma, E. C. (2001). Cultural competence: Cardiovascular medications. *Prog Cardiovasc Nurs 16*(4), 152–160, 169.

Leininger, M. M. (Ed.). (2001). *Culture care diversity and universality: A theory of nursing.* Sudbury, MA: Jones & Bartlett Publishers.

Martin, L., Miracle, A. W., & Bonder, B. R. (2001). *Culture in clinical care.* Thorofare, NJ: Slack, Inc.

Nichols-English, G., & Poirier, S. (2000). Optimizing adherence to pharmaceutical care plans. *J Am Pharm Assoc 40*(4), 475–485.

Richardson, L. G. (2003). Psychosocial issues in patients with congestive heart failure. *Prog Cardiovasc Nurs 18*(1), 19–27.

Sleath, B., & Wallace, J. (2002). Providing pharmaceutical care to Spanish-speaking patients. *J Am Pharm Assoc 42,* 799–801.

Spector, R. E. (2004). *Cultural diversity in health & illness* (6th ed.). Upper Saddle River, NJ: Prentice Hall.

Wick, J. Y. (1996). Culture, ethnicity and medications. *J Am Pharm Assoc 9,* 557–564. Issue(NS36).

Chapter 11

Blumenthal, M. (Ed.). (2000). *Herbal medicine: Expanded commission E monographs.* Austin, TX: American Botanical Council.

Ebadi, M. (2002). *Pharmcodynamic basis of herbal medicine.* Boca Raton, FL: CRC Press.

Eisenberg, D. M., Davis, R. B., Ettner, S. L., Appel, S., Wilkey, S., Van Rompay, M., & Kessler, R. C. (1998). Trends in alternative medicine use in the United States, 1990–1997. *JAMA 280,* 1569–1575.

Fontaine, K. L. (2000). *Healing practices: Alternative therapies for nursing.* Upper Saddle River, NJ: Prentice Hall.

Foster, S., & Hobbs, C. (2002). *A field guide to western medicinal plants and herbs.* Boston and New York: Houghton Mifflin Co.

Goldman, P. (2001). Herbal medicines today and the roots of modern pharmacology. *Ann of Int Med 135*(8), 594–597.

Hardy, M. L. (2000). Herbs of special interest to women. *Am Pharm Assoc 40*(2), 234–242.

Hatcher, T., Dokken, D., & Sydnor-Greenberg, N. (2000). Exploring complementary and alternative medicine in pediatrics: Parents and professionals working together for new understanding. *Pediatr Nurs 26*(4), 383.

Medical Economics Staff (Ed.). (2000). *Physician's desk reference for herbal medicines* (2nd ed.). Montvale: Medical Economics.

Murch, S. J., KrishnaRaj, S., & Saxena, P. K. (2000). Phytopharmaceuticals: Problems, limitations, and solutions. *Sci Rev of Alt Med 4*(2), 33–37.

The review of natural products: 2002. Missouri: Facts and Comparisons®, Publisher.

Scott, G. N., & Elmer, G. W. (2002). Update on natural product-drug interactions. *Am J Health-Sys Pharm 59*(4), 339–347.

Tyler, V. E. (2000). Product definition deficiencies in clinical studies of herbal medicines. *Sci Rev of Alt Med 4*(2), 17–21.

White, L. B., & Foster, S. (2000). *The herbal drugstore.* Emmaus, PA: Rodale.

White House Commission on Complementary and Alternative Medicine Policy. (2000, March) Final report, http://govinfo.library.unt.edu/whccamp/

Chapter 12

Barangan, C. J., & Alderman, E. M. (2002). Management of substance abuse. *Pediatr Rev 23*(4), 123–131.

Chychula, N. M., & Sciamanna, C. (2002). Help substance abusers attain and sustain abstinence. *Nurse Pract 27*(11), 30–47.

Freese, T. E., Miotto, K., & Reback, C. J. (2002). The effects and consequences of selected club drugs. *J Subst Abuse Treat 23*(2), 151–156.

Hardie, T. L. (2002). The genetics of substance abuse. *AACN Clin Issues 13*(4), 511–522.

Haseltine, E. (2001). The unsatisfied mind: Are reward centers in your brain wired for substance abuse? *Discover 22*(11), 88.

Jason, L. A., Davis, M. I., Ferrari, J. R., & Bishop, P. D. (2001). A review of research and implications for substance abuse recovery and community research. *J of Drug Educ 31*(1), 1–28.

Kandel, D. B. (2003). Does marijuana use cause the use of other drugs? *JAMA 289*(4), 482–483.

Manoguerra, A. S. (2001). Methamphetamine abuse. *J of Toxicol: Clinic Toxicol 38*(2), 187.

Naegle, M. A., & D'Avanzo, C. E. (2001). *Addictions and substance abuse: Strategies for advanced practice nursing.* Upper Saddle River, NJ: Prentice Hall.

O'Brien, C. P. (2001). Drug addiction and drug abuse. In J. G. Hardman, L. E. Limbird, & A. G. Goodman (Eds.), *The pharmacological basis of therapeutics* (pp. 621–642). New York: McGraw-Hill.

Sindelar, J. L., & Fiellin, D. A. (2001). Innovations in treatment for drug abuse: Solutions to a public health problem. *Ann Rev of Pub Health 22,* 249.

Tuttle, J., Melnyk, B. M., & Loveland-Cherry, C. (2002). Adolescent drug and alcohol use. Strategies for assessment, intervention, and prevention. *Nurs Clin North Am 37*(3), 443–460, ix.

U.S. Department of Health and Human Services. (1998). *Tobacco use among U.S. racial/ethnic minority groups—African Americans, American Indians and Alaska Natives, Asian Americans and Pacific Islanders, and Hispanics: A report of the surgeon general*. Atlanta: U.S. Department of Health and Human Services, Centers for Disease Control and Prevention, National Center for Chronic Disease Prevention and Health Promotion, Office on Smoking and Health.

Wasilow-Mueller, S., & Erickson, C. K. (2001). Drug abuse and dependency: Understanding gender differences in etiology and management. *J Am Pharm Assoc 41*(1), 78–90.

Chapter 13

Bouchard, R., Weber, A. R., & Geiger, J. D. (2002). Informed decision-making on sympathomimetic use in sport and health. *Clin J Sport Med 12*(4), 209–224.

Cazzola, M., Centanni, S., & Donner, C. F. (1998). Anticholinergic agents. *Pulmon Pharmacol Ther 11*(5–6), 381–392.

Chapple, C. R., Yamanishi, T., & Chess-Williams, R. (2002). Muscarinic receptor subtypes and management of the overactive bladder. *Urology 60* (5 Suppl. 1), 82–88; discussion 88–89.

Cilliers, L., & Retief, F. P. (2003). Poisons, poisoning and the drug trade in ancient rome, www.sun.ac.za

Defilippi, J., & Crismon, M. L. (2003). Drug interactions with cholinesterase inhibitors. *Drugs Aging 20*(6), 437–444.

Herbison, P., Hay-Smith, J., Ellis, G., & Moore, K. (2003). Effectiveness of anticholinergic drugs compared with placebo in the treatment of overactive bladder: Systematic review. *BMJ 19*, 326(7394), 841–844.

Hoffman, B. B., & Taylor, P. (2001). Neurotransmission: The autonomic and somatic motor nervous systems. In J. G. Hardman, L. E. Limbird, & A. G. Goodman (Eds.), *The pharmacological basis of therapeutics* (pp. 115–154). New York: McGraw-Hill.

Kolpuru, S. (2003). Doctor corner: Approach to a case of Down's syndrome. *Pediatric OnCall*™, www.pediatriconcall.com

Lemstra, A. W., Eikelenboom, P., & van Gool, W. A. (2003). The cholinergic deficiency syndrome and its therapeutic implications. *Gerontol 49*(1), 55–60.

McCrory, D. C., & Brown, C. D. (2002). Anti-cholinergic bronchodilators versus beta$_2$-sympathomimetic agents for acute exacerbations of chronic obstructive pulmonary disease. *Cochrane Database Syst Rev 4*, CD003900.

Medical Economics Staff (Ed.). (2000). *PDR for herbal medicines*. Montvale, NJ: Author.

Miller, C. A. (2002). Anticholinergics: The good and the bad. *Geriatr Nurs 23*(5), 286–287.

MSN Health. (2003). Drugs & herbs: Phenylephrine ophthalmic, www.content.health.msn.com

National Toxicology Program, National Institutes of Health. (2001). NTP chemical repository: Phenylephrine, www.ntp-server.hiehs.nih.gov

Rodrigo, G. J., & Rodrigo, C. (2002). The role of anticholinergics in acute asthma treatment: An evidence-based evaluation. *Chest 121*(6), 1977–1987.

Roe, C. M., Anderson, M. J., & Spivack, B. (2002). Use of anticholinergic medications by older adults with dementia. *J Am Geriatr Soc 50*, 836–842.

ThinkQuest On-line Library. (2003). Belladonna, deadly nightshade. *Poisonous Plants and Animals*, www.library.thinkquest.org

Wang, H. E. (2002). Street drug toxicity resulting from opiates combined with anticholinergics. *Prehosp Emerg Care 6*(3), 351–354.

Chapter 14

Baldessarini, R. J. (2001). Drugs and the treatment of psychiatric disorders: Depression and anxiety disorders. In J. G. Hardman, L. E. Limbird, & A. G. Goodman (Eds.), *The pharmacological basis of therapeutics* (pp. 447–484). New York: McGraw-Hill.

Breggin, Peter R. (1999). *Your drug may be your problem: How and why to stop taking psychiatric medications*. Reading, MA: Perseus Books.

Charney, D. S., Mihic, J., & Harris, A. (2001). Hypnotics and sedatives. In J. G. Hardman, L. E. Limbird, & A. G. Goodman (Eds.), *The pharmacological basis of therapeutics* (pp. 399–428). New York: McGraw-Hill.

Fontaine, K. L., & Fletcher, J. S. (1999). *Mental health nursing* (4th ed.). Upper Saddle River, NJ: Prentice Hall.

Gorman, J. N. (2001). Generalized anxiety disorder. *Clin Corner 3*(3), 37–46.

Health A to Z. (2003). Benzodiazepines, www.healthatoz.com

Lippmann, S., Mazour, I., & Shahab, H. (2001). Insomnia: Therapeutic approach. *South Med J 94*(9), 866–873.

Medical Economics Staff (Ed.). (2001). *PDR for nutritional supplements*. Montvale, NJ: Author.

National Institute for Drug Abuse (NIDA). (2001, August). Facts about prescription drug abuse and addiction, 16:3. Bethesda, MD: Author, www.drugabuse.gov

Smock, T. K. (2001). *Physiological psychology: A neuroscience approach*. Upper Saddle River, NJ: Prentice Hall.

United States Drug Enforcement Agency (DEA). (2003). Benzodiazepines, www.usdoj.gov/dea

United States Drug Enforcement Agency (DEA). (2003). Depressants, www.usdoj.gov/dea

Vitiello, M. V. (2000). Effective treatment of sleep disturbances in older adults. *Clin Corner 2*(5), 16–27.

Chapter 15

Beers, M., & Berkow, R. (Eds.). (1999). *Vitamin D deficiency and dependency. Merck manual of diagnosis and therapy* (17th ed.). Whitehouse Station, NJ: Merck Research Laboratories.

Burstein, A. H., Horton, R. L., Dunn, T., et al. (2000). Lack of effect of St. John's wort on carbamazepine pharmacokinetics in healthy volunteers. *Clin Pharmacol and Therap 68*, 6.

Johnson, K. (2002). Epilepsy and pregnancy. *Medscape Ob/Gyn & Women's Health 7*(2).

Murphy, P. A., & Blaylock, R. L. (2001). *Treating epilepsy naturally: A guide to alternative and adjunct therapies*. New York: McGraw-Hill Contemporary Books.

Pack, A. M., & Morrell, M. J. (2003). Treatment of women with epilepsy. *Semin Neurol 22*(3), 289–298.

Patel, P., & Mageda, M. (2002, April). *Vitamin K deficiency*. E-Medicine: Instant Access to the Minds of Medicine, www.emedicine.com

Snelson, C., & Dieckman, B. (2000, June). Recognizing and managing purple glove syndrome. *Critical Care Nurse 20*(3), 54–61.

Tierney, L. M., McPhee, S. J., and Papadakis, M. A. (Eds.). (2002). The nervous system. In M. J. Minoff (Ed.), *Current medical diagnosis and treatment* (ch. 24). New York: Lange Medical Books/McGraw-Hill Medical Publishing Division.

Trimble, M., & Schmitz, B. (Eds.). (2002). *The neuropsychiatry of epilepsy*. New York: Cambridge University Press.

United States National Library, National Institutes of Health. (2003). *Neural tube defects*. Medlineplus Health Information, www.nlm.nih.gov/medlineplus

University of Illinois at Chicago, College of Pharmacy Drug Information Center. (2003). Is there an interaction between phenytoin and enteral feedings? www.uic.edu

Wyllie, E. (2001). *The treatment of epilepsy: Principles and practice* (3rd ed.). Philadelphia: Lippincott, Williams & Wilkins Publishers.

Chapter 16

American Academy of Pediatrics. (2000). Diagnosis and evaluation of the child with attention deficit-hyperactivity disorder. *Pediatrics 105*(5), 1158–1170.

Baldessarini, R. J. (2001). Drugs and the treatment of psychiatric disorders: Depression and anxiety disorders. In J. G. Hardman, L. E. Limbird, & A. G. Goodman (Eds.), *The pharmacological basis of therapeutics* (pp. 447–484). New York: McGraw-Hill.

Bodkin J. A., & Amsterdam, J. D. (2002). Transdermal selegiline in major depression: A double-blind, placebo-controlled study in outpatients. *J Psychiatry, 159*(11), 1869–1875.

Brown, C. S., Markowitz, J. S., Moore, T. R., & Parker, N. G. (1999). Atypical antipsychotics: Part II. Adverse effects, drug interactions, and costs. *Ann Pharmacother 33*, 210–217.

Burns, M. J. (2001). The pharmacology and toxicology of atypical antipsychotic agents. *J of Toxicol: Clin Toxicol 39*(1), 1.

Desai, H. D., & Jann, M. W. (2000). Major depression in women: A review of the literature. *J Am Pharm Assoc 40*(4), 525–537.

Eli Lilly & Company. (2003). *Strattera: Safety information for health care professionals*. Indianapolis, IN: Author, www.strattera.com

Emslie, G. J., & Mayes, T. L. (1999). Depression in children and adolescents: A guide to diagnosis and treatment. *CNS Drugs 11*(3), 181–189.

Janicak, P. (2002). Research report: rTMS vs. ECT in depressed patients. Chicago: University of Illinois.

Lin, K. M. (1982). Cultural aspects in mental health for Asian Americans. In A. Gaw (Ed.), *Cross cultural psychiatry* (pp. 69–73). Boston: John Wright.

Medical Economics Staff (Ed.). (2000). *PDR for herbal medicines*. Montvale, NJ: Author.

Moses, S. (2003). Imipramine. *Family practice notebook*. Lino Lakes, MN: Family Practice Notebook, LLC, www.fpnotebook.com

National Association of State Boards of Education. (2003). The use and abuse of Ritalin. *Policy Update 7*(18). Alexandria VA: Author.

Schellenburg, R. (2001). Treatment for the premenstrual syndrome with agnus castus fruit extract: Prospective, randomized placebo-controlled study. *British Medical Journal 322*(279), 134.

Sifton, D. (Ed.). (2002). *Health care provider's desk reference (PDR)*. Montvale, NJ: Medical Economics Company.

Spector, R. E. (2000). *Cultural diversity in health and illness*. Upper Saddle River, NJ: Prentice Hall Health.

Chapter 17

Bailey, K. (2003). Aripiprazole: The newest antipsychotic agent for the treatment of schizophrenia. *Psychosocial Nursing and Mental Health Services 41*(2), 14–18.

Baldessarini, R. J., & Tarazi, F. I. (2001). Drugs and the treatment of psychiatric disorders: Psychosis and mania. In J. G. Hardman, L. E. Limbird, & A. G. Goodman (Eds.), *The pharmacological basis of therapeutics* (pp. 485–520). New York: McGraw-Hill.

Barclay, L. (2002, July 1). Quetiapine well-tolerated, effective in refractory schizophrenia. *Medscape Medical News*, www.medscape.com

Barthel, R. (2002, October 27). Early interventions in psychosis. *Medscape Medical News*, www.medscape.com

Brown University Child and Adolescent Psychopharmacology Update. (2002, July 19). Drugs in the pipeline: New drugs and indications for children and adolescents, www.medscape.com

Brown University Geriatric Psychopharmacology Update. (2002, December 9). Treating bipolar disorder in older adults: Gaps in knowledge remain, www.medscape.com

Burns, M. J. (2001). The pharmacology and toxicology of atypical antipsychotic agents. *J Toxicol: Clin Toxicol 39*(1), 1.

Cada, D., Levien, T., & Baker, D. (2003). Aripiprazole. *Hospital Pharmacy 38*(3), 247–254.

Kneisl, C. R., Wilson, H.S., & Trigoboff, E. (2004). *Contemporary psychiatric-mental health nursing*. Upper Saddle River, NJ: Prentice Hall.

Markowitz, J. S., Brown, C. S., & Moore, T. R. (1999). Atypical antipsychotics: Part I. Pharmacology, pharmacokinetics, and efficacy. *Ann Pharmacother 33*, 73–85.

Medical Economics Staff (Ed.). (2000). *PDR for herbal medicines*. Montvale, NJ: Author.

Medscape Medical News. (2003, February 13). Dispensing errors reported for serzone and seroquel, www.medscape.com

Vitiello, B. (2001). Psychopharmacology for young children: Clinical needs and research opportunities. *Pediatrics 108*(4), 983.

Wahlbeck, K., Cheine, M., & Essali, M. A. (2002, April 1). Clozapine versus typical neuroleptic medication for schizophrenia. *Cochrane Review Abstracts*, www.medscape.com

Chapter 18

Alzheimer's disease. (2003, April 11). Unraveling the mystery. The search for new treatments, www.alzheimers.org

Alzheimer's disease fact sheet, www.alzheimers.org

Birks, J., Grimley-Evans, J., & Van Dongen, M. (2003). Ginkgo biloba for cognitive impairment and dementia. *Medscape*, www.medscape.com

Brain-cell growth protein shows promise for Parkinson's in early human trial, www.parkinsons-foundation.org

Capozza, K. (2003, April 2). Drug slows progression of Alzheimer's, www.nlm.nih.gov/medlineplus

Cummings, J. L. (2000). Treatment of Alzheimer's disease. *Clinic Corner 3*(4), 27–39.

Dooley, M., & Lamb, H. M. (2000). Donepezil: A review of its use in Alzheimer's disease. *Drugs and Aging 16*(3), 199–226.

Gruetzner, H. (2001). *Alzheimer's: A caregiver's guide and sourcebook* (3rd ed.). Indianapolis: John Wiley & Sons.

Hristove, A. H., & Koller, W. C. (2000). Early Parkinson's disease: What is the best approach in treatment? *Drugs Aging 17*(3), 165–181.

Kahle, P. (2003). *Molecular mechanisms of Parkinson's disease*. Georgetown, TX: Eurekah.com, Inc.

Lambert, D., & Waters, C. H. (2000). Comparative tolerability of the new generation antiparkinson agents. *Drugs and Aging 16*(1), 55–65.

Olanow, C. W., & Tatton, W. G. (1999). Etiology and pathogenesis of Parkinson's disease. *Ann Rev Neurosci 2*, 123–144.

Richter, R. (Ed.). (2003). *Alzheimer's disease: The Physicians guide to practical management*. Totowa, NJ: Human Press.

Standaert, D. G., & Young, A. B. (2001). Treatment of central nervous system degenerative disorders. In J. G. Hardman, L. E. Limbird, & A. G. Goodman (Eds.), *The pharmacological basis of therapeutics* (pp. 549–568). New York: McGraw-Hill.

Chapter 19

Bannwarth, B. (1999). Risk-benefit assessment of opioids in chronic noncancer pain. *Drug Safety 21*(4), 283–296.

Barkin, R. L., & Barkin, D. (2001). Pharmacologic management of acute and chronic pain: Focus on drug interactions and patient-specific pharmacotherapeutic selection. *South Med J 94*(8), 756–812.

Bell, J., Kimber, J., Mattick, R., Ali, R., Lintzers, N., Monhert, B., Quigley, A., Ritter A., & White, J. (2003). Interim clinical guidelines: Use of naltrexone in relapse prevention for opioid dependence (abbreviated version). Washington, DC: Office of Disease Prevention and Health Promotion, United States Department of Health and Human Services, www.health.gov

Broadbent, C. (2000). The pharmacology of acute pain—Part 3. *Nursing Times 96*(26), 39.

Tfelt-Hansen, P., DeVries, P., & Sexena, P. R. (2000). Triptans in migraine: A comparative review of pharmacology, pharmacokinetics, and efficacy. *Drugs 60*(6), 1259–1287.

Diamond, M. (2003). Emergency treatment of headache. Chicago: Internal Medicine Department, Columbus Hospital, www.usdoctor.com

Glajchen, M. (2001). Chronic pain. Treatment barriers and strategies for clinical practice. *J Am Board Fam Pract 14*(3), 178–183.

Guay, D. R. P. (2001). Adjunctive agents in the management of chronic pain. *Pharmacother 21*(9), 1070–1081.

Gunsteuin, H., & Akil, H. (2001). Opioid analgesics. In J. G. Hardman, L. E. Limbird, & A. G. Goodman (Eds.), *The pharmacological basis of therapeutics* (pp. 569–620). New York: McGraw-Hill.

Khouzam, H. R. (2000). Chronic pain and its management in primary care. *South Med J 93*(10), 946–952.

Moses, S. (Ed.). (2002). Sub-arachnoid hemorrhage. *Family Practice Notebook*, www.fpnotebook.com/NEU28.htm

National Reye's Syndrome Foundation, Inc. (2000). Aspirin or salicylate-containing medications. Bryan, OH: Author, www.reyessyndrome.org

Office of Disease Prevention and Health Promotion, United States Department of Health and Human Services. (2003). Section 11: Gastrointestinal system. Washington, DC: Author, www.health.gov

Rialto.com. (2003). Clinical aspects of G6PD deficiency, www.rialto.com

RxList.com. (2003). Bayer ASA side effects & ASA drug interactions, www.rxlist.com

Tepper, S. J., & Rapoport, A. M. (1999). The triptans: A summary. *CNS Drugs 12*(5), 403–417.

Chapter 20

Catterall, W. A., & Mackie, K.(2001). Local anesthetics. In J. G. Hardman, L. E. Limbird, & A. G. Goodman (Eds.), *The pharmacological basis of therapeutics* (pp. 367–384). New York: McGraw-Hill.

Colbert, B. J., & Mason, B. J. (2001). *Integrated cardiopulmonary pharmacology*. New Jersey: Prentice Hall.

Evers, A., & Crowder, C. M. (2001). General anesthetics. In J. G. Hardman, L. E. Limbird, & A. G. Goodman (Eds.), *The pharmacological basis of therapeutics* (pp. 337–366). New York: McGraw-Hill.

KidsHealth for Parents. (2003). Your child's anesthesia. *The Nemours Foundation*, http://www.kidshealth.org

Medline Plus. (2003). General anesthesia. *National Institute of Health*, http://www.search.nlm.nih.gov/medlineplus

Nagelhout, J. J., Nagelhout, K., & Zaglaniczny, V. H. (2001). *Handbook of nurse anesthesia* (2nd ed.). Philadelphia: W. B. Saunders.

Omogui, S. (1999). *Sota Omogui's anesthesia drugs handbook* (3rd ed.). Hawthorne, CA: State of the Art Technologies.

Stoelting, R. K. (1999). *Pharmacology and physiology in anesthetic practice* (3rd ed.). Philadelphia: Lippincott, Williams, & Wilkins.

Waugaman, W. R., Foster, S. D., & Rigor, B. M. (1999). *Principles and practice of nurse anesthesia* (3rd ed.). Upper Saddle River, NJ: Prentice Hall.

Chapter 21

Allergy Resources International. (2003). Angioedema, http://allallergy.net/articles/index.cfm/edeoc/AO

Colbert, B. J., & Mason, B. J. (2001). *Integrated cardiopulmonary pharmacology*. Upper Saddle River, NJ: Prentice Hall.

Hajjar, I. M., Grim, C. E., George, V., & Kotchen, T. A. (2001). Impact of diet on blood pressure and age-related changes in blood pressure in the U.S. population: Analysis of NHANES III. *Archives of Internal Medicine 161*, 589.

Klag, M. J., Wang, N. Y., Meoni, L. A., Brancati, F. L., Cooper, L. A., Liang, K. Y., Young, J. H., & Ford, D. E. (2002). Coffee. Intake and risk of hypertension. The Johns Hopkins Precursors Study. *Arch Intern Med 162*, 657–662.

National Emphysema Foundation. (2003). Grapefruit juice and drugs, http://emphysemafoundation.org

National High Blood Pressure Education Program. National Heart, Lung & Blood Institute. (2003). *JNC–7 Express: The Seventh Report of the Joint National Committee on Prevention, Detection, Evaluation and Treatment of High Blood Pressure*. Bethesda, MD: Author.

National Institutes of Health. (2003). NHLBI issues new high blood pressure clinical practice guidelines. *NIH NEWS*, www.nhlbi.nih.gov

Nurko, S. (2001). At what level of hyperkalemia or creatinine elevation should ACE inhibitor therapy be stopped or not started? *Cleveland Clinic Journal of Medicine 68*, 9, 754–760.

Oates, J. A., & Brown, N. J. (2001). Antihypertensive agents and the drug therapy of hypertension. In J. G. Hardman, L. E. Limbard, & A. G. Goodman (Eds.), *The pharmacological basis of therapeutics* (pp. 871–900). New York: McGraw-Hill.

Poudre Valley Health System. (2003). Herbal medicines and dietary supplements: Information for people with heart disease, www.pvhs.org

Sifton, D. (2002). *The health care provider's desk reference (PDR)* (56th ed.). Montvale, NJ: Medical Economics Company.

Simpson, C. (2003). Autonomic nervous system agents: Adrenergics and adrenergic blocking agents, www.cotc.tech.oh.us

Thadhani, R., Camargo, Jr., C. A., Stampfer, M. J., Curhan, G. C., Willett, W. C., & Rimm, E. B. (2002). Prospective study of moderate alcohol consumption and risk of hypertension in young women. *Arch Intern Med 162*, 569–574.

University of Illinois at Chicago, College of Pharmacy Drug Information Center. (2003). Can angiotensin receptor blockers be administered to patients who develop angioedema while receiving ACE inhibitors? www.uic.edu

Woods, A. D. (2001). Improving the odds against hypertension. *Nursing 2001 31*(8), 36–42.

Chapter 22

Albrant, D. H. (2001). Drug treatment protocol: Management of chronic systolic heart failure. *J Am Pharm Assoc 41*(5), 672–681.

Gomberg-Maitland, M., Baran, D. A., & Fuster, V. (2001). Treatment of congestive heart failure: Guidelines for the primary care health care provider and the heart failure specialist. *Arch Intern Med 161*, 342–352.

Jamali, A. H., Tang, A. H. W., Khot, U. N., & Fowler, M. B. (2001). The role of angiotensin receptor blockers in the management of chronic heart failure. *Arch Intern Med 161*, 667–672.

Ooi, H., & Colucci, W. (2001). Pharmacological treatment of heart failure. In J. G. Hardman, L. E. Limbard, & A. G. Goodman (Eds.), *The pharmacological basis of therapeutics* (pp. 901–932). New York: McGraw-Hill.

Opie, L. H., & Gersh, B. J. (Eds.). (2001). *Drugs for the heart* (5th ed.). Philadelphia: W. B. Saunders.

Paul, S. (2002). Balancing diuretic therapy in heart failure: Loop diuretics, thiazides, and antagonists. *CHF 8*(6), 307–312.

Richardson, L. G. (2003). Psychosocial issues in patients with congestive heart failure. *Progressive Cardiovascular Nursing 18*(1), 19–27.

Sperelakis, N., Kurachi, Y., Terzic, A., & Cohen, M. (Eds.). (2001). *Heart physiology and pathophysiology* (4th ed.). San Diego: Academic Press.

Steering Committee and Membership of the Advisory Council to Improve Outcomes Nationwide in Heart Failure. (1999). Consensus recommendations for the management of chronic heart failure. *Am J Cardiol 83*(2A), 1A–38A.

Van Bakel, A. B., & Chidsey, G. (2000). Management of advanced heart failure. *Clinic Corner 3*(2), 25–35.

Chapter 23

Dayer, M., & Hardman, S. (2002). Special problems with antiarrhythmic drugs in the elderly: Safety, tolerability, and efficacy. *Amer J of Geriatric Cardiol 11*(6), 370–375.

Falk, R. H. (2001). Medical progress: Atrial fibrillation. *N Eng J Med 344*, 1067–1078.

Fenton, J. M. (2001). The clinician's approach to evaluating patients with dysrhythmias. *AACN Clin Issues 12*(1), 72–86.

Haugh, K. H. (2002). Antidysrhythmic agents at the turn of the twenty-first century: A current review. *Crit Care Nurs Clin North Am Mar 14*(1), 53–69.

Huikuri, H. V., Castellanos, A., & Myerburg, R. J. (2001). Medical progress: Sudden death due to cardiac arrhythmias. *N Eng J Med 345*, 1473–1482.

Kudzma, E. C. (2001). Cultural competence: Cardiovascular medications. Progress in Cardiovascular Inderal. Medscape Drug-Info (2003), www.medscape.com/druginfo/

Morrill, P. (2000). Pharmacotherapeutics of positive inotropes. *AORN-Journal 71*(1), 173–178, 181–185.

Podrid, P. J., & Kowey, P. R. (Eds.). (2001). *Cardiac arrhythmia: Mechanisms, diagnosis, and management* (2nd ed.). Philadelphia: Lippincott, Williams, & Wilkins.

Roden, D. M. (2001). Antidysrhythmic drugs. In J. G. Hardman, L. E. Limbard, & A. G. Goodman (Eds.), *The pharmacological basis of therapeutics* (pp. 933–970). New York: McGraw-Hill.

Chapter 24

Alligood, K. A., & Iltz, J. L. (2001). Update on antithrombotic use and mechanism of action. *Prog in Card Nurs 16*(2), 81–85.

HealthSquare.com. (2003). *Coumadin: Prescription drug reference*, www.healthsquare.com

Hiatt, W. R. (2001). Drug therapy: Medical treatment of peripheral arterial disease and claudication. *N Engl J Med 344*, 1608–1621.

Majerus, P. W., & Tollefson, D. M. (2001). Anticoagulant, thrombolytic, and antiplatelet drugs. In J. G. Hardman, L. E. Limbard, & A. G. Goodman (Eds.), *The pharmacological basis of therapeutics* (pp. 1519–1538). New York: McGraw-Hill.

Sifton, D. (Ed.). (2002). *Health care provider's desk reference (PDR)*. Montvale, NJ: Medical Economics Company.

Vasant, B. P., & Moliterno, D. J. (2000). Glycoprotein IIb/IIIa antagonist and fibrinolytic agents: New therapeutic regimen for acute myocardial infarction. *J Invasive Cardiol 12*(B), 8B–15B.

Chapter 25

Ambrose, J., & Dangas, G. (2000). Unstable angina: Current concepts of pathogenesis and treatment. *Arch Int Med 160*, 25–37.

Deedwania, P. C. (2000). Silent myocardial ischemia in the elderly. *Drugs & Aging 16*(5), 381–389.

Kerins, D. M., Robertson, R. M., & Robertson, D. (2001). Drugs used for the treatment of myocardial ischemia. In J. G. Hardman et al. (Eds.), *The pharmacological basis of therapeutics* (10th ed.). New York: McGraw-Hill.

Kreisberg, R. A. (2000). Overview of coronary heart disease and selected risk factors. *Clin Rev* (Spring), 4–9.

Larsen, J. A., Kadish, A. H., & Schwartz, J. B. (2000). Proper use of antiarrhythmic therapy for reduction of mortality after myocardial infarction. *Drugs & Aging 16*(5), 341–350.

Levine, G. N., Ali, M. N., & Schafer, A. I. (2001). Antithrombotic therapy in patients with acute coronary syndromes. *Arch Intern Med 161*, 937–948.

Parchure, N., & Brecker, S. J. (2002). Management of acute coronary syndromes. *Curr Opin Crit Care 8*(3), 230–235.

Priglinger, U., & Huber, K. (2000). Thrombolytic therapy in acute myocardial infarction. *Drugs & Aging 16*(4), 301–312.

Sarti, C., Kaarisalo, M., & Tuomilehto, J. (2000). The relationship between cholesterol and stroke. Implications for antihyperlipidemic therapy in older patients. *Drugs & Aging 17*(1), 33–51.

Staniforth, A. D. (2001). Contemporary management of chronic stable angina. *Drugs & Aging 18*(2), 109–121.

Chapter 26

Baumgartner, J. D., & Calandra, T. (1999). Treatment of sepsis: Past and future avenues. *Drugs 57*(2), 127–132.

Cummins, R. (Ed.). (1999). *Advanced cardiac life support*. Dallas: American Heart Association.

Dellinger, R. P. (2003). Cardiovascular management of septic shock. *Crit Care Med 31*(3), 946–955.

Hasdai, D., Berger, P. B., Battler, A., & Holmes, D. R. (2002). *Cardiogenic shock: Diagnosis and treatment.* Totowa, NJ: Humana Press.

Kolecki, P., & Menckhoff, C. R. (2001, December 11). Hypovolemic shock. *eMedicine Journal 2*(12).

Menon, V., & Fincke, R. (2003). Cardiogenic shock: A summary of the randomized SHOCK trial. *Congest Heart Fail 9*(1), 35–39.

Moser-Wade, D. M., Bartley, M. K., & Chiari-Allwein, H. L. (2000). Shock: Do you know how to respond? *Nursing 30*(10), 34–40.

Von Rosenstiel, N., von Rosenstiel, I., & Adam, D. (2001). Management of sepsis and septic shock in infants and children. *Paediatr Drugs 3*(1), 9–27.

Chapter 27

American Association of Clinical Endocrinologists. (2002). Medical guidelines for clinical practice for the diagnosis and treatment of dyslipidemia and prevention of atherogenesis. Amended version *Endocrine Practice 6*(2), March/April 2000.

Beaird, S. L. (2000). HMG-CoA reductase inhibitors: Assessing differences in drug interactions and safety profiles. *J Am Pharm Assoc 40*(5), 637–644.

Illingworth, D. R. (2000). Management of hypercholesterolemia. *Med Clin North Am 84*(1), 23–42.

Kreisberg, R. A. (2000). Art and science of statin use. *Clin Rev* (Spring), 47–51.

Law, M. (2000). Plant stanol and sterol margarines. *Brit Med J 320*, 861–864.

Mahley, R. W., & Bersot, T. P. (2001). Drug therapy for hypercholesterolemia and dyslipidemia. In J. G. Hardman, L. E. Limbard, & A. G. Goodman (Eds.), *The pharmacological basis of therapeutics* (pp. 971–1002). New York: McGraw-Hill.

Maltin, L. (2002, April 9). Statin drugs may fight Alzheimer's, too. WebMD Medical News. my.webmd.com/content/article/16/1626_50907

Nutrition and Metabolism Advisory Committee, Heart Foundation. (2001) Plant sterols and stanols, a position statement. Melbourne, Australia: Heart Foundation.

Oberman, A. (2000). Role of lipids in the prevention of cardiovascular disease. *Clin Rev* (Spring), 10–15.

Robinson, A. W., Sloan, H. L., & Arnold, G. (2001). Use of niacin in the prevention and management of hyperlipidemia. *Prog Cardiovasc Nurs 16*(1), 14–20.

U. S. Food and Drug Administration Center for Food Safety and Applied Nutrition, Office of Nutritional Products, Labeling, and Dietary Supplements. (2001, February). New dietary ingredients in dietary supplements (updated September 10, 2001).

Young, K. L., Allen, J. K., & Kelly, K. M. (2001). HDL cholesterol: Striving for healthier levels. *Clin Rev 11*(5), 50–61.

Chapter 28

Bailey, L. B., Rampersaud, G. C., & Kauwell, G. P. (2003). Folic acid supplements and fortification affect the risk for neural tube defects, vascular disease and cancer: Evolving science. *J Nutr 133*(6), 1961S–1968S.

Dharmarajan, T. S., Adiga, G. U., & Norkus, E. P. (2003). Vitamin B_{12} deficiency. Recognizing subtle symptoms in older adults. *Geriatrics 58*(3), 30–34, 37–38.

Eden, A. N. (2003). Preventing iron deficiency in toddlers: A major public health problem. *Contemporary Pediatrics 20*(2), 57–67.

Edroso, R. (2003). Understanding HIV fatigue: What's dragging you down? WebMDHealth, http://my.webmd.com

Marcus, R., & Coulston, A. M. (2001). Water-soluble vitamins: The vitamin B complex and ascorbic acid. In J. G. Hardman, L. E. Limbard, & A. G. Goodman (Eds.), *The pharmacological basis of therapeutics* (pp. 1753–1772). New York: McGraw-Hill.

Oh, R., & Brown, D. L. (2003). Vitamin B_{12} deficiency. *Am Fam Health Care Provider 67*(5), 979–986.

Rampersaud, G. C., Kauwell, G. P., & Bailey, L. B. (2003). Folate: A key to optimizing health and reducing disease risk in the elderly. *J Am Coll Nutr 22*(1), 1–8.

Somer, E. (2003). Ironing out anemia. WebMDHealth, http://my.webmd.com

Chapter 29

Celli, B. (2003). *Pharmacotherapy in chronic obstructive pulmonary disease.* New York: Marcel Dekker.

Colbert, B. J., & Mason, B. J. (2001). *Integrated cardiopulmonary pharmacology.* Upper Saddle River, NJ: Prentice Hall.

Drazen, J. M., Israel, E., & O'Bryne, P. M. (1999, January 21). Treatment of asthma with drugs modifying the leukotriene pathway. *N Engl J Med 340*, 197–206.

Fink, J. (2000). Metered dose inhalers, dry powder inhalers and transitions. *Respir Care 45*, 623–635.

Rogers, D. F. (2003). Airway hypersecretion in allergic rhinitis and asthma: New pharmacotherapy. *Curr Allergy Asthma Rep 3*(3), 238–248.

Rosenwasser, L. J. (2002). Treatment of allergic rhinitis. *Am J Med 16*(113, Suppl 9A), 17S–24S.

Stevens, N. (2003). Inhaler devices for asthma and COPD: Choice and technique. *Prof Nurse 18*(11), 641–645.

Undem, B. J., & Lichtenstein, L. M. (2001). Drugs used in the treatment of asthma. In J. G. Hardman, L. E. Limbard, & A. G. Goodman (Eds.), *The pharmacological basis of therapeutics.* New York: McGraw-Hill.

Wheeler, L. (2003, Mar-April). The last word: asthma management in schools. *FDA Consumer 37*(2).

Chapter 30

Capriotti, T. (2001). Monoclonal antibodies: Drugs that combine pharmacology and biotechnology. *MedSurg Nursing 10*(2), 89.

Centers for Disease Control. (2003). Fact Sheet: Racial and ethnic disparities in health care. U.S. Department of Health and Human Services, http://www.cdc.gov/od/oc/media/pressrel/fs020514b/htm

Centers for Disease Control and Prevention. (2003). National Vaccine Program Office: Immunization laws, http://www.cdc.gov/od/nvpo/law.htm

Children's Defense Fund. (2003). Every child deserves a healthy start, www.childrensdefense.org/hs-tp-immuniz.php

Fitzgerald, K. A., O'Neill, L. A., & Gearing, A. J. (Eds.). (2001). *The cytokine factsbook* (2nd ed.). Burlington, MA: Elsevier Science & Technology Books.

Karam, U. S., & Reddy, K. R. (2003). Pegylated interferons. *Clin Liver Dis 7*(1), 139–148.

Krensky, A. M., Strom, T. B., & Bluestone, J. A. (2001). Immunomodulators: Immunosuppressive agents, toleragens, and immunostimulants. In J. G. Hardman, L. E. Limbard, & A. G. Goodman (Eds.), *The pharmacological basis of therapeutics* (pp. 1463–1484). New York: McGraw-Hill.

Neuzil, K. M. (2003). Adult immunizations: A review of current recommendations, www.medscape.com

Santamaria, P. (2003). *Cytokines and autoimmune disease*. New York: Kluwer Academic/Plenum Publishers.

Sur, D. K., Wallis, D. H., & O'Connell, T. X. (2003). Vaccinations in pregnancy. *Am Fam Physician 68*, E299–E309.

Thomson, A. W., & Lotze, M. T. (2003). *The cytokine handbook* (4th ed., vols. 1–2). Burlington, MA: Elsevier Science & Technology Books.

Chapter 31

Baigent, C., & Patrono, C. (2003). Selective cyclooxygenase-2 inhibitors, aspirin, and cardiovascular disease: A reappraisal. *Arthritis Rheum 48*(1), 12–20.

Berger, W. E. (2003). Overview of allergic rhinitis. *Ann Allergy Asthma Immunol 90*(6, Suppl 3), 7–12.

Braunstahl, G., & Hellings, P. W. (2003). Allergic rhinitis and asthma: The link further unraveled. *Curr Opinion in Pulm Med 9*(1), 46–51.

Fitzgerald, G. A., & Patrono, C. (2001). Drug therapy: The coxibs, selective inhibitors of cyclooxygenase-2. *N Engl J Med 345*, 433–442.

Galley, H. F. (2002). *Critical care focus: Vol. 10. Inflammation and immunity*. London: BMJ Books.

Jackson, L. M., & Hawkey, C. J. (2000). COX-2 selective nonsteroidal anti-inflammatory drugs: Do they really offer any advantages? *Drugs 59*(6), 1207–1216.

Nathan, R. A. (2003). Pharmacotherapy for allergic rhinitis: A critical review of leukotriene receptor antagonists compared with other treatments. *Ann Allergy Asthma Immunol 90*(2), 182–190.

Raeburn, D., & Giembycz, M. A. (Eds.). (2001). *Rhinitis: Immunopathology and pharmacotherapy*. Boston: Birkhauser.

Roberts, L. J., & Morrow, J. D. (2001). Analgesic-antipyretic and anti-inflammatory agents employed in the treatment of gout. In J. G. Hardman, L. E. Limbard, & A. G. Goodman (Eds.), *The pharmacological basis of therapeutics* (pp. 687–732). New York: McGraw-Hill.

Sklar, G. E. (2002). Hemolysis as a potential complication of acetaminophen overdose in a patient with glucose-6-phosphate dehydrogenase deficiency. *Pharmacotherapy 22*(5), 656–658.

Chapter 32

Barclay, L. (2003). Linezolid treats resistant gram-positive infections in children. *Pediatr Infect Dis J 23*, 677–685.

Chambers, H. F. (2001). Antimicrobial agents: The aminoglycosides. In J. G. Hardman, L. E. Limbard, & A. G. Goodman (Eds.), *The pharmacological basis of therapeutics* (pp. 1219–1239). New York: McGraw-Hill.

Diekema, D., & Jones, R. (2001). Oxazolidinones: A review. *Drugs 59*(1), 7–16.

Gilbert, D. N., Moellering, R. C., & Sande, M. A. (2001). *The Sanford guide to antimicrobial therapy 2001* (31st ed.). Hyde Park, VT: Antimicrobial Therapy, Inc.

Moran, G. J., & Mount, J. (2003). Update on emerging infections: News from the Centers for Disease Control and Prevention. *Ann Emerg Med 41*(1), 148–151.

Petri, W. A. (2001). Antimicrobial agents: Penicillins, cephalosporins, and other beta-lactam antibiotics. In J. G. Hardman, L. E. Limbard, & A. G. Goodman (Eds.), *The pharmacological basis of therapeutics* (pp. 1189–1218). New York: McGraw-Hill.

Petri, W. A. (2001). Antimicrobial agents: Sulfonamides, trimethoprim-sulfamethasoxazole, quinolones, and agents for urinary tract infections. In J. G. Hardman, L. E. Limbard, & A. G. Goodman (Eds.), *The pharmacological basis of therapeutics* (pp. 1171–1188). New York: McGraw-Hill.

Petri, W. A. (2001). Drugs used in the chemotherapy of tuberculosis, *Mycobacterium avium* complex disease, and leprosy. In J. G. Hardman, L. E. Limbard, & A. G. Goodman (Eds.), *The pharmacological basis of therapeutics* (pp. 1273–1294). New York: McGraw-Hill.

Sheff, B. (2001). Taking aim at antibiotic-resistant bacteria. *Nursing 2001 31*(11), 62–68.

Small, P. M., & Fujiwara, P. I. (2001). Medical progress: Management of tuberculosis in the United States. *N Engl J Med 345*, 189–200.

Spector, R. E. (2000). *Cultural diversity in health & illness*. Upper Saddle River, NJ: Prentice Hall.

Wooten, J., & Sakind, A. (2003). Superbugs: Unmasking the threat. *RN 66*(3), 37–43.

Chapter 33

Bennet, J. E. (2001). Antimicrobial agents: Antifungal agents. In J. G. Hardman et al. (Eds.), *The pharmacological basis of therapeutics* (10th ed.). New York: McGraw-Hill.

Centers for Disease Control and Prevention. (2002). Recommendations of the International Task Force of Disease Eradication. *MMWR*, U.S. Department of Health and Human Services.

Dickson, R., Awasthi, S., Dimellweek, C., & Williamson, P. (2003). Anthelmintic drugs for treating worms in children: Effects on growth and cognitive performance. *Cochrane Review*, http://www.medscape.com

Kontoyiannis, D. P., Mantadakis, E., & Samonis, G. (2003). Systemic mycoses in the immunocompromised host: An update in antifungal therapy. *J Hosp Infect 53*(4), 243–258.

Pray, W. S. (2001). Treatment of vaginal fungal infections. *U.S. Pharmacist 26*(9).

Steile, R. W. (2002). Focus on infection, prevention detection and treatment. Medscape Medical News, http://www.medscape.com

Re, V. L., & Gluckman, S. J. (2003). Prevention of malaria in travelers. *Am Fam Physician 68*, 509–514, 515–516.

Tracy, J. W., & Webster, L. T. (2001). Drugs used in the chemotherapy of protozoal infections: Malaria. In J. G. Hardman et al. (Eds.), *The pharmacological basis of therapeutics* (10th ed.). New York: McGraw-Hill.

Turness, B. W., Beach, M. J., & Roberts, J. M. (2000). Giardiasis surveillance. *MMWR*, Center for Disease Control.

Chapter 34

Almuente, V. (2002). Herbal therapy in patients with HIV. *Medscape Pharmacists 3*(2), 1–4.

Duggan, J., Peterson, W. S., Schutz, M., Khuder, S., & Chakraborty, J. (2001). Use of complementary and alternative therapies in HIV-infected patients. *AIDS Pat Care and STDS 15*, 159–167.

Goldschmidt, R. H., & Dong, B. J. (2001). Treatment of AIDS and HIV-related conditions. *J Am Board Fam Pract 14*(4), 283–309.

Hayden, F. G. (2001). Antimicrobial agents: Antiviral agents (nonretroviral). In J. G. Hardman, L. E. Limbard, & A. G. Goodman (Eds.), *The pharmacological basis of therapeutics* (pp. 1313–1348). New York: McGraw-Hill.

HIV Panel on Clinical Practices for Treatment of HIV Infection. (2000). Guidelines for the use of antiretroviral agents in HIV-infected adults and adolescents. Washington DC: U.S. Department of Health and Human Services, http://www.hivatis.org/guidelines/adult/Feb0501/

Idemyor, V. (2003). Twenty years since human immunodeficiency virus discovery: Considerations for the next decade. *Pharmacotherapy 23*, 384–387.

Kirkbride, H. A., & Watson, J. (2003). Review of the use of neuraminidase inhibitors for prophylaxis of influenza. *Commun Dis Public Health 6*(2), 123–127.

Kuritzkes, D. R., Boyle, B. A., Gallant, J. E., Squires, K. E., & Zolopa, A. (2003). Current management challenges in HIV: Antiretroviral resistance. *AIDS Read 13*(3), 133–135, 138–142.

Lesho, E. P., & Gey, D. C. (2003). Managing issues related to antiretroviral therapy. *Am Fam Physician 68*, 675–686, 689–690.

Ofotokun, I., & Pomeroy, C. (2003). Sex differences in adverse reactions to antiretroviral drugs. *Top HIV Med 11*(2), 55–59.

Raffanti, S. P., & Haas, D. W. (2001). Antimicrobial agents: Antiretroviral agents. In J. G. Hardman, L. E. Limbard, & A. G. Goodman (Eds.), *The pharmacological basis of therapeutics* (pp. 1349–1380). New York: McGraw-Hill.

Walker, B. D. (2002). Immune reconstitution and immunotherapy in HIV infection. Medscape Clin Update, http://www.medscape.com/viewprogram/2435

Chapter 35

Birner, A. (2003). Safe administration of oral chemotherapy. *Clin J of Oncol Nur 2*, 158–162.

Breed, C. D. (2003). Diagnosis, treatment, and nursing care of patients with chronic leukemia. *Semin Oncol Nurs 19*(2), 109–117.

Buzdar, A. U. (2000). Tamoxifen's clinical applications: Old and new. *Arch Fam Med 9*, 906–912.

Chabner, B. A., Ryan, D. P., Paz-Ares, L., Garcia-Carbonero, R., & Calabresi, P. (2001). Antineoplastic agents. In J. G. Hardman, L. E. Limbard, & A. G. Goodman (Eds.), *The pharmacological basis of therapeutics* (10th ed.). New York: McGraw-Hill.

Chemoprevention of Breast Cancer: Recommendations and Rationale, U.S. Preventive Services Task Force. (2003). *Am Fam Physician 67*(6), 1309–1314.

Dalton, R. R., & Kallab, A. M. (2001). Chemoprevention of breast cancer. *South Med J 94*(1), 7–1.

Hood, L. E. (2003). Chemotherapy in the elderly: Supportive measures for chemotherapy-induced myelotoxicity. *Clin J of Oncology Nurs 7*(2), 185–190.

Moran, P. (2000). Cellular effects of cancer chemotherapy administration. *J of Infusion Nur 23*(1), 44.

Rieger, P. (2001). *Biotherapy: A comprehensive overview* (2nd ed.). Sudbury, MA: Jones and Bartlett.

Rugo, H. (2001, October 15). How to succeed with breast cancer adjuvant therapy, http://healthology.com

Smith, B., Waltzman, R., & Rugo, H. (2002, December 10). Living longer with cancer: Preserving quality of life, http://healthology.com

Wood, L. (2001). Antineoplastic agents. *J of Infusion Nurs Innovative 24*(1), 48.

Chapter 36

Hoogerwerf, W. A., & Pasricha, P. J. (2001). Agents used for the control of gastric acidity and treatment of peptic ulcers and gastroesophageal reflux disease. In J. G. Hardman, L. E. Limbard, & A. G. Goodman (Eds.), *The pharmacological basis of therapeutics* (10th ed.). New York: McGraw-Hill.

Huggins, R. M., Scates, A. C., & Latour, J. K. (2003). Intravenous proton-pump inhibitors versus H$_2$-antagonists for treatment of GI bleeding. *Ann Pharmacother 37*(3), 433–437.

Meurer, L. N., & Bower, D. J. (2002). Management of *Helicobacter pylori* infection. *Am Fam Physician 65*, 1327–1336, 1339.

Patel, A. S., Pohl, J. F., & Easley, D. J. (2003). What's new: Proton pump inhibitors and pediatrics. *Pediatr Rev 24*(1), 12–5.

Petersen, A. M. (2003). *Helicobacter pylori*: An invading microorganism? A review. *FEMS Immunol Med Microbiol 36*(3), 117–126.

Sharma, P., & Vakil, N. (2003). Review article: *Helicobacter pylori* and reflux disease. *Aliment Pharmacol Ther 17*(3), 297–305.

Stanghellini, V. (2003). Management of gastroesophageal reflux disease. *Drugs Today 39* (Suppl A), 15–20.

Vanderhoff, B. T., & Tahboub, R. M. (2002). Proton pump inhibitors: An update. *Am Fam Physician 66*, 273–280.

Chapter 37

Glazer, G. (2001). Long-term pharmacotherapy of obesity: A review of efficacy and safety. *Arch Intern Med 161*, 1814–1824.

Gordon, C. R., & Shupak, A. (1999). Prevention and treatment of motion sickness in children. *CNS Drugs 12*(5), 369–381.

Guglietta, A. (2003). *Pharmacotherapy of gastrointestinal inflammation*. Basel, Switzerland: Birkhauser Verlag.

Jafri, S., & Pasricha, P. J. (2001). Agents used for diarrhea, constipation and inflammatory bowel disease; Agents used for biliary and pancreatic disease. In J. G. Hardman, L. E. Limbard, & A. G. Goodman (Eds.), *The pharmacological basis of therapeutics* (10th ed.). New York: McGraw-Hill.

Knutson, D., Greenberg, G., & Cronau, H. (2003). Management of Crohn's disease—A practical approach. *Am Fam Physician 68*, 707–714, 717–718.

Pasricha, P. J. (2001). Prokinetic agents, antiemetics and agents used in irritable bowel syndrome. In J. G. Hardman, L. E. Limbard, & A. G. Goodman (Eds.), *The pharmacological basis of therapeutics* (10th ed.). New York: McGraw-Hill.

Pray, W. S. (2000). Diarrhea: Causes and self-care treatments. *U.S. Pharmacist 25*(11).

Spanier, J. A., Howden, C. W., & Jones, M. P. (2003). A systematic review of alternative therapies in the irritable bowel syndrome. *Arch Intern Med 163*(3), 265–274.

Wald, A. (2003). Is chronic use of stimulant laxatives harmful to the colon? *J Clin Gastroenterol 36*(5), 386–389.

Weigle, D. S. (2003). Pharmacological therapy of obesity: Past, present, and future. *J Clin Endocrinol Metab 88*(6), 2462–2469.

Chapter 38

Bhagavan, N. V. (2002). *Medical biochemistry*. Burlington, MA: Harcourt/Academic Press.

Levine, M., Rumsey, S. C., Daruwala, R., et al. (1999). Criteria and recommendations for vitamin C intake. *JAMA 281*, 1415–1423.

Marcus, R., & Coulston, A. M. (2001). Fat-soluble vitamins: Vitamins A, K and E. In J. G. Hardman, L. E. Limbard, & A. G. Goodman (Eds.), *The pharmacological basis of therapeutics* (10th ed.). New York: McGraw-Hill.

Marcus, R., & Coulston, A. M. (2001). Water-soluble vitamins: The vitamin B complex and ascorbic acid. In J. G. Hardman, L. E. Limbard, & A. G. Goodman (Eds.), *The pharmacological basis of therapeutics* (10th ed.). New York: McGraw-Hill.

McDermott, J. H. (2000). Antioxidant nutrients: Current dietary recommendations and research update. *J Am Pharm Assoc 40*(6), 785–799.

Oh, R. C., & Brown, D. L. (2003). Vitamin B$_{12}$ deficiency. *Am Fam Physician 67*, 979–986, 993–994.

Padayatty, S. J., Katz, A., Wang, Y., Eck, P., Kwon, O., Lee, J. H., Chen, S., Corpe, C., Dutta, A., Dutta, S. K., & Levine, M. (2003). Vitamin C as an antioxidant: Evaluation of its role in disease prevention. *J Am Coll Nutr 22*(1), 18–35.

Perrotta, S., Nobili, B., Rossi, F., Di Pinto, D., Cucciolla, V., Borriello, A., Oliva, A., Della Powers, H. J. (2003). Riboflavin (vitamin B$_2$) and health. *Am J Clin Nutr 77*(6), 1352–1360.

Ragione, F. (2003). Vitamin A and infancy. Biochemical, functional, and clinical aspects. *Vitam Horm 66*, 457–591.

Rampersaud, G. C., Kauwell, G. P., & Bailey, L. B. (2003). Folate: A key to optimizing health and reducing disease risk in the elderly. *J Am Coll Nutr 22*(1), 1–8.

Chapter 39

Demester, N. (2001). Diseases of the thyroid: A broad spectrum. *Clin Rev 11*(7), 58–64.

Farwell, A. P., & Braverman, L. E. (2001). Thyroid and antithyroid drugs. In J. G. Hardman et al. (Eds.), *The pharmacological basis of therapeutics* (10th ed.). New York: McGraw-Hill.

Griffiths, H., & Jordan, S. (2002). Corticosteroids: Implications for nursing practice. *Nurs Stand 17*(12), 43–53.

Holcomb, S. S. (2002). Thyroid diseases: A primer for the critical care nurse. *Dimens Crit Care Nurs 21*(4), 127–133.

Margioris, A. N., & Chrousos, G. P. (Eds). (2001). *Adrenal disorders*. Totowa, NJ: Humana Press.

Parker, K. L. & Schimmer, B. P. (2001). Pituitary hormones and their hypothalamic releasing factors. In J. G. Hardman, L. E. Limbard, & A. G. Goodman (Eds.), *The pharmacological basis of therapeutics* (10th ed.). New York: McGraw-Hill.

Schori-Ahmed, D. (2003). Defenses gone awry. Thyroid disease. *RN 66*(6), 38–43.

Winqvist, O., Rorsman, F., & Kämpe, O. (2000). Autoimmune adrenal insufficiency: Recognition and management. *BioDrugs 13*(2): 107–114.

Chapter 40

American Diabetes Association. (2001). Standards of care. *Diabetes Care 24* (Suppl 1), 33–43.

Bates, N. (2002). Overdose of insulin and other diabetic medication. *Emergency Nurse 10*(7), 22–26.

Bohannon, N. J. V. (2002). Treating dual defects in diabetes: Insulin resistance and insulin secretion. *Am J of Health System Pharmacy 59*, 59.

Bell, D. S. H., & Ovalle, F. (2000). Management of type 2 diabetes. *Clin Rev* (Spring), 93–96.

Chehade, J. M., & Mooradian, A. D. (2000). A rational approach to drug therapy of type 2 diabetes mellitus. *Drugs 60*(1), 95–113.

Chen, S. W. (2002). Editorial: Insulin glargine: Basal insulin of choice? *Am J Health System Pharmacy 59*, 609, 643.

Cole, L. (2002). Unraveling the mystery of acute pancreatitis. *Dimen of Critical Care Nur 21*, 86–91.

Davis, S. N., & Granner, D. K. (2001). Insulin, oral hypoglycemic agents and the pharmacology of the endocrine pancreas. In J. G. Hardman, L. E. Limbard, & A. G. Goodman (Eds.), *The pharmacological basis of therapeutics* (10th ed.). New York: McGraw-Hill.

Gottlieb, S. W. (2003). Just the facts: The importance of diabetic research. *Diabetes Forecast 56*, 39–42.

Harrigan, R. A., Nathan, M. S., & Beattie, P. (2001). Oral agents for the treatment of type 2 diabetes mellitus: Pharmacology, toxicity, and treatment. *Ann of Emer Med 38*(1), 68.

Hjwlm, K., Mufunda, E., Nambozi, G., & Kemp, J. (2003). Preparing nurses to face the pandemic of diabetes mellitus: A literature review. *J of Advanced Nur 41*, 424–435.

Mantis, A. K. et al. (2001). Continuous subcutaneous insulin infusion therapy for children and adolescents: An option for routine diabetes care. *Pediatrics 107*, 351–357.

Mitchell, R. M. S., Byrne, M. F., & Baillie, J. (2003). Pancreatitis. *Lancet 361*, 1447–1456.

Mokdad, A. H., Bowman, B. A., & Ford, E. S. (2001). The continuing epidemics of obesity and diabetes in the United States. *JAMA 286*, 1195–1200.

Chapter 41

Conley, C. (2003). Hormonal therapy for breast cancer: Current issues, http://healthology.com

Frackiewicz, E. J., & Shiovitz, T. M. (2001). Evaluation and management of premenstrual syndrome and premenstrual dysphoric disorder. *J Am Pharm Assoc 41*(3), 437–447.

Kusiak, V. (2002). FDA approves prescribing information for postmenopausal hormone therapies, http://www.premarin.com/hep/html

Leeman, L., Fontaine, P., King, V., Klein, M. C., & Ratcliffe, S. (2003). The nature and management of labor pain: Part II. Pharmacologic pain relief. *Am Fam Physician 68*, 1115–1120, 1121–1122.

Loose-Mitchell, D. S., & Stancel, G. M. (2001). Estrogens and progestins. In J. G. Hardman, L. E. Limbard, & A. G. Goodman (Eds.), *The pharmacological basis of therapeutics* (10th ed.). New York: McGraw-Hill.

Ludwig, M., Westergaard, L. G., Diedrich, K., & Andersen, C. Y. (2003). Developments in drugs for ovarian stimulation. *Best Pract Res Clin Obstet Gynaecol 17*(2), 231–247.

Nelson, A. (2000). Contraceptive update Y2K: Need for contraception and new contraceptive options. *Clinic Corner 3*(1), 48–62.

Olds, S. B., London, M. L., Ladewig, P. A., & Davidson, M. R. (2004). *Maternal-newborn nursing and women's health care* (7th ed.). Upper Saddle River, NJ: Prentice Hall Health.

Shepherd, J. E. (2001). Effects of estrogen on cognition, mood, and degenerative brain diseases. *J Am Pharm Assoc 41*(2), 221–228.

Snyder, P. J. (2001). Androgens. In J. G. Hardman, L. E. Limbard, & A. G. Goodman (Eds.), *The pharmacological basis of therapeutics* (10th ed.). New York: McGraw-Hill.

Understanding the WHI study: Assessing the results. (2003). http://www.premarin.com/pdf/Risk.Tearsheet.pdf

Chapter 42

Brock, G. B. (2003). Tadalafil: A new agent for erectile dysfunction. *Can J Urol 10* (Suppl 1), 17–22.

Carrier, S. (2003). Pharmacology of phosphodiesterase 5 inhibitors. *Can J Urol 10* (Suppl 1), 12–6.

Gordon, A. E., & Shaughnessy, A. F. (2003). Saw palmetto for prostate disorders. *Am Fam Physician 67*(6), 1281–1283.

Padma-Nathan, H., Saenz de Tejada, I., Rosen, R. C., & Goldstein, I. (Eds.). (2001). *Pharmacotherapy for erectile dysfunction*. London: Taylor & Francis Books Ltd.

Kassabian, V. S. (2003). Sexual function in patients treated for benign prostatic hyperplasia. *Lancet 361*(9351), 60–62.

Khastgir, J., Arya, M., Shergill, I. S., Kalsi, J. S., Minhas, S., & Mundy, A. R. (2002). Current concepts in the pharmacotherapy of benign prostatic hyperplasia. *Expert Opin Pharmacother 3*(12), 1727–1737.

Mcleod, D. G. (2003). Hormonal therapy: Historical perspective to future directions. *Urology 61*(2, Suppl 1), 3–7.

Steiner, B. S. (2002). Hypogonadism in men. A review of diagnosis and treatment. *Adv Nurse Pract 10*(4), 22–27, 29.

Susman, E. (2003). ACC: Investigative anti-impotence drug appears with antihypertensive medications. http://www.docguide.com/news/content.nsf/PatientResAllCateg/Erectile%20Dysfunction?OpenDocument#News

Thiyagarajan, M. (2002). Alpha-adrenoceptor antagonists in the treatment of benign prostate hyperplasia. *Pharmacology 65*(3), 119–128.

Chapter 43

Costello-Boerrigter, L. C., Boerrigter, G., & Burnett, J. C. (2003). Revisiting salt and water retention: New diuretics, aquaretics, and natriuretics. *Med Clin North Am 87*(2), 475–491.

Jackson, E. K. (2001). Diuretics. In J. G. Hardman, L. E. Limbard, & A. G. Goodman (Eds.), *The pharmacological basis of therapeutics* (10th ed.). New York: McGraw-Hill.

Josephson, D. L. (1999). *Intravenous fluid therapy for nurses: Principles and practice.* Clifton Park, NY Delmar Publishers.

Chapter 44

Chio, P. T. L., Gordon, Y., Quinonez, L. G., et al. (1999). Crystalloids vs. colloids in fluid resuscitation: A systemic review. *Crit Care Med 27*(1), 200–203.

Rose, B. D. (2000). *Clinical physiology of acid-base and electrolyte disorders* (5th ed.). New York: McGraw-Hill.

Wilmore, D. (2000). Nutrition and metabolic support in the 21st century. *J of Parenteral & Enteral Nutr 4*(1), 1–4.

Chapter 45

American Society for Aesthetic Plastic Surgery. (2003). Your image, http://surgery.org/EFFECTIVE_METHODS.HTML

Dystonia. (2003). *Botulism toxin injections.* Dystonia Medical Research Foundation, http://www.dystonia-foundation.org/treatment/botox.asp

Dystonia. (2003). *Complementary therapy.* Dystonia Medical Research Foundation, http://www.dystonia-foundation.org/treatment/comp.asp

Dystonia. (2003). Dystonia defined. *Dystonia* Medical Research Foundation, http://www.dystonia-foundation.org/defined/

Medlineplus. (2003). *Spasticity.* National Institute of Health, http://www.nlm.nih.gov/medlineplus/ency/article/003297.htm

National Institute of Neurological Disorders and Stroke. (2003). *NINDS spasticity information page.* National Institute of Health, http://nindsupdate.ninds.nih.gov/health_and_medical/disorders/spasticity_doc.htm

Chapter 46

Burke, S. (2001). Boning up on osteoporosis. *Nursing 2001 31*(10): 36–42. October.

Cashman, J. N. (2000). Current pharmacotherapeutic strategies in rheumatic diseases and other pain states. *Clin Drug Invest 19* (Suppl 2), 9–20.

Clemett, D., & Goa, K. L. (2000). Celecoxib. A review of its use in osteoarthritis, rheumatoid arthritis and acute pain. *Drugs 59*(4), 957–980.

Curry, L. C., & Hogstel, M. O. (2002). Osteoporosis. *Am J of Nurs 102*, 26–32.

Jelley, M. J., & Wortmann, R. (2000). Practical steps in the diagnosis and management of gout. *BioDrugs 14*(2), 99–107.

Lacki, J. K. (2000). Management of the patient with severe refractory rheumatoid arthritis. Are the newer treatment options worth considering? *Biodrugs 13*(6), 425–435.

Love, C. (2003). Dietary needs for bone health and the prevention of osteoporosis. *Br J Nurs 12*(1), 12–21.

Marcus, R. (2001). Agents affecting calcification and bone turnover: Calcium, phosphate, parathyroid hormone, vitamin D, calcitonin and other compounds. In J. G. Hardman, L. E. Limbard, & A. G. Goodman (Eds.), *The pharmacological basis of therapeutics* (10th ed.). New York: McGraw-Hill.

Orwoll, E. S. (1999). Osteoporosis in men. *New Dim in Osteopor 1*(5), 2–8, 12.

Prestwood, K. M. (2000). Prevention and treatment of osteoporosis. *Clin Corner 2*(6), 34–44.

Roberts, L. J., Morrow, J. D. (2001). Analgesic-antipyretic and antiinflammatory agents employed in the treatment of gout. In J. G. Hardman, L. E. Limbard, & A. G. Goodman (Eds.), *The pharmacological basis of therapeutics* (10th ed.). New York: McGraw-Hill.

Sanofi-synthelabs. (2003). Hyalgan-sodium hyaluraonte solutions, http://www.sanofi-synthelabous.com

Chapter 47

Feldman, S. (2000). Advances in psoriasis treatment. *Dermat Online 6*(1), 4.

Hooper, B. J. (1999). *Primary dermatologic care.* St. Louis: Mosby, Inc.

Lebwohl, M. (2003). Psoriasis. *Lancet 361*, 1197–1206.

Leung, D. Y., & Boguniewicz, M. (2003). Advances in allergic skin diseases. *J Allergy Clin Immunol 111*(3, Suppl), S805–S812.

Lindow, K. B., & Warren, C. (2001). Understanding rosacea: A guide to facilitating care. *Am J of Nurs 101*, 44–51.

Murphy, K. D., Lee, J. O., & Herndon, D. N. (2003). Current pharmacotherapy for the treatment of severe burns. *Expert Opin Pharmacother 4*(3), 369–384.

Oprica, C., Emtestam, L., & Nord, C. E. (2001). Overview of treatments for acne. *Dermatology Nursing 14*, 242–246.

Roos, T. C., & Merk, H. F. (2000). Important drug interactions in dermatology. *Drugs 59*(2), 181–192.

Smith, G. (2003). Cutaneous expression of cytochrome P-450 CYP25: Individuality in regulation by therapeutic agents for psoriasis and other skin diseases. *Lancet 361*, 1336–1344.

Wyatt, E. L., Sutter, S. H., & Drake, L. A. (2001). Dermatological pharmacology. In J. G. Hardman, L. E. Limbard, & A. G. Goodman (Eds.), *The pharmacological basis of therapeutics* (pp. 1795–1818). New York: McGraw-Hill.

Chapter 48

APhA Drug Treatment Protocols. (2000). Management of pediatric acute otitis media: Introduction by D. H. Albrant. *J Am Pharm Assoc 40*(5), 599–608.

Brook, I. (1999). Treatment of otitis externa in children. *Paediatr Drugs 1*(4), 283–289.

Camras, C. B., Toris, C. B., & Tamesis, R. R. (1999). Efficacy and adverse effects of medications used in the treatment of glaucoma. *Drugs Aging 15*(5), 377–388.

Hoyng, P. F. J., & van Beek, L. M. (2000). Pharmacological therapy for glaucoma. A review. *Drugs 59*(3), 411–434.

Leibovitz, E., & Dagan, R. (2001). Otitis media therapy and drug resistance. Part 1: Management principles. *Infect Med 18*(4), 212–216.

Leibovitz, E., & Dagan, R. (2001). Pediatric infection: Otitis media therapy and drug resistance. Part 2: Current concepts and new directions. *Infect Med 18*(5), 263–270.

Moroi, S. E., & Lichter, P. R. (2001). Ocular pharmacology. In J. G. Hardman, L. E. Limbard, & A. G. Goodman (Eds.), *The pharmacological basis of therapeutics* (10th ed.). New York: McGraw-Hill.

Pray, S. (2001). Swimmer's ear: An ear canal infection. *U.S. Pharmacist 26*(8).

Answers to Critical Thinking Questions

Chapter 7

1. Pyelonephritis is frequently associated with preterm labor in pregnancy. Before initiating antibiotic therapy, the nurse should first determine the patient's gestational age. The potential for a drug to be teratogenic is highest during the first trimester. The nurse should also look up the pregnancy classification of the antibiotic. Selected agents, for example, tetracylines, should not be used during pregnancy. The nurse should address any concerns regarding the drug category with the prescriber.

2. Prior to considering a sedative agent, the patient should be assessed for other physical causes of confusion. For example, in the frail elderly, alterations in electrolytes, drug side effects, and rapid environmental changes can contribute to confusion. Attempts at reorientation should be made. The nurse should determine how diazepam (Valium) is distributed and metabolized. Valium is a fat-soluble drug and, because the elderly have an increase in total body fat, the drug has a much longer half-life. In addition, numerous drugs decrease the metabolism of diazepam and may contribute to an increased half-life and enhanced CNS depression. If sedation is deemed necessary, other drugs should be considered.

3. This question requires the student to go back to Chapter 4 on drug administration and to review techniques for infants. The nurse should consult with the pharmacist regarding the need to repeat the dose. Many oral elixirs are absorbed, to some degree, in the mucous membranes of the oral cavity. Therefore, the nurse may not need to repeat the dose. The nurse should consider using an oral syringe, which is used to accurately measure and administer medications to infants. The syringe tip should be placed in the side of the mouth, not forced over the tongue. Conditions affecting the GI tract, such as gastroenteritis, can impact drug absorption due to the effect on peristalsis.

Chapter 8

1. The purpose of the question is to encourage use of communication skills required for the assessment phase of the nursing process. It is recommended that students consult a nursing diagnosis handbook to support their answers.

The nurse would need to determine that the patient's poor eating habits are related to a nontherapeutic environment. One might be tempted to make this initial judgment due to the mother's appearance. Instead, the nurse should determine if other indicators of noncompliance exist, for example, unused medications, missed medical appointments, and other signs of progression of the disease process may suggest noncompliance. The nurse should also determine if the financial cost of therapy is impacting compliance. He or she should also evaluate the type and quality of diabetic education that the patient and her mother received.

The nurse should use open-ended questions to encourage the patient's mother to verbalize her concerns about her daughter's diagnosis and well-being. He or she should determine if the patient's mother has unrealistic expectations about her daughter's ability to manage her disease process (i.e., diet, medications, exercise).

2. The instructor, depending on what system of nursing diagnosis is being used, could modify this question. The question also assumes that the student has a basic understanding of the pathophysiology of diabetes and the use of the subcutaneous insulin pumps.

Typical nursing diagnoses would include:

Risk for Ineffective Coping related to complex self-care regimen

Risk for Ineffective Therapeutic Regimen Management related to insufficient knowledge of condition and medication regimen

Imbalanced Nutrition: Less Than Body Requirements related to intake less than energy expenditure

Risk for Infection related to site for organism invasion

3. Accountability is the act of being professionally responsible and accountable for one's behavior. The Patient's Bill of Rights states that a patient is entitled to information about drug therapy including name of drug, purpose, action, and potential side effects. The nurse is the professional who is responsible for patient-family education. Failing to teach can impact the patient's ability to safely self-administer medications and may impact compliance with pharmacologic therapy. The nurse should routinely integrate teaching as a critical part of drug administration.

Chapter 9

1. The nurse should be well organized in preparing for drug administration. The medication administration record must be assessed at the beginning of the shift and the nurse should develop a system (i.e., lists of room numbers and times for scheduled drug administration on the report sheet) that will serve as a reminder of when drugs are due.

In most institutions, regularly scheduled drugs may be administered 30 minutes before and 30 minutes after the assigned time. If administered within this time frame, the drugs are considered to have been given "on time." Institutional policies vary and should be consulted.

2. This order as written does not contain an indication for "right dose." Tylenol 3 is a combination drug, acetaminophen and codeine, given orally and the typical mistake is to assume that the healthcare provider meant for the patient to have one tablet by mouth. The nurse should not make this assumption due to the risk of an unintended drug error. Prior to administering the dose, the nurse should consult with the healthcare provider to clarify the intent of the order.

3. A change in prescriptive authority requires an amendment to a state's nurse practice act. This can only be done by "opening" the nurse practice act during a legislative session. A bill for an amendment must be sponsored by a legislator. Any change in the nurse practice act results in a new statute.

4. There are numerous persons potentially "at fault" in this scenario. The nurse is ultimately responsible for the dosage error because a quick check of a drug handbook and a simple dosage calculation might have revealed that the dosage was too high. The prescriber was also responsible for writing the wrong dosage; however, the nurse should have notified the healthcare provider to get the dosage corrected. The pharmacist was also responsible for not checking to see that the dosage was correct for the age and weight of the patient. There are numerous possibilities for error. Nurses must work within an institution's medical error reporting system to ensure that such errors are identified and that mechanisms to prevent subsequent errors can be implemented.

Chapter 10

1. The primary concern for this patient would be the potential for drug-diet interactions. Warfarin (Coumadin) achieves its anticoagulant effect by interfering with the synthesis of vitamin K–dependent clotting factors. The anticoagulant effect of Coumadin can be decreased by a diet high in vitamin K. Fresh greens and tomatoes from the garden are excellent sources of vitamin K. The nurse must include questions related to the dietary intake of these foods. It is common for rural people to "eat out of their gardens" during the growing season. The nurse must also determine if other medications have been added to the patient's regimen that could interfere with the action of Coumadin.

2. As women age, they experience a 10% decrease in total body water. In general, body weight also decreases in this aging population. The nurse should carefully assess the patient's current weight and

compare it to the previously documented weight. In addition, because body weight has decreased, she may also have a decreased serum protein. Because the dose of furosemide is dependent on the degree of protein binding, less serum protein could make the drug more pharmacologically active. The patient may need to have the dosage adjusted.

3. This textbook includes a reference to community health statistics in the United States. Many of the statistics relate to healthcare concerns among rural citizens. These statistics, and the student's own perceptions, can lead to a general discussion about the impact of culture and ethnicity on healthcare. The primary point of any discussion is to emphasize the limited access to care that the culture of poverty creates. This patient is more impacted by poverty and a transient living style than either culture or ethnicity in the matter of managing his own healthcare.

Chapter 11

1. For this question, students should review their resources for information about tamoxifen (Nolvadex). Tamoxifen is a selective estrogen receptor modulator (SERM) that acts by preventing estrogen from binding to the estrogen receptor in breast cells. Therefore, breast cell proliferation is inhibited. Many women assume that because they are taking a SERM, that estrogen replacement is indicated. In fact, tamoxifen's effect in tissues other than the breast is similar to estrogen. Tamoxifen does not cause menopause and does not prevent pregnancy. If the patient takes a "natural" soy product this may interfere with the desired action of tamoxifen. Her concern should be acknowledged but she should be warned not to consume any herbal product without first consulting her healthcare provider.

2. Both garlic and ginseng have a potential drug interaction with the anticoagulant warfarin sodium (Coumadin). It is known that ginseng is capable of inhibiting platelet activity. When taken in combination with an anticoagulant, these herbals are capable of producing increased bleeding potential.

3. The nurse would need to consider the possibility of illicit drug use; however, the nurse should also consider the possibility that the patient is using an ephedra product. These herbals are commonly used as dietary supplements for weight loss. Side effects include those seen in this patient (i.e., hypertension, rapid heart rate, and seizure). Because these preparations are sold in traditional pharmacies as well as health food stores, many consumers believe them to be safe.

Chapter 12

1. The National Institute on Drug Abuse (www.drugabuse.gov/Infofax/ecstasy.html) offers a link entitled Infofax which provides a great deal of information about MDMA. This drug is a neurotoxic agent. When taken in high doses it can produce malignant hyperthermia, which can lead to muscle damage and renal and cardiovascular system failure. Physical symptoms of MDMA use include: muscle tension, nausea, rapid eye movement, faintness, chills, sweating, increase in heart rate and blood pressure and involuntary teeth clenching.

2. The NIDA Infofacts sheet (at www.drugabove.gov) points out that aggression is a common psychiatric side effect of anabolic steroid abuse. Research indicates that users may experience paranoid jealousy, extreme irritability, delusions, and impaired judgment. Other symptoms are extreme mood changes and maniclike symptoms even when the user reports feeling "good."

3. The principal danger associated with prolonged use of barbiturates is tolerance and physical addiction. Barbiturates generally lose their effectiveness as hypnotics within 2 weeks of continued usage. This patient is demonstrating signs of developing tolerance. He needs to gradually discontinue the drug to decrease the risk of complications associated with sudden withdrawal. These symptoms include severe anxiety, tremors, marked excitement, delirium, and rebound rapid eye

movement (REM) sleep. Today, nonbarbiturates are usually prescribed as first line hypnotics.

Chapter 13

1. Terbutaline (Brethine) is a sympathomimetic which was originally prescribed for the treatment of asthma. Terbutaline promotes bronchodilation and therefore reduces bronchospasm by inducing smooth muscle relaxation. Today, terbutaline has found widespread use as a tocolytic because it also produces smooth muscle relaxation in the uterus. Because terbutaline is a sympathomimetic, the nurse should prepare the patient for potential adverse reactions such as nervousness, tremor, and tachycardia. The nurse should also teach the patient to take the medication exactly as directed and on schedule, and instruct on the signs and symptoms of preterm labor should they occur again.

2. Bethanechol is a direct-acting cholinergic agent that works by stimulating the parasympathetic nervous system. The desired effect, in this case, is an increase in smooth muscle tone in the bladder. Any side effects would be related to an overstimulation of the parasympathetic nervous system. Following are suggested nursing diagnoses.

Risk for Injury related to side effects of cholinergic agents (hypotension, bradycardia, and syncope)

Alteration in Comfort related to abdominal cramping, nausea, and vomiting

Risk for Ineffective Individual Therapeutic Management related to side effects and precautions of using cholinergic agents

3. Benztropine (Cogentin) is an anticholinergic. Blocking the parasympathetic nerves allows the sympathetic nervous system to dominate. The drug is given as an adjunct in PD to reduce muscular tremor and rigidity. Anticholinergics affect many body systems and produce a wide variety of side effects. The nurse should monitor for decreased heart rate, dilated pupils, decreased peristalsis, and decreased salivation in addition to decreased muscular tremor and rigidity. Many of the side effects of anticholinergics are dose dependent. Adverse effects include typical signs of sympathetic nervous system stimulation.

Chapter 14

1. Pain is currently emphasized as being the fifth vital sign. The assessment and appropriate management of pain is a nursing function. A nurse might be tempted to give this patient a sleeping medication alone, fearing the side effects that might occur when giving an opioid narcotic in combination. Secobarbital is a short-acting barbiturate. Barbiturates are not effective analgesics and generally do not produce significant hypnosis in patients with severe pain. The barbiturate may intensify the patient's reaction to painful stimuli. Administering a barbiturate with a potent analgesic appears to reduce analgesic requirements by about 50%. The nurse may need to consult with the prescriber regarding lowering or titrating the dose of narcotic.

2. The student may immediately recognize lorazepam (Ativan) as an antianxiety agent. The assumption might be that the purpose of the drug in this case is to control anxiety related to the patient's diagnosis and treatment. After consulting the handbook, the student will discover that lorazepam also has an unlabeled use as an antiemetic prior to chemotherapy. The treatment modality that will control chemotherapy-related nausea must be individualized.

3. The student should consider conducting a thorough assessment of the patient's sleep patterns. In addition, the student should consider nonpharmacologic interventions. In older adults the total amount of sleep does not change; however, the quality of sleep deteriorates. Time spent in REM sleep and stages 3 and 4 NREM sleep shortens. Older adults awaken more often during the night. This can be compounded by the presence of a chronic illness. The alteration in sleep patterns may also be due to changes in the CNS that affect the regulation of sleep. After a thorough assessment, the nurse should discuss age-related issues, health concerns, and environmental factors that may be impacting the quality of sleep.

Chapter 15

1. Carbamazepine (Tegretol) is the second most widely prescribed antiepileptic drug in the United States. Common side effects are drowsiness, dizziness, nausea, ataxia, and blurred vision. Serious and sometimes fatal blood dyscrasias secondary to bone marrow suppression have occurred with carbamazepine. The patient's hematocrit suggests anemia and the petechiae and bruising suggest thrombocytopenia. The nurse practitioner should evaluate the patient for complaints of fever and sore throat which would suggest leukopenia. This patient needs immediate evaluation by the healthcare provider who is responsible for monitoring the seizure disorder.

2. This question requires that the student consult a laboratory reference manual. The therapeutic drug level of phenytoin (Dilantin) is 5 to 20 mg/dl. Patients may become drug toxic and demonstrate signs of CNS depression. Exaggerated effects of Dilantin can be seen if the drug has been combined with alcohol or other agents. Dilantin also, demonstrates dose-dependent metabolism. When hepatic enzymes necessary for metabolism are saturated, any increase in drug concentration results in a disproportionate increase in plasma concentration level.

3. Long-term phenytoin therapy can produce an androgenic stimulus. Reported skin manifestations include acne, hirsutism, and an increase in subcutaneous facial tissue—changes that have been characterized as "Dilantin facies." These changes, coupled with the risk for gingival hypertrophy, may be difficult for the adolescent to cope with. In addition, the adolescent with a seizure disorder may be prohibited from operating a motor vehicle at the very age when driving becomes a key to achieving young adult status. The thoughtful nurse will consider the range of possible support groups for this patient, once she is discharged, and will encourage the patient to discuss her concerns about the drug regimen with her healthcare provider.

Chapter 16

1. Methylphenidate (Ritalin) therapy is usually administered twice a day, with one dose before breakfast and one dose before lunch. A child in school would be required to visit a school nurse in order to receive a dose of Ritalin before lunch. Amphetamine (Adderall) requires once-a-day dosing and may be better accepted by the child and his or her family because treatment can be privately managed at home. Although many children cope effectively with treatment for ADD, a 10-year-old female might be concerned about being "singled out" for therapy. She is old enough at the time of treatment to realize her problems in performance. Children in this age group have their self-esteem tied to success in school. This is characteristic of Erikson's developmental stage of industry versus inferiorty. Children who have difficulty in school perceive themselves as being inferior to peers. Helping the child with ADD pharmacologically may require the healthcare provider to be sensitive to social factors such as dosage regimens.

2. The nurse should teach the patient that it might take 2 to 4 weeks before she begins to note therapeutic benefit. The nurse should help the patient identify a support person or network to help assist as she works through her grief. The nurse also needs to instruct the patient that both caffeine and nicotine are CNS stimulants and will decrease the effectiveness of the medication.

3. The use of any drug during pregnancy must be carefully evaluated. Setraline (Zoloft) is a pregnancy category B drug, which means that studies indicate no risk to animal fetus although safety in humans has not been established. The prescriber must weigh risks and benefits of any medication during pregnancy. The nurse should recognize this patient's risk for ineffective coping as evidenced by her history of depression and help the patient to identify support groups in the community. She may be functioning in some degree of isolation from family or other parenting women, which is typical of women who suffer postpartum depression. Identifying community resources for the patient is one intervention designed to provide more holistic care for the patient.

Chapter 17

1. The patient is exhibiting signs of extrapyramidal symptoms (EPS). Initially the nurse would assess the patient to ensure no recent neck injury, trauma, and so forth, but if the neck spasms started spontaneously, the nurse would then assess for the possibility that this is due to EPS. The patient probably needs to be on a medication such as benztropine (Cogentin) to decrease the EPS effects. The patient should be taught to recognize the symptoms of EPS and to seek medical evaluation when the symptoms occur.

2. The patient is elderly and safety is a priority when taking this medication. Postural hypotension and dizziness are common; therefore, the patient needs to move and change position slowly. Constipation is also a concern while on this medication, especially in the elderly.

3. The nurse should initially assess if the patient has been taking the medication as ordered or has altered the dose in any way. It is not uncommon for a young person to "cheek" the medication or attempt to cut back on the dose because of the lack of desire to take the medication on a continual basis—especially when the patient begins to feel better. It is important that the patient understand the necessity of being on this medication for a lifetime, and not to adjust the dose without consulting a healthcare provider.

Chapter 18

1. The patient should reassess with a healthcare provider the need for regular Mylanta. This drug contains magnesium which may cause increased absorption and therefore toxicity. The patient needs teaching on decreasing foods that contain vitamin B_6 (e.g., bananas, wheat germ, green vegetables), as vitamin B_6 may also cause an increase in the absorption of the medication. Teaching should include information about a potential loss of glycemic control (patient is a diabetic) and safety issues related to postural hypotension.

2. A patient on benztropine (Cogentin) has a decreased ability to tolerate heat. Arizona in July is hot, so the patient should be taught to avoid hot climates if at all possible or to increase rest periods, avoid exertion, and observe for signs of heat intolerance. When symptoms occur, the patient must immediately get out of the heat and rest.

3. The nurse should refer the patient and his wife to a healthcare provider regarding the appropriateness of this medication (this is not a nursing function). The couple should be educated regarding safety issues such as postural hypotension and bradycardia that may occur with this medication. Anorexia is also a potential problem—this patient is diabetic and thus may cause him glycemic issues.

Chapter 19

1. The nurse should initially manage the patient's ABCs (airway, breathing, and circulation—open airway, provide oxygen support) and then stop the PCA pump. Although the nurse will want to go directly to the PCA, it is important to initially manage the patent's airway before stopping the PCA as the nurse does not know how long the patient has been hypoxic. The nurse then needs to obtain naloxone (Narcan), which is a narcotic antagonist to give the patient intravenously. After these initial steps have been completed and the patient is stabilized, the nurse must inform the healthcare provider of this adverse effect of the morphine.

2. Sumatriptan (Imitrex) is not recommended for patients with CAD, diabetes, or hypertension due to the drug's vasoconstrictive properties. The nurse should refer the patient to the healthcare provider for review of medications and possible adverse reactions related to sumatriptan.

3. The patient should be taught not to take any medication, including OTC medications, without the approval of the healthcare provider. This patient is on anticoagulant therapy and aspirin increases bleeding time. The patient needs to be taught how to recognize the signs and symptoms of bleeding related to the anticoagulant therapy. The patient should review with the healthcare provider all her medications, with a possible change of aspirin as the anti-inflammatory medication for arthritis.

Chapter 20

1. The nurse should question the healthcare provider regarding this order. Lidocaine is an appropriate choice for a local anesthesia, but not if it includes epinephrine. Epinephrine has alpha adrenergic properties, is a potent vasoconstrictor, and may cause cardiac dysrhythmias with this elderly patient. Epinephrine is traditionally not used in the areas of "fingers, nose, penis, toes," as these areas may suffer adverse effects from the vasoconstrictive properties of the drug.

2. The nurse understands that this drug is a depolarizing medication and therefore has the potential to increase potassium release. The nurse is aware that this patient is on digoxin (Lanoxin) and has renal failure, and therefore would not be a good candidate for this drug due to the potential hyperkalemia that may result in life-threatening cardiac dysrhythmias.

3. The priority postoperative drug is St. John's wort, as it may prolong the effects of anesthesia as well as opioids in the patient's system, causing depression of the CNS and respiratory system. The patient should also be monitored for postoperative bleeding related to the use of ibuprofen. The digoxin concentration should be at a therapeutic level prior to surgery, to decrease possible adverse effects of the cardiovascular system postoperatively.

Chapter 21

1. Traditionally, any systolic BP that is less than 110 should be held unless verified with the healthcare provider that the dose should be given. The patient is on a low sodium, low protein diet which may contribute to hypotension. Because the patient has mild renal failure, the excretion of the drug may be prolonged and also contribute to the hypotensive effects. If the healthcare provider wants the patient to receive the benazepril (Lotensin), then the BP should be rechecked at 30 minutes and 60 minutes after giving the medication. The patient should be cautioned about postural hypotension.

2. Atenolol (Tenormin) is a beta$_1$-adrenergic blocker medication that works directly on the heart. The nurse and the patient need to be aware that the patient's heart rate will rarely go above 80 due to the action of the medication. Tachycardia is one of the adrenergic signs of hypoglycemia that would not be evident with this patient. Both the nurse and patient need to be aware of the more subtle signs of hypoglycemia (or any other condition that may be recognized by tachycardia) that would not be evident with a patient on beta-blocking medications.

3. The nurse must be careful that the patient's BP is not lowered too dramatically or hypotension can occur. This is an example when 120/80 is not necessarily an ideal BP. Typically the BP is not lowered below 160 systolic—the patient is reevaluated and then (often many hours later) the BP is brought down further. This drip is light sensitive and must remain covered with foil during infusion. Once prepared, the drip is stable only for 24 hours. Nitroprusside is a cyanide by-product; therefore, any patient on this drug must be monitored for cyanide toxicity.

Chapter 22

1. The nurse should first note improved signs of perfusion if this medication is effective. The nurse would evaluate the patent's skin signs, BP, heart rate, and urinary output. If the medication is effec-

tive, all of these will be within normal limits, or at least improved from the patient's baseline. The EKG may show improvement by switching to a normal sinus rhythm once the digoxin (Lanoxin) has reached therapeutic level.

2. The nurse understands that there is a cross sensitivity between sulfa and furosemide (Lasix) and therefore would inform the healthcare provider of the patient's allergy status so a different diuretic may be utilized. Morphine is an appropriate medication for this patient not only for its analgesic and sedative effects but also for the increased venous capacitance that it causes.

3. This diabetic patient needs to be educated about the importance of regular glucose checks as this medication may cause the blood sugar to vary sporadically. Typically, hypoglycemia is more of a problem, so the patient needs to be especially aware of the symptoms and treatment of hypoglycemia. Safety should be emphasized, especially regarding postural hypotension.

Chapter 23

1. Propranolol (Inderal) is a nonselective beta-blocking drug which means that it not only works on the intended system (cardiac) but also acts on the lungs. This may cause the patient to have untoward lung problems such as shortness of breath; therefore, this patient should not be taking propranolol.

2. The patient should be monitored closely for hypotension, especially in the first few weeks of treatment, and should be taught about postural hypotension. Pulmonary toxicity is a major complication of this drug so the patient should be monitored for cough or shortness of breath. Because digoxin (Lanoxin) slows the heart rate as well as amiodarone (Cordarone), the patient must be monitored closely for bradycardia. Safety and pulmonary symptoms are priorities of care for this patient. Amiodarone often increases the effects of digoxin and warfarin (Coumadin) and thus must be closely monitored.

3. Bradycardia is a potential problem for a patient taking verapamil (Isoptin) and digoxin. The patient may exhibit signs of decreased cardiac output, such as pale skin, chest pain, shortness of breath, hypotension, and altered level of consciousness. The patient needs to be taught to recognize the signs of decreasing cardiac output as well as how to assess heart rate.

Chapter 24

1. The nurse should question the healthcare provider about this order. No patient who appears to be having a CVA (brain attack) should have heparin until a CT scan of the brain has been done. Approximately 20% of CVAs are hemorrhagic and this needs to be ruled out before an anticoagulant is given.

2. The major adverse effect of a fibrinolytic drug is bleeding. All tubes (NG, Foley, ETT), blood draws, and IV insertions need to be done prior to the medication being given or they may potentiate bleeding in this patient.

3. Whether the nurse gives this drug or is teaching the patient to self-administer the medication, proper placement in the abdomen is vital. The injection must be given at least 1 to 2 inches away from the umbilicus. There are major blood vessels that run close to the umbilicus and if the LMWH is given near one of these vessels, there is an increased chance of bleeding into the abdomen or a large (and often occult initially) hematoma forming in the abdomen.

Chapter 25

1. The nurse needs to verify blood pressure. A major adverse effect of nitroglycerin is hypotension. If the systolic blood pressure remains under 100, the nurse needs to notify the healthcare provider of the patient's chest pain and blood pressure.

2. Beta-blockers slow the heart rate to a desired 50 to 65 beats per minute (bpm). Many patients suffer from postural hypotension if the heart rate drops below 60 bpm and therefore the nurse needs to educate the patient about the necessity of changing positions slowly. The nurse must be aware that a cardinal sign of decreasing cardiac output is tachycardia—a heart rate >100 bpm for the patient not on beta-blockers. If the patient is on beta-blocking medication, the heart rate may not go above 80 to 85 bpm and is considered tachycardia for this type of patient.

3. Diltiazem (Cardizem) has been given to lower the heart rate and to decrease the myocardial oxygen consumption for this patient with chest pain. The nurse must monitor closely for hypotension as this medication lowers the heart rate but also lowers the BP, and this patient already has a borderline low BP of 100/60. The patient should be on a cardiac monitor with frequent monitoring of BP.

Chapter 26

1. A major action of this vasopressor medication is the positive inotropic action that it has on a damaged myocardium that is having difficulty maintaining a good cardiac output (and therefore BP). The drip must be slowly tapered to a point that the BP is well maintained, normally a systolic BP greater than 100. The nurse must never consider a BP as okay and shut off the vasopressor drip—the patient may immediately become acutely hypotensive.

2. This isotonic solution is appropriate for this patient. Based on history and assessment, the patient is demonstrating signs of being hypovolemic (heart rate of 122) and requires a solution that will meet the intracellular need. The patient must be monitored for hypernatremia and hyperchloremia if more than 3 L of normal saline are given. As the patient responds to the fluid, the nurse will note a corresponding decrease in the heart rate.

3. This is not an appropriate IV solution for a head injury patient. Once this IV solution is infused into the patient, it is considered to be a hypotonic solution that moves fluids into the cells. A patient with an increased ICP cannot tolerate an increase of fluid at the cellular level, as this may cause the brain to herniate and lead to death.

Chapter 27

1. Photosensivity is a major problem with atorvastatin (Lipitor) and the patient must take precautions such as using sunscreen, wearing sunglasses and protective clothing, and staying out of the direct sun as much as possible. This will probably be a lifestyle change for this patient and education with reinforcement is necessary.

2. This medication has the possibility of causing esophageal irritation, so taking the proper fluids or food with this medication is important. Pulpy fruit such as applesauce could be used for dual purposes with this drug as the applesauce works for the esophageal irritation and it also may help prevent the constipation due to the drug.

3. The nurse should advise this patient to seek medical advice before self-medicating—especially as this patient is a diabetic and many drugs affect hyperglycemic medications and blood glucose. Niacin can cause hyperglycemia in this patient and serum glucose should be evaluated. The flushing and hot flashes are normal side effects of this medication.

Chapter 28

1. Chronic renal failure patients often have decreased secretion of endogenous erythropoietin and therefore require a medication such as epoetin alfa (Epogen) to stimulate RBC production and reduce the potential of becoming anemic (or to decrease the effects of anemia).

2. Patients who are receiving filgrastim (Neupogen) should have their vital signs assessed every 4 hours (especially pulse and temperature) to monitor for signs of infection related to a low WBC count. The order to obtain vital signs every shift is not appropriate and the healthcare provider should be notified.

3. Patients taking this drug need to be educated especially about the GI distress that may occur while on iron supplements. This medication may be taken with food to reduce the potential for GI upset. Constipation is a common complaint by patients on this medication, so preventative measures need to be taken. The patient needs to ensure that this medication has a childproof cap and is safely secured, as overdose of iron supplements is a common toxicology emergency for children.

Chapter 29

1. The nurse needs to ensure that the patient understands the potential side effects related to the anticholinergic effects of this medication. The patient (based on age) is at higher risk for urinary retention, glaucoma (or other visual changes), and constipation. These are also common problems for patients who are taking this medication.

2. Although codeine is a more powerful antitussive, it can cause dependence, as well as constipation. Dextromethorphan is a more appropriate choice for this patient initially, with codeine syrup as a potential later choice for more severe cough symptoms.

3. The patient who is taking medication such as beclomethasone (Beconase) utilizes this as an anti-inflammatory medication to prevent exacerbation of lung problems. As with any steroid, the patient's serum glucose must be monitored periodically, as hyperglycemia is a common problem while on this medication.

Chapter 30

1. The nurse should refer the patient to the healthcare provider for information regarding this medication. The nurse is legally not allowed to prescribe drugs, and telling a patient to take any drug not prescribed by a healthcare provider is beyond the nursing scope of practice. The healthcare provider needs to evaluate the patient's current medical condition and what drugs this patient takes prior to agreeing that echinacea would be an appropriate medication at this time.

2. The patient needs the protection of this passive form of immunity after an exposure to such an illness. The gamma globulin will act as a protective mechanism for 3 weeks while the patient is in the window of opportunity of developing hepatitis A. This drug does not stimulate the patient's immune system but will help protect the patient from developing the disease. The nurse should inform the patient that the shot is far less debilitating than developing the disease.

3. Cyclosporine is a toxic medication with many serious adverse effects. The nurse must understand that this drug cannot be given with grapefruit juice; patients who take this medication need their kidney function assessed regularly (not because of the kidney transplant but because cyclosporine reduces urine output). The nurse also must assess if this patient is taking steroids, which are often given concurrently with cyclosporine, as the serum glucose will need to be monitored regularly.

Chapter 31

1. This patient has many potential problems related to the use of prednisone over a sustained period of time. The primary current concern is the hyperglycemia—an adverse effect of the prednisone that can become serious when the patient is diabetic. Blood pressure must be monitored for potential hypertension, which is related to sodium retention and therefore increased water retention caused by the prednisone. The patient is also at high risk for infection while on the prednisone due to suppression of the immune system, which is also related to the diabetes.

2. The nurse should give the patient celebrex (Celecoxib) for the elbow inflammation and pain. This medication should provide adequate relief of the symptoms for this patient. Ensure that the patient is not allergic to sulfa prior to giving this medication. The patient should not take acetaminophen (Tylenol) due to the related potential liver compromise secondary to the alcohol abuse. The patient should not take ibuprofen (Motrin) because of the potential gastric bleeding that may occur (also the stomach is already at risk because of the alcohol abuse and the chance for bleeding is elevated due to the potential liver problems secondary to the alcohol abuse).

3. The nurse should request the patient to stop taking the diphenhydramine (Benadryl) and refer him or her to the healthcare provider for advice regarding treatment for allergy symptoms. Diphenhydramine has the potential to increase intraocular pressure in the patient with glaucoma and should not be used. This medication also has anticholinergic properties and may cause urinary retention (patient already at risk related to enlarged prostate). The patient must also be cautioned about the potential for postural hypotension and hypoglycemia while taking diphenhydramine.

Chapter 32

1. This patient should not be on tetracycline (Achromycin) while pregnant because tetracycline is a category D drug that has teratogenic effects on the fetus. Counseling should be provided for alternate sources of care for her acne as well as the use of drugs when pregnant.

2. No, the nurse should not give the erythromycin, as this medication is metabolized by the liver. An alternate type of antibiotic should be utilized.

3. This medication is typically reserved for more serious infections and has a higher potential for toxicity. A priority assessment for this patient would be renal function. The nurse should monitor urinary output, urine for protein, and the serum BUN and creatinine on a regular basis. A secondary priority would be hearing assessment as ototoxicity is not uncommon for patients on gentamycin.

Chapter 33

1. As always, the ABCs are a priority for any patient; and must be considered. The nurse must monitor the patient's airway for evidence of bronchospasm and/or decreased gas exchange, such as coughing, poor color and decreased oxygen saturation. The nurse must understand that leukopenia is a problem for these patients (related to the amphotericin B and the patient's own depressed immune status) and prevention of infection is always a priority. The patient's renal status (urinary output, serum BUN and creatinine) also must be closely monitored as approximately 30% of patients on this medication suffer renal damage.

2. This patient has vaginal candidiasis and it must be stressed that her partner be treated or reinfection may occur. Alcohol must be avoided while on this medication or profound vomiting may occur. It is important to stress that alcohol is not only found in the traditional manner (alcoholic drinks) but also in products such as cough medicine, vanilla, and at times even application of perfume that is absorbed via the dermis may cause this vomiting effect.

3. This drug can have profound adverse effects and the patient must be carefully screened as well as educated about this drug prior to taking it. The patient must have a baseline physical assessment prior to initiating pharmacotherapy. A priority would be an EKG and blood pressure assessment, liver and renal function tests, and a hearing and visual assessment screening. Because the patient may suffer permanent organ damage while taking this medication, baseline information is crucial.

Chapter 34

1. Famciclovir (Famvir) has the potential to cause digoxin toxicity and the patient must be taught the signs of toxicity and to seek immediate medical attention as needed. The nurse should teach the patient to monitor the pulse for regularity and to watch for visual disturbances. Digoxin level should be monitored on a regular basis.

2. This medication may cause bone marrow suppression. This patient is already immune compromised and the potential for leukopenia is high. The patient should be taught to watch for any evidence of infection, monitor temperature, and have regular lab tests. The patient also needs instruction about the importance of good handwashing and safeguarding against potential sources of infection.

3. The nurse should inform the healthcare provider that the medication needs to be administered over a minimum of 1 hour and the nurse is unable to give the medication as a bolus or "intravenous piggyback" for less than 1 hour. The IV site must be monitored closely while the medication is infusing for potential infiltration. If this occurs, the IV must be stopped immediately.

Chapter 35

1. The patient needs to be taught strategies for coping with the side effects of the chemotherapy regimen. A major focus would be on the nutritional issues: The patient should always take antiemetics 1 hour prior to chemotherapy, eat small frequent meals, drink high-calorie liquids if unable to eat solid food, and increase fluids if diarrhea occurs.

2. The patient and family should be taught about the potential for infection related to immunosuppression. The nurse should stress frequent handwashing, avoiding large crowds, self-assessing temperature accurately at home, and knowing when to call the healthcare provider. Nurses take these basics for granted even though patients often have misconceptions about them.

3. The nurse should remain with the solution and call for someone to bring the chemo spill kit immediately. While waiting for the spill kit, the contaminated fluid may be covered with paper towels (the nurse must not touch the solution without wearing protective equipment). The nurse should clean up the spill and dispose of the waste per hospital protocols. At no time should the chemo spill be left unattended.

Chapter 36

1. Regular use of aluminum hydroxide (Amphojel) may cause hypercalcemia—calcium and phosphorus have a reciprocal relationship in that if the calcium goes up, the phosphorus goes down. A patient with a low serum phosphorus often exhibits signs of increasing weakness. The treatment would be to replace the aluminum hydroxide with a different antacid and take oral phosphorus supplements until serum phosphorus returns to a normal level.

2. The stomach is empty during the sleep cycle and this is the time when the protective protein peptide (TFF2) is most effective at repairing the mucoprotective lining of the stomach. For the TFF2 protein to reach its maximum effectiveness, the person needs a minimum of 6 hours uninterrupted sleep, which is uncommon in people who sleep during the daytime.

3. This patient has a history of peptic ulcer disease and therefore alcohol and smoking are contraindicated as they will exacerbate the condition. This patient is on ranitidine (Zantac) and smoking decreases the effectiveness of the medication. Alcohol is a depressant and can cause increased drowsiness in combination with the ranitidine. This patient should be advised to stop smoking and drinking alcohol if the PUD is to be resolved.

Chapter 37

1. A priority for the nurse would be the potential for dehydration. The nurse would assess the patient for possible hypotension and tachycardia. The cause of this ongoing diarrhea needs to be investigated by the physician.

2. The patient needs to be informed that the prochlorperazine (Compazine) is administered in its own syringe and must not be mixed with any other drug. The nurse could notify the healthcare provider that the patient wants a change of antiemetic to one that could be combined with an analgesic and given in the same syringe.

3. This patient needs to take a contact laxative to stimulate the nerve endings to facilitate a bowel movement as opposed to a bulk-forming laxative, which promotes bowel regularity. The liquid stool may be a result of fecal impaction with only liquid being able to seep out. If this patient has ongoing bowel irregularity problems, the bulk-forming laxative may be helpful at a later date. The nurse should educate the patient to drink plenty of fluids when taking bulk-forming laxatives.

Chapter 38

1. The patient is experiencing a normal reaction to the niacin but should be instructed to follow up with the healthcare provider for guidance on the appropriate amounts of niacin to take.

2. This patient should be instructed to see a healthcare provider for guidance on the appropriate doses of vitamins. Vitamin A can cause increased intracranial pressure which could be the cause of the headaches. Patients need to be instructed on the appropriate amounts of vitamins and about the potential adverse effects—especially when taking megadoses of vitamins.

3. This patient needs to be assessed for possible renal calculi. The patient is taking 500 mg of vitamin C daily to prevent an upper respiratory infection, but vitamin C is contraindicated in a patient with a history of renal calculi as this may exacerbate the problem.

Chapter 39

1. To answer this question the student should refer to a medical-surgical text or a laboratory manual.

A child with diabetes insipidus will produce large amounts of pale or colorless urine with a low specific gravity of 1.001 to 1.005. A daily volume of urine may be 4 to 10 L or more and result in excessive thirst and rapid dehydration. Desmopressin is a synthetic analog of ADH. It may be administered intranasally and therefore may be better tolerated by a child. With pharmacotherapy, there should be an immediate decrease in urine production and an increase in urine concentration. The child's mother or caregiver should be taught to use a urine dipstick to check specific gravity during the initiation of therapy. A normal specific gravity would range from 1.005 to 1.030 and would indicate that the kidneys are concentrating urine. The caregiver also should be taught to monitor urine volumes, color, and odor until a dosing regimen is established.

2. The nurse must be empathetic to the patient's father and allow him to express his concerns. He may feel guilty about contributing to his son's current health crisis. Once the patient's condition begins to improve, the nurse should assess the father's understanding of the asthma regimen. The father and the patient should receive instruction on the side effects of glucocorticoid therapy. Glucocorticoids used for anti-inflammatory purposes can suppress the hypothothalamic-pituitary axis. Abruptly discontinuing a glucocorticoid after long-term therapy (greater than 10 days) can produce cardiovascular collapse. The father needs to be instructed on the dosage regimen for prednisone, which may include an incremental decrease in the drug dosage when discontinuing the drug. An additional concern the nurse might have is related to the economic needs of this family. Referrals to a resource providing medication financial support would be appropriate.

3. This question requires the student to utilize an additional resource such as a drug handbook. In this situation, the parents need to be instructed as follows:

a. Drug action—stimulates growth on most body tissues, especially epiphyseal plates; also increases cellular size

b. How to reconstitute the medication, site selection, and technique for IM or SC injection

c. Dosing schedule—somatropin injections usually scheduled 48 hours apart

d. Pain and swelling at the injection site

e. Importance of regular follow-up with healthcare provider, including checks on height, weight, and bone-age

Chapter 40

1. The nurse should first explain that management of type 1 diabetes is initiated with diet, exercise, and home blood glucose monitoring. Compliance with prescribed regimens may reduce the patient's fasting and postprandial blood glucose values to acceptable levels. Mothers with type 1 diabetes must keep their blood glucose within a very narrow range to prevent the numerous complications that can occur as a result of elevated blood glucose during pregnancy. These complications can range from fetal deformity to fetal macrosomia and its subsequent sequela. Some authorities recommend that the FBS be maintained at or below 100 mg % and the postprandial glucose be below 120 mg %. The nurse should prepare the patient for insulin therapy should diet and exercise fail to maintain control. Oral hypoglycemic agents cross placental membranes and have been implicated as teratogenic agents. Their use is not recommended during pregnancy.

2. Part of the exocrine function of the pancreas is the production of lipase, trypsin, and amylase. These enzymes enter the duodenum to digest fat, protein, and carbohydrate. In cystic fibrosis, the enzyme secretions become so tenacious that they plug the ducts supplied by the acinar cells. The blockage eventually results in atrophy of the acinar cells with loss of the ability to produce digestive enzymes, leading to steatorrhea and subsequent malnutrition. Children with cystic fibrosis require pancreatic enzyme replacement therapy to aid in digestion and improve the child's nutritional state. This patient demonstrated the classic signs of both pulmonary and pancreatic involvement.

3. There is variation in the absorption rates of subcutaneous insulin among various body areas. It is known that the abdomen has the fastest rate of absorption, followed by the arms, thighs, and buttocks. It is also generally accepted that exercise of a body area can increase the rate of insulin absorption. Rotating from arm, to leg, to abdomen for each injection will impact glucose control due to the variation in absorption rates. For this reason, systematic rotation within one area at a time is recommended. The nurse in this situation should review a correct system of rotation for this patient.

Chapter 41

1. The student should be able to use this example to help illustrate neuroendocrine control of the female reproductive system. Leuprolide acetate is a synthetic GnRH agonist that acts by stimulating the anterior pituitary to secrete FSH and LH. The pituitary receptors become desensitized with a resultant decrease in FSH and LH secretion. Consequently, estrogen production, which is dependent on ovarian stimulation, is diminished and the patient's menstrual cycle is suppressed. The goal of suppressing the menstrual cycle is to decrease hormonal stimuli to abnormal endometrotic tissue. It is expected that amenorrhea will result and that there will be a decrease in endometrosis lesions. A decrease in lesions will likely enhance the patient's fertility or improve her level of comfort during menstruation. The patient will remain on this drug therapy for approximately 6 months. Menstrual periods usually resume 2 months after the completion of therapy.

2. Misoprostol (Cytotec) is a prostaglandin that may be prescribed as an antiulcer agent. The drug also has two unlabeled uses, which include cervical ripening prior to induction of labor or termination of pregnancy when used with mifepristone. It is known that prostaglandins have a role in the initiation of labor. This has been demonstrated with the vaginal application of prostaglandin E. Misoprostol is a prostaglandin E analog that has been clearly demonstrated to produce uterine contractions. In this example, the fetus was not tolerating the uterine contractions and the nurse used correct judgment in quickly acting to remove the drug.

3. Oxytocin exerts an antidiuretic effect when administered in doses of 20 mU/minute or greater. This will result in a decrease in urine output and an increase in fluid retention. Most patients begin a postpartum diuresis and are able to balance fluid volumes relatively quickly. However, the nurse should evaluate the patient for signs of water intoxication that include drowsiness, listlessness, headache, and oliguria.

Chapter 42

1. This patient's age puts him at risk for a variety of health problems. Conditions such as renal or hepatic dyfunction may alter the manner in which the drug is metabolized or excreted. Potential impact on patients with coronary artery disease using nitrates has been well documented. Because the patient is requesting a prescription for sildenafil (Viagra), the nurse should ensure that the history includes the following data.

Sexual dysfunction

Cardiovascular disease and use of organic nitrates

Severe hypotension

Renal impairment or hepatic impairment—which requires a decrease in the prescribed dose

Hypertension and use of antihypertensives (concurrent treatment can increase risk of hypotension)

Nurses can be effective in initiating conversations about sexuality. Studies have shown that patients are often forthcoming with concerns about sexual performance when an interviewer is open and professional.

2. According to Erikson's theory of psychosocial development, this young man is in the stage of identity versus isolation. The family has been replaced in its influence, to a large extent, by the adolescent's peer group. This young man's desire to be accepted as an athelete and a team member may produce a willingness to "do what it takes" to fit in. In addition, the young man may have aspirations of a career in sports and recognizes the need to be in optimum physical condition. The young man may not realize that the use of testosterone in immature males has not been associated with significant increases in muscle mass. This has been documented only in mature males. In addition, testosterone can produce premature epiphyseal closure, potentially impacting this young man's adult height.

3. Finasteride (Proscar), an androgen inhibitor, is used to shrink the prostate and relieve symptoms associated with hypertrophy. Finasteride inhibits 5-alpha-reductase, an enzyme that converts testosterone to a potent androgen 5-alpha-dihydrotestosterone (DHT). The prostate gland depends on this androgen for its development, but excessive levels can cause prostate cells to increase in size and divide. A regimen of 6 to 12 months may be necessary to determine patient response. Saw palmetto is an herbal preparation derived from a shrublike palm tree that is native to the southeastern United States. This phytomedicine compares pharmacologically to finasteride in that it is an antiandrogen. The mechanism of action is virtually the same in these two agents. Authorities note no significant adverse effects of saw palmetto extract and no known drug-drug interactions. Just as with finasteride, long-term use is required.

Chapter 43

1. Losartan (Cozaar) is an angiotensin II receptor antagonist commonly prescribed for hypertension. Because some patients do not respond adequately to monotherapy, Hyzaar combines losartan with hydrochlorothiazide, a diuretic. This combination decreases blood pressure initially by reducing blood volume and arterial resistance. Over time, the diuretic is effective in maintaining the desired change in sodium balance with a resultant decrease in the sensitivity of vessels to norepinephrine. Angiotensin II receptor antagonists appear to prevent the hypokalemia associated with thiazide therapy.

2. The nurse should carefully monitor fluid status. Because the primary concern is cardiopulmonary, the nurse should assess and document lung sounds, vital signs, and urinary output. Depending on the patient's condition, a Foley catheter may be inserted to permit the measurement of hourly outputs. Daily weights should be obtained. Edema should be evaluated and documented as well as status of mucous membranes and skin turgor. Because furosemide (Lasix) is a loop diuretic, the nurse would anticipate a rapid and profound diuresis. Therefore, the nurse should also observe for signs of dehydration and potassium depletion over the course of therapy.

3. Cerebral edema occurs as a result of the body's response to an initial head trauma. In this case, the patient sustained a skull fracture and the trauma of required surgery. The nurse should explain to the mother that mannitol (Osmitrol) helps to reduce swelling or cerebral edema at the site of her son's injury. The nurse might explain that the drug helps to "pull" water from the site of injury and carry it to the kidneys where it is eliminated. The patient's mother should understand that the goal of decreasing swelling is to promote tissue recovery. Nurses must be sensitive to the fact that family members may have severe emotional reactions to a patient's injury and need help to focus on short-term goals for recovery when the long-term prognosis is not known.

For additional information on the action or administration of mannitol, students should consult a drug handbook.

Chapter 44

1. Aggressive treatment with loop diuretics is a common cause of hypokalemia. As in this example, hypokalemia can produce a myriad of sequela including a variety of dyshythmias. KCl is indicated for patients with low potassium levels, and is preferred over other potassium salts because chloride is simultaneously replaced.

The nurse administering the KCl must keep in mind several critical concerns to safeguard the patient. The primary concern is the risk of potassium intoxication. High plasma concentrations of potassium may cause death through cardiac depression, arrhythmias, or arrest. The signs and symptoms of potassium overdose include mental confusion, weakness, listlessness, hypotension, and EKG abnormalities. In a patient with heart disease, cardiac monitoring may be indicated during potassium infusion.

Students should consult their drug handbooks and look up the maximum rates for infusing KCl in adults and children.

To prevent potassium intoxication, the nurse should carefully regulate the infusion of IV fluids. Most institutions require that any solution containing KCl be administered using an infusion pump. Prior to beginning and throughout the infusion, the nurse should assess the client's renal function (BUN and creatinine levels). A patient with diminished renal function is more likely to develop hyperkalemia.

2. The student should recognize that this patient is dehydrated from an intravascular standpoint despite her appearance. The patient's elevated H/H is one indication of her degree of "dehydration." Most pregnant women present with dilution anemia. This client does not. The midwife recognizes the need to increase the intravascular fluid compartment to promote renal and uterine perfusion.

Chapter 45

1. The nurse would anticipate a decrease in the patient's spasticity after 1 week of therapy. If there has been no improvement in 45 days, the medication regimen is usually discontinued. In this case, the nurse should evaluate the patient's muscle firmness, pain experience, range of motion, and ability to maintain posture and alignment when in a wheelchair. When spasticity is used to maintain posture, dantrolene should not be used. In this case, the patient's spasticity involved only the lower extremities.

2. Leg and foot cramps have anecdotally been associated with tamoxifen, an antiestrogenic drug. Tamoxifen, which has been shown to reduce the reoccurrence of some breast cancers, has been demonstrated to preserve bone density. Tamoxifen has several side effects that impact lifestyle, including the potential for weight gain and leg cramps. The nurse should assess several factors before responding to this patient's concerns.

- What is the patient's activity level? Muscle cramps are associated with muscle fatigue.
- Does she take exogenous calcium?
- Can she tolerate dietary sources of calcium?

Interventions for leg cramps include:

Stretching exercises before sleep

Daily calcium and magnesium supplements

Increasing dietary calcium intake

Glass of tonic water (containing quinine) at bedtime

This patient needs to relate her concerns to the oncologist. A healthcare provider may consider starting the patient on quinine 200 to 300 mg at bedtime. This is an unlabeled use and requires careful patient evaluation.

3. Cyclobenzaprine (Flexeril) has been demonstrated to produce significant anticholinergic activity. Students should recall that anticholinergics block the action of the neurotransmitter Ach at the muscarinic receptors in the parasympathetic nervous system. This allows the activities of the sympathetic nervous system to dominate. In this case, the result has been a decrease in oral secretions and relaxation of the smooth muscle of the GI tract. Decreased peristalsis and motility can result in constipation. The anticholinergic effect is also responsible for urinary retention by increasing constriction of the internal sphincter.

Chapter 46

1. The student should use a secondary source to answer this question. Alendronate (Fosamax) is poorly absorbed after oral absorption and can produce significant GI irritation. It is important that the patient be educated regarding several elements of drug administration.

To promote absorption, the drug should be taken first thing in the morning with 8 ounces of water before ingesting food, beverages, or any other medications. It has been shown that certain beverages, such as orange juice and coffee, interfere with drug absorption. By delaying eating for 30 minutes or more, the patient is promoting absorption of the drug. Additionally, the patient should be taught to sit upright after taking the drug to reduce the risk of esophageal irritation. Alendronate must be used carefully in patients with esophagitis or gastric ulcer.

If the patient misses a dose, she should be told to skip it and not to double up on the next dose. Alendronate has a long half-life and missing an occasional dose will do little to interfere with the therapeutic effect of the drug.

2. Frail elderly patients may be susceptible to hypocalcemia due to dietary deficiencies of calcium and vitamin D or because of decreased physical activity and lack of exposure to sunshine. This patient has all of these risk factors. She is uninterested in eating, has physical limitations, and is not able to get out of the house into the sunshine without assistance. Orally administered calcium requires vitamin D for absorption to take place. Because this patient does not consume milk, the most recognizable source of vitamin D, she needs to be encouraged to increase her intake of other dietary sources of this vitamin. Vitamin D-rich foods include canned salmon, cereals, lean meats, beans, and potatoes. To promote the effectiveness of calcium supplementation, the nurse must remember the importance of drug-nutrient interactions.

3. The triage nurse should obtain information about the onset of symptoms, degree of discomfort, and frequency of attacks. A familial history of gout can be predictive due to the fact that primary gout is inherited as an X-linked trait. A past medical history of renal calculi may also be predictive of acute gouty arthritis.

The nurse should ask the patient questions about his diet and fluid intake. An attack of gout can be precipitated by alcohol intake (particularly beer and wine), starvation diets, and insufficient fluid intake. In addition, the nurse should obtain information about prescribed drugs and the use of OTC drugs containing salicylates. Thiazide diuretics and salicylates can precipitate an attack.

The nurse should also ask about recent lifestyle events. Stress, illness, trauma, or strenuous exercise can precipitate an attack of gouty arthritis.

4. Raloxifene (Evista) is a selective estrogen receptor modulator. It stimulates estrogen receptors on bone and blocks estrogen receptors on tissues of the breast and uterus. Raloxifene prevents bone loss by increasing bone mineral density and the drug produces a cardioprotective action through its effects on cholesterol. With raloxifene, the total and LDL cholesterol levels are decreased without impacting HDL cholesterol levels or triglycerides. Raloxifene will not reduce hot flashes associated with estrogen deficiency, and may in fact precipitate them. However, the patient will benefit by prevention of osteoporosis and the cardioprotective effect of this drug therapy.

Chapter 47

1. To establish a rapport with the baby's mother, the nurse should first respond to the mother's anxiety. She should validate that the baby's condition is indeed cause for concern and commend the mother for seeking medical guidance. The nursing student should recognize that the availability of OTC preparations can be a temptation to a young mother who wants only to see her infant more comfortable and relieved of symptoms.

However, the student nurse must also recognize that topical use of corticosteroid ointments can be potentially harmful, especially for young children. Corticosteroids, when absorbed by the skin in large enough quantities, over a long period, can result in adrenal suppression and skin atrophy. Children have an increased risk of toxicity from topically applied drugs because of their greater skin surface area to weight ratio compared to that of adults. The student nurse should ensure that the healthcare provider at the public health clinic sees this patient. Once a drug treatment modality is prescribed, the student nurse should make sure that the baby's mother understands the correct method for drug administration.

2. According to Piaget, this 14-year-old patient is capable of formal operations, the highest level of cognitive development. A young person in this age group is able to think logically and make decisions regarding healthcare problems as well as being in control of a treatment regimen. To safely self-medicate, the teenager needs information about the medication, its administration, and side effects to anticipate. Teenagers need clear instructions and often respond to a caregiver outside the family as a resource for information.

The nurse should recognize that this patient is experiencing GI side effects which are common in doxycycline treatment as well as with all tetracyclines. Recent studies have demonstrated cases of esophagitis in teenage patients. To develop an effective teaching plan, the nurse will need to assess the client's dosing regimen as well as current dietary patterns. A teaching plan would include:

Encouraging oral fluids, to maintain hydration, even if nausea occurs

Drinking a full glass of water with the medication to reduce gastric irritation

Sitting up for 30 minutes after the nighttime dose to reduce gastric irritation and reflux

Consuming small frequent meals to ensure adequate nutrition

Taking the drug 1 hour before or 2 hours after meals to promote its absorption and effectiveness (If nausea persists, however, the patient should be encouraged to take the doxycycline with food.) Taking doxycycline with milk products or antacids decreases the absorption of the drug. Therefore, other remedies for GI irritation will need to be discussed with the healthcare provider.

3. This patient's presentation is typical of rosacea. To prevent long-term changes in the skin, therapy should be aggressive despite the fact that this patient is also of childbearing age. Isotretinoin (Accutane) is a pregnancy category X drug and has a picture of a fetus overlaid by the "No" symbol on the package. Reported teratogenic effects include severe CNS abnormalities such as hydrocephalus, microcephalus, cranial nerve deficits, and compromised intelligence scores. This patient needs to understand that she must use contraception while receiving drug therapy and for up to 6 months after therapy is discontinued. She should not begin therapy unless first demonstrating a negative pregnancy test. In addition, she should be taught to begin therapy on the second or third day of her normal menstrual cycle. Teenagers who are on isotretinoin should anticipate monthly pregnancy tests.

Chapter 48

1. Cortisporin Otic is a combination of neomycin, polymyxin B, and 1% hydrocortisone. The technique for instilling this drug applies to most eardrops. The nurse needs to instruct the mother to position her daughter in a side-lying position with the affected ear facing up. The mother needs to inspect the ear for the presence of drainage or cerumen and, if present, gently remove it with a cotton-tipped applicator. Any unusual odor or drainage could be suggestive of a ruptured tympanic membrane and should be reported to the healthcare provider. Next the mother should be taught to straighten the child's

external ear canal by pulling down and back on the auricle, to promote distribution of the medication to deeper external ear structures. After the drops are instilled, the mother can further promote medication distribution by gently pressing on the tragus of the ear. The mother should be taught to keep her daughter in a side-lying position for 3 to 5 minutes after the drops are instilled. If a cotton ball has been prescribed, the cotton ball should be placed in the ear without applying pressure. The cotton ball can be removed in 15 minutes.

2. Timoptic, a beta-adrenergic blocking agent, is contraindicated in individuals with chronic obstructive pulmonary disease. This agent has been known to produce bronchospasm by blocking the stimulation of beta$_2$-adrenergic receptors. When beta$_2$-receptors are stimulated, relaxation of bronchial smooth muscles is facilitated. Timolol is contraindicated in COPD, an air-trapping disorder, and may be contraindicated in chronic asthma. In both cases, the beta-adrenergic blocking effect of timolol could be potentially life threatening. Betaxolol (Betoptic) is also a beta-adrenergic blocking agent, but is considered safer for use in patients with COPD who require treatment for glaucoma.

3. All ophthalmic agents should be administered in the conjunctival sac. The cornea is highly innervated and direct application of medication to the cornea can result in excessive burning and stinging. The conjunctival sac normally holds one or two drops of solution. Following administration of the medication, the patient should be reminded to place pressure on the inner canthus of the eye to prevent the medication from flowing into the nasolacrimal duct. This maneuver helps to prevent systemic absorption of medication and decreases the risk of side effects commonly associated with antiglaucoma agents.

Indexing style is as follows: **Prototype drugs appear in boldface,** <u>generic names are underlined,</u> **<u>generic names of prototype drugs are boldface and underlined,</u>** DRUG CLASSIFICATIONS ARE IN SMALL CAPS, tables have a t and figures have an f after the page number, trade name drugs are referenced back to the generic name, trade names are capitalized, and diseases are in red.

A

A-beta protein, 360

Aδ fibers, pain and, 222, 727

AAP Committee on Drugs. *See* American Academy of Pediatrics Committee on Drugs

<u>abacavir</u>, 486t

abciximab
  actions and uses of, 322
  adverse effects and interactions of, 322
  antiplatelet action of, 321t
  for cardiac disorders, 333t

ABCs, of diarrhea treatment, 539

Abel, John Jacob, 3

Abelcet. *See* **<u>amphotericin B</u>**

Abenal. *See* <u>acetaminophen</u>

Abilify. *See* <u>aripiprazole</u>

Abiplatin. *See* <u>cisplatin</u>

abortion, pharmacologic, drugs for, 610, 612–613, 612t

Abreva. *See* <u>docosanol</u>

abscess, 440t

absence seizure, 158, 727
  drugs used in management of, 159t

absolute neutrophil count, calculation of, 503

absorption, 48–49, 48f, 49f, 727

abstinence syndrome, CNS depressants and, 148

<u>acarbose</u>, 596, 596t, 597

Accolate. *See* <u>zafirlukast</u>

Accupril. *See* <u>quinapril</u>

Accutane. *See* **<u>isotretinoin</u>**

ACE. *See* angiotensin-converting enzyme

ACE INHIBITORS. *See* ANGIOTENSIN-CONVERTING ENZYME (ACE) INHIBITORS

<u>acebutolol</u>, 136t, 741
  breastfeeding and, 71t
  for dysrhythmias, 304t

Acel-Imune. *See* <u>diphtheria, tetanus, and pertussis</u>

<u>acetaminophen</u>, 16t, 230, 231t, 424, 741
  actions and uses of, 425
  adverse effects and interactions of, 425
  in antihistamine combination, 427t
  in antihistimine-decongestant-analgesic combination, 427t
  in combination analgesics, 224
  for fever, 423, 424
  mechanism of action of, 425

metabolism of, ethnic variability in, 424
  versus NSAIDs, 419
  in opioid combination cold medicine, 396t
  for osteoarthritis, 691

<u>acetaminophen-codeine</u>, 744

Acetazolam. *See* **<u>acetazolamide</u>**

<u>acetazolamide</u>, 646, 647t, 718t, 719, 741
  for acute pancreatitis, 598

<u>acetohexamide</u>, 596t, 741

acetyl CoA, in cholesterol synthesis, 360

acetylcholine, 127, 727
  anticholinergics and, 129
  atropine counteracting buildup of, 128
  and cholinergic transmission, 125–126, 125f, 126t
  nerve agent actions on, 23
  synthesis of, 126

acetylcholinesterase, 125, 216, 727
  drugs blocking, 717, 718t

ACETYLCHOLINESTERASE INHIBITORS
  for Alzheimer's disease, 216–217, 216t
    nursing considerations in use of, 217–218
    patient education in use of, 217–218
  mechanism of action of, 217f

<u>acetylcysteine</u>
  for bronchial secretions, 397
  for common cold, 395t

Acetylsalicylic acid. *See* **<u>aspirin</u>**

acetyltransferase, polymorphisms in, 97, 97t

Ach. *See* acetylcholine

AchE. *See* acetylcholinesterase

Achromycin. *See* **<u>tetracycline HCl</u>**

acid-base balance, 661–665
  imbalances in, 661, 662f. *See also* acidosis; alkalosis

acid production
  by stomach, 522–523
    natural defenses against, 523, 523f
    proton pump inhibitors and, 525–526

acidosis, 662f, 727
  metabolic, 663t
    and renal failure, pharmacologic management of, 641t
  pharmacotherapy of, 663. *See also* **<u>sodium bicarbonate</u>**
    nursing considerations in, 663–664
  respiratory causes of, 663t
  sea vegetables for, 664

acinar cells, in pancreas, 597

Aciphex. *See* <u>rabeprazole</u>

<u>acitretin</u>, 710, 712t

<u>aclometasone</u>, 711t

Aclovate. *See* <u>aclometasone</u>

acne vulgaris, 705–706, 727
  burdock root for, 708
  pharmacotherapy of, 706–707
    nursing considerations in, 707
    patient education in, 707

acquired immunodeficiency syndrome. *See* HIV-AIDS

acquired resistance, 727

acromegaly, 570

ACTH. *See* adrenocorticotropic hormone; corticotropin; corticotropin injection

ACTH-40. *See* <u>repository corticotropin</u>

ACTH-80. *See* <u>repository corticotropin</u>

Acthar. *See* <u>corticotropin</u>; <u>corticotropin</u> injection

Actidil. *See* <u>triprolidine</u>

Actifed. *See* <u>pseudoephedrine</u>; <u>triprolidine</u>

Actifed Cold and Allergy. *See* <u>triprolidine-pseudoephedrine</u>

Actifed Cold and Sinus. *See* <u>chlorpheniramine-pseudoephedrine-acetaminophen</u>

Actinomycin-D. *See* <u>dactinomycin</u>

action potential, 727
  cardiac, 300, 301
    ion channels in, 301, 303f

Actiq. *See* <u>fentanyl citrate</u>

Activase. *See* **<u>alteplase</u>**

activated partial thromboplastin time, 315, 727
  in anticoagulation therapy, 317–318

active immunity, 727

active transport, 47

activities of daily living
  antiviral drug side effects affecting, 489
  spasticity and, 673

Actonell. *See* <u>risedronate sodium</u>

Actos. *See* <u>pioglitazone</u>

Actron. *See* <u>ketoprofen</u>

Acuprin. *See* **<u>aspirin</u>**

acute radiation syndrome, 23, 727

<u>acyclovir</u>, 489, 493t, 745
  actions and uses of, 494
  adverse effects and interactions of, 494
  for viral skin lesions, 701

AD. *See* Alzheimer's disease

Adalat. *See* **<u>nifedipine</u>**

Adamsite, 24t

<u>adapalene</u>, 706t, 707

ADD. *See* attention-deficit disorder

Adderall. *See* <u>amphetamine racemic mixture</u>

addiction, 15, 110, 727
  to opioids, 112

Addison's disease, 570t, 581, 727

<u>adefovir dipivoxil</u>, 494, 495t

Adenocard. *See* <u>adenosine</u>

adenohypophysis, 568, 727

Adenoscan. *See* <u>adenosine</u>

<u>adenosine</u>
  direct-acting parasympathomimetics and, 129
  for dysrhythmias, 304t, 309

adenosine diphosphate
  in clotting process, 313

inducing, treatments available. *See*
ANOREXIANTS
in type 2 diabetes mellitus
management, 593
weight monitoirng, in diuretic therapy
loop diuretics, 643
thiazide diuretics, 645
Welchol. *See* colesevelam
Wellbutrin. *See* bupropion
Wellferon. *See* interferon alfa-n1
Westcort. *See* **hydrocortisone**
white blood cells, 370
in myocardial infarction, 339t
whiteheads, 706
whole blood, for shock, 346, 348t
whooping cough, 20t
Winpred. *See* **prednisone**
WinRho SDF. *See* Rh₀(D) immune globulin
withdrawal, 15, 740
withdrawal syndrome, 110–111, 111t, 740
worms. *See* helminthic infections;
helminthes
wrinkling of skin, 701t
Wyamine. *See* **mephentermine**
Wycillin. *See* penicillin G procaine
Wymox. *See* amoxicillin
Wytensin. *See* guanabenz

X

x-rays, cancer risk and, 499
Xalatan. *See* **latanoprost**
Xanax. *See* alprazolam
xanthine oxidase enzyme
allopurinol blocking, 693
uric acid crystals and, 692
Xenical. *See* orlistat
Ximelagatran. *See* exanta
Xolada. *See* capecitabine
Xopenex. *See* levalbuterol HCl
Xylocaine. *See* **lidocaine**
Xylocard. *See* **lidocaine**
xylometazoline, 432t

Y

Yasmin combination oral
contraceptive, 609t
yeasts, 740
as fungal pathogens, 466
tyramine in, 184t
yellow dock, 708
yellow fever, 20t
Yersina pestis, 20t
Yodoxin. *See* iodoquinol
Yutopar. *See* ritodrine; ritodrine HCl

Z

Z-PAM. *See* pralidoxime chloride
zafirlukast, 393t, 395
Zagam. *See* sparfloxacin
zalcitabine, 486t
zanamivir, 493, 494t
Zanosar. *See* streptozocin
Zantac. *See* **ranitidine**
Zapex. *See* oxazepam
Zarontin. *See* **ethosuximide**
Zaroxolyn. *See* metolazone
Zebeta. *See* bisoprolol
Zefazone. *See* cefmetazole
Zelnorm. *See* tegaserod
Zenaflex. *See* tizanidine
Zenapax. *See* daclizumab
Zerit. *See* stavudine
zero tolerance in schools, 189
Zestoretic. *See* **lisinopril**
Zestril. *See* **lisinopril**
Zetia. *See* ezetimibe
Ziac. *See* hydrochlorothiazide-bisoprolol
Ziagen. *See* abacavir
zidovudine, 486t, 487
actions and uses of, 489
adverse effects and interactions
of, 489
clarithromycin interaction with, 450
zileuton, 393t, 395
Zinacef. *See* cefuroxime

zinc
function of, 560t
pharmacotherapy with, 560
RDA of, 560t
supplementation with, 556t
zinc acetate, 556t, 560
zinc gluconate, 556t, 560
zinc sulfate, 556t, 560
Zincate. *See* zinc sulfate
Zingiber officinalis, 102t, 524
active chemicals in, 102
drug interactions with, 106t
standardization of, 103t
ziprasidone, 204t
Zithromax. *See* azithromycin
Zocor. *See* simvastatin
Zofran. *See* ondansetron
Zoladex. *See* goserelin; goserelin acetate
zoledronic acid, 517t
Zollinger-Ellison syndrome, 528, 740
zolmitriptan, 236t
Zoloft. *See* sertraline
zolpidem, 150, 151t, 152, 744
actions and uses of, 152
adverse effects and interactions of, 152
Zometa. *See* zoledronic acid
Zomig. *See* zolmitriptan
Zonegran. *See* zonisamide
zonisamide, 165t
zonisamide, 165, 166
ZORprin. *See* **aspirin**
Zosyn. *See* piperacillin tazobactam
Zovirax. *See* **acyclovir**
Zyflo. *See* zileuton
Zyloprim. *See* allopurinol
Zyprexa. *See* olanzapine
Zyrtec. *See* cetirizine
Zyvox. *See* linezolid